T0419361

CARDIOLOGY RESEARCH AND CLINICAL DEVELOPMENTS

PERCUTANEOUS VALVE TECHNOLOGY

PRESENT AND FUTURE

CARDIOLOGY RESEARCH AND CLINICAL DEVELOPMENTS

Additional books in this series can be found on Nova's website under the Series tab.

Additional E-books in this series can be found on Nova's website under the E-book tab.

CARDIOLOGY RESEARCH AND CLINICAL DEVELOPMENTS

PERCUTANEOUS VALVE TECHNOLOGY

PRESENT AND FUTURE

JOSE LUIS NAVIA
AND
SHARIF AL-RUZZEH
EDITORS

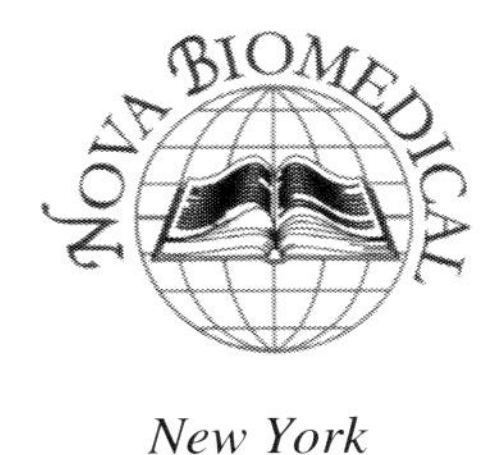

New York

For permission to use material from this book please contact us:
Telephone 631-231-7269; Fax 631-231-8175
Web Site: http://www.novapublishers.com

Library of Congress Cataloging-in-Publication Data

Library of Congress Control Number: 2011946009

ISBN: 978-1-61942-577-4

Published by Nova Science Publishers, Inc. † New York

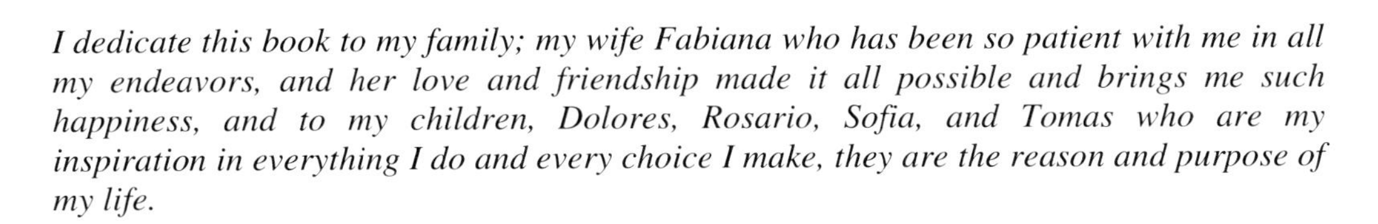

I dedicate this book to my family; my wife Fabiana who has been so patient with me in all my endeavors, and her love and friendship made it all possible and brings me such happiness, and to my children, Dolores, Rosario, Sofia, and Tomas who are my inspiration in everything I do and every choice I make, they are the reason and purpose of my life.

Dr Jose Luis Navia, MD, FACC

May 2012

I dedicate this book to the soul of my beloved father, Mohamed Hasan, who devoted all his life to get me where I am now. I also dedicate this book to my "two eyes" my two sons, Omar and Tarek, and my Wife, Kinda, my faithful, loving and caring companion in this life journey. I also dedicate this book to my sister, Rasha, and my Mother, Enayat, for giving me everlasting love and support.

Dr Sharif Mohamed Hasan Al-Ruzzeh, MD, PhD, FRCS, FRCSEd

May 2012

Contents

Foreword

Advances in the use of percutaneous techniques for the treatment of coronary artery disease have occurred during the last fifty years. In recent years, these advances inspired the percutaneous interventions for the treatment of stenotic valvular lesions as in pulmonary stenosis, rheumatic mitral stenosis, and tricuspid stenosis and finally with calcific aortic stenosis.

Although widespread acceptance is premature, the future of percutaneous valve procedures is of great interest and will likely be embraced. Obvious benefits are avoidance of a major surgical procedure, improved and more rapid recovery, and reduced morbidity and mortality. However, issues regarding proper valve sizing, and native tissue ablation require further attention. Operator experience is still somewhere on the steep learning curve. And most importantly, the longevity of such repairs and replacements and their test against time, is still to be studied and reported. The magnitude of investment by major medical device companies and amount of capital investment will clearly drive this technology forward rapidly.

We believe the book is very much needed at this time. The Percutaneous Valve technology, despite the recent major developments, is at its first days with huge predictions and investments already directed towards it. It is a virgin field where the medical and scientific community is looking ambitiously at. We aimed this book to provide the up-to-date state of art knowledge and practical experience of the rapidly evolving percutaneous valve technology.

The book is divided into thirty-one chapters. The first 7 chapters present an overview of the up-to-date guidelines, anesthesiology implications, imaging of the valves and the biomedical engineering concepts that stand behind this technology. Chapters 8-15 deal with the Aortic valve. Chapters 16-24 deal with the mitral valve. Chapter 25 discusses the endovascular stent as a related technology. Chapters 26 and 27 deal with the tricuspid valve. Chapter 28 deals with the pulmonary valve. Chapter 29 is a unique chapter that addresses the percutaneous valve technology applications in the pediatric patients. Finally, chapters 30 and 31 deal with the industry and marketing sides.

This book is aimed to look into this rapidly evolving technology from all around and into the future by the eyes of the world known experts in fields of Cardiology, Radiology, Anatomy, Surgery, Echo-cardiology, Anesthesiology, Biomedical Engineers and even Industry leaders and Marketers. Opinions, analyses, reviews, predictions, theories, suggestions, plans, pitfalls and designs in addition to invaluable first hand experience of world experts in the field are all coming together in this unique piece of medical literature.

Jose L. Navia MD, FACC
Staff Surgeon
Department of Thoracic and Cardiovascular Surgery
Sydell and Arnold Miller Family Heart and Vascular Institute
Surgical Director
Center for Electrical Therapy in Heart Failure
Staff of the Department of Biomedical Engineering
Lerner Research Institute
Cleveland Clinic
9500 Euclid Avenue / J4-1
Cleveland, OH 44195
United States of America

Sharif Al-Ruzzeh, MD, PhD, FRCS
Staff Project Scientist
Cleveland Clinic Foundation
9500 Euclid Avenue
Cleveland, OH 44195
United States of America

Preface

"It is not the strongest of the species that survive, nor the most intelligent, but the one most responsive to change", a famous quote by Charles Darwin that best describes how to deal with present and future revolution that has been happening in the management of cardiac and vascular disease. There has been an accumulated successful development in application of percutanoeus technology to the treatment of peripheral vascular disease by vascular surgeons and radiologists in the fifties and sixties, then to coronary disease by cardiologists in the seventies and eighties and then to thoracic and abdominal aortic disease by radiologists and cardiovascular surgeons in the nineties and 2000s. Knocking down boundaries between those specialties and creating a new group of "interventialists". All these differently trained physicians were inadvertently helping evolve the same "intravascular percuteous technology" in different domains and directions to treat vascular disease at different locations. This technology is now rising to a new horizon of treating intra-cardiac valves without conventional "open-heart" surgery. It would not difficult to predict that a new "Interventional percutaneous technology specialist" will be a medical specialty on its own in the near future.

Valve repair and or replacement still remains the gold standard treatment for valvular dysfunction and therefore remains the caliber to compare to. While open-heart procedures report short and long term successes, they are still associated with major morbidity and mortality, especially, when you consider the risks of reoperation for valve dysfunction, complications of thromboembolism and anticoagulation and endocarditis. All these have prompted clinicians and researchers to explore a variety of less invasive techniques including valve repairs, minimally invasive surgical approaches, and, more recently, percutaneous approaches toward valve repair or replacement. The safety of this new technology demands certain basic features to be available including optimum imaging, such echocardiography, new CT scan and MRI modalities, of the valve to be treated, hence the need of developed echocardiographic monitoring, the safe ablation of a special material valve and deployment of the valve within or without the native valve using a flexible delivery system, hence the required development in biomedical sciences.

There are technical limitations and challenges of this evolving technology that are being addressed at present including but not limited to the suturing technique of the valve to the scaffold, the expandability of calcified tissue, and proper sizing in both the diameter of the valve and the length; the latter, perhaps more important for aortic valve procedures to avoid obstruction to coronary ostial flow. The preoperative assessment is crucial to guide selection and preparation of the stent-valve prosthesis. Industry has dealt with technical challenges like this in the past and undoubtedly it will succeed this time too.

This is exactly what why we decided to write this book. We aimed to provide the reader with a snap-shot of the current "state of art" of this rapidly evolving technology with a realistic prediction of its course in the future. We have been extremely fortunate that our invitations to the world known experts in percutaneous valve technology, including Cardiologits, Surgeons, Anatomists, Biomedical Engineers, Echo-cardiologits, Anesthesiologists and Industry leaders and marketers, have been accepted and resulted in this unique piece of medical literature that captures this technology from all around.

Jose L. Navia MD, FACC
Staff Surgeon
Department of Thoracic and Cardiovascular Surgery
Sydell and Arnold Miller Family Heart and Vascular Institute
Surgical Director
Center for Electrical Therapy in Heart Failure
Staff of the Department of Biomedical Engineering
Lerner Research Institute
Cleveland Clinic
9500 Euclid Avenue / J4-1
Cleveland, OH 44195
United States of America

Sharif Al-Ruzzeh, MD, PhD, FRCS
Staff Project Scientist
Cleveland Clinic Foundation
9500 Euclid Avenue
Cleveland, OH 44195
United States of America

Contributors

David H. Adams, M.D.
Department of Cardiothoracic Surgery,
Mount Sinai Medical Center, New York, NY, US

Imran N. Ahmad, M.D.
Department of Cardiovascular Medicine, Interventional Cardiology, Heart and Vascular Institute, Cleveland Clinic, Cleveland, OH, US

Turki B. Albacker, M.D., FRCSC
Department of Cardiac Surgery, King Fahad Cardiac Center, College of Medicine, King Saud University,
Riyadh, Saudi Arabia

Andrej Alfirevic, M.D.
Department of Cardiothoracic Anesthesiology, Heart and Vascular Institute, Cleveland Clinic, Cleveland, OH, US

Sharif Al-Ruzzeh, M.D., PhD, FRCS, FRCSEd
Department of Biomedical Engineering, Lerner Research Institute, Cleveland Clinic, Cleveland, OH, US

David G. Anthony, M.D.
Department of Cardiothoracic Anesthesiology, Heart and Vascular Institute, Cleveland Clinic, Cleveland, OH, US

Saif Anwaruddin, M.D.
Section of Interventional Cardiology, Hospital of the University of Pennsylvania, Philadelphia, PA, US

Vasilis Babaliaros, M.D.
Division of Cardiology, Emory Health Care, Emory University Hospital
NE Atlanta, GA, US

Cesare Beghi, M.D.
Cardiac Surgery Unit, Community Hospital, Parma, Italy

Peter Block, M.D.
Division of Cardiology, Emory Health Care, Emory University Hospital
NE Atlanta, GA, US

Nicolas A. Brozzi, M.D.
Department of Thoracic and Cardiovascular Surgery, Heart and Vascular Institute, Cleveland Clinic, Cleveland, OH, US

Xin Chen, M.D,
Department of Thoracic and Cardiovascular Surgery, Nanjing Heart Hospital, Nanjing First Hospital affiliated to Nanjing Medical University, Nanjing, P.R. China

A. Cheung, M.D.
Division of Cardiology, St. Paul's Hospital, University of British Columbia, Vancouver, Canada

Joanna Chikwę, M.D., FRCS
Department of Cardiothoracic Surgery,
Mount Sinai Medical Center, New York, NY, US

Giuliano Chizzola, M.D.
Cardiology Unit, Community Hospital, Brescia, Italy

Domenico Corradi, M.D.
Pathology Unit, Community Hospital, Parma, Italy

Salvatore Curello,M.D.
Cardiology Unit, Community Hospital, Brescia, Italy

Antonio D'Aloia, M.D.
Cardiology Unit, Community Hospital, Brescia, Italy

Giuseppe De Cicco, M.D.
Cardiac Surgery Unit, Brescia, Community Hospital, Italy

Francis G. Duhay, M.D.
Global Medical Affairs, Edwards Lifesciences LLC, Irvine , CA, US

Stephen G. Ellis, M.D.
Department of Cardiovascular Medicine, Section of Interventional Cardiology, Heart and Vascular Institute. Cleveland Clinic, Cleveland, OH, US

Federica Ettori, M.D.
Cardiology Unit, Community Hospital, Brescia, Italy

Pompilio Faggiano, M.D.
Cardiology Unit, Community Hospital, Brescia, Italy

Christopher M. Feindel, M.D.
Division of Cardiovascular Surgery, Peter Munk Cardiac Centre,
Toronto General Hospital, University of Toronto,
Toronto, Ontario, Canada

Claudia Fiorina, M.D.
Cardiology Unit, Community Hospital, Brescia, Italy

Mario Frontini, M.D.
Cardiac Surgery Intensive Care Unit, Community Hospital, Brescia, Italy

Kiyotaka Fukamachi, M.D., PhD.
Department of Biomedical Engineering, Lerner Research Institute, Cleveland Clinic,
Cleveland, OH, US

Sandro Gelsomino, M.D., PhD.
Cardiac Surgery Unit, Community Hospital, Brescia, Italy

Brian P. Griffin, M.D.
Department of Cardiovascular Medicine, Heart and Vascular Institute, Cleveland Clinic,
Cleveland, OH, US

R. Gurvitch, M.D.
Division of Cardiology, St. Paul's Hospital, University of British Columbia,
Vancouver, Canada

Martin Haensig, M.D.
Department of Cardiac Surgery, University of Leipzig Heart Center, Leipzig, Germany

Sandy S. Halliburton, PhD.
Imaging Institute and Heart & Vascular Institute, Cleveland Clinic, Cleveland, OH, US

Stephen A. Hart, M.D.
Department of Cardiovascular Medicine, Heart and Vascular Institute, Cleveland Clinic,
Cleveland, OH, US

David M. Holzhey, M.D.
Department of Cardiac Surgery, University of Leipzig Heart Center, Leipzig, Germany

Eric Horlick, M.D.
Division of Cardiology, Peter Munk Cardiac Centre,
Toronto General Hospital, University of Toronto,
Toronto, Ontario, Canada

Fuhuang Huang, M.D., PhD.
Department of Thoracic and Cardiovascular Surgery, Nanjing Heart Hospital, Nanjing First
Hospital affiliated to Nanjing Medical University, Nanjing, P.R. China

Sarah Huoh
Global Communications, Edwards Lifesciences LLC, Irvine, CA, US

Bernard Iung, M.D.
Cardiology Department, Bichat Hospital, AP-HP, Paris, France

J. Je, M.D.
Division of Cardiology, St. Paul's Hospital, University of British Columbia, Vancouver, Canada

Samir R. Kapadia, M.D.
Department of Cardiovascular Medicine, Section of Interventional Cardiology, Heart and Vascular Institute, Cleveland Clinic, Cleveland, OH, US

Ghassan S. Kassab, PhD.
Department of Biomedical Engineering, Surgery, Cellular and Integrative Physiology, IUPUI, Indianapolis, IN, US

Allan L. Klein, M.D.
Department of Cardiovascular Medicine, Heart and Vascular Institute, Cleveland Clinic, Cleveland, OH, US

Richard A. Krasuski, M.D.
Department of Cardiovascular Medicine, Heart and Vascular Institute, Cleveland Clinic, Cleveland, OH, US

Amar Krishnaswamy, M.D.
Department of Interventional Cardiology, Heart and Vascular Institute, Cleveland Clinic, Cleveland, OH, US

John Kubasiak, B.A.
Division of Cardiac Surgery, Northwestern University Feinberg School of Medicine, Bluhm Cardiovascular Institute, Northwestern Memorial Hospital, Chicago, IL, US

Deborah H. Kwon, M.D.
Department of Cardiovascular Medicine, Heart and Vascular Institute, Cleveland Clinic, Cleveland, OH, US

John Liddicoat, M.D., MBA
Structural Heart, Medtronic Cardiac and Vascular Group, Mounds View, MN, US

David Liff, M.D.
Division of Cardiology, Emory Health Care. Emory University Hospital, NE Atlanta, GA, US

Roberto Lorusso, M.D., PhD.
Cardiac Surgery Unit, Community Hospital, Brescia, Italy

S. Chris Malaisrie, M.D.
Division of Cardiac Surgery, Northwestern University Feinberg School of Medicine, Bluhm Cardiovascular Institute, Northwestern Memorial Hospital, Chicago, IL, US

Eric Manasse, M.D.
C.M.O. Sorin Group, Milan, Italy

Patrick M. McCarthy, M.D.
Division of Cardiac Surgery, Northwestern University Feinberg School of Medicine, Bluhm Cardiovascular Institute, Northwestern Memorial Hospital, Chicago, IL, US

Friedrich W. Mohr, M.D.
Department of Cardiac Surgery, University of Leipzig Heart Center, Leipzig, Germany

Krishna R. Mudimbi,M.D.
Department of Cardiothoracic Anesthesiology, Heart and Vascular Institute, Cleveland Clinic, Cleveland, OH, US

Jose Luis Navia, M.D., F.A.C.C.
Department of Thoracic and Cardiovascular Surgery. Heart and Vascular Institute, Department of Biomedical Engineering, Lerner Research Institute, Cleveland Clinic, Cleveland, OH, US

Mark Osten, M.D.
Division of Cardiology, Peter Munk Cardiac Centre, Toronto General Hospital, University of Toronto, Toronto, Ontario, Canada

Lourdes R. Prieto, M.D.
Department of Pediatric Cardiology, Heart and Vascular Institute, Cleveland Clinic, Cleveland, OH, US

Sharan Ramaswamy, PhD.
Department of Biomedical Engineering, Florida International University, Miami, FL, US

Ardawan J. Rastan, M.D.
Department of Cardiac Surgery, University of Leipzig Heart Center, Leipzig, Germany

L. Leonardo Rodriguez, M.D.
Department of Cardiovascular Medicine, Heart and Vascular Institute, Cleveland Clinic, Cleveland, OH, US

Eric E. Roselli, M.D.
Department of Thoracic and Cardiovascular Surgery, Heart and Vascular Institute, Cleveland Clinic, Cleveland, OH, US

Martin T. Rothman, M.D.
Coronary and Peripheral, Medtronic Cardiac and Vascular Group, Santa Rosa, CA, US

Virna L. Sales, M.D.
Division of Cardiac Surgery, Northwestern University Feinberg School of Medicine, Bluhm Cardiovascular Institute, Northwestern Memorial Hospital, Chicago, IL, US

D. Schmidt, M.D.
Department of Otolaryngology, University of Pittsburgh Medical Center, Pittsburgh, PA, US

Paul Schoenhagen, M.D.
Imaging Institute and Heart & Vascular Institute, Cleveland Clinic, Cleveland, OH, US

William J. Stewart, M.D.
Department of Cardiovascular Medicine, Heart and Vascular Institute, Cleveland Clinic, Cleveland, OH, US

Lars Svensson, M.D., PhD.
Department of Thoracic and Cardiovascular Surgery, Heart and Vascular Institute, Cleveland Clinic, Cleveland, OH, US

Tohru Takaseya, , M.D., PhD.
Department of Biomedical Engineering, Lerner Research Institute, Cleveland Clinic, Cleveland, OH, US

Gilbert H. L. Tang, M.D.,
Division of Cardiovascular Surgery, Peter Munk Cardiac Centre,
Toronto General Hospital, University of Toronto,
Toronto, Ontario, Canada

Andrew C. Y. To, M.D.
Department of Cardiovascular Medicine, Heart and Vascular Institute, Cleveland Clinic, Cleveland, OH, US

E. Murat Tuzcu, M.D.
Department of Cardiovascular Medicine, Section of Interventional Cardiology, Heart and Vascular Institute, Cleveland Clinic, Cleveland, OH, US

Alec Vahanian, M.D.
Cardiology Department, Bichat Hospital, AP-HP, Paris, France

Thomas A. Vassiliades, Jr., M.D., MBA
Structural Heart, Medtronic Cardiac and Vascular Group, Mounds View, MN, US

Enrico Vizzardi, M.D.
Cardiology Unit, Community Hospital, Brescia, Italy

John G. Webb, M.D.
Division of Cardiology, St. Paul's Hospital, University of British Columbia, Vancouver, Canada

Ernest Young, PhD.
Department of Biomedical Engineering, Lerner Research Institute, Cleveland Clinic, Cleveland, OH, US

Melissa Young, PhD.
Department of Biomedical Engineering, Lerner Research Institute, Cleveland Clinic, Cleveland, OH, US

Uygar C. Yuksel, M.D.
Department of Cardiovascular Medicine, Section of Interventional Cardiology, Heart and Vascular Institute. Cleveland Clinic, Cleveland, OH, US

In: Percutaneous Valve Technology: Present and Future
Editors: Jose Luis Navia and Sharif Al-Ruzzeh
ISBN: 978-1-61942-577-4

Chapter I

Overview of Guidelines and Philosophical Medical Implications of Percutaneous Valve Technology

David Liff, Vasilis Babaliaros and Peter Block

Introduction

Valvular heart disease is a serious public health problem. In 2009, more than 24,000 aortic valve replacements and nearly 7,000 mitral valve repairs were performed in the United States [1]. As the population ages, the number of patients affected will increase. Surgery has been the only treatment proven to improve quality of life and survival for patients suffering from most forms of valvular disease.

Percutaneous therapy for stenotic lesions of the pulmonic, aortic, and mitral valves has been available to patients for years; however, the proliferation of novel percutaneous therapies for structural heart disease in the last decade has been unprecedented. Since the first-in-man report of transcatheter aortic valve replacement (TAVR) in 2002 [2], more than 20,000 TAVR have been performed worldwide. In that time, a multi-disciplinary effort, led by cardiologists, cardiothoracic surgeons, and imaging specialists has dramatically improved rates of procedural success, complications, and outcomes.

More percutaneous devices aimed at valvular disorders are developed every year, blurring traditional distinctions between cardiologist and cardiothoracic surgeons. It is yet unclear how to best investigate these devices, what patients should be included in trials, and who ought to be performing these procedures.

Though several professional societies have begun to address these topics through position statements, formal guidelines do not yet exist.

I. How should Percutaneous Valvular Interventions be Studied

A 2005 position statement issued by a consortium of professional societies described the various steps in the clinical development of percutaneous therapies [3]. Testing of an investigational device typically begins in a bench-research setting before being studied in an animal model. Subsequently, small, Phase I trials intended to test the feasibility and safety of the device are performed. Larger clinical trials follow, in which the success of the novel therapy is tested against an accepted clinical standard. Many new devices have undergone, or are currently in, Phase I testing, but only a few have advanced to the stage of advanced clinical evaluation. For aortic stenosis, the Edwards-SAPIEN valve (Edwards Lifesciences, Irvine CA) and the Medtronic CoreValve (Medtronic, Minneapolis MN) have been the subject of various clinical registries. For mitral valve therapies, only the Evalve MitraClip (Abbot Laboratories, Abbot Park, IL) has advanced beyond phase I testing, and in pulmonic interventions, only the Medtronic Melody valve is undergoing clinical investigation. To date, the MitraClip and Edwards-SAPIEN valve are the only devices to have been studied in randomized controlled trials.

Selection of an appropriate reference group with which to compare new devices is difficult. Surgical outcomes for valvular heart disease are excellent. The average mortality for patients undergoing isolated surgical aortic valve replacement (SAVR) is 2.6%, and 1.6% for isolated mitral valve repair (MVR) [4,5]. However, risk varies widely according to patient factors (i.e age) and clinical characteristics (i.e left ventricular ejection fraction, coronary artery disease, and comorbidities). It is unlikely that a new device will be able to significantly improve outcomes in a low risk population, thus investigators of novel percutaneous therapies have two choices: to undertake randomized trials to test superiority in a high-risk cohort, or non-inferiority trials to assess statistical equivalence in average risk cohorts.

Conservatively treated patients with symptomatic aortic stenosis are known to have a dismal prognosis. Balloon aortic valvuloplasty (BAV) does provide temporary relief; however, valvuloplasty registries have found that nearly 25% of patients experience a significant complication and most patients symptoms return by 6 months [6]. The PARTNER trial comparing TAVR to standard medical treatment, including BAV, for inoperable, symptomatic AS patients was designed as a superiority trial. The 20% absolute risk reduction with TAVR says as much about the futility of conservative therapy (49.7% mortality at 1 year) as it does about the efficacy of the Edwards-SAPIEN valve (30.7% mortality at 1 year) [7]. For future comparisons in a healthier cohort, demonstrating a difference between SAVR and TAVR may be difficult, and trials to test non-inferiority may be preferred.

The PARTNER trial also exposed a serious ethical dilemma for leaders of future trials. Poor outcomes in the medical therapy group were expected. Knowing how badly symptomatic patients fare when not offered SAVR, how much of a choice did patients really have when giving consent to participate in the randomization process? Furthermore, given the demonstrated benefit of TAVR in this population, can medical therapy justifiably serve as a standard of care for any future trials? These issues will have to be addressed at several levels including professional societies, regulatory bodies, and at individual institutional review boards.

Percutaneous valve interventions are less invasive and improve acute patient morbidity, an advantage that was illustrated by the EVEREST II trial. This study included patients with a standard indication for surgical MVR, and randomized them to percutaneous placement of the MitraClip or surgical MVR. The study found that reduction in mitral regurgitation was greater after surgery suggesting a more effective therapy. However, after a year, clinical outcomes were similar enough to meet the non-inferiority threshold, and acute morbidity was significantly better in the MitraClip arm [8]. The authors concluded that the MitraClip offers a safer way to achieve an equivalent clinical result to surgical MVR. Similar results may occur in future studies because surgical outcomes are so good, and the less invasive nature of percutaneous therapies is principally intended to improve morbidity. Physicians and patients will have to decide whether they can accept a safer treatment that is slightly less effective. Furthermore, it will be asked whether or not a less morbid percutaneous approach ought to be offered as first-line treatment so long as it doesn't preclude or undermine future surgical options. Settling these controversies will be a major task for authors of future guidelines.

Major questions remain regarding the the long-term durability of percutaneous devices. Cardiac surgeons have been performing valve replacement for 50 years, and over time, both mechanical and bioprosthetic valves have displayed excellent durability. In contrast, the longest follow up of a percutaneously placed aortic valve is < 7 years. Long-term follow up of currently placed percutaneous devices is needed before a true comparison with surgery can be complete. The need for post-marketing registries and serial assessment of percutaneous therapies is of paramount importance in assessing their utility.

Percutaneous interventions that are clinically effective without imposing significant morbidity will provide greater options for patients and significantly increase the number of patients eligible for treatment. According to STS statistics, the number of AVR's has increased by roughly 2.5x since 2001 with a similar increase in mitral valve repairs [1]. While these figures reflect the aging population, they also give pause when considering the potential costs of treating these patients with novel and expensive percutaneous devices. While current efforts are focused on expanding and improving percutaneous therapies, future cost-benefit analysis will help further define their role in patient care.

II. Patient Selection and Procedural Planning

In the absence of specific guidelines, a multi-disciplinary approach including cardiologists, surgeons, and referring physicians ought to be applied to patient selection. Studies have found that as many as 30-50% of elderly patients with symptomatic AS are not referred for surgery, and a number of patients seen by surgeons will be declined because of prohibitive operative risk [9,10]. But how do we determine that someone is inoperable, and how do we define "high risk"?

In all the TAVR registries to date, operative risk has been estimated using the logistic EuroSCORE or the Society of Thoracic Surgery Predicted risk of mortality score (STS-PROM). The logistic EuroSCORE was derived from an analysis of patients undergoing any cardiac surgery [11]. Coronary artery bypass comprised the majority of cases entered in the database, skewing risk estimates for other cardiac surgeries, including valve operations, significantly higher. Several studies have shown that the logistic EuroSCORE significantly overstates the risk of aortic valve surgery, as much as three-fold [12,13]. The STS-PROM index was derived in a similar fashion to the EuroSCORE, however, it reviewed significantly more cases and had a more even distribution of valve cases. For high-risk valve surgery, including isolated aortic valve replacement, the STS-PROM score is highly accurate [13]. However, the score fails to consider several factors, including patient frailty and impaired mobility, that may have a significant impact on outcomes.

While accurately gauging the risk of surgery is important, estimating the likelihood of meaningful clinical benefit is just as significant. As noted in a recent review of current TAVR outcomes, "the disappointing late survival in some very high-risk groups begs the question as to whether some elderly patients with comorbidities who may be able to tolerate this therapy may not derive significant benefit from it [14]." It also raises the issue of appropriate outcome measures in the elderly and medically frail population. The average age of patients in the PARTNER trial was 83 years old and the average STS-PROM score was 11%. Perhaps quality of life measurements would be a more meaningful endpoint in this population than mortality. Because percutaneous therapies are less invasive and better tolerated, these questions are broadly applicable. Future guidelines will not only have to determine indications for percutaneous procedures, they also need to provide insight as to who is ineligible due to an inevitable lack of benefit.

The suitability of patients for various percutaneous therapies is closely related to several anatomic variables. The MitraClip is designed to address the problem of excessive leaflet motion (i.e prolapse), coronary sinus devices for mitral regurgitation rely on the proximity of the coronary sinus to the mitral annulus, and transcatheter aortic valves are approved only for use in stenotic, trileaflet valves. Complicating the issue further, devices have been used in ways not initially intended. The MitraClip was originally studied in only those patients with leaflet prolapse in the central portion of the valve [15]; however, in the EVEREST II trial, patients with functional regurgitation made up 20% of the study population and had similar outcomes compared to patients with prolapsing valves. In the same way, the Edwards-SAPIEN valve has been placed in failed prosthetic valves, both in the aortic and mitral positions. This creative use adds another set of considerations for authors of guidelines.

Perhaps the greatest obstacle for percutaneous valve therapies is the large profile of delivery systems. Their size is related to high rates of vascular complications, and may preclude a percutaneous option for patients with peripheral artery disease, or necessitate an alternative access approach for safe placement.

For TAVR, pre-procedure evaluation should seek to answer several questions including (i) ilio-femoral vessel size, calcification, and tortuosity (ii) anatomic details of the aortic valve leaflets (iii) and annulus, sinotubular and sinus of valsalva dimensions. Failure to accurately perform this assessment can lead to vascular injury, annular rupture, paravalvular leak, valve embolization, and coronary obstruction. At our institution, left heart catheterization, lower extremity angiography, CT of the chest, abdomen, and pelvis, and transthoracic echocardiography (TTE) are used to assess each patient prior to TAVR.

Similar planning is required prior to placement of the Melody pulmonic valve. Before valve deployment, pulmonary artery angiography is needed for sizing. Balloon valvuloplasty timed with coronary angiography is also necessary to confirm that the coronary arteries will not be affected when the Melody valve is deployed.

Most percutaneous therapies currently use intra-procedure transesophageal echocardiography (TEE) to guide operators. High-quality images and communication between imaging specialists and operators is mandatory to achieve optimal results.

Patient selection involves risk assessment, estimation of expected clinical benefit, pre-procedure and intra-procedure imaging, and suitable anatomy. Guidelines will help to standardize the approach to the various percutaneous interventions improving their effectiveness and safety.

III. Who should Perform Percutaneous Interventional Procedures

Percutaneous interventional procedures are currently performed in high volume centers by a team consisting of interventional cardiologists familiar with structural heart interventions, imaging specialists, cardiac anesthesiologists and surgeons experienced in high-risk valve surgery. However, as devices get smaller and easier to use, it is expected that more centers will begin performing percutaneous valvular interventions.

A steep learning curve has been observed for the MitraClip procedure and TAVR, suggesting a certain number of procedures is needed for competency. Novel devices often require unique technical skills and procedural considerations unfamiliar to inexperienced physicians. For centers wishing to perform percutaneous valve interventions, proctoring by specialists experienced with each specific device is a prudent idea.

As the field grows, the creation of a new sub-specialty with dedicated teaching programs and standards for accreditation is afoot. The Society for Cardiac Angiography and Interventions recently released a consensus statement outlining the basic training requirements for physicians wishing to participate in percutaneous "structural and adult congenital heart disease interventions" [16]. Several training programs are beginning to offer dedicated training in the field.

Valvular interventions combine aspects of interventional cardiology with cardiac surgery. The ideal facility in which to perform these procedures is not clear, but several professional societies have suggested that a "hybrid" catheterization laboratory is best. These rooms should include high-quality fluoroscopic capabilities with hemodynamic monitoring, capabilities for cardiopulmonary bypass and ventricular assist devices, and be large enough to accommodate anesthesiologists and TEE machines.

Conclusion

The proliferation of devices for percutaneous valvular interventions represents a paradigm shift in the treatment of structural heart disease. Many, but not all, patients will benefit from percutaneous therapies that provide improved, or equivalent, outcomes to surgery but with less morbidity. Determining which percutaneous therapies are effective and which patients will benefit are difficult questions which can be answered only with further study and more results.

References

[1] https://www.sts.org/sections/stsnatinaldatabase/publications/executive/article. accessed 12/29/2010

[2] Cribier A, Eltchaninoff H, Bash A, et al. Percutaneous transcatheter implantation of an aortic valve prosthesis for calcific aortic stenosis: first human case description. *Circulation* 2002;106(24):3006-8.

[3] Vassiliades TA, Jr., Block PC, Cohn LH, et al. The clinical development of percutaneous heart valve technology: a position statement of the Society of Thoracic Surgeons (STS), the American Association for Thoracic Surgery (AATS), and the Society of Cardiovascular Angiography and Intervention (SCAI). *Catheter Cardiovasc Interv* 2005;65(1):73-9

[4] Brown JM, O'Brien SM, Wu C et al. Isolated aortic valve replacement in North America comprising 108,687 patients in 10 years: changes in risks, valve types, and outcomes in STS database. *J Thoracic Cardiovasc Surg* 2009;137:82

[5] O'Brien SM, Shahian DM, Filardo G, et al. The Society of Thoracic Surgeons 2008 Cardiac Surgery Risk Models: Part 2, Isolated Valve Surgery. *Annals Thoracic Surgery* 2009;88;S23

[6] NHLBI balloon valvuloplasty registry participants. Percutaneous Balloon Aortic Valvuloplasty: acute and 30-day follow-up results in 674 patients from the NHLBI Balloon Valvuloplasty RegistryPercutaneous balloon aortic valvuloplasty. Acute and 30-day follow-up results. *Circulation* 1991;84:2383

[7] Leon MB, Smith CR, Mack M, et al. Transcatheter aortic-valve implantation for aortic stenosis in patients who cannot undergo surgery. *N Engl J Med* 2010;363:1597

[8] Feldman, Ted (2010). EVEREST II Randomized Clinical Trial: safety and efficacy, 2 year results, outocomes in functional and degenerative MR. [Power Point Presentation-ACC/i2], Atlanta, GA

[9] Bramstedt KA. Aortic valve replacement in the elderly: frequently indicated yet frequently denied. *Gerontology* 2004;49:46

[10] Iung B, Baron G, Butchart EG, et al. A prospective survey of patients with valvular heart disease in Europe: the Euro Heart Survey on valvular heart disease. *Eur Heart J* 2003;24:1231

[11] Roques F, Michel P, Goldstone AR, et al. The logistic EuroSCORE. *Eur Heart J.* 2003;24(9):882

[12] Thourani VH, Ailawadi G, Szeto WY, et al. Outcomes of surgical aortic valve replacement in high-risk patients: a multinational study. *Ann Thorac Surg* 2011;91:49

[13] Wendt D, Osswald BR, Kayser K, et al. Society of Thoracic Surgeons score is superior to the EuroSCORE in determining mortality in high risk patients undergoing isolated aortic valve replacement. *Ann Thorac Surg* 2009;88:468

[14] Webb J, Cribier A. Percutaneous transarterial aortic valve implantation: what do we know? *Eur Heart J;* published online December 4, 2010

[15] Feldman T, Wasserman HS, Herrmann HC, et al. Percutaneous mitral valve repair using the edge-to-edge technique: six-month results of the EVEREST Phase I Clinical Trial. *J Am Coll Cardiol* 2005;46(11):2134

[16] Ruiz CE, Feldman TE, Hijazi ZM, et al. Interventional fellowship in structural and congenital heart disease for adults. *J Am Coll Cardiol Intv* 2010;3:e1-15

In: Percutaneous Valve Technology: Present and Future
ISBN: 978-1-61942-577-4
Editors: Jose Luis Navia and Sharif Al-Ruzzeh

Chapter II

The Role of Echocardiography in the Development of Percutaneous Aortic/Mitral Valve Technology – 3D Echocardiography

L. Leonardo Rodriguez

Traditionally echocardiography has played a predominant role in the evaluation of valvular heart disease. This technology has multiples advantages:

- -Real time imaging with good temporal and spatial resolution
- -Portability
- -Ability to assess anatomy and function.

Transthoracic echocardiography is usually enough for clinical management, however, in selected cases transesophageal echo offers superior image quality and is particularly useful in the evaluation of the mitral valve.

With the development of new percutaneous treatments for valvular heart disease, an expanded role of echocardiography has ensued [1-6]. Greater anatomic precision and better understanding of the pathophysiology of the lesions are now required. Similar to what occurred in the operative room, echocardiography has become an important tool in guiding procedures in the catheterization laboratory, assessing immediate post procedural results and diagnosis of complications.

The primary example of the preeminent role of echocardiography during percutaneous valvular procedures is the Eclip mitral valve repair [4, 5, 7, 8].

The availability of real time 3D echocardiography has increased our diagnostic capabilities and has added an important dimension in the detailed evaluation of the mitral valve [9-13].

The current 3D ultrasound equipment uses matrix-array technology with 2500 elements. It is now possible to acquire real time 3D rendered images as well as simultaneous biplane or multiplane 2D images.

Miniaturization has allowed this technology to be adapted for transesophageal probes and is now possible the recording of high spatial resolution images.

3D rendered images can be acquired in real time with the ability of choosing an area of interested and manipulate its orientation in real time. It can also be acquired as full volume over several beats for off-line analysis.

For procedural real time guidance the biplane and the real time 3D sector focused are the most utilized.

Real time 3D has expanded our understanding of the mitral and aortic valve anatomy and function and aortic-mitral valve coupling [14](Figure 1).

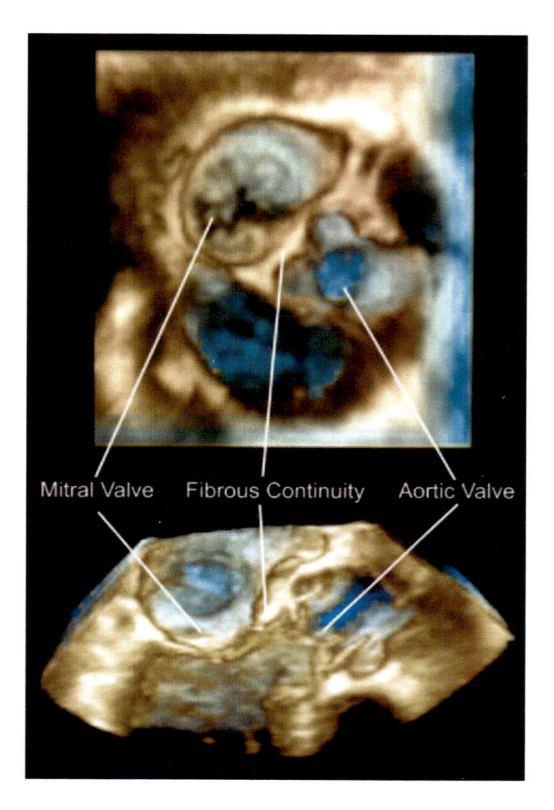

Figure 1. 3D anatomical relationship between the aortic and mitral valves.[14].

Mitral Valve

The mitral valve apparatus is a complex structure that includes the mitral valve annulus, leaflets and subvalvular apparatus. A systematic echocardiographic approach allows visualization of all segments of the mitral valve and constitutes part of the routine examination of patients with mitral valve disease [9, 15, 16]). TEE offers more detailed anatomical information with greater spatial resolution and without interference of chest structures. In patients with mechanical mitral valves TEE is often required when mitral regurgitation is suspected.

Real time 3D TEE has represented a significant advance in the evaluation of the mitral valve. It offers a unique en-face view of the mitral from the left atrium or left ventricle that allows simultaneous visualization of all its segments. Individual scallops and commissures are easily seen [9] [11] (Figures 2,3,4,5). In patients with degenerative valve, prolapsing scallops or rupture chordae can be accurately identified. The 3-D image is often rotated from its initial position to show the "surgeon's" view with the aorta anteriorly and the left atrial appendage to the left of the screen (Figure3).

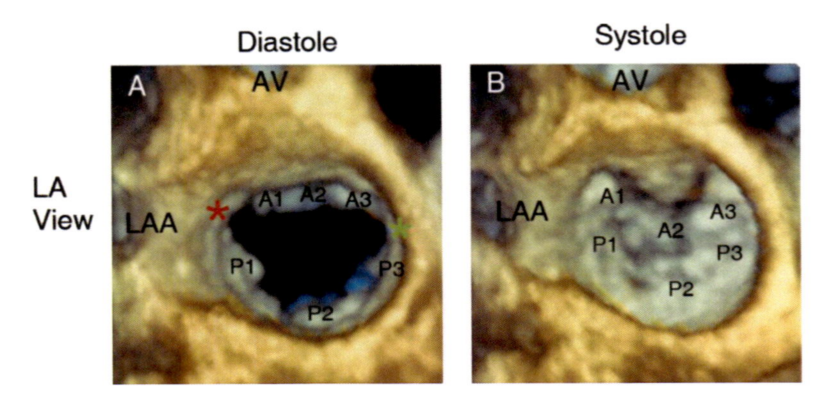

Figure 2. En-face view of the mitral valve from the left atrium in diastole and systole.[11].

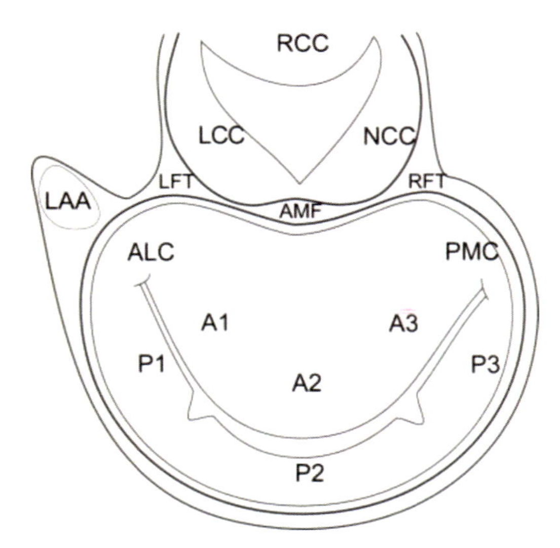

Figure 3. Schematic of the en face 3D TEE view of the mitral valve from the left atrium.[11].

Although there is only limited experience, it appears also possible to guide complex mitral valve interventions using real time 3D echocardiography by accurately directing catheters and devices to specific parts of the mitral valve.

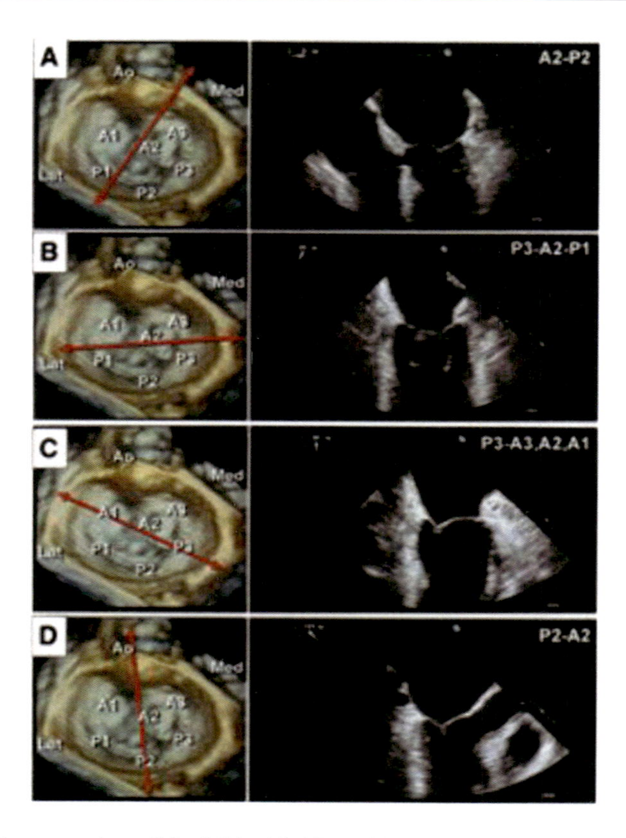

Figure 4. Systematic Interrogation of the MV with 2D and 3D TEE.[9].

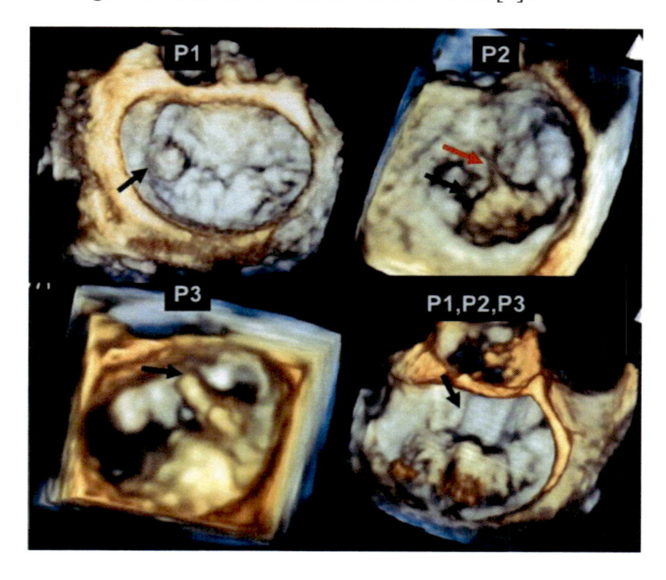

Figure 5. En face view of the mitral valve showing examples of mitral valve prolapse and ruptured chordae (red arrow).[9].

Specific Mitral Valve Procedures

Mitral Balloon Valvuloplasty

Echocardiography is useful at every stage of this procedure: Patient selection: anatomic features of the mitral are powerful predictors of the success and are widely used for patient selection [17-23].

One of the commonly used echocardiographic scores [17-22]) developed to evaluate suitability of patients for balloon valvuloplasty includes the following elements:

1) Degree of valvular thickening
2) 2-Valvular calcification
3) 3-Leaflet immobility
4) 4-Subvalvular involvement.

In addition, commissural morphology has been related to post procedural mitral regurgitation [24, 25].

TEE is also used in selected cases to rule out severe mitral regurgitation or left atrial thrombus, both potential contraindications for this procedure.

Procedural guidance: Echocardiography can also be used to help guiding the transeptal puncture and balloon placement. After each balloon inflation it is possible to evaluate the degree of commisural splitting and presence and severity of mitral regurgitation. Recently it has been shown the prognostic value of unilateral vs. bilateral commissural splitting [26].

The role of echo in mitral balloon valvuloplasty has been summarized in the ASE guidelines for Echocardiography-Guided Interventions

> "Echocardiography provides significant benefit in percutaneous balloon valvuloplasty for mitral stenosis and is recommended for the assessment of patient selection and to assess the adequacy of results. Online intraprocedural echocardiography offers significant advantages compared with fluoroscopic guidance, in monitoring procedural efficacy and monitoring for complications. TEE can also be used to guide the procedure. TTE is recommended for procedural guidance, monitoring for complications, and to assess the adequacy of results, when preprocedural TEE has already been performed. ICE can be used for procedural guidance and provides imaging that is comparable with TEE." [27]

Role of 3D echo: Using TTE or 3D TEE is possible assess the degree of commissural splitting after the procedure. In his early experience using 3D TEE, Zamorano et al. showed a better agreement with the Gorlin formula for estimation of mitral valve area before and after valvuloplasty [13, 28]. However, in this initial experience the mean time to acquire and analyze the images was up to 33 minutes in those in atrial fibrillation, impacting on the practical application of this technique. It is likely that with further experience and advances in imaging processing this time could significantly reduce. Other authors have also confirmed the superiority of 3D echo in the assessment of the anatomy and severity of mitral stenosis [29, 30].

The advent of real time 3D TEE has offered new potential for the routine intraprocedural guidance using this technology [31, 32] (Figure 6). It can also provide immediate feedback regarding commissural splitting [33]. (Figure 7)

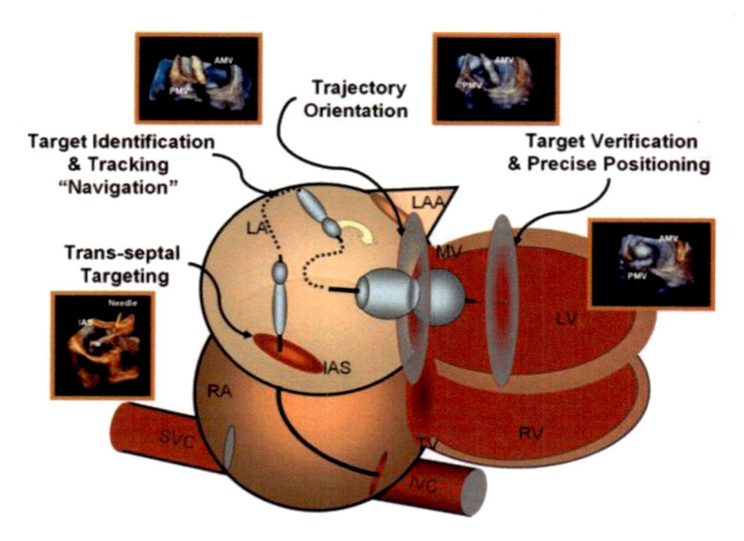

Figure 6. Schematic of interventional imaging process using 3D guidance for mitral valve balloon valvuloplasty (MVBV). Selection of suitable site for septal puncture. Navigation in the left atrium (LA) by tracking the balloon catheter and visualization of the maneuvering margin, sparing the posterior wall (PW) and other structures from damage. Positioning the balloon over the mitral valve (MV) orifice. Trajectory orientation within a 3D frame of reference simplifies alignment centering utilizing a single view. AMV = anterior mitral valve; IVC = inferior vena cava; LAA = left atrial appendage; LV = left ventricle; PMV = posterior mitral valve; RV = right ventricle; RA = right atrium; SVC = superior vena cava; TV = tricuspid valve.[31].

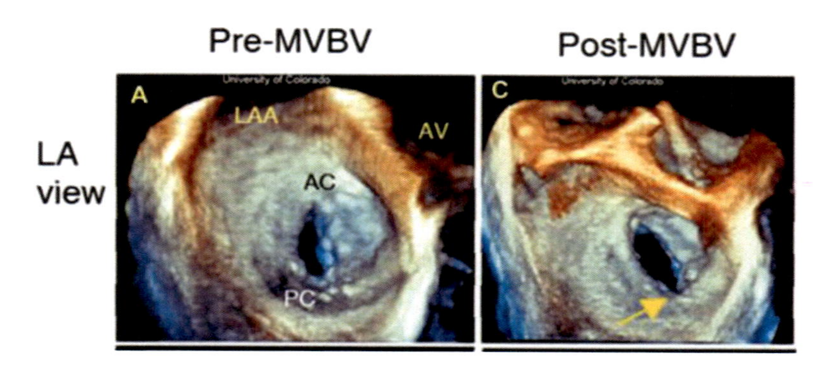

Figure 7. 3D TEE before and after balloon valvuloplasty showing increased in the mitral valve orifice and fissured posterior commissure.[31].

Although severe complications are infrequent during this procedure echocardiography helps in the prompt diagnosis and management. Cardiac tamponade is easily recognized as well as severe mitral valve regurgitation.

Percutaneous Paravalvular Leak Closure

Paravalvular regurgitation is a potential complication after valvular replacement. When severe, it can lead to severe hemolysis, heart failure or both. Traditionally, surgery has been the only option and usually carried a higher operative risk due to the underlying anatomical. Recently, techniques have been developed to close paravalvular regurgitations percutaneously. These techniques require carefully and accurately mapping of sewing ring to precisely locate the origin of the leak. Initial experience has demonstrated the utility of real time 3D-TEE in determining the location and number of leaks and in guiding the procedure [34-38] (Figure 8 [39]).

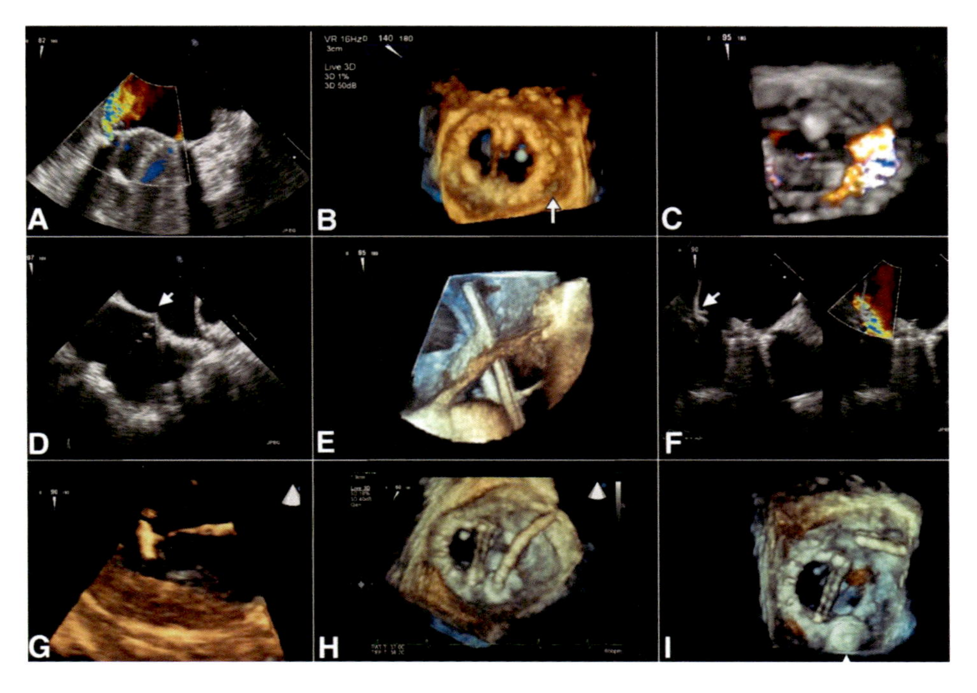

Figure 8. 3D-TEE guidance of percutaneous closure of perivalvular mitral regurgitation in a patient with a mechanical valve. JACC Cardiovascular imaging, Vol. 2 No. 6 2009 June 2009 – 771 – 3.

Future advances in device design and delivery system may position percutaneous closure as the procedure of choice in patients with paravalvular regurgitation. Real time 3D-TEE will be and essential tool in the diagnosis and management of this patients.

Percutaneous Mitral Valve Repair

A long standing goal of interventional cardiology has been the possibility of repairing mitral regurgitation. Significant advances have occurred in this field and the last few years. Several devices have been developed for this purpose involving either leaflet manipulation or mitral annular reduction through the coronary sinus and have been discussed in other chapters.

Percutaneous Edge-to-Edge Technique

This technique reviewed in detail in another section of this book, involves the placement of a sophisticated clip that approximates the middle portion of the anterior and posterior leaflets creating a double mitral valve orifice. It use requires intensive use echocardiography for guidance. This technique is without doubt the most echo-demanding percutaneous valvular procedure available at the present time. The Eclip technique involves transseptal catheterization, accurate steering of the device to the affected segment, clip alignment and delivery. Transesophageal echo is also essential for immediate evaluation of the results and helping in determining the need for a second clip. A randomized trial in percutaneous repair using E-Clip technology has been successfully completed.

Echocardiography is critical at all phases of this procedure from patient selection to procedural guidance to long term follow up.

Echocardiography in Patient Selection

The Eclip device has been designed to treat centrally originating mitral regurgitation and this can be accurately determined using color. In addition, focal calcification at the middle tip of the leaflets can be identified which is considered a contraindication for this procedure as they may be dislodged by the clip. Patients with mitral stenosis or opening restriction can be also identify and excluded from this procedure. Patients with functional mitral regurgitation and severe apical leaflet displacement with little tissue apposition during systole are suboptimal candidates for the procedure.

The basic 2D echocardiographic guidance involves the following views:

1) Mid esophageal short-axis view (multiplane angle of approximately 30–60 degrees) at the base of the heart is used to guide transseptal catheterization and catheter manipulation, monitor system translation, and avoid contact with the lateral structures such as the lateral left atrial wall and left atrial appendage.
2) Mid esophageal commissural or "2-chamber" view (multiplane angle of approximately 60 degrees) is used for medial lateral and axial adjustments of the system.
3) Mid esophageal long axis (LVOT) (multiplane angle of approximately 120–150 degrees) is used for anterior–posterior system adjustments.
4) Transgastric short axis (multiplane angle 0–30 degrees) at the mitral valve level and in the left ventricle is used for alignment of the clip arms perpendicular to the line of coaptation.

Role of 3D Echo

In the planning stages, 3DTEE is helpful in aiding in patient selection. As mentioned before, the clip has been designed to be placed in the central portion of the mitral valve leaflets. The en-face view allows precise anatomical visualization of the posterior mitral valve scallops and anterior mitral valve segments and their pathology (Figures 9a and 9b).

During procedural guidance the biplane mode is used more commonly with one pane at 60°-80°and the other at 110°-150° (steps 2 and 3 from above). 3D volume rendered images can show the site of the transeptal puncture, the course of the catheter and the alignment of the open clip arms perpendicular to the coaptation line (Figure 9b).

The alignment of the clip arms perpendicular to the line of coaptation can be difficult and has typically required either a transgastric view (not available in all patients) or changing to a transthoracic echocardiogram to obtain a short axis view. 3D can be particularly useful in this stage [31, 40]. Again using the en face view either from the atrial or ventricular side the whole line of coaptation can be visualized and the clip rotated accordingly. The final result of the procedure is a double orifice mitral valve (Figures 9b, 10).

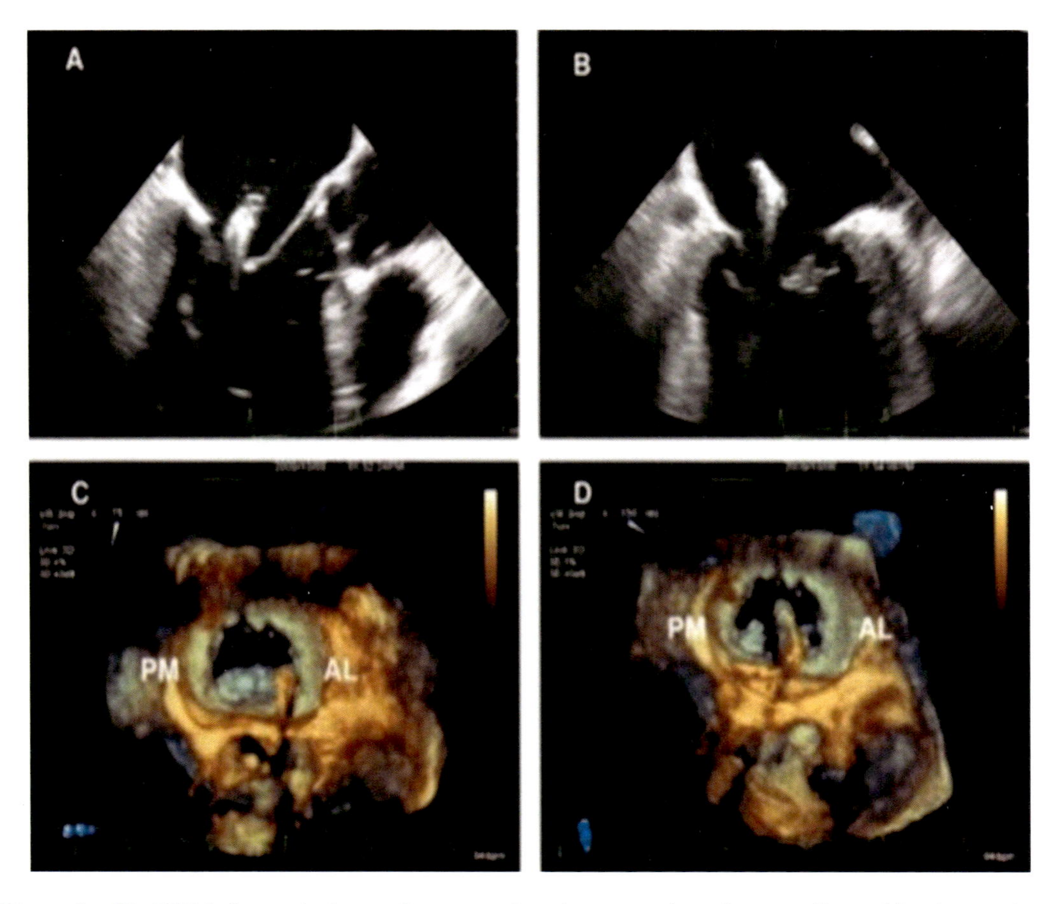

Figure 9a. 2D. TEE left ventricular outflow tract view demonstrating adequate clip position in anterior-posterior direction, (B) 2D TEE with intercommissural view demonstrating adequate clip position in medial-lateral direction. (C) RT 3D TEE with 3D zoom mode demonstrating nonoptimal, too lateral position of the clip delivery system. (D) RT 3D TEE demonstrating optimal position of the clip in anterior-posterior as well as medial-lateral direction after performing the necessary adjustments (A and B). AL = anterolateral; PM = posteromedial; RT = real-time; TEE = transesophageal; 3D = 3-dimensional; 2D = 2-dimensional.[45].

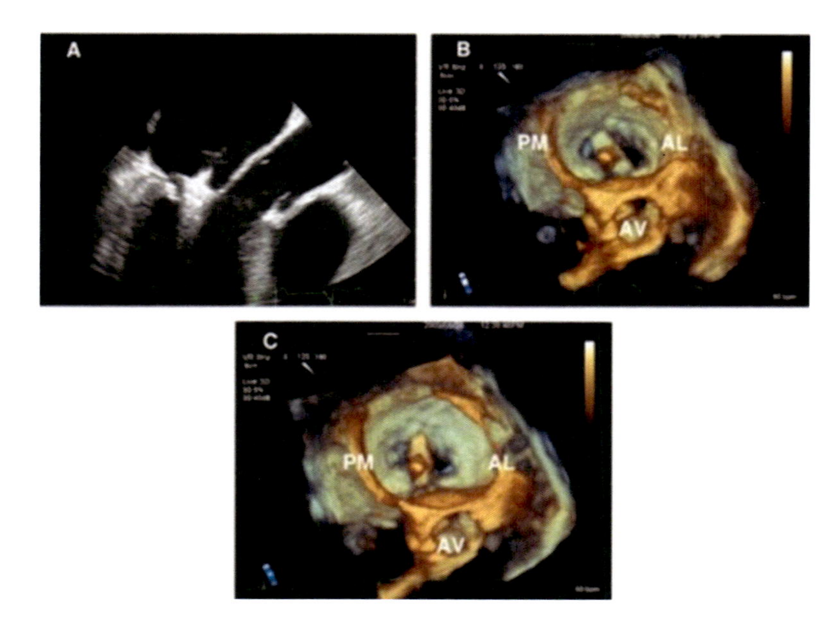

Figure 9b. (A) 2D TEE left ventricular outflow tract image. Clip arms are open clip perpendicular to the commissural line, (B) RT 3D images demonstrating nonoptimal perpendicularity. (C) RT 3D TEE image from the left atrium of the opened clip showing adequate perpendicularity to the commissural line after adjustment of the clip arms using RT 3D TEE. AV = aortic valve.[45].

Figures 9a and 9b. [45]3D-TEE guidance of Eclip percutaneous mitral valve repair. Note that the images have not been rotated and they are presented as their initially appear when captured: aorta is posterior and left atrial appendage is at the right of the image.

Complications, although rare, can also be visualized by 3D TEE. [41].

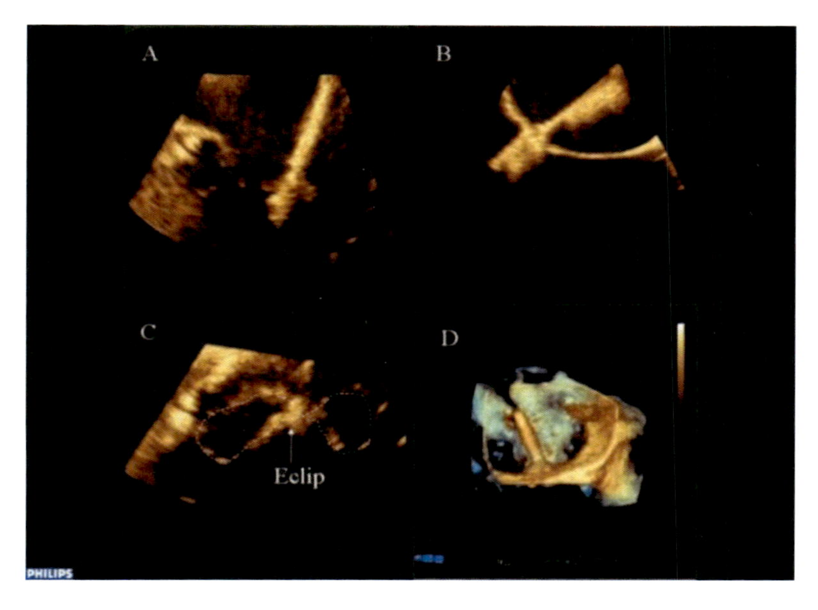

Figure 10. Multiplanar reconstruction of the clip closed but before releasing. A and B showing the anterior and posterior leaflets grasped by the clip. (C) The typical double orifice and (D) 3D rendering.

Trans-Coronary Sinus Repair

The proximity of the coronary sinus to the posterior mitral annulus makes this structure of potential use for percutaneous mitral valve repair. There has been a considerable effort to develop percutaneous annuloplasty devices and multitude of ingenious prototypes has been created. Some of these devices have been implanted in clinical trial is a limited number of patients. The coronary sinus can be seen by echo but is better visualized using computer tomography and angiography. Although echocardiography appears more limited in the guidance of this type of devices still will be extremely helpful in providing immediate feedback regarding the amount of residual regurgitation. Some of these devices allow adjustments to decrease the annular diameter if mitral regurgitation is still present and this titration will have to be done in real time monitored by echocardiography. Conceivable intracardiac echo could also be used for this purpose.

Aortic Valve Procedures

The percutaneous options for treatment of aortic valve pathology are more limited. Aortic balloon valvuloplasty is a palliative procedure done under fluoroscopic guidance. However, the introduction of percutaneous aortic valve replacement has opened an exciting chapter in the treatment of aortic stenosis.

The imaging aspect of this procedure is very important from patient selection and procedural planning (Computer tomography and echocardiography), procedural guidance (Fluoroscopy, angiography and transesophageal echo) and immediate results evaluation and followup (echocardiography).

Patient selection: This technology is currently used in high risk patients with severe aortic stenosis. Echocardiography is used for evaluation of left ventricular function, presence and severity of aortic regurgitation and other valvular lesions. For the Sapiens-Edwards valve the measurement of the aortic annulus is important in selecting the size of the aortic prosthesis. This has been done typically by measuring the antero-posterior diameter in the parasternal long axis or transesophageal long axis view and assumes a circular geometry. Comparative results between transthoracic and transesophageal [42]views and between echocardiography and computer tomography have demonstrated suboptimal agreement [43]It appears to be now clear that in some patients, and may be in most of them, the geometry is not circular but rather oval. That explains in part the discrepancy between echo and CT. The use of 3D echo could improve accuracy by reconstructing a true short axis view at the annular level allowing measurement of the largest diameter (Figure 11). Preliminary data has shown a better agreement with of 3D TEE annulus with CT derived measurements [44].

Procedural guidance. This is dominated by fluoroscopy and angiography. However, echo is a useful adjunct to theses techniques. Although the insertion points of the leaflets is clearly seen by transesophageal echo, the visualization of the stent is more difficult. The stent is mounted on a collapse balloon with some residual angiographic contrast. The interface between the balloon and the stent is hard to discern even after adjusting gains and other settings. In addition, heavily calcified annulus may also obscure the stent. In experienced hands it is possible to identify the stent and help in reaching the optimal position. The stent valve is usually positioned 50-60% in the LVOT and 40-50% in the aortic side. Alternatively, the distal (ventricular) edge of stent can aligned with the hinge point of the anterior mitral leaflet. Immediately after deployment is when the echocardiogram is more useful. Information regarding proper position, leaflet motion and degree of aortic regurgitation can be rapidly provided.

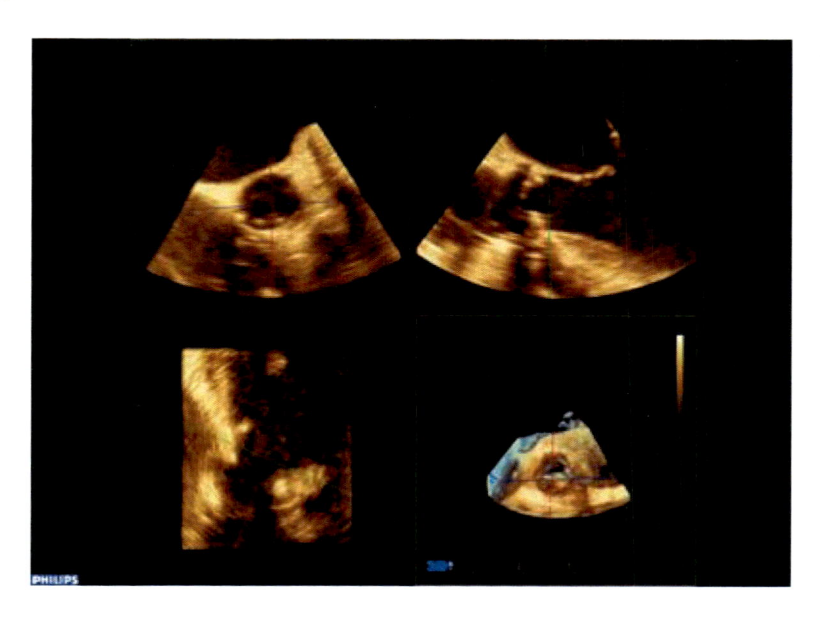

Figure 11. Multiplanar reconstruction of the left ventricular outflow tract in a patient being considered for percutaneous aortic valve implantation. On the image in the upper left corner diameters and area by planimetry can be obtained.

Role of 3D: The utility of 3D echocardiography is more limited in this procedure but the initial experience has been positive (). 3D appears to be better suited to measure the left ventricular outflow tract more accurately. 3D color mapping can also be used to more precisely evaluate number and location of residual regurgitant jets.

Challenges: The field of percutaneous intervention for structural valvular disease is expanding at a fast pace. The interaction between echocardiographers and interventionists and surgeons during these procedures is also evolving. One important lesson learned from the Eclip trial is that proper communication between members of the teams is essential.

Dedicated personal with expertise in this technique is not widely available. In addition, it is imperative to involve both cardiovascular surgeons and interventional cardiologist in learning and getting familiar with the different views that may allow procedural guidance. The use of real time 3D echocardiography during valvular procedure is in its initial stages. The limitation of poor image quality will also apply to 3D echo.

It is important to develop a standard set of images for each particular procedure and for interventionists and surgeon to learn those views. They need to learn how to navigate catheters and instruments in real time 3D echocardiographic space. It is conceivable that the routine use of 3D echo may significantly reduce procedural time and fluoroscopy exposure and make these procedures safer with more accurate catheter manipulation.

References

[1] Van Mieghem, N.M., et al., Anatomy of the mitral valvular complex and its implications for transcatheter interventions for mitral regurgitation. *J Am Coll Cardiol.* 56(8): p. 617-26.

[2] Christofferson, R.D., et al., Emerging transcatheter therapies for aortic and mitral disease. *Heart,* 2009. 95(2): p. 148-55.

[3] Piazza, N. and R. Bonan, Transcatheter mitral valve repair for functional mitral regurgitation: coronary sinus approach. *J Interv Cardiol,* 2007. 20(6): p. 495-508.

[4] Feldman, T., et al., Percutaneous mitral valve repair using the edge-to-edge technique: six-month results of the EVEREST Phase I Clinical Trial. *J Am Coll Cardiol,* 2005. 46(11): p. 2134-40.

[5] Feldman, T., et al., Percutaneous mitral repair with the MitraClip system: safety and midterm durability in the initial EVEREST (Endovascular Valve Edge-to-Edge REpair Study) cohort. *J Am Coll Cardiol,* 2009. 54(8): p. 686-94.

[6] Kim, J.H., et al., Mitral cerclage annuloplasty, a novel transcatheter treatment for secondary mitral valve regurgitation: initial results in swine. *J Am Coll Cardiol,* 2009. 54(7): p. 638-51.

[7] Silvestry, F.E., et al., Echocardiographic guidance and assessment of percutaneous repair for mitral regurgitation with the Evalve MitraClip: lessons learned from EVEREST I. *J Am Soc Echocardiogr,* 2007. 20(10): p. 1131-40.

[8] Feldman, T., Intraprocedure guidance for percutaneous mitral valve interventions: TTE, TEE, ICE, or X-ray? *Catheter Cardiovasc Interv,* 2004. 63(3): p. 395-6.

[9] O'Gara, P., et al., The role of imaging in chronic degenerative mitral regurgitation. *JACC Cardiovasc Imaging,* 2008. 1(2): p. 221-37.

[10] Lang, R.M., et al., Live three-dimensional transthoracic echocardiography: case study world atlas. *Echocardiography,* 2005. 22(1): p. 95-8.

[11] Salcedo, E.E., et al., A framework for systematic characterization of the mitral valve by real-time three-dimensional transesophageal echocardiography. *J Am Soc Echocardiogr,* 2009. 22(10): p. 1087-99.

[12] Hirata, K., et al., Clinical utility of new real time three-dimensional transthoracic echocardiography in assessment of mitral valve prolapse. *Echocardiography,* 2008. 25(5): p. 482-8.

[13] Zamorano, J., et al., Real-time three-dimensional echocardiography for rheumatic mitral valve stenosis evaluation: an accurate and novel approach. *J Am Coll Cardiol,* 2004. 43(11): p. 2091-6.

[14] Veronesi, F., et al., A study of functional anatomy of aortic-mitral valve coupling using 3D matrix transesophageal echocardiography. *Circ Cardiovasc Imaging,* 2009. 2(1): p. 24-31.

[15] Omran, A.S., et al., Intraoperative transesophageal echocardiography accurately predicts mitral valve anatomy and suitability for repair. *J Am Soc Echocardiogr,* 2002. 15(9): p. 950-7.

[16] Monin, J.L., et al., Functional assessment of mitral regurgitation by transthoracic echocardiography using standardized imaging planes diagnostic accuracy and outcome implications. *J Am Coll Cardiol,* 2005. 46(2): p. 302-9.

[17] Wilkins, G.T., et al., Percutaneous balloon dilatation of the mitral valve: an analysis of echocardiographic variables related to outcome and the mechanism of dilatation. *Br Heart J,* 1988. 60(4): p. 299-308.

[18] Reid, C.L. and S.H. Rahimtoola, The role of echocardiography/Doppler in catheter balloon treatment of adults with aortic and mitral stenosis. *Circulation,* 1991. 84(3 Suppl): p. I240-9.

[19] Reid, C.L., et al., Influence of mitral valve morphology on double-balloon catheter balloon valvuloplasty in patients with mitral stenosis. Analysis of factors predicting immediate and 3-month results. *Circulation, 1*989. 80(3): p. 515-24.

[20] Rahimtoola, S.H., et al., Current evaluation and management of patients with mitral stenosis. *Circulation,* 2002. 106(10): p. 1183-8.

[21] Abascal, V.M., et al., Prediction of successful outcome in 130 patients undergoing percutaneous balloon mitral valvotomy. *Circulation,* 1990. 82(2): p. 448-56.

[22] Abascal, V.M., et al., Echocardiographic evaluation of mitral valve structure and function in patients followed for at least 6 months after percutaneous balloon mitral valvuloplasty. *J Am Coll Cardiol,* 1988. 12(3): p. 606-15.

[23] Abascal, V.M., et al., Mitral regurgitation after percutaneous balloon mitral valvuloplasty in adults: evaluation by pulsed Doppler echocardiography. *J Am Coll Cardiol,* 1988. 11(2): p. 257-63.

[24] Padial, L.R., et al., Echocardiography can predict the development of severe mitral regurgitation after percutaneous mitral valvuloplasty by the Inoue technique. *Am J Cardiol,* 1999. 83(8): p. 1210-3.

[25] Padial, L.R., et al., Echocardiography can predict which patients will develop severe mitral regurgitation after percutaneous mitral valvulotomy. *J Am Coll Cardiol,* 1996. 27(5): p. 1225-31.

[26] Messika-Zeitoun, D., et al., Impact of degree of commissural opening after percutaneous mitral commissurotomy on long-term outcome. *JACC Cardiovasc Imaging,* 2009. 2(1): p. 1-7.

[27] Silvestry, F.E., et al., Echocardiography-guided interventions. *J Am Soc Echocardiogr,* 2009. 22(3): p. 213-31; quiz 316-7.

[28] Zamorano, J., et al., Non-invasive assessment of mitral valve area during percutaneous balloon mitral valvuloplasty: role of real-time 3D echocardiography. *Eur Heart J,* 2004. 25(23): p. 2086-91.

[29] Anwar, A.M., et al., Validation of a new score for the assessment of mitral stenosis using real-time three-dimensional echocardiography. *J Am Soc Echocardiogr.* 23(1): p. 13-22.

[30] Chu, J.W., et al., Assessing mitral valve area and orifice geometry in calcific mitral stenosis: a new solution by real-time three-dimensional echocardiography. *J Am Soc Echocardiogr,* 2008. 21(9): p. 1006-9.

[31] Eng, M.H., et al., Implementation of real time three-dimensional transesophageal echocardiography in percutaneous mitral balloon valvuloplasty and structural heart disease interventions. *Echocardiography,* 2009. 26(8): p. 958-66.

[32] Perk, G., et al., Use of real time three-dimensional transesophageal echocardiography in intracardiac catheter based interventions. *J Am Soc Echocardiogr,* 2009. 22(8): p. 865-82.

[33] Gill, E.A., M.S. Kim, and J.D. Carroll, 3D TEE for evaluation of commissural opening before and during percutaneous mitral commissurotomy. *JACC Cardiovasc Imaging,* 2009. 2(8): p. 1034-5; author reply 1035-6.

[34] Horton, K.D., B. Whisenant, and S. Horton, Percutaneous closure of a mitral perivalvular leak using three dimensional real time and color flow imaging. *J Am Soc Echocardiogr.* 23(8): p. 903 e5-7.

[35] Karthik, S., et al., Intraoperative assessment of perivalvular mitral regurgitation: utility of three-dimensional echocardiography. *J Cardiothorac Vasc Anesth,* 2008. 22(3): p. 431-4.

[36] Garcia-Fernandez, M.A., et al., Utility of real-time three-dimensional transesophageal echocardiography in evaluating the success of percutaneous transcatheter closure of mitral paravalvular leaks. *J Am Soc Echocardiogr,* 2010. 23(1): p. 26-32.

[37] Azran, M.S., et al., Echo rounds: application of real-time 3-dimensional transesophageal echocardiography in the percutaneous closure of a mitral paravalvular leak. *Anesth Analg,* 2010. 110(6): p. 1581-3.

[38] Little, S.H., et al., Three-dimensional transesophageal echocardiogram provides real-time guidance during percutaneous paravalvular mitral repair. *Circ Heart Fail,* 2008. 1(4): p. 293-4.

[39] Hamilton-Craig, C., et al., The role of 3D transesophageal echocardiography during percutaneous closure of paravalvular mitral regurgitation. *JACC Cardiovasc Imaging,* 2009. 2(6): p. 771-3.

[40] Swaans, M.J., et al., Three-dimensional transoesophageal echocardiography in a patient undergoing percutaneous mitral valve repair using the edge-to-edge clip technique. *Eur J Echocardiogr,* 2009. 10(8): p. 982-3.

[41] Pedrazzini, G.B., et al., Complications of Percutaneous Edge-to-Edge Mitral Valve Repair: The Role of Real-Time Three-Dimensional Transesophageal Echocardiography. *J Am Soc Echocardiogr.*

[42] Moss, R.R., et al., Role of echocardiography in percutaneous aortic valve implantation. *JACC Cardiovasc Imaging,* 2008. 1(1): p. 15-24.

[43] Messika-Zeitoun, D., et al., Multimodal assessment of the aortic annulus diameter: implications for transcatheter aortic valve implantation. *J Am Coll Cardiol,* 2010. 55(3): p. 186-94.

[44] Ng, A.C., et al., Comparison of aortic root dimensions and geometries before and after transcatheter aortic valve implantation by 2- and 3-dimensional transesophageal echocardiography and multislice computed tomography. *Circ Cardiovasc Imaging.* 3(1): p. 94-102.

[45] Altiok, E., et al., Real-Time 3D TEE Allows Optimized Guidance of Percutaneous Edge-to-Edge Repair of the Mitral Valve. *JACC Cardiovasc Imaging,* 2010. 3(11): p. 1196-8.

In: Percutaneous Valve Technology: Present and Future
Editors: Jose Luis Navia and Sharif Al-Ruzzeh
ISBN: 978-1-61942-577-4

Chapter III

3-Dimensional Computed Tomographic (CT) Imaging in the Context of Transcatheter Valvular Interventions

Paul Schoenhagen and Sandy S. Halliburton

Abstract

Less invasive surgical and transcatheter procedures for valvular and structural heart disease are characterized by limited direct exposure of the operative field. Therefore pre-procedural planning and intra-operative decision-making increasingly relies on image guidance.

The need for pre- and intra- operative visualization has been met by novel 3-dimensional imaging approaches. Pre-procedural 3-D imaging provides detailed understanding of the operative field for surgical/interventional planning. Subsequent integration of imaging during the procedure allows real-time guidance.

This chapter describes the emerging experience with computed tomography for interventional guidance of valvular procedures. Other modalities allowing 3-D imaging, including rotational angiography (C-arm CT), echocardiography, and MRI are briefly compared, but are discussed in more detail in other chapter of the book.

I. Introduction

Less invasive surgical and transcatheter procedures for valvular and structural heart disease are characterized by limited direct exposure of the operative field. Therefore pre-procedural planning and intra-operative decision-making increasingly relies on image guidance.

The need for pre- and intra- operative visualization has been met by novel 3-dimensional imaging approaches. Pre-procedural 3-D imaging provides detailed understanding of the operative field for surgical/interventional planning. At least theoretically, it provides an advantage over direct intra-operative inspection, because the cardiac structures are seen under physiologic condition rather than in the collapsed state after initiation of cardiopulmonary bypass. Subsequent integration of imaging during the procedure allows real-time guidance.

This chapter describes the emerging experience with computed tomography for interventional guidance of valvular procedures. Other modalities allowing 3-D imaging, including rotational angiography (C-arm CT), echocardiography, and MRI are briefly compared, but are discussed in more detail in other chapter of the book.

II. 3-D Imaging with Multi-Detector Computed Tomography (MDCT)

The following paragraphs will describe basics of CT scanner technology, image acquisition, and image analysis with particular focus on imaging in the context of valvular imaging.

Scanner Technology

Multi-detector row computed tomography scanners house one or two x-ray tubes mounted on a gantry, which rotates rapidly around the patient table. The attenuated x-rays are detected on the opposite side of the gantry by multiple rows of detectors, segmented by collimators.

The use of MDCT for 3-D cardiovascular imaging has become possible due to fast gantry rotation time and a large number of detector rows arranged with narrow collimated widths. [1,2] A 360° rotation of the x-ray tube requires between 270 to 350 ms with state-of-the-art scanners, and determines the temporal resolution. The best temporal resolution (75 ms) can be achieved using dual-tube technology.[2]

Data covering the entire heart, synchronized to the heartbeat, are acquired within a single breath hold. Scanners with extended anatomical coverage along the patient's long axis or extended z-coverage (e.g. 320 detector row scanners) acquire up to 16cm per gantry rotation and can cover the entire heart in one rotation. [1] Images are reconstructed with slice thickness ranging from 0.5 to 3 mm depending on the specific cardiac application. Spatial resolution in the axial image plane is typically 0.5 mm x 0.5 mm.

Because of the extensive and rapid motion of valvular structures during the cardiac cycle, use of state-of-the-art scanners (at a minimum 64-slice technology) is critical for imaging in the context of valvular interventions.

Image Acquisition

Acquisition Parameters and Acquisition Protocols

Important basic parameters for the acquisition of cardiac CT data include gantry rotation time, collimated detector-row width, longitudinal or z-coverage, pitch (for helical data acquisition only), x-ray tube voltage, x-ray tube current, and axial versus helical mode. These parameters are optimized for specific clinical indications. Imaging in the context of valvular interventions often requires advanced protocols with superior spatial and temporal resolution. In the following text it will be described that such protocols are associated with increased radiation exposure, which must be justified for individual patients. [3]

Gantry Rotation Time

The time required for the x-ray tube/detector system to rotate 360° around the patient (gantry rotation time) determines the temporal resolution. Because only approximately 180° of projection data are required by cardiac algorithms to reconstruct each image, the temporal resolution is about one-half the gantry rotation time for single x-ray source CT scanners, and one-fourth the gantry rotation time for dual x-ray source scanners. Faster gantry rotation (minimum values between 270 ms and350 ms with current scanners) results in improved temporal resolution, but decreases the number of x-ray photons available (for a given x-ray tube voltage and tube current), resulting in increased image noise. Therefore, in order to limit noise, faster rotation time requires increasing x-ray tube output and is associated with increased radiation exposure [4].

Collimation Size and Z-Coverage

The z-coverage per rotation is defined by the width and number of detector rows. The collimated width of one detector row slice determines the minimum reconstruction slice thickness. State-of-the-art CT systems have minimum detector row widths of 0.5 mm or 0.625 mm wide detector rows at the center of rotation. Although thinner reconstructed slices widths offer improved z-axis spatial resolution, fewer x-ray photons contribute to the reconstructed image (for a given x-ray tube voltage and tube current) resulting in increased image noise. This increased noise can be overcome by increasing the x-ray tube current, or less common, the tube voltage. However, this is associated with increased radiation exposure. Therefore reconstruction of submillimeter slices should be reserved for coronary artery imaging and other small structures. For imaging of larger cardiovascular anatomy without need the for high spatial resolution, data acquired using several of these small detectors can be combined during image reconstruction so more photons contribute to the reconstructed image (i.e., thicker slices can be reconstructed) and the desired image noise achieved with decreased radiation exposure.

A greater number of detector rows in a multi-detector array increase z-coverage per rotation and subsequently decrease scan time. The z-coverage with state-of-the-art scanners ranges from approximately 2 cm to 16 cm per rotation. It is important to note that the number of detector rows does not necessarily equal the number of slices that can be acquired per rotation; some scanners sample each detector twice per rotation such that the number of slices acquired per rotation is two times the number of detector rows used [5].

Pitch

For helical imaging (see below) a related parameter is pitch, which describes patient table movement with respect to gantry rotation and is defined as:

$$\frac{\text{Table movement (mm) per 360o rotation of the gantry}}{\text{Total nominal scan length (mm)}}$$

A pitch of 1 indicates acquisition of contiguous data slabs. A pitch less than 1 indicates acquisition of overlapping data slabs, while a pitch greater than 1 indicates gaps in the acquisition of successive data slabs. Pitch values much less than 1, typically 0.2 to 0.5, are required for cardiac data acquisition to insure continuity in z-coverage between images sets reconstructed from consecutive cardiac cycles. Lower pitch values, however, result in increased radiation exposure and increased total scan time [4].

It should be mentioned that recent developments with dual-source technology allow high-pitch cardiac imaging. [6] With the use of two x-ray sources and two data detection systems, spiral CT scans can be acquired using pitch values up to 3.2, without loss of data coverage in a limited field of view in patient with low heart rate. Data from the entire heart is acquired during the diastolic phase of a single heartbeat. The ECG-triggered high-pitch helical scan mode appears to be associated with lower radiation dose than other cardiac scan techniques on the same DSCT equipment (25% and 60% dose reduction compared to ECG-triggered sequential step-and-shoot and ECG-gated helical with tube current modulation).

Tube Voltage

Discrete values for peak x-ray tube voltage (80 - 140 kVp) are selectable on CT systems. A peak tube voltage of 120 kVp is standard for cardiac imaging. Because of the increase in both the energy and number of x-ray photons, selection of a higher tube voltage results in increased x-ray penetration and decreased image noise. However, this benefit comes at the expense of increased radiation exposure to the patient. Additionally, image contrast is compromised with the selection of higher voltage values because within the diagnostic CT energy range, differences in attenuation among body tissues decrease with increasing x-ray photon energy. More recently, lower voltage, specifically 100 kVp, is frequently used in patients with a low body mass index (e.g.< 30 kg/m^2) because of significant reduced radiation dose [7,8].

Tube Current

A continuous range of tube currents (50 to 300 mA) is available on clinical CT systems. Because an increase in x-ray tube current increases the number of x-ray photons produced per unit time, selection of a higher x-ray tube current decreases image noise, but is associated with increased radiation exposure to the patient. Therefore, the lowest x-ray tube current that meets the image noise requirements of the clinical application is desired. Lower tube currents are appropriate in smaller patients and for clinical indications requiring reconstruction of only thicker (> 1.5 mm) slices.

Axial and Helical Acquisition Mode

For most cardiovascular indications, imaging is synchronized to the cardiac cycle. This is necessary to focus data acquistion/reconstrution on a period in the cardiac cycle with minimal motion (to reduce motion artifact) and in order to align blocks of images from subsequent gantry rotations with limited z-coverage (to avoid “step”- artifacts). Synchronization can be performed with different modes of data acquisition. The two basic approaches are axial (sequential, "step and shoot") and helical (spiral) imaging.

With axial acquisition, data are acquired during rotation of the gantry around a stationary patient. [7] Data acquisition is prospectively triggered by the ECG signal during the desired cardiac phase. If necessary to cover the anatomy of interest, the patient table is incremented to a new position between periods of data acquisition. The major advantage of the axial technique for cardiac imaging is reduced x-ray exposure, because exposure occurs only during a narrow, pre-specified window of the cardiac cycle (with the x-ray tube turned off for the remainder of the cardiac cycle). However, this precludes reconstruction during multiple phases of the cardiac cycle. Other potential limitations of the axial mode include increased sensitivity to arrhythmia due to prospective referencing of the ECG signal and increased examination times due to the increment of the patient table between data acquisitions. Currently, axial imaging is only feasible for patients with low and regular heart rates, but is increasingly used in order to reduce radiation exposure.

With the helical mode, data are acquired continuously during simultaneous rotation of the gantry and translation of the patient table, with simultaneous recording of the ECG signal. Most often, data are then retrospectively referenced to the simultaneously recorded ECG signal after the acquisition and reconstructed during one or more cardiac phases. Typically images are initially reconstructed in a diastolic window. Because only data during a limited pre-specified portion of the cardiac cycle is typically used for reconstruction, reduction of the tube current (to 4-20% of the maximum value) outside the pre-specified phase, tube current modulation, can be used with significantly reduced radiation exposure [9-11]. Helical data acquisition permits reconstruction of overlapping slices and reconstruction during multiple cardiac phases for dynamic 4-D display of cardiac and valvular motion. Advantages of the helical technique are faster anatomic coverage and less sensitivity to arrhythmia. However, the helical mode is associated with higher patient radiation doses because of continuous x-ray exposure during the entire cardiac cycle.

Alternatively, helical data acquisition can be prospectively triggered by the ECG signal. Prospectively ECG-triggered helical scanning, similar to ECG-triggered, axial scanning, switches the x-ray tube on and off to acquire data from only the target cardiac phase during continuous movement of the patient table. [12] For prospective ECG-triggered, high-pitch helical imaging, data acquisition is triggered by the ECG signal to occur during a diastolic window of a single cardiac cycle. [2,6] Because of the rapid acquisition, this technique is associated with a lower radiation dose compared to retrospective ECG-gated helical imaging.

Radiation Dose

There is increasing debate about the rising radiation exposure from medical imaging and its potential long-term effects [13,14]. The specialized protocols used in the context of valvular interventions are frequently associated with high levels of radiation exposure. Therefore, careful individual planning of the imaging protocol and consideration of potential alternative imaging modalities is important to control radiation exposure.[3]

Balancing diagnostic yield and radiation exposure requires adjusting acquisition parameters to patient characteristics and the specific clinical question. Strategies associated with lower dose for cardiovascular CT imaging include prospectively ECG-triggered imaging techniques, tube current modulation with retrospective ECG-gated helical imaging, and use of low x-ray tube voltage (e.g., 100 kVp).[15,16]

Radiation dose describes the radiation energy absorbed by a patient and is expressed in the standard international (SI) units of Gray (Gy) [conventional units are Roentgen Equivalent in Man (rem) where 1 Gy = 100 rem]. Because radiation dose is difficult to measure directly, radiation exposure [SI unit: Coulomb/kg; conventional unit: Roentgen] is typically measured and converted to radiation dose [11]. The CT dose index (CTDI) parameter $CTDI_{100}$ describes the radiation exposure from a single axial scan integrated over a 100 mm length ionization chamber inserted into a plexiglass phantom [11]. The measured exposure is converted to absorbed dose in the phantom and used as an approximation of the radiation energy absorbed by a patient. The average radiation dose of a three-dimensional slab of a patient's body can be derived from a $CTDI_{100}$ value and expressed as $CTDI_{vol}$ in units of Gy. $CTDI_{vol}$ values reflect x-ray properties (tube voltage, tube current) but are independent of scan length. Therefore, estimates of the total radiation energy absorbed by a patient's body must be obtained by integrating the $CTDI_{vol}$ along the scan length (DLP = $CTDI_{vol}$ x scan length). The resulting value is the dose-length product (DLP), expressed in units of mGy x cm where DLP = CTDIvol x scan length, expressed in units of mGy x cm where DLP = CTDIvol x scan length.

The DLP is useful for estimating the radiation energy absorbed by a patient during a CT scan and is related to the biologic effects of the radiation dose received. However, biologic effects depend not only on the magnitude of the radiation dose but also on the biological sensitivity of the irradiated tissue. Therefore a weighting factor is assigned to each tissue in the body based on its radiosensitivity and relative contribution to radiation risk and the sum of the weighted absorbed doses in all irradiated tissues is defined as the effective dose (E), expressed in units of milliseverts (mSv). Effective dose can be estimated directly from organ measurement within an anthropomorphic phantom or calculated (Monte Carlo methods) [11]. A simpler method for obtaining a reasonable approximation of the effective dose was proposed by the European Working Group for Guidelines on Quality Criteria in Computed Tomography that groups tissues into body regions and assigns a single coefficient to each region based on the radiosensitivies of all tissues within the region [17]. The effective dose for cardiovascular imaging can then be calculated using the equation E = DLP x k, where k = 0.014 mSv x mGy^{-1} x cm^{-1} for the chest.

Estimates of effective dose describe risk for a specific scan but are limited for an individual patient to the extent the patient differs from the actual or virtual phantom employed in dose estimation. Effective dose estimates are indicators of biologic risk and allow to comparison of risk among sources of exposure (e.g., nuclear stress test versus coronary CT angiography.

Recent multi-center studies show that effective dose values vary over wide ranges for the same clinical indication [15,16] reflecting local differences in acquisition parameters (e.g., tube current, tube voltage). For CT imaging in general and for imaging in the context of valvular intervention specifically, it is important to reach a consensus about appropriate use of imaging modalities and standardization of specific acquisition protocols.

Summary: Scanner Technology and Acquisition Protocols for Imaging in the Context of Valvular Interventions

Because of the extensive and rapid motion of valvular structures during the cardiac cycle, use of state-of-the-art scanners (at a minimum 64-slice technology) is critical for imaging in the context of valvular interventions. Advanced protocols with superior spatial and temporal resolution are typically required. Most experience to date is based on retrospectively ECG-gated helical acquisitions (typically with use of tube current modulation but a wide dose modulation window). If 4-D imaging is not necessary, prospective ECG-triggered axial acquisitions focused on a specific phase in the cardiac cycle are a viable alternative, with significantly lower radiation exposure. The minimum gantry rotation time should be used to optimize temporal resolution. The need for high spatial resolution requires minimal collimated detector row width, and sufficient x-ray tube voltage and tube current output. Such protocols are usually associated with increased radiation exposure. Therefore limiting z-coverage strictly to the valvular region (e.g. aortic root only rather than entire heart) is critical to reduce radiation exposure. However, radiation exposure has to be considered in the context of patient specific characteristics (age, gender) and underlying clinical condition. [3,14]

Image Formation, Reconstruction, and Analysis

CT projection data are used to reconstruct two-dimensional pixels, corresponding to three-dimensional voxels within the patient. Each image pixel displays the average attenuation of x-rays within each corresponding patient voxel. Standard reconstruction algorithms use filtered backprojection. More recently implementation of computationally intensive iterative reconstruction algorithms has been introduced for CT imaging. [18] Compared to standard reconstruction of data acquired using a given amount of radiation, equivalent image noise can be achieved with iterative reconstruction of data acquired with less radiation.

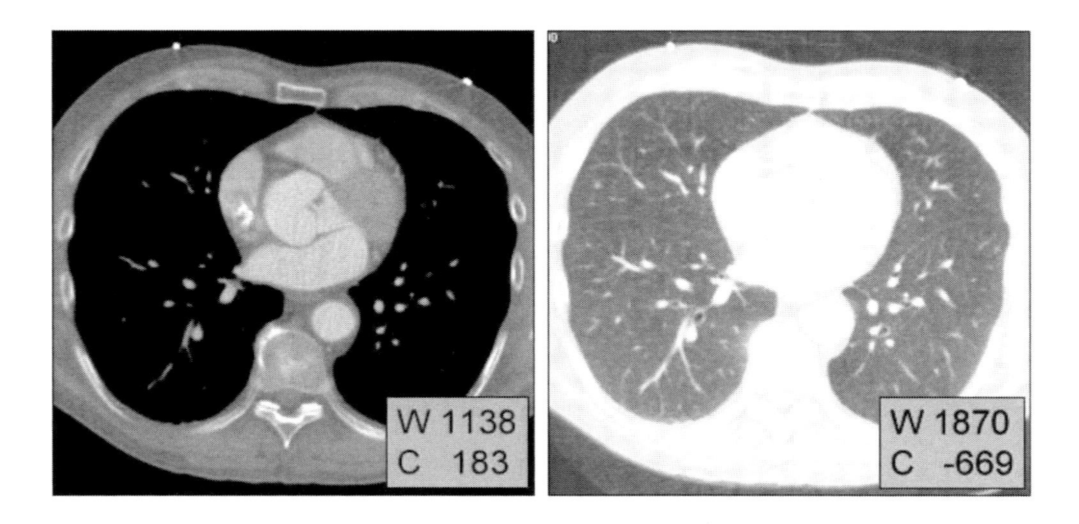

Figure 1. Axial Images and Window Levels. This figure shows axial image of the chest at the level of the aortic root. A 'soft-tissue window' (left panel) and a 'lung window' (right panel) are shown. 'Windowing' of CT images is important to facilitate detection of small changes in grey scales in the tissue of interest.

The x-ray attenuation coefficient for a given voxel of tissue defines the CT number of the corresponding image pixel. CT numbers are described in Hounsfield Units (HU) and typically range from -1000 to 3000 HU. Water has a CT number of zero. Tissues with attenuation coefficients less than that of water, such as air spaces or fatty tissues, have negative CT numbers and appear dark on the CT image, while tissues with attenuation coefficients greater than water, such as dense soft tissue or bone, appear bright. For image display, CT numbers are assigned gray levels. To facilitate detection of small changes in CT numbers, viewing is limited to a portion of the available range of CT numbers through a technique called windowing. The specific range of CT numbers displayed depends on the tissue of interest (e.g. soft tissue window, lung window) (Figure1). The CT number assigned to the center of the gray scale (window level or window center, WC) is typically determined by the average CT number of the tissue of interest. The available number of gray levels (e.g. 256) are then assigned only to a limited range of CT numbers above and below the center CT number. The complete range of CT numbers above and below the center CT number is the window width (WW). The window level and window width can be manipulated to change the appearance of the image but do not alter the value of the CT numbers.

Image Transfer and Access

3-D imaging results in large data sets and requires significant storage capacity and computing power during reconstruction and analysis. Images are transferred from the scanner to archiving systems (PACS), servers, and individual workstations. High-end workstations are traditionally stationed in dedicated 'reading rooms' (e.g. in the Radiology Department). However, in particular when images are reviewed at several locations, client-server models are increasingly used. Such servers provide simultaneous access to multiple users at multiple locations. Because image storage and data analysis takes place at the server level, the system requirements of the individual user interface at the point of care are less. These systems also allow future access by mobile and hand-held devices for bed-side review. [19,20]

The availability of the imaging data at the point-of-care is particularly important for use in the context of valvular interventions, where the CT data has to be available in the operating room.

Image Review and Post-Processing

An initial systematic review includes an assessment of image quality including the presence of artifacts, which requires access to the axial images and in some cases, the un-reconstructed raw data. The initial review also focuses on cardiac and extra-cardiac structure, which are not the primary clinical focus. For example, a CT scan of the chest, abdomen, and pelvis performed to assess vascular access and aortic anatomy in the context of TAVI requires a complete assessment of chest and abdominal anatomy.

Imaging Artifacts

Common artifacts include cardiac motion artifacts, respiratory motions artifacts, partial volume averaging, beam hardening, and noise. Recognition of these artifacts is critical for accurate image interpretation.

Motion Artifact

Movement of the heart and great vessels during data acquisition leads to cardiac motion artifacts. Cardiac motion can result in misregistration of the reconstructed data and blurriness or streaks in the cross-sectional image. Further, the z-axis coverage of most current scanners requires several gantry rotations to image the entire scan range. This results in a three-dimensional volume comprised of data from multiple cardiac cycles. Heart beat irregularities can cause misregistration of adjacent image sets and a "stair-step" appearance in off-axis orientations. Cardiac motion artifacts are minimized by lowering patient heart rate and heart rate variability.

The small size and rapid motion of normal valve leaflets limits their visibility with CT. Pathologic valve leaflets are better visualized if the disease process is associated with thickening, calcification, and restricted motion (e.g. calcified aortic stenosis). In contrast imaging of valve pathology associated with redundant mobile leaflets (e.g. prolaps) is limited with CT.

Respiratory Motion

Inability of the patient to maintain a breath hold during CT data acquisition can lead to respiratory motion artifacts similar in appearance to cardiac motion artifacts. Unlike misregistration of data due to cardiac motion, misregistration due to respiratory motion involves the chest wall. Respiratory motion artifacts are eliminated with shorter scan times that permit complete breath-holding.

Volume Averaging

Highly attenuating tissues such as calcium and materials such as iodine or surgically implanted metallic objects can give rise to several types of image artifacts. Overestimation of the size of such dense objects results from partial volume averaging and is commonly referred to as the "blooming artifact" [21]. The attenuation value assigned to each image pixel is a weighted average of the attenuation of all tissue within the corresponding patient voxel. Therefore, the presence of even a small amount of dense material within a voxel will dominate the attenuation value of the pixel. Partial volume averaging is reduced with smaller pixel size and thinner slices.

These artifacts affect imaging of densely calcified valvular structures and imaging of prosthetic valves containing metal parts. However, using modern scanners, neither is a contraindication for CT imaging.

Beam Hardening

Artificially lowered CT numbers (i.e. dark spots or streaks) adjacent to highly attenuating objects result from beam hardening. In general, lower energy x-rays are preferentially attenuated such that the x-ray beam exiting the imaged object contains a lower percentage of low energy photons with respect to the incident x-ray beam. The transmitted x-ray beam is described as hardened. X-ray beams passing through highly attenuating objects are excessively hardened. Because of the disproportionately large number of high-energy photons in this beam, the reconstruction algorithm assumes the beam passes through a low attenuating object and assigns low CT numbers to pixels adjacent to the dense object. This is a problem at valve leaflets and surrounding annular ring and can be difficult to differentiate from pannus [22,23]. (Figure 2)

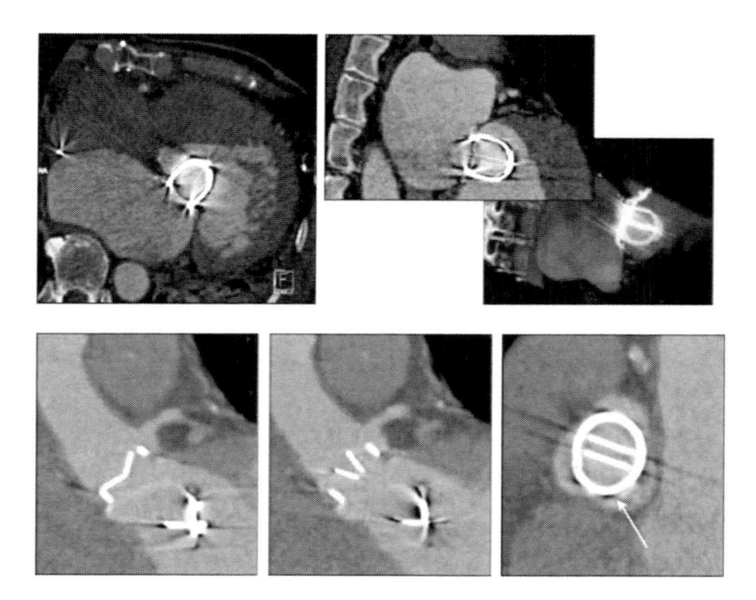

Figure 2. Prosthetic Valves and Beam-Hardening. This figure shows a ball-in-cage mitral valve and a tilting disc aortic valve prosthesis, with beam hardening (arrow). Beam hardening describes an artifact resulting in artificially lowered CT numbers (i.e., dark spots or streaks) adjacent to highly attenuating objects. This is a problem at valve leaflets and surrounding annular ring and can be difficult to differentiate from pannus.

In addition, streaks of high CT numbers sometimes radiate from dense objects because of severely reduced transmission of x-rays, also known as photon starvation.

Noise

CT images sometimes have a grainy appearance with large variation in pixel values within a homogeneous region as a result of image noise. CT image noise is inversely proportional to the number of photons contributing to the reconstructed image [4]. For obese patients, the selected tube voltage and tube current may not allow sufficient x-ray photon penetration thereby preventing absorption of attenuated photons by the detectors and increasing image noise. In addition, acquisition of projection data during a shorter time duration (i.e., higher temporal resolution) or reconstruction of thinner slices (i.e., higher z-axis spatial resolution) results in fewer photons contributing to the reconstructed image and increased noise for a given tube voltage and tube current compared to longer acquisition times or thicker slices. Image noise can be decreased for larger patients or for faster rotation times and thinner slices by increasing the tube current, but at the expense of increased radiation exposure.

Analysis

After the initial systematic review by an image specialist/ radiologist the images are further processed for a more focused review by the interventionalist/ surgeon. Dedicated advanced software allows image processing and display that is increasingly optimized for the specific clinical application. However, because post-processing can be associated with loss of information and introduction of artifacts, the post-processed image should be analyzed in the context of a systematic review of the entire data set.

Axial Images

During systematic review of the axial images (Figure 1) experienced readers synthesize a virtual 3-dimensional impression. Advanced software programs are used to display actual 3-D images, which can be stored and shared between users.

Multiplanar Reformation

Multiplanar reformation (MPR) describes creation of thin cut planes through the 3-D volume. [Figure 3] These images provide detailed 2-D views and are used extensively. An unlimited number of planes can be visualized in any orientation, including planes similar to standard views with echocardiography or angiography. However, in contrast to angiographic projections, e.g. coronary angiography, where the projected images reflects a summation of data from the entire vessels depth, the MPR image is a thin cut plane through the vessel. Therefore, scrolling through a stack of these thin tomographic images is necessary to cover the entire depth of a vascular structure.

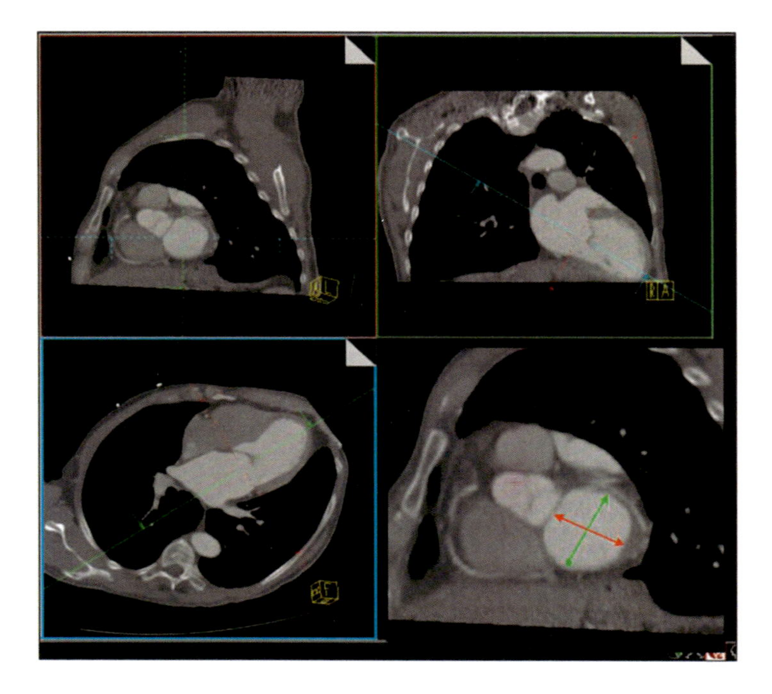

Figure 3. Multi-planar Reconstruction (MPR). Multiplanar reformation describes creation of thin cut planes through the 3-D volume, e.g. planes similar to standard views with echocardiography. This figure shows an example of a double-oblique reconstruction of the mitral annulus. The colored lines in each image correspond to the cut-plane shown in the panel framed in the same color. The right lower panel shows a double-oblique reconstruction at the level of the mitral annulus with diameter measurements.

Maximum-Intensity Projection

In order to display CT data in a format that resembles a conventional angiogram, maximum-intensity projection (MIP) images are created. MIP images are orthogonal or oblique planes/slabs with increased thickness, basically displaying the information contained within a stack of MPR images. However, the display is weighted towards voxels with increased Hounsfield unit (HU) values; a MIP image displays only the maximum intensity voxels encountered in a 2D projection through a slab of the imaged volume. These images provide more comprehensive assessment of vascular structures, similar to conventional angiograms. However, increasing thickness is associated with overlapping of the adjacent structures.

Volume Rendered Technique, Surface-Shaded Display, and Virtual Endoscopy

Volume rendered (VR) techniques assign a specific color and opacity value to every voxel inside a volume of interest. [Figure 4] By changing color and opacity settings, the user can interactively highlight groups of voxels for display e.g. the LV versus the chest wall and vice versa. It is important to consider that the appearance of VR images is determined by the specific image settings, which can for example change the appearance of luminal stenosis severity. It is therefore critically important to analyze VR images in the context of the information obtained from the review of the original axial images and reformatted MPR/MIP images.

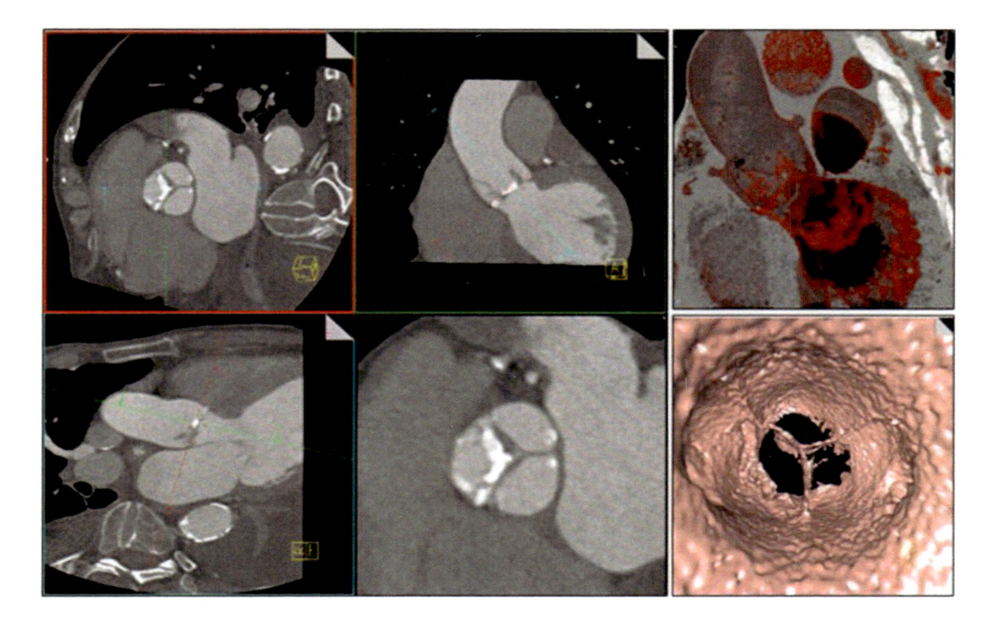

Figure 4. Volume Rendered Imaging (VRI). This figure shows MPR and VR images of the aortic root. The left panels show MPR images reconstructed at the level of the aortic valve. The upper right panel shows a longitudinal VRI images of the aortic root. The lower right panels shows an 'endoscopic view' into the aortic root.

4-D Image Reconstruction

Images acquired using a retrospectively ECG-gated helical mode can be reconstructed at multiple phases throughout the cardiac cycle (e.g. at 5% or 10% intervals). These reconstructions can subsequently be viewed as a cine-loop and provide functional assessment of valvular structures with limited temporal resolution compared to echocardiography.

Segmentation and Image Fusion/ Co-Registration

Segmentation involves isolating the data from specific regions of interest (e.g. aorta for endovascular stenting, the left atrium and pulmonary vein for pulmonary vein ablation (PVI). Various segmentation techniques exist beyond manual segmentation, including threshold-based segmentation and region-growing segmentation. [24]

An exciting area of investigation is image fusion. This can involve registration of images from two imaging modalities (e.g. CT and angiography) or of images from one imaging modality and one functional data set (e.g. EPS electroanatomical mapping).

Summary: Image Formation, Reconstruction, and Analysis

The acquired CT images typically undergo an initial systematic review of all cardiac and extracardiac findings and are then further processed for more focused use in the context of valvular intervention.

If images are reviewed at several locations, client-server models are increasingly used. Such servers provide simultaneous access to multiple users at multiple locations. Because image storage and data analysis takes place at the server level, the system requirements of the individual user interface at the point of care are less.

There is an increasing number of software programs allowing dedicated reconstructions for visualization and also fusion of CT data with other imaging modalities, including conventional angiography. These solutions provide increasing integration of the CT data into the interventional procedure.

However, it is critical to understand the limitations of CT in general and advanced image processing in order to avoid misinterpretation.

III. Clinical Application in the Context of Valvular Intervention

Conventional Cardiothoracic Surgery

Imaging is a critical component for planning of conventional surgical valvular repair and replacement, with echocardiography being the standard method to assess valve anatomy and function.

In addition, specific findings of chest anatomy have been identified in particular with CT that can influence the surgical approach. Examples are extensive calcification of the ascending aorta ("porcelain aorta") and close proximity or adhesion of cardiothoracic structures including coronary bypass grafts to the sternum. The pre-operative identification of these high-risk anatomic findings allows preventive surgical strategies, in particular for patients undergoing re-operative cardiothoracic surgery (RCS). [25-27] (Figure 5) Preventive surgical strategies include non-midline incision, deep hypothermic circulatory arrest, initiation of peripheral cardiopulmonary bypass, or extrathoracic vascular exposure prior to incision. Previous non-randomized studies demonstrated a positive impact of pre-surgical CT imaging on outcomes after RCS. [28]

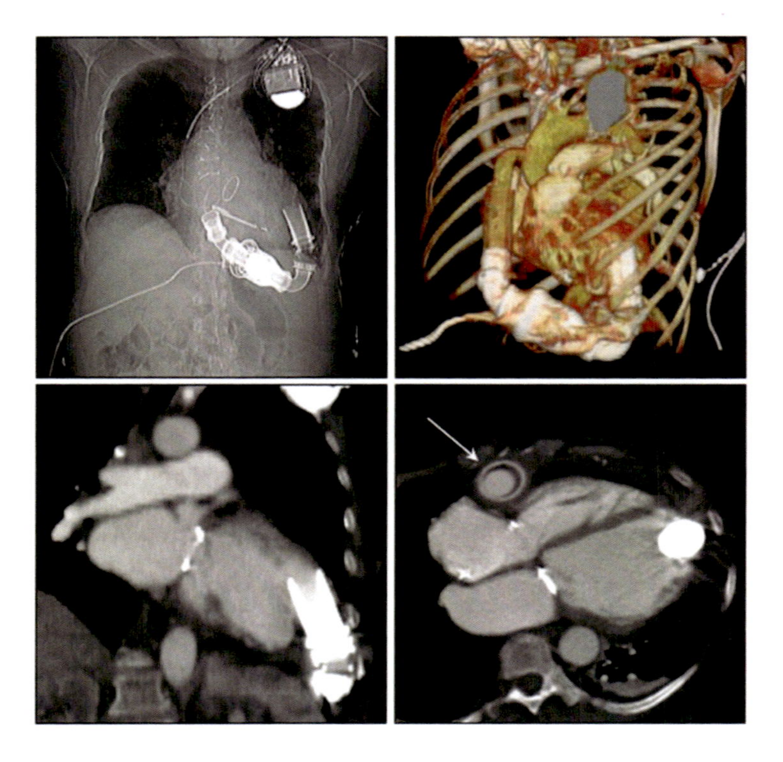

Figure 5. Pre-operative Assessment of Chest Anatomy. The pre-operative identification of high-risk anatomic findings allows preventive surgical strategies, in particular for patients undergoing re-operative cardiothoracic surgery. This figure shows the complex chest anatomy in a patient with history of LVAD placement for DCM, who is evaluated for heart transplantation. The outflow-cannula lies immediately behind the sternum (arrow). In the lower panels, the position of the inflow cannula in the LV apex is identified.

More recently, pre-operative assessment has been used in the context of minimally invasive and robotic assisted surgery, which are associated with decreased direct visualization and novel approaches of vascular access. [20,39] For example, robotic surgery establishes cardiopulmonary bypass by retrograde perfusion via the common femoral vessels, and absence of atherosclerotic disease is important to reduce the risk of cerebral embolism or retrograde aortic dissection. Therefore, pre-operative aortic imaging with CT angiography of the pelvic vessels is frequently used to evaluate vascular access. (Figure 6)

The experience with imaging for standard and minimally invasive surgical procedures demonstrates the importance of image guidance, and has been the basis for use of imaging guidance for transcatheter valve procedures.

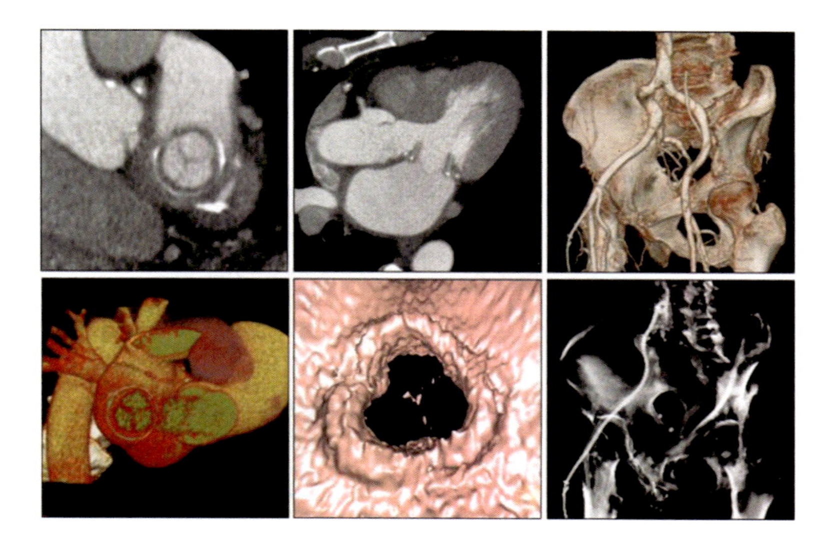

Figure 6. Minimally Invasive and Robotically Assisted Surgery. The left panels show images after robotically assisted mitral valve replacement. The bio-prosthetic valve is identified. The right-sided images show the pre-operative anatomy of iliac arteries, with image acquisition after intra-arterial injection of 15 ml contrast material.

Transcatheter Valve Procedures

Image guidance has a significant impact on emerging transcatheter valve procedures. Data demonstrate the benefit of preoperative understanding of valvular apparatus for planning of procedural detail. However, there is a lack of data evaluating the clinical impact of imaging modalities, e.g. the impact of assessment of the annulus diameter on eligibility for the procedure and choice of the device size. [31] Further evaluation and correlation between planar and 3-D imaging modalities is necessary. The emerging experience of CT imaging in the context of aortic, mitral, and pulmonic valve procedures is described in the following paragraphs.

Transcatheter Aortic Valve Implantation (TAVI)

The complex anatomy of the aortic root provides the framework within which the aortic valve leaflets are suspended. Implantation of a stent/valve has complex and incompletely understood consequences for these structures and their relationships. [Figure 7] CT imaging allows evaluation these relationships before the procedure. [31-36] MDCT with 4-D reconstruction also provides limited insight into the changes of root geometry throughout the cardiac cycle and allows reconstruction at specific positions in the R-R interval. [37,38]

The aortic annulus describes the interface between the LVOT and the aortic root and is defined by the hinge-point/commisures of the aortic valve leaflets. The commisures extend upward into the aortic root describing the shape of a crown, similar to the struts of a bioprosthetic valve. In clinical imaging, the level of the annulus is defined at the lowest point of the valve hinge-point ("inferior virtual basal ring"). Detailed 3-D analysis demonstrates that this clinical defined annulus is typically elliptical. [34, 39, 40]

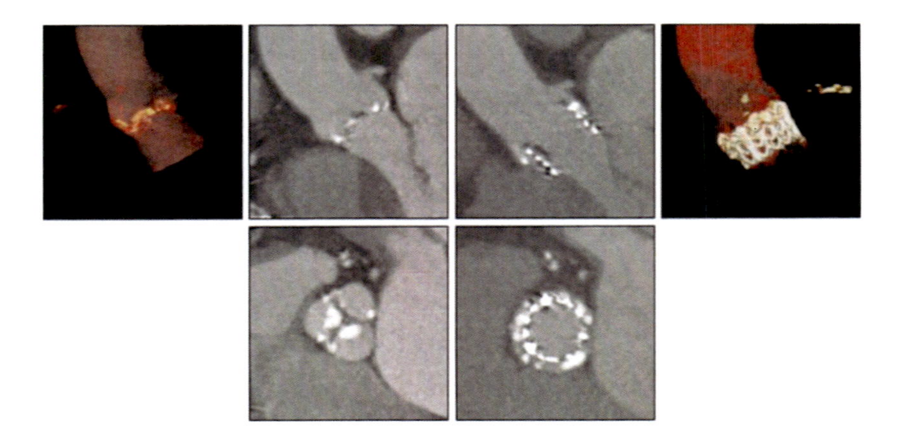

Figure 7. Transcatheter Aortic Valve Implantation. The panels on the left and right show pre- and post-implantation double-oblique reconstructions and VR images at the level of the aortic valve/root in a patient with severe aortic stenosis.

Visualization of a plane at the tip of the leaflets at different times during the cardiac cycle allow determination the maximal opening of the aortic valve during the cardiac cycle by planimetry (typically mid-late systole). [41] Direct planimetry of AVA with CT has been shown to provide reproducible results in comparison to transesophageal echocardiography and magnetic resonance imaging. [42-46] Similarly, planimetry of the regurgitant orifice area in patients with aortic regurgitation has been examined. [47,48] An advantage of the direct observation of the aortic valve opening area is the ability to correlate the pattern of valve opening with leaflet anatomy.

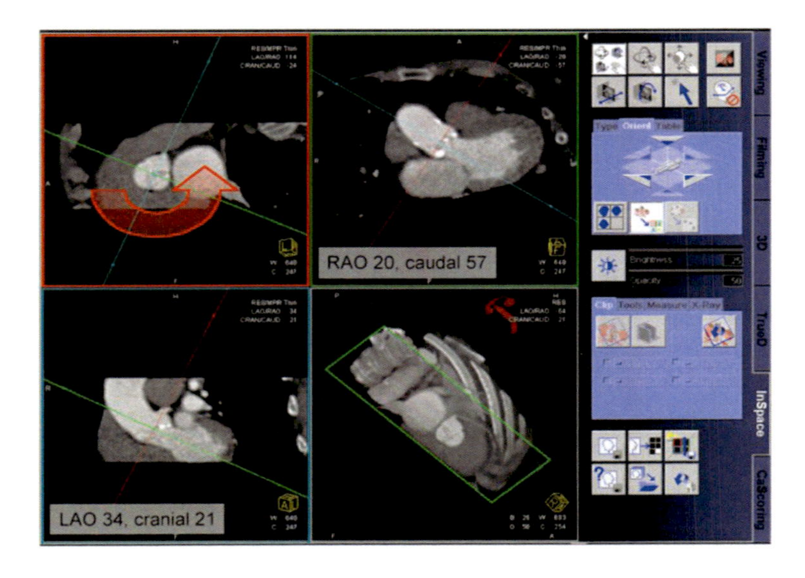

Figure 8. Prediction of Angiographic Planes for TAVI (1). This and the next figure show the use of CT for prediction of angiographic angulations for correct placement during the TAVI procedure. In a double oblique reconstructed image, the cross-hair of the cut-planes is centered on the aortic valve (left upper panel) and rotated to obtain images of the aortic root, described in angiographic coordinates/planes (right upper panel).

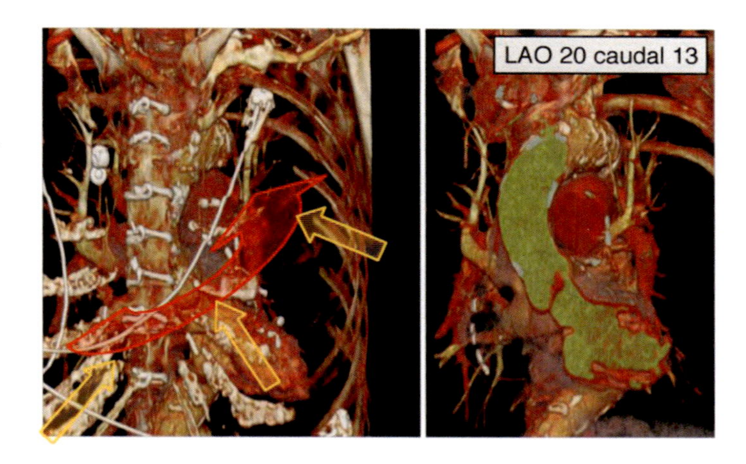

Figure 9. Prediction of Angiographic Planes for TAVI (2). This figure shows volume rendered images of the aortic root in an angiographic plane orthogonal to the aortic root.

Detailed analysis allows assessment of the location of calcification, leaflet thickening, fusion, geometry and symmetry of the opening area. [41,49] Importantly, CT also allows description of the relationship of the leaflet calcification to the coronary artery ostia. [33,34,35,39,50,51]. Based on emerging data, the detailed evaluation of aortic root anatomy appears important for successful deployment of the percutaneous valve prosthesis. [52-55]

3-D analysis also allows description the relationship of the aortic root relative to the body axis for planning of surgical or interventional access planes [Figure 8,9]. [56] A recent paper describes prediction of 2-D angiographic projections orthogonal to the aortic valve area, simplifying the subsequent implantation of the percutaneous valve. [57]

Transcatheter Mitral Valve and Pulmonic Valve Procedures

In the context of transcatheter valve procedures [58] 3-dimensional imaging in general allows a detailed understanding of the mitral valve apparatus including the mitral annulus, valve leaflets, and chordae tendinae/papillary muscles. Real-time 3D, full-volume acquisition with transesophageal echocardiography allows imaging of the entire annular volume including the valve over full cardiac cycles. The complex anatomic structure of the mitral annulus determines valve function but the interactions are incompletely understood. [59-62] Imaging of the mitral apparatus has been extensively described with echocardiography [61-68]. For example, pioneering echocardiographic work with 3-dimensional (3D) reconstruction defined the complex "saddle shape," geometry of the mitral annulus. [69,70] These data have significantly influenced surgical and interventional approaches for mitral valve repair.
Using CT, assessment of the mitral valve leaflets is limited due to their rapid motion. [71] Most of the emerging CT data therefore describes mitral annular anatomy. (Figure 10-12) Accurate definition of MA geometry is critical for preoperative planning in the context of recently introduced transcatheter approaches for ring annuloplasty. [72-74] The goal of these devices, which are placed in the coronary sinus, is displacing the posterior mitral valve leaflet forward in an attempt to change the anterior-posterior dimension of the mitral valve and reduce MR severity. A recent study [75] showed the feasibility of percutaneous reduction in functional MR with a novel CS-based mitral annuloplasty device in patients with heart failure, and was associated with an improvement in quality of life and exercise tolerance.

In this context, assessment of the annulus and its surrounding structures has been described with CT. The data shows nonplanar shape of the mitral annulus and substantial dynamic changes of the shape, size, and motion throughout the cardiac cycle, with significant differences between healthy subjects and patients with cardiomyopathy. [76] In patients with DCM, the MA area was significantly larger as compared with normals, but the change of MA area throughout the cardiac cycle was significantly smaller.

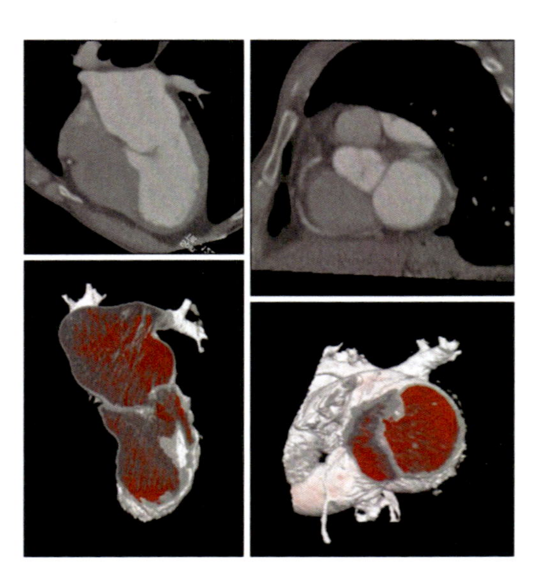

Figure 10. Visualization of the Mitral Annulus (1). This figure shows MPR and VR images of the mitral annulus. Because of the complex saddle-shaped configuration of the mitral annulus, representation in a single MPR can be challenging.

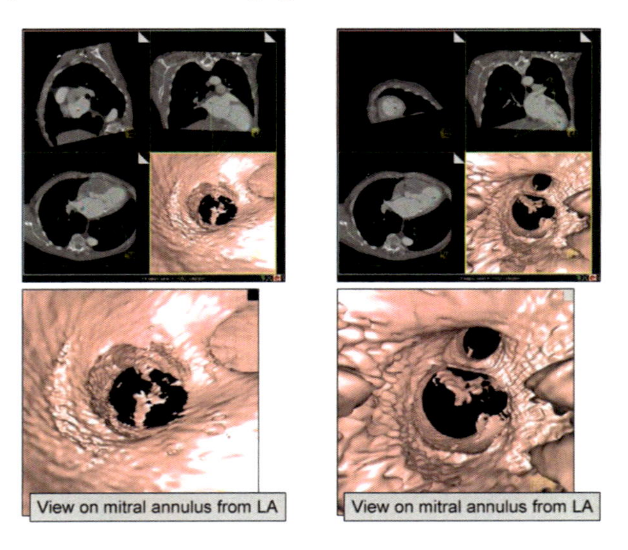

Figure 11. Visualization of the Mitral Annulus (2). This figure shows VR images (endoscopic views) of the mitral annulus, as seen from the left atrium (left panels) and left ventricle (right panel).

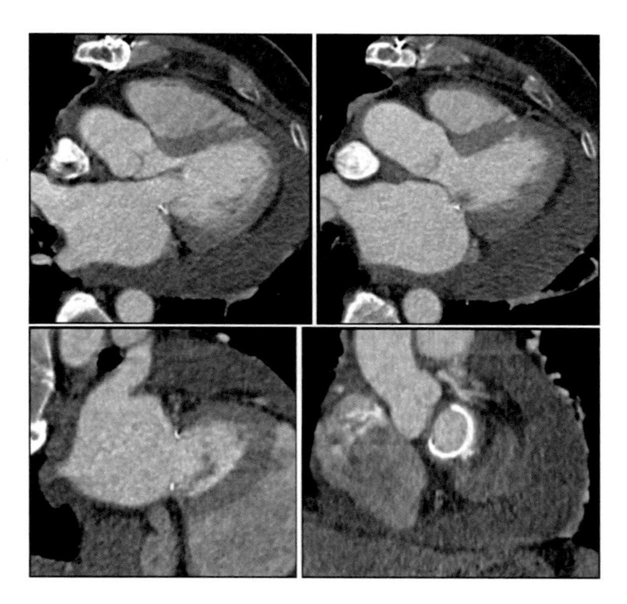

Figure 12. Visualization of the Mitral Annulus (3). In comparison, this figure shows the position of a surgically placed C-shaped mitral annular ring.

A major concern is the close proximity of the CS to the left circumflex artery (LCX), and the potential risk of CS-based devices potentially impinging on the LCX. [77] CT studies described the in vivo anatomical relationships between mitral annulus (MA) and coronary sinus (CS) as well as CS and left circumflex coronary artery (Figure 13). [78] In a small number of normal individuals and patients with severe MR due to mitral valve prolapse, separation between MA and CS was measured and the anatomical relation of LCX and CS were determined. There was significant variance of CS to MA separation. The left circumflex artery crossed between CS and MA in 80% of patients at a variable distance from the ostium of CS. In a larger study [79] of 102 normal patients and 27 patient with ischemic severe MR, the LCX initially crossed under the coronary sinus/great cardiac vein (CS/GCV) in 74% to 97% in normal patient, depending on cornary dominance. In patients with ischemic severe MR, the LCX initially crossed under the CS/GCV in 96%. In addition, obtuse marginal branches and posterolateral branches were also in a position to potentially be compressed by a device placed within the CS. These data raise concern for potential coronary ischemia induced by a CS-based device and emphasize the need to evaluate the relationship between the CS/GCV and LCX is an important factor in determining the safety of CS-based devices.

Other recent application of CT have been described in the context of valve-in-valve implantation [80]. Clinical studies describe safety, procedural success, and short-term effectiveness for transcatheter pulmonic valve replacement in patients with dysfunctional right ventricular outflow tract conduits and pulmonary regurgitation (PR) [81]. However, the current literature about CT imaging in the context of transcatheter pulmonic valve replacement is limited. A recent study describes implantation of a new percutaneous pulmonary valve into a dilated pulmonary trunk, using patient specific data to influence the design of the device and ensure patient safety. [82] In the context of CT imaging and radiation exposure, it is important to consider differences in the patient populations undergoing aortic versus mitral/pulmonic procedures. The current patient population undergoing TAVI is typically older with more significant co-morbidities than patients evaluated for mitral/pulmonic valve procedures. As described above patient characteristics affect long-term adverse effects of radiation exposure. [14] Therefore choice of imaging modality and imaging protocol should consider these differences. [3]

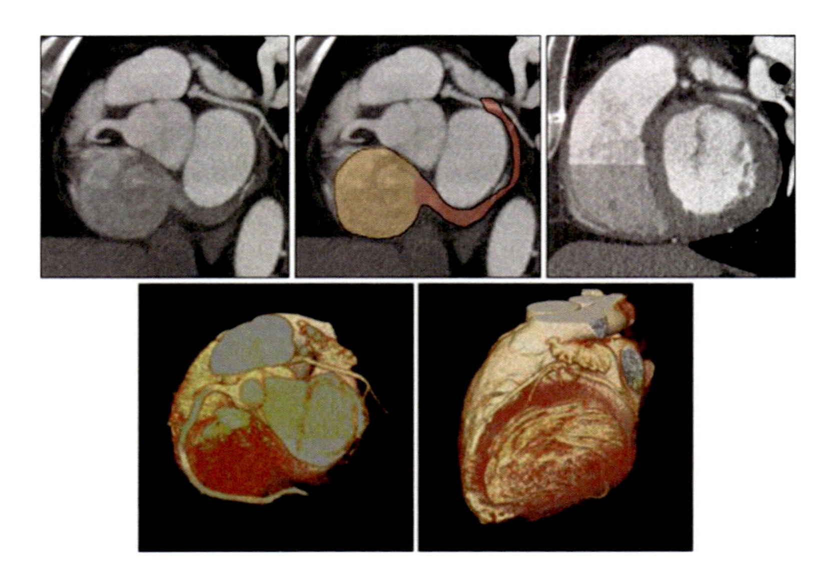

Figure 13. Visualization of the Coronary Sinus. Accurate definition of the mitral annulus and coronary sinus geometry is critical for preoperative planning in the context of recently introduced transcatheter approaches for ring annuloplasty. This figure shows the right atrium (orange) and coronary sinus (red), in relationship to the LCX (upper middle panel).

Role of 3-D Imaging for Endovascular Device Design

Beyond its value for clinical decision-making in the individual patient, 3-D data sets are increasingly used for device design. [83] Traditionally, device design has relied mainly on bench and animal testing followed by human clinical trials. [84] Advances in medical imaging and computational modeling allow simulation of physiological conditions in patient-specific 3-D vascular models. [85] Such models can account for the unique features of the human circulation with appropriate 3-D anatomical and physiological input data to define relevant boundary conditions. This approach will allow prospective design of devices that can withstand the force variations in the cardiovascular system.

C-Arm CT (Rotational Angiography)

For practical purposes and associated significant contrast and radiation exposure, CT is limited to a single pre-interventional scan for procedural planning. While fusion of CT with procedural angiographic images is becoming a reality, it is limited by e.g. differences in patient positioning, interval changes in heart rate, etc. Therefore CT-like data acquisition during the procedure would be attractive.

C-arm CT (rotational angiography) describes the use of CT-like acquisition and reconstruction techniques with C-arm based x-ray angiography systems to obtain 3D data. The C-arm is rotated over a wide arc (180°+ 2xfan-angle) with or without continuous contrast injection, acquiring multiple views of the cardiovascular structure in order to reconstruct a 3D image. [86] For ECG-referenced cardiac imaging, identical alternating forward and backward rotations are triggered by the ECG signal to acquire projections covering the entire acquisition range at a similar cardiac phase.

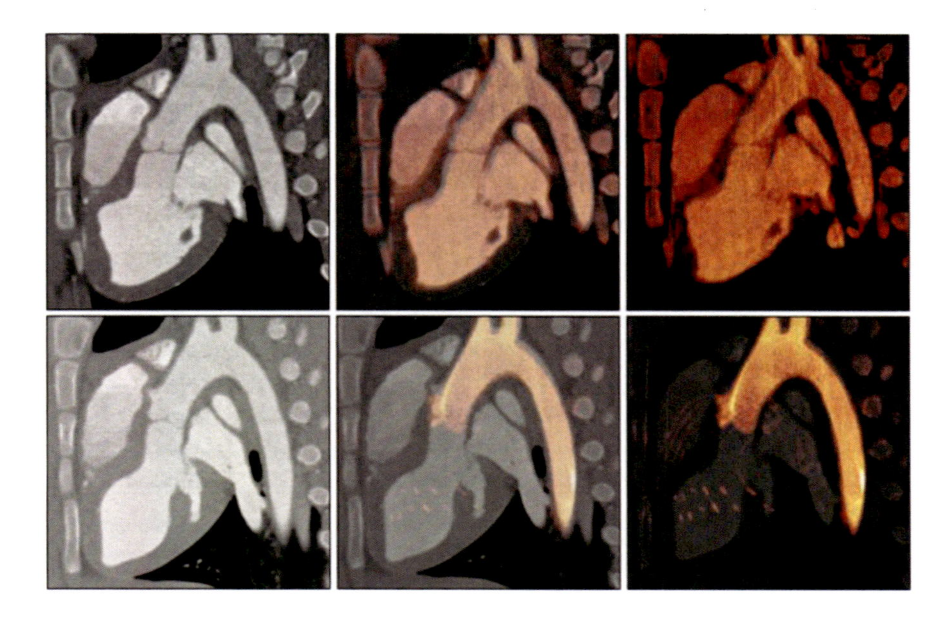

Figure 14. C-Arm CT (Rotational Angiography) and Fusion Imaging in an Animal Model. This figure shows examples of images fusing CT and C-Arm CT. The left panels show 100% CT images. In the middle and right panels CT and C-arm CT are fused (50-50% middle panels, and 70-30% right panels).

The acquisition of 3D data directly from the angiography system may facilitate registration with data from a 3-D modality. C-arm CT can be used to obtain volumetric 3D data that may be more easily registered registered to the 2D fluoroscopy images obtained using the same system. [Figure 14] Additionally, the availability of current 3D anatomical information from the patient along with the possibility to use this information for real time guidance during interventions may offer advantages beyond those of pre-procedural images in some instances. C-arm CT has shown potential for use during various cardiovascular interventional procedures including EVAR (87), PVI [88], and PCI [89,90]. In a recent study, feasibility of C-arm CT acquisition with automatic 3D reconstruction was demonstrated. [90]

Non-Invasive Procedural Imaging with 3-D Echocardiography and MRI

Because of the exposure to radiation and iodinated contrast material associated with both CT and C-arm CT, repeat real time monitoring during the procedure is limited with these modalities. In contrast, 3D-echocardiography [91-93] and interventional cardiovascular magnetic resonance (iCMR) [94,95] have the potential for real-time procedural image guidance during minimally invasive and catheter-based therapies.

3-D transthoracic or transoesophageal echocardiography has become possible with rectangular (or matrix) array transducers. A 3-D pyramidal data volume is collected in real-time. [92,96-103]. Depending on the field of view of the probe, a series of smaller 3D ultrasound sub-volumes acquired over a series of cardiac cycles are combined. These 'fused' subvolumes are subject to motion artifact if there are alterations in position of the heart during the acquisition of the component images. Recently introduced systems allow acquisition of full 90°×90° volume data in real-time. Similar to CT, the 3-D data can be reconstructed after the acquisition. Multiple 2D cut planes can be applied to display structures of interest from different perspectives. [104] This approach is used to ensure that 2D images are on axis and is a valuable tool for measurement e.g. of the aortic annulus.

Initial experience with real-time 3D trans-esophageal echocardiography (TOE) demonstrates its value in the clinical evaluation of structural heart disease [96, 101, 102, 105-110], intraoperative assessment, and guidance of interventional procedures that require real-time imaging. [98,100,111,112].

Examples of cardiovascular CMR-guided procedures are catheter-based endovascular interventions of the aorta and transcatheter aortic valve implantation [113,114]. (Figure 15) Using MRI, multiple concurrent slices can be displayed in 3D to indicate their relative location and orientation. Alternatively, computer algorithms can locate and even automatically reposition the scan plane to show the entire region of interest in 3 dimensions. Fusion or co-registration of angiographic and magnetic resonance imaging, referred to as XFM (X-ray fused with magnetic resonance imaging), overlays MR images to enhance otherwise-difficult X-ray fluoroscopy procedures. In hybrid operating rooms, imaging with conventional angiography and cardiovascular MR is possible during the same procedure. On-line co-registration allows that the 3-D contours of cardiovascular structures from MR are overlaid on live X-rays. Views update as the C-arm or table position changes. Catheter position can be computed from two X-ray projections and back-displayed on a 3D MR roadmap. This multimodality approach has applied to complex procedures including transcatheter valve repair. [115]

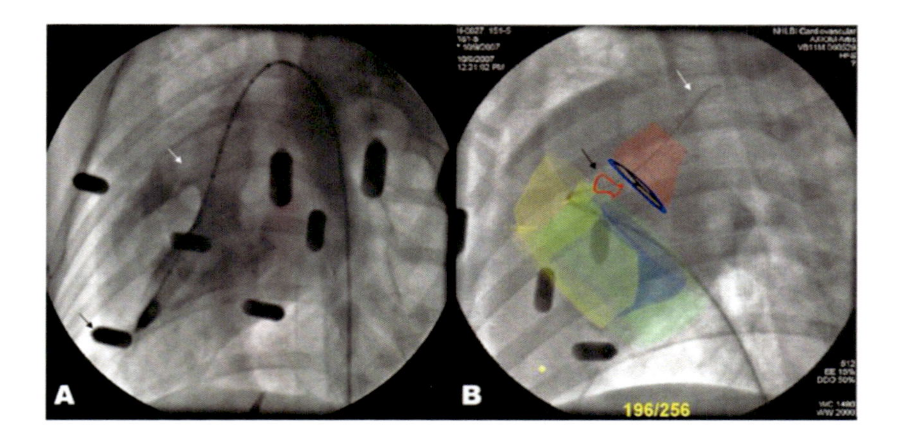

Figure 15. Interventional MRI and Angiographic Fusion. This figure shows the potential use of interventional applications of MRI allowing real-time fusion of angiographic and MRI images in hybrid MRI/angiographic suites, for direct procedural guidance Image courtesy Dr. Lederman; Adapted with permission from: Ratnayaka K, et al. JACC Cardiovasc Interv. 2009;2:224-30.

Conclusion

Precise pre- and intra-operative imaging is critical for valvular interventional procedures. Complementing standard echocardiography and catheterization, novel 3-D imaging modalities, including CT, MRI, and 3-D echocardiography acquire volumetric datasets, and allow subsequent 3-D display and visualization in unlimited planes.

The data described above suggests an emerging role of 3-D imaging for novel surgical and transcatheter approaches including device design. However, there is a lack of prospective data, comparing the utility of different imaging modalities and demonstrating clinical impact of image guidance in the context of these procedures. Eventually, evidence-based data demonstrating favorable risk/benefit impact on clinical outcome in controlled clinical trials is necessary.

References

[1] Rybicki FJ, Otero HJ, Steigner ML, Vorobiof G, Nallamshetty L, Mitsouras D, Ersoy H, Mather RT, Judy PF, Cai T, Coyner K, Schultz K, Whitmore AG, Di Carli MF. Initial evaluation of coronary images *Int J Cardiovasc Imaging* 2008;24:535-46.

[2] Achenbach S, Marwan M, Ropers D, Schepis T, Pflederer T, Anders K, Kuettner A, Daniel WG, Uder M, Lell MM. Coronary computed tomography angiography with a consistent dose below 1 mSv using prospectively electrocardiogram-triggered high-pitch spiral acquisition. *Eur Heart J* 2010;31:340-6.

[3] Halliburton SS, Schoenhagen P. Cardiovascular imaging with computed tomography *JACC Cardiovasc Imaging*. 2010;3:536-40.

[4] Primak AN, McCollough CH, Bruesewitz MR, Zhang J, Fletcher JG. Relationship between Noise, Dose, and Pitch in Cardiac Multi–Detector Row CT. *RadioGraphics* 2006; 26: 1785-1794.

[5] Flohr T, Stierstorfer K, Raupach R, Ulzheimer S, Bruder H. Performance evaluation of a 64-slice CT *Rofo*. 2004;176:1803-10.

[6] Flohr TG, Leng S, Yu L, Aiimendinger T, Bruder H, Petersilka M, Eusemann CD, Stierstorfer K, Schmidt B, McCollough CH. Dual-source spiral CT with pitch up to 3.2 and 75 ms temporal resolution: image reconstruction and assessment of image quality. *Med Phys*. 2009 ;36:5641-53.

[7] Husmann L, Valenta I, Gaemperli O, Adda O, Treyer V, Wyss CA, Veit-Haibach P, Tatsugami F, von Schulthess GK, Kaufmann PA. Feasibility of low-dose coronary CT angiography: first experience with prospective ECG-gating. *Eur Heart J* 2007;29:191–7.

[8] Hausleiter J, Meyer T, Hadamitzky M, Huber E, Zankl M, Martinoff S, Kastrati A, Schömig A. Radiation dose estimates from cardiac multislice computed tomography in daily practice: impact of different scanning protocols on effective dose estimates. *Circulation* 2006; 113:1305-10.

[9] Jakobs T, Becker CR, Ohnesorge B, Flohr T, Suess C, Schoepf UJ, Reiser MF. Multislice helical CT of the heart with retrospective ECG gating: reduction of radiation exposure by ECG-controlled tube current modulation. *Eu Radiol* 2002; 12:1081-1086.

[10] Leschka S, Scheffel H, Desbiolles L, Plass A, Gaemperli O, Valenta I, Husmann L, Flohr TG, Genoni M, Marincek B, Kaufmann PA, Alkadhi H. Image quality and reconstruction intervals of dual-source CT coronary angiography: recommendations for ECG-pulsing windowing. *Invest Radiol.* 2007; 42(8):543-9.

[11] Morin RL, Gerber TC, McCollough CH. Radiation Dose in Computed Tomography of the Heart. *Circ* 2003; 107: 917-922.

[12] DeFrance T, Dubois E, Gebow D, Ramirez A, Wolf F, Feuchtner GM. Helical prospective ECG-gating in cardiac computed tomography *Int J Cardiovasc Imaging.* 2010;26:99-107.

[13] Brenner DJ, Hall EJ. Computed tomography - an increasing source of radiation exposure. *N Engl J Med.* 2007;357:2277-84

[14] Einstein AJ, Henzlova MJ, Rajagopalan S. Estimating risk *JAMA.* 2007;298:317-23.

[15] Hausleiter J, Meyer T, Hermann F, Hadamitzky M, Krebs M, Gerber TC, McCollough C, Martinoff S, Kastrati A, Schömig A, Achenbach S. Estimated radiation dose associated with cardiac CT angiography. *JAMA* 2009;301:500-7.

[16] Bischoff B, Hein F, Meyer T, Hadamitzky M, Martinoff S, Schömig A, Hausleiter J. Impact of a reduced tube voltage on CT *JACC Cardiovasc Imaging.* 2009;2:940-6.

[17] European Commission: European Guidelines on Quality Criteria for Computed Tomography, EUR 16262EN. Luxembourg: Office for Official Publications of the European Communities 2000. Available at: www.drs.dk/guidelines/ct/quality/main index.htm. Accessed October 30, 2008.

[18] Prakash P, Kalra MK, Digumarthy SR, Hsieh J, Pien H, Singh S, Gilman MD, Shepard JA. Radiation *J Comput Assist Tomogr.* 2010;34:40-5.

[19] LaBounty TM, Kim RJ, Lin FY, Budoff MJ, Weinsaft JW, Min JK. Diagnostic accuracy of coronary computed tomography *JACC Cardiovasc Imaging.* 2010;3:482-90.

[20] Toomey RJ, Ryan JT, McEntee MF, Evanoff MG, Chakraborty DP, McNulty JP, Manning DJ, Thomas EM, Brennan PC. Diagnostic efficacy of handheld devices *AJR Am J Roentgenol.* 2010;194:469-74.

[21] Kroft LJM, de Roos A, Geleijns J. Artifacts in ECG-Synchronized MDCT Coronary Angiography. *Am. J. Roentgenol* 2007; 189:581-591.

[22] LaBounty TM, Agarwal PP, Chughtai A, Bach DS, Wizauer E, Kazerooni EA. Evaluation of mechanical heart valve size and function with ECG-gated 64-MDCT. *AJR Am J Roentgenol.* 2009;193:W389-96.

[23] Symersky P, Budde RP, de Mol BA, Prokop M. Comparison of multidetector-row computed tomography *Am J Cardiol.* 2009;104:1128-34.

[24] Zheng Y, Barbu A, Georgescu B, Scheuering M, Comaniciu D. Four-chamber heart modeling and automatic segmentation for 3-D cardiac CT volumes using marginal space learning and steerable features. *IEEE Trans Med Imaging* 2008;27:1668–81.

[25] Gasparovic H, Rybicki FJ, Millstine J, Unic D, Byrne JG, Yucel K, Mihaljevic T. Three dimensional computed tomographic imaging in planning the surgical approach for redo cardiac surgery after coronary revascularization. *Eur J Cardiothorac Surg* 2005;28:244-9.

[26] Aviram G, Sharony R, Kramer A, Nesher N, Loberman D, Ben-Gal Y, Graif M, Uretzky G, Mohr R. Modification of surgical planning based on cardiac multidetector computed tomography in reoperative heart surgery. *Ann Thorac Surg* 2005;79:589-95.

[27] Kamdar AR, Meadows TA, Roselli EE, Gorodeski EZ, Curtin RJ, Sabik JF, Schoenhagen P, White RD, Lytle BW, Flamm SD, Desai MY. Multidetector computed tomographic angiography in planning of reoperative cardiothoracic surgery. *Ann Thorac Surg* 2008;85:1239-45.

[28] Maluenda G, Goldstein MA, Lemesle G, Weissman G, Weigold G, Landsman MJ, Hill PC, Pita F, Corso PJ, Boyce SW, Pichard AD, Waksman R, Taylor AJ. Perioperative outcomes in reoperative cardiac surgery *Am Heart J* 2010;159:301-306.

[29] Nifong, L.W., Chitwood, P.S., Pappas, C.R., Smith, C.R., Argenziano, V.A., Starnes, P.M. Robotic mitral valve surgery: A United States multicenter trial. *J. Thorac Cardiovasc Surg* 2005;129:1395-1404.

[30] Falk V, Mourgues F, Adhami L, Jacobs S, Thiele H, Nitzsche S, Mohr FW, Coste-Maniere E. Cardio navigation: planning, simulation, and augmented reality in robotic assisted endoscopic bypass grafting. *Ann Thorac Surg* 2005;79:2040-7.

[31] Messika-Zeitoun D, Serfaty JM, Brochet E, Ducrocq G, Lepage L, Detaint D, Hyafil F, Himbert D, Pasi N, Laissy JP, Iung B, Vahanian A. Multimodal assessment of the aortic annulus diameter. Implication for transcatheter aortic valve implanation. *J Am Coll Cardiol* 2009;2010;55:186-94.

[32] Schoenhagen P, Tuzcu EM, Kapadia SR, Desai MY, Svensson LG. Three-dimensional imaging of the aortic valve and aortic root with computed tomography: new standards in an era of transcatheter valve repair/implantation. *Eur Heart J* 2009;30:2079-86

[33] Tops LF, Wood DA, Delgado V. Noninvasive Evaluation of the Aortic Root with Multislice Computed Tomography: Implications for Transcatheter Aortic Valve Replacement. *J Am Coll Cardiol Img* 2008;1:321-330.

[34] Akhtar M, Tuzcu EM, Kapadia SR, Svensson LG, Greenberg RK, Roselli EE, Halliburton S, Kurra V, Schoenhagen P, Sola S. Aortic Root Morphology in Patients Undergoing Percutaneous Aortic Valve Replacement. Evidence of Aortic Root Remodeling. *J Thorac Cardiovasc Surg* 2009;137:950-6

[35] Del Valle-Fernández R, Jelnin V, Panagopoulos G, Dudiy Y, Schneider L, de Jaegere PT, Schultz C, Serruys PW, Grube E, Ruiz CE. A method for standardized computed tomography *Eur Heart J.* 2010 May 25. [Epub ahead of print]

[36] Ng ACT, Delgado V, van der Kley F, Shanks M, van de Veire NRL, Bertini M, Nucifora G, van Bommel RJ, Tops LF, de Weger A, Tavilla G, de Roos A, Kroft LJ, Leung DY, Schuijf J, Schalij MJ, Bax JJ. Comparison of Aortic Root Dimensions and Geometries Before and After Transcatheter Aortic Valve Implantation by 2-and 3-Dimensional Transesophageal Echocardiography and Multislice Computed Tomography *Circ Cardiovasc Imaging.* 2010; 3:94-102

[37] Kazui T, Izumoto H, Yoshioka K, Kawazoe K. Dynamic morphologic changes in the normal aortic annulus during systole and diastole. *J Heart Valve Dis* 2006;15:617-21.

[38] Kazui T, Kin H, Tsuboi J, Yoshioka K, Okabayashi H, Kawazoe K. Perioperative dynamic morphological changes of the aortic annulus during aortic root remodeling with aortic annuloplasty at systolic and diastolic phases. *J Heart Valve Dis* 2008;17:366-70.

[39] Tops LF, Wood DA, Delgado V. Noninvasive Evaluation of the Aortic Root with Multislice Computed Tomography: Implications for Transcatheter Aortic Valve Replacement. *J Am Coll Cardiol Img* 2008;1:321-330.

[40] Doddamani S, Grushko MJ, Makaryus AN, Jain VR, Bello R, Friedman MA, Ostfeld RJ, Malhotra D, Boxt LM, Haramati L, Spevack DM. Demonstration of left ventricular outflow tract eccentricity by 64-slice multi-detector CT. *Int J Cardiovasc Imaging* 2009;25:175-81.
[41] Willmann JK, Weishaupt D, Lachat M, Kobza R, Roos JE, Seifert B, Lüscher TF, Marincek B, Hilfiker PR. Electrocardiographically gated multi-detector CT for assessment of valvular morphology and calcifications in aortic stenosis. *Radiology* 2002;225:120-8
[42] Okura H, Yoshida K, Hozumi T, Akasaka T, Yoshikawa J. Planimetry and transthoracic two-dimensional echocardiography in noninvasive assessment of aortic valve area in patients with valvular aortic stenosis. *J Am Coll Cardiol* 1997;30:753-9.
[43] John AS, Dill T, Brandt RR, Rau M, Ricken W, Bachmann G, Hamm CW. Magnetic resonance to assess the aortic valve area in aortic stenosis. *J Am Coll Cardiol* 2003;42:519 -26.
[44] Shah RG, Novaro GM, Blandon RJ, Wilkinson L, Asher CR, Kirsch J. Mitral valve *AJR Am J Roentgenol.* 2010;194:579-84.
[45] Shah RG, Novaro GM, Blandon RJ, Whiteman MS, Asher CR, Kirsch J. Aortic valve *Int J Cardiovasc Imaging.* 2009;25:601-9.
[46] Feuchtner GM, Dichtl W, Friedrich GJ, Frick M, Alber H, Schachner T, Bonatti J, Mallouhi A, Frede T, Pachinger O, zur Nedden D, Müller S. Multislice computed tomography for detection of patients with aortic valve stenosis and quantification of severity. *J Am Coll Cardiol* 2006;47:1410-7
[47] Alkadhi H, Desbiolles L, Husmann L, Plass A, Leschka S, Scheffel H, Vachenauer R, Schepis T, Gaemperli O, Flohr TG, Genoni M, Marincek B, Jenni R, Kaufmann PA, Frauenfelder T. Aortic regurgitation: assessment with 64-section CT. *Radiology* 2007;245:111-21.
[48] Zeb I, Mao SS, Hamirani YS, Raina S, Kadakia J, Elamir S, Budoff MJ. Central aortic valve *Int J Cardiovasc Imaging.* 2010 May 26.
[49] Morgan Three dimensional volume quantification of aortic valve calcification using multislice computed tomography. *Heart* 2003;89:1191-4.
[50] Knight J, Kurtcuoglu V, Muffly K, Marshall W Jr, Stolzmann P, Desbiolles L, Seifert B, Poulikakos D, Alkadhi H. Ex vivo and in vivo coronary ostial locations in humans. *Surg Radiol Anat.* 2009 Mar 14.
[51] Stolzmann P, Knight J, Desbiolles L, Maier W, Scheffel H, Plass A, Kurtcuoglu V, Leschka S, Poulikakos D, Marincek B, Alkadhi H. Remodelling of the aortic root in severe tricuspid aortic stenosis: implications for transcatheter aortic valve implantation. *Eur Radiol.* 2009 Feb 4. [Epub ahead of print]
[52] John D, Buellesfeld L, Yuecel S, Mueller R, Latsios G, Beucher H, Gerckens U, Grube E. Correlation of Device Landing Zone Calcification and Acute Procedural Success in Patients Undergoing Transcatheter Aortic Valve Implantations With the Self-Expanding CoreValve Prosthesis. *J Am Coll Cardiol Intv.* 2010; 3:233-243
[53] Latsios G, Gerckens U, Buellesfeld L, Mueller R, John D, Yuecel S, Syring J, Sauren B, Grube E. "Device landing zone" calcification, assessed by MSCT, as a predictive factor for pacemaker implantation after TAVI. *Catheter Cardiovasc Interv.* 2010 Mar 26. [Epub ahead of print];

[54] Delgado V, Ng ACT, van de Veire NR, van der Kley F, Schuijf JD, Tops LF, de Weger A, Tavilla G, de Roos A, Kroft LJ, Schalij MJ, Bax JJ. Transcatheter Aortic Valve Implantation: Role of Multi-Detector Row Computed Tomography to Evaluate Prosthesis Positioning and Deployment in Relation to Valve Function. *European Heart Journal.* 2010; 8:113-123

[55] Jilaihawi H, Chin D, Spyt T, Jeilan M,Vasa-Nicotera M, Bence J, Logtens E, Kovac J. Prosthesis-Patient Mismatch After Transcatheter Aortic Valve Implantation with the Medtronic-Corevalve Bioprosthesis. *European Heart Journal.* 2009;119:1034-1048

[56] Ammar R, Porat E, Eisenberg DS, Uretzky G. Utility of spiral CT in minimally invasive approach for aortic valve replacement. *Eur J Cardiothorac Surg* 1998;14 Suppl 1:S130-3.

[57] Kurra V, Kapadia SR, Tuzcu EM, Halliburton SS, Svensson L, Roselli EE, Schoenhagen P. Pre-procedural imaging of aortic root orientation and dimensions: comparison between X-ray angiographic planar imaging and 3-dimensional multidetector row computed tomography. *JACC Cardiovasc Interv* 2010;3:105-13.

[58] Feldman T, Kar S, Rinaldi M, Fail P, Hermiller J, Smalling R, Whitlow PL, Gray W, Low R, Herrmann HC, Lim S, Foster E, Glower D; EVEREST Investigators. Percutaneous mitral repair with the MitraClip system: safety and midterm durability in the initial EVEREST (Endovascular Valve Edge-to-Edge REpair Study) cohort. *J Am Coll Cardiol.* 2009;54:686-94.

[59] Salgo IS, Gorman JH, Gorman RC, Jackson BM, Bowen FW, Plappert T, St John Sutton M, Edmunds LH. Effect of annular shape on leaflet curvature in reducing mitral leaflet stress. *Circulation.* 2002;106: 711–717.

[60] Timek TA, Miller DC. Experimental and clinical assessment of mitral annular area and dynamics: what are we actually measuring? *Ann Thorac Surg.* 2001;72:966–974.

[61] Boltwood CM, Tei C, Wong M, Shah PM. Quantitative echocardiography of the mitral complex in dilated cardiomyopathy: the mechanism of functional mitral regurgitation. *Circulation.* 1983;68:498–508.

[62] Flachskampf FA, Chandra S, Gaddipatti A, Levine RA, Weyman AE, Ameling W, Hanrath P, Thomas JD. Analysis of shape and motion of the mitral annulus in subjects with and without cardiomyopathy by echocardiographic 3-dimensional reconstruction. *J Am Soc Echocardiogr.* 2000;13:277–287.

[63] Ormiston JA, Shah PM, Tei C, Wong M. Size and motion of the mitral valve annulus in man. I. A two-dimensional echocardiographic method and findings in normal subjects. *Circulation.* 1981;64:113–120.

[64] Ormiston JA, Shah PM, Tei C, Wong M. Size and motion of the mitral valve *Circulation.* 1982;65:713-9.

[65] Dall'Agata A, Taams MA, Fioretti PM, Roelandt JR, Van Herwerden LA. Cosgrove-Edwards mitral ring dynamics measured with transesophageal three-dimensional echocardiography. *Ann Thorac Surg.* 1998;65:485–490.

[66] Pai RG, Tanimoto M, Jintapakorn W, Azevedo J, Pandian NG, Shah PM. Volume-rendered three-dimensional dynamic anatomy of the mitral annulus using a transesophageal echocardiographic technique. *J Heart Valve Dis.* 1995;4:623–627.

[67] Kaplan SR, Bashein G, Sheehan FH, Legget ME, Munt B, Li XN, Sivarajan M, Bolson EL, Zeppa M, Arch MZ, Martin RW. Three dimensional echocardiographic assessment

of annular shape changes in the normal and regurgitant mitral valve. *Am Heart J.* 2000;139:378–387.

[68] Komoda T, Hetzer R, Uyama C, et al. Mitral annular function assessed by 3D imaging for mitral valve surgery. *J Heart Valve Dis.* 1994;3:483–490.

[69] Levine RA, Handschumacher MD, Sanfilippo AJ, Hagege AA, Harrigan P, Marshall JE, Weyman AE. Three-dimensional echocardiographic reconstruction of the mitral valve, with implications for the diagnosis of mitral valve prolapse. *Circulation.* 1989;80:589–598.

[70] Levine R, Stathogiannis E, Newell J, Harrigan P, Weyman A. Reconsideration of echocardiographic standards for mitral valve prolapse: lack of association between leaflet displacement isolated to the apical four chamber view and independent echocardiographic evidence of abnormality. *J Am Coll Cardiol.* 1988;11:1010-9.

[71] Feuchtner GM, Alkadhi H, Karlo C, Sarwar A, Meier A, Dichtl W, Leschka S, Blankstein R, Gruenenfelder J, Stolzmann P, Cury RC. Cardiac CT angiography for the diagnosis of mitral valve prolapse: comparison with echocardiography. *Radiology.* 2010;254:374-83.

[72] Maselli D, Guarracino F, Chiaramonti F, et al. Percutaneous mitral annuloplasty: an anatomic study of human coronary sinus and its relation with mitral valve annulus and coronary arteries. *Circulation.* 2006;114:377–380.

[73] Kaye DM, Byrne M, Alferness C, Power J. Feasibility and short-term efficacy of percutaneous mitral annular reduction for the therapy of heart failure-induced mitral regurgitation. *Circulation* 2003;108:1795–1797.

[74] Tops LF, Van de Veire NR, Schuijf JD, de Roos A, van der Wall EE, Schalij MJ, Bax JJ. Noninvasive evaluation of coronary sinus anatomy and its relation to the mitral valve annulus: Implications for percutaneous mitral annuloplasty. *Circulation* 2007;115:1426–1432.

[75] Schofer J, Siminiak T, Haude M, Herrman JP, Vainer J, Wu JC, Levy WC, Mauri L, Feldman T, Kwong RY, Kaye DM, Duffy SJ, Tübler T, Degen H, Brandt MC, Van Bibber R, Goldberg S, Reuter DG, Hoppe UC. Percutaneous mitral annuloplasty for functional mitral regurgitation: Results of the CARILLON Mitral Annuloplasty Device European Union Study. *Circulation* 2009;120:326–333.

[76] Alkadhi H, Desbiolles L, Stolzmann P, Leschka S, Scheffel H, Plass A, Schertler T, Trindade PT, Genoni M, Cattin P, Marincek B, Frauenfelder T. Mitral annular shape, size, and motion in normals and in patients with cardiomyopathy: evaluation with computed tomography. *Invest Radiol.* 2009;44:218-25.

[77] Maselli D, Guarracino F, Chiaramonti F, Mangia F, Borelli G, Minzioni G. Percutaneous mitral annuloplasty: An anatomic study of human coronary sinus and its relation with mitral valve annulus and coronary arteries. Circulation 2006;114:377–380.

[78] Choure AJ, Garcia MJ, Hesse B, Sevensma M, Maly G, Greenberg NL, Borzi L, Ellis S, Tuzcu EM, Kapadia SR. In vivo analysis of the anatomical relationship of coronary sinus to mitral annulus and left circumflex coronary artery using cardiac multidetector computed tomography: implications for percutaneous coronary sinus mitral annuloplasty. *J Am Coll Cardiol.* 2006;48:1938-45.

[79] Gopal A, Shah A, Shareghi S, Bansal N, Nasir K, Gopal D, Budoff MJ, Shavelle DM. The role of cardiovascular computed tomographic angiography for coronary sinus mitral annuloplasty. *J Invasive Cardiol.* 2010;22:67-73.
[80] Webb JG, Wood DA, Ye J, Gurvitch R, Masson JB, Rodes-Cabau J, Osten M, Horlick E, Wendler O, Dumont E, Carere RG, Wijesinghe N, Nietlispach F, Johnson M, Thompson CR, Moss R, Leipsic J, Munt B, Lichtenstein SV, Cheung A. Transcatheter Valve-in-Valve Implantation for Failed Bioprosthetic Heart Valves. *Circulation.* 2010; 121:1634-1636
[81] Zahn EM, Hellenbrand WE, Lock JE, McElhinney DB. Implantation of the melody transcatheter pulmonary valve in patients with a dysfunctional right ventricular outflow tract conduit early results from the US Clinical trial. *J Am Coll Cardiol.* 2009;54:1722-9.
[82] Schievano S, Taylor AM, Capelli C, Coats L, Walker F, Lurz P, Nordmeyer J, Wright S, Khambadkone S, Tsang V, Carminati M, Bonhoeffer P. First-in-man implantation of a novel percutaneous valve: a new approach to medical device development. *EuroIntervention.* 2010 ;5:745-50.
[83] Schoenhagen P, Hill A. Transcatheter aortic valve implantation and potential role of 3D imaging. *Expert Rev Med Devices* 2009;6:411-21.
[84] Abel DB, Dehdashtian MM, Rodger ST, Smith AC, Smith LJ, Waninger MS. Evolution and future of preclinical testing for endovascular grafts. *J Endovasc Ther* 2006;13:649–659.
[85] Zarins CK, Taylor CA. Endovascular device design in the future: transformation *J Endovasc Ther* 2009;16,Suppl 1:I12-21. Review.
[86] Tommasini G, Camerini A, Gatti A, Derchi G, Bruzzone A, Vecchio C. Panoramic coronary angiography. *J Am Coll Cardiol* 1998; 31: 871–877.
[87] Biasi L, Ali T, Thompson M. Intra-operative dynaCT in visceral-hybrid repair of an extensive thoracoabdominal aortic aneurysm. *Eur J Cardiothorac Surg* 2008;34:1251-1252.
[88] Nölker G, Gutleben KJ, Marschang H, Ritscher G, Asbach S, Marrouche N, Brachmann J, Sinha AM. Three-dimensional left atrial and esophagus reconstruction using cardiac C-arm computed tomography with image integration into fluoroscopic views for ablation of atrial fibrillation: accuracy of a novel modality in comparison with multislice computed tomography. *Heart Rhythm* 2008;5:1651-1657.
[89] Garcia JA, Chen SY, Messenger JC, Casserly IP, Hansgen A, Wink O, Movassaghi B, Klein AJ, Carroll JD. Initial clinical experience of selective coronary angiography using one prolonged injection and a 180 degrees rotational trajectory. *Catheter Cardiovasc Interv* 2007; 70: 190–196.
[90] Neubauer AM, Garcia JA, Messenger JC, Hansis E, Kim MS, Klein AJ, Schoonenberg GA, Grass M, Carroll JD. Clinical Feasibility of a Fully Automated 3D Reconstruction of Rotational Coronary X-Ray Angiograms. *Circ Cardiovasc Interv* 2010;3:71-9
[91] Johri AM, Passeri JJ, Picard MH. Three dimensional echocardiography: approaches and clinical utility. *Heart* 2010;96:390-397.
[92] Hung J, Lang R, Flachskampf F, et al. 3D Echocardiography: a review of the current status and future directions. *J Am Soc Echocardiogr* 2007;20:213–33.

[93] Balzer J, Kelm M, Kühl HP. Real-time three-dimensional transoesophageal echocardiography for guidance of non-coronary interventions in the catheter laboratory. *J Echocardiogr* 2009;10:341-9.

[94] Guttman MA, Ozturk C, Raval AN, Raman VK, Dick AJ, DeSilva R, Karmarkar P, Lederman RJ, McVeigh ER. Interventional cardiovascular procedures guided by real-time MR imaging: an interactive interface using multiple slices, adaptive projection modes and live 3D renderings. *J Magn Reson Imaging* 2007; 26:1429–1435.

[95] Elgort DR, Wong EY, Hillenbrand CM, Wacker FK, Lewin JS, Duerk JL. Real-time catheter tracking and adaptive imaging. *J Magn Reson Imaging* 2003;18:621–626.

[96] Balzer J, Kuhl H, Rassaf T, Hoffmann R, Schauerte P, Kelm M, Franke A. Real-time transesophageal three-dimensional echocardiography for guidance of percutaneous cardiac interventions: first experience. *Clin Res Cardiol* 2008;97(9):565–574

[97] Handke M, Heinrichs G, Moser U, Hirt F, Margadant F, Gattiker F, Bode C, Geibel A. Transesophageal real-time three-dimensional echocardiography methods and initial in vitro and human in vivo studies. *J Am Coll Cardiol* 2006;48(10):2070–2076

[98] Pothineni KR, Inamdar V, Miller AP, Nanda NC, Bandarupalli N, Chaurasia P, Kirklin JK, McGiffin DC, Pajaro OE. Initial experience with live/real time three-dimensional transesophageal echocardiography. *Echocardiography* 2007;24:1099–1104

[99] Sugeng L, Shernan SK, Salgo IS, Weinert L, Shook D, Raman J, Jeevanandam V, Dupont F, Settlemier S, Savord B, Fox J, Mor-Avi V, Lang RM. Live 3-dimensional transesophageal echocardiography initial experience using the fully-sampled matrix array probe. *J Am Coll Cardiol* 2008; 52:446–449

[100] Scohy TV, Ten Cate FJ, Lecomte PV, McGhie J, de Jong PL, Hofland J, Bogers AJ. Usefulness of intraoperative real-time 3D transesophageal echocardiography in cardiac surgery. *J Card Surg* 2008; 23:784–786

[101] Sugeng L, Shernan SK, Weinert L, Shook D, Raman J, Jeevanandam V, DuPont F, Fox J, Mor-Avi V, Lang RM. Real-time three-dimensional transesophageal echocardiography in valve disease: comparison with surgical findings and evaluation of prosthetic valves. *J Am Soc Echocardiogr* 2008; 21:1347–1354

[102] Grewal J, Mankad S, Freeman WK, Click RL, Suri RM, Abel MD, Oh JK, Pellikka PA, Nesbitt GC, Syed I, Mulvagh SL, Miller FA. Real-time three-dimensional transesophageal echocardiography in the intraoperative assessment of mitral valve disease. *J Am Soc Echocardiogr* 2009; 22: 34–41

[103] Bouzas-Mosquera A, Alvarez-Garcia N, Ortiz-Vazquez E, Cuenca-Castillo JJ Role of real-time 3-dimensional transesophageal echocardiography in transcatheter aortic valve implantation. *Eur J Cardiothorac Surg* 2009; 35:909

[104] Iwakura K, Ito H, Kawano S, Okamura A, Kurotobi T, Date M, Inoue K, Fujii K. Comparison of orifice area by transthoracic three-dimensional Doppler echocardiography versus proximal isovelocity surface area (PISA) method for assessment of mitral regurgitation. *Am J Cardiol 2006*;97:1630–7.

[105] Sharma R, Mann J, Drummond L, Livesey SA, Simpson IA. The evaluation of real-time 3-dimensional transthoracic echocardiography for the preoperative functional assessment of patients with mitral valve prolapse: a comparison with 2-dimensional transesophageal echocardiography. *J Am Soc Echocardiogr* 2007;20:934–940

[106] Pepi M, Tamborini G, Maltagliati A, Galli CA, Sisillo E, Salvi L, Naliato M, Porqueddu M, Parolari A, Zanobini M, Alamanni F. Head-to-head comparison of two-

and three-dimensional transthoracic and transesophageal echocardiography in the localization of mitral valve prolapse. *J Am Coll Cardiol* 2006;48:2524–30.

[107] Otsuji Y, Handschumacher MD, Liel-Cohen N, Tanabe H, Jiang L, Schwammenthal E, Guerrero JL, Nicholls LA, Vlahakes GJ, Levine RA. Mechanism of ischemic mitral regurgitation with segmental left ventricular dysfunction: three-dimensional echocardiographic studies in models of acute and chronic progressive regurgitation. *J Am Coll Cardiol* 2001;37:641–8.

[108] Sugeng L, Shernan SK, Weinert L, Shook D, Raman J, Jeevanandam V, DuPont F, Fox J, Mor-Avi V, Lang RM. Real-time three-dimensional transesophageal echocardiography in valve disease: comparison with surgical findings and evaluation of prosthetic valves. *J Am Soc Echocardiogr* 2008;21:1347–54.

[109] Lang RM, Mor-Avi V, Dent JM. Three-dimensional echocardiography: is it ready for everyday clinical use? *J Am Coll Cardiol Img* 2009;2:114–117

[110] Grewal J, Suri R, Mankad S, Tanaka A, Mahoney DW, Schaff HV, Miller FA, Enriquez-Sarano M. Mitral Annular Dynamics in Myxomatous Valve Disease: New Insights With Real-Time 3-Dimensional Echocardiography. *Circulation.* 2010; 121:1423-1431

[111] Détaint D, Lepage L, Himbert D, Brochet E, Messika-Zeitoun D, Iung B, Vahanian A. Determinants of Significant Paravalvular Regurgitation After Transcatheter Aortic Valve: Implantation Impact of Device and Annulus Discongruence. *JACC Cardiovasc Interv.* 2009; 2(9):821-827

[112] Daimon M, Shiota T, Gillinov AM, Hayase M, Ruel M, Cohn WE, Blacker SJ, Liddicoat JR. Percutaneous mitral valve repair for chronic ischemic mitral regurgitation: A real-time three-dimensional echocardiographic study in an ovine model. *Circulation* 2005;111:2183–2189.

[113] Eggebrecht H, Kuhl H, Kaiser GM. Feasibility of real-time magnetic resonance-guided stent-graft placement in a swine model of descending aortic dissection. *Eur Heart J* 2006;27:613–620.

[114] Kuehne T, Yilmaz S, Meinus C. Magnetic resonance imaging-guided transcatheter implantation of a prosthetic valve in aortic valve position: feasibility study in swine. *J Am Coll Cardiol* 2004;44:2247–2249.

[115] Kim JH, Kocaturk O, Ozturk C, Faranesh AZ, Sonmez M, Sampath S, Saikus CE, Kim AH, Raman VK, Derbyshire JA, Schenke WH, Wright VJ, Berry C, McVeigh ER, Lederman RJ. Mitral cerclage annuloplasty, a novel transcatheter treatment for secondary mitral valve regurgitation: initial results in swine. *J Am Coll Cardiol* 2009;54:638-51.

In: Percutaneous Valve Technology: Present and Future ISBN: 978-1-61942-577-4
Editors: Jose Luis Navia and Sharif Al-Ruzzeh

Chapter IV

General Concepts on Transcatheter Cardiovascular Therapies

Nicolas Brozzi, Eric Roselli, Sharif Al-Ruzzeh and Jose Luis Navia

Introduction

Development of transcatheter therapies has revolutionized the surgical treatment of cardiovascular disease. The less invasive nature of these approaches has improved recovery and expanded surgical indications to higher risk patients. Since the early days of coronary angioplasty transcatheter therapies have been developed for the treatment of numerous structural cardiac and vascular diseases. The development of these procedures has required impressive technical advances not only for the design of implantable devices, but also the tools to deliver them such as wires, sheaths, and catheters; and the imaging systems which have made it all possible. The development of hybrid operating rooms has brought all these technologies together creating an optimal environment for transcatheter cardiovascular interventions. This chapter presents an overview of the basic knowledge required to perform most transcatheter therapies, including description of instruments, sheath, wires, catheters, and devices, as well as diagnostic and intraoperative imaging.

Pathologies

A wide range of pathologies is currently treated with transcatheter therapies, including congenital structural heart disease, acquired structural heart disease, coronary heart disease, and peripheral vascular disease. Discussion of technical aspects regarding individual pathologies is beyond the scope if this chapter and is included in subsequent chapters. Some of the pathologies currently treated with transcatheter therapies include:

1) Congenital structural heart disease
    a) Patent foramen ovale

   b) Atrial septal defect
   c) Ventricular septal defect
   d) Aortic stenosis
   e) Pulmonic stenosis
2) Acquired structural heart disease
   a) Coronary artery disease
   b) Ischemic ventricular septal defect
   c) Traumatic atrial or ventricular septal defect
   d) Aortic valve stenosis / insufficiency
   e) Pulmonary valve stenosis / insufficiency
   f) Tricuspid valve insufficiency
   g) Mitral valve stenosis / insufficiency
3) Peripheral vascular disease
   a) Aortic coarctation
   b) Aortic aneurysm
   c) Aortic dissection (acute or chronic)
   d) Traumatic aortic transection
   e) Aortic occlusive disease
   f) Peripheral arterial occlusive disease
   g) Peripheral arterial aneurysm / pseudoaneurysm
   h) Peripheral arterial / venous thrombosis
   i) Arterio-venous fistulae / malformations

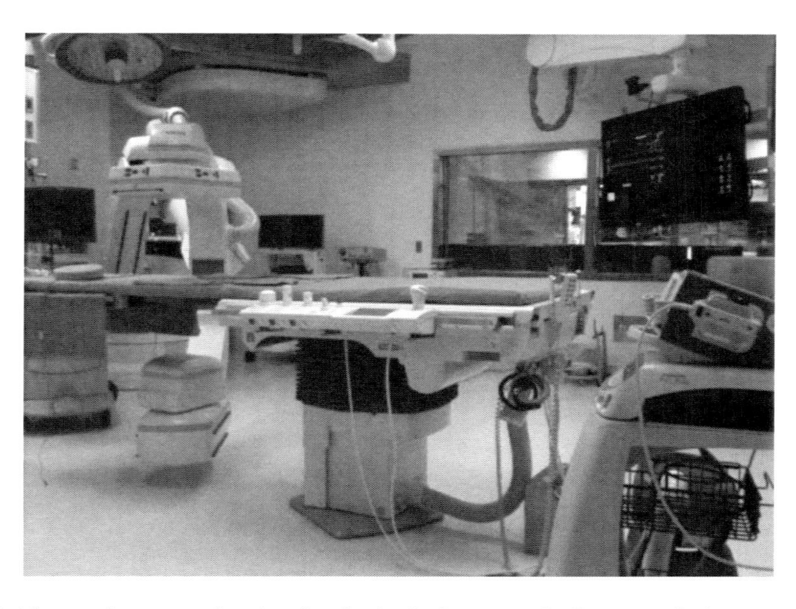

Figure 1. Hybrid operating room showing fixed robotic fluoroscopic C-arm, radio lucent operating table, TEE monitor, and multi parametric display monitor. Control desk is identified behind the radiation protective glasses in the back.

Role of Imaging Systems in Transcatheter Terapies

Imaging systems play a critical role when performing any transcatheter cardiac or vascular procedure. While the conduct of the procedure usually involves several physicians with specialized knowledge in each area, the surgeon should be familiar with the basic concepts of ultrasound systems and proficient in the management of fluoroscopy. Operative planning also requires the surgeon to be familiar with analysis of cross sectional imaging like CT scan reconstruction as well.

Preoperative Imaging

Imaging is crucial for patient evaluation, device selection in correlation with the anatomy of the lesion, as well as formulation of a plan for the intervention. Recent advances in imaging technologies, in part inspired by advancements in stent-graft technology, have drastically changed the character and role of pre-procedural imaging. The accepted diagnostic gold standard, digital subtraction angiography, is now being challenged by the state-of-the-art computed tomography angiography (CTA), magnetic resonance angiography (MRA) and transoesophageal echocardiography (TEE). These techniques provide information not only on the aortic lumen but also on the wall and surrounding mediastinal structures. Technological advancements of multidetector computed tomography have optimized the balance between spatial and temporal resolution and invasiveness, becoming the most used diagnostic imaging modality.

Multidetector computed tomographic angiography allows the comprehensive evaluation of thoracic aortic lesions in terms of morphological features and extent, presence of thrombus, relationship with adjacent structures and branches as well as signs of impending or acute rupture, and is routinely used in these setting particularly when planning transcatheter procedure.[1]

Intraoperative Imaging

Fluoroscopy

Transcatheter therapies require intermitent intraoperative monitoring with radioscopic systems. These can range in complexity from a basic portable C-arm with recording capabilities and a radiolucent operating table to a fixed C-arm mounted on the operating room floor or ceiling with remote activation controls, and a movable tabletop. While portable radioscopic systems are cheaper and can be moved from one operating room to the other, fixed systems present greater imaging capabilities providing superior image quality and additional measuring capabilities. A higher tube heat capacity allows fixed radioscopic systems to be used for longer periods of time.

While the patient is the person most exposed to primary radiation that comes directly out of the tube housing during a trans-catheter intervention, the members of the surgical team are repeatedly exposed to scattered radiation that spreads up to 6 feet away from the source. Every person involved in the procedure should wear lead shields as the amount of radiation accumulated in the body increases over subsequent exposures. Every effort is made to reduce exposure to radiation including use of collimators, reducing the distance from the source to the image intensifier, using intermittent fluoroscopy, and adding filtration shields. Ultrasound technology has contributed to optimize accuracy in the conduct of the procedures, and minimize exposure to radiation in recent years.

Several contrast agents are available to use during the procedures. (See Table 1) The standard iodine containing dye is most frequently used diluted with normal saline in a proportion 50:50.

In contrast to ionic contrast agents, non-ionic agents do not dissociate in solution, avoiding hypertonicity. Non-ionic agents present a higher ratio of iodine per osmotic particle, and a lower osmolality, which have been related to lower side effects when compared to ionic agents.

Table 1. Comparison and properties of commonly used radiocontrast agents *

Type and osmolality	Name (Trade name)	Viscocity CPS at 37° C	Iodine content mg/ml
High osmolar >12,000 mOsm/kg	Diatrizoate meglumine (Gastrograffin)	5.0	306
	Iothalamate sodium (Glofil)	2.75	325
Low osmolar 500-700 mOsm/kg	Ioxaglate meglumine (Hexabrix)	7.5	320
	Ioxaglate sodium (Hexabrix)	7.5	320
	Iohexol (Omnipaque)	6.3	300
	Ioversol (Optiray)	5.5	300
	Iopamidol (Isovue)	4.7	300
	Iopromide (Ultravist)	4.6	300
Iso-osmolar 300 mOsm/kg	Iodixanol (Visipaque)	11.4	320
	Iotrolan (Isovist)	8.1	300

*Adapted from Al-Ghonaim et al. Prevention and treatment of contrast-induced nephropathy. Tech Vasc Interventional Rad 2006;9:42-9.

Contrast media have cytostatic, cytotoxic and apoptotic effects on endothelial cells. These effects are more evident with ionic contrast media, in particular highly osmolar agents. Contrast media-induced endothelial injury may play a role in the pathophysiology of adverse effects including hemodynamic instability, thrombosis, and pulmonary edema.

Nephropathy induced by contrast media is one of the most frequent complications of parenteral administration of contrast, and is the third leading cause of hospital-acquired acute renal failure accounting for 12% of cases.[2] It is usually recognized by an acute deterioration in renal function 2 to 7 days following contrast administration, occurring in the absence of other identifiable causes of acute reanl failures, with a rise in serum creatinine over 25% of preprocedural values.

Most frequently patients present reversible non-oliguric renal failure with complete recovery of renal function within 14 days of contrast administration.[3] However, this complication is associated with significant economic and clinical consequences including increased length of hospitalization, acute dialysis requirement, major adverse cardiovascular events, and death.[4] Hospital mortality in the range of 22% to 37% has been reported for patients developing renal insufficiency after coronary angiography.[5]

Important patient risk factors for contrast-induced nephropathy include chronic kidney disease, diabetes mellitus, heart failure, older age, anemia, and left ventricular systolic dysfunction.

Non-patient related risk factors include high-osmolar contrast, ionic contrast, contrast viscosity, and contrast volume. In addition to minimizing the volume of contrast employed during the procedure, several preprocedural prophylactic strategies have been described to prevent or attenuate the effect of contrast agents in kidney function including hydration, bicarbonate, N-acetylcysteine, and ascorbic acid.

Determining serum creatinine levels before the procedure in high-risk patients contributes to identify those patients that may benefit from these strategies. Patients at risk for contrast-induced nephropathy should receive iso- or low-osmolar contrast agents, and every effort should be made to minimize the volume of contrast administered during the procedure. Adecuate postprocedural hydration additionally contributes to the elimination of the contrast agent.

Role of Carbon Dioxide as Contrast Agent

CO_2 can be used as intra-arterial contrast as it represents a safe, effective, and inexpensive alternative to the relatively toxic ionic contrast agents.[6] When injected in the blood stream, CO_2 reduces the attenuation of the blood vessel compared with soft tissue and fat. The most serious safety concern is related to neurotoxicity that has been reported when injected CO_2 has refluxed into vertebral arteries causing seizures.[7] Endovascular stent-grafting has been performed in the abdominal aorta with acceptable rates of success, but intraarterial CO_2 should not be used above the diaphragm and it is absolutely contraindicated for cerebral and upper limb angiography. Additionally, intravenous CO_2 should not be used in patients with right to left intracardiac shunt.[8,9]

Role of Ultrasound in Transcatheter Cardiovascular Therapies

Transesophageal Echocardiogram

Transesophageal echocardiogram (TEE) has become a standard of care in many cardiac procedures as it provides excellent structural and hemodynamic information that assists the surgical team along the conduct of the procedures. Additionally, TEE is extensively used when performing transcatheter therapies of structural heart pathologies.[10]

TEE has gained importance in the diagnosis and treatment of thoracic aortic pathologies as well. It presents high sensitivity for the diagnosis of aortic dissections and provides high quality images of the ascending and descending aorta. Imaging of the aortic arch is usually limited by the anatomic disposition and interposition of the airway.

During the conduct of aortic transcatheter procedures TEE provides information regarding the position of the vascular stent-grafts, identifies endoleaks, and the blood flow within the true and false lumens by Doppler ultrasound.[11]

TEE has proven to be particularly useful during the implantation of percutaneous aortic valves as it provides accurate information of the aortic annulus and native valve anatomy that is necessary for selecting the size and the area of deployment of the prosthetic valve, and it also provides information on the function of the implanted valve.

Intravascular Ultrasound

The intravascular ultrasound (IVUS) probe can be inserted in the vascular system through a sheath and navigated over most frequently used guidewires to any anatomic location within the vascular tree. It is limited by lack of Doppler capabilities. But it provides high definition images of the arterial walls, origin of collaterals, characteristics of dissection flaps, entry and reentry tears, and atherosclerotic plaques.[12]

Several recent studies have reported the utility of IVUS imaging to identify endoleaks and evaluate deployed stents, providing the opportunity to perform corrective interventions that correlate with better long-term outcomes.

Postoperative Imaging

Patients that have received cardiac devices are usually followed up by transthoracic echocardiogram. Doppler ultrasound is useful in the evaluation of cardiac valves and intracardiac shunts, as well as the diagnosis of peripheral vascular pathologies including arterial stenosis, and pseudoaneurysms. Patients receiving transcatheter therapies for aortic pathology are followed up within the first six months and then annually with physical exam and computed tomographic scan of the affected areas. Of note, follow up CT scans should include arterial and venous phases to provide complete images and accurate diagnosis of endoleaks, and assess the false lumen for delayed blood flow.

Conduct of the Procedure

The following sections will discuss general aspects related to the instruments generally employed during transcatheter therapies. While we do not intend to discuss any specific procedure in detail, we present general basic knowledge that apply to the conduct of all transcatheter procedures.

Vascular Access

Many procedures can be performed by obtaining vascular access with a percutaneous puncture and subsequent introduction of dilators and introducers. Some others may require a groin incision with open dissection of the femoral artery, and arteriotomy for introduction of large sheaths to deploy aortic stent-grafts or aortic valve prosthesis.

Occasionally, patients may present severe peripheral vascular disease precluding safe conventional approach through the groin with femoral dissection, and alternative routes need to be used.

These include retroperitoneal approach with dissection of an iliac artery or the distal aorta itself, subclavian approach with dissection of the axillary artery, or median sternotomy / hemisternotomy with direct approach through the ascending aorta. When accessing a large artery a Dacron graft (8-14 mm) is frequently anastomosed on the side of the artery and used as a conduit to perform the procedure without interrupting arterial blood flow to distal areas of the body.

While the latter routes require a more complex approach, they still present advantage in terms of invasiveness and complexity when compared to conventional surgical treatment of complex cardiac and vascular pathologies. In general, the patient receives intravenous heparin at a dose of 100 units/kg, to obtain anticoagulation with an activated clotting time > 300 seconds.

Needles

Initial access to the arterial or venous system can be obtained by a wide range of needles from a 21 gauge micro puncture needle that allows for the introduction of a thin .018" flexible wire, to a larger 18 gauge "pink" needle that allows the introduction of 0.032" to 0.038" wires for subsequent exchange of dilators and introducers.

Ultrasound can be of great help to perform an accurate puncture of the vessel, particularly in patients with large amount of adipose tissue, and those with scars from previous incisions, or hemathomas.

Vascular Sheaths

The vascular sheaths are introduced in the vessels on top of a wire and will maintain open access to the vessel throughout the procedure. The wall of the sheaths is constructed from teflon, and some of them present a braided shaft design that provides strength, flexibility, and resistance to kinking.

A radiopaque marker at the end of the sheath provides visualization by fluoroscopy, which can be particularly important for stent delivery. They most often present a hemostatic valve on the end that is exposed on the surface of the patient.

The structure of the sheath is described in terms of length and caliber, referring to the inner diameter of the sheath described in French units (1F = 0.33 mm).

A wide range of sheath are commercially available, going from 4 F to 24 F in diameter. (Figures 2 A, and 2 B) Sheaths usually present a side conduit connected to the main lumen that allows the extraction of blood samples, measurement of blood pressure, and injection of contrast agents in the blood stream. The length of the sheath can vary in the range of 5.5 cm to 90 cm for specific applications.

All sheath come with at least one dilator that is placed inside the sheath to facilitate advancement of the sheath over the guide wire to introduce it in the vessel and to navigate areas of angulation or stenosis within the vessels. Larger sheath present several dilators of progressive bigger diameters to facilitate vessel instrumentation.

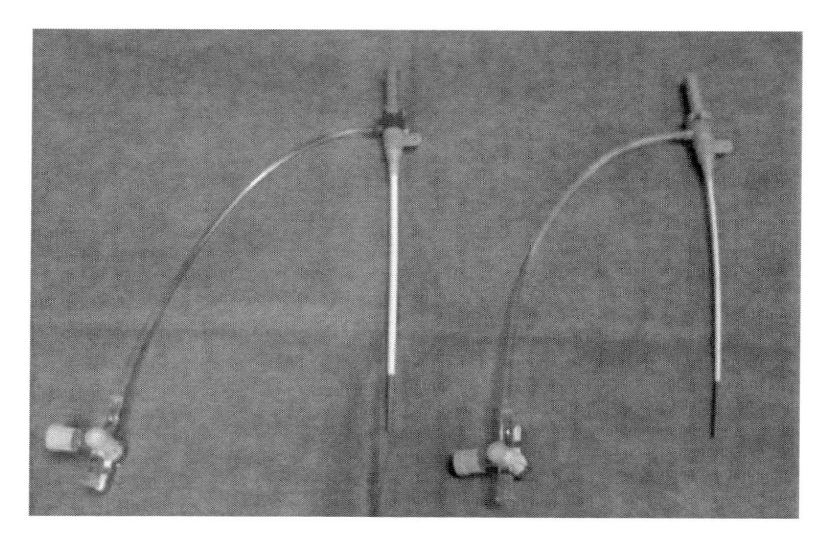

Figure 2 A. Small vascular access sheaths (5 F and 4 F) provide vascular access for wires and catheters.

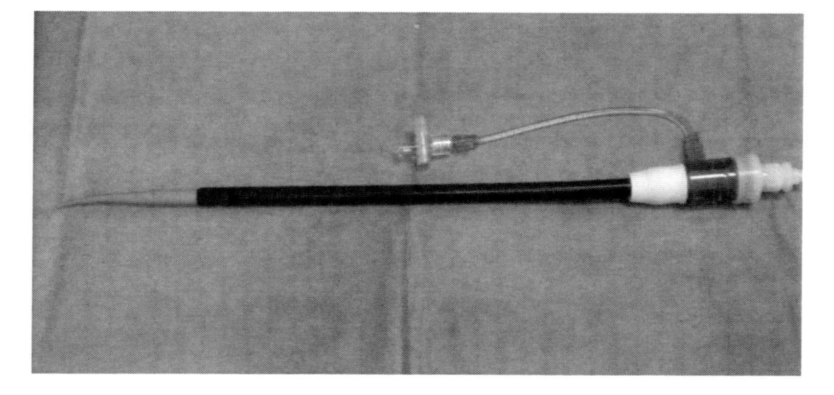

Figure 2 B. 24 F sheath provide vascular access for introduction of large vascular devices like an aortic stent-graft.

There is a universal color coding system that facilitates differentiation of sheath during the procedure:

- 4 F : red
- 5 F : gray
- 6 F ; green
- 7 F : orange
- 8 F : blue
- 9 F : black
- 10 F : violet
- 11 F : yellow

While smaller sheath will be placed percutaneously with a modified Seldinger's technique, sheaths larger that 12 F may require a cut down with direct arteriotomy for safe access of a major artery.

Guide Wire Anatomy

The wires constitute railways inside the blood vessels, and are manufactured in a wide range of calibers, lengths, and stiffness. The structure of the guide wire presents a core body and a tip. The tip presents a flexible non-traumatic end that is inserted in the blood vessel, and the core body provides each particular wire the performance characteristics.

Guide wires are constructed in a jacketed composite design with stainless steel and nitinol. The stainless steel provides support to the wire, and the stiffness will depend on the diameter of the core body. A layer of nitinol covering the core body provides flexibility, memory and kink resistance, while tapered grinds additionally enhance the performance of the wire. The flexible tip is usually constructed with a central area of platinum or gold that provides radiopacity, is resistant to the pressure provided by the body of the wire, and is non-traumatic to the vessel walls. Many wires present a silicon or Teflon external coating that provides them hydrophilic properties, enhancing the navigability/maneuverability inside the blood vessels.

Guide wire dimensions are described in terms of the outer diameter or the main body and the tip, both measured in inches, and length of the wire which is measured in centimeters.

Guide wires can be stiff, intermediate, or floppy depending on the materials employed, the diameter of the core body, the grind, and the tip performance. Handling wires and catheters during a transcatheter procedure is equivalent to tying knots and handling instruments in open surgery. Attention must be focused to never lose control of a wire that is inserted in the patient by controlling the access sheath. Wires must always be kept clean and wet. Several aspects need to be kept in mind when selecting a guide wire for a specific purpose. Like any other surgical instrument, the different features of each guide wire will provide it individual characteristics for specific applications.

Diameters of .035 to .038 are most frequently employed in peripheral wires used as starter wires, selective wires, exchange wires, and specialty wires.

Smaller diameter wires of .014 to .018 inches are commonly used in the treatment of occlusive disease in vessels of more than 1 mm in diameter.

When choosing the length of the guide wire, we need to consider the following distances:

1) From sheath hub to the insertion site
2) From sheath insertion site to therapy site, or the catheter length, which ever is longer.
3) Length of wire needed distal to the therapy target to secure safe access.
4) Length needed to place a torque device.

Standard length of guide wires include 145 cm, 175/180 cm, 260 cm, and 300 cm.

Regarding the characteristics of the guide wire tip, four major models are available, including:

1) Soft tip
   a) Consists of inner core end to end combined with tip shaping capabilities.
   b) Is more aggressive in crossing tight lesions.
2) Floppy tip
   a) Has no inner core to the tip of the wire and is usually comprised of a ribbon of stainless steel, nitinol, gold, or platinum, which allows to shape the wire.
   b) Allows for safe, non traumatic selective navigation of vessels.
3) "J" tip
   a) Inner core end to end with a pre-formed "J" shape soft tip.
   b) Allows for safe passage of wires through irregular lesions or stents, by keeping the wire in the "true lumen" and not through the struts.
4) Angled tip
   a) Selectively used to steer wire because of tip angle.
   b) It is the tip usually present on selective wires.

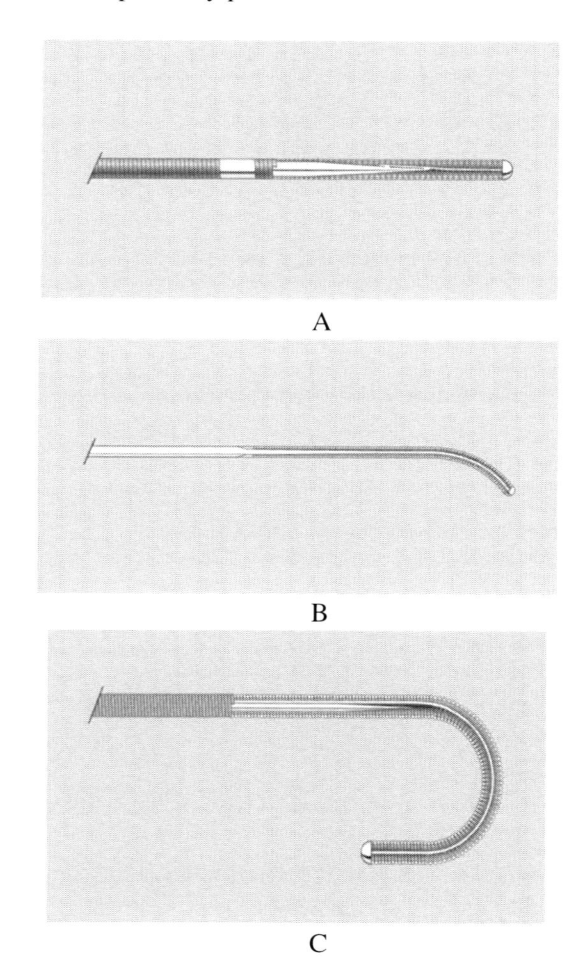

Figure 3. Guide wire tips present variable shapes and stiffness, including: 3A: soft tip; 3B: angled tip; 3C: "J" tip.

The structural characteristics of the wires will make each wire useful for specific parts of the operation. Additional criteria that we need to consider when selecting a specific guide wire are related to the goal of the procedure, the location of the vascular access being used, the device that will be delivered over the wire (whether diagnostic catheter or a therapeutic device), and finally the compatibility between the guide wire and the device with respect to size, length, and coating characteristics.

Guide wires are provided by the manufacturer in sterile packages with coating preservation solutions so they need to be prepared and flushed with normal saline on the scrub table before they can be used in the patient.

Catheters

The catheters are used to assist in directing guide wires through target lesions, to inject contrast agents in specific regions, and to provide shaped support when delivering therapeutic devices to target lesions.

The material employed in the construction of catheters provides specific features to each model (figure 4). Polyethylene catheters are usually pliable and present good shape memory. Polyurethane catheters are softer, more pliable, and follow guide wires easier, but have a higher degree of friction. Nylon is the most frequent material employed for catheters as they are stiffer and tolerate higher flow rates. Finally Teflon represents the stiffest material, ideal for dilators and sheaths. Both catheters and sheaths may be manufactured in braided and non-braided designs, and present specific features like hydrophilic coating, radio opaque tips, and radio opaque markers.

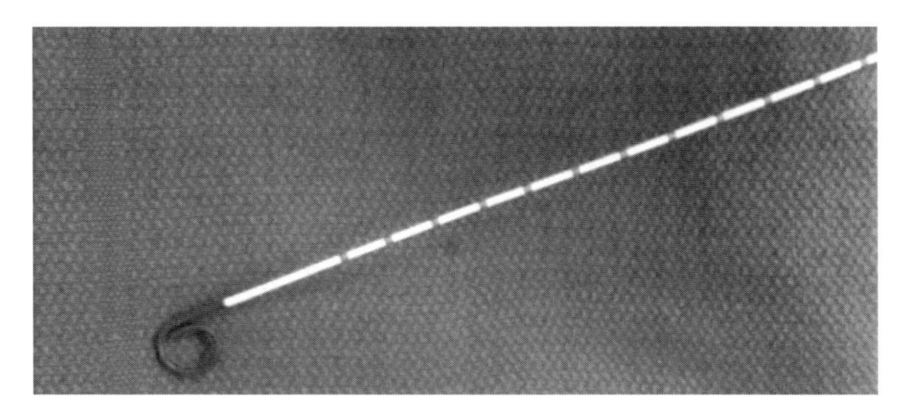

Figure 4. Diagnostic angiographic catheter with radio opaque markers.

They are manufactured in a wide range of calibers and length for specific purposes. The outer diameter of commercially available catheters goes from 3 F to 12 F, and the length can vary from 40 to 150 cm.

The shape of the tip of the catheter is designed for specific purposes. There are catheters commonly employed to guide wires, to exchange wires, to inject contrast agents, and some others are more specifically designed to be used in the cerebral, coronary, or visceral arteries.

Devices

A. Baloons

Transcatheter balloons can be used to open stenotic lesions, to deliver mounted stents, or to secure stents or stent-grafts after delivery (Figure 5). They are inserted inside a catheter and directed over a wire to reach the target area. Baloons are usually inflated with contrast agent diluted in normal saline to identify them under fluoroscopic control. Some balloons are very compliant (profile ballooning) and adapt to the vascular anatomy requiring lower pressure to inflate them; some are semi-compliant (profile/therapeutic baloonig); and other balloons (ie, angioplasty balloons) are non-compliant and require a pressure syringe to inflate them with higher pressures and open stenotic lesions. Stents are usually mounted on soft, compliant balloons.

Balloon size is described by diameter in millimeters, and length in centimeters. The pressure needed to inflate a balloon is measured in atmospheres_and is often described with a particular nominal and burst pressure limits. The rated burst pressure is the pressure at which 1% of all manufacturer's tested balloons burst.

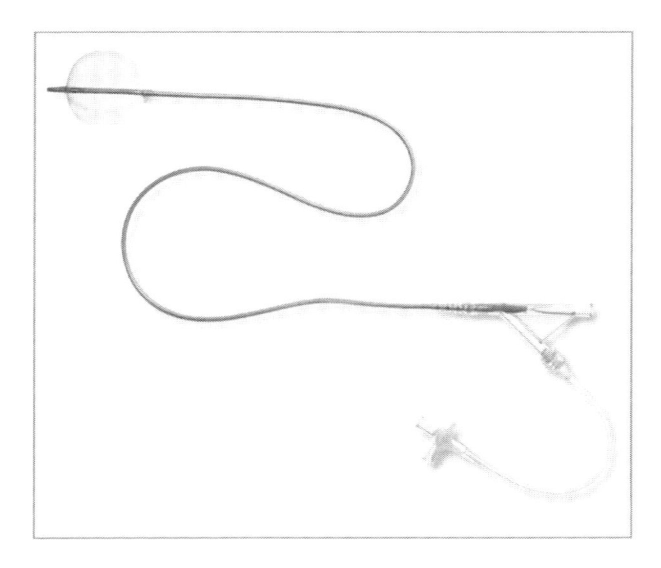

Figure 5. Angioplasty balloon.

B.Vascular Stents, and Stent-Grafts

Palmaz introduced stents into clinical use in 1987.[13] Pioneering work by Parodi and colleagues in 1991 using a handcrafted covered stent showed that endovascular techniques were feasible to repair abdominal aortic aneurysms.[14]

Conventional stent materials, such as stainless steel or cobalt-based alloys, exhibit a limited elastic deformation behavior with approximately 1% linear elongation with strain, which is distinctly different from that of the structural materials of the living body. Natural materials, such as hair, tendon, and bone, can be elastically deformed, in some cases up to 10% strain in a non-linear way. When the deforming stress is released, the strain is recovered at lower stresses. Nitinol alloys present a similar behavior to natural materials.[15] Nitinol stents can be completely compressed (crushed) flat and will return to their original diameter when the deforming force is removed.

Self-expanding Nitinol stents are selected to fit a diameter larger than that of the target vessel. A unique feature of Nitinol stents is their temperature dependent stiffness. Their transformation temperature is typically set to 30°C. They feel quite weak when squeezed or crushed at room or lower temperature, and can be easily crimped and placed in a delivery system. To prevent premature expansion during delivery into the body the stent is constrained by a retractable sheath or by other means. At the treatment site it is released from the delivery system and expands until it hits the vessel wall and conforms to it. At body temperature the stent is superelastic, conforming to the anatomy of the target vessel.[16]

To improve the radiopacity of Nitinol stents, markers are often attached to the stent struts. Markers are typically made from high-density materials such as gold, platinum, or tantalum.

Kink resistance is an important feature of Nitinol for stents in superficial vessels that could be deformed through outside forces. The carotid artery is a prime example. There is a perceived risk for balloon-expandable stents in carotid arteries to be permanently deformed through outside pressure resulting in a partially or completely blocked vessel, once the buckling strength of the stent is exceeded. Although Nitinol stents typically do not have the buckling strength of stainless steel stents, they cannot be permanently deformed through outside forces.

C. Valves in stents

Following the development of stent-grafts, the next natural development was to approach the cardiac valves. The first successful treatment of aortic valve pathology was reported by Cribier et al in 2002, who deployed a prosthetic valve composed of 3 bovine pericardial leaflets mounted within a balloon-expandable stent.[17] These was followed by development of several valve models with the same concept of pericardial leaflets mounted on balloon-expandable stent that have been approved for use in surgically high risk patients.

Similar concepts are being applied for the development of valve prosthesis mounted on stents that can be delivered over a guidewire in the mitral and tricuspid position as well as transcatheter devices designed to repair these valves.

Additional Endovascular Tools

A. Embolization Coils

Embolization coils and microcoils work by promoting localized thrombosis. They are usually used in endovascular therapies aimed at thrombosing aneurysms (commonly intracerebral), arteriovenous fistulas, pseudoaneurysms, and perforations. Additionally, coils are also usefull to generate thrombosis in proximal segments of by-passed arteries as well as in areas of endoleak.

The coils are typically made of metal, such as stainless steel, platinum, or platinum-tungsten alloy, which induces thrombosis and ultimately fibrosis.[18]

This process is not significantly inhibited by systemic heparinization. The basic design of an embolization coil involves a wire (usually of steel or platinum) that is wound tightly into a straight primary coil, and then formed into a secondary structure of various designs (such as three-dimensional loops, helices, and spheres). The coil is usually then packaged into a delivery device and upon extrusion resumes its preformed shape. Platinum coils come in various shapes and sizes, such as helical, conical, diamond, tornado, cloverleaf, straight, J-shape, C-shape, and other complex three-dimensional shapes.[19]

The use of some of these coils requires specialized microcatheters and small selective catheters with sufficient internal lumen diameter, while others require specialized equipment such as coil pushers and coil-positioning catheters which allow repositioning and withdrawal of the coils prior to coil release.

Techniques for coil embolization to some degree are dependent on the device and the manufacturer. Most modern coils have device-specific instructions for deployment. However, some general techniques include using the delivery or guide catheter for the necessary support to deliver and form a dense coil mass; using high radial force coils as a scaffold upon which small softer coils are delivered to create a dense coil mass; and deploying part of the coil in a branch vessel as an anchor, and then deploying the rest of the coils in the target vessel using the anchor as support. The branch vessel is sacrificed.

Important complications associated with the use of embolization coils include coil dislodgement and inadvertent embolization of a non targeted vessel. Other technical considerations include appropriate matching of the helical diameter of the coil to the diameter of the target vessel. If the coil is too large, the coil may elongate and protrude back into the healthy part of the vessel. If too small, the coil may dislodge and migrate distally. Displacement or dislodgement of the delivery catheter can result in misplacement of the coils.[20]

B. Snares

Several wires present the working end with one to three loops that can be placed around another wire under fluoroscopic guidance, and snared to retrieve second wire to the entry site of the snare wire. (Figure 6)

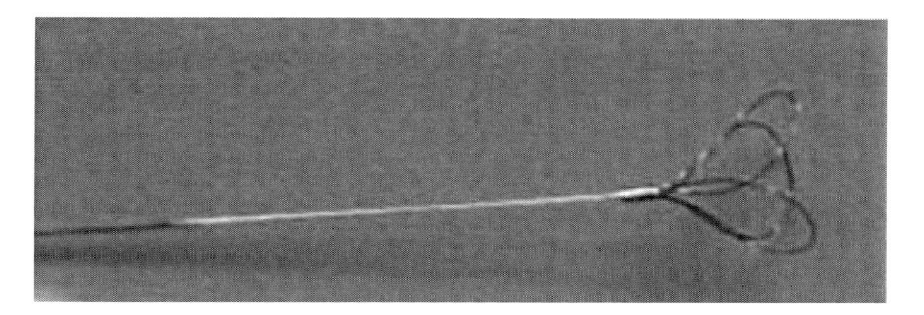

Figure 6. Snare device.

Similar techniques have been reported to recover catheter or wire tips that have dislodged and embolized in the vascular tree.[21]

C. Arterial Closure Devices

Common femoral artery puncture remains the mainstay for arterial access in cardiac and vascular diagnosis and intervention. It provides reliable and convenient access in the majority of patients. When the access is obtained with a percutaneous puncture, hemostosis at the end of the procedure has traditionally been achieved by manual compression at the arteriotomy site during 10 minutes, followed by bed rest with local groin compression for a period of 4-6 hours, depending on the size of the sheath and catheter used, as well as the clinical characteristics of the patient. However, several complications can arise from the arterial puncture site including hemorrhage, pseudoaneurysm formation, arterio-venous fistula, arterial dissection, and thrombosis.[22]

Numerous arterial closure devices have been developed with the goal of reducing time to primary hemostasis, ambulation, and hospital discharge. Four principles have been applied in the development of vascular closure devices, which relate to their mode of action (Table 2).

Table 2. Current available vascular closure devices†

Collagen Plug / Sponge Devices	Suture Mediated Devices	Staple / Clip Devices	Patch / Pad Technology
Angio-Seal (St Jude Medical)	Perclose (Abbott Vascular)	Starclose (Abbott Vascular)	Syvek Patch (Marine Plimer Technologies)
Vasoseal (Datascope Corp.)	Prostar XL (Abbott Vascular)	EVS Vascular Closure System (Angiolink)	Clo-Sur Pad (Scion Cardio-Vascular)
Duett (Vascular Solutions)	SuperStitch (Sutura)	-	Chito-Seal Pad (Abbott Vascular Devices)
Quickseal (Sub-Q Inc)	X-Press (X-Site Medical)	-	D-Stat (Vascular Solutions)

† Adapted from Madigan et al. Arterial closure devices: A review. J Cardiovasc Surg 2007;48:607-24.

Collagen based vascular closure devices deploy a collagen plug outside the vessel wall on the arteriotomy site. (Figure 7) This exogenous collagen material forms an extracellular lattice, which triggers a hemosatic cascade by promoting platelet aggregation, adherence, and activation. Secondary, upon contact with blood, the collagen expands its physical mass resulting in mechanical occlusion of the vessel punctue site and tissue tract.[23] The collagen plugs are reabsorbed within 4 to 6 weeks. They are usually indicated for closure of access sites of 4 to 9 F.

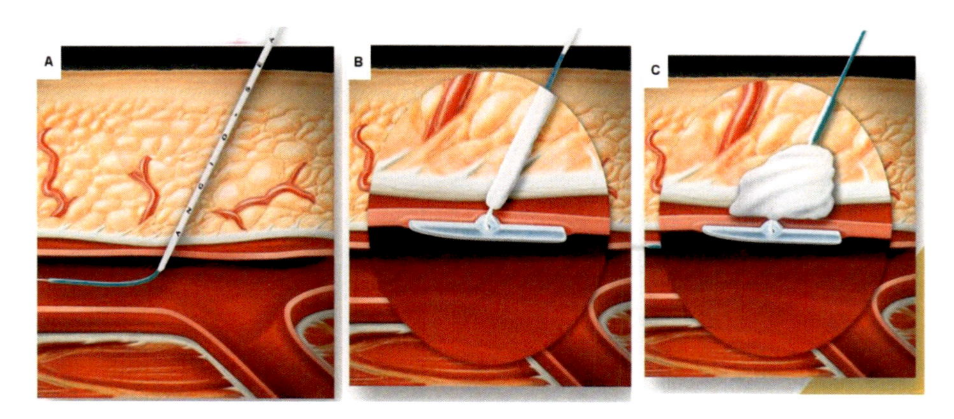

Figure 7. Collagen based vascular closure device, deploys and intraluminal anchor and a collagen plug that seal the arterial access site. Both the anchor and the collagen plug are absorbed within 30 days. (Images provided courtesy of St.Jude Medical).

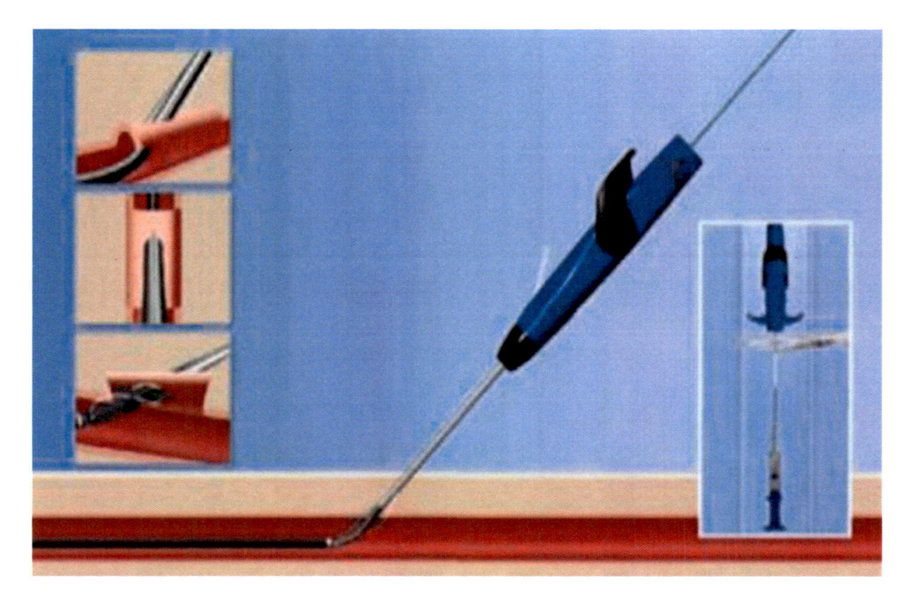

Figure 8. Suture based vascular closure device. Sutures are deployed around the arteriotomy and pulled from the device outside the skin where the knots are tied and pushed down with a knot pusher. (Images provided courtesy of Abbott Vascular).

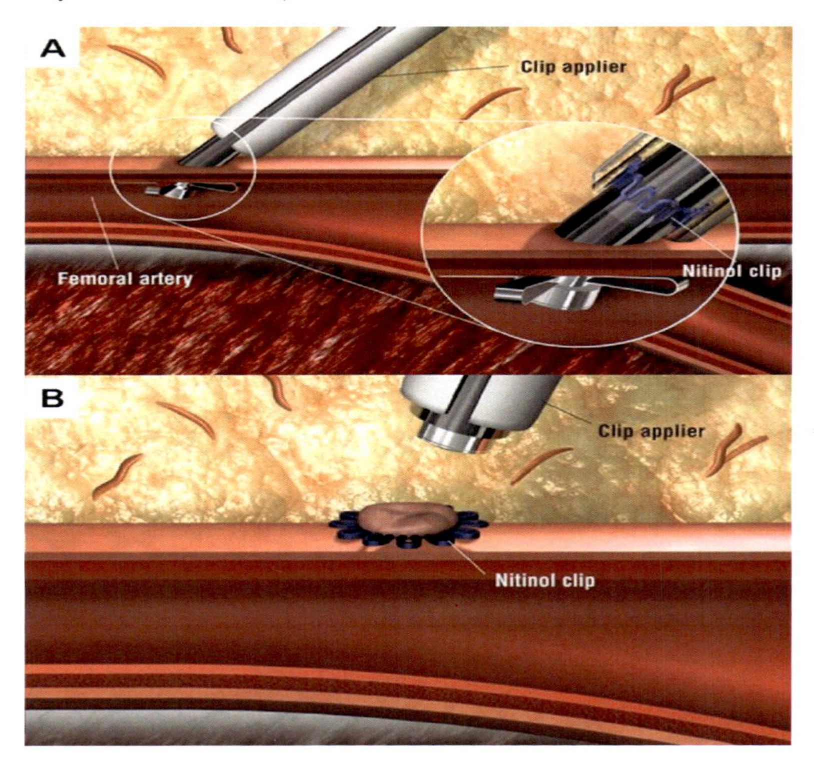

Figure 9. (A-B). Metal clip vascular closure device. A nitinol clip is deployed outside the arterial puncture site to approximate adventitia that will seal the arterial wall. (Images provided courtesy of Abbott Vascular).

Suture based vascular closure devices deploy sutures which are tied to form a surgical knot to close the arteriotomy. (Figure 8) The knot is tied by a built-in mechanism within the closure device, but can also be tied manually if necessary. They are employed after using arterial sheaths of 5 to 12 F.

Metal clip vascular closure devices deploy either a metal or nitinol staple or clip that penetrates the vessel wall to achieve hemostasis. (Figure 7C) Upon deployment, the metal clip or staple remains in situ over the vessel wall and forms a geometric configuration that approximates adventitial vessel layers to close the arterial hole. These devices are not reabsorbed by the body. They are employed in arteriotomies of 4 to 10 F.

Another vascular access closure strategy involves the application of patches and pads chemically impregnated with a procoagulant material that is applied with manual compression to the puncture site.

Most of the products based on collagen plugs, sutures and clips are limited in their application by procedural sheath size. This has implications for punctures where procedural equipment requires a large access site, for example for the deployment of covered aortic stents. Although some authors have reported closure of large arteriotomy incisions using 2 or more vascular closure devices, the safety and long term efficacy of this practice has not been proven. The more conservative approach is to perform a small groin incision with arteriotomy and direct closure with continuous sutures when using large arterial sheath (20-24 F) required for most aortic stent-graft procedures.

The use of vascular closure devices has been associated with a significant shorter time to hemostasis and may shorten recovery time, particularly after diagnostic procedures. However, the use of vascular closure devices may also be associated with an increased risk of infection, lower limb ischemia or arterial stenosis, and device entrapment in the artery requiring vascular surgery for arterial complications.[24]

Conclusion

In summary, technological advances have resulted in the development of multiple devices that are currently deployed in minimally invasive surgery using transcatheter based techniques. The development of newer surgical techniques may result in benefits in terms of lower postoperative complications than conventional surgery, and improved recovery particularly for high surgical risk patients.

As the application of transcatheter therapies expand, it is essential for the surgeons to be familiar with these new technologies, and actively participate in the teams that will offer less invasive surgical treatments to patients with cardiovascular pathologies.

References

[1] Rousseau H, Chabbert V, Maracher MA, et al. The importance of imaging assessment before endovascular repair of thoracic aorta. *Eur J Vasc Endovaasc Surg* 2009;38:408-21.

[2] Nash K, Hafeez A, Hou S. Hospital-acquired renal insufficiency. *Am J Kidney Dis.* 2002;39:930-6.

[3] Gleeson TG, Bulugahapitiya S: Contrast-induced nephropathy. *AJR Am J Roentgenol* 2004;183(6):1673-1689.

[4] McCullough PA, Wolyn R, Rocher LL, et al: Acute renal failure after coronary intervention: incidence, risk factors, and relationship to mortality. *Am J Med* 103(5):368-375, 1997

[5] Levy EM, Viscoli CM, Horwitz RI: The effect of acute renal failure on mortality. A cohort analysis. *JAMA* 1996;275(19):1489-1494.

[6] Hawkins IF. Carbon dioxide digital subtractionarteriography. *AJR Am J Roentgenol* 1982;139:19-24.

[7] Ehrman KO, Taber TE, Gaylord GM, et al. Comparison of diagnostic accuracy with carbon dioxide versus iodinated contrast material in the imaging of hemodiálisis access fistulas. *J Vasc Interv Radiol* 5:771-5.

[8] Shaw DR, Kessel DO. The current status of the use of carbon dioxide in diagnostic and interventional angiographic procedures. *Cardiovasc intervet Radiol* 2006;29:323-31.

[9] Bush RL, Lin PH, Bianco DD, et al. Endovascular aortic aneurysm repair in patients with renal dysfunction or severe contrast allegry: Utility of imaging modalities without iodinated contrast. *Ann Vasc Surg* 2002;16:537-44.

[10] Berry C, Oukerraj L, Asgar A, et al. Role of transesophageal echocardiography in percutaneous aortic valve replacement with the Core Valve Revalving System. *Echocardiography* 2008;25(8):840-8.

[11] Rapezzi C, Rocchi G, Fattori R, et al. Usefulness of transesophageal echocardiographic monitoring to improve the outcome of stent-graft treatment of thoracic aortic aneurysms. *Am J Cardiol* 2001;87:315-19.

[12] Bartel T, Eggebrecht H, Müller S, et al. Comparison of diagnostic and therapeutic value of transesophageal echocardiography, intravascular ultrasonic imaging, and intraluminal phased-array imaging in aortic dissection with tear in the descending thoracic aorta (Type B). *Am J Cardiol* 2007;99:270-4.

[13] Plamaz JC, Richter GM, Noldge G, et al. Intraluminal Palmaz stent implantation. The first clinical case report on a balloon-expanded vascular prosthesis. *Radiol* 1987;27:560-3.

[14] Parodi JC, Palmaz JC, Barone HD. Transfemoral intraluminal graft implantation for abdominal aortic aneurysms. *Ann Vasc Surg* 1991;5:491-99.

[15] Shabalovskaya S. On the nature of the biocompatibility and medical applications of NiTi shape memory and superelastic alloys. *Bio Med Mat Eng* 1996;6:267.

[16] Stoeckel D, Pelton A, Duerig T. Self-expanding nitinol stents; material and design considerations. *Wur Radiol* 2004;14:292-301.

[17] Cribier A, Eltchaninoff H, Bash A, et al. Percutaneous transcatheter implantation of an aortic valve prosthesis for calcific aortic stenosis. *Circulation* 2002;106:3006-8.

[18] Byrne JV, Hope JK, Hubbard N, et al. The nature of thrombosis induced by platinum and tungsten coils in saccular aneurysms. *Am J Neuroradiol* 1997;18:29-33.

[19] Yeo KK, Rodgers JH, Laird JR, Use of stent grafts and coils in vessel rupture and perforation. *J Interven Cardiol* 2008;21:86-99.

[20] Chuang VP, Wallace S, Gianturco C, et al. Complications of coil embolization: prevention and management. *Am J Roentgenol* 1981;137:809-13.

[21] Cantarelli MJ, de Paola Ade A, Alves CM, et al. Percutaneous retrieval of intravascular foreign bodies. *Arq Bras Cardiol* 1993;60:171-5.

[22] Koreny M, Riedmuller E, Nikfardjam M, et al. Arterial puncture closing devices compared with Standard manual compression after cardiac catheterization: systematic review and meta-analysis. *JAMA* 2004;291:350-7.

[23] Bechara CF, Annambhotla S, Lin PH. Access site management with vascular closure devices for percutaneous transarterial procedures. *J Vasc Surg* 2010;52:1682-96.

[24] Biancari F, D'Andrea V, Di Marco C, et al. Meta-analysis of randomized trials on the efficacy of vascular closure devices alter diagnostic angiography and angioplasty. *Am Heart J* 2010;159:518-31.

In: Percutaneous Valve Technology: Present and Future
Editors: Jose Luis Navia and Sharif Al-Ruzzeh
ISBN: 978-1-61942-577-4

Chapter V

Anesthetic Implications of Percutaneous Valve Procedures

Andrej Alfirevic, David G. Anthony and Krishna R. Mudimbi

Abstract

Valvular heart disease represents a growing public health problem correlating with the increase in older age population. Periprocedural as well as long term morbidity and mortality after conventional surgical procedures are still significant in high risk surgical candidates. In addition, a good percentage of patients do not get operated on because of the presence of patients' co-morbidities, old age and other factors. Advances in technology enabled evolution of different percutaneous minimally invasive procedures reserved to decrease the risk of perioperative morbidity and mortality from conventional surgical procedures.

The anesthetic management of percutaneous valve procedures involves non-traditional operating room settings including remote locations with confined space as well as exposure to radiation and requires detailed knowledge of sequence of events pertained to the specific technique and potential complications associated with it. Anesthesiologists are involved in the preoperative, intraoperative and postoperative care of these patients. Meticulous preparedness and communication between all members of the team is crucial for the success.

Newer techniques such as aortic and mitral valve trans-catheter procedures are becoming alternative treatment options to wide variety of patients while techniques such as balloon valvuloplasties are trying to redefine their positions. Percutaneous approach to paravalvular regurgitation is also becoming an interesting minimally invasive alternative technique avoiding complications of conventional re-operation surgery. Percutaneous procedures are performed in the catheterization lab or hybrid operating rooms under the guidance of fluoroscopic angiography as well as trans-esophageal echocardiography both requiring management expertise from the involved anesthesiologist.

Introduction

Valvular heart disease represents a growing public health problem correlating with the increase in older age population.[1] The data is supported by hospital in-patient survey and electrographic study,[2-4] which may introduce selection bias, but also from the well characterized population samples.[1] The prevalence of the valvular heart disease has been reported to be 2.5% in overall adult patient population and 13.2% in patients 75 years of age and older.[1] Mitral valve regurgitation (MR) represents most common valve disorder followed by aortic valve stenosis (AS).[1,4,5]

Current guidelines suggest surgical aortic valve replacement (AVR) as a recommended treatment option for the symptomatic patient as well as in some asymptomatic patients with AS.[6] Without the surgical AVR, survival of elderly patients with severe AS was shown to be significantly decreased.[7,8] Even though approximately 50,000 patients undergo AVR each year, in US alone, about 27-41% of patients with symptomatic AS do not get operated on for variety of reasons, primarily due to significant co-morbidities increasing the risk of operation which significantly impacts survival.[5-7,9,10] Old age (>75), neurological dysfunction, heart failure, artrial fibrillation (AF) and decreased left ventricular (LV) ejection fraction (EF) pertain increased calculated risk of conventional surgical AVR, reflected in a logistical EUROSCORE risk $\geq$ 20% or STS_PROM score $\geq$ 10%.[6,11] Other important risk factors, such as end-stage liver disease, frailty, significant abnormalities of other valves peripheral and aortic vascular disease, "porcelain aorta", previous chest radiation, which are not included in risk-score analysis, may significantly contribute to early and late mortality after transcatheter aortic valve implantation (TAVI) and surgical AVR.

Prevalence of mitral valve disease, particularly MR is shown to directly correlate with the increase in age.[1] In addition, operative mortality in patients with degenerative MR older than 75 years of age is higher than in their younger counterparts who are < 65 years of age (adjusted OR 5.4, 95% CI 1.5-19.6; P=0.01) despite improvements in surgical techniques leading to overall decrease in postoperative mortality across all age groups.[12] According to ACC/AHA Task Force recommendations patients with moderate-to-severe or severe MR who are symptomatic or asymptomatic with moderate-to-severe or severe MR with compromised LV function (EF<50% or LV end-systolic diameter >45mm) are amenable for surgical correction.[6]

Advances in technology enabled evolution of different percutaneous minimally invasive procedures reserved to decrease the risk of perioperative morbidity and mortality from conventional surgical procedures. The invention of expandable stent-valves for AVR and different types of MV clips and annuloplasty rings placed by cardiologists in cardiology suite via femoral vessel access avoids opening patient's sternum and initiation of cardio-pulmonary bypass (CPB). In addition, recent research has shown encouraging success with valve-in-valve implantation in patients with failed bioprosthetic valves not only in aortic but also in mitral, tricuspid and pulmonic position.[13] The anesthesiologists providing care to these patients are faced with different challenges some including remote location and confined working space, exposure to radiation and procedure related hemodynamic challenges. In this chapter we are discussing anesthetic concerns pertinent to the management of patients having TAVI, percutaneous MV implantation (PMVI), AV and MV balloon valvuloplasty and percutaneous closures of paravalvular leaks.

Aortic Valve

Patients undergoing isolated surgical AVR have fairly low overall operative mortality of <5%, depending upon the surgical experience and patients' co-morbidities.[14] Nevertheless, 30-day post-procedural mortality after AVR in octagenerians with decreased LV function is reported to be 12% and increases to 17% in nonagenerians.[15,16] The role of TAVI is to reduce the impact of invasive surgical procedure, including sternotomy as well as CPB and its potential detriments on different organ systems. The studies comparing AVR to TAVI primarily used operative morbidity and mortality as well as 30-day mortality as outcome measures. Three techniques of TAVI have been described (see Figure 1): 1) antegrade venous trans-septal approach (not in use anymore)[17]; 2) retrograde trans-femoral approach (TFAVI)[18]; 3) antegrade trans-apical approach (TAAVI).[19-22]

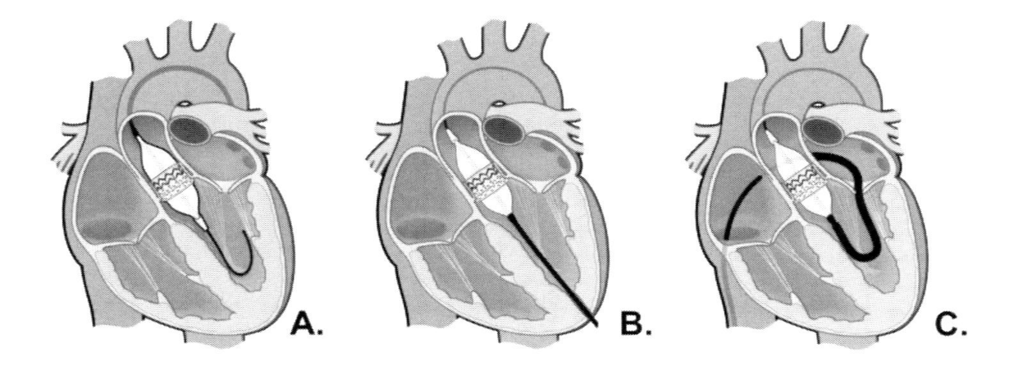

Figure 1. Illustration of different trans-catheter aortic valve implantation techniques: A) Image illustrates retrograde trans-femoral implantation technique; B} Image illustrates antegrade trans-apical implantation technique; C) Image illustrates antegrade venous trans-septal implantation technique.

Anesthetic Implications for Trans-Femoral Aortic Valve Implantation (TFAVI)

Suggested procedural technique used for TFAVI has been described in details in the designated chapters of this book as well as in the previously published journal articles.[17,23-26] In majority of cases balanced general anesthesia techniques are used, even though reports exist of TFAVI procedures performed using local anesthetic infiltration of the peripheral venous access sites with addition of intravenous sedation.[27-30] In general, anesthesiologists are faced with the challenges of providing anesthesia to high acuity patient population at the remote locations such as cardiac catheterization lab.

Preoperative

Patients undergoing TFAVI are symptomatic and have severe AS. Patients who are considered high risk surgical candidates or inoperable because of the severe symptomatic heart disease and clinically significant co-morbidities may be candidates for a less invasive procedures such as TFAVI.[28,29,31] The co-morbidities usually include previous neurological events such as stroke or TIAs, chronic renal insufficiency (CRI), different degrees of hepatic dysfunction as well as decreased respiratory reserve. Even though there are no strict exclusion criteria, patients with significant cognitive dysfunction due to Alzheimer's dementia, concomitant severe mitral disease, Child's B hepatic cirrhosis and very poor physical condition may not be suitable candidates for TAVI.[31] In addition, strictly procedure-related contraindications to TFAVI include an AV annulus that is too small (<18mm) or too large (>26mm) to accommodate currently available prosthesis as well as severe peripheral vascular disease (atherosclerosis, arterial aneurysm).[26,32,33] Procedure unrelated contraindications are not very clearly defined at this point. Presence of LV dysfunction and non-revascularized coronary disease, MR>2+, tricuspid valve regurgitation >2+, coagulopathy, uncontrolled atrial fibrillation, previous thoracotomy, severe chronic obstructive pulmonary disease (COPD) and pulmonary hypertension, "porcelain aorta" all represent relative contraindications and make management of these patients very challenging.[26,32,33] Recent evidence has shown the predictors of 1-year cumulative mortality in patients having either TFAVI or TAAVI to be pulmonary hypertension (PH), need for hemodynamic support , sepsis and COPD.[34] In addition, 30-day mortality was predicted by preoperative presence of severe MR and PH but not increased ST-PROM score or presence of "porcelain aorta".[34] Thorough evaluation and optimization of each one of these organ systems during the perioperative assessment is crucial for the final success of the procedure. The evaluation and decision process of offering the patient PAVI is best made by the multidisciplinary team approach consisting of cardiologists, cardiac surgeons, internists and anesthesiologists.[31]

Preoperative evaluation doesn't significantly differ from the usual preoperative assessment of the patient scheduled for AVR. Some additional procedure specific details need attention though.

Transthoracic (TTE) or transesophageal echocardiography (TEE) will provide assessment of the AS severity and structural and functional assessment of the other valves, LV and right ventricle (RV). It is useful to obtain a baseline electrocardiogram to compare it to the post-procedural one should the myocardial ischemia or arrhythmia occur during the post-operative time. Coronary angiography provides structural and risk assessment of the coronary artery lesions. Computerized tomography (CT) scan of the chest and pelvis is important to obtain the assessment of the atherosclerotic and/or aneurysmatic disease of the aorta and more peripheral arteries in the femoral area. In patients with previous open heart surgery, CT scan of the chest with angiographic contrast is important to look for the position of the heart and coronary grafts and their location underneath the sternum which may change the vascular cannullation strategy should the need for rescue CPB occurs. Beside history and physical examination neurological status is assessed by CT or MRI of the brain. Duplex ultrasound of the carotid arteries is also part of the screening process. Laboratory work up should include assessment of the kidney function as a baseline value since the majority of patients present with some degree of chronic insufficiency. Additionally, patients will receive intravenous contrast dye during the procedure which may result in deterioration of the kidney function postoperatively. The assessment of liver function is focused on coagulation profile with additional blood workup including hemoglobin, glucose and type and crossmatch of two units of packed red blood cells. Patients with respiratory problems will have pulmonary function tests, chest-X-ray and arterial blood gases obtained to assess the pattern and severity of the disease process. Careful evaluation of the airway status is important not only to avoid possible unexpected difficult airway but also to select patients who may be better served with general anesthesia by securing the airway in advance as opposed to dealing with the potentially difficult airway should the need for obtaining the airway occurs during the procedure. The list of preoperative medications should be reviewed and patient instructed to continue medications as they would for any other surgical procedure. TAVI specific medications may include aspirin and clopidogrel. Aspirin, in a dose of 75-300 mg is usually started before the procedure and continued indefinitely afterwards.[27-29,33,35] No clear guidelines exist about the need and duration of anti-platelet medication regimen. Thus, different regimens vary regarding the use of clopidogrel, which is given as a bolus of 75-300 mg preoperatively and continued for 1-12 months after the procedure.[27-29,33,35]

Table 1. Advantages and disadvantages of general anesthesia technique versus local anesthetic infiltration with additional intravenous sedation. CBF- cerebral blood flow; RVP- rapid ventricular pacing

Intraoperative		
	Advantages	Disadvantages
Balanced General Anesthesia	Necessity of using TEE throughout the procedure; Secured airway at all times; Ability to decrease respiratory translocation of the heart during the deployment;	Airway manipulation and potential damage; Potential for prolonged intubation;
Local Anesthetic Infiltration and iv. Sedation	Avoidance of airway manipulation; Quicker emergence and potential recovery;	Procedural need for lying in one position for prolonged period of time; Intolerance of decrease in CBF with RVP; A need for securing the airway during the procedure should the hemodynamic instability ensues; Local anesthetic toxicity;

Balanced general anesthesia (BGA) techniques have been utilized in the majority of cases, even though some authors report successful use of local anesthetic infiltration of the femoral vessels in addition with intravenous sedation.[27,28,36] Table 1. summarizes advantages and disadvantages of both techniques. In authors' opinion, the abundance of potential advantages and minimal associated risks associated with BGA makes it a preferable anesthesia technique. Anesthetic care comprises similarities with the care of a high risk patient undergoing surgical AVR but is also tailored towards early extubation at the end of the procedure, bearing in mind patient's old age, co-morbidities and hemodynamic goals. Prior to induction, large bore peripheral intravenous line and radial arterial line (either arm is suitable) for continuous blood pressure monitoring is placed in addition to standard monitors. In the situation of pre-existing LV and/or RV failure with pulmonary hypertension central venous introducer and pulmonary artery catheter (PAC) may be placed pre-induction. Approximately 1 liter of crystalloid is given to optimize preload and compensate for the NPO status (slower preload optimization in patients with RV failure guided by PAC values). Anesthetic induction is carried out with the hemodynamic goals of maintaining intravascular preload, contractility and afterload. After induction, single lumen endotracheal and the TEE probe are placed followed by a large bore central-venous multi-lumen introducer sheath and PAC to obtain baseline hemodynamic parameters (pulmonary artery systolic, diastolic and mean pressures; cardiac output and index; wedge pressure). In the anticipation of the hemodynamic compromise after the rapid ventricular pacing (RVP) periods, infusions of inotropic and vasopressor medications, such as epinephrine and norepinephrine, are prepared and connected. Antibiotic prophylaxis which usually consists of 1.5 g of cefuroxime is given at this point and urinary catheter inserted. Anesthesia is maintained with a balanced technique using volatile anesthetics such as isoflurane or sevoflurane, intermediate acting muscle relaxants such as rocuronium or cis-atracurium and smaller intermittent doses of fentanyl or infusions of remifentanyl, alfentanyl and sufentanyl.[27,29,36] Profound muscle paralysis is definitely not needed for the whole duration of the procedure but it is important to avoid any patient movement during valvuloplasty and stent-valve deployment. External defibrillation pads are placed in proper locations on the patient's chest. The bilateral femoral/iliac arterial and venous sites are used for introduction of the device introducer sheath as well as for placement of the temporary pacemaker wire for RVP. Those are usually not very stimulating events. Patient is maintained in the supine position for the duration of the procedure with the arms above the head to avoid shadowing artifacts from the interaction between X-ray beams and patient's arm bone structure when lateral biplane C-arm fluoroscopy is used (see Figure 2). Meticulous padding of the pressure points and making sure the arms are not overly stretched out is important in prevention of peripheral nerve injury. As mentioned earlier, patients are usually given 75-300 mg bolus of clopidogrel preoperatively in addition to aspirin which increases the risk of blood and blood product transfusion. In addition, procedural anticoagulation is achieved by administering 70 IU/kg of unfractionated heparin (UFH) to maintain activated clotting time (ACT) level >250 seconds after the exposure of the femoral artery and before crossing the AV with the wire. ACT levels are checked every 30 minutes and additional doses of UFH administered if needed. After the successful deployment and evaluation of the stent-valve the sheath and wires are removed from the femoral access sites and residual heparin is reversed with protamine in a 1:1 ratio.

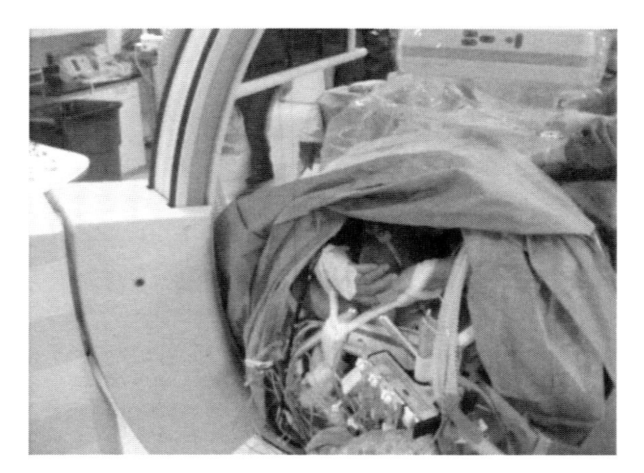

Figure 2. Positioning of the patient for the trans-femoral aortic valve implantation with the arms placed above patient's head. Note the relationship of the multi-axis bi-plane C-arm (lateral cameras not depicted) to the patient and operating table.

Guidance during TFAVI is provided by fluoroscopic angiographic imaging with the TEE and intracardiac echocardiography (ICE) having important complimentary roles.[37-39] As mentioned in the preoperative paragraph echocardiographic evaluation is focused on the AV leaflet mobility, calcification and the grade of severity of stenosis. Functional assessment of LV, morphology and functionality of MV as well as evaluation of thoracic aorta for atheroslerosis need to be obtained prior to balloon valvuloplasty and deployment.[37] The measurement of the AV annular diameter is important in determining the size of the implanted prosthesis and may be different depending which modality is used. In the study by Moss and colleagues, the mean difference in AV annulus dimension was 1.36 mm larger imaged by TTE then by TEE, but if 2 standard deviations of mean were used the range between -4.48 and +1.75 mm may result in the change of stent-valve that is deployed.[38] TEE is also helpful in assessing the leaflet mobility and severity of aortic insufficiency (AI) after balloon valvuloplasty (see Figure 3). TEE serves as an adjunct modality to fluoroscopy for accurate positioning of the stent-valve. Clear visualization of the stent-valve in relation to the AV annulus may be limited from shadowing artifact in patients with severe AV calcification. The prosthesis is placed in the proper position if more than the half of the prosthesis remains on the LV side in relation to the junction point of the native AV leaflets and annulus (see Figure 4 and 5).[38,39] Post-deployment TEE provides immediate assessment of stent-valve leaflets mobility and gradation of the severity of intra- and/or para-valvular AI (see Figure 6).[37-39]

Majority of patients would have a trivial to mild paravalvular regugitation detected by TEE immediately after the stent-valve deployment, which either improves or remains the same in severity[25,38,40] Native AV annular calcification is a most common factor predisposing for development of the paravalvular regurgitation.[25,40] Early device complications, such as migration (discussed below), and concomitant LV and RV dysfunction, severe MV regurgitation and pericardial effusion are easily assessed by TEE.[37-39]

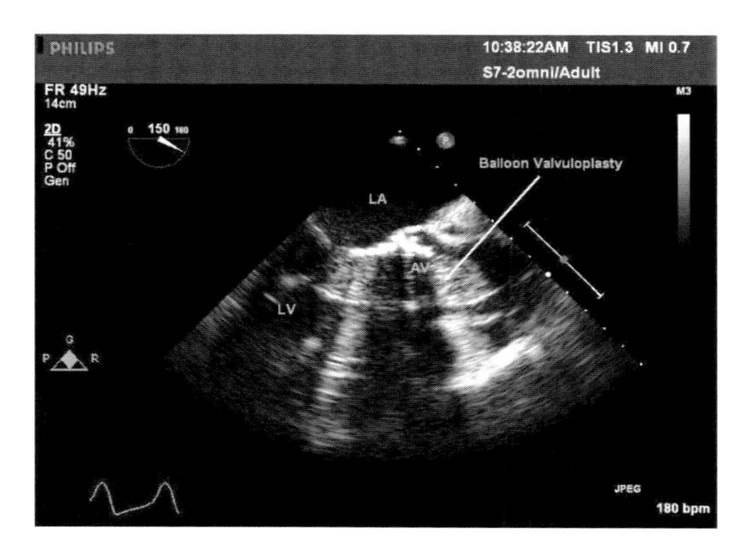

Figure 3. Mid-esophageal long axis TEE view showing inflated valvuloplasty balloon across the aortic valve.

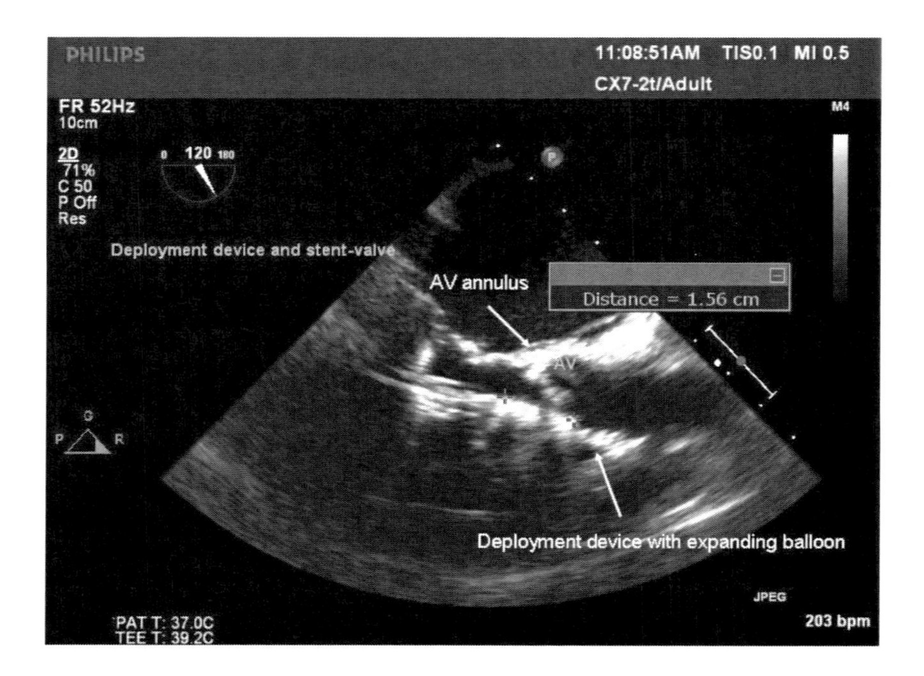

Figure 4. Mid-esophageal long axis TEE view showing proper positioning of the stent- valve in relation to AV annulus.

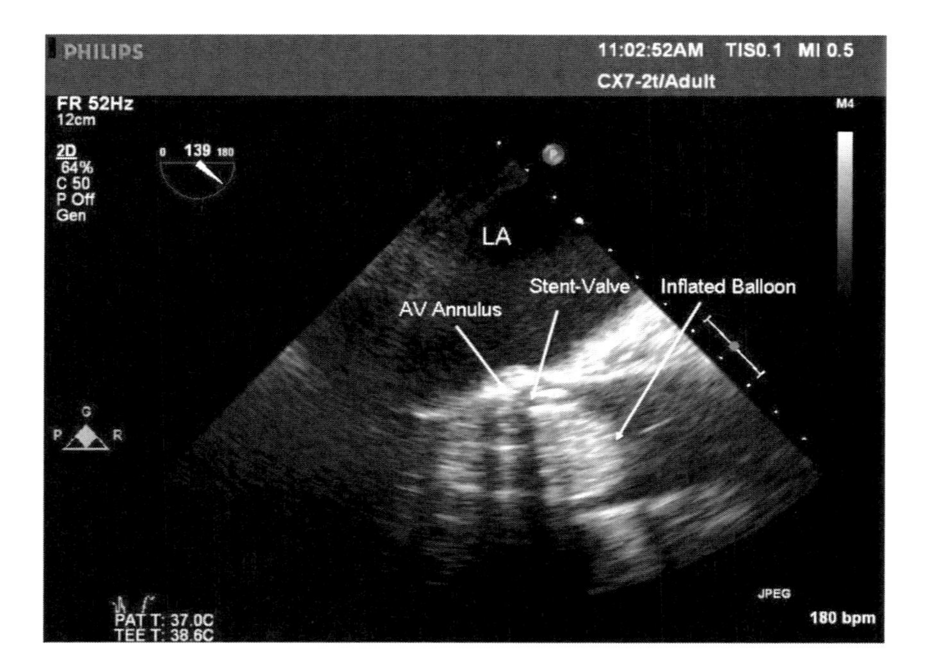

Figure 5. Mid-esophageal long axis TEE view describing inflation of the balloon with the stent-valve positioned on top of it.

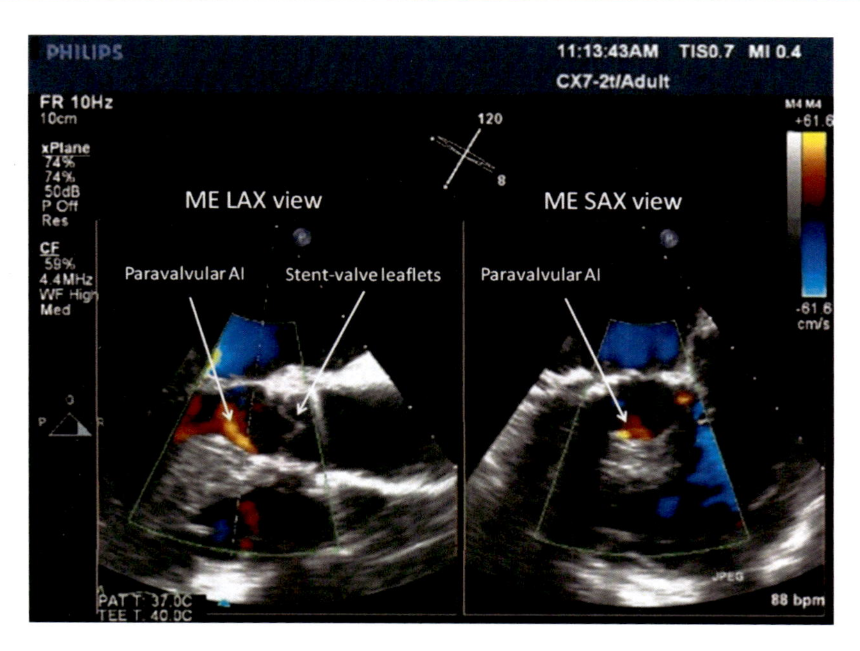

Figure 6. TEE image - orthogonal X-plane color flow Doppler images of the aortic valve – left side of the image mid-esophageal long axis view depicting trivial paravalvular leak in the anterior aspect of the valve; right side of the picture depicting mid-esophageal short axis view with trivial paravalvular leak at 6 o'clock.

RVP in the rate of 180-220 bpm is used to limit the chance of balloon migration during valvuloplasty and stent-valve deployment as s result of it being pushed forward by the stroke volume of the beating heart (see Figure 7 and 8). RVP has negative hemodynamic effect since it decreases myocardial oxygen supply by decreasing cardiac output and therefore coronary perfusion pressure and increases oxygen demand due to tachycardia. Thus it is important to limit the duration of RVP to minimum possible (10-15 seconds) and provide adequate time for re-perfusion of the heart between subsequent RVP episodes. Also, preemptive administration of boluses of phenylephrine may be necessary for circulatory support. In majority of cases patient's heart rate, normal sinus rhythm and blood pressure return to baseline levels spontaneously after RVP episode (see Figure 9).

In the situation of inadequate return of hemodynamic parameters to baseline, aggressive support of the circulation may be required using boluses and/or infusions of epinephrine and norepinephrine.[29] In addition to ischemia from RVP, moderate and severe grades of either intravalulvular or paravalvular AI result in an acute increase in left ventricular end-diastolic pressure (LVEDP) further diminishing myocardial oxygen supply. Circulatory support at that point is very challenging without speedy decision making process in determining the need for mechanical circulatory support or possibility of stent-valve re-expansion or deployment of the new one. Perfusionist with CPB machine on stand-by should be ready in the room.

Anesthesiologists should have clear communication with the cardiologist, surgeon and perfusionist and up-front planning made about cannullation strategy should the need for emergent CPB occurs. Additional theoretical immediate post-valvuloplasty or post-deployment complications include obstruction of the coronary ostia, dislodgement of the valve-stent, pericardial tamponade and hemodynamically significant ventricular arrhythmias.[9,25,26,28,29,33,35]

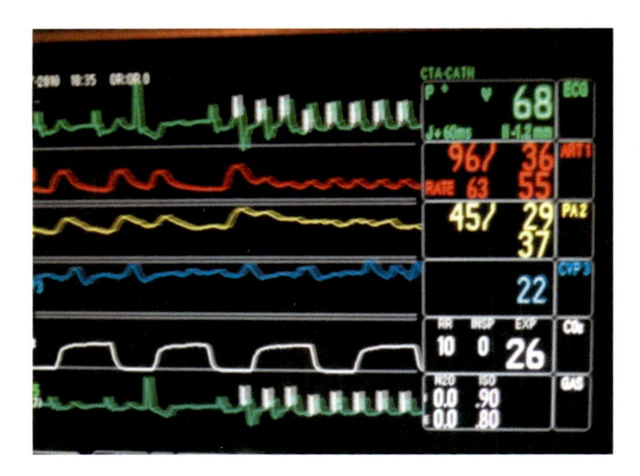

Figure 7. Initiation of rapid ventricular pacing – pacemaker spikes seen on EKG tracing.

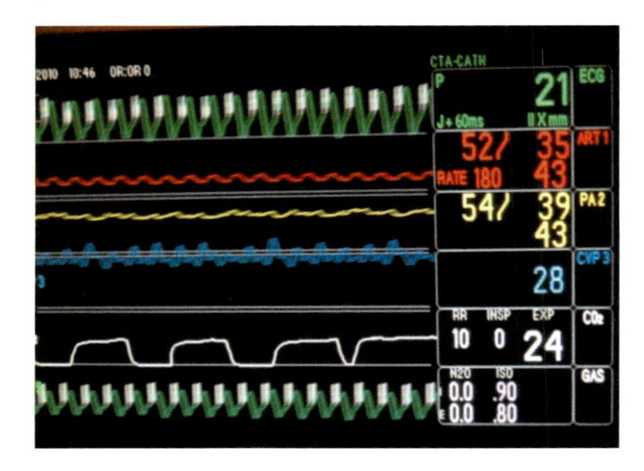

Figure 8. Hemodynamics during rapid ventricular pacing – systemic arterial pressure waveform in red; pulmonary artery waveform in yellow; central venous pressure waveform in blue.

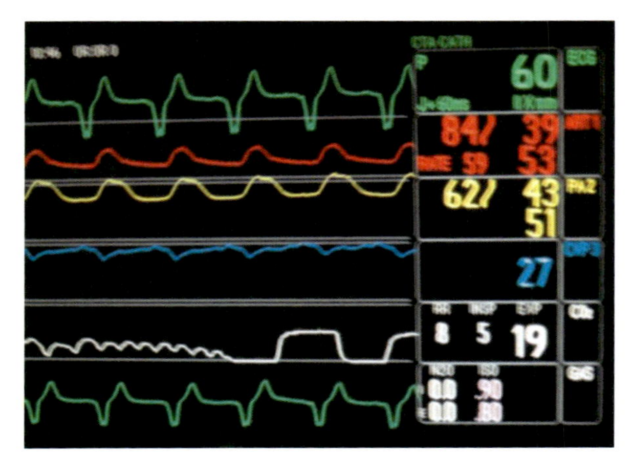

Figure 9. Spontaneous return of the circulation towards the baseline and re-initiation of the ventilatory support.

Obstruction of the coronary ostia is a theoretical concern and may occur due to either obstruction of the ostial orificies with bulky native valve leaflets, stent-valve malposition/embolisation and calcium deposits embolization.[41] The acute appearance of regional wall motion abnormalities on TEE and acute rise in pulmonary artery pressures in addition to ST-T segment changes on EKG should increase the suspicion of coronary ischemia event. The management consists of the circulatory support with inotropes and vasopressors as well as mechanical support including CPB, intra-aortic balloon pump (IABP) and ECMO. Secondary to either lack of reporting and/or accuracy in deployment of the stent-valve reports from the most experienced centers do not suggest coronary ostial obstruction to be of profound clinical significance.[25,33]

With the improvement in procedural learning curve, malposition of the stent-valve is seen fairly rarerly.[33,35,38] Nevertheless, it is an emergency situation which in addition to the prompt circulatory support frequently requires either re-implantation of the second valve-stent or conversion to open surgical procedure. As discussed previously RVP is the method used to decrease the risk of stent-valve dislocation immediately after the deployment. The ability to control the patient's ventilation enables suspension of the ventilatory support during the deployment process which reduces translocation of the heart in the chest cavity.

Pericardial tamponade and aortic dissection are primarily complications of multiple efforts to position the wire and deployment device across the AV traversing in a retrograde fashion in the aorta. The incidence of both complications may be decreased by softer "pig-tail" wiring technology,[29,33] while adequate fluoroscopic imaging and TEE monitoring may result in accurate diagnosis and initiation of a prompt management strategy.

Hemodynamically significant ventricular arrhythmias occur relatively infrequently after valvuloplasty and valve-stent deployment.[25,28,29] Pathophysiological mechanisms include a decrease in cardiac output secondary to RVP for prolonged period of time as well as exacerbation of the AI. Immediate implementation of the ACLS algorithm with defibrillation and chest compression and clear communication with the team members is important. Preemptive boluses of phenylephrine and/or epinephrine before balloon valvuloplasty and stent-valve deployment, as previously discussed, may decrease the incidence. Clinically significant atrio-ventricular conduction block develops in 4-19%[26,28,29] with 4.4-7% of patients requiring permanent pacemaker.[25,29] If the conduction block persists after the procedure temporary pacemaker wire needs to be left in the femoral access site of relocated to the internal jugular venous site.

Intravascular fluid management is tailored according to patient's NPO status, insensible losses and surgical bleeding. In majority of cases crystalloids and colloids are sufficient for adequate optimization of the intravascular volume status but blood and blood product transfusion may be required with profound bleeding. Incidence of the blood transfusion vary from 11.6% of patients reported by Webb and colleagues[25] to 23% and 50% reported by Guinot and colleagues[29] and Covello and colleagues,[28] respectively. Significant blood loss may be enquired during the introduction and removal of the deployment device sheath from the femoral vascular access sites. Contrast dye injection guided fluoroscopy is used to assess for possible arterial dissection or leakage sites requiring vascular stent implantation or major vascular repair.[29] Normotermia is maintained by fluid warming as well as warm forced-air garments.

In majority of cases (81%) emergence from anesthesia is achieved at the end of the procedure in the catheterization suite[29], unless there are contraindication to it in which case patient is transported to the intensive care unit intubated. If extubated, patients are often transported with minimal oxygen support via nasal cannula or face mask. Post-operative nausea and vomiting prophylaxis with ondansentron is administered as well as full reversal of muscle relaxants. Postoperative analgesia is managed initially with intermittent boluses of intravenous narcotics (fentanyl or morphine) and oral tramadol or acetaminophen depending on patient's needs and institutional preferences.[29] Unless femoral vascular access was surgically obtained incisional pain is fairly minimal particularly if infiltrated with local anesthetic (lidocaine, bupivacaine or ropivacaine). In addition, patients are typically given dual anti-platelet therapy throughout peri-operative period, leading to potential bleeding problems if regional anesthesia techniques are being used.

Postoperative

The experience and success rate of the TFAVI technology has constantly been on the rise since the initial world-wide attempts. Current procedural success rates, depending which author and institution is looked at, vary in the range of 86-100%.[23,25,26,28,29,31,33,34,42] At the same time procedural and 30-day mortality have declined to 2-3%[26,29,32,35] and 8-12%,[25,26,29,33,34,42] respectively. Improvement in patient's cardiovascular and NYHA status is directly related to the success of the procedure with the improvement in trans-aortic mean pressure gradients, aortic valve area and ejection fraction.[25,26,32,33,40] In their report comparing TAVI to surgical AVR using stented or stentless valves, Clavel and coleeagues showed superior hemodynamic performance in terms of trans-prosthetic gradients and lower incidence of severe prosthesis-patient mismatch in patients with TAVI.[40]

Most common complications related to the procedure seen during post-operative period are related to vascular access injury. The incidence is reported to be in the range from 8% described by Webb and colleagues,[25] to 28% and 35% described by Covello and colleagues[28] and Guinot and colleagues[29], respectively. This also relates to the increase in risk of blood and blood product transfusion ranging from 11.6% in the study by Webb and colleagues to 23% and 50% reported by Guinot and colleagues[29] and Covello and colleagues,[28] respectively. Improvements in technology and procedural experience tend to decrease in risk of peripheral vascular injury.[25]

The prevalence of the periprocedural stroke has been reported to be within a 1-10% range amongst different institutional studies.[25,29,32,33,35] As a comparison, the risk of perioperative stroke in patients $\geq$ 80 years of age, after CABG or combined AVR and CABG, has been documented to be in 10-15% range.[43] Thus, TFAVI may benefit patients who are at higher risk of developing stroke. Nevertheless, the stroke prevalence of 10% after TFAVI may not be acceptable in the lower risk patient population. The etiology of cerebrovascular events in patients after TFAVI is still speculative and remains to be determined. Manipulation of the wire in the ascending aorta, arch and AV in the retrograde fashion may dislodge the atherosclerotic particles resulting in embolization and so can AV balloon valvuloplasty as well as stent-valve deployment. The role of preoperative CT scan is to purposely distinguish patients with more significant atherosclerotic disease who may be better candidates for transapical AV implantation (TAAVI). In addition, minimization of wire manipulation at the native AV level, careful de-airing of the deployment device may potentially decrease the risk of cerebrovascular events.[29]

Worsening of the renal failure after conventional AVR occurs in 24%[44] of patients and is associated with the increase in short- and long-term mortality.[45] Pre-existing chronic renal insufficiency (CRI) is one of the factors for the patients to be considered for TFAVI or TAAVI in the first place. TAVI procedures involve administration of the contrast dye, retrograde wire manipulation in the atherosclerosis diseased aorta and periods of profound hypotension during RVP, all of which are risk factors for development of acute renal insufficiency (ARI). The incidence of ARI is reported as 4.4% in patients after TFAVI with no patients requiring temporary hemodialysis.[25] Beside transapical approach, preoperative CRI was found to be a predictor of mortality at the late follow-up.[25] In the study of patients after TFAVI by Guinot and colleagues, ARI (defined as serum creatinine values >200µmol/L) developed in 5% of with the rest of patients having no change in their serum creatinine levels or creatinine clearance.[29] Aregger and colleagues reported much higher incidence of (28%) of ARI with 7.4% of patients requiring temporary hemodialysis.[46] Risk factors for ARI included transapical approach, post-procedural thrombocytopenia, number of blood transfusions and increase in C-reactive protein.[46] In the largest study so far, specifically designed to compare the occurrence of ARI in TAVI versus surgical AVR, Bagur and colleagues reported 11.7% incidence of ARI with 1.4% requiring hemodialysis. A history of preoperative hypertension, chronic obstructive pulmonary disease and perioperative blood transfusion were risk factors for ARI.[47] ARI was an independent risk factor of mortality, associated with greater than four-fold increase in the risk of post-procedural mortality. Compared to surgical AVR patients, the incidence of ARI in patients who underwent TAVI was lower (OR: 0.33, 95% CI: 0.13-0.79, P =0.014 after propensity score adjustment) even though the patients in TAVI group were older, had higher logistic EuroSCORE and lower pre-procedural glomerural filtration rates.[47] In addition, the amount of contrast dye and number of RVP runs were not associated with occurrence of ARI.[47] In conclusion, patients with CRI may benefit from decreasing the incidence of ARI when undergoing TAVI as opposed to surgical AVR.

Anesthetic Implications for Trans-Apical Aortic Valve Implantation (TAAVI)

TAAVI approach shares similar peri-operative anesthetic considerations as described in the previous paragraphs on TFAVI. Nevertheless, differences exist and are tailored by the antegrade approach which includes insertion of the wire, sheath and deployment device through the apex of the beating heart. Details of the surgical techniques have been described in this book as well as in previously published papers.[19,20,29,48] Although initial TAAVI procedures were performed with the cardiopulmonary-bypass support,[21,49] the increase in experience resulted in performing the procedure with the femoral vessels exposed and accessed should the need for emergent initiation of CPB occurs.[20,49] Left anterior mini-thoracotomy approach determines performing these procedures in the hybrid cardiac operating rooms equipped with fluoroscopic angiographic capability.

Preoperative

The candidates for TAAVI belong to the high risk surgical patient group based on the logistic EuroSCORE and STS-PROM score. Patients undergoing TFAVI and particularly TAAVI present with additional risk factors which are not included in risk score analysis. Traditionally, STS mortality risk-prediction model doesn't include patient's frailty, "porcelain aorta", end-stage liver disease, significant peripheral vascular or aortic disease or prior chest wall radiation. Those factors have to be taken into consideration when assessing the risk of the TAVI as well as surgical AVR. Patients for TAAVI (as opposed to either TFAVI or surgical AVR) are usually selected if any of the following criteria is present: diameter of femoral or iliac arteries < 7mm (if a 23mm valve is used) or <8mm (if a 26mm valve is used); peripheral vascular disease, severe calcification of both ilio-femoral arteries, "porcelain aorta" and horizontal ascending aorta.[31,34,50] Pre-operative assessment consists of the evaluation of heart disease severity as well as severity of damage of other organ systems as described in the previous paragraphs on TFAVI. In addition to thorough history and previous vascular surgery operative reports, detailed assessment of the extent of aortic and peripheral vascular disease usually includes different imaging modalities such as multi-slice CT angiography. This will guide the cannullation approach strategy in case of emergent need for initiation of CPB. As of this point, contraindications for the TAAVI are not clearly defined.[31]

Intraoperative

TAAVI procedures are performed under BGA, with the placement of either single-lumen (SLT) or duble-lumen endotracheal tube (DLT).[19-21,25,49] The surgical approach involves an approximately 8 cm long left anterior thoracotomy incision performed in the 5th or 6th inter-costal space. Since the lower lobe of the left lung can be easily moved aside by the surgeon searching for the access to the LV apex, placement of the DLT or bronchial blocker present only a relative indication for one-lung ventilation (OLV). Even though patients are maintained is supine position throughout the procedure, OLV is maintained without complications in the majority of patients but may result in quick desaturation in patients with severe pulmonary disease and minimal reserve. Induction of anesthesia is performed in the same manner and with same hemodynamic goals as with TFAVI. The risk of bleeding during the procedure is higher than with TFAVI since it involves surgical placement of the deployment device sheath through the LV apex. Therefore, large bore peripheral intravenous and multilumen central venous PAC are placed. It is important to verify presence of current type and cross-match of packed red-blood cells. The arterial line is preferentially placed in the right radial artery to leave the left brachial artery free for potential insertion of a pigtail catheter served to obtain aortic root aortography and fluoroscopic imaging of AV leaflets' nadir.[19,20] The pigtail catheter is preferentially introduced via femoral artery in the absence of severe peripheral vascular disease. Choosing the vascular access cannullation site should the CPB has to be initiated is of utmost importance. Patients may have a history of peripheral re-vascularization surgery where arterial cannullation through the grafts are not possible and/or are contraindicated. Other options for arterial cannullation include direct cannullation of the aorta through the anterior thoracotomy incision or left brachial/axillary artery. Venous drainage is obtained via direct cannullation of the femoral veins. RVP is obtained by placement of the pacemaker wire through femoral venous access or direct epicardial stimulation. It is important to maintain adequate LV preload and to bleed all parts of deployment device sheath in order to prevent air entry into the heart cavity.[19,20] Intraprocedural anticoagulation and subsequent AV balloon valvuloplasty and stent-valve deployment are performed in the similar fashion as with TFAVI. Hemodynamic stability and the need for optimization of the intravascular fluid status is assessed and monitored invasively and with TEE.[37,38]

Immediate Post-Procedural Complications

The return of hemodynamic parameters toward the baseline is achieved spontaneously in majority of patients after valvuloplasty as well as after stent-valve deployment. It is not clear whether large and stiff deployment device introduced through LV apex introduces additional change in LV geometry which may potentially lead to exacerbation of LV dysfunction and/or MR due to tethering effect. The report by Webb and colleagues, has shown an upward trend in the emergent need for CPB in patients after TAAVI versus TFAVI.[25] The recent report from Ye and colleagues has shown patients with preoperative MR grades 3+ and 4+ to tolerate TAAVI well with the post-procedural MR grades staying the same or diminishing.[50] Utilization of invasive monitors and TEE for detecting LV and RV dysfunction, assessment of the MR, tricuspid regurgitation and residual AI are of utmost importance. Immediate post-procedural and longer term echocardiographic evaluation shows the likely presence of trivial to mild paravalvular AI in majority of patients and was clinically insignificant and remained stable during the 3-year follow up.[50] Embolization of the stent-valve has been reported,[20] like in patients with TFAVI and results in profound hemodynamic instability. On the other hand, better coaxial alignment with the native AV annulus and stabilization of the stent-valve during the deployment because of the short and straight line from the apex can be achieved with TAAVI resulting in potentially decreasing the chance of stent-valve embolization.[50] Since the LV apex is surgically accessed the incidence of blood transfusion can be as high as 29%,[22] but did not reach statistically significant difference when compared to TFAVI procedures.[25,29] Preparation for management of blood transfusion is important and includes large bore vascular access and availability of cell-saver and blood. Initial learning curve of LV apex puncturing technique may be responsible for the increase in early patients' mortality and with the improvements in technique, such as use of pledgeted suturing material, early mortality significantly decreased.[50] During the manipulation of the wire and deployment of device it is possible to damage MV, LV free wall and aorta leading to pericardial tamponade and acute hemodynamic deterioration. Ventricular arrhythmias develop with the same incidence as in patients with TFAVI,[25,29] but the incidence of atrial fibrillation is reported to be higher with TAAVI.[25,29] The incidence of atrio-ventricular conduction block after TAAVI has been reported in the range of 8-12%,[29,51] with 4-7.3% of patients needing permanent pacemaker placement.[25,29]

Emergence of anesthesia is tailored by patient's co-morbidities and ability to maintain hemodynamic stability throughout the procedure. When compared to TFAVI, patients during TAAVI received larger doses of longer acting narcotics.[29] They also had lower rates of extubations in the catheterization suite (81% vs. 25%, $p<0.001$) and longer duration of mechanical ventilation (505 vs. 220 minutes, $p<0.001$), despite having shorter procedure times (97 vs. 120 minutes, $p<0.001$).[29] Because of the observational character of the study this may just represent selection bias in terms of TAAVI patients being "sicker" and procedures being performed though thoracotomy approach, which may preclude early extubation is mind of some anesthesiologists. Even though majority of cases are performed under BGA, TAAVI procedure has been performed in the awake patient using thoracic epidural analgesia which was also used for post-operative pain control.[52] Majority of TAAVI patients are given anti-platelet medication regimen (clopidogrel and aspirin) during the preoperative evaluation, contraindicating central neuroaxial anesthesia technique. Minimization of the surgical incision and intercostal nerve blockade, under direct surgical vision, using bupivacaine or ropivacaine provides adequate analgesia.[49] Analgesia is additionally maintained with supplemental boluses of intravenous narcotics and/or IVPCA and continuation of oral medications when possible.

Postoperative

As with TFAVI experience and advances in technology associated with TAAVI resulted in improvement in the success rate of the procedure as well as patients' outcome. Success rate of almost 100% establishes confidence for future development of the technique.[19,20,25,49,50] In addition, patients are experiencing improvements in their NYHA status mean AV gradients and AV area.[20,25,49] At the same time, 30-day mortality has been in decline since the initial procedural experience.[25,50] The 30-day TAAVI mortality has been reported to be 25% with a decline to 11.1% after the initial learning curve.[25] Similar rate of decline from 33% to 12.5% has been reported by Ye and colleagues.[50] Both approaches, TAAVI and TFAVI are associated with comparable early and late mortality despite a very high-risk patient profile.34 Amongst the patients who survived first 30 days, 24- and 36-month survival rates were 79.8% and 69.8 %, respectively with rare valve-related complications.[50]

Despite peripheral vascular disease as well as "porcelain aorta" being frequent co-morbidity in patients with TAAVI, peri-procedural stroke has been reported to be of lesser incidence (0-5%[20,25,29]) compared to patients with TFAVI.[25,29] The risk of stroke is inherent to both procedures involving manipulation of the aorta and calcific AV resulting in embolization of the aortic atheroma and/or valvular calcified debris. This risk may be higher with the retrograde TFAVI approach without any other known identifiable factor.[25,29]

Some reports associated TAAVI with an increased risk for ARI[25,29] with statistically significant increase in incidence of temporary hemodialysis when compared with TFAVI.[25] Recent data, specifically describing incidence of ARI, noted a trend of TAAVI being an independent risk factor.[47] Even though 48% of patients had TAVI performed via trans-apical approach, predictive factors of ARI included hypertension (P=0.01), COPD (P=0.038), peri-procedural blood transfusion (P=0.005) with a trend of ARI in TAAVI operated patients (64% vs 46%, P=0.093).[47] Rodes-Cabau and colleagues reported no indication that the approach, TAAVI versus TFAVI, being of prognostic value in acute and late outcomes.[34]

Mitral Valve

Anesthetic Implications for Percutaneous Mitral Regurgitation Repair

Prevalence of moderate and severe mitral regurgitation (MR) increases with age, similar to AS, making the MR most common valvular disease in elderly population.[1] Surgical treatment of severe MR remains the gold standard, with the repair rather than replacement being a preferred method. If performed by a surgeon with great experience in MV repairs, repair techniques showed excellent long term success as well as low reoperation rates even in elderly patients with degenerative MR.[53] Because of the complex functional anatomy of MV and its subvalvular apparatus wide varieties of different etiological entities result in MR, best described by Carpentier classification.[54] Following the trend of minimally invasive surgical procedures, several different procedural techniques have been developed for percutaneous MR treatment.[55,56] These techniques are designed to either change mitral annular geometry or to reduce MR by so called edge-to-edge technique which mimics Alfieri's well renowned suturing technique.[57,58] In addition some techniques addressed the importance of LV geometry as the etiology factor in patients with MR in an attempt to provide "remodeling" of the LV.[57] Since MitraClip (Evalve, Menlo Park, CA) edge-to-edge device technology advanced the furthest into human experience we will base our anesthetic considerations toward that technique.

Preoperative

Patients ≥ 75 years of age presenting for conventional MV surgery secondary to ischemic MR have more advanced symptoms of heart failure, atrial-fibrillation, coronary artery disease needing CABG as opposed to their younger counterparts.[12] Operative morbidity and mortality as well as freedom from significant recurrent MR needing re-operation is decreased in patients with ischemic MR.[59,60] Open heart procedure carries higher risks in elderly patients who present with variety of co-morbidities.[61] In addition, up to 50% of patients with severe symptomatic MR are denied surgery primarily due to patients' co-morbidities.[5] Percutaneous MV procedures have been developed to decrease the invasiveness of the heart surgery in higher-risk surgical candidates with both degenerative and functional MR.[62]

Perioperative evaluation consists of the non-invasive and invasive assessment of the severity and mechanism of MR, LV and RV function and associated pulmonary hypertension. Patients with long standing MR present with different grades of LV remodeling which can be a result of either organic (primary) leaflet disease process or functional (secondary) ischemic disease. In chronic MR, LV function is typically underestimated by load-dependant measurement techniques such as ejection fraction evaluated with echocardiography. This decrease in systolic LV function is because of the unloading of the blood volume into the compliant left atrium which serves as a preload "boost" during diastole, optimizing Frank-Starling curve of the LV and masking the underlying dysfunction.[63] The mechanism and severity of the MR is evaluated and determined with TTE, TEE and MRI of the heart. The increase in left atrial pressure with chronic MR results in pulmonary hypertension, severity of which is measured by right heart catheterization invasively or by echocardiography non-invasively. Echocardiographic evaluation of RV function and the degree of tricuspid valve regurgitation (TR) severity is particularly important. Decrease in RV function associated with higher grades of TR may result in liver congestion decreasing the metabolic capabilities of the liver. Of particular importance are potential decrease in hepatically metabolized anesthetics prolonging or exacerbating their effect and a decrease in production of coagulation factors leading to increased risk of peri-procedural bleeding. Increase in left atrial pressure results in an increase in left atrial volume predisposing for atrial fibrillation associated with higher risk of stroke and complications of chronic anticoagulation regimen. Patients with functional MR have underlying cardiomyopathy most commonly ischemic in origin. Preoperative coronary angiography determines the location and severity of coronary obstruction and the need for revascularization. Preoperative medications such as beta-blokers, ACE-inhibitors and angiotensin receptor blockers are continued throughout the peri-procedural period.

Since these procedures are offered to the patients under investigational terms certain inclusion criteria need to be met. Those include patients with symptomatic moderate or severe MR with EF >25%and LV end-systolic diameter (LVID) ≤ 55mm or asymptomatic with 1 or more of the following: LV EF >25% to 60%; LVID ≥ 40-50mm; new onset atrial-fibrillation; pulmonary hypertension.[62] In addition, successful repair is more common if the coaptation length and depth are, ≥ 2mm and <11mm, respectively. If a flail leaflet exists, the flail gap must be ≤ 10mm and the flail width ≤ 15mm to have sufficient leaflet tissue for mechanical coaptation with the MitraClip device.[62]

Intraoperative

The procedural details have been described previously in this book and in published EVEREST (Endovascular Valve Edge-to-Edge Repair Study) trial.[62,64] Briefly, mimicking Alfieri's edge-to-edge suturing, stearable MitraClip (Evalve Inc, Menlo Park, CA) is inserted via the guide catheter, through percutaneous femoral venous antegrade trans-septal approach (see Figure 10 and 11). The clip is stearable in both antero-posterior as well as medio-lateral directions (see Figure 12). Once positioned perpendicular to the MV leaflet coaptation line, the V-shaped clip grasps and coapts the leaflets during the systole of the beating heart (see Figure 13A and B and 14). The procedure is commonly performed under BGA with the fluoroscopy and TEE guidance although using conscious sedation in addition to local anesthesia in the femoral region has been reported as well.[62,64,65] The advantages of BGA are similar as in TAVI, which include having secured airway if emergent hemodynamic instability ensues, patient paralysis and control of ventilation to reduce patient movement and heart translocation during device deployment, use of TEE throughout the procedure, decreasing patient's discomfort from lying down for the long periods of time and decreasing pain from insertion of the large deployment device.

After placement of standard monitors and peripheral intravenous line, a radial arterial line is placed prior to induction of BGA. Hemodynamic goals during the induction and maintenance of anesthesia are to maintain myocardial contractility and preload without the need for aggressive volume optimization prior to induction due to increase chance of pulmonary edema formation. Afterload is usually decreased by anesthetic induced decrease in systemic vascular resistance, promoting the forward flow of blood form the LV to aorta. Infusions of sodium-nitroprusside and nitroglycerin are readily available if optimization of the systemic vascular tone is needed. After securing the airway with endotracheal tube, introducer with PAC is placed through the right internal-jugular vein followed by insertion of TEE probe. In authors' institution, infusions of inotropic and vasopressor medications are readily available in case of hemodynamic instability which may result from incidental peripheral vascular injury during wire and device introduction, heart injury during wire manipulation as well as trans-septal introduction of the deployment device.

Patient's femoral vascular access is prepared for emergent CPB cannullation with perfusionist readily available. Antibiotic prophylaxis, which usually consists of 1.5 g of cefuroxime is given at this point and urinary catheter inserted. Procedural anticoagulation is achieved with intravenous heparin which is given before trans-septal puncture to achieve ACT>250 sec.

Since the trans-septal approach is utilized, careful de-airing of the device is needed to avoid introduction of air to the left side of the heart and systemic circulation. TEE is very useful not only for accurate determination of the jet origin and its severity but also for guiding and monitoring different stage of the procedure.

Determination of the accurate clip position as well as monitoring hemodynamics during and after the procedure is provided by TEE imaging.[39,66] The puncture of the superior and posterior portion of the intra-atrial septum is guided by TEE.[39,66] In addition, TEE helps in determining the decision to release the positioned clip in case of suboptimal MV leaflet capture or if the closure of the clip is abandoned in cases of minimal MR reduction.[39,66] Addition of real-time 3D echocardiography to 2D imaging enables another aspect of improving accuracy and success in device deployment.[67,68]

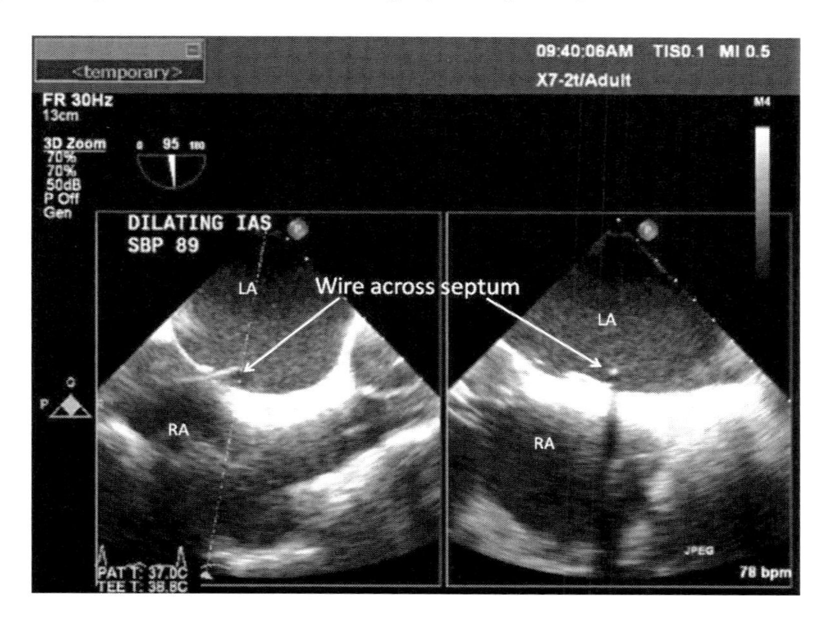

Figure 10. X-plane orthogonal TEE views of the inter-atrial septum (IAS) with the wire traversing from right atrium (RA) to left atrium (LA) dilating IAS.

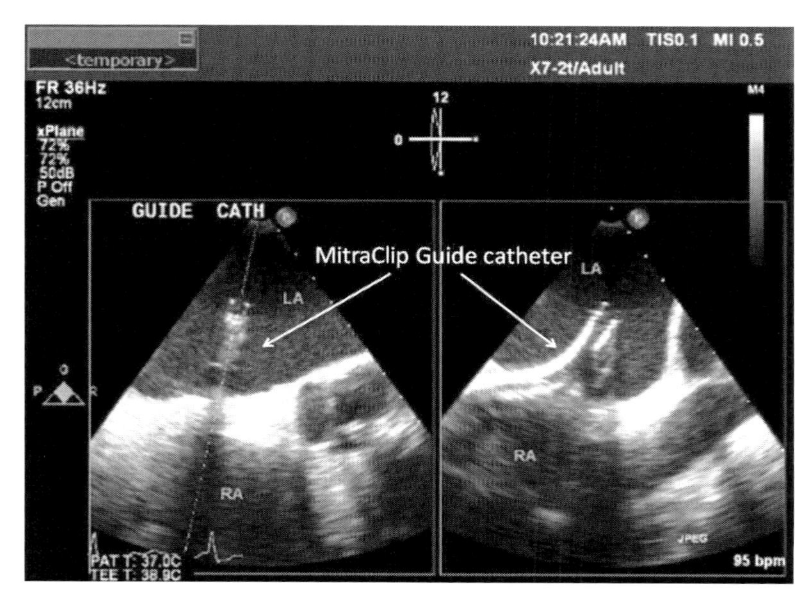

Figure 11. X-plane orthogonal TEE views of the inter-atrial septum (IAS) after introduction of MitraClip guide catheter.

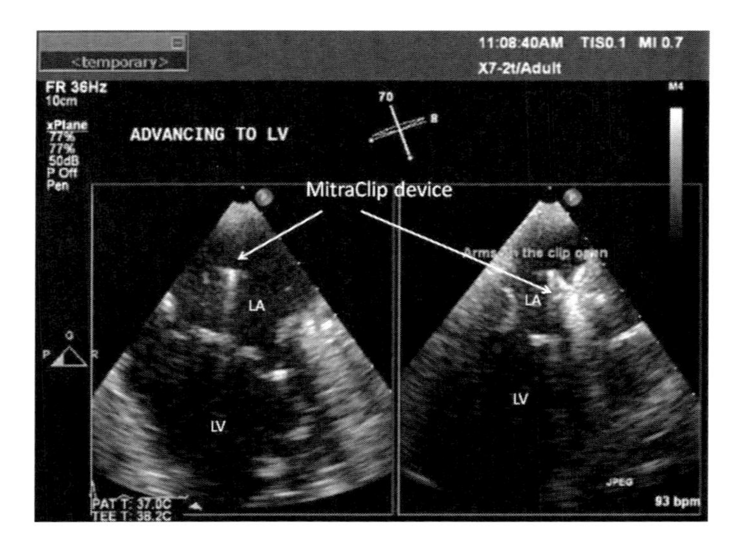

Figure 12. X-plane orthogonal TEE views of the left atrium (LA) with the clip device approaching MV.

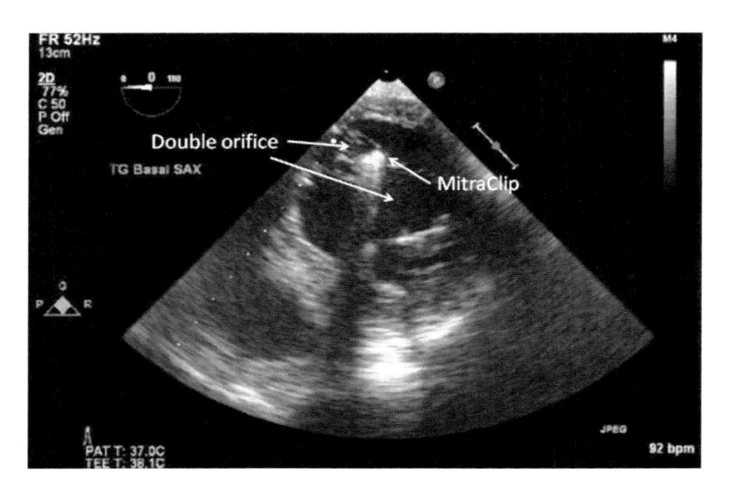

Figure 13A. TEE trans-gastric short axis view of the mitral valve with the edge-to-edge clip placed.

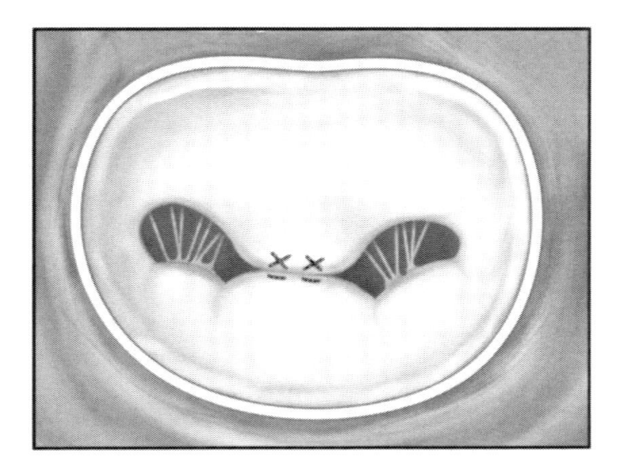

Figure 13B. Illustration of the edge-to-edge suturing producing double orifice of the mitral valve.

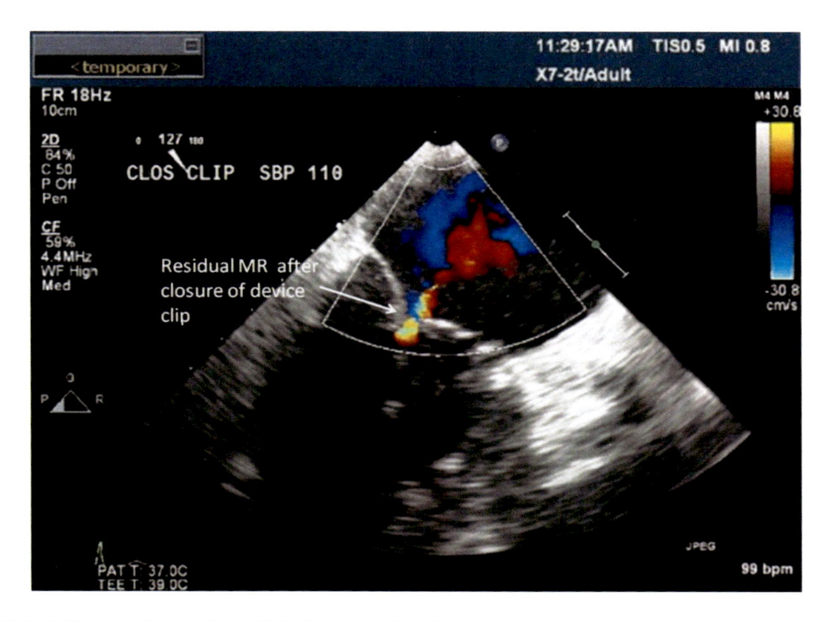

Figure 14. TEE Mid-esophageal modified long-axis view with color-flow Doppler of the residual mitral regurgitation.

Immediate post-procedural complications:

Trans-septal approach to MV may result in the injury to the inter-atrial septum (IAS) increasing the incidence of paradoxical embolism involving air or thrombus and the need for repair.[62] Throughout the peri-procedural period, particular attention is given in careful de-airing of all the central venous catheters and stopcocks as well as delivery system catheters. Once the clip-delivery system is retracted proper echocardiographic evaluation by 2D, color-flow Doppler and saline-in-blood agitated solution is undertaken to rule-out any residual blood flow across the IAS. Additionally, wire and device manipulation may result in an injury to heart chambers and subsequent hemodynamic instability due to cardiac tamponade. Clinical diagnosis of tamponade is supported by TEE evaluation and monitoring of pericardial effusion accumulation. The increased risk of cardiac tamponade and injury to the peripheral venous access sites contribute to the indication for peri-procedural blood transfusion. The incidence of blood transfusion is reported to be about 3.7% of cases.[62] Even though embolization of the MitraClip pertains only a theoretical concern, partial clip detachment has been reported in 9% of patients[62] during the peri-procedural time but was not associated with urgent intervention. Grasping and pulling of the MV leaflets during the clip positioning usually doesn't result in significant exacerbation of the MR severity.[62] Nevertheless, increase in grade of MR severity, may acutely increase left atrial and pulmonary artery pressure leading to RV dysfunction and TR. Communication with the surgeon and cardiologist is important as well as support of the ventricular function with the inotropic medications.

Maintenance of anesthesia is tailored toward quick emergence at the conclusion of the procedure, which is achieved by BGA using Isoflurane or Sevoflurane and intermittent boluses of fentanyl and rocuronium. Infusions of remi-fentanyl may be used as well as total-intravenous technique using propofol infusion. Heparin is reversed by protamine in a standard way. Prior to extubation, nausea and vomiting prophylaxis is administered according to individual risk and muscle relaxant is adequately reversed. Since no standardization protocol exits at this point, patients enrolled in EVEREST trials received aspirin 325mg daily for 6 months and clopidogrel 75mg daily for 30 days.[62]

Postoperative

Acute procedural success reported from EVEREST trial defined as a MR ≤ 2+, is 74% with 64% discharged with MR ≤ 1+ and one in-hospital death (non-procedure related).[62] Successful decrease in severity of MR to ≤ 2+ was achieved by using one clip in 61% and with two clips in 29% of patients (in 10% of patients percutaneous trans-septal approach was unable to reduce the degree of MR).[62] Subsequent report from Argenziano and colleagues analyzed 32/107 (30%) of patients from the EVEREST cohort who had MV surgery following attempted percutaneous MitaClip repair.[69] The study included patients in whom: 1. MitraClip devices was not deployed due to inability to reduce; 2. One or two MitraClips deployed without reduction of MR ≤ 2+, assessed by TEE at discharge; 3. The initial success was documented but followed by recurrent MR > 2+; 4. There was another indication for surgery (ASD repair as a result of trans-septal puncture). Overall, in 21/32 (67%) patients, successful surgical MV repair was possible despite observed damage to the leaflet tissue and/or chordae from the previous MitraClip repair.[69]

Even though post-procedural ARI is of theoretical concern its incidence has not been reported in the literature.

Anesthetic Considerations for Percutaneous Mitral Valve Valvuloplasty

Percutaneous valvuloplasty procedures offer a minimally invasive therapeutic treatment option for patients with predominantly stenotic valvular disease. Originally developed for patients at increased risk of complications following open surgical intervention or with extensive coexisting disease, percutaneous techniques have been adapted for use in an ever-expanding patient population.[70] Essential for success is an understanding of underlying pathophysiology, patient comorbidities, and conduct of the procedure. Aortic valve balloon valvuloplasty has been reserved as a "palliative" therapeutic treatment effort in patients at high for morbidity and mortality related to the conventional surgical replacement. Nevertheless, due to the high re-stenosis rates[71,72] and with the development of the new stent-valve procedures, described above, balloon valvuoplasty became just part of the stent-valve implantation procedure. Therefore, this paragraph will review relevant anesthetic considerations in patients undergoing percutaneous valvuloplasty procedures for mitral valve stenosis.

Mitral Valve Stenosis

Rheumatic heart disease with resultant inflammatory changes represents the leading cause of mitral valve stenosis. Less frequent etiologies include malignant carcinoid disease, structural changes following therapeutic radiation treatment, systemic lupus erythematosus, rheumatoid arthritis, Whipple Disease, and rare connective tissue disorders. Patients typically experience symptoms at rest when mitral valve area decreases to less than 1.5 cm^2.[73]

Appropriate patient selection for balloon valvuloplasty is based upon mitral valve morphology and coexisting disease. Characteristics of the mitral valve which correlate with successful balloon valvuloplasty were elucidated by Wilkins and colleagues.[74] This group devised a scoring system or splitability index based on echocardiographic assessment of the mitral valve (see Table 2). Echocardiographic measures in the index include degree of calcification, amount of thickening, valve leaflet mobility, and amount of subvalvular thickening. A score below eight is associated with improved outcome.[55,74]

Table 2. Splitability Index

Grade	Calcification	Subvalvular Thickening	Leaflet Mobility	Thickening
1	Single Area	Minimal thickening below leaflets	Highly mobile with leaflet tip restriction	Near normal thickness (4-5 mm)
2	Scattered areas limited to leaflet margins	Thickening extending to one third chordal length	Leaflet mid & base portions have normal mobility	Margin thickening (5-8 mm)
3	Brightness extending into leaflet midportion	Thickening extending to distal third of chords	Normal valve movement in diastole, from base	Thickening of entire leaflet (5-8 mm)
4	Brightness throughout most of leaflet tissue	Thickening of entire chordae extending to papillary muscle	No or minimal valve movement in diastole	Considerable thickening of entire leaflet (>8-10 mm)

Modified from Wilkins GT, Weyman AE, Abascal VM et al. Percutaneous balloon dilation of the mitral valve: an analysis of echocardiographic variables related to outcome and the mechanism of dilatation. Br heart J 1988;60(4):299-308

Underlying anatomic and physiologic derangements in patients with mitral stenosis depend on the severity and duration of disease. A stenotic mitral valve creates an increased pressure gradient between the left atrium and left ventricle. Left atrial dilation is common as this chamber is subjected to chronic pressure overload. This dilation predisposes patients to atrial fibrillation. A tendency for low-flow of blood within the atrium also places patients at increased risk of intracardiac thrombosis, particularly within the left atrial appendage. If mitral stenosis is severe or long-standing, the increased pressure in the left atrium can be transmitted to the pulmonary vasculature and subsequently lead to right ventricular failure.[75]

Anesthetic Management of Mitral Valve Balloon Valvuloplasty

Anesthetic management for a patient undergoing mitral valve balloon valvuloplasty begins with a thorough evaluation of the etiology, severity, and chronology of the patient's mitral stenosis. A detailed past medical history should be elicited to determine if management of coexisting disease is optimal or if consultation with specialists is required. As with any cardiac procedure, particular attention is directed to the cardiopulmonary system with review of previous interventions and current degree of debility.

Mitral valve balloon valvuloplasty is most often performed by cardiologists in the catheterization laboratory or in the interventional procedural suite. Since this is a percutaneous technique with device access obtained through the femoral vein, optimal procedural conditions are usually achieved with sedative medications and local anesthetics. However, if a patient will be unable to lie still for the duration of the procedure or if concomitant disease requires more intense monitoring and management, a dedicated anesthesia provider may be required in the peri-procedural period.[30] If a balloon valvuloplasty is to be performed outside the realm of the anesthesia provider's normal working environment, a fully functional anesthesia machine, emergency equipment, access to necessary medications and supplies, and available backup personnel should be accounted for. The fluoroscopy and catheterization equipment used for this procedure occupy a significant area in the procedure room; optimal planning usually requires airway and intravenous line extensions to provide enough room for the additional procedural equipment and to allow ready access to the patient as necessary.

Valvulopasty is performed with either a single-balloon Inoue or double balloon technique. In either case, the balloon is introduced into the femoral vein and guided up into the right atrium. It is then passed through the atrial septum and threaded into the annulus of the mitral valve. Maximal amount of inflation is determined according to geometric formulas standardized to body surface area. Following balloon inflation, left ventriculography is used to assess the amount of mitral regurgitation. Moderate to severe mitral insufficiency is a contraindication to balloon valvuloplasty as regurgitation is expected to increase by one grade following the procedure.[73]

In terms of outcomes, Cubeddu and colleagues report a follow-up on 844 patients that underwent percutaneous mitral valve balloon valvuloplasty.[55] Mean follow-up time was 4.2 years post-procedure. There were 110 deaths, 234 patients required mitral valve replacement, and 54 patients had a second valvuloplasty. On follow-up, the highest proportion of patients who were classified as New York Heart Association Class I or II, were those with an Echo Score of less than eight.[55]

Anesthetic Consideration for Transcatheter Paravalvular Leak Closures

The ever increasing number of procedures being performed in the modern day cardiac catheterization laboratory (CCL) include cardiac catheterizations, coronary artery stent placements, closure of septal defects, patent foramen ovale, prosthetic paravalvular leaks (PVLs), valve repairs and replacements, ablations of atrial and ventricular arrythmias and AICD placements.[76] This increase in both the variety and complexity of procedures being performed in the CCL, the general remoteness of the CCL, the inadequacy of ancillary support and the stress of working in an unfamiliar and non standardized anesthetizing location all combine to make the provision of anesthesia to these patients with sometimes significant cardiac dysfunction in the CCL very challenging.[76]

Prosthetic valve replacement surgery is performed in approximately 21000 patients annually.[77] Anywhere from 3% to 12.5% of replaced prosthesis will eventually demonstrate a clinically significant paravalvular leak.[77] Common causes of PVLs include infection, suture disruption and tissue damage around the annulus.[78] In patients with mechanical prosthesis limitation of disc mobility by thrombi or vegetations may also be seen.[78] Patient factors, like old age, malnutrition, renal insufficiency and anatomic factors like annular calcification, endocarditis, large atria, the type of valve used, the valve location and the suture technique are all risk factors for the development of a PVL.[79] Clinically significant PVLs seem to affect the mitral and aortic valve more than other valves with mitral being most commonly affected.[77] PVLs lead to symptoms related to valve regurgitation (chamber enlargement, exercise intolerance and congestive heart failure) and/or hemolysis (leading to anemia, heart failure and renal failure).[77] Since medical management of PVLs is merely palliative and surgical treatment of PVLs is fraught with all the risks of a re-operation, percutaneous transcatheter closure is an exciting alternative.[77] Increased availability of live 3D TEE and the development of dedicated occlusion devices are dramatically improving the success of transcatheter PVL closures. Contraindications for percutaneous closure of PVLs include the presence of active infection, vegetations, thrombi, large defects and PVLs located close to point of maximal leaflet excursions.[79] Currently, a variety of make-shift devices like the Amplatzer septal occluder, the Amplatzer duct occluder, the Amplatzer coil and the Gianturco coil are being used for this purpose.[80]

Preprocedure Evaluation

As with any cardiac surgical/interventional procedure, a thorough history, physical examination and relevant laboratory and imaging work should precede the administration of an anesthetic. The patient's functional status, the reason for the original valve surgery, type of the prior valve surgery and valve used should be ascertained. Signs and symptoms usually include fatigue, dyspnea, orthopnea, arrythmias and cyanosis which are all related to the different degrees of the blood volume regurgitation.[81]

In addition, same symptoms may be a result of hemolytic anemia, renal failure and repeated blood transfusions frequently seen in patients with paravalvular insufficiency. Important preoperative investigations include comprehensive metabolic panel to detect and treat electrolyte abnormalities such as hyperkalemia resulting from hemolysis and renal failure, complete blood count to detect the severity of anemia, coagulation profile since the patients are usually on anticoagulants, liver function tests, EKG, chest X-ray to detect pleural effusions and pulmonary edema which are common in this patient population and an echocardiogram to determine the extent and locations of the PVLs. Increasingly, 3D TEE is being utilized to accurately assess the location, shape and extent of the PVLs. Since these patients have extensive cardiac history, their medication regimen can be complex and should be reviewed.[81]

Intraprocedure Evaluation

Standard ASA monitors, an arterial line, TEE and fluoroscopy (to facilitate the procedure) are commonly used. Since the procedure is performed on a fluoroscopy table surrounded by fluoroscopy equipment, access to the patient is very limited once the procedure commences.

A central venous line is usually placed both for access and monitoring purposes in addition to peripheral venous access. Since the fluoroscopy table moves on a regular basis during the procedure (oftentimes without prior notice) and since the anesthesia machine is far removed from the fluoroscopy table, it is important to have long intravenous lines and breathing circuits with plenty of slack but at the same time avoid possible kinking.[76] While the procedures can be performed under sedation technique, possibility of having extended duration of the procedure and difficulty in accessing patient's airway during the procedure, general anesthesia with the establishment of a secure airway is the preferred alternative. Hemodynamic goals for the procedure are similar to the goals that would be required if the patient were to have the procedure performed surgically.

They involve avoidance of augmentation of preload in patients with signs of heart failure, avoidance of bradycardia and maintenance of high normal heart rate to minimize blood volume regurgitation fraction, normal contractility and afterload reduction. Patient extubation at the end of the procedure should be the goal of the anesthetic regardless of the technique used.[81] Since the procedure is not very stimulating, the anesthetic can be conducted with a relatively small dose of narcotics used.

Induction with midazolam, fentanyl and propofol, intubation using succinylcholine or rocuronium and maintenance with an inhalational agent and rocuronium with full reversal of neuromuscular blockade at the end of the procedure is generally considered acceptable. A total intravenous anesthetic using propofol and remifentanil is a good alternative.

Intraprocedure TEE

Since analysis of the PVL with TTE is suboptimal, intraprocedure TEE is pivotal to the success of transcatheter PVL closure. Though two-dimensional TEE is still the standard echo modality used and is essential to fully characterize the PVL, it has several limitations including an inability to simultaneously image multiple imaging planes, to visualize the catheter tip continuously and to characterize the 3D anatomy of the PVL (2).[82] These problems can be circumvented by the use of 3D TEE. Since a three dimensional understanding of the anatomy of the PVL is pivotal to the success of the procedure, the availability of 3D echocardiography can be a huge advantage. The echocardiographer must work very closely with the interventional cardiologist and be able to communicate the location of the leak relative to landmarks seen on fluoroscopy.[82] Live 3D echo and 3D color-flow Doppler can greatly improve the detection of multiple leaks and help characterize the size, shape and location of the leaks.[83]

In addition, TEE can also be used to evaluate possible adverse effects of a device or catheter on valve function like interference with leaflet motion, cardiac tamponade due to perforation and aortic dissection.[83]

Post-Procedure Considerations

Some of the potential complications encountered during the post-procedural time include myocardial ischemia, dysrhythmias, electrolyte abnormalities, pain, nausea, and procedural complications like femoral artery / venous access site hematomas/ruptures and cardiac tamponade. Pain in the PACU is managed with intermittent narcotic boluses that are later transitioned to oral medications. Early discharge from the PACU is to be expected.

Hybrid Operating Room

Developments in cardiac surgery have led toward minimally invasive procedures, which usually incorporate some form of trans-catheter technique. To enable the conduct of these procedures they need to incorporate a fluoroscopic angiography system, which has been traditionally used in the cardiology catheterization suites. The development of the hybrid cardiac operating rooms bridges the gap between interventional cardiology and cardiac surgery and enables an integrated way in patient's management. The hybrid operating room integrates imaging devices such as high-power semi-mobile multi-axis biplane or monoplane C-arm fluoroscopy machine.[84] These machines are usually bulky and occupy a good portion of the operating room. A meticulous planning strategy needs to be applied into designing process, which incorporates positioning of the anesthesia machine, poles, TEE machine in order to have functioning setup (see Figure 15A and B and 16).

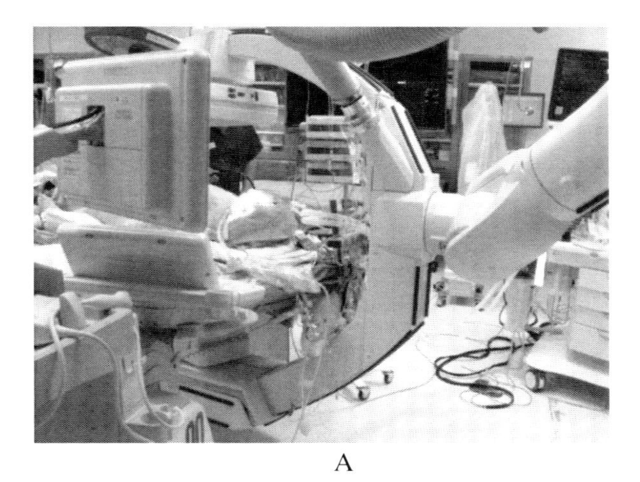

A

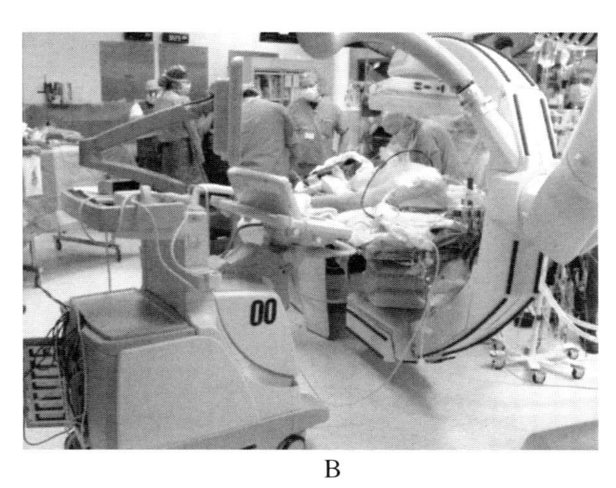

B

Figures 15. A and B. Images depict locations of the anesthesia equipment around the operating table and fluoroscopy C-arm in the hybrid operating room.

Mobility of any of these machines is important to maintain flexibility in adaptation to different procedural situations. Since different procedures require different variety of imaging views, the ability to freely move C-arm around the patient is very important to obtain accurate images. For example, a 3D CT-like imaging of the heart is performed by 1 or 2 sweeps of up to 220° around the patient. Positioning the patient on the table is also procedure specific. If the biplane C-arm with lateral axis is used to obtain images patient's arms are placed above the head to avoid interference between X-ray beams and patient's arm bones. It is important to assure adequate padding of the arms and avoidance of excessive traction of the brachial plexus to avoid peripheral nerve injury.

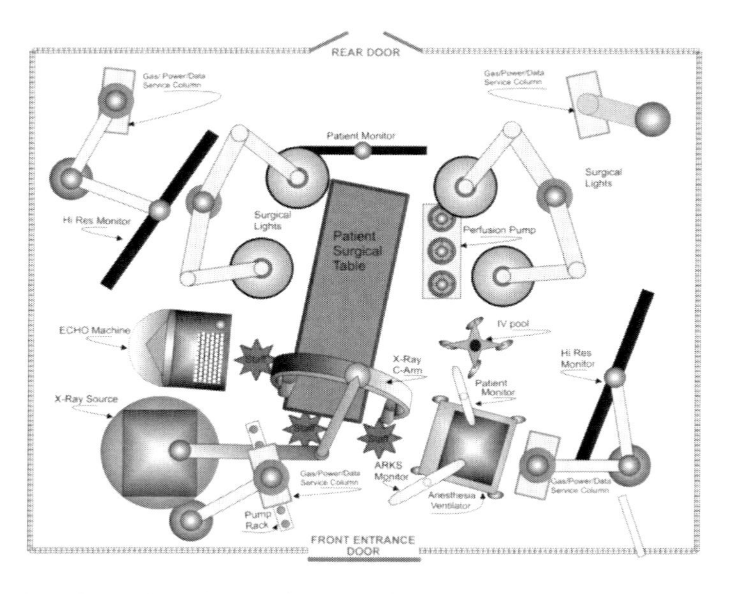

Figure 16. Illustration of the orientation and location of the anesthesia staff and equipment in relation to the operating table and C-arm in the hybrid operating room.

This wide range of C-arm motion requires modification of the usual anesthesia setups and also limits free access to the patient. The anesthesia machine is usually moved away from the patient to accommodate for the C-arm movement particularly if a bi-plane machine is used. That requires longer breathing circuits theoretically resulting in increase in dead space, which is easily overcome by the increase in gas flow volume rate. Clinically more important is a potential for kinking and damaging long circuit tubings. In addition, all intravenous tubings need to have extensions to enable safe mobility of the C-arm around the patient. Additionally, operating room table is manipulated by the surgeon/cardiologist so sudden unexpected movements can be encountered. The table is made of carbon to enable radiolucency and should allow for wide range of movements.[84] Typically used anesthesia equipment may not be readily available in the remote locations. Care should be taken to supply the remote anesthetic locations with the additional carts in the situation of difficult airway or emergent need for vasoactive medications.

The radiation dose emitted from fluoroscopy machine is reported to be rather small.[84] Hybrid operating rooms are isolated and control area with the workstation is shielded from to prevent radiation leakage.[76] Radiation injury to the body can happen in two ways.[85] One is dose-independent way of DNA injury resulting in increase in incidence of cancer and is related to lifetime cumulative dosage received. Second one is dose-dependent injury causing cellular death leading to bone marrow suppression, desquamation, erythema, gonadal injury with sterility and fibrosis. Radiation exposure dose in the cine mode is 10-fold higher than with intermittent fluoroscopy.[85] Exposure to radiation is attenuated by the square of distance from the source.[85] Collimation of the X-ray beam and copper filters help reduce exposure to the team members. To decrease radiation exposure properly positioned acrylic shield lead aprons, thyroid collars and protective eyeglasses need to be worn by everyone in the operating room.[85] Radiation exposure of the patient is decreased by collimation of the X-ray beam, pulsed fluoroscopic use, copper filters, limiting magnified views and direct shielding of gonads keeping the source-to-image distance as narrow as possible.[85]

Conclusion

TFAVI has been internationally recognized as an effective minimally invasive procedure, which improves symptoms and functional capacity in very high risk patient population. Patents with severe AS and peripheral vascular disease are given an option of TAAVI resulting in an improvement in functional status with lessened incidence of morbidity and mortality than with conventional surgical management. Furthering the experience and advancing the technology may result in TAVI becoming a standard procedure offered to selective high risk or even lower risk patients.

PMVI is an option for patients at higher risk of morbidity and mortality from conventional surgical technique. For the younger with low surgical risk and no major co-morbidities, a 74% success rate of PMVI may not be optimal as of yet.

Further advances in technology and experience with different repair modalities may enable non-surgical options for wide variety of patients. Distinguishing whether patients with functional or organic MV disease are better served with PMVI is still in progress. Nevertheless, surgical treatment options still persist after incomplete or unsuccessful percutaneous attempt.

Older techniques, such as AV and MV balloon valvuloplasty remain an option to selective patients but it remains to be seen if they resist the challenge of advancing technology and find their space in management algorithms.

Anesthetic management will follow procedural advances along with the need for flexibility in providing best possible environment for the procedural success without jeopardizing patients' safety.

TEE remains one of the most reliable modalities used to determine patients' procedural eligibility, offering guidance during the procedure and evaluating the success of the procedure.

Anesthesiologists maintain their crucial role in the "triangle of success" maintaining and optimizing patient's hemodynamics as well as providing TEE expertise. Challenges of remote location and hybrid operating rooms and constantly developing technologies should be overcome by vigilance, meticulous preparedness and communication between all members involved.

Acknowledgment

Special thanks to Mr. Dave Schumick from the Department of Medical Illustration and to Mr. Mike Lapic from the CTA Section of Clinical Engineering at Cleveland Clinic for their help with making the illustrations and obtaining photos from the operating room.

References

[1] Nkomo VT, Gardin JM, Skelton TN, Gottdiener JS, Scott CG, Enriquez-Sarano M: Burden of valvular heart diseases: a population-based study. *Lancet* 2006; 368: 1005-11

[2] Jones EC, Devereux RB, Roman MJ, Liu JE, Fishman D, Lee ET, Welty TK, Fabsitz RR, Howard BV: Prevalence and correlates of mitral regurgitation in a population-based sample (the Strong Heart Study). *Am J Cardiol* 2001; 87: 298-304

[3] Lindroos M, Kupari M, Heikkila J, Tilvis R: Prevalence of aortic valve abnormalities in the elderly: an echocardiographic study of a random population sample. *J Am Coll Cardiol* 1993; 21: 1220-5

[4] Iung B, Vahanian A: Valvular heart diseases in elderly people. *Lancet* 2006; 368: 969-71

[5] Iung B, Baron G, Butchart EG, Delahaye F, Gohlke-Barwolf C, Levang OW, Tornos P, Vanoverschelde JL, Vermeer F, Boersma E, Ravaud P, Vahanian A: A prospective survey of patients with valvular heart disease in Europe: The Euro Heart Survey on Valvular Heart Disease. *Eur Heart J* 2003; 24: 1231-43

[6] Bonow RO, Carabello BA, Kanu C, de Leon AC, Jr., Faxon DP, Freed MD, Gaasch WH, Lytle BW, Nishimura RA, O'Gara PT, O'Rourke RA, Otto CM, Shah PM, Shanewise JS, Smith SC, Jr., Jacobs AK, Adams CD, Anderson JL, Antman EM, Faxon DP, Fuster V, Halperin JL, Hiratzka LF, Hunt SA, Lytle BW, Nishimura R, Page RL, Riegel B: ACC/AHA 2006 guidelines for the management of patients with valvular heart disease: a report of the American College of Cardiology/American Heart Association Task Force on Practice Guidelines (writing committee to revise the 1998 Guidelines for the Management of Patients With Valvular Heart Disease): developed in collaboration with the Society of Cardiovascular Anesthesiologists: endorsed by the Society for Cardiovascular Angiography and Interventions and the Society of Thoracic Surgeons. *Circulation* 2006; 114: e84-231

[7] Varadarajan P, Kapoor N, Bansal RC, Pai RG: Survival in elderly patients with severe aortic stenosis is dramatically improved by aortic valve replacement: Results from a cohort of 277 patients aged > or =80 years. *Eur J Cardiothorac Surg* 2006; 30: 722-7

[8] Kojodjojo P, Gohil N, Barker D, Youssefi P, Salukhe TV, Choong A, Koa-Wing M, Bayliss J, Hackett DR, Khan MA: Outcomes of elderly patients aged 80 and over with symptomatic, severe aortic stenosis: impact of patient's choice of refusing aortic valve replacement on survival. *Qjm* 2008; 101: 567-73

[9] Kapadia SR, Goel SS, Svensson L, Roselli E, Savage RM, Wallace L, Sola S, Schoenhagen P, Shishehbor MH, Christofferson R, Halley C, Rodriguez LL, Stewart W, Kalahasti V, Tuzcu EM: Characterization and outcome of patients with severe

symptomatic aortic stenosis referred for percutaneous aortic valve replacement. *J Thorac Cardiovasc Surg* 2009; 137: 1430-5

[10] Bach DS, Cimino N, Deeb GM: Unoperated patients with severe aortic stenosis. *J Am Coll Cardiol* 2007; 50: 2018-9

[11] Vahanian A, Alfieri O, Al-Attar N, Antunes M, Bax J, Cormier B, Cribier A, De Jaegere P, Fournial G, Kappetein AP, Kovac J, Ludgate S, Maisano F, Moat N, Mohr F, Nataf P, Pierard L, Pomar JL, Schofer J, Tornos P, Tuzcu M, van Hout B, Von Segesser LK, Walther T: Transcatheter valve implantation for patients with aortic stenosis: a position statement from the European association of cardio-thoracic surgery (EACTS) and the European Society of Cardiology (ESC), in collaboration with the European Association of Percutaneous Cardiovascular Interventions (EAPCI). *EuroIntervention* 2008; 4: 193-9

[12] Detaint D, Sundt TM, Nkomo VT, Scott CG, Tajik AJ, Schaff HV, Enriquez-Sarano M: Surgical correction of mitral regurgitation in the elderly: outcomes and recent improvements. *Circulation* 2006; 114: 265-72

[13] Webb JG, Wood DA, Ye J, Gurvitch R, Masson JB, Rodes-Cabau J, Osten M, Horlick E, Wendler O, Dumont E, Carere RG, Wijesinghe N, Nietlispach F, Johnson M, Thompson CR, Moss R, Leipsic J, Munt B, Lichtenstein SV, Cheung A: Transcatheter valve-in-valve implantation for failed bioprosthetic heart valves. *Circulation;* 121: 1848-57

[14] Astor BC, Kaczmarek RG, Hefflin B, Daley WR: Mortality after aortic valve replacement: results from a nationally representative database. *Ann Thorac Surg* 2000; 70: 1939-45

[15] Edwards MB, Taylor KM: Outcomes in nonagenarians after heart valve replacement operation. *Ann Thorac Surg* 2003; 75: 830-4

[16] Vaquette B, Corbineau H, Laurent M, Lelong B, Langanay T, de Place C, Froger-Bompas C, Leclercq C, Daubert C, Leguerrier A: Valve replacement in patients with critical aortic stenosis and depressed left ventricular function: predictors of operative risk, left ventricular function recovery, and long term outcome. *Heart* 2005; 91: 1324-9

[17] Cribier A, Eltchaninoff H, Bash A, Borenstein N, Tron C, Bauer F, Derumeaux G, Anselme F, Laborde F, Leon MB: Percutaneous transcatheter implantation of an aortic valve prosthesis for calcific aortic stenosis: first human case description. *Circulation* 2002; 106: 3006-8

[18] Webb JG, Chandavimol M, Thompson CR, Ricci DR, Carere RG, Munt BI, Buller CE, Pasupati S, Lichtenstein S: Percutaneous aortic valve implantation retrograde from the femoral artery. *Circulation* 2006; 113: 842-50

[19] Lichtenstein SV, Cheung A, Ye J, Thompson CR, Carere RG, Pasupati S, Webb JG: Transapical transcatheter aortic valve implantation in humans: initial clinical experience. *Circulation* 2006; 114: 591-6

[20] Svensson LG, Dewey T, Kapadia S, Roselli EE, Stewart A, Williams M, Anderson WN, Brown D, Leon M, Lytle B, Moses J, Mack M, Tuzcu M, Smith C: United States feasibility study of transcatheter insertion of a stented aortic valve by the left ventricular apex. *Ann Thorac Surg* 2008; 86: 46-54; discussion 54-5

[21] Walther T, Simon P, Dewey T, Wimmer-Greinecker G, Falk V, Kasimir MT, Doss M, Borger MA, Schuler G, Glogar D, Fehske W, Wolner E, Mohr FW, Mack M:

Transapical minimally invasive aortic valve implantation: multicenter experience. *Circulation* 2007; 116: I240-5

[22] Ye J, Cheung A, Lichtenstein SV, Pasupati S, Carere RG, Thompson CR, Sinhal A, Webb JG: Six-month outcome of transapical transcatheter aortic valve implantation in the initial seven patients. *Eur J Cardiothorac Surg* 2007; 31: 16-21

[23] Cribier A, Eltchaninoff H, Tron C, Bauer F, Agatiello C, Sebagh L, Bash A, Nusimovici D, Litzler PY, Bessou JP, Leon MB: Early experience with percutaneous transcatheter implantation of heart valve prosthesis for the treatment of end-stage inoperable patients with calcific aortic stenosis. *J Am Coll Cardiol* 2004; 43: 698-703

[24] Grube E, Laborde JC, Gerckens U, Felderhoff T, Sauren B, Buellesfeld L, Mueller R, Menichelli M, Schmidt T, Zickmann B, Iversen S, Stone GW: Percutaneous implantation of the CoreValve self-expanding valve prosthesis in high-risk patients with aortic valve disease: the Siegburg first-in-man study. *Circulation* 2006; 114: 1616-24

[25] Webb JG, Altwegg L, Boone RH, Cheung A, Ye J, Lichtenstein S, Lee M, Masson JB, Thompson C, Moss R, Carere R, Munt B, Nietlispach F, Humphries K: Transcatheter aortic valve implantation: impact on clinical and valve-related outcomes. *Circulation* 2009; 119: 3009-16

[26] Webb JG, Pasupati S, Humphries K, Thompson C, Altwegg L, Moss R, Sinhal A, Carere RG, Munt B, Ricci D, Ye J, Cheung A, Lichtenstein SV: Percutaneous transarterial aortic valve replacement in selected high-risk patients with aortic stenosis. *Circulation* 2007; 116: 755-63

[27] Billings FTt, Kodali SK, Shanewise JS: Transcatheter aortic valve implantation: anesthetic considerations. *Anesth Analg* 2009; 108: 1453-62

[28] Covello RD, Maj G, Landoni G, Maisano F, Michev I, Guarracino F, Alfieri O, Colombo A, Zangrillo A: Anesthetic management of percutaneous aortic valve implantation: focus on challenges encountered and proposed solutions. *J Cardiothorac Vasc Anesth* 2009; 23: 280-5

[29] Guinot PG, Depoix JP, Etchegoyen L, Benbara A, Provenchere S, Dilly MP, Philip I, Enguerand D, Ibrahim H, Vahanian A, Himbert D, Al-Attar N, Nataf P, Desmonts JM, Montravers P, Longrois D: Anesthesia and Perioperative Management of Patients Undergoing Transcatheter Aortic Valve Implantation: Analysis of 90 Consecutive Patients With Focus on Perioperative Complications. *J Cardiothorac Vasc Anesth*

[30] Haas S, Richter HP, Kubitz JC: Anesthesia during cardiologic procedures. *Curr Opin Anaesthesiol* 2009; 22: 519-23

[31] Rodes-Cabau J, Dumont E, De LaRochelliere R, Doyle D, Lemieux J, Bergeron S, Clavel MA, Villeneuve J, Raby K, Bertrand OF, Pibarot P: Feasibility and initial results of percutaneous aortic valve implantation including selection of the transfemoral or transapical approach in patients with severe aortic stenosis. *Am J Cardiol* 2008; 102: 1240-6

[32] Cribier A, Eltchaninoff H, Tron C, Bauer F, Agatiello C, Nercolini D, Tapiero S, Litzler PY, Bessou JP, Babaliaros V: Treatment of calcific aortic stenosis with the percutaneous heart valve: mid-term follow-up from the initial feasibility studies: the French experience. *J Am Coll Cardiol* 2006; 47: 1214-23

[33] Grube E, Schuler G, Buellesfeld L, Gerckens U, Linke A, Wenaweser P, Sauren B, Mohr FW, Walther T, Zickmann B, Iversen S, Felderhoff T, Cartier R, Bonan R:

Percutaneous aortic valve replacement for severe aortic stenosis in high-risk patients using the second- and current third-generation self-expanding CoreValve prosthesis: device success and 30-day clinical outcome. *J Am Coll Cardiol* 2007; 50: 69-76

[34] Rodes-Cabau J, Webb JG, Cheung A, Ye J, Dumont E, Feindel CM, Osten M, Natarajan MK, Velianou JL, Martucci G, DeVarennes B, Chisholm R, Peterson MD, Lichtenstein SV, Nietlispach F, Doyle D, DeLarochelliere R, Teoh K, Chu V, Dancea A, Lachapelle K, Cheema A, Latter D, Horlick E: Transcatheter aortic valve implantation for the treatment of severe symptomatic aortic stenosis in patients at very high or prohibitive surgical risk: acute and late outcomes of the multicenter Canadian experience. *J Am Coll Cardiol;* 55: 1080-90

[35] Ree RM, Bowering JB, Schwarz SK: Case series: anesthesia for retrograde percutaneous aortic valve replacement--experience with the first 40 patients. *Can J Anaesth* 2008; 55: 761-8

[36] Behan M, Haworth P, Hutchinson N, Trivedi U, Laborde JC, Hildick-Smith D: Percutaneous aortic valve implants under sedation: our initial experience. *Catheter Cardiovasc Interv* 2008; 72: 1012-5

[37] Berry C, Oukerraj L, Asgar A, Lamarche Y, Marcheix B, Denault AY, Laborde JC, Cartier R, Ducharme A, Bonan R, Basmadjian AJ: Role of transesophageal echocardiography in percutaneous aortic valve replacement with the CoreValve Revalving system. *Echocardiography* 2008; 25: 840-8

[38] Moss RR, Ivens E, Pasupati S, Humphries K, Thompson CR, Munt B, Sinhal A, Webb JG: Role of echocardiography in percutaneous aortic valve implantation. *JACC Cardiovasc Imaging* 2008; 1: 15-24

[39] Naqvi TZ: Echocardiography in percutaneous valve therapy. *JACC Cardiovasc Imaging* 2009; 2: 1226-37

[40] Clavel MA, Webb JG, Pibarot P, Altwegg L, Dumont E, Thompson C, De Larochelliere R, Doyle D, Masson JB, Bergeron S, Bertrand OF, Rodes-Cabau J: Comparison of the hemodynamic performance of percutaneous and surgical bioprostheses for the treatment of severe aortic stenosis. *J Am Coll Cardiol* 2009; 53: 1883-91

[41] Kapadia SR, Tuzcu EM: Transcatheter aortic valve implantation. *Curr Treat Options Cardiovasc Med* 2009; 11: 467-75

[42] Piazza N, Grube E, Gerckens U, den Heijer P, Linke A, Luha O, Ramondo A, Ussia G, Wenaweser P, Windecker S, Laborde JC, de Jaegere P, Serruys PW: Procedural and 30-day outcomes following transcatheter aortic valve implantation using the third generation (18 Fr) corevalve revalving system: results from the multicentre, expanded evaluation registry 1-year following CE mark approval. *EuroIntervention* 2008; 4: 242-9

[43] Alexander KP, Anstrom KJ, Muhlbaier LH, Grosswald RD, Smith PK, Jones RH, Peterson ED: Outcomes of cardiac surgery in patients > or = 80 years: results from the National Cardiovascular Network. *J Am Coll Cardiol* 2000; 35: 731-8

[44] Del Duca D, Iqbal S, Rahme E, Goldberg P, de Varennes B: Renal failure after cardiac surgery: timing of cardiac catheterization and other perioperative risk factors. *Ann Thorac Surg* 2007; 84: 1264-71

[45] Ihle BU: Acute renal dysfunction after cardiac surgery: still a big problem! *Heart Lung Circ* 2007; 16 Suppl 3: S39-44

[46] Aregger F, Wenaweser P, Hellige GJ, Kadner A, Carrel T, Windecker S, Frey FJ: Risk of acute kidney injury in patients with severe aortic valve stenosis undergoing transcatheter valve replacement. *Nephrol Dial Transplant* 2009; 24: 2175-9

[47] Bagur R, Webb JG, Nietlispach F, Dumont E, De Larochelliere R, Doyle D, Masson JB, Gutierrez MJ, Clavel MA, Bertrand OF, Pibarot P, Rodes-Cabau J: Acute kidney injury following transcatheter aortic valve implantation: predictive factors, prognostic value, and comparison with surgical aortic valve replacement. *Eur Heart J*; 31: 865-74

[48] Ye J, Cheung A, Lichtenstein SV, Carere RG, Thompson CR, Pasupati S, Webb JG: Transapical aortic valve implantation in humans. *J Thorac Cardiovasc Surg* 2006; 131: 1194-6

[49] Fassl J, Walther T, Groesdonk HV, Kempfert J, Borger MA, Scholz M, Mukherjee C, Linke A, Schuler G, Mohr FW, Ender J: Anesthesia management for transapical transcatheter aortic valve implantation: a case series. *J Cardiothorac Vasc Anesth* 2009; 23: 286-91

[50] Ye J, Cheung A, Lichtenstein SV, Nietlispach F, Albugami S, Masson JB, Thompson CR, Munt B, Moss R, Carere RG, Jamieson WR, Webb JG: Transapical transcatheter aortic valve implantation: follow-up to 3 years. *J Thorac Cardiovasc Surg*; 139: 1107-13, 1113 e1

[51] Ye J, Cheung A, Lichtenstein SV, Altwegg LA, Wong DR, Carere RG, Thompson CR, Moss RR, Munt B, Pasupati S, Boone RH, Masson JB, Al Ali A, Webb JG: Transapical transcatheter aortic valve implantation: 1-year outcome in 26 patients. *J Thorac Cardiovasc Surg* 2009; 137: 167-73

[52] Mukherjee C, Walther T, Borger MA, Kempfert J, Schuler G, Mohr FW, Ender J: Awake transapical aortic valve implantation using thoracic epidural anesthesia. *Ann Thorac Surg* 2009; 88: 992-4

[53] Johnston DR, Gillinov AM, Blackstone EH, Griffin B, Stewart W, Sabik JF, 3rd, Mihaljevic T, Svensson LG, Houghtaling PL, Lytle BW: Surgical repair of posterior mitral valve prolapse: implications for guidelines and percutaneous repair. *Ann Thorac Surg;* 89: 1385-94

[54] Carpentier A, Chauvaud S, Fabiani JN, Deloche A, Relland J, Lessana A, D'Allaines C, Blondeau P, Piwnica A, Dubost C: Reconstructive surgery of mitral valve incompetence: ten-year appraisal. *J Thorac Cardiovasc Surg* 1980; 79: 338-48

[55] Cubeddu RJ, Palacios IF: Percutaneous techniques for mitral valve disease. *Cardiol Clin;* 28: 139-53

[56] Rajagopal V, Kapadia SR, Tuzcu EM: Advances in the percutaneous treatment of aortic and mitral valve disease. *Minerva Cardioangiol* 2007; 55: 83-94

[57] Alqoofi F, Feldman T: Percutaneous approaches to mitral regurgitation. *Curr Treat Options Cardiovasc Med* 2009; 11: 476-82

[58] Alfieri O, Maisano F, De Bonis M, Stefano PL, Torracca L, Oppizzi M, La Canna G: The double-orifice technique in mitral valve repair: a simple solution for complex problems. *J Thorac Cardiovasc Surg* 2001; 122: 674-81

[59] Grossi EA, Bizekis CS, LaPietra A, Derivaux CC, Galloway AC, Ribakove GH, Culliford AT, Esposito RA, Delianides J, Colvin SB: Late results of isolated mitral annuloplasty for "functional" ischemic mitral insufficiency. *J Card Surg* 2001; 16: 328-32

[60] McGee EC, Gillinov AM, Blackstone EH, Rajeswaran J, Cohen G, Najam F, Shiota T, Sabik JF, Lytle BW, McCarthy PM, Cosgrove DM: Recurrent mitral regurgitation after annuloplasty for functional ischemic mitral regurgitation. *J Thorac Cardiovasc Surg* 2004; 128: 916-24

[61] Trichon BH, Glower DD, Shaw LK, Cabell CH, Anstrom KJ, Felker GM, O'Connor CM: Survival after coronary revascularization, with and without mitral valve surgery, in patients with ischemic mitral regurgitation. *Circulation* 2003; 108 Suppl 1: II103-10

[62] Feldman T, Kar S, Rinaldi M, Fail P, Hermiller J, Smalling R, Whitlow PL, Gray W, Low R, Herrmann HC, Lim S, Foster E, Glower D: Percutaneous mitral repair with the MitraClip system: safety and midterm durability in the initial EVEREST (Endovascular Valve Edge-to-Edge REpair Study) cohort. *J Am Coll Cardiol* 2009; 54: 686-94

[63] Carabello BA: The current therapy for mitral regurgitation. *J Am Coll Cardiol* 2008; 52: 319-26

[64] Feldman T, Wasserman HS, Herrmann HC, Gray W, Block PC, Whitlow P, St Goar F, Rodriguez L, Silvestry F, Schwartz A, Sanborn TA, Condado JA, Foster E: Percutaneous mitral valve repair using the edge-to-edge technique: six-month results of the EVEREST Phase I Clinical Trial. *J Am Coll Cardiol* 2005; 46: 2134-40

[65] Ussia GP, Barbanti M, Tamburino C: Feasibility of percutaneous transcatheter mitral valve repair with the MitraClip(R) system using conscious sedation. *Catheter Cardiovasc Interv* 2009

[66] Kahlert P, Plicht B, Janosi RA, Kamler M, Kuhl H, Eggebrecht H, Sack S, Buck T, Konorza T, Erbel R: The role of imaging in percutaneous mitral valve repair. *Herz* 2009; 34: 458-67

[67] Perk G, Lang RM, Garcia-Fernandez MA, Lodato J, Sugeng L, Lopez J, Knight BP, Messika-Zeitoun D, Shah S, Slater J, Brochet E, Varkey M, Hijazi Z, Marino N, Ruiz C, Kronzon I: Use of real time three-dimensional transesophageal echocardiography in intracardiac catheter based interventions. *J Am Soc Echocardiogr* 2009; 22: 865-82

[68] Silvestry FE, Rodriguez LL, Herrmann HC, Rohatgi S, Weiss SJ, Stewart WJ, Homma S, Goyal N, Pulerwitz T, Zunamon A, Hamilton A, Merlino J, Martin R, Krabill K, Block PC, Whitlow P, Tuzcu EM, Kapadia S, Gray WA, Reisman M, Wasserman H, Schwartz A, Foster E, Feldman T, Wiegers SE: Echocardiographic guidance and assessment of percutaneous repair for mitral regurgitation with the Evalve MitraClip: lessons learned from EVEREST I. *J Am Soc Echocardiogr* 2007; 20: 1131-40

[69] Argenziano M, Skipper E, Heimansohn D, Letsou GV, Woo YJ, Kron I, Alexander J, Cleveland J, Kong B, Davidson M, Vassiliades T, Krieger K, Sako E, Tibi P, Galloway A, Foster E, Feldman T, Glower D: Surgical revision after percutaneous mitral repair with the MitraClip device. *Ann Thorac Surg;* 89: 72-80; discussion p 80

[70] Wong MC, Clark DJ, Horrigan MC, Grube E, Matalanis G, Farouque HM: Advances in percutaneous treatment for adult valvular heart disease. *Intern Med J* 2009; 39: 465-74

[71] Otto CM, Mickel MC, Kennedy JW, Alderman EL, Bashore TM, Block PC, Brinker JA, Diver D, Ferguson J, Holmes DR, Jr., et al.: Three-year outcome after balloon aortic valvuloplasty. Insights into prognosis of valvular aortic stenosis. *Circulation* 1994; 89: 642-50

[72] Lieberman EB, Bashore TM, Hermiller JB, Wilson JS, Pieper KS, Keeler GP, Pierce CH, Kisslo KB, Harrison JK, Davidson CJ: Balloon aortic valvuloplasty in adults: failure of procedure to improve long-term survival. *J Am Coll Cardiol* 1995; 26: 1522-8

[73] Reginelli JP, Griffin B: The challenge of valvular heart disease: when is it time to operate? *Cleve Clin J Med* 2004; 71: 463-5, 469-70, 472 passim

[74] Wilkins GT, Weyman AE, Abascal VM, Block PC, Palacios IF: Percutaneous balloon dilatation of the mitral valve: an analysis of echocardiographic variables related to outcome and the mechanism of dilatation. *Br Heart J* 1988; 60: 299-308

[75] Chen G DT: Periperative Care in Cardiac Anesthesia and Surgery Lippincott, *Williams and Wilkins,* 2005

[76] Shook DC, Gross W: Offsite anesthesiology in the cardiac catheterization lab. *Curr Opin Anaesthesiol* 2007; 20: 352-8

[77] Latson LA: Transcatheter closure of paraprosthetic valve leaks after surgical mitral and aortic valve replacements. *Expert Rev Cardiovasc Ther* 2009; 7: 507-14

[78] Swiatkiewicz I, Chojnicki M, Woznicki M, Gierach J, Fiszer R, Sielski S, Kubica J: Percutaneous closure of mitral perivalvular leak. *Kardiol Pol* 2009; 67: 762-4

[79] Shapira Y, Vaturi M, Sagie A: Hemolysis associated with prosthetic heart valves: a review. *Cardiol Rev* 2009; 17: 121-4

[80] Kim MS, Casserly IP, Garcia JA, Klein AJ, Salcedo EE, Carroll JD: Percutaneous transcatheter closure of prosthetic mitral paravalvular leaks: are we there yet? *JACC Cardiovasc Interv* 2009; 2: 81-90

[81] Hensley FA: A Practical Approach to Cardiac Anesthesia. 2003

[82] Cortes M, Garcia E, Garcia-Fernandez MA, Gomez JJ, Perez-David E, Fernandez-Aviles F: Usefulness of transesophageal echocardiography in percutaneous transcatheter repairs of paravalvular mitral regurgitation. *Am J Cardiol* 2008; 101: 382-6

[83] Garcia-Fernandez MA, Cortes M, Garcia-Robles JA, Gomez de Diego JJ, Perez-David E, Garcia E: Utility of real-time three-dimensional transesophageal echocardiography in evaluating the success of percutaneous transcatheter closure of mitral paravalvular leaks. *J Am Soc Echocardiogr;* 23: 26-32

[84] Nollert G, Wich S: Planning a cardiovascular hybrid operating room: the technical point of view. *Heart Surg Forum* 2009; 12: E125-30

[85] Bashore TM, Bates ER, Berger PB, Clark DA, Cusma JT, Dehmer GJ, Kern MJ, Laskey WK, O'Laughlin MP, Oesterle S, Popma JJ, O'Rourke RA, Abrams J, Bates ER, Brodie BR, Douglas PS, Gregoratos G, Hlatky MA, Hochman JS, Kaul S, Tracy CM, Waters DD, Winters WL, Jr.: American College of Cardiology/Society for Cardiac Angiography and Interventions Clinical Expert Consensus Document on cardiac catheterization laboratory standards. A report of the American College of Cardiology Task Force on Clinical Expert Consensus Documents. *J Am Coll Cardiol* 2001; 37: 2170-214

In: Percutaneous Valve Technology: Present and Future
Editors: Jose Luis Navia and Sharif Al-Ruzzeh
ISBN: 978-1-61942-577-4

Chapter VI

Transcatheter Heart Valves: Development and Evaluation

Ernest Young and Melissa Young

Abstract

This chapter focuses on the engineering behind transcatheter heart valves (THV), both in scientific terms and in way of thought. It begins with a brief history of the development of artificial heart valves, encompasses the major advances along its path, and escalates to its current evolution. Each aspect of the THV implantation procedure, from crimping to valve implantation and function, is assessed for possible and proven risks and hazards. They are analyzed using the international standards for heart valve development and testing, in order to show the approach by which an engineer tackles the design and improvement of transcatheter heart valves. The chapter progresses on to materials currently used in THV applications, specifically conversing the advantages and obstacles of each material. Similarly, the material science behind balloon and self-expanding valve technology is summarized. Corrosion and biocompatibility are discussed to demonstrate the utmost need for proper material processing and stent design, followed by description of the tissue component, how it is modified, designed, and optimized. Lastly, the engineering evaluation of the THV is explained through the use of the international standards in order to shed light on additional clinical and engineering challenges required to develop a successful THV design.

1.0. Introduction

Surgically implanted artificial heart valves have a long history with more than half a century of development, industry support, academic research, clinical data and regulatory experience. These factors have created a large knowledge base for the engineering and design of surgical heart valves, which has driven the growth and understanding of artificial heart valves. Transcatheter heart valves (THV) is a relatively new term for a new technology, and is defined as artificial heart valve prosthesis that is delivered to the therapeutic site via catheter delivery. The available knowledge base on THV is relatively small in comparison, partly due to the relative infancy of THV development and partly because there is considerable overlap between surgical and transcatheter heart valves. Yet, the differences between the two heart valves types are significant and must be accounted for when developing a new THV.

This chapter will focus on the process of designing, engineering and testing an artificial heart valve, specifically transcatheter heart valves. This discussion will have a specific emphasis on the differences between surgical and transcatheter heart valve design considerations and the in vitro testing and in vivo evaluation requirements.

2.0. History of Heart Valve Development

The history of surgical cardiac valve implants dates back to Dr. Charles Hufnagel's implantation of caged ball valves in the descending aorta in 1952 [1,2]. After the invention and introduction of cardiopulmonary bypass in the 1960's the field of artificial cardiac valves was galvanized by the ability to perform surgery on the open heart [3-6]. Significant effort and engineering has gone into the evolution of this field with the result of two types of surgically implanted artificial heart valves: those of purely mechanical components and those made of xenograft material.

The first artificial heart valve type to be implanted and heavily developed was the purely mechanical valve design. Starting from the first Starr-Edwards ball-and-cage valve in 1960 [7] and evolving later into the tilting-disk valves in 1969 [8] and now to modern bileaflet designs introduced in 1978 [9]. These improvements have been made in an effort to develop better hemodynamic performance and to reduce thromboembolic complications seen in earlier designs [10]. Mechanical valves have many advantages including high durability, which makes them suitable for young patients. On the other hand, several undesirable traits of mechanical valves include the patient's increased risk of blood clotting and the need for anticoagulant therapies [11-12]. There are other concerns pertaining to the possible wear of the surface coatings on the mechanical components, and although uncommon, if they do fail it is typically a catastrophic failure [13].

The field of biological artificial valves initially started with homografts such as the Ross procedure and later on as allograft implants from cadavers. The field did not fully expand until a method of chemical fixation for both allograft and xenograft tissue was established which prevented host antigenic responses. This happened in 1969 with the modification of porcine aortic valves by glutaraldehyde fixation techniques [6]. The early bioprothestic valves were porcine aortic valves that had been treated with glutaraldehyde with rigid structural support (Hancock 1972, Medtronic, Minneapolis, USA; Carpentier Edwards Porcine 1970/1976, Edwards Lifesciences, Irvine, Ca). Subsequent advances included the use of fixed bovine pericardium in a flat sheet configuration as a leaflet substitute to make a fully manufactured pericardial bioprosthesis that could be engineered to exact specifications (Ionescu 1971) [14]. This approach allowed for specific leaflet geometries to be cut out and form pericardial valve designs, thus allowing a deviation from the set anatomy of the porcine aortic valve. Earlier versions of the pericardial bioprosthesis showed encouraging hemodynamics but poor fatigue life [15]. Improvements on the pericardial design (Carpentier-

Edwards Pericardial Valve 1980, Edwards Lifesciences) showed the same hemodynamic performance with improved durability and clinical performance [16-18]. Later trends in xenograft bioprosthesis saw the development of "stentless" porcine aortic valves technology with the driving force of improving hemodynamics. Although the developmental history of surgically implanted artificial heart valves spans back nearly six decades the history of transcatheter heart valves does not even cover half that distance. Conceptually the idea of an implanted catheter delivered heart valve dates back to 1965 when Davies tested catheter delivered valves for relief of aortic insufficiency in animal models [19]. Many early designs of catheter delivered valves were focused on relief or aortic regurgitation and were not applicable for permanent implantation.[20-21] That is until Dr. Henning Andersen designed and tested the first permanent catheter delivered aortic valve and implanted it into an animal model in 1989 [22]. The initial valve designed by Andersen consisted of a metal stent made from stainless steel wires normally used in thoractomy and a porcine cardiac valve sutured within the stent. [22, 23]

The progression after this point was slow, with its maturation most likely coinciding with concurrent advances in metallic stent processing technology as well as the rising therapeutic use and industry interest in endovascular stent technology. The first human implant of a THV wasn't until 2000 when Dr. Bonhoeffer implanted a stented valve (predecessor to the Medtronic Melody Valve) within the pulmonary valve position [24]. Soon after this in 2002, Dr. Alain Cribier implanted the predecessor to the Edwards SAPIEN transcatheter aortic valve in the human aortic position [25-26]. The interest of the medical community and industry has increased steadily to the point that there are now three commercially available catheter delivered bioprosthetic heart valves in Europe: the Medtronic CoreValve and Medtronic Melody (Figures 1c & 1d) (Medtronic, Minneapolis, MN, USA) and the Edwards Lifesciences Edwards SAPIEN and its successor the SAPIEN XT [27], (Edwards Lifesciences, Irvine, CA, USA) (Figure 1a & 1b).

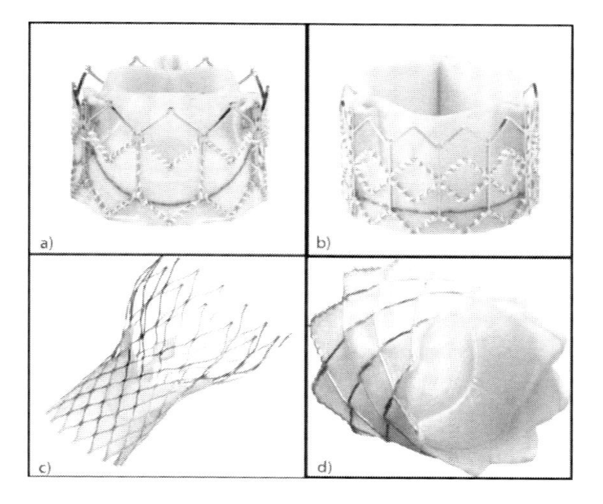

Figure 1a. Edwards SAPIEN with bovine pericardium leaflets and stainless steel stent frame. 1b) Edwards SAPIEN XT with bovine pericardium leaflets and cobalt-chromium stent frame (Pictures courtesy of Edwards Lifesciences, Irvine, CA, USA). 1c) Medtronic CoreValve with porcine pericardium leaflets and nitinol frame. 1d) Medtronic Melody transcatheter pulmonary valve made of bovine jugular vein valve and platinum-iridium stent(Courtesy of Medtronic, Minneapolis, MN, USA).

Many more different novel designs and second generation devices are being developed and some have already undergone clinical first-in-man implantations [28-35].

Similar to the first generation endovascular stents, the originally implanted transcatheter heart valves, the Bonhoeffer and Cribier designs, were balloon expanded designs that required a saline filled vavuloplasty balloon to expand the stented valves to the final diameter [24, 25]. Soon after this the Medtronic CoreValve had their first implant in 2006 by Grube et al, using a self-expanding shape-memory alloy, made a valve design that did not rely on balloon expansion [36-37]. Because of the continued demand for smaller device sizes, there has been a rising trend towards shape-memory self expanding designs in transcatheter valve research.

3.0. Designing a Transcatheter Heart Valve - Risks

The outcome of years of surgical heart valve research and clinical results has lead to the generation of regulatory guidance documents such as the FDA Draft Replacement Heart Valve Guidance [38] and the International Standard ISO 5840 on Cardiovascular implants – cardiac valve prosthesis [39]. These documents are a mixture of recommendations andguidelines that provide minimal functional requirements for artificial heart valves. However, their most important role is to provide a recommended process by which a medical device developer may take an early stage concept for a heart valve and create the documentation, conduct in vitro testing, preclinical in vivo and clinical studies necessary to start clinical trials. Thus lying down the groundwork toward eventual product regulatory approval and commercialization. These guidance documents usually contain nonbinding recommendations, in order to leave the guidelines flexible and to ensure that they do not restrict technological advancement.

The FDA Draft Guidance for Industry and FDA Staff on Heart Valves - Investigational Device Exemption (IDE) and Premarket Approval (PMA) was released on January of 2010 and represents an update from the previous version which was released in 1994 and withdrawn in 2005. The differences are many, but the current document presents the FDA's recommendations on cardiac valves that are either in addition or contrast to the recommendations in the International Organization for Standardization (ISO), ISO 5840:2005 "Cardiovascular Implants – Cardiac Valve Prosthesis." ISO 5840:2005 (which is an update from the 1996 version) is an internationally accepted standard that utilizes both clinical and academic data to create guidelines for in vitro, in vivo testing procedures and specifications as well as outlining recommendations for manufacturing, labeling and clinical investigations.

One of the key differences in both of these documents from their earlier versions is an emphasis on implementation of a risk-based approach towards all aspects of cardiac valve prosthesis development. Specific methods of risk analysis are outlined in ISO 5840:2005 and the current FDA Draft Guidance references the ISO 5840:2005 risk assessment methods and recommends their use (both documents also allow use of other equivalent risk analysis/assessment methods). The goal of this approach is to allow a flexible and adapting method to identify possible failure modes and hazards that can then be evaluated and mitigated by the heart valve developer. Methods of risk analysis such as that outlined in ISO 5840:2005 such as hazard analysis, failure mode and effect analysis (FMEA), and methods for estimating probability and severity of risk are also mentioned. An example of a hazard analysis based on ISO 5840:2005 and the risks discussed in this chapter is in Table 1.

Table 1. Example of Hazards, failure modes, mitigations and evaluation methods table, adopted from ISO 5840:2005

Hazard	Possible Failure Mode	Possible Mitigation Strategies	Possible In Vitro Evaluation Methods
Structural Degradation (Tissue)	Acutely: Crimp Damage Stent Surface Deformity	Crimper Design Implant Procedure Stent Processing	In vitro delivery system testing
	Chronically: Leaflet abrasion High Stress	Achieve Desired Geometry Accurately Model Patient anatomy	Hydrodynamic Testing Accelerated Wear Testing Computational Modeling In vivo animal studies Clinical Evaluation
Paravavlular Leak	Incorrect positioning	Implant Procedure Implant Design	In vitro delivery system testing In vivo animal studies
	Patient-Bioprosthesis Mismatch	Implant Design (Stent) Clinical Protocol Valve Size Specifications	In vitro delivery system testing Hydrodynamic Testing Clinical Evaluation
	Lack of Sealing	Additional Sealing Zone Additional Devices	Hydrodynamic Testing In vivo animal studies Clinical Evaluation
Cardiac Conduction Block	Low Implantation Excessive Oversizing	Implant Procedure Implant Design Clinical Protocol Valve Size Specifications	In vitro delivery system testing In Vivo animal studies

Ideally the risk-based approach starts early in the design phase when the product is still not in its final configuration. This risk assessment/analysis approach will help in the designing of the product, identification of the necessary functional testing (in vitro and in vivo), creation of design specifications, and help spur ongoing improvement of device design and function. Another goal is to encourage the communication and collaboration between medical device developers and regulatory bodies in the process of evaluating the necessary requirements to demonstrate the product's safety and efficacy.

As can be seen from the emphasis on risk analysis and management in the developmental process of cardiac valves, it is very important in the designing of transcatheter heart valves to identify and analyze the risks in all aspects of the device including but not limited to: the body's anatomy and biological response, valve design, and implantation procedure. The following sections will endeavor to identify some of these risks in the generic THV system particularly where they are unique to THV. Where possible some evaluation methods are suggested for risk mitigation but further discussion occurs later in the chapter. The explanation is not exhaustive and does not include much of the design of the delivery system, instead it is meant to shed light on the differences in certain risks between surgical and transcatheter cardiac valves and how to approach them from a valve design and engineering perspective.

The example template is a generic THV procedure as explained in literature: the THV is made of a metallic stent with tissue leaflets, it is crimped down to a smaller diameter upon a catheter, it is introduced into the vascular system through a small access point via introducer sheath, and it is delivered to the therapeutic site where it expands and functions.

Most of the current THV technologies currently being investigated or developed have been generated with the indication of aortic stenosis in mind [25-27, 36]. Aortic stenosis is one of the most common valvular diseases in Western society and its prevalence is growing with the aging population. [40, 41] Aortic stenosis is the indication for usage of THV in Europe and in investigational trials worldwide in select patient populations. [42]. The difference between surgical aortic valve replacement (AVR) and transcatheter aortic valve implantation (TAVI) for the treatment of aortic stenosis is that surgical AVR removes the calcified native aortic valve while TAVI implants the transcatheter aortic valve within the native aortic valve. Examining each procedural step of the transcatheter heart valve implantation we can evaluate the risks inherent to the steps. These steps are: the crimping of the valve, the delivery of the valve, the expansion of the valve, and finally the functioning of the valve. Each step will be explained in terms of engineering challenges both in designing the system and also the analysis of the risks associated with each step.

3.1. Crimping the Transcatheter Heart Valve

In the current field for THV there is a push towards miniaturization, namely the reduction in crimp profile of the device that must be introduced into the vascular system (the first generation Edwards SAPIEN was crimp profile 22 and 24 French evolving to second generation of 18 and 22 French, the first generation CoreValve was 25 French changing to a 21 than 18 French device in its current configuration). One of the main driving factors is the peripheral vascular disease seen in the patient population group, which limits the maximal size of a catheter that can have vascular access (Figures 2a & 2b). [37, 43-44] A decrease in crimp profile of the valve and catheter system will then increase the amount of patients that can be treated by including smaller and more tortuous vascular access sites. A reduction of crimp profile will also reduce the invasiveness of the procedure, decrease the probability of vascular complications and decrease procedural complexity and morbidity.

One of the important factors and engineering challenges in modifying crimp profile of the THV is the support scaffold which gives the valve its rigid structure. In almost all current first and second generation THV designs the rigid structure and collapsibility of the THV is due to the use of a metallic stent as the outer scaffold. [30, 46-47]

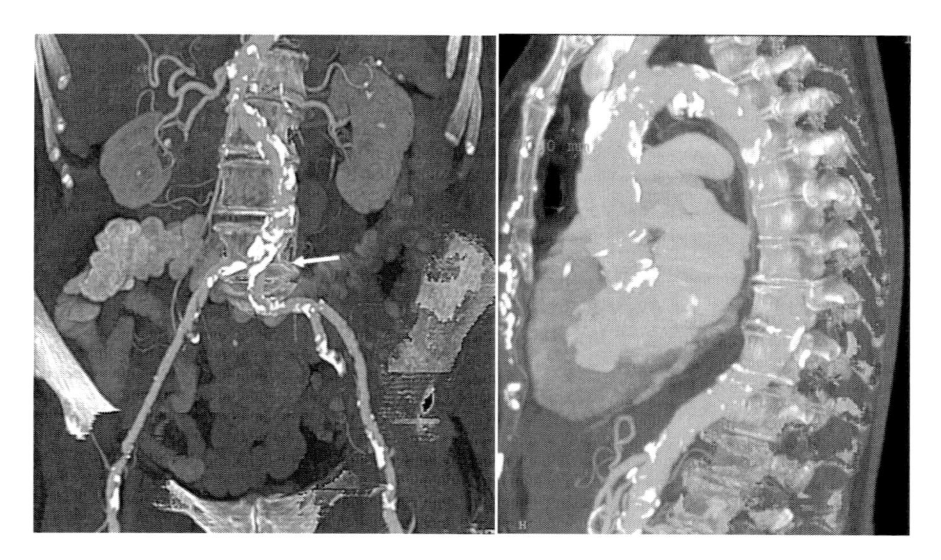

Figure 2a. CT angiogram of the abdominal aorta and the iliac/femoral arteries. Note the excessive wall calcification, as well as the high grade bilateral stenosis at the aortic bifurcation (arrow).] 2b) CT showing severe calcification of the ascending aorta starting 7 cm above the aortic valve level. The left subclavian artery is also unsuitable for TAVI. Reproduced with permission of author [60].

The use of a stent is intuitive as it is specifically designed to collapse into a smaller diameter for delivery and then expanded at the therapeutic site. The stent's design makes it capable of this change in geometry. Stents are generally manufactured from smaller diameter tubing, lasercut to form a pattern, expanded to the final diameter size, heat treated, and further processed to enhance biocompatibility and surface characteristics. The stent acts as a support scaffold for the valve components, which are attached to create a functional design. To modulate the final crimp profile, different stent designs, tube (stent) thicknesses, stent materials and internal valvular components can be and have been used. The material aspect of deciding the stent properties is detailed later in this chapter.

3.1.1. Crimp Damage

There are changes, perhaps irreversible, that the crimping procedure has on the valve components. Unlike a surgical BAV the implantation procedure of a THV requires a reduction in internal cross sectional area within the actual valve. [47] This "crimping" of the actual valve tissue has no precedence in the history of surgical BAVs, thus the THV must be engineered in such a way that crimping does not affect its future hydrodynamic and long term performance. Theoretically there is risk that crimping could cause damage to the leaflets (Figure 3), leaflet attachments or other nonvalvular components such as the delivery device it must be crimped upon [48]. This could cause compression or even "scissor" or shear like damage that can occur as the struts of the stent/scaffold collapse and come in or near direct apposition of each other. The design is thus crucial in minimizing this damage while still achieving the desired crimp profile. This may also include external devices that protect the components of the valve during the act of crimping.

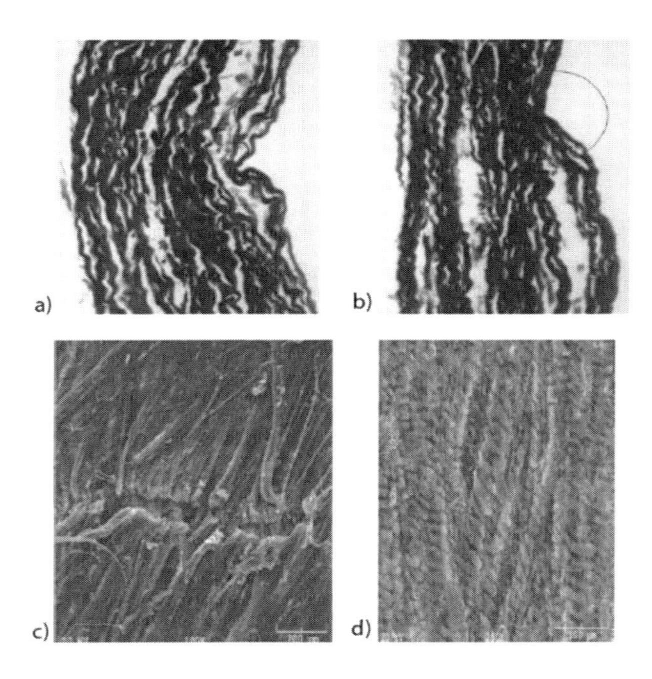

Figure 3. Damage to collagen fibers in leaflet tissue in a prototype valve under optical microscope 3a) slight damage and 3b) crease in circle due to crimp. SEM images of leaflet damage 3c) when compared to a normal leaflet 3d). Reprinted with permission of author [48].

3.1.2. Crimp Procedure

The way each valve is crimped is also important to the repeatability of the procedure. Thus the design of the crimping method should take into account the damage to valve components. During radial compression the materials within the THV (delivery system, leaflets, cloth, suture, etc.) may resist the compression with an outward force. This is important since after the removal of the crimping force, if done before the valve has reached the therapeutic site, may cause the instant relief of this outward force which will manifest itself as "recoil." Thus the intended crimp profile will not be achieved, despite the effort and control of the crimping procedure. If the recoil is known and accounted for in the procedure than it may be possible to still achieve the intended crimp profile by modifying the crimp procedure such as crimping to a smaller diameter (with the risk of increasing severity of any preexisting compression damage).

3.1.3. Symmetrical Crimp

The crimping procedure should be designed not just to achieve the desired crimp profile but also to confirm the valve is not asymmetrically crimped. This is an issue for balloon expanded THV models since self-expanding THV models will theoretically regain their original symmetry on self-expansion. Off-axis crimp with the stent/valve no longer in a cylindrical shape will affect the final expanded dimensions and also change the coaptation of the leaflets; affecting long term vavular hemodynamics of the expanded valve. Asymmetrical crimping may also cause unequal stress concentrations within the stent and the residual stress may cause damage to the frame affecting the strength of expansion and also the long term fatigue.

The risk for short term damage such as balloon puncture, delivery failure, leaflet tears, suture rips, etc. must also be accounted for and considered during the design of the THV and delivery system and procedure for crimping. The way to evaluate possible insidious long term damage would be in vivo and in vitro durability and wear testing that is explained later on this chapter. An example of a crimper used in the clinical field is in Figure 4

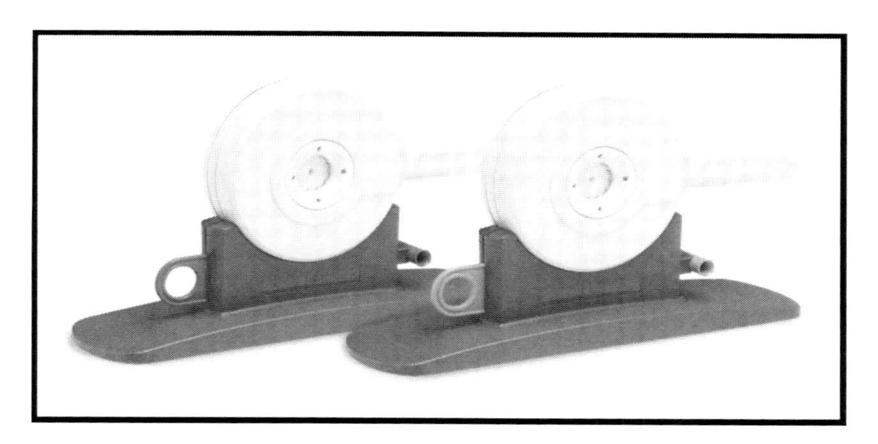

Figure 4. Crimpers used to crimp the Edwards SAPIEN. "O" ring attachments on the left help size the balloon and the gauge to the right help confirm the size of the crimped valve and delivery system. (Pictures courtesy of Edwards Lifesciences, Irvine, CA, USA).

3.2. Transcatheter Heart Valve Delivery

3.2.1. Vascular Injury

Once the valve has been crimped upon the catheter or delivery device it must now enter the vascular system. Many of the current THV systems utilize introducer sheath systems similar to other vascular entry devices, with corresponding dilators to increase size of the access site in order that larger sheaths can eventually be entered into the system [27, 36, 49-51]. Ideally the entry system should be done in the least traumatic method available without need for further surgery and reduction of complications such as vascular injury [52-55]. The force required to advance the catheter in the cardiovascular environment and through the introducer sheath should be minimized in order to prevent trauma and facilitate ease of use.

3.2.2. Dislodgement from Delivery System

The crimped THV is subject to friction forces and other pulsatile forces which may cause it to dislodge or move upon the delivery system . A system should account for this possibility because this can affect both the final expansion of the valve but also its placement at the therapeutic site. The design should be engineered in a way to secure the valve and assure that the valve will be delivered and expanded safely.

While tracking the device to the site the delivery system design must account for possibilities of traumatic complications. Recent literature has shown issues with the guidewire tips possibly causing tamponade by piercing the cardiac wall [37, 44]. Therefore the use of even normally available and frequently used devices such as guidewires and inflators should be accounted for in the design of the delivery system.

3.2.3. Accessing Implant Location

The environment of the calcified aortic valve varies significantly between patients [56-58] and the calcified pathology makes entry via retrograde means theoretically difficult [49, 59]. Early procedures of accessing the aortic valve used the antegrade approach using a tran-septal delivery route [25, 26[. Current procedures use a retrograde delivery and the challenges of this entry way have been already addressed but bear contemplating upon. Many of these calcified aortic valves have small and fused orifices that make it difficult to cross a delivery system across [59] (Figure 5).

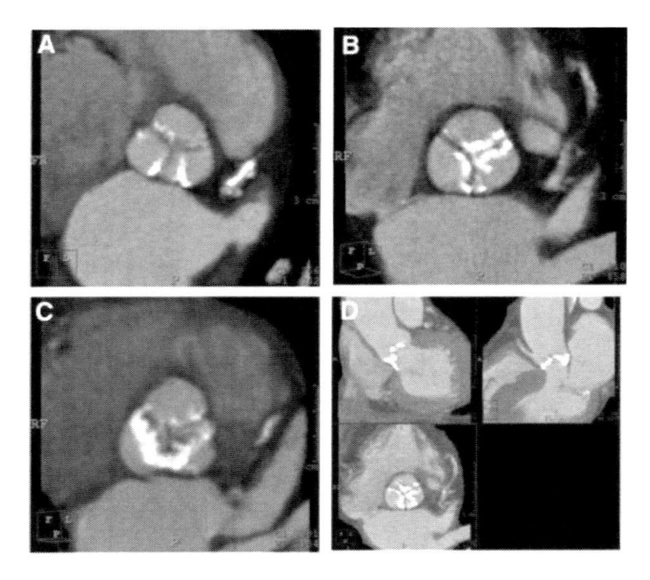

Figure 5. Variable calcification of the aortic annulus graded as: 5a) mild calcification, 5b) moderate calcification, 5c) heavy calcification, 5d) massive calcification with large calcific mass above the annulus. Reprinted with permission of the author [56].

This is especially true if the delivery system has large changes in geometry such as the differences in diameter between a guidewire and catheter and the large cylinder of an exposed crimped valve [49, 59]. Thus it is possible that the delivery system or valvemay not cross the stenosed valve. Another possibility is that crossing the stenosed valve may cause movement of the crimped valve upon the delivery system or damage the delivery system.

Current designs and engineering workarounds for this issue have been the development of delivery system modifications that use a cone nose-tip to help cross the valve into the left ventricle, thus reducing the sudden change of geometry (Figure 6) and by reducing the crimp profile. In addition most TAVI procedures pre-prepare the aortic valve with a standard balloon vavuloplasty before attempting to transverse the aortic valve with the delivery system and stent.

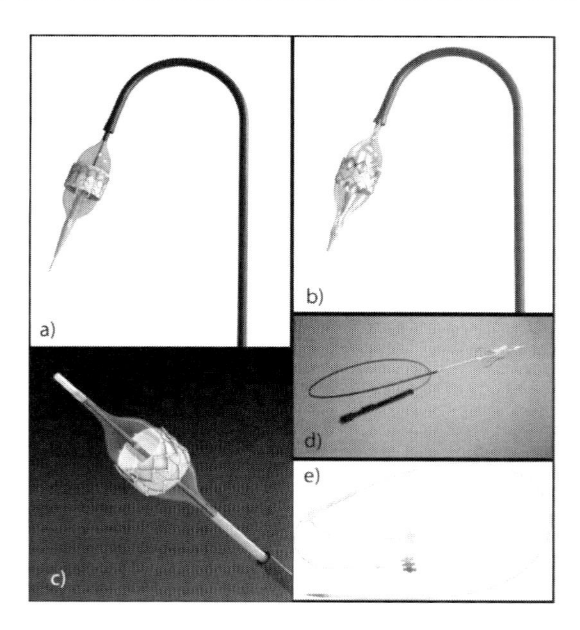

Figure 6a. Novaflex delivery system with 23mm Edwards SAPIEN XT 18 French delivery system. 5b) Retroflex III delivery system (22 French) with Edwards SAPIEN, 6c) Ascendra II transapical delivery system (24 French) for Edwards SAPIEN XT, 6d) Accutrack delivery system (18 French) for CoreValve, 6e) Ensemble delivery system (18, 20, 22 French) for Melody. Design demonstrates curving catheter to navigate the aortic arch as well as pointed tip distal catheter point for navigating through the calcific aortic valve retrograde. (Courtesy of Edwards Lifesciences, Irvine, CA, USA. Courtesy of Medtronic, Minneapolis, MN, USA).

3.3. Transcatheter Heart Valve Expansion

3.3.1. Expansion to Desired Geometry

Currently there are two possible transcatheter heart valve expansion methods: balloon expansion and self expansion. Balloon expansion is typically done with liquid with the stented THV crimped upon the balloon. The challenges behind designing a balloon expanded valve are assuring that the balloon expands the THV to the desired diameter or geometry from which it was designed to function. This means the balloon must have the proper amount of pressure to overcome the resistance to expansion from the THV stent/scaffold and any additional radial resistance such as that from the native cardiac valve leaflets at the implantation site. The risks of underdeployment and nonconcentric geometry have already been reported in clinical reports [55, 58, 61-63]. There is additional risk that the balloon my burst, a complication that has already been documented. The causes of this bursting can theoretically be the calcified nature of the aortic annulus, overinflation of the balloon, and sharp geometry of the THV stent, damage caused during crimping or damage that pre-existed in the balloon catheter. The balloon expansion method therefore should incorporate these design challenges and evaluate whether this failure mode is caused by the balloon device or the THV.

The self-expanding THV designs have utilized the shape memory alloy, nitinol, and do not require a forced expansion with a balloon. Instead the nitinol stent, which will be discussed later in this chapter, is constrained within the delivery device and at the implantation site they are slowly deployed via the exposure of the device from an inner sheath [36, 46]. The self expansion is an inherent property of nitinol and the final geometry, radial expansion force and other material properties can be modified.

Another difference in expansion between balloon expanded and self-expanding THV models has been a difference in the time needed for deployment (Balloon expansion expands the whole valve and takes seconds and is irreversible [49, 59], self-expansion can be deployed segmentally and can be prolonged to help positioning [64]. The final geometry after deployment is not reliant on the balloon expansion or balloon geometry but on the design of the nitinol stent and the anatomical variance at the aortic valve. Incidentally the risk for non-ideal configurations such as underexpansion can also occur with self-expanding models; therefore proper risk assessment of this occurrence should be implemented in the design and the expansion procedure [61].

In both balloon and self expansion of the valve, the expanding valve must overcome the constraints of the pathological anatomy to achieve the desired THV geometry. There have also been documented studies showing the existence large nodule calcifications in the aortic annulus, in the leaflet commissures, and even in the left ventricular outflow tract (LVOT) [56-58]. How these large solitary nodules affect the expanded valve has not been studied but remains a known environmental factor that should be considered in the integrity and ultimately the durability of the valve. [55, 58, 61-63] This point has been underscored by the known stent fracture issue of the pulmonary transcatheter valve, Medtronic Melody [65]. This stent fracture has now been theoretically attributed to a lack of correlation between the geometry of the stent when evaluated in vitro testing and computational modeling when compared to the actual geometry clinically [66].

3.3.2. Paravalvular Leak

Clinically there is a known issue of paravalvular leak which can persist long term. [37, 44, 53, 67-69] From a valve expansion standpoint this leak can be caused by the presence of calcium preventing complete sealing between stent and valve leaflet/annulus or the valve may be incompletely or improperly expanded. This is due to the implantation zone which can be highly variable due to presence of severe calcification or a nonconcentric left ventricular outflow tract (LVOT) [56-58, 70-71]. Most currently performed TAVI procedures include post-dilation of the valve after expansion (in both self-expanding and balloon-expanded models) to try and reduce the amount of improper sealing [72-74]. Self-expanding THV designs like the CoreValve are approached clinically via a "wait and see" approach since nitinol is known to expand slowly after deployment allowing for the possibility of reduction or regurgitation over time [64].

Another cause for paravalvular leak could be a prosthesis-patient mismatch. This is not wholly a valve design issue and currently is mitigated clinically by oversizing and thorough native valve size identification [75]. Paravalvular leak can also be caused by implantation of a valve that descends to far into the ventricle. All current valve designs have leaflets that coapt at a certain level of the whole valve; beneath this coaptation is the "sealing zone" which denotes a zone which lets through minimal blood if the valve is closed. However if the valve is placed too low in the native valve than blood can exit through the frame of the stent and when the valve coapts and back into the ventricle as regurgitation [76]. The current clinical approach if this occurs, is to either insert another THV into the previous THV ("Valve-in-

Valve") [76-81] or in the case of the CoreValve, a snaring procedure to grasp the distal portion of the device and move it towards the ascending aorta [82].

The clinical risks of the non-resolving paravavular leak are currently unknown even though it is currently well tolerated [83]. Yet lack of knowledge does not make it any less undesirable. From a valve design approach, two aspects of the valve that can be modified to prevent paravalvular leak is the stent and the sealing zone. From the stent there must be a trade off between rigidity and compliance. The stent must be rigid enough to have the radial strength to resist the external forces of the aortic annulus and calcification yet not too rigid so as to leave gaps between calcified native leaflets and the circular stent. Overly rigid balloon expandable stents are also prone to recoil which could lead to paravavular leak. The stent should also be compliant enough to allow for some conformity to the natural shape of the native environment, allowing for proper sealing. Yet, too much compliance can cause a reduction in fatigue strength and susceptibility to external forces.

Increasing the sealing zone will also help prevent paravavular leak as increasing this zone creates a larger portion of the stent that will not allow leakage. This adaptation is already seen in current designs with CoreValve which hasa porcine pericardial tissue sealing zone and the Edwards SAPIEN which has a polyethylene terephthalate "skirt." Another possible adaptation is the addition of a compliant and sealing buffer that attaches to the outside of the valve. Such a buffer would not only help smooth the areas of irregularity between the native annulus and valve but would prevent leakage. A previous design of the Edwards SAPIEN had such an adaptation[84]. Such a sealing device would increase the crimp profile of the valve and so would be less than ideal in a device that requires a minimum crimp profile to be therapeutically available.

Any such engineering design that addresses the risk of paravavular leak would need to adequately model the pathological anatomy to evaluate its function. In the case of sealing devices that require coagulation and wound healing to reduce leakage, only an in vivo evaluation would adequately minic this.

3.3.3. Accurate Positioning within Implant Zone

Complications with placing the THV in a position above the native valve include aortic dissection into the ascending aorta [85], blocking the coronary ostia with the stent or calcified leaflets, and the migration of the whole valve after expansion [44, 53]. Complications of low placement include cardiac conduction problems as the stent impinges on the conduction anatomy [86], perforation of the membranous interventricular septum [87], and even possible damage to the mitral valve due to direct abrasion against the THV stent. These complications are both an aspect of not just the implantation and expansion/placement procedure but are also due to the respective lengths of the THV designs. Longer designs would be more likely to cause complications such as those described above in areas farther from its intended therapeutic site (the native aortic valve in this case). The design should also recognize that a short valve design which would make accurate placement more technically difficult and might also lack the proper integrity. These complications with a "longer" THV design are difficult to evaluate outside the clinical or animal model arena and as such are harder to design for. This underscores the importance of accurate placement.

The shorter Edwards SAPIEN facilitates an accurate placement by using rapid ventricular pacing [89] during balloon expansion to prevent the movement of the THV. The Medtronic CoreValve uses its ability to stepwise deploy without pacing, readjustment using a snaring catheter and some mode of retrievability to mitigate the possibility of misplacement [64, 85]. These adaptations again are all clinical, the engineering challenge is to design a valve that can be accurately placed and that requires both an ability to reposition the placement of the valve once it is deployed and/or to ultimately retrieve a valve that has been improperly deployed. Some of the next generation valves such as the Lotus Valve (Sadra Medical Inc, Saratoga CA, USA) are in the process of addressing the issues if adjustability and retrievability [30].

3.4. Transcatheter Heart Valve Function

Historically the performance and long term characteristics of the surgical artificial valve and its' components has been documented and known hazards such as frame fracture, thromboembolism, paravalvular leak, etc. have all been well defined in the ISO 5840:2005 and FDA Heart Valve guidances. Therefore the in vitro, in vivo, and clinical testing required to fully characterize these issues as it pertains to surgical artificial valves has been well established [38-39].

However, when faced with the prospect of a transcatheter heart valve there are specific unique considerations that must be taken into account which will change the approach towards valve performance testing and characterizing. These include: a nonconcentric or underdeployed final geometry of the valve, the forces acting upon the valve, and the tenuous position of the valve within the pathological aortic valve. All these considerations must be analyzed both in terms of hydrodynamic performance impact and possible long term durability for performance implications.

3.4.1. Designing the Transcatheter Heart Valve for Irregular Anatomy

Noncircular final valve geometry has already been demonstrated in the literature [55, 58, 61-63, 90]. However, the possible geometries do not extend to just noncircular but also to any variance in geometry away from the designed intended shape, such as over and under deployments or even the hourglass shapes seen in some cases [62]. This would rarely if ever happen in a surgical valve which is designed in a certain shape and implanted non-deformed in the heart. Therefore it is imperative that the THV be designed to accommodate a variety of shapes after deployment and still maintain its hydrodynamic and durability performance. The hydrodynamic performance of the valve relies on the proper coaptation of the leaflets and accurate leaflet mechanics [62]. Non ideal geometry obtained during deployment of a transcatheter valve could result in lack of coaptation leading to central leakage through the valve and thus regurgitation and valve insufficiency. Also valve performance markers such as transvalvular pressure gradient and effective orifice area (EOA) would differ from that originally designed. The effects of noncircular geometry have not been well studied but changes that decrease diameter would theoretically lead to increase in pressure gradients across the valve and a decrease in EOA [90].

There would also be an effect on long term durability of the valve [91] and its components. One possible outcome is that the valve would fail faster than expected due to large and non-uniformly distributed stresses upon the leaflets. Large mechanical stresses have been documented to cause increase calcification and lead to valve failure [92-94]. These stresses could theoretically be caused by the improper coaptation of a valve due to non-circular geometry where one or multiple leaflets may be affected [58]. An underdeployment may also cause premature failure modes due to the excess leaflet material in the valve. These leaflet redundancy failure modes include increase abrasion of the leaflets against the surrounding metallic stent support and suture attachment weakening or tears at high stress locations due to the change in mechanics of the leaflet behavior. Leaflet abrasion may eventually lead to increased calcification or leaflet delamination that can cause a loss of durability in the implant or even failure via leaflet tearing [95-97].

The effects on the valve components are something that has not been well established, but the main concern for the implant durability remains to be the stent. It is recommended to use finite element analysis (FEA) to help accurately model the stent and valve design in order to identify the weakest area of the design, and determine if that design will provide the structural integrity needed for the valve support frame [38, 98]. If the difference in final deployment geometry is not taken into account the stresses that the stent actually experiences may be outside the tolerable range and could eventually lead to fatigue failure [66]. Likewise the use of FEA has been shown to be a useful tool in designing whole valves and valve leaflets [99-100]

These issues may be accounted for by designing the stent and valve to function in a variety of diameters and in a variety of shapes. It can also be approached by designing and controlling the deployment. For example, many current clinical procedures conduct a balloon vavuloplasty before implantation in order to break up the fused calcified valve and make the leaflets more compliant, reducing the risk that the native calcifiedleaflets would force the valve geometry into a undesired shape. This clinical adaptation could spur the movement towards creating and evaluating a vavuloplasty balloon that would work specifically with the device and achieve more desirable results.

There is currently a need to properly understand the native valve anatomy. Knowing the properties such as the force required to expand the leaflets, the hardness of the calcified nodules, the pulsatile force caused by the compliant contraction of the aorta with the heart, etc.; all this knowledge would give insight on the environment that the valve must contend with. Specifically when one runs a fatigue test on structural components of the valve (such as the stent), knowing what the forces the stent will see and experience is absolutely critical [66, 98]. The same can be said about any finite element modeling of the valve design which is usually used to help determine areas of high stress and therefore modify the design during the design phase. Validation of the FEA model is necessary since computational modeling requires many assumptions and approximations. The validation of the model can be done in numerous ways depending on design, but traditionally confirming fatigue performance and location of failure are used to assess the accuracy of the model predictions. Studies evaluating the interaction between the valve design and the calcified aortic annulus in cadavers or in a model may also help elucidate key features and risks. Knowing the extremes of calcification such as the large nodule size and density in the aortic annulus, can help provide input into analysis of failure modes and also aid in implementation of any dynamic failure mode (DFM) testing.

3.4.2. Migration of the Transcatheter Heart Valve

Migration is a very important concept that will be discussed because it is a key concern for transcatheter heart valves. Transcatheter heart valves do not have anchoring sutures that ground the implant like traditional surgical heart valve replacements, and therefore rely on the stent- annulus interface. Migration is a failure mode that has already been documented within surgical heart valves but the situation takes on a different meaning when the valve is not sutured within the annulus. In THV the implant instead sits within the aortic annulus and relies on an "interference fit." This "interference fit" is the combination of compressive radial forces of the anatomy, the opposing radial strength of the THV stent and friction between the stent and the possibly calcified surface of the annulus to cause the fixation of the expanded THV within the native valve. For balloon expanded valves, the expanded THV must retain its geometry and be able to resist the radial compressive force to ensure the maximum amount of the outer stent surface is in contact with the aortic annulus. Maximizing this surface contact increases the amount of "interference" leading to a tighter fit and less risk for migration but would also theoretically cut down on possible paravalvular leak. Self-expanding valves interact with their aortic annulus environments to the same degree except there is a "chronic outward force" due to their material properties and stent design which causes the stent structure to not just resist the radial compressive force but to combat it with its own outward force which can cause a gradual increase in valve diameter over time. This not only increases "interference" with the native valve, but also has a chance of increasing interference over time and possibly reducing paravalvular leak given time (thus the "wait and see" tactic explained earlier).

Another issue associated with valve migration is the positioning of the THV as explained earlier. If valves are designed to sit squarely within the annulus then placing the valve either too high or too low would decrease the amount of the outer stent that is in contact with the native aortic valve components. This is complicated by the high pulsatile pressures of the beating heart which can cause the valve to embolize into the ascending aorta or down into the left ventricle. The risk of this occurring can be addressed in both design and in procedure. For example, the self-expanding CoreValve has a modifiable step wise deployment allowing for accurate placement into the proper segment of the aortic annulus and also adds additional adjusting capabilities through "bail-out" procedures. This reduces the risk of an improper placement and thus the risk of migration [64, 85]. The CoreValve also further decreases the risk of migration by its valve design which has two areas of "interference fit" between its stent support and the anatomy, one in the aortic annulus and one in the ascending aorta, thus making the possibility of migration less likely. Even with these modifications, accidental improper placements still happens and migration can occur. Embolism of the valve, especially into the ventricle, is an indication for emergency corrective surgery, and thus considering that TAVI is only indicated for patients who cannot undergo traditional AVR; its occurrence must be strenuously avoided.

The long term possibility of migration must also be mentioned briefly. To date, during patient post procedure follow-up there has been no evidence of THV migration clinically, but the risk still remains. Theoretically the constant and cyclic pressure during the cardiac cycle could cause the valve to migrate down into the left ventricle. However this rarely happens theoretically due to the tight interference fitting of the THV designs within the aortic annulus, and due to long term tissue ingrowth into the THV, especially into regions that promote tissue ingrowth. This tissue ingrowth or wound healing process should theoretically cause an increase in the bond between the THV and its environment overtime, making the risk of valve migration less likely with time.

In summary, the whole valve function is heavily dependent on its final geometry, its placement within the aortic annulus and long term factors contributing to its durability. Some of these issues were briefly described in light of their current clinical equivalents in the literature. It is imperative that design and the procedure of the transcatheter heart valve being developed consider these technical challenges and reduce the probability of their occurrence.

4.0. Material Design Consideration

The field of transcatheter heart valves is technically very young, with many designs being developed and with very few commercially available designs. The literature therefore on the development of THV designs is sparse and long term data is not readily available. In many ways the THV, which is in the most general description is a stented heart valve, shares the similar technological history and knowledge base with intravascular stents and artificial bioprosthetic heart valves especially in reference to material considerations. Their experiences will serve as a background when discussing the selection of materials available for developing a THV.

The materials detailed in this chapter are those being proposed in literature and their relevant material properties will be discussed. The components of the transcatheter heart valve (THV) include: the metallic stent, leaflets and accessory sealing components. Due to the lack of long term and comparative studies of the available designs, many of the pros and cons of the material selections are either theoretical or currently unknown. Where available the known material properties of particular components will be discussed in direct comparison.

4.1. Metallic Stent

The stent structure of the transcatheter heart valve is one of the most critical components. It is the crux to the THV's ability to be delivered via catheter and it also serves as a support scaffold for the intravalvular components, including the leaflets. There are currently two types of stents being used in the field today and these are balloon expanded and self-expanding stents. The balloon expanded stent should be able to be crimped down for delivery, expanded plastically at the therapeutic site, and the expanded valve/stent should maintain its geometry in the delivered position. A self-expanding stent should be able to be crimped into a delivery device as well but should have enough elasticity to not only expand at the therapeutic site but be able to overcome radial compressive forces in order to achieve its desired shape. The general traits for a THV stent scaffold is that it must have: minimal crimp profile to allow vascular access and crossing of stenosed valves, adequate expansion at the site in order to push aside native leaflets/diseased anatomy and achieve desired geometry, conformity to the therapeutic site so that there is minimal paravalvular leak, and sufficient radial hoop strength and negligible recoil such that the expanded valve will be able to maintain its geometry and not be deformed by compressive forces. The stent must also have acceptable radiopacity/magnetic resonance imaging compatibility for assistance during in vivo implantation and must be thromboresistive to prevent blood clotting and embolism. The traits related to crimping and expansion are related not only to the material selection but also the design of the THV and the method of expansion. The radiopacity, MRI compatibility, and thromboresistive traits are more inherent to the metallic stent material used. [102, 103]

There are four transcatheter heart valves currently marketed in Europe. Three of them are indicated for aortic stenosis (Edwards SAPIEN & Edwards SAPIEN XT, Edwards Lifesciences, Ca, USA and CoreValve, Medtronic, Minneapolis, MN, USA) and one of them is indicated for pulmonary valve/conduit stenosis (Melody, Medtronic, Minneapolis, MN, USA). All four of these valves use different metallic stent materials: Edwards SAPIEN uses a Stainless Steel material [25], SAPIEN XT utilizes a Cobalt Chromium frame [27], CoreValve has a superelastic nitinol stent [36], and the Melody has a Platinum-Iridium scaffold [24]. These metals all have historic use in medical devices, specifically in endovascular stent products. Because of the similarities in design and desired function the extensive literature and clinical history relating to the performance of these materials in stents is applicable to this discussion as a stent scaffold for a THV.

4.1.1. Stainless Steel

Stainless steel is one of the most commonly used biomaterials for medical implant applications. It has a long history of use in dental, orthopedic and recently in endovascular stents [10, 104]. It is the most common material used for balloon expanded endovascular stents, and is historically the material used for the first FDA approved endovascular stent, the Palmaz-Schatz stent, which is now used as an industry standard. The most common of the stainless steels used in endovascular implants is the stainless steel alloy 316LVM ("L" denotes low carbon content, "VM" for vacuum melted) which is detailed under ASTM F138 [105]. The low carbon content and the vacuum melting creates an alloy with minimal voids and contaminants and a reduction in carbide precipitates that reduce corrosion resistance in other stainless steel alloys [11, 106]The addition of elements such as Mo, Cr and Mn and low amounts of sulphur and phosphorus also add to its corrosion resistance.

The material properties are well established (Table 2) and its history makes it one of the most widely known biomaterials with regulatory bodies as well as being widely available from manufacturers. The disadvantages of stainless steel 316LVM in endovascular stent include its poor MRI and fluoroscopic compatibility and issues with its biocompatibility. The 316LVM is 60-65 wt% pure Fe and thus is ferromagnetic which theoretically makes it non-MRI compatible and also has low density making it hard to view on fluoroscopy. The biocompatibility of stainless steel is related to the release of ions from the implant such as nickel, chromate and molybdenum which has been shown to activate inflammatory reactions leading to restenosis in endovascular applications [107].

However, all these above disadvantages are from the endovascular stent application of 316LVM. The Edwards SAPIEN balloon-expanded transcatheter heart valve is made of a stainless steel stent scaffold with sizes ranging in the 23mm-26mm range. These large sizes make the low density not a concern for fluoroscopic visualization of transcatheter heart valves in this size range as clinical studies have shown; the Edwards SAPIEN is visible under fluoroscopy [56]. As for biocompatibility the concern of nickel and other ion leeching is always a concern if the patient has allergic reactions to nickel [108]. However, the issue of restenosis is not as much a concern in the transcatheter replacement of heart valves as it is with endovascular stenting, as the implant site is not subject to intimal hyperplasia. Although theoretically a poor biocompatibility response in a stainless steel THV device may cause an increase in tissue ingrowth and pannus overgrowth [109] which may lead to long term valvular failure. The Edwards SAPIEN valve made of stainless steel, and is currently the

THV with the longest implant history to date and it has shown acceptable biocompatibility, fluoroscopic compatibility, and corrosion resistance. [42, 53]

Table 2. Material Properties of different metallic options for THV stent. Properties from tubing stock [130-131] Reprinted with permission of author [130]

	Density (gr/cm3)	Elastic ModulusS (GPa)	Ultimate Tensile Strength (MPa)	0.2% Yield Strength (MPa)	UTS - Yield (MPa)	Elong (%)	Elastic Range (%)*
Stainless Steels							
Fe-18Cr-14Ni-2.5Mo "316LVM" ASTM F138	7.95	193	670	340	330	48	0.17
Cobalt Alloys							
Co-20Cr-35Ni-10Mo "MP35N" ASTM F 562	8.43	233	930	414	516	45	0.18
Co-20Cr-16Ni-16Fe-7Mo "Phynox" ASTM F 1058	8.30	221	950	450	500	45	0.20
Precious							
Pt-10Ir	21.55	150	340	200	140	25	0.13
Nitinol							
Martensitic	6.45	40	1200	200-300	900-1000	25	1.9
Cold Worked 40%	6.45	40	1450	NS	NS	12	4-6
Superelastic ASTM F2063	6.45	90	1137	-	-	10	6-8

*Elastic range denotes maximum recoverable strain and quantifies the superelastic behavior of nitinol.

4.1.2. Cobalt-Chromium

Cobalt-Chromium alloys have an extensive history in implants similar to stainless steel. Like stainless steel Co-Cr alloys also consisted of many blood contacting implants such as endovascular stents, stent grafts, and pacemaker leads. In endovascular stent design there was a shift towards thinner struts after the ISAR-STEREO clinical trial showed that stent designs with thinner strut thicknesses caused lower restenosis rates [110]. This caused a push towards finding higher strength stent materials that would allow balloon expanded stents to be designed with reduced strut thickness but with comparable strength. The rational was that the reduced thickness would result in less vascular trauma [111] but also that the reduced thickness would lead to a more flexible device that had a smaller diameter that could cross through smaller diameter lesions. It is this same push towards reducing device profile and strut thicknesses without sacrificing material properties that has driven the same shift in Transcatheter Heart Valves. Most notably the second generation balloon expanded aortic THV the Edwards SAPIEN XT which is made from a cobalt chromium alloy stent. The push in this case is the diameter of the access site, as patients with severe peripherally vascular disease are thus unable to undergo the less traumatic vascular access procedures.

Cobalt chromium alloys have already been used in the surgical heart valve industry for many years. The use of Elgiloy (ASTM F1058 [112]) a Co-Cr alloy has been used as the metal of choice for metallic wireforms in surgical bioprosthetic heart valves for decades with good durability and clinical performance [113]. This same Co-Cr alloy has also been used in the self-expanding Wallstent (Boston scientific Corp., Natick, Ma) for many years. However both of these applications use Elgiloy wireform which is different than the tubing required to laser cut endovascular stents and more to the point, transcatheter heart valve stents. The two Co-Cr alloys currently used in endovascular balloon-expandable stents are the L605 alloy (ASTM F90 [114]) used in the Multi-Link Vision coronary stent (Abbott Laboratories, Abbott Park, IL) and the MP35N alloy (ASTM F562 [115]) used in the Driver coronary stent (Medtronic Inc., Minneapolis, MN). Both of these alloys show increased strength compared to stainless steel (Table 2) [116]. Additional advantages to the use of Co-Cr is that it has a high density and is non-ferromagnetic making it radiopaque and MRI-compatible. It also has high strength, high elastic modulus and good corrosion resistance (table 2).

4.1.3. Platinum Iridium

Platinum 90% - Iridium 10% has been used as pacemaker electrodes medical devices, and as radiopaque coatings and markers, and has garnered some interest in the endovascular stent world [121-124]. This is due to its excellent radiopacity and corrosion resistance [124]. The Platinum-Iridium alloy is currently used in the pulmonary transcatheter heart valve (Melody, Medtronic Inc., Minneapolis MN) although the 2nd generation model uses gold reinforcements at the weld points for additional mechanical support. The disadvantages to this alloy are its relatively lower mechanical properties (Table 2) compared to the other metals, especially its ultimate tensile strength (UTS). This would indicate not only lower material strength and fatigue performance, but also that larger struts would be necessary for adequate strength and thus a sacrifice of crimp profile would be needed. The clinical data on the Melody valve which has spanned more than half a decade and includes several hundred human implants and commercial availability in Europe, suggests adequate blood-contacting biocompatibility of the material in the pulmonary valve position [125]. However the data base and literature on this alloy for use in blood-contacting devices is still for the most part unexplored.

4.1.4. Nitinol

Nitinol is a nickel titanium alloy composed of near equitomic mixture of nickel and titanium with 49.7-57.5 % nickel depending on desired material properties. Nitinol is capable of solid state phase transformations which can be induced by temperature change ("Shape Memory") or by stress ("Superelasticity"). What this means generally speaking is that nitinol is capable of achieving large elastic deformations of up to 10% before being plastically deformed giving the stress strain curve a pronounced hysteresis that is very similar to physiological materials (Figure 7). The mechanical properties and unique features of nitinol will be explained later in this chapter but it is important to note that nitinol is used in the only self-expanding THV, CoreValve (Medtronic). It is self expanding due to its shape memory effect which is already been utilized in numerous approved nitinol stents. Nitinol is processed in such a way that the parent phase (Austenite which is less deformable and more ordered) exists at body temperature and the other phase (Martensite which is highly deformable) exists at a lower temperature. Thus a nitinol transcatheter heart valve or endovascular stent would be designed to be at a smaller diameter at low temperatures during the crimping procedure and have a large diameter when at body temperature and deployed into the body. [125-127]

Nitinol therefore is self-expanding and does not theoretically require a balloon catheter in order to expand the valve to its operational diameter within the annulus. The material itself has good corrosion resistance [128] and it is generally accepted that processing of the material changes the corrosion characteristics of the material. Processing, specifically surface passivation and electropolishing effects nickel release and biocompatibility. The clinical data on the CoreValve to date does not show any issues with thrombogenicity or lack of biocompatibility of nitinol stent within the aortic annulus. Additionally, although some nitinol stents are not fluoroscopically visible [129] due to their small size, there has been no issue with the CoreValve which is a very large stent exclusively deployed under fluoroscopic guidance.

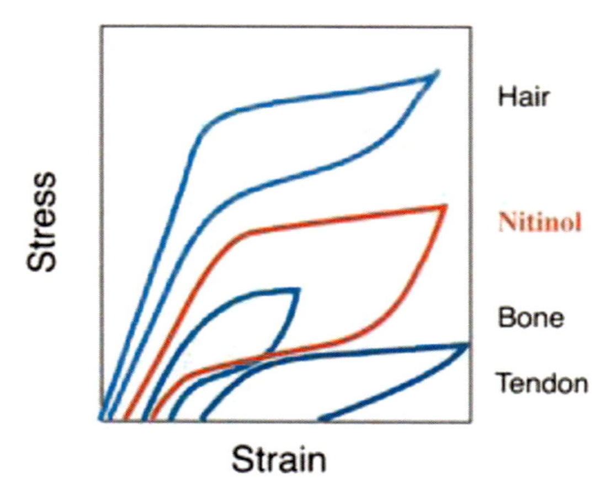

Figure 7. Characteristic stress-strain curve with deformation similar to other physiological tissues. Reprinted with permission of author [126].

4.1.5. Comparison of Properties

The material selection process requires some scrutiny when embarking on the beginning stages of design. The properties listed here are the Young's modulus (E), ultimate tensile strength (σ_{UTS}), UTS – yield or yield strength (σ_y), 0.2% yield strength (0.2% σ_y), percent elongation at break (% Elongation,) and elastic range.

The concept of stress is defined as the force per unit area (such as N/m^2 or psi). The definition therefore of yield strength (σ_y) is the stress value at which the material experiences irreversible and plastic deformation. The ultimate tensile strength (σ_{UTS}) is the highest stress that the material can handle before failing. Strain on the other hand is a measurement of deformation that the material experiences while under stress. The relationship between given amounts of stress and its respective strain is called the Young's Modulus (E) which is a measure of stiffness.

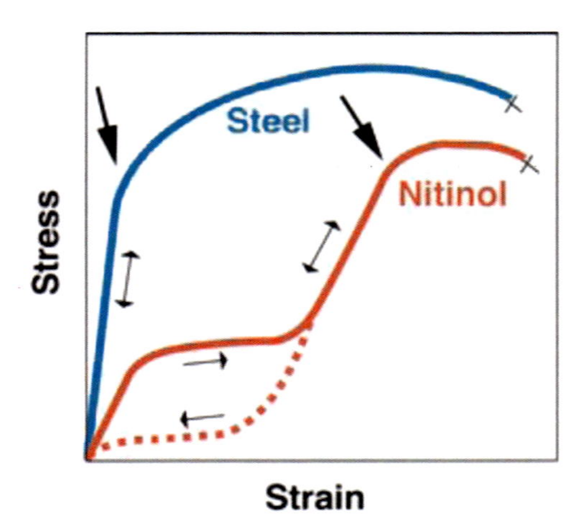

Figure 8. Stress-strain curve for nitinol and Stainless Steel. Nitinol curve shows characteristic loading/unloading curves with large deformations (strains) without significant increase in stress. Arrows show difference location of relative yield strengths of the two materials. Reprinted with permission of author [126].

In the traditional stress strain curve of a material, stress is on the vertical axis and strain on the horizontal axis. For a given amount of stress there will be a proportional amount of strain. The slope of the relationship will be linear up to the point of the yield strength (σ_y); the slope of the linear portion is generally denoted as the Young's Modulus. Conceptually a large Young's Modulus would mean for a given amount of stress there is less strain, and the material would be "stiffer." The percent elongation to break is instead a measure of ductility. The elastic range is mainly applicable to nitinol and demonstrates the maximum recoverable elastic strain that the material can withstand before plastic deformation. This is a measure of the "superelasticity" of nitinol that can withstand from 8-10% strain without permanent deformation unlike most metals that are plastically deformed after less than 1%. (Figure 8) [126, 132]

4.2. Translation to Stent Design

The usefulness of each mechanical property depends greatly on the application, anatomy and delivery method of the transcatheter heart valve being designed, but there is some knowledge to be gained from comparing values of different materials. However, the materials need to be separated by application as stent components of balloon expanded transcatheter heart valves have different requirements than self-expanding heart valves.

4.2.1. Balloon-Expanded Transcatheter Heart Valves

For balloon-expanding valves it is given that the valve must be crimped upon a balloon and then expanded by a balloon at the site via plastic deformation. In both of these instances the material is plastically altered, first by crimping and then by balloon expansion, therefore relatively low yield strength is necessary for this to occur. High yield strength would necessitate very large forces to crimp the valve and very large pressures within the balloon to expand the valve. The force required to plastically deform an expanded stent is called *Hoop strength* and it is the force that must be over come to crimp the valve, expand the valve, and ultimately the force that would be overcome if the anatomical forces would later deform the implanted valve.

The Young's Modulus (E) is important to this discussion as it denotes the slope of the stress/strain curve and thus the ease (the amount of stress needed) by which the hoop strength is overcome to cause plastic deformation. A low Modulus (E) would facilitate expansion due to its larger strain per unit stress. The downside is that when the valve is expanded, a high Modulus (E) would resist any elastic/plastic deformation due to its very small strain per unit stress. The Modulus (E) value would also indicate the degree of elastic recoil after the balloon is deflated. A material with a large Modulus (E) would be predicted to have larger recoil as greater amounts of the stent component had not reached its yield strength and therefore still reside in the elastic region, causing elastic recoil. Thus a stent with a high elastic modulus would be difficult to crimp and expand, and also might have high elastic recoil after balloon expansion, yet the high Modulus (E) would make the stent very resistive to deformation by external forces once implanted. [102, 132]

The ultimate tensile strength (σ_{UTS}) is important to the overall radial strength and resistance to fatigue. A high σ_{UTS} would also indicate that less material can be used in the stent design overall, which is beneficial for the THV since it would indicate a reduction in strut thickness leading to improved crimp profile. The difference between σ_{UTS} and 0.2% σ_y is important for balloon expanded THV designs since it demonstrates the slope of the work hardening curve which affects the forces required for deployment and the strength of the deployed/implanted stent. The concept of work hardening is summarized as an increase of the yield stress (σ_y) of the material caused by plastic deformation. Plastic deformation causes permanent strain in a material and also increases the stress at which a subsequent deformation can be achieved. Therefore a balloon expanded material would want a sufficiently large difference in the σ_y and σ_{UTS} as this would mean that an expanded valve would have higher *hoop strength* and not compromise integrity by being too close to the failure point, σ_{UTS}. Similarly the ductility of the material (denoted here as % elongation to break) is an important factor as it denotes the amount of deformation (and thus the amount of relative expansion) the material can see before it fractures.

How this discussion relates to the materials currently used for balloon expanded transcatheter heart valves really is a debate of compromise and desired outcomes;where tradeoffs between material properties must be balanced with the desired therapeutic effect and performance.

The materials currently used: Stainless Steel, Cobalt-Chromium, and Platinum-Iridium can be compared. Stainless steel has a very long history in the use of endovascular stents and its choice is a good balance of properties in terms of modulus, yield strength, ductility and cost. The advantages of cobalt chrome comparatively to stainless steel is a higher density, Young's Modulus, yield strength, difference between its yield strength and ultimate tensile strength all while having a similar ductility to stainless steel. The higher tensile strength makes it desirable due to the ability to reduce strut thickness and overall crimp profile. However the higher yield strength and modulus would potentially mean higher necessary forces to deform the valve during crimping and expansion, and also larger recoil.

Platinum-iridium has comparatively lower values in almost all categories except density (the major reason it is used in many radiopaque markers). The benefit to the lower modulus and yield strength means lower pressures needed to crimp and expand and thus easier plastic deformation of a stent that would likely conform to the anatomy of the implant site. The lower modulus allows for crimping the device manually, without the aid of a mechanical crimper machine. However, the low UTS combined with the smaller difference between yield strength and UTS means that the material has a weaker fatigue resistance necessitates larger strut widths for adequate radial strength and has a yield strength that is close to its UTS, which increases the risk for failure during deformation. However, it is not just the material properties that are important in the material choice as will be explained later on in this chapter. [130]

4.2.2. Self-Expanding Transcatheter Heart Valves

Self-expanding transcatheter heart valve designs such as the CoreValve and many proposed second generation designs are made up of nitinol. The unique mechanical properties of nitinol bear a more detailed explanation due to its difference from other metals. The ability of nitinol to undergo solid-state phase transformations due to increased strain or change in temperature leads to a unique stress and strain relationship. The response to stress is called "superelastic" and refers to the ability of nitinol to yield to an applied stress by changing its molecular crystal structure i.e. phase shifting from an austenite to martensitic phase. This is demonstrated by nitinol's reversible elastic deformation of up to 10% [126]. This can be seen on the stress-strain curve (Figure 8) which is more similar to biological materials than metallic. In contrast, materials such as stainless steel only have up to 1% elastic strain before the material is irreversible deformed.

The thermal response is called "shape memory" and it is a result of a phase transformation due to changes in temperature of the material. When nitinol is cooled below its transformation temperature it changes molecular crystal structure from austenite to martensite. The martensitic phase can be easily plastically deformed into different shapes via external forces, however upon heating the material above its transition temperature it regains its previous "memorized" shape. This is the property which is utilized in nitinol transcatheter heart valves as the nitinol support stent is cooled below its transformation temperature in a cold environment, crimped (plastically deformed) down to a smaller diameter and placed within a restraining catheter. Once inside the body the nitinol reaches body temperature at which point, if the nitinol's transition temperature is below body temperature, it would want to achieve its original diameter and thus release of the stent from the catheter causes it to regain its original shape. The transition temperature is also dependent on material processing such as heat treatments, thus it is usual methodology for stents is to have the transition temperature be below body temperature.

The unique properties of nitinol stents are explained by the terms "radial resistive force" and "chronic outward force." The self-expansion of nitinol can be explained by the unloading curve of the stress-strain curve, as the reduced diameter (compressed) stent, unloads its stress down the unloading curve it expands (relieves strain) back to its original geometry. However if one were, during unloading, to try and re-crimp or compress the stent it will resist this deformation due to a shift to the loading plateau of the stress-strain curve. In practice this means that the stent will resist compression from external sources such as pulsatile movements of vasculature of the heart. This is unlike hoop stress which involves the yield strength of traditional metals and is a resistance to permanent plastic (yield) deformation of the metallic stent; instead the nitinol stent resists compression with "radial resistance force."

In the event that the radial resistance force is overcome and the stent is deformed, the deformation will be elastic (unless the strain exceeds the maximum allowable).

The "chronic outward force" is not the force by which the nitinol resists compression but the force by which the nitinol expands outwards. This force is only present when the nitinol is being compressed ("Strained") so that the stent exerts force outwards toward the constraining environment. This force is "chronic" because it exists so long as the nitinol is not in its shape ingrained in its "shape memory." Thus it is important that the nitinol transcatheter Heart valve be implanted into valve annulus smaller than its natural diameter such that the nitinol is compressed and thus the "chronic outward force" can resist migration and shear stresses via its tight friction fit with the surrounding environment. [133] In some clinical cases the nitinol CoreValve even continued to expand outwards after implantation which theoretically created a tighter seal between the non-homogenous surface of the calcified valve and the CoreValve and reducing paravalvular leak [63].

Figure 9 explains the crimping and expanding of a nitinol superelastic stent and thus can be related to the nitinol CoreValve. The graph represents crimping with the axis switches from stress and strain to hoop force and stent diameter, the mode is compression. The explanation will be given in terms of a self-expanding transcatheter heart valve. A THV stent larger than the valve annulus to be implanted in (point a) is crimped into its delivery system to a constrained diameter (point b, original diameter not on scale, expansion of the valve goes towards a).

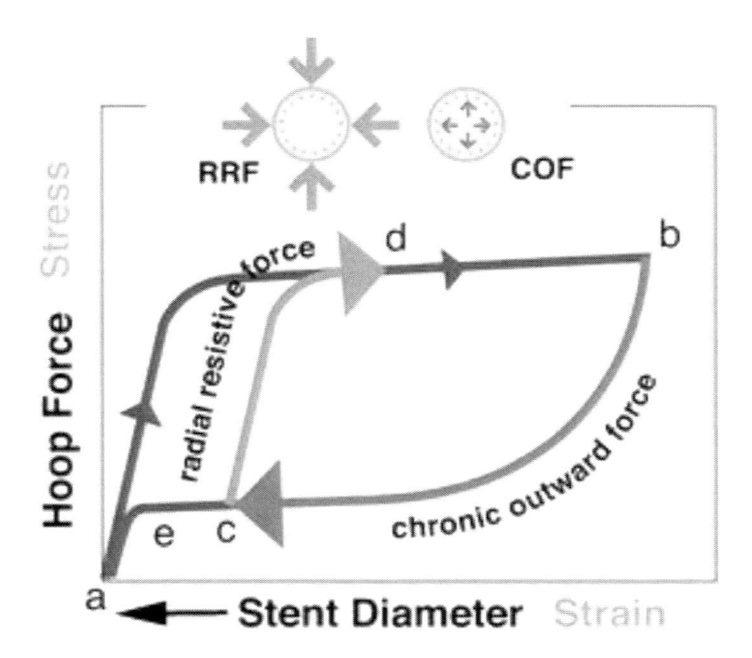

Figure 9. Nitinol stent deployment with radial resistive force and chronic outward force.

After accessing the implantation site the THV is released where it unloads until reaching the native valve at point "c." At this point the valve is constrained and has still not achieved its natural diameter and thus exerts a "chronic outward force" on the constraining native valve in a effort to unload its strain (towards point "e" and "a" and beyond). This is the "chronic outward force" that is by design continue to increase the diameter of the THV and thus achieve better geometry and better sealing with the native valve. Additionally, any external force that then acts on the THV to compress it (such as pulling of the stent inwards by the closing valve) as well as any recoil force will be resisted by the "radial resistive force" (from point "c" to "d"). This radial resistive force travels up a steeper slope than the chronic outward force and is thus stronger (however once the radial resistive force is overcome and the hoop-force and diameter curve is on the loading plateau the THV will than deform). [126]

In light of this explanation of the mechanics of nitinol the material properties cannot be looked upon in the same light as the traditional metals of balloon expanded valves. The elastic modulus of nitinol is small yet the range is large due to the superelasticity that causes an increased strain without increased force due to phase transformations. It also has comparatively high yield and tensile stress. Different mixtures of nitinol alloy containing variable amounts of Nickel and Titanium are also capable of different mechanical properties that are vastly different than the archetypical superelastic and shape memory version that is currently used in transcatheter heart valves. [130]

Nitinol is a promising metal for THV applications. Oversizing, the act of putting a larger THV into a smaller valve, increases the chronic outward force of the THV thus pushing aside the native valve and also sealing the stent against any irregularities in the native annulus. There is no concern for recoil like in balloon-expanded THV. Additionally the superelasticity allows for great amounts of deformation without plastically yielding the material, allowing the elastic crimping of the valve down to very small crimp profile. Its shape memory properties allow the configuration of THV shapes that could not be expanded on a cylindrical expandable balloon, and its superelasticity allows those shapes to be crimped without permanent strain.

5.0. Corrosion

Metallic biomaterials are subject to corrosion, an electrochemical reaction which causes chemical dissolution of the surface of the material [134-136]. The environment of the body is a known corrosive environment due to a high concentration of aggressive ions, facilitating molecules and elevated temperatures [11, 137]. The corrosion process itself is influenced by the local biological environment as well as the bulk and surface properties of the metal. The materials discussed in this chapter, stainless steel 316LVM, Co-Cr alloys, nitinol and platinum-iridium have a long history of use in medical implants and their corrosion properties can be discussed herein for the purposes of developing a corrosion resistant THV stent support.

The need for protection against corrosion in the biological environment has narrowed down the metallic biomaterial choice to metals that are either noble or passivated. The noble materials such as platinum-iridium are a standard for excellent corrosion resistance due to their highly ranked position within the electrochemical series. Passivation is the spontaneous formation of a thin oxide layer on the surface of certain metals (such as chromium and titanium) in the nanometer or micrometer range that act as a protective barrier between the bulk metal and the corrosive biological environment [11, 135, 139]. The effectiveness of this barrier depends on the rate of ion transfer through the barrier, stability, chemical composition, structure, thickness, as well as environmental conditions. Of the passivating metals discussed, both stainless steel (316LVM) and cobalt-chromium alloys contain chromium (Cr) which creates a Cr_2O_3 oxide layer whereas the titanium in nitinol produces a titanium oxide (TiO_2) layer [139-142].

The chemical composition of Stainless steel, as specified in ASTM F138, consists of 18% Chromium, 14% Nickel, 2.5% Molybdenum and 0.03% carbon content. Cr is responsible for its formation of a chromium oxide passivated layer that protects it from corrosive damage [11]. The molybdenum also adds to this protective layer. [135, 140] High carbon content greater than 0.03% could cause formation of chromium-carbides at the grain boundaries and deplete the Cr_2O_3 layer. **This process called "sensitization", could cause intergranular** corrosion and lead to potential fractures. Typically, the material should have >30% cold work to improve yield strength, UTS (ultimate tensile strength), and fatigue.

Cobalt-chromium alloys used in biomedical applications for stents use approximately 20% chromium (ASTM F90, ASTM F562, and ASTM F1058) which enhance its corrosion resistance via a spontaneously occurring passivation layer [143]. This oxide layer is also unique for its high interfacial strength and scratch resistance making cobalt chromium one of the frequently chosen metals for orthopedic applications [144]. Nitinol containing varying mixtures of around 50% titanium naturally generates a titanium oxide resistive layer just like other titanium alloy biomaterials. [142]

There are many different types of corrosion that the metallic implant can undergo including pitting corrosion, crevice corrosion, stress-corrosion cracking, fretting, galvanic corrosion and integranular corrosion [135]. Pitting corrosion is a localized corrosion that is caused by the local dissolution of the passive surface film, thus exposing the bulk metal which actively corrodes, causing cavities to form around the intact passivated surface. [145] Crevice corrosion is related to pitting and it occurs on areas where mass transfer is limited such as cracks and precipitates. The local environment in these areas promotes the aggregation of corrosive ions and the depletion of oxygen leading to corrosion. Fretting corrosion, although traditionally associated with orthopedic implants, occurs when two closely fitting surfaces touch and are subjected to constant wear and joint corrosion action. This process actively destroys the passive film which cannot protect the bulk motel from corrosion. Fretting corrosion, unlike pitting and crevice which has to do with material properties, has more to do with implant design, contacting surface materials, and location and thus should be considered. Galvanic must be considered in designs using more than one type of metal.

There are many different types of corrosion tests described in literature using solutions such as plasma/saliva analogs, Hanks solution, phosphate buffered saline solution, etc. and different test methodologies. [142, 146-148] This variance of the testing reflects the evolution of metallic biomaterial uses. Presently small implants such as stents and heart valve wireforms fall under the corrosion testing guidance ASTM F2129. ASTM F2129 uses a cyclic potentiodynamic polarization measurement to determine corrosion susceptibility and it requires the use of the implant in its final and finished form. [149]

In addition it has been shown that the morphology, thickness and composition of the surface layer are all important in determining the corrosion resistance of the metal. [150-153] **The morphology of the metal's surface is important in the formation** of the passive surface oxide layer. An uneven and precipitate and impurity-riden surface will result in an uneven covering of the passive layer. [154] The uneven non-homogeneous surfaces of the stent can be dictated by raw material processing and post processing steps. For example, when lasercutting the geometrical pattern into a stent, if the temperature rises above the critical transformation point of the metal, a recast non uniform layer is formed that is often referred to as the heat affected zone, or HAZ. The options for surface morphology modifications are extensive and rely on multiple factors encompassing not just corrosion but also biocompatibility and durability. An example of some surface modification techniques used for the improvement of corrosion resistance in metallic biomaterials includes electropolishing and passivation treatments. Electropolishing is a technique by which the metal is immersed in an electrolyte and subjected to a direct current (Figure 10). The metal implant in question becomes the anode which polarizes and loses metal ions at a controlled rate to the cathode. [155] The previous oxide layer is removed, surface morphology is smoothed and a new, more uniform, oxide layer is formed with new chemical composition. [142, 153, 156, 164] Passivation treatments augment the protective surface oxide layer by exposing it to a highly oxidizing condition such as nitric acid. This process has been shown to create a surface oxide layer that has a chemical composition that increases corrosion resistance [142, 140, 152, 159]

The processing steps and methodology in modifying surface passivation layers is delicate process that depends on implant design as well as material composition. For example the electropolishing process which removes material from the surface to create the new oxide layer must be tightly controlled when processing a small metallic implant such as a THV stent where the struts are on the order of millimeters; overpolishing can cause a reduction in strength and possibly even fatigue life [163]. The actual thickness of the surface oxide is also important as overly thick oxide layers can fracture during the strain caused by the crimping and expansion process of a THV stent or during normal pulsatile strain leading to corrosion [141, 165].

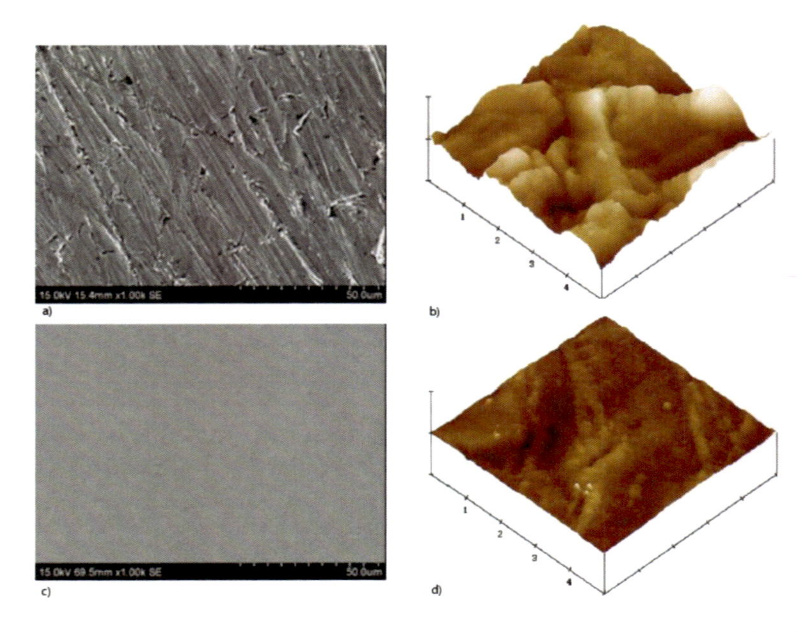

Figure 10. SEM and AFM pictures of unmodified nitinol (10a & b) and electropolished nitinol (10c & d) Reprinted with Permission from author [230].

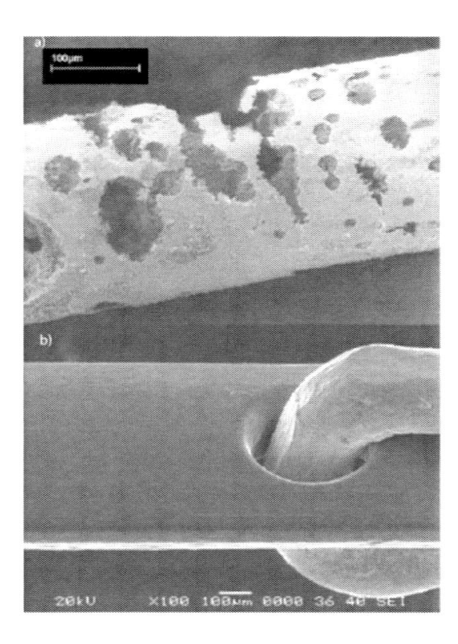

Figure 11. a. Corroded nitinol explants with oxide thickness 0.2-0.3 µm and E_{bd} of 280mV (5 months) 11b) Non-corroded electropolished explants with oxide thickness of 0.01 µm and E_{bd} > 900mV (12 months). This demonstrates the need for proper stent surface modification and processing. Reprinted with permission from author [126].

This is especially important for nitinol which can undergo 8% strain in its superelastic range during implantation and later during pulsatile cardiac stresses [166, 167]. It is also established that the uniformity of the surface oxide layer is more important that its thickness (Figure 11 & 12) [150].

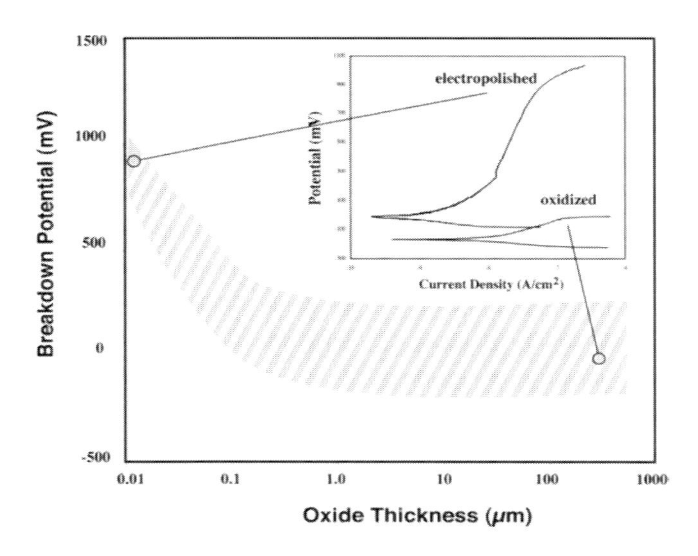

Figure 12. Breakdown potential as function of oxide thickness on nitinol (oxide layer modified by heat treatment variations). Inset: results of potentiodynamic corrosion tests of nitinol samples with electropolished or oxidized surface treatments and their respective oxide thickness layers. Thicker oxide thickness correlates with low breakdown potential and thus low corrosion resistance. Reprinted with permission from author [126].

Thus it is important that the surface finish process be engineered to prevent corrosion while considering the implant design, material and function. There are guidelines under the ASTM standards (i.e. ASTM E1558, B912 and ASTM F86) for appropriate treatments for metallic implants to ensure adequate passivity [161-163].

Important in the engineering of appropriate corrosion resistant implants is the technique used to test its corrosion. The ASTM F2129 test, recognized by the FDA as an accelerated assessment of corrosion resistance, gives quantitative data on corrosion resistance in the form of E_{BD} or breakdown potential at which the device undergoes pitting corrosion [149]. It is pitting corrosion which is the most important to cardiovascular implants unless the THV design consists of articulating metal surfaces (fretting and stress corrosion) or consists of different metals (galvanic corrosion). Testing the corrosion of the transcatheter heart valve component brings up the question of what amount of corrosion resistance is tolerable and what is safe. A possible route to assess corrosion acceptance would be to compare the breakdown potential to a known device in the field with proven clinical durability and long term data in vivo which experiences similar biological and implant conditions, such as vascular stents [126].

It is also crucial to recognize the amount of manufacturing and implant steps (crimping, expanding, etc.) that the metallic component of the THV must experience before ending in its final deployed configuration within a patient. Therefore, to ensure quality and device safety, the worst case scenario implant steps should be performed on the stent prior to corrosion testing, or other in vitro tests to provide a more realistic representation of the in vivo conditions. Unlike vascular stents, the manufacturing process of a transcatheter heart valve requires suturing cloth and leaflets to a metallic stent, likely with metallic needles. Scratches from manufacture could lead to corrosion. The crimping procedure could also introduce scratches if the process is not controlled. Additionally it is known that the surface modification procedures such as electropolishing may have problems polishing non exposed or hard to reach areas such as the lateral surfaces of a collapsed stent [149]. This is equally important for THV stents which may have small holes for suturing or other small geometry metallic surfaces.

The corrosion of the metallic biomaterials discussed above has been researched extensively. The literature is confusing and sometimes contradictory on the corrosion of small cardiovascular implants such as stents. This is partially due to lack of adequate stent geometries used during corrosion testing, non-uniform or characterized surface modification samples, and the use of a many different types of "corrosion tests." [149, 168] However, the existence of many commercially approved vascular stent devices made from these metals, as well as minimal cases reported for stent corrosion in vivo points to their general acceptable corrosion resistance in the cardiovascular environment regardless of the metal chosen (at least for endovascular stents).

Some of the current clinical reports bring up the possibility of different types (other than pitting) corrosion. There haven't been any recorded cases of structural failure or corrosion but the "bail out" procedures bear some consideration. The use of another THV ("valve-in-valve") [76-81] within another THV brings up the question of fretting corrosion and fatigue. Ideally one would avoid such a situation where you could get micro movements across two metal surfaces. Additionally, the implantations of THV into a failing bioprothesis ("valve-in-bioprothesis") [169-173] bring up the situation of galvanic corrosion when stent materials are of different metal composition. (Galvanic corrosion is tested via ASTM G71). [175]

6.0. Biocompatibility

The biocompatibility of the metal chosen is intricately woven with its corrosion performance, and in particular its release of metal ions and other corrosion breakdown products into the biological environment. It is understood in the body's corrosive environment that even with the presence of a passive layer, there exists a constant partial dissolution and repreciptation of the surface oxide layer causing metal ion release [176]. This release of these metal ions has been studied extensively in the context of orthopedic and dental implants [177-184]. The release of metal ions and corrosion products has been associated with tissue swelling, inflammation, allergic reactions, remote tissue accumulation and even clinical implant failure [181-182, 185]. In both dental and orthopedic implants there is a known history of corrosion damage due to breakdown of surface oxide layers by fretting wear and micromotion between articulating implant surfaces and bone [182, 187-189]. This increased oxide layer breakdown leads to increased metal release [190].

However, the applicability of this research towards cardiovascular implants, which are decidedly smaller than orthopedic implants and are not subject to the same fretting or stress corrosion conditions, is still be fully characterized [191,192]. What is known is that each metal, except platinum-iridium, has oxide layers of different compositions that release different ions within the body environment. Stainless steel and cobalt chromium alloys both rely on chromium oxide passivation layers but their actual compositions vary. Stainless steel oxide layer consists of iron, chromium, nickel, molybdenum and manganese [193]. Cobalt chromium alloy surface oxide layer consists of cobalt and chromium oxides with some molybdenum depending on the alloy. [194] Nitinol's passive oxide layer consists mainly of titanium oxide [142, 156, 195]. Yet the actual release of ions from these metals is different than their respective oxide layer compositions and the bulk metal composition. This preferential release of ions [176] means that the amount and type of metal ion released from the implant is not a function of the bulk material composition. For example, stainless steel preferentially releases nickel and manganese ions compared to iron and chromium (despite stainless steel being mostly iron and chromium). [177, 196, 197] Cobalt chromium alloys release chromium, cobalt and nickel in varying amounts [177, 179, 180, 197] and nitinol releases mainly nickel [142, 198].

Of these ions released the ones with cytotoxic and carcinogenic effects have been hexavalent chromium, cobalt, and nickel [176, 199-205]. Attempts at preventing the release of metal ions from the implants has lead down the same path as corrosion resistance towards surface oxide layer modification. It is now known that the amount of metal ion release depends on the strength, composition, thickness and uniformity of the oxide layer as well as the biological environmental considerations (implant location etc.) [176-177, 197, 206-210] This finding has been the most evident in the work on nitinol which has shown that surface treatments such as mechanical polishing can lead to increased amount of nickel ions within the titanium surface oxide leading to an increased release of nickel. This in contast to eletropolished surfaces which create an enriched titanium oxide layer depleted of most of its nickel [212, 214]. Similar studies on stainless steel and Co-Cr alloys have shown that surface processing can reduce the amount of nickel within the mostly titanium (nitinol) or chromium (Co-Cr and Stainless Steel) oxide layers (table 3). Other processing techniques such as electropolishing and passivation on nitinol, stainless steel and cobalt chromium should lead to a decrease in ion release (Figure 13) and an increase in corrosion resistance [157, 176-177, 197, 211].

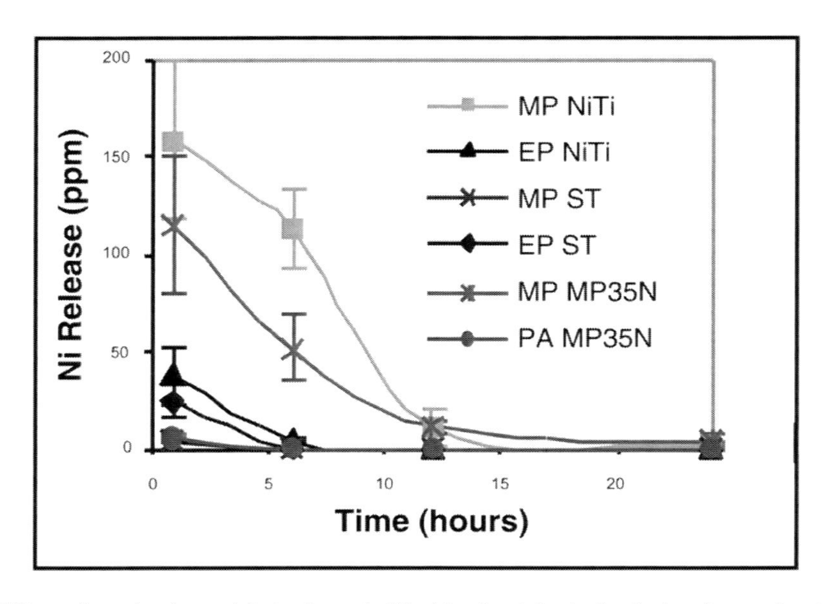

Figure 13. Effect of passivation: nickel release in Hank's physiological solution for mechanically polished (MP) stainless steel (MP ST), NiTi (MP NiTi) and MP35N (MP MP35N); electropolished stainless steel (EP ST) and NiTi (EP NiTi); and acid passivated MP35N (PA MP35N). Reprinted with permission by author [210].

Table 3. Ratio of nickel to titanium and chromium in surface oxide layers for different surface treatments of nitinol (ASTM F2063), MP35N (Co-Cr-Ni-Mo alloy ASTM F562) and Stainless steel (ASTM F138). Reproduced with Permission by authors [126, 210]

Material	Surface Condition	Ni:Ti	Ni:Cr
Nitinol	Mechanically Polished	0.18	—
Nitinol	Electropolished	0.14	—
MP35N	Mechanically Polished	—	0.4
MP35N	Passivated	—	0.08
316LSS	Mechanically Polished	—	0.11
316LSS	Electropolished	—	0.07

For cardiovascular stents there has been a concern that nickel release from stents could lead to restenosis from local inflammatory reactions and hypersensitivity to nickel or molybdenum [213-214]. Nickel in particular has shown to induce soft tissue inflammation at subtoxic concentrations through an inflammatory response [215-216] which may in turn cause increased corrosion of the metallic device. Hypersensitivity to metal ions released by metallic implants has been documented as being correlated to higher rates of restenosis when patients are shown sensitive to nickel and molybdenum on a skin patch test [213, 217]. Although it is estimated that roughly 10% of the general population have metal sensitivities to Co, Cr and Ni ions the actual clinical correlation towards restenosis has not materialized and even the correlation between skin patch test and restenosis is still under dispute [218-220]. Meanwhile the concern about nickel release in cardiovascular stents has also not stopped the continual commercial approval of new stents consisting of the same metals. This speaks not only to the improvement of stent surface processing to reduce nickel and other metal ion release but also the corrosion resistance of these surfaces.

Thrombogenicity is always an issue for blood contacting materials, especially metals which are naturally thrombogenic. It has been shown that for endovascular stent materials the higher the roughness the more thrombogenic the material thus arguing for the need for a polishing surface modification [221-222]. Work on stent metal materials that have been electropolished and surface modified have shown decreased thrombogenicity and decreased neointimal hyperplasia [223-224]. The uniformity of the oxide layer is also important as surface irregularities caused by plastic deformation during crimping and expanding the stent have shown to be thrombogenetic [228].

Although this is a very brief summary of the biocompatibility and corrosion properties of the metals chosen for endovascular stents and in turn transcatheter heart valves, the definition of biocompatibility implies that the material perform appropriately in its intended location and function [228]. The appropriate requirements for biocompatibility of the stent component of the transcatheter heart valve have yet to be fully defined. Despite its similarities to vascular stents, there is no concern for neointima hyperplasia and restenosis as there is in vascular stents as of this date. In reality however, any transcatheter heart valve, component or whole implant, must undergo biocompatibility tests outlined under International Standard ISO-10993, "Biological Evaluation of Medical Devices" as well as preclinical in vivo tests to confirm the biocompatibility and hemocompatibility of the device [229]. This does not include any additional testing that regulatory bodies or risk analysis may require during implant development. The long term clinical data on currently marketed transcatheter heart valves is still to be determined due the relative infancy of this technology, thus the burden of proving the biocompatibility of the technology falls upon the manufacturer.

7.0. Tissue Design Considerations

The tissue valve in a THV is a critical component for durability and functional implant performance. The tissue valve must not evoke thrombosis, infection, abnormal healing, or hemolysis, and as such tissue processing advancements over the years have been immeasurable. The majority of tissue valves are xenografts, or animal tissue valves. The most common animal tissues used are bovine and porcine, and therefore will be discussed thoroughly in this chapter.

Several commercially available surgical heart valves are made from porcine aorta roots including the Carpentier Edwards (Edwards Lifesciences, Irvine, Ca, USA) and the Medtronic Mosaic valves (Medtronic, Minneapolis, MN, USA). Porcine root tissue has not been utilized yet for transcatheter heart valves probably due to the crimp profile considerations for the THV (current applications are approximately < 24 French), and also because the native porcine aortic valve contains innate features (i.e. sinus, non-coronary leaflets, commissural junctions) that do not flatten smoothly; making it become more difficult for catheter deliverability. However, pericardial tissue shows promise since it is processed flat, thin, and therefore can ultimately achieve an acceptable crimp profile. A typical pericardial leaflet thickness for a size 23mm surgical valve is 0.4mm, but for a similar size transcatheter valve the leaflet thickness may be about 0.25mm, which is a 40% reduction in thickness [47]. Equine, bovine, and porcine pericardial tissue has been observed in THV products. Porcine pericardial tissue is used for the leaflet assembly in the Medtronic CoreValve, while the Edwards SAPIEN and its successor the SAPIEN XT are constructed with bovine pericardial tissue leaflets (but the predecessor (the Cribier Edwards PHV was made of equine pericardial tissue).

There are many reasons to opt for either bovine or porcine pericardial tissue for THV products since both have unique viscoelastic characteristics. The advantage of using bovine pericardial tissue includes good biocompatibility and clinical data showing more than 20 years durability in surgical heart valve applications (i.e. the Carpentier Edwards Perimount Pericardial valve). On the other hand, because crimp profile is one of the driving factors for a THV design, porcine pericardial tissue may be a good alternative. Generally porcine pericardial tissue is found to be thinner compared to the bovine pericardial tissue [47,231], however if a detailed thickness selection manufacturing process is in place then either bovine or porcine pericardial tissue may be sufficient, expecting perhaps a higher yield loss for picking only the thinnest regions of the bovine pericardial tissue sac.

It is important to acknowledge that there is a relationship between increased tissue thickness and lower valve peak stresses. Thicker tissue increases the surface area of the leaflet and distributes stress loads more effectively, making the leaflets feasibly stronger and more durable. Additionally, porcine pericardial tissue has been shown to be statistically stiffer and less extensible compared to thicker bovine pericardium due to the structural differences including higher levels of type II collagen and higher degrees of cross-linking observed in biochemical analysis testing [231]. Also, despite tissue orientation (radial or circumferential), FEA modeling results has exhibited that bovine pericardial leaflets have a lower maximum principal stress compared to porcine pericardial leaflets [47]. For THV designs, the drive for smaller crimp profile may require thinner leaflet thickness but this drive must be balanced for the need for tissue that is thick enough to endure long term physiological pressures. Regardless of the mechanical behavioral differences between both bovine and porcine pericardial tissue, both have shown promising results in current THV applications.

When engineering a transcatheter valve, common failure modes of bioprosthetic tissue heart valves such as calcification need to be considered. Calcification can be accelerated by age, increased mechanical stress, and valve factors such as the glutaraldeyhde fixation treatment [92]. This is why it is essential to establish tissue processing techniques that will mitigate valve failure modes like calcification. However, because of the intrinsic anisotropy of the pericardial tissue, the process engineering behind tissue valve development remains remarkably complex due to a variety of elements that are difficult to control. Many manufacturers implement stringent screening that involves tissue selection based on leaflet orientation, thickness, extensibility, and surface characteristics [48]. Processing techniques for "tissue clean down," fixation, cutting the leaflet shape, and manufacturing assembly have been carefully established. The tissue clean down process can be quite manually intensive and requires removing fat, scarring, and loose fibers to obtain a smooth tissue surface. The "tissue clean down" prepares the tissue for the chemical fixation process, which stabilizes the biological tissue by crosslinking covalent chemical bonds between proteins in the tissue. Chemical fixation time can depend on the concentrations of the crosslinking fixatives used, temperature, tissue thickness and other variables including fixturing/tooling technique. The fixturing technique may aid to improve mechanical properties in the tissue, since scientists have demonstrated that applications of strain, pressure, tethering, and other approaches during crosslinking may produce tissue with more desirable isotropic properties [232-235].

Additional tissue processing steps including leaflet shape cutting and manufacturing assembly will only be discussed briefly because they are directly dependent on the valve and stent design. Leaflet shape cutting can be performed by standard die cut or lasercutting the leaflet pattern from the tissue. Lasercutting might provide a smoother edge, however laser parameters have to be determined to demonstrate that the tissue is not denatured or that the heat from the laser will not produce irreversible changes in the tissue structure [236]. Manufacturing assembly is perhaps one of the most important steps toward achieving good tissue mechanics and valve design. Since there is a loss of resistance to rupture on tissue with sutures [237], the seam type and methods of tissue attachment to the stent need to be carefully tested. There are many seams that could potentially be used to assemble the leaflet geometry for example a whip stitch, running stitch, or blanket stitch all of which will provide different resulting mechanical strength characteristics. But it is not only the tissue and seam type that determine the strength of the valve design, it is also dependent on the suture material and suture size. For a transcatheter heart valve a suture that lays flat like a monofilament suture, and a seam design that maintains a small crimp profile will be worthy candidates. Collectively, suture materials such as polytetrafluoroethylene (PTFE) have been used in heart valve assembly with wonderful success. Ultimately, accelerated wear testing (as discussed later in this chapter) will help evaluate which seams and manufacturing assembly methods are appropriate for the valve design.

The tissue valve leaflet geometry plays a distinct role in distribution of overall valve stresses, and therefore a good leaflet geometrical design will improve fatigue performance. The leaflet motion is very challenging to depict, however the leaflets must remain sufficiently compliant and coapted when apposed, which is a bi-directional response [238]. One method of capturing the movement and predicting the leaflet stresses is by computational model simulations (Figure 14). For most leaflet designs, analysis efforts have detected that the highest tensile stresses are located in the vicinity of the commissure regions [47, 239-240]. And it has been shown that pattern of stresses at the frame depend strongly on method of tissue attachment [241]. Surgical bioprothesis have shown that flexible leaflet attachment to stent reduces the peak stress on the leaflets, but for a transcatheter valve many tubular structures limit the amount of stent deflection [48]. Therefore, besides controlling leaflet shape, in order to reduce high stresses (which could potentially lead to abrasion, tears, or wear issues) advanced assembly concepts can be contrived to include leaflet folding/padding or external support structures. Most commonly these ridged support structures that provide leaflet and tissue structural reinforcement are found at the commissures [48], as observed in the Edwards SAPIEN transcatheter aortic valve design.

Transcatheter heart valve leaflet designs need to account for the possibility of over and under expansion since all patients' diseased vessels are unique due to the frequency, location, size, hardness, thickness of the calcification present. Zegdi *at el.* revealed that the aortic leaflets ventricular surface was almost always irregular, and calcification almost certainly crossed the stent frame, [58]. If the valve is overexpanded past the intended design diameter, then the individual leaflets will not coapt completely. The gap in the middle of the leaflets could lead to central leakage and make it difficult for the pressures across the valve to be maintained. Likewise, if the valve is underexpanded or deployed into a non-concentric environment it could be equally detrimental to the valve performance. The leaflets might not close with synchronicity, and possibly will be skewed because of the valve position within the physiological setting of the patient. The non-uniform closure of the leaflets could lead to poor quality hydrodynamic performance, or worse, premature valve failure. But there are several ways engineering the leaflet shape could reduce these risks, for example the valve design might include an initial slight leaflet redundancy at the free edge to over accommodate and ensure valve closure. The valve designer must optimize the leaflet geometry adequately because too much leaflet redundancy could be problematic, instigating a constant leaflet to leaflet abrasion. Moving forward, it will be critical for the engineering design team to work closely with the surgeons and cardiologist to understand the patient anatomy during the development of transcatheter heart valve replacements.

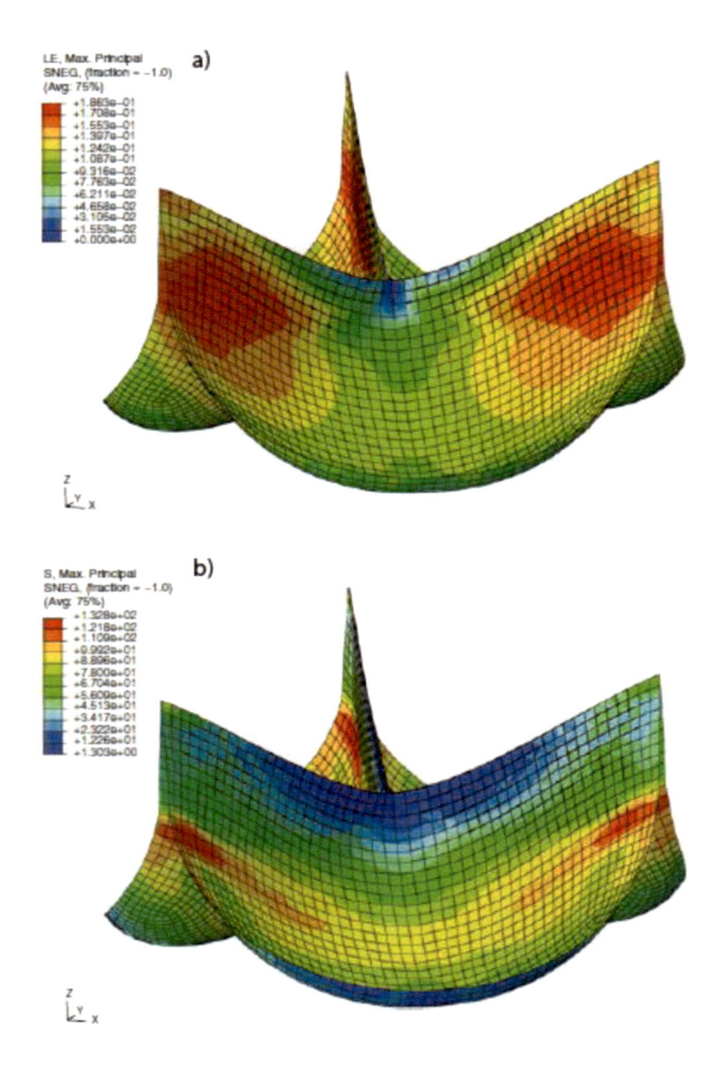

Figure 14. Finite element analysis (FEA) model of a Transcatheter Heart Valve leaflet design with a) Maximum principal strains and 14b) Maximum principal stresses. Reprinted with permission of author [47].

8.0. Transcatheter Heart Valve in Vitro and in Vivo Evaluation

Just as the engineering concepts and knowledge behind prosthetic heart valves has evolved and developed over time so too has the standardization of its performance evaluation. Early in the history of prosthetic heart valves there lacked the long term clinical data to help engineers and physicians correlate the properties of the valve to clinical outcomes. As data eventually was released, areas of improvement were discovered and encorporated into the engineering process. It also became necessary to show that newer enhancements actually offered clear advantages to the patient. It was this environment that spurred the creation of standardized tests that would allow newly developed heart valves to be compared to those already on the market. These standards, when available, also gave minimum performance requirements on certain key properties of the heart valves. The outcome was performance standards that serve as a guideline for heart valve developers for use in planning the in vitro and in vivo performance evaluation of bioprosthetic and mechanical heart valves.

The current guidelines for in vitro and in vivo evaluation of artificial heart valves are encapsulated in the FDA (Food and Drug Administration) Draft Replacement Heart Valve Guidance [39] and the International Standard ISO 5840 on Cardiovascular implants [38]. These two documents have been modified extensively over the years as the understanding of heart valve science expands and as fresh technology enters the field. As of this date, neither of these documents holds transcatheter heart valve specific tests or guidelines. The current draft of the FDA Heart Valve Guidance (issued January 2010)[29] states that the guidance "also applies to percutaneously delivered valves; however, different or additional *in vitro, in vivo* preclinical, and clinical studies may be appropriate for such devices, depending on the specific device design, the proposed indications for use, and the results of your risk analysis. We recommend you contact the Circulatory and Prosthetics Devices Branch to discuss planned submissions for percutaneously delivered valves." Implicit in this statement is that the guidance encompassed percutaneous heart valves (THV) when applicable to bioprosthetic valves, but that additional testing would most likely be needed. This indicates that an open communication between the heart valve developer and the regulatory bodies would help elucidate the testing pathway required to reach clinical trials. The FDA guidance explains that the guidance document is meant to act as a FDA specific supplement to the ISO 5840:2005 guidance. Thus the draft guidance is meant to be used in conjunction with the ISO 5840 guidance or any other standard equivalent to ISO 5840.

Also the FDA draft guidance document refers to the FDA guidance, Non-Clinical Tests and Recommended Labeling for Intravascular Stents and Associated Delivery Systems [98] when referring to additional testing. This guidance document covers all extracranial intravascular stents, balloon and self expanding versions as well as their delivery systems. It is fitting that the transcatheter heart valve which relies heavily on intravascular stent technology would also be covered by the FDA intravascular stent guidance.

From a broader viewpoint these standards, although detailed in their testing and study methodology, provide direction to ensure quality assurance and good manufacturing practices in the production of the device. This makes the standards invaluable for heart valve developers aiming at bringing a final design to market. However they may also be too constraining and time consuming for verification of new designs and concepts that have yet to be solidified. Thus a balance must be struck especially in the experimental phase of product development.

In summary all three of these documents, the FDA draft guidance on Heart Valves, the FDA guidance on Intravascular Stents and ISO 5840 should be used to guide the in vitro and in vivo evaluation of transcatheter heart valves. However, the FDA guidance documents carry FDA specific requirements that may not be necessary for application to regulatory bodies outside the United States. If approval within the US is not the first goal, than following other standards (ISO 5840 is generally accepted in the EU) should be satisfactory.

The rest of this section will summarize and detail where appropriate, the in vitro and in vivo evaluation process of a transcatheter heart valve. In particular these evaluations will be split up into both in vitro and in vivo segments and stent and whole heart valve segments.

8.1. In Vitro Stent Evaluation

The FDA guidance on Intravascular Stents outlines many different in vitro tests for both stent and delivery system. A non-exclusive list of available stent in vitro tests and evaluations are in table 4.

Table 4. An outline describing many of the required stent in vitro tests and evaluations. [38-39, 98]

In vitro engineering tests	
Stent Component	Whole valve
Material Composition Shape Memory and Superelasticity Stent Corrosion Resistance Dimensional Verification Percent Surface Area Foreshortening Stent Recoil (Balloon Expandable Stents) Stent Integrity Radial Stiffness and Radial Strength Radial Outward Force Mechanical Properties Stress/Strain Analysis Fatigue Analysis Accelerated Durability Testing Radiopacity MRI Safety and Compatibility	Hydrodynamic Testing Steady Forward Flow Steady Back-flow Leakage Pulsatile Flow Testing Verification of Bernoulli Relationship Flow Visualization Accelerated Wear Testing Dynamic Failure Mode Testing
Other Testing	
Biocompatibility Sterility/Packaging Shelf Life Delivery System Testing	

Many of these tests are covered in multiple national or international guidances (such as corrosion) and thus it is up to the developer to choose the appropriate guidance to follow. Additionally the use of risk analysis methods drives the required performance specifications that must be met for each test. For example in order to confirm final material properties of the stent component, many samples would be selected from multiple finished lots in order to statistically show confidence and reliability that the properties meet the required design and drawing specifications which were defined by risk analysis.

Most of these stent evaluations are stent specific and would therefore not be completed in the testing of a surgical bioprosthetic valve. These tests also are just guidelines and are meant to accommodate intravascular stent designs. THV stent designs that are unorthodox may be subject to additional testing per the manufacturers risk analysis or by recommendation of a regulatory body. Some of these tests and their relation to THV will be explained.

Material Composition is covered in all three guidance documents. Reference to material standards is suggested such as ASTM F138 for stainless steel, etc. Testing should be done to confirm and verify the material certification from the supplier, especially if any processing of the stent material occurs after the certification has been issued.

Shape memory and superelasticity is a nitinol stent specific evaluation. This evaluation defines the temperature relationship at which the nitinol stent changes its phase (shape memory) as well as its response to strain (superelasticity). Both ASTM standards F2004 and F2082 are suggested as they are accepted guidelines on how to test nitinol material either with a bend free recovery method or a differential scanning calorimeter. [242-243]

Stent Corrosion analysis was explained in detail earlier but the testing methodology bears explaining. As mentioned earlier, ASTM standard F2129 [149] should be used to determine the pitting and crevice corrosion potential of the THV stent component. The guidance recommends that the stent to be tested be the finished product and in the case of the THV, most likely after the THV has been fully assembled (the manufacturer would have to remove all tissue/suture material to test the stent component for corrosion), crimped, and expanded similar to in vivo implantation. It is also recommended that the stents used in durability testing (either stent fatigue or whole valve durability) be tested for corrosion and that the stents be analyzed under Scanning Electron Microscopy (SEM) for microscopic details, or damage. Aged stent components are also required to be tested up through 10 years equivalent.

Percent surface area is a test that uses dimensions recorded through ASTM F2081 [244] to properly calculate the area of the stent that contacts the implant site. The applicability of this test, especially in the aortic valve site, is questionable since the purpose of the test was to help quantify the interaction of the stent and vessel due to possible unwanted biological responses. This was seen in the ISAR-STEREO study for intravascular stents [110], where larger struts and percent surface area caused more restenosis. However this may not be true for the aortic stenosis THV indication since the tissue that is contact with the stent is heavily calcified leaflet tissue and not all of the THV stent may actually be in contact with the leaflet.

The recoil for balloon expandable THV stent designs is very important for the clinical sizing of the THV during implantation. This is important in light of the discussion on how the stiffness (elastic modulus) of the material affects the amount of recoil. Recoil is recommended to be measured through ASTM F2079 [246]. When quantified the amount of recoil will help the physician determine the final diameter of the valve after balloon dilation and allow for appropriate sizing algorithms. This is vital for balloon expandable THV stents which rely on apposition with the irregular implant anatomy for an "interference fit" to prevent migration. It has been observed that typical interference fits for current THV devices range from 1-3mm, or up to 15% radial interference. Thus if recoil is not taking into consideration, migration could be a failure mode.

Stent integrity is an analysis of the defects and flaws that can be seen under microscopy. The justification for such analysis is to examine any damage left from the manufacturer or from the crimping and expansion process. Defects such as sharp edges could lead to damage of a balloon meant for valve expansion or damage to the suture material that is in contact after valve construction. Other defects such as cracks or pits could lead to undesirable corrosion or fatigue resistance.

Radial stiffness and radial strength are both balloon-expanded stent properties. In balloon-expanded THV designs the balloon expands the stent into a rigid position from which it must then resist any external forces such as the pulsatile contraction of the heart around the aortic annulus. Radial stiffness is the relationship between the diameter of the stent and a uniformly applied external radial pressure whereas radial strength is the pressure at which the stent undergoes irreversible plastic deformation. Both of these quantities rely on material selection and stent design.

Radial outward force is a property of self-expanding stents and is related to the chronic outward force exerted by the self-expanding nitinol THV stent as it strives to achieve its native shape/diameter. This force is recommended to be measured at different sizes/diameters and at different parts of the stent if the stent is designed or indicated to have different forces at different segments (Such as the Medtronic CoreValve).

The stress/strain analysis is a vital test meant to provide not just stress and strain relationships within the device but also help define long term durability. The test specimens should undergo similar processing steps as the final device in order to provide an accurate representation. The FDA guidance recommends the use of computational modeling such as finite element analysis. Computational modeling can be a powerful tool that simulates the in vivo loading and boundary conditions along the stent itself. FEA can establish expansion characteristics of novel stent designs, laser-cut from advanced engineering materials such as nitinol, and also incorporate plastic deformation characteristics of more traditional materials, such as stainless steel and cobalt chromium [247]. The computational simulations should include loading, deploying, and deforming the stent in a manner that is intended to mimic deployment into the therapeutic site and deformation seen in vivo. The actual process of creating the computational model is long and involved and requires the proper analysis of the "stress/strain history" including all the stresses built into the system during manufacturing (such as heat-treatment and electropolishing processes), crimping, expansion, recoil and the physiological conditions it will experience. The mechanical properties of the stent material will also be inputted into the system. The output of this test will be the stress and strain characterization of the entire THV stent and thus the areas of maximum tensile and compressive stresses and strains can be visualized. This test, if not the final product can also serve as a tool to design a THV stent that further reduces stress/strain. In view of the importance and effort put into the computational modeling it is equally if not more important to validate the computational model. Validation involves direct experimental testing, both of the real device and, if possible, the specific physiological anatomy to be implanted in, such that the inputs into the system can be validated. The example used in the guidance is the use a radial loading test on the stent in order to validate the correlation between force and displacement in the real device and a simulation of radial loading within the FEA model.

Fatigue Analysis is also derived from the computational modeling as the mean and alternating stresses/strains output from the FEA test combined with mechanical properties of the stent will help estimate the fatigue life of the THV stent component using a Goodman analysis or other equivalent tool. It is also recommended that safety factors are worked into the equation and design.

Accelerated Durability Testing is the culmination and longest in vitro test procedure for the stent component. It is the validation of the fatigue analysis performed from outputs of the FEA model. This is testing of the real stent samples in physiological loading conditions under pulsatile flow. (see Figure 15a) The inputs into the testing (the loading conditions) will depend on the FEA analysis as well as any safety factor that is considered. In the FDA stent guidance it recommends the testing of up to 10 years equivalent which is roughly 400 million cycles. However the heart valve guidance, ISO 5840 and the FDA Draft guidance both recommend that the stent support of a heart valve be tested for 600 million cycles (15 years equivalent). The minimum amount of time this test will take is 6 months to 1 year. This testing will evaluate the long term failure modes such as fretting, abrasion, wear and fatigue fracture. It will be able to identify and expose conditions that the computational model could not.

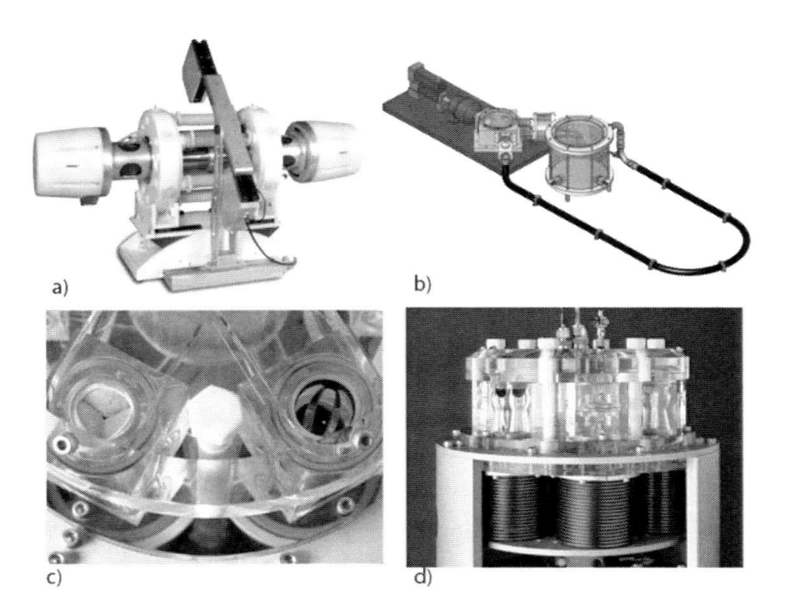

Figure 15. Transcatheter & Surgical Valve Testing Equipment, example of commercially available testers. 15a) Bose ElectroForce Stent/Graft Tester Model 9150 for in vitro fatigue testing of stents (Courtesy of Bose Corporation, Eden Prairie, MN, USA). 15b) Dynatek Dalta MP3 Pulse Duplicator system for hydrodynamic testing. 15c & d) Dynatek Dalta M6 Heart Valve Tester for Accelerated Wear Testing of artificial heart valves. (Courtesy of Dynatek Dalta, Galena, Mo, USA).

8.2. In Vitro Whole Valve Evaluation

Most of the tests outlined in this section are traditional artificial heart valve in vitro evaluations that have evolved and modified over the years into the current forms of ISO 5840 and the FDA Draft Heart Valve Guidance. They are broken up into both hydrodynamic (hemodynamic) and durability tests. The ideal heart valve from the hemodynamic point of view should have the following qualities: 1) produce minimal pressure gradient, 2) yield relatively small regurgitation, 3) minimize production of turbulence, 4) not induce regions of high shear stress and 5) contain no stagnation or separation regions in its flow field [247]. These qualities are all adequately evaluated in the in vitro evaluations covered in the guidance, but there are unique properties to THV that may add to the evaluation or even require innovative test procedures.

The key distinction here to make before any in vitro testing is performed is how the THV's performance is to be represented. Unlike a surgical valve which is sutured and fixated into place and virtually unaffected by its surrounding, the THV relies heavily on its implanted anatomy [248]. The question becomes how will the THV's in vitro performance be evaluated, in a fixture that is meant to mimic its future environment or will it be tested like a traditional heart valve? For example a traditional bioprosthetic heart valve's leakage is usually thought as mostly being central with minimum paravalvular leak, whereas THV applications have already shown a penchant for large amounts of paravalvular leak due to improper sealing with its implant site. The answer as of now seems to be a mixture of both test methods and will rely on the design, clinical input, and communication with regulatory bodies.

Steady flow testing is a mainstay of artificial heart valve testing and involves steady forward flow across the open prosthesis and then steady back flow/pressure upon the closed prosthesis. For the forward flow the significance of this test is to measure pressure gradient across the valve, as this pressure gradient needs to be low across a wide range of flows. The steady back-flow/pressure test not only measures the integrity of the valve against large static pressures but also any leakage that may slip through during static fluid load. For the THV the steady forward and back flow also can theoretically serve as tests of migration resistance to both the shear stress of fluid during forward flow [249] and the pressure during back flow.

Testing in physiological pulsatile testers is the gold standard tests for valve hydrodynamics and there are several commercially available testers such as the one in Figure 15b. These testers are meant to evaluate the in vitro hemodynamic performance of the valve over a range of pressure, heart rate and flow ratings [39]. This ranges from hypotensive to extreme hypertensive conditions and allows the valve's full performance to be characterized. Some of these tests may also be helpful in determining the migration characteristics of a THV if the extreme ranges of the pressure are used. It is required to use a reference control device so that not only the THV being analyzed can be compared to a known commercial quantity but also to help identify any deviations in the system.

Since one of a valve's main tasks is to allow blood flow through without significant impediment the pressure gradient across the open valve is important. Data points such as the effective orifice area (EOA) quantify this ability or lack thereof to allow flow unimpeded. A large EOA corresponds to small pressure drops and thus a smaller energy loss and is therefore desirable [10]. EOA can be quantified using the Gorlin equation via collection of variables during normotensive conditions (70 beats per minute, mean differential pressure across the closed valve of 95 mmHg, 5 liters per minute cardiac output and a 35% forward flow systolic ratio) [10, 39]. EOA is one of the few properties that have minimum requirements per valve size in ISO 5840. Another significant factor in pulsatile testing is the amount regurgitation allowed. Regurgitation is defined as the reverse flow back across the closed valve which is usually very small in bioprosthetic valves (on the range of 0.2-3%) [10]. It is also important to create an in vitro model of the implant anatomy in order to test the in vitro propensity for paravalvular leak due to its current clinical importance and correlation.

As in stent testing, the durability testing of the whole THV is the test of the longest duration. Also known as accelerated wear testing (Figure 15c & 15d), the heart valves undergo cyclic back pressures (defined by FDA as being between 125 and 150 mmHg) under pulsatile flow conditions for 200 million cycles (for bioprosthetic valves) or roughly 5 years equivalent.

The maximum cycle rate is dependent on the system and other constraints on the waveforms of the pressure curve set in the standards. At a rate of 1200 cycles per minute [250], 200 million cycles would be achieved in less than 6 months ignoring the need to take the valves out periodically to test their hydrodynamic performance and inspect them as detailed in the ISO and FDA guidances [38-39].

Thus for such a long term test it is important that all possible durability concerns are evaluated. For a THV as detailed earlier in this chapter, there is possible concern for damage: to the leaflets caused by the crimping and expanding of the valve, to the sutures that must undergo tension and compression cycles against the metallic stent surface, possible stent fretting corrosion and fatigue, and the stent itself (since the stent durability testing is not performed on the whole valve, it does not take into consideration stent deflection caused by leaflet closure during pressure) [48].

This list is not exclusive and different designs and delivery system will have various "risks" to the durability of the whole THV's integrity. There is no available information on the durability on THV, both in the in vitro setting and clinically. Even in the absence of such data it is a requirement that new designs and/or changes of previous designs have proven durability. The requirement to complete accelerated wear testing is deemed as necessary before any clinical testing may be started in the US [38-39].

8.3. In Vivo Whole Valve Preclinical Evaluation

Preclinical animal studies serve not only as validation of in vitro testing but to determine biological factors that could not be simulated in vitro. This includes biocompatibility, implant procedure and other clinical factors. The requirements and details on how to design such a study are in the FDA and ISO heart valve guidances and will not be detailed in this chapter. However it is important to note that there is a need to recreate the proper anatomic model for in vivo evaluations. The THV which was designed to treat aortic stenosis, needs a animal model that mimics aortic stenosis.

However creation of such a model is difficult since the animals always tend to be young and healthy. Studies implanting currently available THV models into the porcine aortic model have been unsuccessful as the THVs tended to migrate. The possible explanation was that the porcine aortic model in its compliant and noncalcific state, did not serve as a proper implantation area for the THV which relies on rigid and calcific implantation areas for fixation and support against migration. [248, 251]

Thus it becomes very important for the THV developer to create an appropriate model to test the acute implantation and fixation of the device and the chronic performance of the device while eliminating the possibility of migration. Future THV technology that desire to correct other valve pathologies should also be concerned on how other valve pathologies can be modeled in the animal.

8.4. Prototype Testing

Although most if not all of the testing explained in the preceding sections may be required for clinical studies to be approved, it may not fit in the schedule or scope for devices that still have not achieved their final design. For a developer who has made their first prototype sample and has crimped and expanded it for the first time, it may not help to put the valve in a durability tester to find out the results in several months. Computational modeling, especially finite element analysis has shown to be useful in determining THV designs [47]. Pulsatile testing is useful in determining valve function quickly and the range of settings available per the ISO guidance may allow for extreme condition testing exploring possible failure modes. Accelerated Wear Testing at extreme conditions under Dynamic Failure Mode settings prescribed in the FDA and ISO guidance can also help elucidate failure modes and areas of improvement in a short amount of time.

Conclusion

This chapter endeavored to elucidate the science and engineering behind transcatheter heart valve technology and the challenges faced during the development and evaluation phase. It also demonstrated how important physicians are to the innovation and improvement of transcatheter heart valves both in understanding their clinical knowledge, as well as supporting the design efforts. The focus on the risk analysis and the description of the in vitro and in vivo test evaluation process summarized the process that each new design must go through in order to reach commercial approval. FDA and ISO guidance documents offer guidelines for conducting the engineering testing, but many in vitro evaluation methods still need to be perfected to provide a more accurate model. Not covered in this chapter, although very important to the engineering of transcatheter heart valves and all medical devices is the concepts of design control and quality assurance. Furthermore, additional advanced concepts in THV technology not in this chapter such as fatigue, stent design, and valve design are currently being researched, and add to the many factors that influence the performance of a transcatheter heart valve. The future work of transcatheter valve replacements will reinforce the need for collaborative initiatives involving physicians and all disciplines of engineering to create a successful product that will last a lifetime.

References

[1] Hufnagel, CA; Harvey, WP. The surgical correction of aortic regurgitation. Preliminary report. *Bull Georgetown Univ Med Center,* 1953;6:3–6.

[2] Hufnagel CA. Basic concepts in the development of cardiovascular prostheses. *Am J Surg* 1979;137:285–300.

[3] Harken, D.; Soroff, H.; Taylor, W.; Lefemine, A.; Gupta, S.; Lunzer, S.; Partial and complete prostheses in aortic insufficiency, *J Thorac Cardiovasc Surg.* 1960;40(6):744–762.

[4] Braunwald, NS.; Cooper, T.; Morrow, AG., Complete replacement of the mitral valve. Successful clinical application of a flexible polyurethane prosthesis, *J Thorac Cardiovasc Surg* 1960:40, pp. 1–11.

[5] O'Brien, M.; Clarebrough, J.; Heterograft aortic valve translantation for valve disease, *Med J Aust* 1966: 2, pp. 228–232.

[6] Carpentier, A.; Lemaigre, G.; Robert, L., Carpentier, S; Dubost, C., Biological factors affecting long-term results of valvular heterografts, *J Thorac Cardiovasc Surg* 58 1969: 4, pp. 467–483.

[7] Starr, A.; Edwards, ML. Mitral replacement: clinical experience with a ball-valve prosthesis, *Ann Surg* 1961: 154, pp. 726–740.

[8] Bjork,VO., Aortic valve replacement with the Bjork-Shiley tilting disc valve prosthesis, *Br Heart J* 1971: 33 (Suppl), pp. 42–46.

[9] Emery, RW., Mettler, E., Nicoloff, DM;, A new cardiac prosthesis: the St. Jude Medical cardiac valve: in vivo results, *Circulation* 1979: 60 (2, Part 2), pp. 48–54.

[10] Yoganathan AP, Leo HL, Travis B, Teoh S.-H, Heart Valve Prosthesis. *Comprehensive Structural Integrity*, 2007, Chapter 9.07, Pages 297-328

[11] Ratner BD, Hoffman AS, Shoen FJ, Lemons JE. *Biomaterials Science: an Introduction to Materials in Medicine*. San Diego: Elsevier/Academic Press; 2004

[12] Butchart, EG; Bodnar, E. *Thrombosis, Embolism and Bleeding*, 1st Edition. London: ICR Publishers; 1992. p. 160–171

[13] Giddens, DP.; Yoganathan, AP.; Schoen, FJ.; Prosthetic cardiac valves. *Cardiovasc. Pathol.*, 1993: 2(suppl. 3), 167s-177s.

[14] Ionescu, MI.; Tandon, AP; Mary, DAS.; Abid, A.; Heart valve replacement with the Ionescu-Shiley pericardial xenograft, *J Thorac Cardiovasc Surg.*, 1977: 73, pp. 31–42.

[15] Nistal, F.; Carcia-Satue, E.; Artinano, E.; Duran, CMG.; Gallo, I.; Comparative study of primary tissue valve failure between Ionescu-Shiley pericardial and Hancock porcine valves in the aortic position, *Am J Cardiol.*, 1986;57:161–164.

[16] Gabbay, S.; Frater, RWM.; In vitro comparison of the newer heart valve bioprostheses in the mitral and aortic positions Proceedings of the Second International Symposium. In: LH Cohn and V Gallucci, Editors, *Cardiac prostheses.*, Yorke Medical Books, Stoneham, Mass. 1982, pp. 456–468.

[17] Cosgrove, DM; Lytle, BW; CC Gill, CC; Golding, LA; Stewart, RW; Loop, FD; Williams, GW. In vivo hemodynamic comparison of porcine and pericardial valves, *J Thorac Cardiovasc Surg.* 1985; 89, pp. 358–368.

[18] Pellerin, M; Mihaileanu, S; Couetil, JP; Relland, JY; Deloche, A; Fabiani, JN; Jindani, A; Carpentier, AF. Carpentier-Edwards pericardial bioprosthesis in aortic position: Long-term follow-up 1980 to 1994, *Ann Thorac Surg* 1995: 60 (Suppl), pp. S292–S295 discussion S295–6.

[19] Davies, H. Catheter-mounted valve for temporary relief of aortic insufficiency. *Lancet* 1965;1:250.

[20] Moulopoulos, SD; Anthopoulos, L; Stamatelopoulos, S; Stefadouros, M. Catheter-mounted aortic valves. *Ann Thorac Surg* 1971;11: 423–30.

[21] Matsubara, T; Yamazoe, M; Tamura, Y; Ohshima, M; Yamazaki, Y; Suzuki, M; Izumi, T; Shibata, A. Balloon catheter with check valves for experimental relief of acute aortic regurgitation. *Am Heart J* 1992;124:1002–8.

[22] Andersen, HR; Knudsen, LL; Hasenkam, JM. Transluminal implantation of artificial heart valves. Description of a new expandable aortic valve and initial results with implantation by catheter technique in closed chest pigs. *Eur Heart J* 1992;13:704–8.

[23] Knudsen, LL; Andersen, HR; Hasenkam, JM. Catheter-implanted prosthetic heart valves. Transluminal catheter implantation of a new expandable artificial heart valve in the descending thoracic aorta in isolated vessels and closed chest pigs. *Int J Artif Organs* 1993;16:253–62.

[24] Bonhoeffer, P; Boudjemline, Y; Saliba, Z; Hausse, AO; Aggoun, Y; Bonnet, D; Sidi, D; Kachaner, J. Percutaneous replacement of pulmonary valve in a right-ventricular to pulmonary-artery prosthetic conduit with valve dysfunction. *Lancet* 2000;356:1403–5

[25] Cribier, A; Eltchaninoff, H; Bash, A; Borenstein, N; Tron, C; Bauer, F; Derumeaux, G; Anselme, F; Laborde, F; Leon, MB. Percutaneous transcatheter implantation of an aortic valve prosthesis for calcific aortic stenosis: first human case description. *Circulation* 2002;106:3006–8.

[26] Cribier, A; Eltchaninoff, H; Tron, C; Bauer, F; Agatiello, C; Sebagh, L; Bash, A; Nusimovici, D; Litzler, PY; Bessou, JP; Leon, MB. Early experience with percutaneous transcatheter implantation of heart valve prosthesis for the treatment of end-stage inoperable patients with calcific aortic stenosis. *J Am Coll Cardiol* 2004;43:698 –703.

[27] Webb, JG; Altwegg, L; Masson, JB; Al Bugami, S; Al Ali, A; Boone, RA. A new transcatheter aortic valve and percutaneous valve delivery system. *J Am Coll Cardiol.* 2009 May 19;53(20):1855-8.

[28] Del Valle-Fernández, R; Martinez, CA; Ruiz, CE. Transcatheter aortic valve implantation. *Cardiol Clin.* 2010 Feb;28(1):155-68.

[29] Low, RI; Bolling, SF; Ebner, A. Direct Flow medical percutaneous aortic valve: proof of concept. *EuroIntervention* 2008; 4. (2): 256-261

[30] Buellesfeld, L.; Gerckens, U; Grube, E: Percutaneous implantation of the first repositionable aortic valve prosthesis in a patient with severe aortic stenosis. *Catheter Cardiovasc Interv* 2008;71. 579-584.

[31] Paniagua, D; Condado, JA; Besso, J; Vélez, M; Burger, B; Bibbo, S; Cedeno, D; Acquatella, H; Mejia, C; Induni, E; Fish, RD. First human case of retrograde transcatheter implantation of an aortic valve prosthesis. *Tex Heart Inst J* 2005;32. 393-398.

[32] Falk, V; Schwammenthal, EE; Kempfert, J; Linke, A; Schuler, G; Mohr, FW; Walther, T. New anatomically oriented transapical aortic valve implantation. *Ann Thorac Surg.* 2009 Mar;87(3):925-6.

[33] Martens, S; Ploss, A; Sirat, S; Miskovic, A; Moritz, A; Doss, M.: Sutureless aortic valve replacement with the 3f Enable aortic bioprosthesis. *Ann Thorac Surg.* 2009 Jun;87(6):1914-7.

[34] Shrestha, M; Khaladj, N; Bara, C; Hoeffler, K; Hagl, C; Haverich, A. A staged approach towards interventional aortic valve implantation with sutureless valve: initial human implants. *Thorac Cardiovasc Surg.* 2008 Oct;56(7):398-400

[35] Ferrari, M; Figulla, HR; Schlosser, M; Tenner, I; Frerichs, I; Damm, C; Guyenot, V; Werner, GS; Hellige, G. Transarterial aortic valve replacement with a self expanding stent in pigs. *Heart.* 2004 Nov;90(11):1326-31.

[36] Grube, E; Laborde, JC; Zickmann, B; Gerckens, U; Felderhoff, T; Sauren, B; Bootsveld, A; Buellesfeld, L; Iversen, S. First report on a human percutaneous

transluminal implantation of a self-expanding valve prosthesis for interventional treatment of aortic valve stenosis. *Catheter Cardiovasc Interv*. 2005 Dec;66(4):465-9.

[37] Grube, E; Schuler, G; Buellesfeld, L; Gerckens, U; Linke, A; Wenaweser, P; Sauren, B; Mohr, FW; Walther, T; Zickmann, B; Iversen, S; Felderhoff, T; Cartier, R; Bonan, R. Percutaneous aortic valve replacement for severe aortic stenosis in high-risk patients using the second- and current third-generation self-expanding CoreValve prosthesis: device success and 30-day clinical outcome. *J Am Coll Cardiol* 2007;50:69 –76.

[38] FDA Draft Guidance for Industry and FDA Staff: Heart Valves - Investigational Device Exemption (IDE) and Premarket Approval (PMA) Applications – Jan 20, 2010. Available online: http://www.fda.gov/MedicalDevices/DeviceRegulationandGuidance/GuidanceDocuments/ucm193096.htm

[39] Cardiovascular Implants – Cardiac Valve Prosthesis. EN ISO 5840:2005 (E); 2005

[40] Iung, B; Baron, G; Butchart, EG; Delahaye, F; Gohlke-Bärwolf, C; Levang, OW; Tornos, P; Vanoverschelde, JL; Vermeer, F; Boersma, E; Ravaud, P; Vahanian, A. A prospective survey of patients with valvular heart disease in Europe: The Euro Heart Survey on Valvular Heart Disease. *Eur Heart J*. 2003 Jul;24(13):1231-43.

[41] Nkomo ,VT; Gardin, JM; Skelton, TN; Gottdiener, JS; Scott, CG; Enriquez-Sarano, M. Burden of valvular heart diseases: a population-based study. *Lancet*. 2006 Sep 16;368(9540):1005-11.

[42] Yan, TD; Cao, C; Martens-Nielsen, J; Padang, R; Ng, M; Vallely, MP; Bannon, PG. Transcatheter aortic valve implantation for high-risk patients with severe aortic stenosis: A systematic review. *J Thorac Cardiovasc Surg*. 2010 Jun;139(6):1519-28.

[43] Webb, JG; Pasupati, S; Humphries, K; Thompson, C; Altwegg, L; Moss, R; Sinhal, A; Carere, RG; Munt, B; Ricci, D; Ye, J; Cheung, A; Lichtenstein, SV. Percutaneous transarterial aortic valve replacement in selected high-risk patients with aortic stenosis. *Circulation*. 2007 Aug 14;116(7):755-63.

[44] Cribier, A; Eltchaninoff, H; Tron, C; Bauer, F; Agatiello, C; Nercolini, D; Tapiero, S; Litzler, PY; Bessou, JP; Babaliaros, V. Treatment of calcific aortic stenosis with the percutaneous heart valve: mid-term follow-up from the initial feasibility studies: the French experience. *J Am Coll Cardiol*. 2006 Mar 21;47(6):1214-23.

[45] Bolling, SF; Rogers, JH; Babaliaros, V; Piazza, N; Takeda, PA; Low, RI; Block, PC.: Percutaneous aortic valve implantation utilising a novel tissue valve: preclinical experience. *EuroIntervention*. 2008 May;4(1):148-53.

[46] Chiam, PT; Ruiz, CE. Percutaneous transcatheter aortic valve implantation: Evolution of the technology. *Am Heart J*. 2009 Feb;157(2):229-42.

[47] Li, K; Sun, W. Simulated thin pericardial beioprosthetic valve leaflet deformation under static pressure-only loading conditions: implications for percutaneous valves. *Ann Biomed Eng. 2010* Aug;38(8):2690-701.

[48] Laske, T; Denton, M; Eberhardt, C. *The development of transcatheter heart valves: opportunities and challenges*, 31st Annual International Conference of the IEEE EMBS Minneapolis, Minnesota, 2009.

[49] Cribier, A; Litzler, PY; Eltchaninoff, H; Godin, M; Tron, C; Bauer, F; Bessou, JP. Technique of transcatheter aortic valve implantation with the Edwards-Sapien heart valve using the transfemoral approach. *Herz*. 2009 Aug;34(5):347-56.

[50] Lichtenstein, SV; Cheung, A; Ye, J; Thompson, CR; Carere, RG; Pasupati, S; Webb, JG.Transapical transcatheter aortic valve implantation in humans: initial clinical experience. *Circulation*. 2006 Aug 8;114(6):591-6.

[51] Walther, T; Falk, V; Borger, MA; Dewey, T; Wimmer-Greinecker, G; Schuler, G; Mack, M; Mohr, FW. Minimally invasive transapical beating heart aortic valve implantation—proof of concept. *Eur J Cardiothorac Surg*. 2007 Jan;31(1):9-15.

[52] Serruys, P.W.: Keynote address–EuroPCR 2008, Barcelona, May 14th, 2008. Transcatheter aortic valve implantation: state of the art. *EuroIntervention*. 2009; 4(5): 558-565.

[53] Webb, JG; Pasupati, S; Humphries, K; Thompson, C; Altwegg, L; Moss, R; Sinhal, A; Carere, RG; Munt, B; Ricci, D; Ye, J; Cheung, A; Lichtenstein, SV.: Percutaneous transarterial aortic valve replacement in selected high-risk patients with aortic stenosis. *Circulation*. 2007 Aug 14;116(7):755-63.

[54] Spargias, K; Manginas, A; Pavlides, G; Khoury, M; Stavridis, G; Rellia, P; Smirli, A; Thanopoulos, A; Balanika, M; Polymeros, S; Thomopoulou, S; Athanassopoulos, G; Karatasakis, G; Mastorakou, R; Lacoumenta, S; Michalis, A; Alivizatos, P; Cokkinos, D. Transcatheter aortic valve implantation: first Greek experience. *Hellenic J Cardiol*. 2008 Nov-Dec;49(6):397-407.

[55] Webb, JG; Chandavimol, M; Thompson, CR; Ricci, DR; Carere, RG; Munt, BI; Buller, CE; Pasupati, S; Lichtenstein, S.Percutaneous aortic valve implantation retrograde from the femoral artery. *Circulation*. 2006 Feb 14;113(6):842-50.

[56] John, D; Buellesfeld, L; Yuecel, S; Mueller, R; Latsios, G; Beucher, H; Gerckens, U; Grube, E. Correlation of Device landing zone calcification and acute procedural success in patients undergoing transcatheter aortic valve implantations with the self-expanding CoreValve prosthesis. *JACC Cardiovasc Interv*. 2010 Feb;3(2):233-43.

[57] Latsio,s G; Gerckens ,U; Buellesfeld, L; Muelle,r R; John, D; Yuecel, S; Syring, J; Sauren, B; Grube, E. "Device landing zone" calcification, assessed by MSCT, as a predictive factor for pacemaker implantation after TAVI. *Catheter Cardiovasc Interv*. 2010 Mar 26

[58] Zegdi, R; Ciobotaru, V; Noghin, M; Sleilaty, G; Lafont, A; Latrémouille, C; Deloche, A; Fabiani, JN. Is it reasonable to treat all calcified stenotic aortic valves with a valved stent? Results from a human anatomic study in adults. *J Am Coll Cardiol*. 2008 Feb 5;51(5):579-84.

[59] Eltchaninoff, H; Zajarias, A; Tron, C; Litzler, PY; Baala, B; Godin, M; Bessou, JP; Cribier, A. Transcatheter aortic valve implantation: technical aspects, results and indications. *Arch Cardiovasc* Dis. 2008 Feb;101(2):126-32.

[60] Latsios, G; Gerckens, U; Grube, E. Transaortic transcatheter aortic valve implantation: a novel approach for the truly "no-access option" patients. *Catheter Cardiovasc Interv*. 2010 Jun 1;75(7):1129-36.

[61] Ussia, GP; Barbanti, M; Tamburino, C. Consequences of underexpansion of a percutaneous aortic valve bioprosthesis. *J Invasive Cardiol*. 2010 May;22(5):E86-9.

[62] Zegdi, R; Blanchard, D; Achouh, P; Lafont, A; Berrebi, A; Cholley, B; Fabiani JN. Deployed Edwards Sapien prosthesis is always deformed. *J Thorac Cardiovasc Surg*. 2010 Apr 15 (Epub ahead of print)

[63] Zegdi, R; Lecuyer, L; Achouh, P; Didier, B; Lafont, A; Latrémouille, C; Fabiani, JN. Increased radial force improves stent deployment in tricuspid but not in bicuspid stenotic native aortic valves. *Ann Thorac Surg*. 2010 Mar;89(3):768-72.

[64] Grube, E; Buellesfeld, L; Mueller, R; Sauren, B; Zickmann, B; Nair, D; Beucher, H; Felderhoff ,T; Iversen, S; Gerckens, U. Progress and current status of percutaneous aortic valve replacement: results of three device generations of the CoreValve Revalving system. *Circ Cardiovasc Interv*. 2008 Dec;1(3):167-75.

[65] Nordmeyer, J; Khambadkone, S; Coats, L; Schievano, S.; Lurz, P; Parenzan, G; Taylor, AM; Lock, JE; Bonhoeffer, P. Risk stratification, systematic classification, and anticipatory management strategies for stent fracture after percutaneous pulmonary valve implantation. *Circulation*. 2007;115(11):1392–1397.

[66] Schievano, S; Taylor, AM; Capelli, C; Lurz, P; Nordmeyer, J; Migliavacca, F; Bonhoeffer, P. Patient specific finite element analysis results in more accurate prediction of stent fractures: Application to percutaneous pulmonary valve implantation. *J Biomech*. 2010 Mar 3;43(4):687-93.

[67] Clavel, MA; Webb, JG; Pibarot, P; Altwegg, L; Dumont, E; Thompson, C; De Larochellière, R; Doyle, D; Masson, JB; Bergeron, S; Bertrand, OF; Rodés-Cabau, J.. Comparison of the hemodynamic performance of percutaneous and surgical bioprostheses for the treatment of severe aortic stenosis. *J Am Coll Cardiol*. 2009 May 19;53(20):1883-91.

[68] Walther, T; Simon, P; Dewey, T; Wimmer-Greinecker, G; Falk, V; Kasimir, MT; Doss, M; Borger, MA; Schuler, G; Glogar, D; Fehske, W; Wolner, E; Mohr, FW; Mack, M. Transapical minimally invasive aortic valve implantation: Multicenter experience. *Circulation*. 2007 Sep 11;116(11 Suppl):I240-5.

[69] Rodés-Cabau, J; Dumont, E; De LaRochellière, R; Doyle, D; Lemieux, J; Bergeron, S; Clavel, MA; Villeneuve, J; Raby, K; Bertrand, OF; Pibarot, P. Feasibility and initial results of percutaneous aortic valve implantation including selection of the transfemoral or transapical approach in patients with severe aortic stenosis. *Am J Cardiol*. 2008 Nov 1;102(9):1240-6.

[70] Tops, LF; Wood, DA; Delgado, V; Schuijf, JD; Mayo, JR; Pasupati, S; Lamers, FP; van der Wall, EE; Schalij, MJ; Webb, JG; Bax, JJ. Noninvasive evaluation of the aortic root with multislice computed tomography: implications for transcatheter aortic valve replacement. *JACC Cardiovasc Imaging*. 2008 May;1(3):321-30.

[71] Piazza, N; de Jaegere, P; Schultz, C; Becker, AE; Serruys, PW; Anderson, RH. Anatomy of the aortic valvar complex and its implications for transcatheter implantation of the aortic valve. *Circ Cardiovasc Interv*. 2008 Aug;1(1):74-81.

[72] Piazza, N; Grube, E; Gerckens, U; den Heijer, P; Linke, A; Luha, O; Ramondo, A; Ussia, G; Wenaweser, P; Windecker, S; Laborde, JC; de Jaegere, P; Serruys, PW. Procedural and 30-day outcomes following transcatheter aortic valve implantation using the third generation (18F) CoreValve ReValving System—Results from the multicenter, expanded evaluation registry 1-year following CE mark approval. *EuroIntervention*. 2008 Aug;4(2):242-9.

[73] Rajani, R; Kakad, M; Khawaja, MZ; Lee, L; James, R; Saha, M; Hildick-Smith, D. Paravalvular regurgitation one year after transcatheter aortic valve implantation. *Catheter Cardiovasc Interv*. 2010 May 1;75(6):868-72.

[74] Zahn, R; Schiele, R; Kilkowski, C; Zeymer, U. Severe aortic regurgitation after percutaneous transcatheter aortic valve implantation: on the importance to clarify the underlying pathophysiology. *Clin Res Cardiol.* 2010 Mar;99(3):193-7.

[75] Tzikas, A; Piazza, N; Geleijnse, ML; Van Mieghem, N; Nuis, RJ; Schultz, C; van Geuns, RJ; Galema, TW; Kappetein, AP; Serruys ,PW; de Jaegere ,PP. Prosthesis-patient mismatch after transcatheter aortic valve implantation with the medtronic CoreValve system in patients with aortic stenosis. *Am J Cardiol.* 2010 Jul 15;106(2):255-60.

[76] Piazza, N; Schultz, C; de Jaegere, PP; Serruys, PW. Implantation of two self-expanding aortic bioprosthetic valves during the same procedure-Insights into valve-in-valve implantation ("Russian doll concept"). *Catheter Cardiovasc Interv.* 2009 Mar 1;73(4):530-9.

[77] Ruiz, CE; Laborde, JC; Condado, JF; Chiam, PT; Condado, JA. First percutaneous transcatheter aortic valve-in-valve implant with three year follow-up. *Catheter Cardiovasc Interv* 2008;72:143–148

[78] Clavel, MA; Dumont, E; Pibarot, P; Doyle, D; De Larochellière, R; Villeneuve, J; Bergeron, S; Couture, C; Rodés-Cabau, J. Severe valvular regurgitation and late prosthesis embolization following percutaneous aortic valve implantation. *Ann Thorac Surg. 2009 Feb;87(2):618-21.*

[79] Ussia, GP; Mulè, M; Tamburino, C. The valve-in-valve technique: Transcatheter treatment of aortic bioprothesis malposition. *Catheter Cardiovasc Interv.* 2009 Apr 1;73(5):713-6.

[80] Ng, AC; van der Kley, F; Delgado, V; Shanks, M; van Bommel, RJ; de Wege,r A; Tavilla, G; Holman, ER; Schuij, JD; van de Veire, NR; Schalij, MJ; Bax, JJ. Percutaneous valve-in-valve procedure for severe paravalvular regurgitation in aortic bioprosthesis. *JACC Cardiovasc Imaging.* 2009 Apr;2(4):522-3.

[81] Rodés-Cabau, J; Dumont, E; Doyle, D. "Valve-in-valve" for the treatment of paravalvular leaks following transcatheter aortic valve implantation. *Catheter Cardiovasc Interv.* 2009 Dec 1;74(7):1116-9.

[82] Latib, A; Michev, I; Laborde, JC; Montorfano, M; Colombo, A. Post-implantation repositioning of the CoreValve percutaneous aortic valve. *JACC Cardiovasc Interv.* 2010 Jan;3(1):119-21.

[83] Walther, T; Falk, V. Hemodynamic evaluation of heart valve prostheses paradigm shift for transcatheter valves?. *J Am Coll Cardiol.* 2009 May 19;53(20):1892-3..

[84] Walther, T; Kempfert, J; Borger, MA; Fassl, J; Falk, V; Blumenstein, J; Dehdashtian, M; Schuler, G; Mohr, FW.. Human minimally invasive off-pump valve-in-a-valve implantation. *Ann Thorac Surg.* 2008 Mar;85(3):1072-3.

[85] Zahn, R; Schiele, R; Kilkowski, C; Klein, B; Zeymer, U; Werling, C; Lehmann, A; Layer, G; Saggau, W. There are two sides to everything: two case reports on sequelae of rescue interventions to treat complications of transcatheter aortic valve implantation of the Medtronic CoreValve prosthesis. *Clin Res Cardiol.* 2010 Apr 20.

[86] Piazza, N; Onuma, Y; Jesserun, E; Kint, PP; Maugenest, AM; Anderson, RH; de Jaegere, PP; Serruys, PW. Early and persistent intraventricular conduction abnormalities and requirements for pacemaking after percutaneous replacement of the aortic valve. *JACC Cardiovasc Interv.* 2008 Jun;1(3):310-6.

[87] Tzikas, A; Schultz, C; Piazza, N; van Geuns, RJ; Serruys,PW; de Jaegere, PP. Perforation of the membranous interventricular septum after transcatheter aortic valve implantation. *Circ Cardiovasc Interv*. 2009 Dec;2(6):582-3.
[88] Wong, DR; Boone, RH; Thompson, CR; Allard, MF; Altwegg, L; Carere, RG; Cheung, A; Ye, J; Lichtenstein, SV; Ling, H; Webb, JG. Mitral valve injury late after transcatheter aortic valve implantation, *J Thorac Cardiovasc Surg*. 2009 Jun;137(6):1547-9.
[89] Webb, JG; Pasupati, S; Achtem, L; Thompson, CR. Rapid pacing to facilitate transcatheter prosthetic heart valve implantation. *Catheter Cardiovasc Interv*. 2006 Aug;68(2):199-204.
[90] Schultz, CJ; Weustink, A; Piazza, N; Otten, A; Mollet, N; Krestin, G; van Geuns, RJ; de Feyter, P; Serruys, PW; de Jaegere, P. Geometry and degree of apposition of the CoreValve ReValving system with multislice computed tomography after implantation in patients with aortic stenosis. *J Am Coll Cardiol*. 2009 Sep 1;54(10):911-8.
[91] Thubrikar, M; Piepgrass, WC; Shaner, TW; Nolan, SP. The design of the normal aortic valve. *Am J Physiol*. 1981 Dec;241(6):H795-801.
[92] Schoen, FJ; Levy, RJ; Calcification of tissue heart valve substitutes: progress toward understanding and prevention. *Journal of Ann Thorac Surg*, 2005; 79:1072-80
[93] Thubrikar, MJ; Deck, JD; Aouad, J; Nolan, SP. Role of mechanical stress in calcification of aortic bioprosthetic valves. *J Thorac Cardiovasc Surg*. 1983 Jul;86(1):115-25.
[94] Moczar, M; Houël, R; Ginat, M; Clérin, V; Wheeldon, D; Loisance, D. Structural changes in porcine bioprosthetic valves of a left ventricular assist system in human patients. *J Heart Valve Dis*. 2000 Jan;9(1):88-95; discussion 95-6.
[95] Schoen, FJ. Pathologic findings in explanted clinical bioprosthetic valves fabricated from photooxidized bovine pericardium. *J Heart Valve Dis*. 1998 Mar;7(2):174-9.
[96] Purinya, B; Kasyanov, V; Volkolakov, J; Latsis, R; Tetere, G. Biomechanical and structural properties of the explanted bioprosthetic valve leaflets. *J Biomech*. 1994 Jan;27(1):1-11.
[97] Mako, WJ; Shah, A; Vesely, I. Mineralization of glutaraldehyde-fixed porcine aortic valve cusps in the subcutaneous rat model: analysis of variations in implant site and cuspal quadrants. *J Biomed Mater Res*. 1999 Jun 5;45(3):209-13.
[98] FDA guidance, Non-Clinical Tests and Recommended Labeling for Intravascular Stents and Associated Delivery Systems – April 18 2010. Available online: *http://www.fda.gov/MedicalDevices/DeviceRegulationandGuidance/GuidanceDocuments/ucm071863.htm*
[99] Sacks, MS; Merryman, WD; Scmidt, D. On the biomechanics of heart valve function. *J Biomech*. 2009 Aug 25;42(12):1804-24.
[100] Sacks, MS; Mirnajafi, A; Sun, W; Schmidt, P. Bioprosthetic heart valve heterograft biomaterials: structure, mechanical behavior and computational simulation. *Expert Rev Med Devices*. 2006 Nov;3(6):817-34.
[101] Ishihara, T; Ferrans, VJ; Jones, M; Boyce, SW; Roberts, WC. Occurrence and significance of endothelial cells in implanted porcine bioprosthetic valves. *Am J Cardiol*. 1981 Sep;48(3):443-54.
[102] Duerig, TW; Wholey, M. A Comparison of balloon-and self-expanding stents. *Min Invas Ther & Allied Techno*l 2002: 11(4): 173-178

[103] Dyet, JF; Watts, WG; Ettles, DF; Nicholson, AA. Mechanical properties of metallic stents: how do these properties influence the choice of stent for specific lesions? *Cardiovasc Intervent Radiol.* 2000 Jan-Feb;23(1):47-54.

[104] Mani, G; Feldman, MD; Patel, D; Agrawal, CM. Coronary stents: a materials perspective. *Biomaterials.* 2007 Mar;28(9):1689-710.

[105] ASTM Standard F138, 2008 – Standard Specification for Wrought 18Chromium-14Nickel-2.5Molybdenum Stainless Steel Bar and Wire for Surgical Implants, *ASTM International*, West Conshohocken, PA, 2008 DOI: 10.1520/F0138-08, www.astm.org.

[106] Hudson, RM; Joniec, RJ; Shatynski, SR. Pickling of iron and steel In: W.H. Cubberly, Editors, Metals Handbook (ninth ed.), *American Society for Metals,* Metals Park, Ohio (1982), p. 68.

[107] Köster, R; Vieluf, D; Kiehn, M; Sommerauer, M; Kähler, J; Baldus, S; Meinertz, T; Hamm, CW. Nickel and molybdenum contact allergies in patients with coronary in-stent restenosis. *Lancet.* 2000 Dec 2;356(9245):1895-7.

[108] Haudrechy, P.; Foussereau, J.; Mantout, B.; Baroux, B. Nickel release from 304 and 316 stainless steels in synthetic sweat. Comparison with nickel and nickel-plated metals. Consequences on allergic contact dermatitis. *Corros Sci.* 1993: 35(1-4):329–336.

[109] Bortolotti, U; Gallucci, V; Casarotto, D; Thiene, G. Fibrous tissue overgrowth on Hancock mitral xenografts: a cause of late prosthetic stenosis. *Thorac Cardiovasc Surg.* 1979 Oct;27(5):316-8.

[110] Kastrati, A; Mehilli, J; Dirschinger, J; Dotzer, F; Schühlen, H; Neumann, FJ; Fleckenstein, M; Pfafferott, C; Seyfarth, M; Schömig, A. Intracoronary stenting and angiographic results: strut thickness effect on restenosis outcome (ISAR-STEREO) trial. *Circulation.* 2001 Jun 12;103(23):2816-21.

[111] Briguori, C; Sarais, C; Pagnotta, P; Liistro, F; Montorfano, M; Chieffo, A; Sgura, F; Corvaja, N; Albiero, R; Stankovic, G; Toutoutzas, C; Bonizzoni, E; Di Mario, C; Colombo, A. In-stent restenosis in small coronary arteries: impact of strut thickness. *J Am Coll Cardiol.* 2002 Aug 7;40(3):403-9.

[112] ASTM Standard F1058, 2008 – Standard Specification for Wrought 40Cobalt-20Chromium-16Iron-15Nickel-7Molybdenum Alloy Wire and Strip for Surgical Implant Applications, *ASTM International*, West Conshohocken, PA, 2008 DOI: 10.1520/F1058-08, www.astm.org.

[113] Poirer, NC; Pelletier, LC; Pellerin, M; Carrier, M. 15-year experience with the Carpentier-Edwards pericardial bioprosthesis. *Ann Thorac Surg. 1998* Dec;66(6 Suppl):S57-61.

[114] ASTM Standard F90, 2009 – Standard Specification for Wrought Cobalt-20Chromium-15Tungsten-10Nickel Alloy for Surgical Implant Applications, *ASTM International*, West Conshohocken, PA, 2009 DOI: 10.1520/F0090-09, www.astm.org.

[115] ASTM Standard F562, 2007 – Standard Specification for Wrought Cobalt-20Chromium-15Tungsten-10Nickel Alloy for Surgical Implant Applications, *ASTM International*, West Conshohocken, PA, 2007 DOI: 10.1520/F0562-07, www.astm.org.

[116] Kereiakes, DJ; Cox, DA; Hermiller, JB; Midei, MG; Bachinsky, WB; Nukta, ED; Leon, MB; Fink, S; Marin, L; Lansky, AJ; Usefulness of a cobalt chromium coronary stent alloy. *Am J Cardiol.* 2003 Aug 15;92(4):463-6.

[117] Escalas, F; Galante, J; Rostoker, W; Coogan, PH. MP35N: a corrosion resistant, high strength alloy for orthopedic surgical impants: bio-assay results. *J Biomed Mater Res.* 1975 May;9(3):303-13.

[118] Marti, A. Cobalt-base alloys used in bone surgery. *Injury*. 2000 Dec;31 Suppl 4:18-21.

[119] Poncin, P; Millet C; Chevy J; Proft JL Comparing and optimizing Co-Cr tubing for stent applications. *Mater & Processes for Medical Devices Conferences* 2004 25-27.

[120] Teitelbaum, G.; Bradley, W.; Klein, B. MR imaging artifacts, ferromagnetism, and magnetic torque of intravascular filters, stents, and coils. *Radiology. 1988 Mar;166(3):657-64.*

[121] Hijazi, ZM; Homoud, M; Aronovitz, MJ; Smith, JJ; Faller, GT.. A new platinum balloon-expandable stent (Angiostent) mounted on a high pressure balloon: acute and late results in an atherogenic swine model. *J Invasive Cardiol.* 1995 Jun;7(5):127-34.

[122] Bhargava, B; De Scheerder, I; Ping, QB; Yanming, H; Chan, R; Soo Kim, H; Kollum, M; Cottin, Y; Leon, MB.. A novel platinum–iridium, potentially gamma radioactive stent: evaluation in a porcine model. *Catheter Cardiovasc Interv*. 2000 Nov;51(3):364-8.

[123] Trost, DW; Zhang, HL; Prince, MR; Winchester, PA; Wang, Y; Watts, R; Sos, TA. Three-dimensional MR angiography in imaging platinum alloy stents. *J Magn Reson Imaging*. 2004 Dec;20(6):975-80.

[124] Park, JB; Kim, YK; Park, JB; Bronzino; J.D. *Biomaterials principles and applications.* Boca Raton: CRC Press, 2003.

[125] Lurz, P; Bonhoeffer, P; Taylor, AM. Percutaneous pulmonary valve implantation: an update. *Expert Rev Cardiovasc Ther.* 2009 Jul;7(7):823-33

[126] Stoeckel, D; Pelton, A; Duerig, T. Self-expanding nitinol stents: material and design considerations. *Eur Radiol.* 2004 Feb;14(2):292-301.

[127] Hoh, DJ; Hoh, BL; Amar, AP; Wang, MY. Shape memory alloys: metallurgy, biocompatibility, and biomechanics for neurosurgical applications. *Neurosurgery.* 2009 May;64(5 Suppl 2):199-214; discussion 214-5.

[128] Trepanier, C; Venugopalan, R; Pelton, AR; Yahia, LH. *Shape memory implants.* New York: Springer, 2000

[129] Schürmann, K; Vorwerk, D; Kulisch, A; Stroehmer-Kulisch, E; Biesterfeld, S; Stopinski, T; Günther, RW.Experimental arterial stent placement. Comparison of a new nitinol stent and wallstent. *Invest Radiol.* 1995 Jul;30(7):412-20.

[130] Poncin, P.; Proft, J. Stent tubing: Understanding the desired attributes, Proc. *Materials & Processes for Medical Devices Conference*, 8–10 Sept 2003, Anaheim, CA, US, ASM International (2003), pp. 253–259.

[131] Nitinol Superelastic Tubing Stock from Minitubes Inc., Grenoble, France *http://www.minitubes.com/images/brochure/PRD019A.pdf*

[132] Whittaker, DR; Fillinger, MF. The engineering of endovascular stent technology: a review. *Vasc Endovascular Surg*. 2006 Mar-Apr;40(2):85-94.

[133] Duerig, TW; Tolomeo, DE; Wholey, M. An overview of superelastic stent design. *Minim Invasive Ther Allied Technol*. 2000;9(3-4):235-46.

[134] Kruger, J. Fundamental aspects of corrosion of metallic implants. In: *Corrosion and degradation of implant materials* ASTM STP 684. BC Syrett; A Acharya; Eds., American Society for Testing and Materials; 1979. P. 107–113

[135] Fraker, AC. Corrosion of metallic implants and prosthetic devices. In: *ASM Metals handbook*; 9th Ed. Vol 13. Metals Park, OH: ASM International; 1987. p. 1324–3

[136] Leclerc, MF. Surgical Implants. In: *ASTM Metals Handbook* 9th Ed. Vol 2. Metals Park, OH: ASM International; 1987, p. 164-80

[137] Oyane, A; Kim, HM; Furya, T; Kokubo, T; Miyazaki, T; Nakamura, T. Preperation and assessment of revised simulated body fluids. *J Biomed Mater Res A*. 2003 May 1;65(2):188-95.

[138] Virtanen, S; Milosev, I; Gomez-Barrena, E; Trebse, R; Salo, J; Konttinen, YT. Special modes of corrosion under physiological and simulated physiological conditions. *Acta Biomater*. 2008 May;4(3):468-76.

[139] Schultze, JW; Lohrengel, MM. Stability, reactivity and breakdown of passive films. Problems of recent and future research. *Electrochim Acta*. 2000;45:2499–2513.

[140] Milosev, I; Strehblow, HH. The behavior of stainless steels in physiological solution containing complexing agent studied by X-ray photoelectron spectroscopy. *J Biomed Mater Res*. 2000 Nov;52(2):404-12.

[141] Milosev, I; Strehblow, HH. The composition of the surface passive film formed on CoCrMo alloy in simulated physiological solution. *Electrochim Acta*. 2003;48:2767–2774.

[142] Wever, DJ; Veldhuizen, AG; de Vries, J; Busscher, HJ; Uges, DRA; van Horn, JR. Electrochemical and surface characterization of a nicken-titanium alloy. *Biomaterials*. 1998 Apr-May;19(7-9):761-9.

[143] Asphahani, AI. Corrosion of cobalt base alloys. In: ASM Metals handbook, vol. 13. 9th ed. Metals Park, OH: *ASM International*; 1987. p. 658-68

[144] Goldberg, JR; Gilbert, JL. The Electrochemcial and Mechanical Behavior of Passivated and TiN/AIN coated CoCrMo and TiAl4V Alloys. *Biomaterials*. 2004 Feb;25(5):851-64.

[145] Zsklarska-Smialowska, Z. Pitting Corrosion of Metals. Houston, Tx: *National Association of Corrosion Engineers*; 1986

[146] Souto, RM; Burstein, GT. A preliminary investigation into the microscopic depassivation of passive titanium implant materials. *J Mater Sci*. 1996;7:337–43.

[147] Gurappa, I. Characterization of different materials for corrosion resistance under simulated body fluid conditions. *Materials Characterization*. 2002 Aug; 49(1): 73-79

[148] Walke, W; Paszenda Z; Ziębowicz A: Corrosion behaviour of Co-Cr-W-Ni alloy in diverse body fluids. *Archives of Materials Science and Engineering*. 2007; 20(5):293-296.

[149] ASTM Standard F2129, 2008 – Standard Test Method for Conducting Cyclic Potentiodynamic Polarization Measurements to Determine the Corrosion Susceptibility of Small Implant Devices, *ASTM International*, West Conshohocken, PA, 2008 DOI: 10.1520/F2129-06, www.astm.org.

[150] Trépanier, C; Tabrizian, M; Yahia, LH; Bilodeau, L; Piron, DL. Effect of modification of oxide layer on NiTi stent corrosion resistance. *J Biomed Mater Res*. 1998; 43: 433-440,

[151] Sohmura, T. Improvement in Corrosion resistance in Ti-Ni shape memory alloy for implant by oxide film coating. *World Biomaterial Congress Proceedings*, Kyoto, Japan; 1988:574

[152] Wallinder, D; Pan, J; Leygraf, C; Delblanc-Bauer, A. Eis and XPS study of surface modification of 316LVM stainless steel after passivation. *Corrosion Science*. 1998 Feb; 41(2):275-289

[153] Weldon, LM; McHugh, PE; Carroll, W; Costello, E; O'Bradaigh, C. The influence of passivation and electropolishing on the performance of medical grade stainless steels in static and fatigue loading. *Journal of Materials Science: Materials in Medicine*. 2005 Jan; 16(2):107 – 117

[154] Shabalovskaya, S; Anderegg, J; Rondelli, G; Xiong, J. The Effect of Surface Particulates on the Corrosion Resistance of Nitinol Wire, *Proceedings of the SMST*, Asilomar, A. Pelton and T. Duerig, Ed., 2003, p 399–408

[155] Hensel, KB. Electropolishing. *Metal Finishing*, 1999; 97(1): 447-448,450-452,454-455

[156] Thierry, B; Trabrizian, M; Trepanier, C; Savadogo, O; Yahia, L'H. Effect of Surface treatment and sterilization processes on the corrosion behavior of NiTi memory alloy. *J Biomed Mater Res*. 2000;51:685-693

[157] O'Brien, B; Carroll, W; Kelly, M: Passivation of Nitinol wire for vascular implants – a demonstration of the benefits. *Biomaterials*. 2002;23: 1739-1748

[158] Kerber, SJ; Tverberg, J. Stainless steel surface analysis. *Adv Mater Process* 2000; 11:33-6

[159] Cisse, O; Savagodo, O; Wu, M; Yahia,L. Effect of surface treatment of NiTi alloy on its corrosion behavior in Hank's solution, *J Biomed Mater Res,* 2002; 62: 339–345.

[160] Zhu, L; Trepanier, C; Fino, J; Pelton, AR. Oxidation of Nitinol and its Effect on Corrosion Resistance. *Proceedings of the SMST, Asilomar, A. Pelton and T. Duerig, Ed.,* 2003: 367–375.

[161] ASTM Standard F86, 2004 (2009) – Standard Practice for Surface Preparation and Marking of Metallic Surgical Implants, *ASTM International,* West Conshohocken, PA, 2009 DOI: 10.1520/F0086-04R09, www.astm.org.

[162] ASTM Standard E1558, 2009 – Standard Guide for Electrolytic Polishing of Metallographic Specimens, *ASTM International*, West Conshohocken, PA, 2009 DOI: 10.1520/E1558-09, www.astm.org.

[163] ASTM Standard B912, 2002e1 (2008) – Standard Specification for Passivation of Stainless Steels Using Electropolishing, *ASTM International*, West Conshohocken, PA, 2008 DOI: 10.1520/B0912-02R08E01, www.astm.org.

[164] Trigwell, S; Selvaduray, G. Effects of surface finish on the corrosion of NiTi alloy for biomedical applications. In: *Pelton AR, Hodgson 0, Russell SM. Duerig T, editors. Proceedings 2nd International Conference on Shape Memory and Superelastic Technologies (SMS7); Pacific Grove: MIAS.* 1997: 383-8.

[165] Raval, A; Choubey, A; Engineer, C; Kothwala, D. Development and assessment of 316LVM cardiovascular stents. *Materials Science and Engineering A*, 2004; Nov 25; 386(1-2): 331-343.

[166] Rondelli, G; Vicentini, B. Evaluation by electrochemical tests of passive film stability of equiatomic Ni–Ti alloy also in the presence of stress induced martensite. *J Biomed Mater Res, 2000;* 51:47–54.

[167] Heβing, C; Frenzel, J; Pohl, M; Shabalovskaya, S. Effect of martensitic transformation on the performance of coated NiTi surfaces. *Mater Sc Eng A*, 2007; July 15; 486 (1-2): 461-469.

[168] Shabalovskya, S; Anderegg, J; Van Humbeeck, J. Critical Overview of Nitinol surfaces and their modifications for medical applications. *Acta Biomaterialia*,2008; 4: 447-467.

[169] Wenaweser, P; Buellesfeld, L; Gerckens, U; Grube E. Percutaneous aortic valve replacement for severe aortic regurgitation in degenerated bioprosthesis: the first valve in valve procedure using the Corevalve Revalving system. *Catheter Cardiovasc Interv.*, 2007; Nov 1;70(5):760-4.

[170] Bruschi, G; DeMarco, F; Oreglia, J; Colombo, P; Fratto, P; Lullo, F; Paino, R; Martinelli, L; Klugmann, S. Transcatheter aortic valve-in-valve implantation of a CoreValve in a degenerated aortic bioprosthesis. *J Cardiovasc Med (Hagerstown)*, 2010; 11(3):182-5.

[171] Khawaja, MZ; Haworth, P; Ghuran, A; Lee, L; de Belder, A; Hutchinson, N; Trivedi, U; Laborde, JC; Hildick-Smith, D. Transcatheter aortic valve implantation for stenosed and regurgitant aortic valve bioprostheses CoreValve for failed bioprosthetic aortic valve replacements. *J Am Coll Cardiol.*, 2010;55(2):97-101.

[172] Seiffert, M; Franzen, O; Conradi, L; Baldus, S; Schirmer, J; Meinertz, T; Reichenspurner, H; Treede, H. Series of transcatheter valve-in-valve implantations in high-risk patients with degenerated bioprostheses in aortic and mitral position. *Catheter Cardiovasc Interv.*, 2010: Apr 30.

[173] Kempfert, J; Van Linden, A; Linke, A; Borger, MA; Rastan, A; Mukherjee, C; Ender, J; Schuler, G; Mohr, FW; Walther ,T. Transapical off-pump valve-in-valve implantation in patients with degenerated aortic xenografts. *Ann Thorac Surg.*, 2010; 89(6):1934-41.

[174] Platt, JA; Guzman, A; Zuccari, A; Thornburg, DW; Rhodes, BF; Oshida, Y; Moore, BK. Corrosion behavior of 2205 duplex stainless steel. *Am J Orthod Dentofacial Orthop.*, 1997;112(1):69-79.

[175] ASTM Standard G71, 1981 (2009) – Standard Guide for Conducting and Evaluating Galvanic Corrosion Tests in Electrolytes, *ASTM International*, West Conshohocken, PA, 2008 DOI: 10.1520/G0071-81R09, www.astm.org.

[176] Hanawa T. Metal ion release from metal implants. *Mater Sci Eng*, 2004; C24:745-52.

[177] Okazaki, Y; Gotoh, E. Comparison of metal release from various metallic biomaterials in vitro. *Biomaterials*, 2005; 26:11-21.

[178] Wapner, KL. Implications of metallic corrosion in total knee arthroplasty. *Clin Orthop Relat Res*, 1991; 271:12-20.

[179] Pazzaglia, UE; Minola, C; Ceciliani, L; Riccardi, C. Metal determination in organic fluids of patients with stainless steel hip arthroplasty. *Acta Orthop Scand*, 1983; 54:574–579.

[180] Michel, R; Nolte, M; Reich, M; Loer, F. Systemic effects of implanted prostheses made of cobalt–chromium alloys. *Arch Orthop Trauma Surg*, 1991; 110: 61–74.

[181] Jacobs, JJ; Skipor, AK; Black, J; Urban, R; Galante, JO. Release and excretion of metal in patients who have a total hip-replacement component made of titanium-base alloy. *J Bone Jt Surg.*, 1991; 73-A: 1475–1486.

[182] Jacobs, JJ; Silverton, C; Hallab, NJ; Skipor, AK; Patterson, L; Black, J; Galante, JO. Metal release and excretion from cementless titanium alloy total knee replacements. *Clin Orthop Relat Res, 1999;* 358:173–180.

[183] Wataha, J; Craig, R; Hanks, C. The release of elements of dental casting alloys into cell-culture medium. *J Dent Res*, 1991;70: 1014–1018.

[184] Wataha, J. Biocompatibility of dental casting alloys: A review. *The Journal of Prosthetic Dentistry*, 2000; 83 (2): 223-234.

[185] Brune, D. Metal release from dental biomaterials, *Biomaterials*, 1986; 7: 163–175.

[186] Steinemann, SG. Metal implants and Surface Reactions. *Injury*, 1996;27 Suppl 3:SC16-22.

[187] Okazaki, Y. Effect of friction on anodic polarization properties of metallic biomaterials. *Biomaterials, 2002; 23:* 2071–2077.

[188] Khanm, A; Williams, R; Williams, DF. In vitro corrosion and wear of titanium alloys in the biological environment. *Biomaterials,* 1996; 17: 2117–2126.

[189] Agins, HJ; Alcock, NW; Bansal, M; Salvati, EA; Wilson, PD; Pellicci, PM; Bullough, PG. Metallic wear in failed titanium-alloy total hip replacements. *J Bone Jt Surg.*, 1988; 70-A:347–356.

[190] Healy, KE; Ducheyne, P. The mechanisms of passive dissolution of titanium in a model physiological environment. *J Biomed Mater Res.*, 1992; 26: 319–338.

[191] Bertrand, OF; Sipehia, R; Mongrain, R; Rodés, J; Tardif, JC; Bilodeau, L; Côté, G; Bourassa, MG. Biocompatibility aspects of new stent technology. *J Am Coll Cardiol*, 1998; 32(3):562-71.

[192] O'Brien, B; Carroll, W. The evolution of cardiovascular stent materials and surfaces in response to clinical drivers: A review. *Acta Biomaterialia*, 2009; 5(4): 945-958.

[193] Hanawa, T; Hiromoto, S; Yamamoto, A; Kuroda, D; Asami, K. XPS Characterization of the Surface Oxide Film of 316L Stainless Steel Samples that were Located in Quasi-Biological Environments. *Mater. Trans.*, 2002; 43:3088.

[194] Hanawa, T; Hiromoto, S; Asami, K. Characterization of the surface oxide film of a Co–Cr–Mo alloy after being located in quasi-biological environments using XPS. *Appl. Surf. Sci.*, 2001; 183:68.

[195] Shabalovskaya, SA; Anderegg, JW. Surface spectroscopic characterization of TiNi nearly equiatomic shape memory alloys for implants. *J. Vac. Sci. Technol. A*, 1995; 13(5): 2624-2632.

[196] Sasada, T; Morita, M; Mabuchi, K. Evaluation of Wear Toxicity for Implant Materials Through Cell Culture Method. *Yokohomo Proc. Internatl Triibology Conference.* 1995; 1957.

[197] Okazaki,Y; Gotoh, E. Metal release from stainless steel, Co–Cr–Mo–Ni–Fe and Ni–Ti alloys in vascular implants. *Corrosion Science*, 2008; 50(12): 3429-3438.

[198] Cui, Z; Man, H; Yang, X. The corrosion and nickel release behavior of laser surface-melted NiTi shape memory alloys in Hanks solution. *Surf Coat Technol*, 2005; 192: 347–353.

[199] Sun, Z; Wataha, J; Hanks C. Effects of metal ions on osteoblastlike cell metabolism and differentiation. *J Biomed Mater Res*, 1997;34:29–37.

[200] Rae, T. The action of cobalt, nickel, and chromium on phagocytosis and bacterial killing by human polymorphonuclear leukocytes; Its relevance to infection after total joint arthroplasty. *Biomaterials,* 1983;4:175–180.

[201] Rae, T. A study on the effects of particulate metals of orthopaedic interest on murine acrophages in vitro. *J Bone Joint Surg Br*, 1975;57:444–450.

[202] Howie, DW; Rogers, SD; McGee, MA; Haynes, DR. Biological effects of cobalt chrome in cell and animal models. *Clin Orthop*, 1996;329S:S217–S232.

[203] Shettlemore, MG; Bundy, KJ. Toxicity measurement of orthopedic implant alloy degradation products using a bioluminescent bacterial assay. *J Biomed Mater Res.*, 1999; 45(4):395-403.

[204] Hayes, R. The carcinogenicity of metals in human. *Cancer Causes and Control*, 1997; 8:321–327.

[205] Vahey, JW; Simonian, PT; Conrad, EU. Carcinogenicity and metallic implants. *Am J Orthop,* 1995;24:319–324.

[206] Browne, M; Gregson, PJ. Surface modification of titanium alloy implants. *Biomaterials,* 1994; 15:894–898.

[207] Okazaki, Y; Tateishi, T; Ito, Y. Corrosion resistance of implant alloys in pseudo-physiological solution and role of alloying elements in passive films. *Mater Trans JIM,* 1997; 38: 78–84.

[208] Wisbey, A; Gregson, PJ; Peter, LM; Tuke, M. Effect of surface treatment on the dissolution of titanium-based implant materials. *Biomaterials,* 1991; 12:470-473.

[209] Lausmaa, J; Mattsson, L; Rolander, U; Kasemo, B. Chemical composition and morphology of titanium surface oxides. *Mater. Res. Soc. Symp.*, 1986; Proc. 55: 351-359.

[210] Trepanier, C; Venugopolan, R; Messer, R; Zimmerman, J; Pelton, AR. Effect of passivation treatments on nickel release from Nitinol. *Proc Soc Biomater, 2000*; 1043.

[211] Clarke, B; Carroll, W; Rochev, Y; Hynes, M; Bradley, D; Plumley, D. Influence of nitinol wire surface treatment on oxide thickness and composition and its subsequent effect on corrosion resistance and nickel ion release. *J Biomed Mater Res,* 2006; 79A:61–70.

[212] Shabalovskaya, S; Anderegg, J; Laabs, F; Thiel, P; Rondelli, G. Surface conditions of nitinol wires, tubing, and as-cast alloys: the effect of chemical etching, aging n boiling water, and heat treatment. *J Biomed Mater Res*, 2003; 65B:193–203.

[213] Köster, R; Vieluf, D; Kiehn, M; Sommerauer, M; Kähler, J; Baldus, S; Meinertz, T; Hamm, CW. Nickel and molybdenum contact allergies in patients with coronary in-stent restenosis. *Lancet*, 2000; 365:1895–1897.

[214] Kobayashi, Y; Honda, Y; Christie, L; Teirsten, P; Bailey, S; Brown, Cl; Matthews, RV; De Fanco, AC; Schwartz, RC; Goldberg, S; Popma, JJ; Yock, PG; Fitzgerald, PJ. Long-term vessel response of self-expending coronary stent: a serial volumetric intravascular ultrasound analysis from the ASSURE trial. *J Am Coll Cardiol*, 2001; 37(5):1329–1334.

[215] Wataha, JC; Lockwood, PE; Marek, M; Ghazi, M. Ability of Ni-containing biomedical alloys to activate monocytes and endothelial cells in vitro. *J Biomed Mater Res.* 1999; 45:251–257.

[216] Wataha, JC; Ratanasathien, S; Hanks, CT; Sun, Z. In vitro IL-1 beta and TNF-alpha release from THP-1 monocytes in response to metal ions. *Dent Mater*, 1996;12:322–327.

[217] Gimenez-Arnau, A; Riambau, V; Serra-Baldrich, E; Camarasa, JG. Metal-induced generalized pruriginous dermatitis and endovascular surgery. *Contact Dermatitis*, 2000;43:35–40.

[218] Hillen, U; Haude, M; Erbel, R; Goos, M. Evaluation of metal allergies in patients with coronary stents. *Contact Dermatitis*, 2002; 47: 353-356.

[219] Keane, F; Morris, S; Smith, H; Rycroft, RJ. Allergy in coronary in-stent restenosis. *Lancet*, 2001; 357:1205-1206.

[220] Norgaz, T; Hobikoglu, G; Serdar, ZA; Aksu, H; Alper, AT; Ozer, O; Narin, A. Is there a link between nickel allergy and coronary stent restenosis? *Tohoku J Exp Med.* Jul 2005;206(3):243-6.

[221] DePalma, VA; Baier, RE; Ford, JW; Gott, VL; Furuse, A. Investigation of three-surface properties of several metals and their relation to blood compatibility, *J Biomed Mater Res 6,* 1972; 4: 37–75.

[222] Hecker, J; Scandrett, L. Roughness and thrombogenicity of the outer surfaces of intravascular catheters, *J Biomed Mater Res 19, 1985; 4:381-395.*

[223] Scheerder, ID; Sohier, J; Wang, K; Verbeken, E; Zhou, XR; Frooyen, L; Humebeeck, JV; Van de Werf, F. Metallic surface treatment using electrochemical polishing decreases thrombogenicity and neointimal hyperplasia after coronary stent implantation in a porcine model. *JACC,* 1998; 31(Suppl. 1): 227A.

[224] Sheth, S; Litvack, F; Fishbein, MC; Forrester, JS; Eigler, NL. Reduced thrombogenicity of polished and unpolished nitinol vs. stainless steel slotted-tube stents in a pig coronary artery model. *JACC*; 1996. Abstracts-Poster: 197A.

[225] Thierry, B; Merhi, Y; Bilodeau, L; Trépanier, C; Tabrizian,M. Nitinol versus stainless steel stents: acute thrombogenicity study in an ex vivo porcine model. *Biomaterials*, July 2002; 23(14): 2997-3005.

[226] Tepe, G; Schmehl, J; Wendel, HP; Schaffner, S; Heller, S; Gianotti, M; Claussen, C; Duda, SH. Reduced thrombogenicity of nitinol stents—In vitro evaluation of different surface modifications and coatings. *Biomaterials*, 2006; 27(4): 643-650.

[227] Hehrlein, C; Zimmermann, M; Metz, J; Ensinger, W; Kubler, W. Influence of surface texture and charge on the biocompatibility of endovascular stents, *Coron Artery Dis*, 1995; 6(7): 581–586.

[228] Williams, DF. Definitions in biomaterials, *Elsevier*, Amsterdam, 1987.

[229] Biological evaluation of medical devices. ISO 10993/EN 30993, *International Organization for Standardization*, Genève, Switzerland.

[230] Simka, W; Kaczmarek, M; Baron-Wiecheć, A; Nawrat, G; Marciniak, J; Żak, J. Electropolishing and passivation of NiTi shape memory alloy. *Electrochimica Acta*, 2010; 55(7): 2437-2441.

[231] Naimark, W; Lee, MJ; Limeback,, H; Cheung, D. Correlation of structure and viscoelastic properties in the pericardia of four mammalian species. *The American Physiological society, AJP-Heart and Circulatory Physiology*, Oct 1992; 263(4): H1095.

[232] Langdon, S; Chernecky, R; Pereira, C; Abdulla, D; Lee, M. Biaxial mechanical/structural effects of equibiaxial strain during crosslinking of bovine pericardial xenograft materials. *Journal of Biomaterials*; 1999; 20: 137-153.

[233] Butterfield, M; Fisher, J; Davies, GA; Kearney, JM. Leaflet geometry and function in porcine bioprostheses. *Eur. J Cardio-thorac,* 1991; 5: 27-33.

[234] Lee, M; Corrente, R; Haberer, S. The bovine pericardial xenograft II: effect of tethering or pressurization during fixation on the tensile viscoelastic properties of bovine pericardium. *Journal of Biomedical Materials Research*, 1989; 23: 477-489.

[235] Lee, M; Ku, M; Haberer, S. The bovine pericardial xenograft: III. effect of uniaxial and sequential biaxial stress during fixation on the tensile viscoelastic properties of bovine pericardium. *Journal of Biomedical Materials Research*,1989; 23: 491-506.

[236] Gudra, T; Muc, S. Some problems of ultrasonic and laser cutting of biological structures. *Eur. Phys. J. Special Topics*, 2008; 154: 85–88.

[237] Paez, G; Herrero, J; Sanmartin, A; Millian, I; Cordon, A; Maestro, M; Rocha, A; Arenaz, B; Castillo-Olivares, JL. Comparison of the mechanical behaviors of biological tissues subjected to uniaxial tensile testing: pig, calf and ostrich pericardium sutured with Gore-Tex. *Biomaterials 2003;* 24:1671-1679.

[238] Merryman, WD; Engelmayr, GC; Lio, J; Sacks, M. Defining biomechanical endpoints for tissue engineered heart valve leafets from native leaflet properties, *Pediatric Cardiology* 2006; 21:153-160.

[239] Sun, W; Abad, A; Sacks, M. Simulate bioprosthetic heart valve deformation under quasi-static loading, *Journal of Biomechanical Engineering*, Nov 2005; 127:905-914.

[240] Ford, S; Denton, M. Tapping into digital design tools, *Journal of Medical Device and Diagnostics*, 2009; Jan: 92-101.

[241] Black, M; Howard, IC; Huang, X; Patterson, EA. A three-dimensional analysis of a bioprosthetic heart valve. *J. Biomechanics,* 1991; 24(9): 793-780.

[242] ASTM Standard F2004, 2004 (2005) – Standard Test Method for Transformation Temperature of Nickel-Titanium Alloys by Thermal Analysis, *ASTM International*, West Conshohocken, PA, 2005 DOI: 10.1520/F2004-05, www.astm.org.

[243] ASTM Standard F2082, 2006 – Standard Test Method for Determination of Transformation Temperature of Nickel-Titanium Shape Memory Alloys by Bend and Free Recovery, *ASTM International*, West Conshohocken, PA, 2006 DOI: 10.1520/F2082-06, www.astm.org.

[244] ASTM Standard F2081, 2006 – Standard Guide for Characterization and Presentation of the Dimensional Attributes of Vascular Stents, *ASTM International,* West Conshohocken, PA, 2006 DOI: 10.1520/F2081-06, www.astm.org.

[245] ASTM Standard F2079, 2009 – Standard Test Method for Measuring Intrinsic Elastic Recoil of Balloon-Expandable Stents, *ASTM International*, West Conshohocken, PA, 2009 DOI: 10.1520/F2079-09, www.astm.org.

[246] Farnoush, A; Qing, L. Three dimensional nonlinear finite element analysis of the newly designed cardiovascular stent. *5th Australasian Congress on Applied Mechanics, ACAM 2007*, Dec 2007.

[247] Giddens, P; Yoganathan, AP; Shoen, FJ. Prosthetic Cardiac Valves. *Pathol.*, 1993; 2: 167S-177S.

[248] Walther, T; Dewey, T; Wimmer-Greinecker, G; Doss, M; Hambrecht, R; Schuler, G. Transapical approach for sutureless stent-fixed aortic valve implantation: experimental results. *Eur J Cardiothorac Surg.* 2006;29:703-8.

[249] Dwyer, HA; Matthews, PB; Azadani, A; Ge, L; Guy, TS; Tseng, EE. Migration forces of transcatheter aortic valves in patients with noncalcific aortic insufficiency. *J Thorac Cardiovasc Surg.* Nov 2009;138(5):1227-33.

[250] Strope, E. Design considerations for the in vitro testing of cardiovascular prosthesis. *International Society for Artificial Organs, 1986 Annual Meeting.* Available Online: http://www.dynatekdalta.com/papers_archive_032_doc.htm.

[251] Dewey, TM; Walther, T; Doss, M; Brown, D; Ryan, WH; Svensson, L; Mihalievic, T; Hambrecht, R; Schuler, G; Wimmer-Greinecker, G; Mohr, FW; Mach, MJ. Transapical aortic valve implantation: an animal feasibility study. *AnnThorac Surg,* 2006;82:110-6.
[252] Flameng, W; Meuris, B; Yperman, J; De Visscher, G; Herijgers, P; Verbeken, E. Factors influencing calcification of cardiac bioprostheses in adolescent sheep. *J Thorac Cardiovasc Surg*, 2006;132:89– 98.

In: Percutaneous Valve Technology: Present and Future ISBN: 978-1-61942-577-4
Editors: Jose Luis Navia and Sharif Al-Ruzzeh

Chapter VII

Biomechanics of Heart Valves

S. Ramaswamy, D. Schmidt and G. S. Kassab

Abstract

Each year, approximately 250,000 procedures are performed to repair or replace damaged heart valves, and 50,000 aortic valve replacements are performed annually to treat severe stenosis of the aortic heart valve. Clearly, biomechanical forces play a major role in the physiology and pathophysiology of heart valves. The objective of this chapter it to provide an overview of biomechanics of heart valves with emphasis on the interaction between tissue, blood and engineered devices. Future prospects in tissue engineered heart valves, multi-scale computational modeling and percutaneous approaches are also highlighted.

Introduction

Approximately 250,000 procedures are performed to repair or replace damaged heart valves [1] each year. Aortic valve disease is generally treated by replacement with either a mechanical or a bioprosthetic valve [2]. Approximately 50,000 aortic valve replacements are performed annually to treat severe aortic stenosis (a narrowing of the valve which obstructs the flow of blood from the heart to the aorta) [3–5]. Many of the complications of prosthetic heart valves are related to the fluid dynamics of the replacement valve [1]. In this chapter, we will outline the composition and structure of aortic valves and their mechanical properties. The biomechanics of heart valves will be discussed to reflect the inherent structure-mechanical properties-function relation. In this context, the utility and application of biomechanical computational modeling will be outlined to enhance our understanding of valve physiology and patho-physiology. Furthermore, we will review the methodology, approaches and sources of tissue engineered heart valves including percutaneous heart valve devices. Finally, we will outline some recommendations and speculations on future directions in this highly clinically-relevant area of research.

Native Heart Valve Composition and Structure

Soft biological tissue is composed of cellular and non-cellular entities. The latter serves a complex structural function by supporting the cells. This extracellular matrix (ECM) is also adaptive to the functional requirements of the tissue and is a major determinant of mechanical properties. In heart valve tissue, the ECM is composed of proteoglycans and structural proteins.

Proteoglycans are an ECM constituent associated with tissue regulation, maintenance and hydration. The structural proteins, collagen and elastin, are seminal to the transmission of mechanical loads and tissue elasticity [6]. As compared to elastin, valve collagen is relatively stiff in a tensile environment and is considered the primary load bearing constituent. The ECM elastin component may serve as a restoring feature once the load is removed (7). Collagen and elastin are the primary constituents of valve ECM accounting for 50% and 13% of the composition, respectively [8].

Valve leaflets exhibit a tri-layer structure: fibrosa, spongiosa, and ventricularis [9-13]. Each layer is composed of varied amounts of collagen, elastin, glycosaminoglyans (GAG's) and valve interstitial cells.

The structure and composition of each layer is distinctly different. A highly organized collagen fiber network characterizes the fibrosa layer. Elastin and unorganized collagen fibers dominate the ventricularis composition. The spongiosa layer separates the fibrosa and ventricularis and consists mainly of GAGs. Investigators believe that the spongiosa serves to dampen leaflet vibration. Total leaflet thickness is approximately 300 to 700 μm with 45% of the thickness stemming from the fibrosa layer. The spongiosa and ventricularis comprise 35% and 25% of the thickness, respectively.

In the context of gross biomechanical response, the structure and organization of the fibrillar collagen network governs leaflet behavior. The arrangement and density of collagen fibers is the primary mechanism responsible for leaflet mechanical strength. Properties of this fiber structure are directly correlated with tissue function and response to mechanical stimuli. The highly aligned and organized fibers of the fibrosa layer are the dominant contributors to the mechanical behavior.

Examination of a decellularized tissue specimen highlights the complex nature of the fiber network. There are clear differences in radial and circumferential arrangement. Collagen fiber bundles of the fibrosa layer are predominantly aligned in the circumferential direction. Regional differences in fiber structure combined with directional and preferential alignment create a non-homogeneous anisotropic material property. This fiber alignment accommodates the radial expansion required for effective leaflet union and valve closure.

Biomechanics of Soft Tissues

In a planar tension mode, valve leaflet biomechanical response can be characterized as highly nonlinear and anisotropic. A typical response to biaxial tension is illustrated in Fig. 1 [11-13]. The nonlinear nature of this response is attributed to the fibrillar microstructure, and specifically, to the fiber kinematics; i.e., the straightening and rotation of collagen fibers.

This behavior, referred to as fiber recruitment, is characterized by the accumulation of straightened fibers. As fibers transition from a crimped to a straightened state their load bearing quality significantly increases. The aggregate effect of this fiber scale behavior creates a tissue level nonlinear response. Investigators have observed that fiber crimp period and magnitude is distributed within a narrow band and rapidly changes with transvalvular pressure [14]. The difference between circumferential and radial response is attributed to the strong alignment of the fibers with circumferential leaflet direction in the fibrosa layer. The nature of this anisotropy is required to produce a large radial deformation to ensure leaflet coaptation.

The preferred alignment of the fiber architecture in the circumferential direction dominates the tissue response. This registration provokes rapid recruitment of fibers for load bearing.

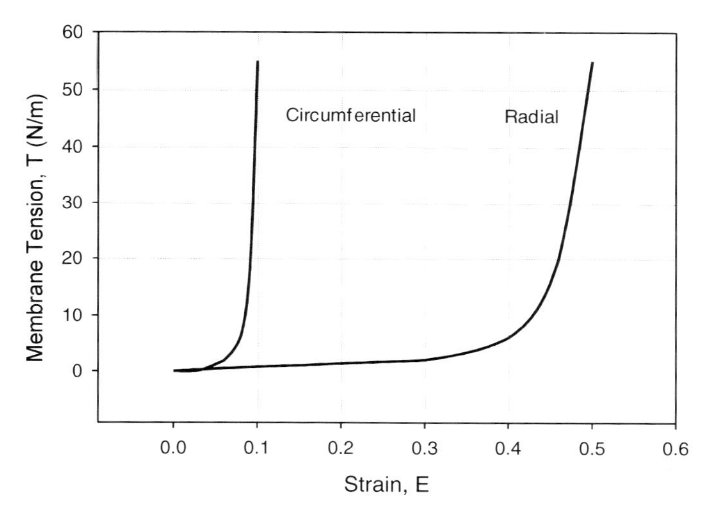

Figure 1. Biaxial response of native porcine aortic valve leaflet (adapted from (6)). Properties of leaflet fibrillar microstructure produce a highly nonlinear anisotropic response. Differences in the directional response are attributed to the fibrosa layer tight fiber alignment and orientation with the circumferential direction.

The fiber load bearing state, under large strains, is defined as fibers acting in a straightened geometry. At the tissue level, this characteristic produces a sharp transition to circumferential stiffness at relatively small strain (less than 5%). This gradual but increased fiber recruitment observed in the radial region stems from less ordered nature of the fiber alignment. The nature of this distinct anisotropy is critical for proper valve function. A relatively sharp circumferential stiffness accommodates the transvalvular pressure while a more compliant radial response allows the leaflets to remain coapted under load.

Application of Soft Tissue Mechanical Models to Valves

Soft biological tissue constitutive model development has been an active area of research for several decades. Researchers have introduced a broad spectrum of soft tissue constitutive models starting with the pioneering work introduced by Fung [15] in 1979. In general, these models have been application specific and can be classified as either phenomenological or structural. The term "structural" has been used to identify models which characterize material response in terms of underlying tissue constituents. Researchers have successfully demonstrated the reliable and robust nature of these models in applications involving cardiac tissue, skin, blood vessels and the tissue of eye lens capsule [16-20]. Although various approaches have been employed, the primary model goal has focused on accurate representations of the tissue fibrillar network. Regardless of application, the collagen fiber network is considered to be the dominant contributor to the mechanical response. Therefore, many of the soft tissue constitutive models presented in the literature involve features that can be applied to heart valve models.

In 1974, Lanir and Fung established the biaxial response of soft tissues through a series of mechanical protocols on rabbit skin [13]. Based on observations of these stress-strain relationships, Fung and co-workers later proposed a strain energy function to describe the highly nonlinear anisotropic material response exhibited in the artery wall [12]. Investigators have used variations of the phenomenological "Fung-type" strain energy model to address a broad spectrum of soft tissue applications [17-25]. The success and acceptance of the Fung model can be attributed to its robust ability to capture highly nonlinear experimentally derived data over a wide strain range. Convexity and material stability issues, however, limit the reliability of Fung-type models in a generalized computational framework.

While phenomenological models have been successfully applied to a broad spectrum of soft tissue applications, they do not capture the mechanisms of tissue behavior. An understanding of the relation between microstructure and physiological functions is central to the development of meaningful constitutive models. A model based on microstructural architecture is necessary to understand pathological remodeling and to engineer artificial tissue. Thus, the primary motivation of structurally-based heart valve models is to characterize macro-level tissue response in terms of fibrillar scale properties [17-20].These models are based on physiological microstructural features quantified through experiential means. Key tissue features such as fiber orientation and crimp period should be incorporated into the models.

In their work related to arterial wall mechanics, Holzapfel et al. proposed a constitutive model which can be considered as "hybrid" in the structural sense [26]. This model considers a family of fibers embedded in an isotropic ground-matrix. A concept common to other structurally-based approaches is the influence of non-fiber ECM components that are characterized by a incompressible isotropic hyperelastic strain energy function [27]. The contributors to the strain energy from decoupled fiber families are described by an exponential function. Although the Holzapfel model addresses microstructure by discrete fiber families, the fiber response is characterized by a phenomenological form that satisfies the convexity condition.

In general, soft tissue models for heart valve mechanics focus on a planar tension mode of deformation. They seek to reproduce and predict the nature of the high strain anisotropic response. Many of the mechanisms that affect low strain behavior are not considered. In low strain regimes, the non-fiber components of the ECM are the dominant contributors to mechanical response. In valve mechanics, the bending mode characterizing an opening or closure event is governed by low strain phenomenon as maximum surface strains are $< 7\%$ [28]. Under these conditions the fiber recruitment and rotation behavior that dominate the high strain response are not present. To date, investigators have used common isotropic hyperelastic models to describe non-fibrillar behavior but structural-based low strain approaches remain a challenge.

Structurally-guided material models are not limited to the study of soft biological tissues. The textile industry has leveraged this model type in understanding woven and non-woven fabric under loads [29-30]. Recruitment mechanisms play an important role in the mechanical response of fabric materials. Similar to soft tissue mechanics, fiber crimp period and fiber-to-fiber interactions are primary micro-scale properties that contribute to micro-scale response. Recent work related to engineered tissue scaffolds used a textile-motivated modeling approach to describe the mechanical characteristics of a non-woven scaffold tissue [31].

In recent years, the suitability of soft tissue models within a computational framework has been a central focus in the biomechanics community. As the field embraces the challenges of developing robust models suitable for computational implementation, issues such as convexity and stability have motivated researchers to recast models into forms which support a continuum nature [32]. Current trends focus on the development of constitutive form with increased computational efficiency using established models while other research highlights on the underlying physiological mechanisms. For computational models to realize their full potential, there is a need to link organ-scale phenomenon to fibrillar and cellular response since mechanisms associated with pathology and engineered tissue are rooted in this length scale. Thus, further structurally-based model developments offer the greatest potential for translational utility.

Structure-Based Modeling

In the context of soft tissue biomechanical models, fibrillar microstructure is typically idealized as a collection of independently acting fibers. Furthermore, interactions with the surrounding ECM, adjacent interstitial cells and other fibers are ignored. An idealized region at a scale of approximately 100 μm, referred to as a representative element, is presented in Fig. 2. Affine transformation assumptions apply to the fiber level strain state where fiber level strains can be developed from tissue deformation. This method of describing the fiber network is fundamental to quantify the nature of fiber orientation and the development of structurally based constitutive models. Common to these goals is the concept of the fiber "ensemble". The ensemble defines a group of fibers with similar orientation that attributes relative to the representative element scale. As compared to the organ and cell length scales, the fiber ensemble can be classified as a meso-scale.

Based on concepts introduced by Lanir [16-17,33], a class of soft tissue constitutive models based on the properties of the fibers has evolved. The description of the spatial state of the fibers, such as orientation and crimp, however, are cast in terms of statistical distributions due to a microstructure complexity that prohibits individual representation. This stochastic description is based on data homogenized at the scale depicted in Fig. 2. At this length-scale, characterization of the fiber microstructure is relative to the fiber ensemble. For example, a fiber angular distribution function describes the dominant fiber alignment direction in an ensemble framework. In addition to the spatial state of the fibers, experimental data that temporally captures the fiber kinematics must be incorporated into the model to accurately predict the stress-strain response of the tissue.

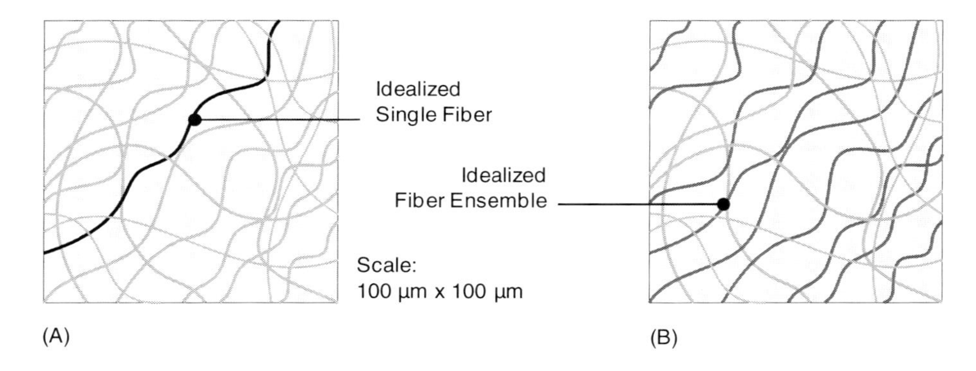

Figure 2. Idealization of the collagen fiber microstructure: (a) single fiber, (b) fiber ensemble (a group of fibers sharing a common orientation).

The framework established by the early work of Lanir was given practical relevance to soft tissue modeling with the introduction of an experimentally derived form for fibrillar orientation by Sacks [18]. This work used data collected using small angle light scattering techniques to develop analytical functions suitable for direct implementation into the context of a structural model [14,19-20]. Structural models treat the contributions of fibrillar and non-fibrillar constituents to the strain energy independently. The fiber network and ground-matrix are described in terms of finite strain fiber-reinforced continuum mechanics [21]. A tissue strain energy function is thereby characterized by the uncoupled sum of isotropic and anisotropic contributors.

Tissue Engineered Heart Valves (TEHVS)

Surgical intervention for severely diseased heart valves normally involves replacing the organ with a prosthetic device that is either made purely of artificial materials (metals, polymers, ceramics) known as mechanical valves or one that consists of fixed bovine or porcine tissue; i.e., bio-prosthetic valves. A third option in fewer cases, involves an autologous valve implant which consists of replacement of the aortic valve with the pulmonary valve, in a surgical method known as the Ross procedure. The primary limitation of mechanical valves is the associated risk of thromboembolism and the lifelong anticoagulation therapy required to minimize that risk. Bio-prosthetic valves on the other hand, are prone to calcification and structural breakdown. In both cases, more than one prosthetic valve replacement surgery may be required during the lifetime of the patient and the number increases if the individual was initially treated at a younger age. Trauma associated with multiple surgeries is difficult to quantify but adds further risks. This has led to efforts in developing minimally invasive surgical protocols for valve implantation [22-24]. Despite the shortcomings, current treatments to treat heart valve disease with a prosthetic device have an expected patency of 15 or more years [25]. Thus, the choice of valve implant is largely a function of the intended recipient's age and the individual's health history.

Independent of the unique features of currently available prosthetic valve devices, none offer the potential to accommodate the growth of the patient [34]. Heart valves are unique organs in that they are susceptible to extensive remodeling if the hemodynamics are altered. Indeed, follow-up studies from the Ross procedure have demonstrated remodeling of the pulmonary valve after implantation in the aorta to suggest aortic-valve like characteristics [35]. This fact provides inspiration for appropriately treated TEHVs that can leverage *in vivo* remodeling processes and hence integrate with the body and function as a normal valve. The opportunity for growth and tissue remodeling thus make TEHVs especially appealing to pediatric patients suffering from severe congenital valve disease and/or anomalies.

Fundamentally, the biomechanics play a significant role in maintaining normal behavior in valves. From a biomimetic perspective, the biomechanics have to be transferred to an *in vitro* environment and their effects on various potential i) cell source(s) and ii) scaffolds have to determined. A growing body of evidence [36-44] has suggested that biomechanical, *in vitro* pre-conditioning of the engineered construct is necessary to promote the necessary degree of tissue formation, in order to sufficiently withstand the dynamic native valve environment. However, many questions remain regarding the exact nature and time frame of *in-vitro* conditioning that is necessary for optimal tissue formation. We focus some attention on the basics of tissue formation; i.e., cells and scaffolds.

Cell Sources for TEHVS

Early TEHV approaches for pediatric valve replacements focused on the use of primary, autologous vascular smooth muscle and endothelial cells [37,39,45]. The results seemed promising in demonstrating proof-of-concept; i.e., that valve-like tissue retaining dense cellularity and that a superficial endothelial lining could be formed [46]. Given the limitation of vascular harvests and possible risks, these types of studies were largely abandoned.

More recently, fetal and embryonic progenitor cell sources have demonstrated significant potential in supporting the valve phenotype. As shown by the work of Schmidt et al [47], human umbilical cord derived progenitor cells (HUC-DPCs) possess specific multi-lineage potential for valves. In particular, the Warton's-jelly myofibroblast (WMF) sub-population of the HUC-DPCs has shown phenotypic profiles very similar to valvular interstitial cells [48]. The blood derived endothelial progenitor cell (EPC) sub-population of HUC-DPCs differentiates to functional endothelial layers on surfaces of tissue engineered leaflets [49]. Similar positive results were possible using amniotically derived embryonic cells [50-51]. As a cell source, the choice of fetal and embryonic cells seems to be very plausible, which enables harvest from the umbilical cord at birth or from the amniotic fluid which is the earliest time at which autologous cells for TEHV development can be utilized after detection of a valve anomaly. These sources are extremely limited in supply, however, and have strong ethical considerations. In addition, as alluded to earlier, normal tissue remodeling continues to occur after birth, during which time, the local hemodynamics surrounding the TEHV are altered and the native cell populations can no longer be considered fetal or embryonic. Thus, in this context, adult progenitor cell sources need to be aggressively explored.

Success with adult bone-marrow (BMSCs) and peripheral-blood derived endothelial progenitor cells (EPCs) for other applications (such as cardiovascular revascularization, generation of nonthrombogenic vascular grafts) and the development of efficient stem cell delivery systems offer practical approaches to vascularize engineered tissues and promoted interest in the TEHV research community. BMSCs are relatively accessible and have the potential to exhibit the desired pluripotency for tissue engineering of cardiovascular organs [38,52-54]. In particular, Sutherland et al [54] completed studies confirming that BMSCs derived from sheep expressed vimentin and α-SMA phenotype markers (evidence of vascular phenotype) throughout the lengthy tissue engineering process. To date, it has not been conclusively demonstrated that BMSCs can differentiate preferentially towards *both* endothelial and smooth muscle cell type lineages and regionally distribute on the TEHV surface and interstitium respectively (i.e., evidence of true valvular phenotype). Recently, peripheral blood derived EPCs that were seeded onto tri-leaflet scaffold valve conduits did positively express markers for both these cell types [55], albeit mechanical conditioning was not considered in the study. Clearly, the effects of mechanical environments on BMSCs and EPCs need to be further investigated so that the quantity and quality of engineered tissue grown *in vitro* can be maximized for subsequent usage in *in vivo* studies. Table 1 summarizes the main considerations in selecting appropriate cell sources in functional TEHV development.

Table 1. Pros and Cons of Various Cell Sources Used in Heart Valve Tissue Engineering

Autologous Cell Type	Primary Advantage(s)	Primary Disadvantage(s)
Primary vascular smooth muscle, fibroblast and endothelial cells	-Phenotypically compliant.	-Not widely available
Embryonic and fetal cells; embryonic stem cells, umbilical and amniotically-derived cell sources	-Pluripotent capability -Demonstrated differentiation to valve-like cells from a single cell source	-Ethical concerns -Sufficient cell numbers may not always be possible -Potential cost issues
Adult progenitor cells (BMSCs, EPCs)	-Omnipotent capability -Minimally invasive -Available in sufficient cell quantities	-Yet to conclusively show cell differentiation and engineered tissue formation supportive of valve-like phenotype and tissue morphology

Scaffolds for TEHVS

To mimic native substrates requires adequate dynamic range in material properties. Although only polymer materials are able to accomplish this task, there is little consensus on which polymers are specifically suited for TEHVs. Traditionally, reviews in the heart valve tissue engineering arena have focused on polymer scaffolds that are synthetically made or naturally derived [56-57]. A more appropriate grouping would be a consideration of the degradable versus nondegradable nature of the materials. Even though degradable materials have generally been thought to be ideal, the ability to guide tissue remodeling with chemically and/or mechanically treated permanent scaffold materials that form a backbone for the new tissue has yet to be fully explored. An important criterion in this approach is the need for excellent biotolerence combined with the ability of the scaffold to be completely encapsulated by new tissue that continues to deform in a native valve-like manner. The advantage herein is that the uncertainty associated with tissue formation and scaffold degradation rates will not factor into the equation since the construct's deformation characteristics will primarily be dictated by the scaffold material properties, which will not change if the scaffold is non-degradable.

The next consideration in scaffold design has to be the material properties of the polymer itself and the associated manufacturing technique that will enable the necessary micro and meso-scale architecture that is conducive to *de novo* tissue formation. Several polymer processing techniques exist for this purpose and many still have yet to be explored for the TEHV application. Several works thus far have focused on natural, decellularized native ECM scaffold [58-62], and nonwoven fabrics [54,63-65] consisting of degradable polymers or co-polymers such a poly-L-lactic acid-polyglycolic acid. More recent attention has focused on elastomeric materials [65] for TEHV scaffolds created via electrospinning which has enabled the creation of microstructures permitting cells to easily attach to the substrate material. Electrospinning also permits the creation of anisotropy in the scaffold fabric that can mimic native valve bi-directional mechanical properties.

Need for Mechanistic Studies in TEHVS

In comparison to tissue engineered skin, blood vessels and cartilage, efforts in engineered heart valve tissue growth have been relatively more recent. Central to this effort is the notion of simulating physiological environments that native heart valves are subjected to. It was a decade ago that Hoerstrup et al [40] first reported the need for custom-made devices or bioreactors capable of providing mechanical environments to *in vitro* culture systems that may enhance engineered heart valve tissue properties. In their research study, they reported on the use of a pulse duplicator system to condition tissue engineered valves at ramping pressure conditions from 30 to 55 mm Hg over a 28 day period. Although they found substantial increases in the net collagen and DNA content of their conditioned constructs over controls; they utilized primary myofibroblasts and endothelial cells in their study which are not practical for clinical translation. Nonetheless, they were able to importantly define three fundamental requirements of a bioreactor: 1) sterile culture environments, 2) ease of use and 3) physiologically realistic surroundings.

The sterility requirement is commonsensical while simplicity in design was intended as a practical criterion to facilitate translation from *in vitro* to *in vivo* settings. The third requirement attempts to provide bio-mimetic stress environments to evolving valve substitutes and innately, heart valves are subjected to flexural, tensile and fluid-induced stresses [58]. Thus, a pulsatile flow system that would enable continuous dynamic stimulation of the TEHVs would provide insights into the coupled effects of these stresses during the conditioning process. The need for such a system has thus far prompted several bioreactor developments [36,39,42,67] that can provide valve-relevant mechanical conditioning. These systems, similar in design to pulsatile loops used in hydrodynamic prosthetic valves testing were built to provide TEHV leaflets with a dynamic conditioning environment that replicates hemodynamic parameters such as arterial pressure and flow conditions while being housed in a sterile location, such as a standard cell culture incubator [36,40,42,67-68]. Very few studies have reported on the actual usage of these types of devices, however, in tissue engineering experiments which can be very expensive, time-consuming and cumbersome to carry out. As a result, most investigations have utilized simple pulsatile flow loops without consideration of simulation of pressure and flow magnitudes/waveforms and phase differences between the two. Even in these studies, improvements such as increased cell viability [69] and graded cell/tissue layering with cells orientated with the flow direction [39-40] were observed. As an example, Mol et al [42] reported on enhanced tissue formation in bioreactor-conditioned leaflets where the nature of the flow was at a very low magnitude (4 ml/min) and the valve was conditioned only during the diastolic phase of the cardiac cycle. More recently, it was shown that dynamically conditioned TEHVs at normal pulmonary artery pressure conditions resulted in increased collagen formation rates and enhanced retention of DNA levels over time. Furthermore, the cross-sectional shape of the leaflets was found to be cylindrical in nature during closure [56].

The ideal *in vitro* conditioning protocol has still yet to be identified. In this regard, it is not clear if the exact reproduction of every aspect of native valve dynamics is possible or for that matter, required to maximize both quantity and quality of engineered tissue growth. Since optimal regimens essential to the overall success of the implant are still largely unknown, there is still an unmet need to develop bioreactors that can provide an avenue to delineate the specific effects of unique stress states on engineered tissue formation [8]. Thus, mechanistically, a precursor to valve conditioning studies may require the development of a device capable of efficiently evaluating individual and coupled effects of the flow, stretch and flexural (FSF) stress states. Such a device was built by Engelmayr *et al* [70-71] where their bioreactor could impart these stresses either individually or coupled onto several rectangular-shaped scaffold specimens at one time. Although the fluid-induced stresses were found to be sub-physiological [71], coupled flexure and sub-physiological levels of flow prompted significantly higher levels of collagen formation by BMSCs than each individual stress state.

In a related study using BMSCs at the tri-leaflet valve scale, Ramaswamy *et al* [64] showed that the fluid stresses likely played a dominant role in eliciting robust tissue formation than solid (flexural and tensile) stresses since the scaffold used could only allow for modest (up to 7%) strains. In particular, there was a high degree of oscillatory fluid shear stress associated with rectangular–shaped specimen deformation, i.e., cyclical bending, which was noted to be similar to the cylindrical shape associated with the closure of the TEHV leaflet. This finding implied that the oscillatory nature of the shear stress was critical in triggering appropriate BMSC signaling events that led to upregulation of tissue formation even in cases where the magnitude of shear stresses was sub-physiological.

Studies in the literature [72-74] have already shown that oscillatory shear stresses do regulate the differentiation capabilities of BMSCs such as the osteogenic, adipogenic and chondrogenic pathways. While FSF stress environments are coupled for the native heart valve, it may not be practically possible for this environment to routinely be applied as a precursor to implantation. Instead, further understanding of the specific role of biomechanical cues such as oscillatory shear stresses on tissue production and cell differentiation from suitable cell sources such as BMSC and EPCs is necessary. A bioreactor system can then be designed to accommodate the tri-leaflet heart valve geometry while maximizing the mechanistic effects that provide optimal engineered heart valve tissue growth.

Computational Predictive Models

There is growing recognition of the potential clinical impact of computational fluid dynamics (CFD) to develop improved diagnostic tools for predicting aortic dilatation in bicuspid aortic valve patients [76]. To obtain a predictive model of the aortic valve, it is necessary to account for the two-way nature of the interaction of the elasticity of the valve leaflets and the fluid dynamics of the blood. The valve leaflets move at the local velocity of the blood, but at the same time they apply forces to the blood that drastically alter the fluid motion. The primarily normal forces prevent backflow when the valve is closed, and the primarily tangential forces shear the forward flow when the valve is open to create vortices that are believed to aid in valve closure. Hence, a predictive aortic valve model requires a FSI approach.

Computer simulation can help design prostheses to maximize flow rates while minimizing shear stresses which cause hemolysis. Simulation can also be used to study and ultimately, optimize percutaneous valve replacement or procedures to repair or replace the aortic root [77-78]. Using predictive computational-based modeling, the influence of key engineered tissue characteristics on organ level response can be evaluated. Simulation results can serve to integrate insights of basic biomechanical mechanisms into tissue engineering paradigms. Figure 3 illustrates a model guided approach to scaffold design for a tissue engineered heart valve. The primary aim of the model shown was to quantify and bind a practical design space relating permutations of scaffold properties (geometry, thickness, and magnitude of anisotropy) with anticipated organ level performance. Simulated design iterations achieved a configuration exhibiting uniform leaflet circumferential strain (Fig. 3a). Mechanisms influencing valve cycling were explored (Fig. 3b) and conditions promoting efficient opening transition were identified. Without sufficient anisotropy, leaflet response in the radial direction cannot develop the strain magnitude required to permit free edge engagement with adjacent leaflets. Through modeling, a coaptation quality was improved by tailoring radial and circumference compliance (Fig. 3C-D).

Delineation of fluid and solid stresses will require additional computational developments. Two critical components are required for accurate quantification and interpretation of the stress field: i) accurate, 3-dimensional (3D) geometric reconstruction and ii) suitable methodologies to simulate 3D spatial + 1-dimensional temporal, i.e., 4-dimensional (4D) events (e.g. heart valve leaflet position over a cardiac cycle). Very few studies thus far have focused on TEHV modeling in comparison to native valves. Primarily, lack of available experimental data has limited the ability to build and validate robust computational models. This database has to consist of more than a conventional mechanical stiffness value or a tensile test. Imaging studies will be needed to capture the representative TEHV geometry and deformation. These metrics will need to subsequently be incorporated in a recognized constitutive modeling framework for fiber-reinforced soft tissues.

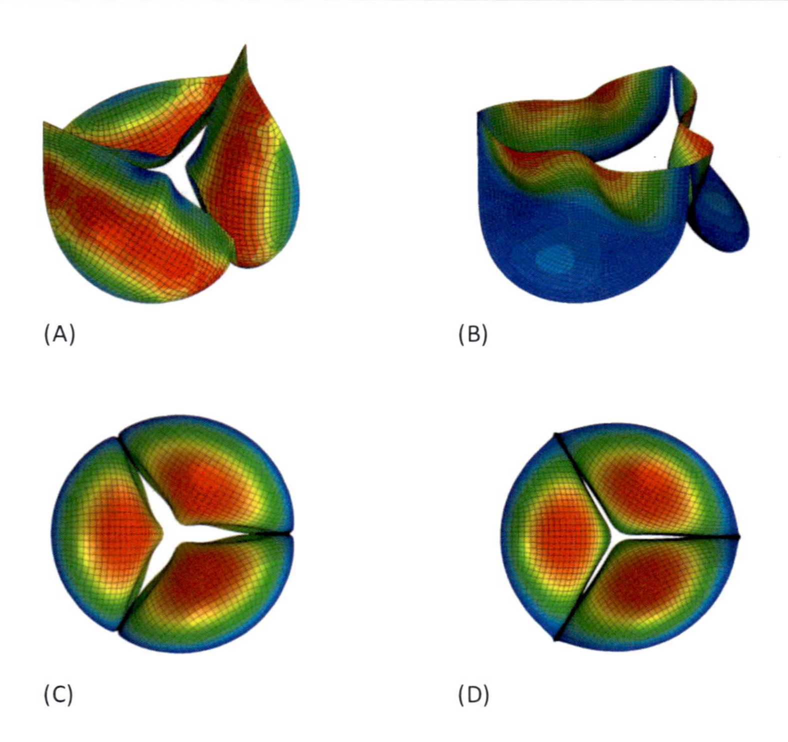

Figure 3. Computational Biomechanical Modeling of Tissue Engineered Aortic Valve Leaflets. (A) Strain distributions within the leaflet, red contours illustrate the relatively high circumferential strain required to accommodate coaptation. (B) Leaflet strain developed during valve cycling. (C,D) Comparison of leaflet coaptation quality between two design parameter sets.

Medical images obtained from computer assisted tomography and magnetic resonance imaging (MRI) techniques can be processed to obtain 4D point cloud data sets from which a meshing program can be used to create the 3D geometry. A 4D analysis can be approached broadly through either a moving boundary approach or a fluid-structure interaction approach. Both of these techniques have a sound theoretical framework but implementation is not trivial. Indeed, several such computational research efforts involve streamlining this implementation so that a real-time clinical diagnosis can be made. Nonetheless, the ability to provide quantitative understanding of mechanistic conditioning events in optimizing engineered heart valve tissue remains an integral part of the development process.

Although computational models of the aortic valve have been developed which include coupling between the blood and the elastic aortic valve leaflets and sinuses [79-85], most of these models [79-81, 83-84] make simplifying assumptions about the symmetry of the flow [86-87] and none use experimentally-based constitutive laws [88-92] to describe the elasticity of both the valve and the root. Hence, much remains to be done in developing validated multi-scale patient specific models of heart valves. Future studies should focus on patient-specific vessel valve anatomy and flow boundary conditions using MRI or other imaging methods with sufficient spatial and temporal resolution. The patient specific models can be used to understand normal and pathophysiological flows within the aortic valve and root.

Percutaneous Heart Valves

Percutaneous aortic valve replacement is a new minimally-invasive procedure for selected patients with severe aortic stenosis in which a prosthetic valve is implanted via a catheter. In this procedure, a stented transcatheter valve is implanted within the diseased valve, or failed bioprosthetic valve [93-95]. Percutaneous aortic valve replacement is rapidly becoming a viable option for selected patients requiring aortic valve replacement who are unable or unwilling to undergo traditional surgical aortic valve replacement [5]. Realistic simulation of the dynamics of such valve prostheses is therefore a topic with potentially significant clinical impact. These patient-specific models described above should be extended to simulate and design the fluid dynamical effects of percutaneous aortic valve replacement. Specifically, the model should be used to study the effect of changes to the axial position and rotational orientation of the implanted valve prosthesis on both overall valve performance and also the flow within the aortic sinuses. The characterizations of the performance of the valve in terms of transvalvular pressure gradient, stroke volume, and regurgitant volume are essential. Optimal performance will likely be obtained when the commissures of the transcatheter valve are aligned with those of the diseased valve. The validated models can also be used to study procedures in which the flow of blood in the aortic sinuses is altered or restricted, or in which the sinuses are replaced.

Different classes of patients, including those with bicuspid aortic valves [96-97] and Marfan syndrome [78] suffer from loss of vascular tissue elasticity and may develop aortic root dilatation which can lead to aortic dissection. Valve sparing aortic root replacement is indicated under certain conditions [77-78]. To guide the decision making for these and other clinically relevant issues, a number of issues regarding percutaneous valves can be addressed through validated computational models including: For which patients should aortic root replacement actually be performed? What are the fluid dynamic effects of percutaneous valve replacement? Is it possible to design a more efficient prosthetic valve for such procedures? Should different designs be used for different patients? Is it important for the graft geometry to reproduce particular anatomical features of the natural aortic root? Should the vascular grafts mimic the compliance of natural aortic sinuses? A better understanding of these and other issues will clearly provide for better device designs and a better clinical outcome.

Conclusion

Development of a functional TEHV will ultimately require a biomimetic approach whereby the mechanical properties and deformation of the individual leaflets closely match those of the native heart valve. Initial efforts are likely to target the severely diseased pediatric pulmonary valve. BMSCs and EPCs are two adult progenitor cell sources that deserve further investigation. Concomitantly, both suitable degradable and nondegradable scaffold materials need to be identified. Cellular and tissue level mechanobiology in the pursuit of functional engineered tissue promises to be an exciting research area not only in the context of TEHVs but has broader impact in the field or cardiovascular regenerative medicine. The design and manufacture of custom built bioreactors for the study of mechanical regulators of cells and tissue coupled to predictive 4D computational models may hold the key in translating TEHV treatment strategies including percutaneous approaches from benchtop to bedside.

References

[1] P. Yoganathan, Z. M. He, and S. C. Jones. Fluid mechanics of heart valves. *Annu Rev Biomed Eng*, 6:331–362, 2004.

[2] J. A. Carr and E. B. Savage. Aortic valve repair for aortic insufficiency in adults: A contemporary review and comparison with replacement techniques. *Eur J Cardio Thorac Surg*, 25(1):6–15, 2005.

[3] R. V. Freeman and C. M. Otto. Spectrum of calcific aortic valve disease: Pathogenesis, disease progression, and treatment strategies. *Circulation*, 111(24):3316–3326, 2005.

[4] R. O. Bonow, B. A. Carabello, K. Chatterjee, A. C. de Leon, D. P. Faxon, M. D. Freed, W. H. Gaasch, B. W. Lytle, R. A. Nishimura, P. T. O'Gara, R. A. O'Rourke, C. M. Otto, P. M. Shah, and J. S. Shanewise. ACC/AHA 2006 guidelines for the management of patients with valvular heart disease. *Circulation*, 114(5):E84–E231, 2006.

[5] M. Singh, M. H. Shishehbor, R. D. Christofferson, E. M. Tuzcu, and S. R. Kapadia. Percutaneous treatment of aortic valve stenosis. *Cleve Clin J Med*, 75(11):805–812, 2008.

[6] Fung YC. Biomechanics: Mechanical Properties of Living Tissues. New York*: Springer-Verlag*; 1981.

[7] Vesely I. The role of elastin in aortic valve mechanics. *Journal of Biomechanics* 1998;31(2):115-123.

[8] Bashey RI, Jimenez SA. Collagen in heart valves. In: Nimni ME, editor. Collagen. Volume 1. Boca Raton: *CRC Press*; 1988. p 258-274.

[9] Thubrikar M. The Aortic Valve. Boca Raton: *CRC;* 1990. 221 p.

[10] Schoen FJ. Aortic valve structure-function correlations: role of elastic fibers no longer a stretch of the imagination. *J Heart Valve Dis* 1997;6(1):1-6.

[11] Billiar KL, Sacks MS. Biaxial mechanical properties of the native and glutaraldehyde-treated aortic valve cusp: Part II--A structural constitutive model. *J Biomech Eng* 2000;122(4):327-335.

[12] Chuong CJ, Fung YC. Three-dimensional stress distribution in arteries. *J Biomech Eng* 1983;105(3):268-274.

[13] Lanir Y, Fung YC. Two-dimensional mechanical properties of rabbit skin. II. Experimental results. *J Biomech* 1974;7(2):171-182.

[14] Joyce EM, Liao J, Schoen FJ, Mayer JE, Jr., Sacks MS. Functional collagen fiber architecture of the pulmonary heart valve cusp. *Ann Thorac Surg* 2009;87(4):1240-1249.

[15] Y. C. Fung KF, P. Patitucci. Pseudoelasticity of arterties and the choice of its mathematical experssion. *The American Physiological Society* 1979.

[16] Lanir Y. Plausibility of Structural Constitutive-Equations for Isotropic Soft-Tissues in Finite Static Deformations. *J Appl Mech-T Asme* 1994;61(3):695-702.

[17] Lanir Y. Plausibility of structural constitutive equations for swelling tissues--implications of the C-N and S-E conditions. *J Biomech Eng* 1996;118(1):10-16.

[18] Sacks MS. Incorporation of experimentally-derived fiber orientation into a structural constitutive model for planar collagenous tissues. *J Biomech Eng* 2003;125(2):280-287.
[19] Sacks MS, Smith DB, Hiester ED. The aortic valve microstructure: effects of transvalvular pressure. *J Biomed Mater Res* 1998;41(1):131-141.
[20] Sacks MS, Smith DB, Hiester ED. A small angle light scattering device for planar connective tissue microstructural analysis. *Ann Biomed Eng* 1997;25(4):678-689.
[21] Spencer A. Deformations of fibre-reinforced materials. *Glasgow: Oxford university press;* 1972. 128 p.
[22] Folliguet T, Dibie A, Laborde F. Future of cardiac surgery: minimally invasive techniques in sutureless valve resection. *Future Cardiol* 2009;5(5):443-452.
[23] Raja SG, Navaratnarajah M. Impact of minimal access valve surgery on clinical outcomes: current best available evidence. *J Card Surg* 2009;24(1):73-79.
[24] Tabata M, Khalpey Z, Shekar PS, Cohn LH. Reoperative minimal access aortic valve surgery: minimal mediastinal dissection and minimal injury risk. *J Thorac Cardiovasc Surg* 2008;136(6):1564-1568.
[25] Rahimtoola SH. The next generation of prosthetic heart valves needs a proven track record of patient outcomes at > or =15 to 20 years. *J Am Coll Cardiol* 2003;42(10):1720-1721.
[26] Holzapfel GA, Gasser TC. A new constitutive framework for arterial wall mechanics and a comparative study of material models. *Journal of Elasticity* 2000;61:1-48.
[27] Einstein DR, Reinhall P, Nicosia M, Cochran RP, Kunzelman K. Dynamic finite element implementation of nonlinear, anisotropic hyperelastic biological membranes. *Comput Methods Biomech Biomed Engin* 2003;6(1):33-44.
[28] Merryman WD, Huang H-YS, Schoen FJ, Sacks MS. The effects of cellular contraction on aortic valve leaflet flexural stiffness. *J Biomech* 2006;39(1):88-96.
[29] Kabla A, Mahadeven, L. Nonlinear mechanics of soft fibrous networks. *Journal of the Royal Society Interface* 2006;4:7.
[30] Nader B, Papadopoulos, P., Steigmann, D. Multiscale Constitutive Modeling and Numerical Simulation of Fabric Material. *International Journal of Solids and Structures* 2006.
[31] Engelmayr GC, Jr., Sacks MS. A structural model for the flexural mechanics of nonwoven tissue engineering scaffolds. *J Biomech Eng* 2006;128(4):610-622.
[32] Wilber JP, Walton JR. The convexity properties of a class of constitutive models for biological soft tissues. *Mathematics and mechanics of solids* 2002;7:217-236.
[33] Lanir Y. Constitutive Equations for Fibrous Connective Tissues. *Journal of biomechanics* 1983;16:1-12.
[34] Kirklin J, Smith D, Novick W, Naffel D, Kirklin J, Pacifico A, Nanda N, Helmcke F, Bourge R. Longterm function of cyropreserved aortic homografts: Ten year study. *J Thorac Cardiovasc Surg* 1993;106(154-166).
[35] Rabkin-Aikawa E, Aikawa M, Farber M, Kratz JR, Garcia-Cardena G, Kouchoukos NT, Mitchell MB, Jonas RA, Schoen FJ. Clinical pulmonary autograft valves: pathologic evidence of adaptive remodeling in the aortic site. *J Thorac Cardiovasc Surg* 2004;128(4):552-561.
[36] Dumont K, Yperman J, Verbeken E, Segers P, Meuris B, Vandenberghe S, Flameng W, Verdonck PR. Design of a new pulsatile bioreactor for tissue engineered aortic heart valve formation. *Artif Organs* 2002;26(8):710-714.

[37] Engelmayr GC, Jr., Rabkin E, Sutherland FW, Schoen FJ, Mayer JE, Jr., Sacks MS. The independent role of cyclic flexure in the early in vitro development of an engineered heart valve tissue. *Biomaterials* 2005;26(2):175-187.

[38] Hoerstrup SP, Kadner A, Melnitchouk S, Trojan A, Eid K, Tracy J, Sodian R, Visjager JF, Kolb SA, Grunenfelder J, Zund G, Turina MI. Tissue engineering of functional trileaflet heart valves from human marrow stromal cells. *Circulation* 2002;106(12 Suppl 1):I143-150.

[39] Hoerstrup SP, Sodian R, Daebritz S, Wang J, Bacha EA, Martin DP, Moran AM, Guleserian KJ, Sperling JS, Kaushal S, Vacanti JP, Schoen FJ, Mayer JE, Jr. Functional living trileaflet heart valves grown In vitro. *Circulation* 2000;102(19 Suppl 3):III44-49.

[40] Hoerstrup SP, Sodian R, Sperling JS, Vacanti JP, Mayer JE, Jr. New pulsatile bioreactor for in vitro formation of tissue engineered heart valves. *Tissue Eng* 2000;6(1):75-79.

[41] Jockenhoevel S, Zund G, Hoerstrup SP, Schnell A, Turina M. Cardiovascular tissue engineering: a new laminar flow chamber for in vitro improvement of mechanical tissue properties. *Asaio J* 2002;48(1):8-11.

[42] Mol A, Driessen NJ, Rutten MC, Hoerstrup SP, Bouten CV, Baaijens FP. Tissue engineering of human heart valve leaflets: a novel bioreactor for a strain-based conditioning approach. *Ann Biomed Eng* 2005;33(12):1778-1788.

[43] Mol A, Bouten CV, Zund G, Gunter CI, Visjager JF, Turina MI, Baaijens FP, Hoerstrup SP. The relevance of large strains in functional tissue engineering of heart valves. *Thorac Cardiovasc Surg* 2003;51(2):78-83.

[44] Perry TE, Kaushal S, Sutherland FW, Guleserian KJ, Bischoff J, Sacks M, Mayer JE. Thoracic Surgery Directors Association Award. Bone marrow as a cell source for tissue engineering heart valves. *Annals of Thoracic Surgery* 2003;75(3):761-767; discussion 767.

[45] Rabkin E, Hoerstrup SP, Aikawa M, Mayer JE, Jr., Schoen FJ. Evolution of cell phenotype and extracellular matrix in tissue-engineered heart valves during in-vitro maturation and in-vivo remodeling. *The Journal of heart valve disease* 2002;11(3):308-314; discussion 314.

[46] Sodian R, Hoerstrup SP, Sperling JS, Daebritz S, Martin DP, Moran AM, Kim BS, Schoen FJ, Vacanti JP, Mayer JE, Jr. Early in vivo experience with tissue-engineered trileaflet heart valves. *Circulation* 2000;102(19 Suppl 3):III22-29.

[47] Schmidt D, Mol A, Odermatt B, Neuenschwander S, Breymann C, Gossi M, Genoni M, Zund G, Hoerstrup SP. Engineering of biologically active living heart valve leaflets using human umbilical cord-derived progenitor cells. *Tissue engineering* 2006;12(11):3223-3232.

[48] Messier RH, Jr., Bass BL, Aly HM, Jones JL, Domkowski PW, Wallace RB, Hopkins RA. Dual structural and functional phenotypes of the porcine aortic valve interstitial population: characteristics of the leaflet myofibroblast. *The Journal of surgical research* 1994;57(1):1-21.

[49] Asahara T, Murohara T, Sullivan A, Silver M, van der Zee R, Li T, Witzenbichler B, Schatteman G, Isner JM. Isolation of putative progenitor endothelial cells for angiogenesis. *Science* (New York, NY 1997;275(5302):964-967.

[50] Schmidt D, Achermann J, Odermatt B, Breymann C, Mol A, Genoni M, Zund G, Hoerstrup SP. Prenatally fabricated autologous human living heart valves based on

amniotic fluid derived progenitor cells as single cell source. *Circulation* 2007;116(11 Suppl):I64-70.

[51] Schmidt D, Achermann J, Odermatt B, Genoni M, Zund G, Hoerstrup SP. Cryopreserved amniotic fluid-derived cells: a lifelong autologous fetal stem cell source for heart valve tissue engineering. *J Heart Valve Dis* 2008;17(4):446-455; discussion 455.

[52] Kadner A, Hoerstrup SP, Zund G, Eid K, Maurus C, Melnitchouk S, Grunenfelder J, Turina MI. A new source for cardiovascular tissue engineering: human bone marrow stromal cells. *Eur J Cardiothorac Surg* 2002;21(6):1055-1060.

[53] Perry TE, Kaushal S, Sutherland FW, Guleserian KJ, Bischoff J, Sacks M, Mayer JE. Thoracic Surgery Directors Association Award. Bone marrow as a cell source for tissue engineering heart valves. *The Annals of thoracic surgery* 2003;75(3):761-767; discussion 767.

[54] Sutherland FW, Perry TE, Yu Y, Sherwood MC, Rabkin E, Masuda Y, Garcia GA, McLellan DL, Engelmayr GC, Jr., Sacks MS, Schoen FJ, Mayer JE, Jr. From stem cells to viable autologous semilunar heart valve. *Circulation* 2005;111(21):2783-2791.

[55] Sales VL, Mettler BA, Engelmayr GC, Jr., Aikawa E, Bischoff J, Martin DP, Exarhopoulos A, Moses MA, Schoen FJ, Sacks MS, Mayer JE, Jr. Endothelial progenitor cells as a sole source for ex vivo seeding of tissue-engineered heart valves. *Tissue Eng Part A* 2010;16(1):257-267.

[56] Mendelson K, Schoen FJ. Heart valve tissue engineering: concepts, approaches, progress, and challenges. *Ann Biomed Eng* 2006;34(12):1799-1819.

[57] Rabkin-Aikawa E, Mayer JE, Jr., Schoen FJ. Heart valve regeneration. *Adv Biochem Eng Biotechnol* 2005;94:141-179.

[58] Dohmen PM, da Costa F, Yoshi S, Lopes SV, da Souza FP, Vilani R, Wouk AF, da Costa M, Konertz W. Histological evaluation of tissue-engineered heart valves implanted in the juvenile sheep model: is there a need for in-vitro seeding? *J Heart Valve Dis* 2006;15(6):823-829.

[59] Hong H, Dong N, Shi J, Chen S, Guo C, Hu P, Qi H. Fabrication of a novel hybrid scaffold for tissue engineered heart valve. *J Huazhong Univ Sci Technolog Med Sci* 2009;29(5):599-603.

[60] Tudorache I, Cebotari S, Sturz G, Kirsch L, Hurschler C, Hilfiker A, Haverich A, Lichtenberg A. Tissue engineering of heart valves: biomechanical and morphological properties of decellularized heart valves. *J Heart Valve Dis* 2007;16(5):567-573; discussion 574.

[61] Vincentelli A, Wautot F, Juthier F, Fouquet O, Corseaux D, Marechaux S, Le Tourneau T, Fabre O, Susen S, Van Belle E, Mouquet F, Decoene C, Prat A, Jude B. In vivo autologous recellularization of a tissue-engineered heart valve: are bone marrow mesenchymal stem cells the best candidates? *J Thorac Cardiovasc Surg* 2007;134(2):424-432.

[62] Yang M, Chen CZ, Wang XN, Zhu YB, Gu YJ. Favorable effects of the detergent and enzyme extraction method for preparing decellularized bovine pericardium scaffold for tissue engineered heart valves. *J Biomed Mater Res B Appl Biomater* 2009;91(1):354-361.

[63] Freed LE, Vunjak-Novakovic G, Biron RJ, Eagles DB, Lesnoy DC, Barlow SK, Langer R. Biodegradable polymer scaffolds for tissue engineering. *Biotechnology* (N Y) 1994;12(7):689-693.

[64] Ramaswamy S, Gottlieb D, Engelmayr GC, Jr., Aikawa E, Schmidt DE, Gaitan-Leon DM, Sales VL, Mayer JE, Jr., Sacks MS. The role of organ level conditioning on the promotion of engineered heart valve tissue development in-vitro using mesenchymal stem cells. *Biomaterials* 2010;31(6):1114-1125.

[65] Sacks MS, Schoen FJ, Mayer JE. Bioengineering challenges for heart valve tissue engineering. *Annu Rev Biomed Eng* 2009;11:289-313.

[66] Sacks MS, Yoganathan AP. Heart valve function: a biomechanical perspective. *Philos Trans R Soc Lond B Biol Sci* 2008;363(1502):2481.

[67] Hildebrand DK, Wu ZJ, Mayer JE, Jr., Sacks MS. Design and hydrodynamic evaluation of a novel pulsatile bioreactor for biologically active heart valves. *Ann Biomed Eng* 2004;32(8):1039-1049.

[68] Barron V, Lyons E, Stenson-Cox C, McHugh PE, Pandit A. Bioreactors for cardiovascular cell and tissue growth: a review. *Ann Biomed Eng* 2003;31(9):1017-1030.

[69] Sodian R, Hoerstrup SP, Sperling JS, Daebritz SH, Martin DP, Schoen FJ, Vacanti JP, Mayer JE, Jr. Tissue engineering of heart valves: in vitro experiences. *Ann Thorac Surg* 2000;70(1):140-144.

[70] Engelmayr GC, Jr., Sales VL, Mayer JE, Jr., Sacks MS. Cyclic flexure and laminar flow synergistically accelerate mesenchymal stem cell-mediated engineered tissue formation: Implications for engineered heart valve tissues. *Biomaterials* 2006;27(36):6083-6095.

[71] Engelmayr GC, Jr., Soletti L, Vigmostad SC, Budilarto SG, Federspiel WJ, Chandran KB, Vorp DA, Sacks MS. A novel flex-stretch-flow bioreactor for the study of engineered heart valve tissue mechanobiology. *Ann Biomed Eng* 2008;36(5):700-712.

[72] Arnsdorf EJ, Tummala P, Kwon RY, Jacobs CR. Mechanically induced osteogenic differentiation--the role of RhoA, ROCKII and cytoskeletal dynamics. *J Cell Sci* 2009;122(Pt 4):546-553.

[73] Arnsdorf EJ, Tummala P, Jacobs CR. Non-canonical Wnt signaling and N-cadherin related beta-catenin signaling play a role in mechanically induced osteogenic cell fate. *PLoS One* 2009;4(4):e5388.

[74] Li YJ, Batra NN, You L, Meier SC, Coe IA, Yellowley CE, Jacobs CR. Oscillatory fluid flow affects human marrow stromal cell proliferation and differentiation. *J Orthop Res* 2004;22(6):1283-1289.

[75] Driessen NJ, Mol A, Bouten CV, Baaijens FP. Modeling the mechanics of tissue-engineered human heart valve leaflets. *J Biomech* 2007;40(2):325-334.

[76] P. M. den Reijer, D. Sallee III, P. van der Velden, E. R. Zaaijer, W. J. Parks, S. Ramamurthy, T. Q. Robbie, G. Donati, C. Lamphier, R. P. Beekman, and M. E. Brummer. Hemodynamic predictors of aortic dilatation in bicuspid aortic valve by velocity-encoded cardiovascular magnetic resonance. *J Cardiovasc Magn Reson*, 12(4), 2010. In press (doi:10.1186/1532-429X-12-4).

[77] G. R. Veldtman, H. M. Connolly, T. A. Orszulak, J. A. Dearani, and H. V. Schaff. Fate of bicuspid aortic valves in patients undergoing aortic root repair or replacement for aortic root enlargement. *Mayo Clin Proc*, 81(3):322–326, 2006.

[78] J. J. J. Aalberts, T. W. Waterbolk, J. P. van Tintelen, H. L. Hillege P. W. Boonstra, and M. P. van den Berg. Prophylactic aortic root surgery in patients with Marfan syndrome: 10 years' experience with a protocol based on body surface area. *Eur J Cardio Thorac Surg*, 34(3):589–594, 2008.

[79] J. de Hart, G. W. M. Peters, P. J. G. Schreurs, and F. P. T. Baaijens. A three-dimensional computational analysis of fluid-structure interaction in the aortic valve. *J Biomech*, 36(1):102–112, 2003.

[80] J. de Hart, F. P. T. Baaijens, G. W. M. Peters, and P. J. G. Schreurs. A computational fluid-structure interaction analysis of a fiber-reinforced stentless aortic valve. *J Biomech*, 36(5):699–712, 2003.

[81] J. de Hart, G. W. M. Peters, P. J. G. Schreurs, and F. P. T. Baaijens. Collagen fibers reduce stresses and stabilize motion of aortic valve leaflets during systole. *J Biomech*, 37(3):303–311, 2004.

[82] M. A. Nicosia, R. P. Cochran, D. R. Einstein, C. J. Rutland, and K. S. Kunzelman. A coupled fluid-structure finite element model of the aortic valve and root. *J Heart Valve Dis*, 12(6):781–789, 2003.

[83] E. J. Weinberg and M. R. Kaazempur-Mofrad. Transient, three-dimensional, multiscale simulations of the human aortic valve. *Cardiovasc Eng*, 7(4):140–155, 2007.

[84] E. J. Weinberg and M. R. Kaazempur-Mofrad. A multiscale computational comparison of the bicuspid and tricuspid aortic valves in relation to calcific aortic stenosis. *J Biomech*, 41(16):3482–3487, 2008.

[85] E. Griffith, X. Luo, D. M. McQueen, and C. S. Peskin. Simulating the fluid dynamics of natural and prosthetic heart valves using the immersed boundary method. *Int J Appl Mech*, 1(1):137–177, 2009.

[86] L. Ge, C. Jones, F. Sotiropoulos, T. M. Healy, and A. P. Yoganathan. Numerical simulation of flow in mechanical heart valves: Grid resolution and the assumption of flow symmetry. *J Biomech Eng*, 125(5):709–718, 2003.

[87] L. P. Dasi, L. Ge, H. A. Simon, F. Sotiropoulos, and A. P. Yoganathan. Vorticity dynamics of a bileaflet mechanical heart valve in an axisymmetric aorta. *Phys Fluid*, 19(6):Art. No. 067105, 2007.

[88] H. Kim, K. B. Chandran, M. S. Sacks, and J. Lu. An experimentally derived stress resultant shell model for heart valve dynamic simulations. *Ann Biomed Eng*, 35(1):30–44, 2006.

[89] H. Kim, J. Lu, M. S. Sacks, and K. B. Chandran. Dynamic simulation of bioprosthetic heart valves using a stress resultant shell model. *Ann Biomed Eng*, 36(2):262–275, 2007.

[90] N. Gundiah, K. Kam, P. B. Matthews, J. Guccione, H. A. Dwyer, D. Saloner, T. A. M. Chuter, T. S. Guy, M. B. Ratcliffe, and E. E. Tseng. Asymmetric mechanical properties of porcine aortic sinuses. *Ann Thorac Surg*, 85(5):1631–1638, 2008.

[91] N. Gundiah, P. B. Matthews, R. Karimi, A. Azadani, J. Guccione, T. S. Guy, D. Saloner, and E. E. Tseng. Significant material property differences between the porcine ascending aorta and aortic sinuses. *J Heart Valve Dis*, 17(6):606–613, 2008.

[92] K. May-Newman, C. Lam, and F. C. P. Yin. A hyperelastic constitutive law for aortic valve tissue. *J Biomech Eng*, 131(8):081009 (7 pages), 2009.

[93] T. Walther, V. Falk, T. Dewey, J. Kempfert, F. Emrich, B. Pfannm¨ uller, P. Br¨oske, M. A. Borger, G. Schuler, M. Mack, and F. W. Mohr. Valve-in-a-valve concept for

transcatheter minimally invasive repeat xenograft implantation. *J Am Coll Cardiol*, 50(1):56–60, 2007.

[94] T.Walther, J.Kempfert, M. A. Borger, J. Fassl, V. Falk, J. Blumenstein, M. Dehdashtian, G. Schuler, and F.W. Mohr. Human minimally invasive off-pump valve-in-a-valve implantation. *Ann Thorac Surg*, 85(3):1072–1073, 2008.

[95] J. Ye, J. G. Webb, A. Cheung, J.-B. Masson, R. G. Carere, C. R. Thompson, B. Munt, R. Moss, and S. V. Lichtenstein. Transcatheter valve-in-valve aortic valve implantation: 16-month follow-up. *Ann Thorac Surg*, 88(4):1322–1324, 2009.

[96] S. Nistri, M. D. Sorbo, M. Marin, M. Palisi, R. Scognamiglio, and G. Thiene. Aortic root dilatation in young men with normally functioning bicuspid aortic valves. *Heart*, 82(1):19–22, 1999.

[97] L. G. Svensson, K.-H. Kim, B. W. Lytle, and D. M. Cosgrove. Relationship of aortic cross-sectional area to height ratio and the risk of aortic dissection in patients with bicuspid aortic valves. *J Thorac Cardiovasc Surg*, 126(3):892–893, 2003.

Aortic Valve

In: Percutaneous Valve Technology: Present and Future ISBN: 978-1-61942-577-4
Editors: Jose Luis Navia and Sharif Al-Ruzzeh

Chapter VIII

Cardiology Perspective of Aortic Valve Disease – The Potential Role of Percutaneous Technology

Andrew C. Y. To and William J. Stewart

Aortic valve disease management remains challenging for clinicians despite advances in medical imaging and surgical techniques.

With the advent of percutaneous management strategies for diseases of the aortic valve, the imaging cardiologist has several important roles.

Firstly, the role of percutaneous technology in individual patients with different types of aortic valve diseases should be considered in the context of existing treatment options such as surgical replacement vs. medical therapy.

Secondly, the imaging cardiologist has the fundamental role in assessing the suitability of patients undergoing percutaneous aortic valve replacement, as well as in the intraoperative guidance of the procedure.

This chapter will be divided into two parts.

1) The medical aspects of aortic valve diseases will be considered, with discussion on the etiology, natural history and current management strategies. The emphasis will be on how transcatheter aortic valve implantation (TAVI) using percutaneous technology fit with the current management of aortic valve disease.
2) The role of imaging in the assessment of potential TAVI candidates and peri-procedural echocardiography in the guidance of TAVI will be discussed.

How Percutaneous Technology Fits in the Current Management Strategies of Aortic Valve Disease

Aortic Stenosis

Aortic stenosis (AS) has a prevalence of 2-4% in adults over 65 [1] and is more common in older individuals. [2] With the aging population, surgical AVR volume has been increasing in recent years, however, many patients are not good candidates for surgery. In addition, many patients who would be surgical candidates do not end up having surgery because they are not referred to a surgical center. The EURO heart survey showed that a third of patients over the age of 75 were deemed unsuitable for surgical AVR because of poor surgical risk. [3] For these patients, the role of TAVI could be enormous.

Etiology

So far, TAVI has been studied in patients who are not surgical candidates and high risk surgical patients. Calcific degenerative AS is the predominant cause of AS encountered in these patients. In the pre-procedural workup of patients for TAVI, it is important to carefully establish AS etiologies, as other etiologies are generally not amenable to TAVI. (Table 1) Valvular AS is the most common type of AS. Degenerative calcific AS results from an atherosclerosis-like process that includes lipid and inflammatory cell infiltration, fibrosis, progressive leaflet calcium deposition, and gradual restriction in leaflet excursion that eventually leads to stenosis usually in the 6th to 8th decade of life [4]. Rheumatic AS has a declining incidence and occurs as a result of late effects of inflammation from rheumatic fever that leads to commissural thickening and fusion. Congenital AS mainly results from bicuspid aortic valve that has an incidence of 1-2% in the general population. Rarely, these patients have such leaflet distortion that they present with significant stenosis in infancy. More commonly, bicuspid valve patients who are younger have no stenosis through many decades of life. [5] However, the long-standing turbulent flow through the structurally abnormal bicuspid valve leads to progressive leaflet calcification, fibrosis and subsequent stenoses, usually in the 4th to 6th decade of life. About 10 to 20% of these patients come to surgery primarily because of aortic regurgitation (AR). Bicuspid valve patients commonly have concurrent aortopathy with dilated aortic root and/or ascending aorta that may develop before or after the onset of significant valvular stenosis.

Subvalvular AS results from fibromuscular membrane in the left ventricular outflow tract, that causes subaortic flow obstruction. The resulting turbulent flow onto the aortic valve leaflets commonly results in associated valvular aortic regurgitation. Supravalvular AS is the least common form of AS which results from the congenital narrowing of the ascending aorta distal to the sinuses of Valsalva, associated with features such as peripheral pulmonary stenosis, hypercalcemia and Elfin facies. Diagnosing subvalvular and supravalvular AS relies on the careful characterization of the subaortic area, aortic root and ascending aorta with echocardiography, often with transesophageal echocardiography. Both conditions require surgical excision and are not amenable to treatment with TAVI.

Table 1. Etiologies of AS

Etiologies
• Valvular AS
o Degenerative
o Rheumatic
o Congenital – bicuspid, unicuspid, quadricuspid
• Supravalvular AS
• Subvalvular AS

Pathophysiology and Clinical Presentation

Typically in valvular AS, aortic leaflet mobility decreases gradually over time, in a slow process that increases the degree of outflow obstruction and decreases the valve orifice area. Progressive left ventricular outflow tract (LVOT) obstruction causes progressive left ventricular (LV) pressure overload and a compensatory increase in LV wall thickness. The LV responds to the increased afterload by hypertrophy, which is a mechanism to normalize wall stress by Laplace's law. However, left ventricular hypertrophy also increases the challenge of diastolic coronary perfusion, as LV diastolic pressure increases toward the level of diastolic coronary pressure and the distance from the epicardial coronaries to the endocardium increases. Patients become symptomatic after a long latent period without symptoms. Although ejection fraction and systolic function are maintained until late in the disease course, diastolic dysfunction develops earlier, related to the myocardial hypertrophy and fibrosis. The LV end-diastolic pressure is often elevated. The increase in myocardial muscle mass leads to an increased demand in coronary artery blood flow, which is often inadequate in advanced cases so that coronary flow reserve is limited especially endocardially.

The above factors of LVOT obstruction, LV diastolic and systolic dysfunction and impaired coronary artery blood flow combine to cause the classic symptoms of angina, syncope and dyspnea. Symptoms are often provoked by exercise as mechanical outflow obstruction prevents cardiac output from augmenting by increasing stroke volume, but rather, relying on an increased heart rate instead. Late in the course of the disease, LV dilation and systolic impairment become inevitable, as the progressive LV hypertrophy no longer matches the increased LV afterload. Severe heart failure and ultimately death ensue.

When valvular AS is mild or moderate in severity, the prognosis of patients in the asymptomatic latent period is excellent.

Surgical AVR is not required until later, often after symptoms develop. In the latent period, careful periodic clinical monitoring is necessary as aortic valve area decreases on average about 0.1 cm^2/year, with an accompanying average increase in mean transaortic gradient of about 7 to 10 mmHg/year. [4] The main predictors of progression include older age, male gender, hypercholesterolemia, smoking, hypertension, and diabetes; that is, most of the atherosclerotic risk factors. A peak aortic jet velocity of >4m/s and/or an increase in peak aortic jet velocity of >0.3m/s/year on echocardiography have been found to be independent markers of rapid progression, [4,6] although significant individual variations remain.

Current Management Strategies

Surgical intervention is typically recommended when symptoms develop because of the high incidence of symptomatic deterioration and sudden death once patients become symptomatic. [7,8] Table 2 outlines the current ACC/AHA recommendations for surgical intervention for AS. Of note, the frequent co-existence of coronary artery disease and AS often poses difficulties in clinical decision-making. The presence of significant coronary stenosis confounds the assessment of whether aortic stenosis is symptomatic or not. In addition, patients with coronary artery disease undergoing CABG may need concurrent aortic valve replacement if they have incidentally noted concurrent moderate or severe AS that is otherwise asymptomatic. [9,10]

Table 2. Current ACC/AHA recommendations for aortic valve replacement for aortic stenosis

Class I
1. AVR is indicated for symptomatic patients with severe AS.* (Level of Evidence: B)
2. AVR is indicated for patients with severe AS* undergoing coronary artery bypass graft surgery (CABG). (Level of Evidence: C)
3. AVR is indicated for patients with severe AS* undergoing surgery on the aorta or other heart valves. (Level of Evidence: C)
4. AVR is recommended for patients with severe AS* and LV systolic dysfunction (ejection fraction less than 0.50). (Level of Evidence: C)
Class IIa
1. AVR is reasonable for patients with moderate AS* undergoing CABG or surgery on the aorta or other heart valves. (Level of Evidence: B)
Class IIb
1. AVR may be considered for asymptomatic patients with severe AS* and abnormal response to exercise (e.g., development of symptoms or asymptomatic hypotension). (Level of Evidence: C)
2. AVR may be considered for adults with severe asymptomatic AS* if there is a high likelihood of rapid progression (age, calcification, and CAD) or if surgery might be delayed at the time of symptom onset. (Level of Evidence: C)
3. AVR may be considered in patients undergoing CABG who have mild AS* when there is evidence, such as moderate to severe valve calcification, that progression may be rapid. (Level of Evidence: C)
4. AVR may be considered for asymptomatic patients with extremely severe AS (aortic valve area less than 0.6 cm2, mean gradient greater than 60 mm Hg, and jet velocity greater than 5.0 m per second) when the patient's expected operative mortality is 1.0% or less. (Level of Evidence: C)
Class III
1. AVR is not useful for the prevention of sudden death in asymptomatic patients with AS who have none of the findings listed under the Class IIa/IIb recommendations. (Level of Evidence: B)

Careful observation with periodic noninvasive testing is recommended for asymptomatic AS patients. The frequency of monitoring has to be individually tailored, depending on AS severity and other clinical factors; with the aim of detecting early clinical deterioration before adverse clinical events and irreversible ventricular remodeling. Because of AS severity is such strong determinant of clinical deterioration and future progression, groups have advocated the early surgical management of patients who have critical asymptomatic AS. In the ACC/AHA valve disease guidelines, surgical AVR is a class IIb indication for asymptomatic individuals who has a high likelihood of rapid progression or has extremely severe AS on echocardiographic criteria (peak aortic jet velocity of >5m/s, mean transaortic gradient of >60mmHg, or a calculated aortic valve area of <0.60cm2). [1] Objective assessment of exercise capacity on exercise testing may be useful in selected cases of severe AS, in order to confirm the self-reported symptom status. [11] Figure 1 summarizes the suggested decision-making algorithm for patients with severe AS from the ACC/AHA valvular disease guidelines.

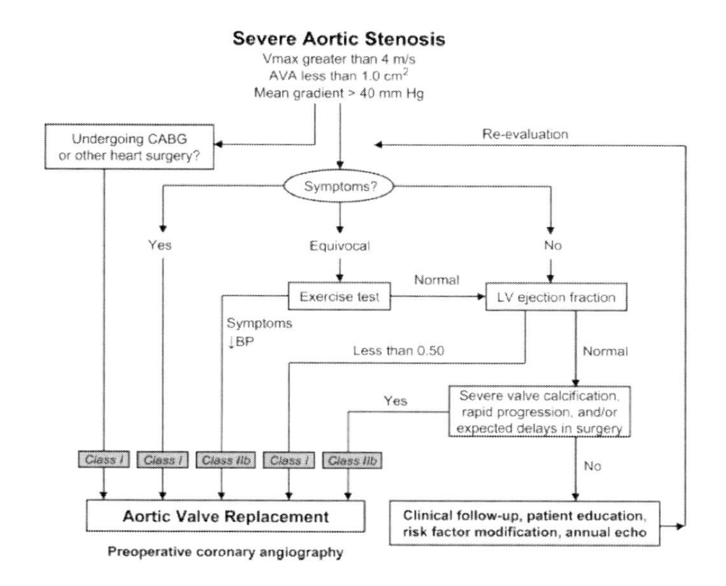

Figure 1. Management strategy for patients with severe aortic stenosis. (Reproduced from Bonow et al.) [1].

The Role of TAVI in the Management of AS

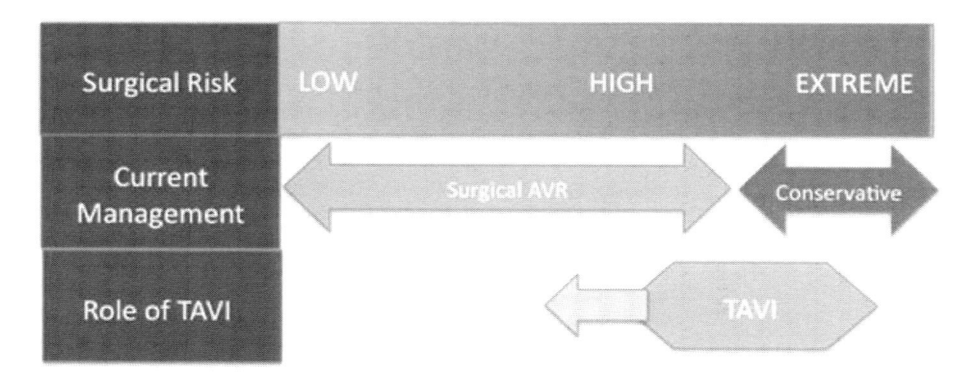

Figure 2. The evolving role of TAVI in the management of AS.

Extreme Risk Candidates – As Alternative to Palliative Management

The current and potential roles of TAVI in the management of AS are outlined in Figure 2. For the great majority of patients, surgical AVR is the established treatment of severe symptomatic AS because of the low peri-operative mortality and its proven value in improving survival. [12-15] The overall 30-day mortality rate has been estimated to be 1-4% for the overall population undergoing surgical AVR. [16] Long term survival after surgical AVR is excellent, with event-free survival similar to age-expected survival rates. [17] Currently, clinical data on TAVI is published in patients who are deemed too high risk to be safe surgical AVR candidates. [18-24] In these patients who otherwise would have been managed palliatively, significant improvement in both 30-day and 1-year mortality were noted, as well as other end-points such as cardiac symptoms and hospitalizations.

Surgical risk assessment takes into account many variables that were shown to increase perioperative morbidity and mortality. These include age, gender, cardiac factors such as LV function and endocarditis, operative factors such as reoperation and emergency surgery, and the presence of co-morbid diseases such as diabetes, renal, cerebrovascular, pulmonary and peripheral vascular diseases. Commonly used risk scores include the EuroSCORE (European System for cardiac operative risk evaluation) [25,26], the STS score (Society of thoracic surgery predicted risk of mortality) [27,28] and the Ambler score [29]. An array of factors was used in regression models to estimate perioperative mortality risk. Readers are referred to the websites www.euroscore.org and www.sts.org for details of the models. It is important to note that risk assessment should be individualized to individual patient's unique history, as factors such as frailty and other rarer conditions such as history of mediastinal irradiation, mediastinitis, cirrhosis, and porcelain (calcified) aorta are not included in these scores.

In the United States, TAVI has been approved by the FDA. From the recently published Partner trial "cohort B" deemed inoperable due to extreme surgical risk, patients had an average STS score of 12% and Logistic EuroScore of 28%. [18] In Europe, guidelines jointly developed by the European Association of Cardio-Thoracic Surgery, European Society of Cardiology and European Association of Percutaneous Cardiovascular Interventions in 2008 put emphasis on clinical judgment in conjunction with objective scores. Expected mortality of >20% with the Logistic EuroScore and >10% with STS score were considered suitable candidates for TAVI in the trial. [30]

The threshold at which patients should be considered poor surgical candidates is currently uncertain. This is also likely a dynamic threshold, depending on the relative efficacy and risks of TAVI vs. surgery in various patient populations.

Advances in surgical techniques and post-operative care means that more high-risk patients can be operated with lower mortality. Several modern surgical series of cardiac surgery in octogenarians have demonstrated surprisingly low surgical mortality, with patients having significantly improved quality of life compared to conservative therapy. [31-34] These series are undoubtedly highly selected groups, but as surgical risk decreases in the high-risk population, the threshold for surgery will continue to decline, therefore the threshold for TAVI may shift upwards.

On the other hand, the threshold at which patients should be considered too high a risk even for TAVI is also uncertain. At some very high level of risk, patients should be treated with palliation.

The availability of TAVI pushes that threshold to a higher level. Currently, clinical trials commonly include "life expectancy of <12 months due to noncardiac co-morbidities" as an exclusion criteria, which is loosely defined and requires clinical judgment of each individual patient. The patient selection criteria for TAVI will be further refined as clinical experience in this new technique increases.

High Risk Candidates – As Alternative to Surgical AVR

In patients who are operative candidates, data from clinical trials are still being accumulated to address whether TAVI is a viable alternative to surgical AVR. Recently, results from "cohort A" of the PARTNER trial were presented at the American College of Cardiology Conference 2011. This cohort included 699 AS patients deemed eligible for surgery, but thought to be high risk by the treating physicians. TAVI is noninferior to traditional surgical AVR in terms of all-cause mortality.

The 1-year mortality of this cohort is high at 26% regardless of the type of treatment. Several important differences are also noted between the groups. TAVI group had a higher incidence of stroke and vascular complications, while the surgical group had a higher incidence of major bleeding and new-onset atrial fibrillation. As further studies will clarify the relative importance of these differences, the different risk profiles of these two distinct procedures will likely become important considerations for individual patients in choosing between the two strategies. However, although long-term durability data is unavailable, the preliminary data from cohort A of the PARTNER trial are promising. Future studies are likely to refine the suitability of TAVI in treating these high-risk patients with severe AS. In particular, as discussed before, continued improvement in surgical techniques such as minimally invasive and robotic surgeries [35] will lower surgical risk and continue to shift the threshold for recommending TAVI as an alternative to surgical AVR.

With maturation of the technology, several specific clinical scenarios may become suitable for TAVI as alternative to surgical AVR and are worth discussing.

- In patients with concurrent coronary artery disease where operative mortality is significantly higher than isolated valvular replacement or isolated CABG, hybrid TAVI and PCI may be considered instead of combined AVR/CABG. Similarly, patients who had prior CABG and subsequently developed symptomatic AS may also opt for TAVI rather than the higher risk re-do surgical AVR.
- Patients with AS and significant LV dysfunction have high operative risk from AVR. TAVI may be considered a medium term strategy in this situation. Even if TAVI was not proven equivalent to surgical AVR, it could potentially be adopted as a bridging procedure for patients with severe LV dysfunction, similar to the occasional use of balloon aortic valvuloplasty as a bridging procedure to see if LV function may improve sufficiently to allow reconsideration for surgical AVR.
- The availability of TAVI as an alternative to surgical AVR may also raise the threshold at which concurrent AVR in patients undergoing CABG who has moderate AS that would otherwise be asymptomatic.

Aortic Regurgitation

To date, the use of TAVI in patients with AR has not been studied in the United States. While calcific degenerative aortic valve disease in the elderly can present with mixed AS and AR, these patients have thus far been excluded from the TAVI trials discussed above. Therefore, little is known about the efficacy and risk of TAVI in patients with significant AR.

Etiology

AR results from either valve leaflet disease or aortic root dilation. The spectrum of valve leaflet pathology for AR is different from those of AS. Vavular etiologies include congenital valvular disorders such bicuspid aortic valve and congenital fenestration, rheumatic disease, myxomatous valve, or endocarditis. Disorders that cause aortic root dilation are varied but include idiopathic aortic root dilation, hypertensive aortopathy, Marfan's syndrome and other connective tissue disease related aortopathy. Aortic annulus dilation leads to disruption of proper leaflet coaptation and hence AR. Many of the above conditions occur in patients who are younger with less co-morbidities. As TAVI is currently targeted to patients with high surgical risk, TAVI is likely to play a limited role in managing AR. In the group of patients with aortic root dilation, concurrent aortic root and/or ascending aortic replacement is often needed. Even when root dilation is less severe and not reaching surgical criteria, the proper deployment of percutaneous devices may be challenging if the landing zone of the device is larger, increasing the risk of post-procedural paravalvular AR. A dilated aortic annulus is a common exclusion criterion in TAVI trials. Bicuspid aortic valves are similarly excluded from these trials, also because of the often asymmetric aortic root increasing the risk of paravalvular AR. The intricate relationship between the etiology of the AR and the anatomy of the aortic root has an impact on how TAVI might be applied in the management of AR.

Pathophysiology, Clinical Presentation and Current Management Strategies

Chronic AR results in both LV volume and pressure overload because the increased total LV stroke volume from the regurgitation is accompanied by a compensatory increase in LV afterload, eccentric LV hypertrophy and LV dilation. Similar to other valvular heart disease, many patients remain asymptomatic until systolic dysfunction develops. Surgical AVR timing, therefore, depends on the development of symptoms or incipient systolic dysfunction indicated by excessive ventricular dilation and/or deterioration in contractile function.

At present, the major challenge in managing severe asymptomatic AR is in determining if incipient systolic dysfunction is present, at which point, prompt surgery is likely to be more beneficial than further delay in treatment. The ACC/AHA valvular heart disease guidelines for surgical AVR recommended a threshold of an LV ejection fraction below 50% or an LV end-systolic diameter above 50-55 mm. Obviously, such threshold is derived from balancing the risk from surgery and the risk of clinical deterioration. As the technology of TAVI matures, the different procedural risk profile to that of surgery may ultimately alter the timing of intervention so that patients with lesser degree of ventricular remodeling may be intervened earlier.

The Role of TAVI in the Management of AR

As previously discussed, the etiologies, demographics and natural history of native valve AR limit the use of TAVI. Studies on the role of TAVI in native valve AR are sparse. Researchers, however, have identified a unique group of patients with prosthetic valve AR where TAVI may be used, in so-called "valve-in-valve" implantations. Patients with prosthetic valve AR tend to be older, frailer, with high predicted perioperative mortality. If conservative therapy is pursued, quality of life is often limited, with high morbidity and mortality. Most of these reports are isolated case reports utilizing the CoreValve percutaneous system in patients with degenerative changes in bio-prosthetic valve cusps that rupture or prolapse, [36-40] rather than paravalvular aortic regurgitation [41]. In one case report, the CoreValve percutaneous sytem is also used successfully for native valve endocarditis with severe regurgitation. [42] Future studies are needed to determine the exact role TAVI plays in this special group of patients.

Pre-Procedural Work-up and Peri-Procedural Management

The pre-procedural work-up and peri-procedural management of patients undergoing TAVI is as important as patient selection. Pre-procedural imaging work-up assesses the feasibility of TAVI and excludes those who have contraindications, while peri-procedural imaging guides interventionist in the successful device implantation and monitors for post-implantation complications.

Pre-Procedural Imaging Work-up

Pre-procedural imaging work-up of TAVI candidates assesses feasibility and excludes contraindications of TAVI. Prior to imaging tests, careful history and physical examination should identify many conditions that are absolute or relative contraindications to TAVI. These include recent cerebrovascular accidents and transient ischemic attacks, active peptic ulcer or gastrointestinal bleeding, renal insufficiency, allergy to aspirin, ticlopidine, clopidogrel or heparin; as well as significant non-cardiac co-morbidities limiting life expectancy. Table 3 summarizes the routine investigations performed in our institution and the relevant information that is obtained with each.

Coronary angiography is routinely performed prior to TAVI to diagnose coronary artery disease. The management of TAVI patients needing coronary revascularization is challenging. Concurrent valvular heart disease and coronary artery disease significantly increases peri-procedural risks, both for surgical AVR/CABG and percutaneous options. Individualized decisions have to be made as to whether such revascularization should be performed surgically or percutaneously and how this should be best combined with the planned TAVI. In addition, pre-procedural catheterization and aortograms are useful in determining the relative position of the coronary arteries, aortic valve and aortic root. This information is important in determining the risk of peri-procedural coronary artery occlusion, although in many cases, information from CT suffices.

Echocardiography, transthoracic and/or transesophageal, is the primary tool by which clinicians screen for existing cardiac conditions that may deem the patients unsuitable for TAVI. Depending on local expertise and regional guidelines, these may include the items listed in Table 3.

Table 3. Pre-procedural imaging work-up

Coronary angiography		
•	concomitant coronary artery disease	
Echocardiography		
•	assessment of aortic annulus anatomy – morphology and dimension	
•	assessment of aortic valve anatomy	
	o	unicuspid or bicuspid aortic valve
	o	concomitant aortic regurgitation
•	assessment of potential contraindications to TAVI	
	o	severe mitral regurgitation
	o	severe left ventricular dysfunction
	o	concomitant cardiomyopathy not related to the valvular dysfunction, e.g. hypertrophic cardiomyopathy
	o	intracardiac mass, thrombus, or vegetation
Computer tomography		
•	assessment of aortic annulus anatomy – morphology and dimension	
	o	relationship between coronary artery ostia and aortic valve leaflets
	o	relationship between anterior mitral valve leaflet and aortic annulus
•	assessment of aorta and iliofemoral arteries	
	o	presence of aneurysm, tortuosity, excessive atheroma, or stenosis
	o	size of the aorta and iliofemoral arteries – minimal diameter

In clinical trials, patients with bicuspid valves are excluded, partly because of concern over the asymmetric geometry of the aortic root and the subsequent risk of incomplete device expansion and deployment leading to paravalvular regurgitation. In addition, information on LV and RV systolic function as well as co-existent valvular abnormalities are also invaluable in peri-procedural anesthetic care and potentially impact on the choice of anesthetic agents and inotropic support.

Aortic Root and LVOT Anatomy

Assessing aortic root and LVOT anatomy is crucial in the pre-procedural work-up of TAVI patients. The correct positioning and sizing of the percutaneous device determine procedural success. The commonly used balloon expandable valve, Edwards-Sapien prosthesis (Edwards Lifesciences Inc.), comes in either a 23mm device for use when annulus diameter is between 18 and 21mm, or a 26mm device for use when annulus diameter is between 21 and 24mm. The commonly used self-expandable valve, CoreValve prosthesis (CoreValve, Irvine, California), comes in either a 26mm device for use when annulus diameter is between 20 and 23mm, or a 29mm device for use when annulus diameter is between 23 and 27mm.

Under-sizing prosthesis relative to the aortic annulus can lead to paravalvular regurgitation of varying severity, or, in severe cases, inadequate support for the stent frame causing valve embolization. Over-sizing prosthesis has the potential of causing annular and aortic root erosion and rupture, although these complications are rare. In the PARTNER trial investigating the Edwards-Sapiens valve, patients with a native aortic annulus size of under 16mm or over 24mm were excluded. For the self-expandable CoreValve system, patients with annulus size of under 20mm and over 27mm are considered ineligible. Similarly, aortic root dimension is also important and in self-expandable prostheses, an aortic root diameter of over 45mm is considered a contraindication.

Aortic root and LVOT annulus sizing is commonly performed by TTE and/or TEE. CT also complements this assessment. Interestingly, recent comparative studies between CT and echocardiography demonstrated the elliptical geometry of the aortic annulus, leading to systematic difference between the modalities in measuring the LVOT annulus. [43] (Fig 2) Further studies are needed to clarify how these measurements are best interpreted to more accurately matching the individual variations in LVOT annulus geometry to the available prosthesis. Understanding of the variations in LVOT annulus geometry is also likely to lead to improvement in device design.

The length of the Edwards-Sapien prosthesis measures 14mm and 16mm for the 23mm and 26mm devices respectively, while the CoreValve device measures 50mm including the self-expandable metal stent frame. Correct device positioning is an important factor for procedural success.

Although rare, the ventricular end of the device has the potential of damaging the anterior mitral valve leaflet and interfering mitral valve function. On the other hand, the aortic end of the prosthesis may interfere with coronary artery flow, resulting from the compression of coronary artery ostia by the calcified native leaflets post device expansion. For the latter, a careful study of the spatial relationship between the often bulky calcified aortic leaflets, coronary ostia and the aortic root and annulus geometry may identify at risk patients for coronary artery occlusion. In our institution, this is performed using both TEE and CT.

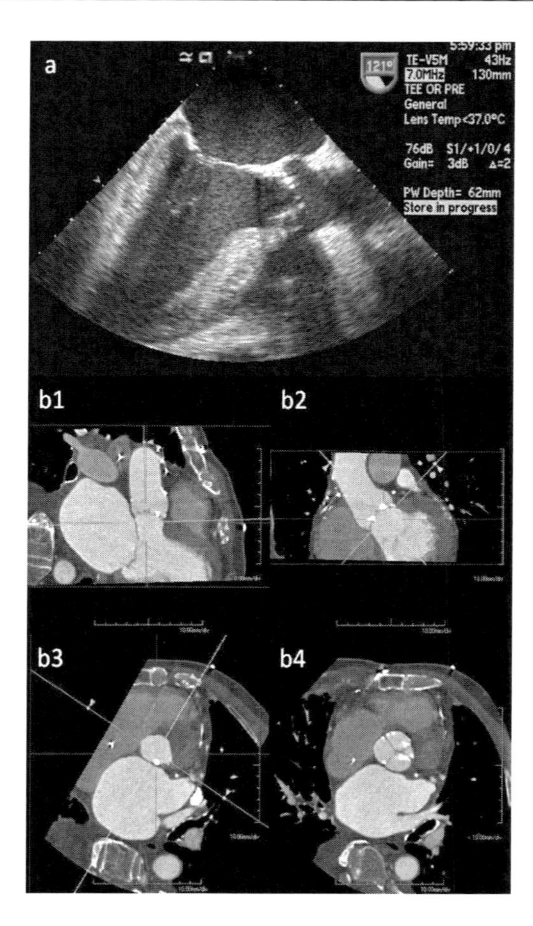

Figure 3. LVOT annulus dimension and geometry. (a) TEE image of the LVOT annulus along the long axis, taken in the mid-esophageal view at 121°. (b) CT assessment of LVOT geometry by multi-planar reconstruction in the same patient, demonstrating that by aligning the aortic root along the long axes (b1, b2), the shape of the LVOT is elliptical (b3), in a patient with normal trileaflet aortic valve (b4).

Pre-procedural TEE has the advantage of assessing the dynamic LVOT anatomy and mitral valve with high temporal resolution, as well as being the modality used for peri-implantation imaging guidance. CT, however, provides a true 3-dimensional dataset for accurate measurements and is especially useful in those with difficult or inconclusive TEEs. Often, CT image acquisitions include a retrospectively gated dataset through the aortic valve and LVOT so that 3-dimensional multi-planar reconstruction can be made at different phases of the cardiac cycle. This accurately studies these anatomical relationships in both diastole and systole, albeit at a lower temporal resolution than that of echocardiography.

Assessment of Aorta and Iliofemoral Arteries

Assessing the descending thoracic and abdominal aorta and iliofemoral arteries is important in determining the patient suitability in undergoing the transfemoral vs. the transpical approach. The choice between the transfemoral and transapical approaches should be individualized to patient condition and local expertise. The major determinant is significant aortic and iliofemoral artery disease. When this prohibits safe passage of the delivery systems through the arterial system to the ascending aorta for the transfemoral approach, the best option is transpical implantation. Currently, the minimal vessel diameter needed to permit the delivery system is 7mm for the Edwards-Sapien system and 6mm for the CoreValve system, although smaller devices will likely be developed in the future.

Aside from vessel dimension, the presence of aneurysm, tortuosity, excessive atheroma or calcifications also determines feasibility. This is especially important in the region of the aortic bifurcation where maneuvering the delivery system can be significantly hindered by the presence of tortuous vessels with significant calcifications. Significant atherosclerotic plaques and/or mural thrombus in the aorta and ilio-femoral arteries also predispose patients to embolic complications in the peripheral and renal vessels. Similarly, significant atheroma in the ascending aorta and aortic arch predisposes to post-procedural strokes. In these patients, the transapical approach may be preferable.

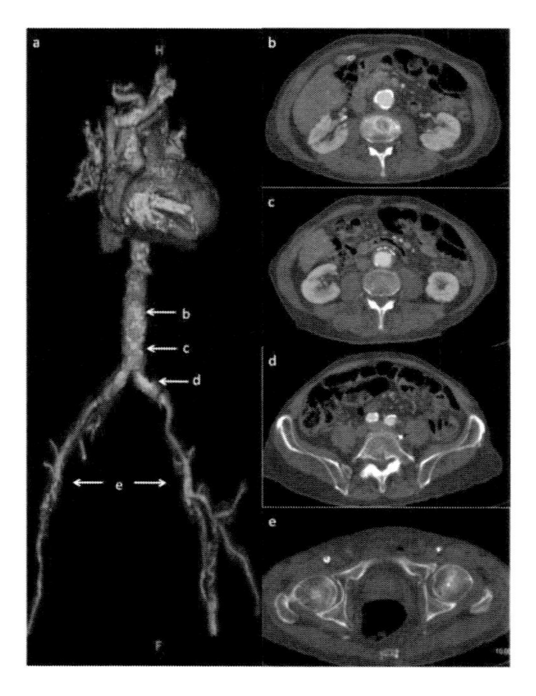

Figure 4. CT assessment of aorta and iliofemoral arteries prior to TAVI. This patient has significant abdominal aortic and ilio-femoral calcific atherosclerotic diseases, illustrated in the volume-rendered image of the arterial tree (a). There is mild aneurysmal dilation of the infrarenal abdominal aorta with moderate calcific atherosclerosis (b,c); severely calcified common iliac artery (d), especially at the origins of the external iliac artery where luminal diameters were only 6mm; and severely calcified common femoral arteries with luminal diameters of 4mm on the left and 5mm on the right (e).

The assessment of the aorta and ilio-femoral arteries is mainly using CT. (Fig 3) While TEE can also diagnose thoracic aortic atheroma, acoustic shadowing from the trachea often obscures parts of the ascending aorta. In our institution, pre-procedural CT of the thoracic and abdominal aorta is routinely performed, with or without the use of iodinated contrast. Non-contrast CT has the potential disadvantage of not identifying non-calcific plaques and mural thrombus, although it may remain the best option for those who have significant renal impairment. Alternatively, dedicated lower abdominal and pelvic CT may be performed using an intra-arterial contrast injection with a smaller volume of contrast, using an arterial pigtail catheter left in the infrarenal abdominal aorta after coronary angiography.

Peri-Procedural Imaging

Peri-procedural TEE is crucial for the successful implantation of the aortic prosthesis. The two main roles of TEE are in guiding device implantation, and detecting post-implantation complications. (Table 4)

Table 4. Role of peri-procedural TEE in TAVI

1)	Guidance of device implantation
a)	Pre-procedural imaging of LVOT for prosthesis sizing
b)	Guiding placement of transcatheter wire
c)	Positioning of the valve within the annulus
2)	Detection of post-implantation complications
a)	Assessing valve position after device expansion
b)	Quantitating post-implantation regurgitation
c)	Documenting the change in transaortic gradient
d)	Excluding new wall motion abnormalities
e)	Excluding hemopericardium
f)	Excluding intracardiac thrombus

Aortic prosthesis positioning is crucial to procedural success. Useful TEE views include the mid-esophageal view at 120-135° for the long-axis view of the LVOT; mid-esophageal view at 35-60° for the short-axis view of the aortic valve. Along the long-axis, the echocardiographer ensures that the device is neither too ventricular nor too aortic in position, which may cause complications of mitral valve damage and coronary artery ostia obstruction respectively. In addition, an aortic prosthesis that is too aortic in position also has a higher likelihood of incomplete apposition of the stent frame onto the aortic annulus, causing paravalvular regurgitation. On the short axis views of the aortic valve, it is important to ensure that both the guidewire and subsequently the device catheter be positioned at the central orifice of the aortic valve, rather than be in an off-centre position near the edge of the commissures. From this regard, biplane views available on 3-dimensional TEE systems are invaluable in providing simultaneous real-time views of both the long-axis and short axis images. Real-time 3-dimensional views are also useful in demonstrating the relations between the prosthetic valve, balloon and the aortic valve leaflets.

In the balloon-expandable devices, the valve portion of the device is identified as an echogenic rectangular structure in sharp profile to the underlying balloon. (Figure 5) The general recommendation is that two-thirds of the valve should be ventricular to the aortic valve leaflets and one-thirds of the valve should rest on the aortic side prior to balloon expansion. The Corevalve, a self-expandable device, can also be visualized by echo (Figure 6). It is important to identify full expansion at the LV rim, waist, and aortic rim of the device by diameter measurements. Proper device placement is accomplished with a combination of fluoroscopic and TEE guidance.

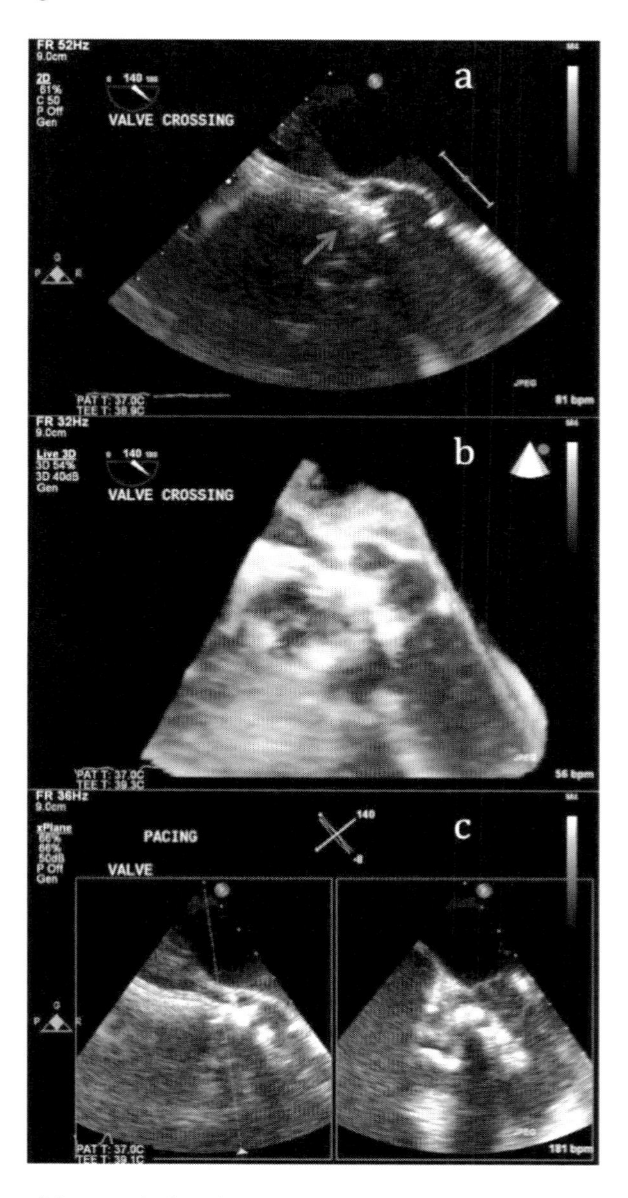

Figure 5. Identification of the prosthetic valve within the inflatable balloon of the Edwards Sapien Valve. (a) In this 95-year-old patient who underwent transfemoral TAVI, the echo density representing the Edwards Sapien valve, measured to be 15mm in length, can be seen with a rectangular profile (arrow) across the LVOT in this mid-esophageal long-axis view. (b) In the same patient, 3D live view of the prosthetic valve assists in the localization of the device in relation to the valve leaflets and LVOT. (c) With the help of biplane views, the position of the stent valve in relation to the LVOT can be assessed simultaneously in orthogonal views.

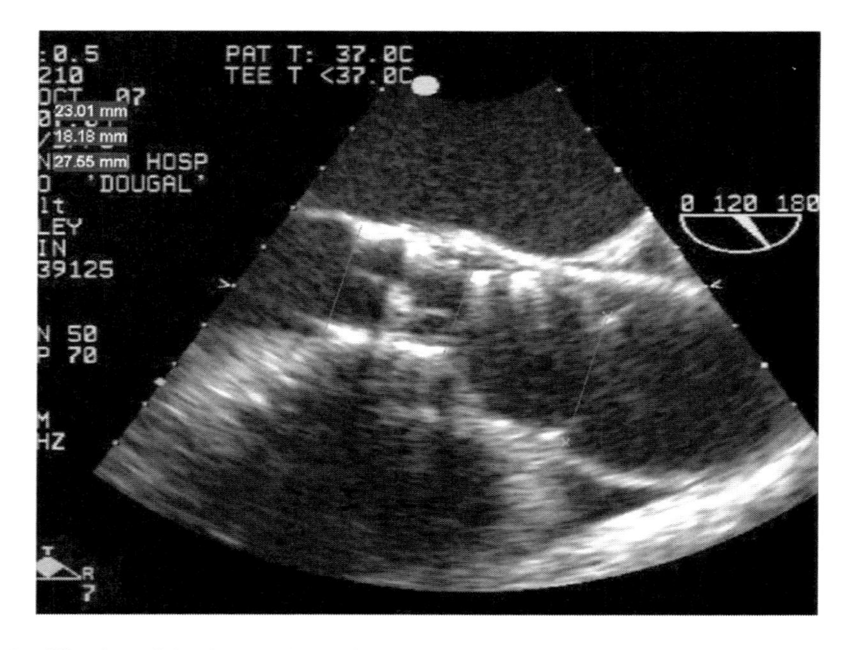

Figure 6. Identification of the CoreValve self-expandable TAVI. This is a fully deployed 29 mm CoreValve with suboptimal expansion, with measrements (red lines) of LV rim diameter 23, waist 18, and aortic rim 28 mm. reprinted from Chin D, European Journal of Echocardiography ; Volume 10, Issue 1; Pp. i21-i29.

Performing TEE during the TAVI procedure can often be technically challenging for a variety of reasons. Proper probe positioning in relation to the LVOT is crucial in ensuring that the views provided to the interventionist are truly along the long axis of the LVOT and across the short axis of the aortic valve. Acoustic shadowing from both the calcified aortic leaflets and the prosthetic device sometimes make it difficult for the echocardiographers to accurately gauge the position of the prosthetic device. Diagnosing valvular and paravaular aortic regurgitation can also be very challenging if there is significant acoustic shadowing.

One of the most important roles of peri-procedural TEE is the detection of complications. Mild paravalvular regurgitation is common after device deployment (Fig 6) and diagnosis is straightforward in most cases unless there is severe acoustic shadowing. The short axis view of the aortic valve is most useful view for localizing the regurgitant jet, so that the interventionists can determine if additional adjustment is necessary. Severe valvular regurgitation immediately post-deployment usually results from dysfunctional valve cusps that fail to coapt properly. This could be due to incomplete expansion or damage to the prosthetic leaflets during the deployment. Furthermore, valvular regurgitation may be exacerbated by the presence of the large-bore delivery catheter in the prosthetic valve orifice that interferes with valve leaflet function. In these cases, removing the delivery catheter leads to significant improvement. In cases with severe AR, persistent hypotension is often present. Very severe valvular regurgitation from dysfunctional valve cusps may be difficult to diagnose, not showing the typical aliasing on color Doppler, because of the brevity of the intense, early diastolic flow. Two-dimensional views of leaflet movement provide useful clues to such dysfunction. Other supplementary information on the AR can be obtained from pulsed Doppler of diastolic flow reversal in the ascending or descending thoracic aorta, or continuous wave Doppler from the deep transgastric view.

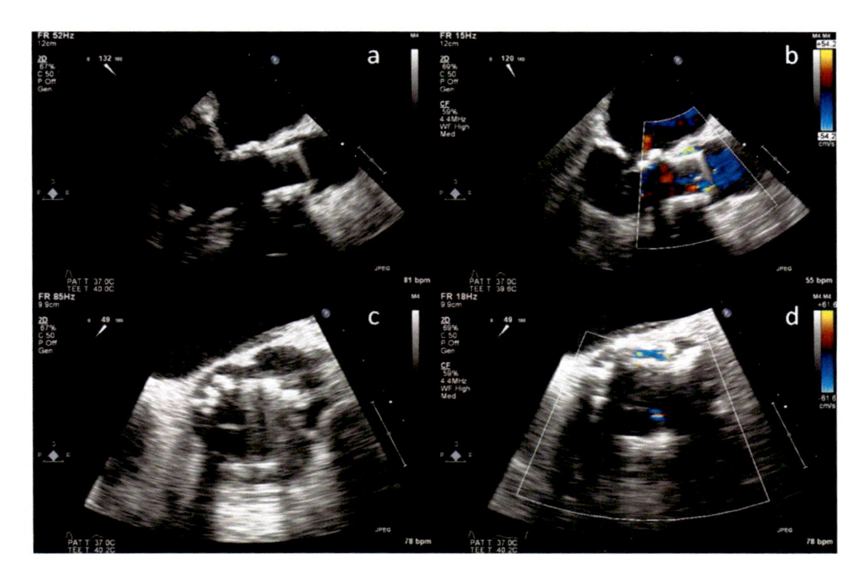

Figure 7. Appearance of the Edwards-Sapien valve post-implantation. Long-axis views are shown in (a,b) and short-axis views are shown in (c,d). After the removal of the balloon, there is trivial residual paravalvular aortic regurgitation (shown in color) along the posterior aortic annulus, between the non-coronary and left coronary sinuses. There is no significant intra-valvular regurgitation.

Other causes of hypotension post-valve deployment include LV dysfunction that could either be global or regional, as well as cardiac tamponade secondary to perforation or rupture. Global LV dysfunction is often due to myocardial stunning from the rapid ventricular pacing and transient outflow obstruction during balloon inflation and device implantation. New regional LV dysfunction results from coronary ostial obstruction post-valve deployment, which may require immediate coronary artery stenting. When that possibility is anticipated by preoperative TEE and CT testing, a wire is placed in the coronary artery prior to valve deployment. Transgastric views are often useful in the diagnosis of regional LV systolic dysfunction, especially for direct comparison with the same views taken prior to valve deployment. Mid-esophageal views are more prone to foreshortening and misalignment, unless probe positioning is optimal. Cardiac tamponade is a rare but treatable complication. Causes include perforation by the multiple guidewires and catheters, as well as aortic root rupture from device oversizing. Diagnosis can be difficult because the pericardial effusions can be small. Multiple TEE views, including the transgastric views and high-midesophageal views, may be necessary to make this diagnosis.

Finally, TEE monitors thrombus formation during the procedure from the multiple instrumentations, despite heparin anticoagulation. In these patients, meticulous management of subsequent anticoagulation is needed to avoid potentially devastating embolic complications such as stroke.

References

[1] Bonow RO, Carabello BA, Chatterjee K, et al. ACC/AHA 2006 guidelines for the management of patients with valvular heart disease: a report of the American College of

Cardiology/American Heart Association Task Force on Practice Guidelines (writing Committee to Revise the 1998 guidelines for the management of patients with valvular heart disease) developed in collaboration with the Society of Cardiovascular Anesthesiologists endorsed by the Society for Cardiovascular Angiography and Interventions and the Society of Thoracic Surgeons. *J Am Coll Cardiol* 2006;48:e1-148.

[2] Nkomo VT, Gardin JM, Skelton TN, Gottdiener JS, Scott CG, Enriquez-Sarano M. Burden of valvular heart diseases: a population-based study. *Lancet* 2006;368:1005-11.

[3] Iung B, Cachier A, Baron G, et al. Decision-making in elderly patients with severe aortic stenosis: why are so many denied surgery? *Eur Heart J* 2005;26:2714-20.

[4] Otto CM, Burwash IG, Legget ME, et al. Prospective study of asymptomatic valvular aortic stenosis. Clinical, echocardiographic, and exercise predictors of outcome. *Circulation* 1997;95:2262-70.

[5] Roberts WC. Anatomically isolated aortic valvular disease. The case against its being of rheumatic etiology. *Am J Med* 1970;49:151-9.

[6] Rosenhek R, Binder T, Porenta G, et al. Predictors of outcome in severe, asymptomatic aortic stenosis. *N Engl J Med* 2000;343:611-7.

[7] Ross J, Jr., Braunwald E. Aortic stenosis. *Circulation* 1968;38:61-7.

[8] Turina J, Hess O, Sepulcri F, Krayenbuehl HP. Spontaneous course of aortic valve disease. *Eur Heart J* 1987;8:471-83.

[9] Hochrein J, Lucke JC, Harrison JK, et al. Mortality and need for reoperation in patients with mild-to-moderate asymptomatic aortic valve disease undergoing coronary artery bypass graft alone. *Am Heart J* 1999;138:791-7.

[10] Pereira JJ, Balaban K, Lauer MS, Lytle B, Thomas JD, Garcia MJ. Aortic valve replacement in patients with mild or moderate aortic stenosis and coronary bypass surgery. *Am J Med* 2005;118:735-42.

[11] Das P, Rimington H, Chambers J. Exercise testing to stratify risk in aortic stenosis. *Eur Heart J* 2005;26:1309-13.

[12] Kvidal P, Bergstrom R, Horte LG, Stahle E. Observed and relative survival after aortic valve replacement. *J Am Coll Cardiol* 2000;35:747-56.

[13] Connolly HM, Oh JK, Orszulak TA, et al. Aortic valve replacement for aortic stenosis with severe left ventricular dysfunction. Prognostic indicators. *Circulation* 1997;95:2395-400.

[14] Murphy ES, Lawson RM, Starr A, Rahimtoola SH. Severe aortic stenosis in patients 60 years of age or older: left ventricular function and 10-year survival after valve replacement. *Circulation* 1981;64:II184-8.

[15] Tarantini G, Buja P, Scognamiglio R, et al. Aortic valve replacement in severe aortic stenosis with left ventricular dysfunction: determinants of cardiac mortality and ventricular function recovery. *Eur J Cardiothorac Surg* 2003;24:879-85.

[16] Edwards FH, Peterson ED, Coombs LP, et al. Prediction of operative mortality after valve replacement surgery. *J Am Coll Cardiol* 2001;37:885-92.

[17] Craver JM, Weintraub WS, Jones EL, Guyton RA, Hatcher CR, Jr. Predictors of mortality, complications, and length of stay in aortic valve replacement for aortic stenosis. *Circulation* 1988;78:I85-90.

[18] Leon MB, Smith CR, Mack M, et al. Transcatheter aortic-valve implantation for aortic stenosis in patients who cannot undergo surgery. *N Engl J Med* 2010;363:1597-607.

[19] Cribier A, Eltchaninoff H, Tron C, et al. Early experience with percutaneous transcatheter implantation of heart valve prosthesis for the treatment of end-stage inoperable patients with calcific aortic stenosis. *J Am Coll Cardiol* 2004;43:698-703.

[20] Cribier A, Eltchaninoff H, Tron C, et al. Treatment of calcific aortic stenosis with the percutaneous heart valve: mid-term follow-up from the initial feasibility studies: the French experience. *J Am Coll Cardiol* 2006;47:1214-23.

[21] Grube E, Laborde JC, Gerckens U, et al. Percutaneous implantation of the CoreValve self-expanding valve prosthesis in high-risk patients with aortic valve disease: the Siegburg first-in-man study. *Circulation* 2006;114:1616-24.

[22] Grube E, Schuler G, Buellesfeld L, et al. Percutaneous aortic valve replacement for severe aortic stenosis in high-risk patients using the second- and current third-generation self-expanding CoreValve prosthesis: device success and 30-day clinical outcome. *J Am Coll Cardiol* 2007;50:69-76.

[23] Webb JG, Pasupati S, Humphries K, et al. Percutaneous transarterial aortic valve replacement in selected high-risk patients with aortic stenosis. *Circulation* 2007;116:755-63.

[24] Webb JG, Chandavimol M, Thompson CR, et al. Percutaneous aortic valve implantation retrograde from the femoral artery. *Circulation* 2006;113:842-50.

[25] Nashef SA, Roques F, Michel P, Gauducheau E, Lemeshow S, Salamon R. European system for cardiac operative risk evaluation (EuroSCORE). *Eur J Cardiothorac Surg* 1999;16:9-13.

[26] Roques F, Michel P, Goldstone AR, Nashef SA. The logistic EuroSCORE. *Eur Heart J* 2003;24:881-2.

[27] Dewey TM, Brown D, Ryan WH, Herbert MA, Prince SL, Mack MJ. Reliability of risk algorithms in predicting early and late operative outcomes in high-risk patients undergoing aortic valve replacement. *J Thorac Cardiovasc Surg* 2008;135:180-7.

[28] Grossi EA, Schwartz CF, Yu PJ, et al. High-risk aortic valve replacement: are the outcomes as bad as predicted? *Ann Thorac Surg* 2008;85:102-6; discussion 107.

[29] Ambler G, Omar RZ, Royston P, Kinsman R, Keogh BE, Taylor KM. Generic, simple risk stratification model for heart valve surgery. *Circulation* 2005;112:224-31.

[30] Vahanian A, Alfieri O, Al-Attar N, et al. Transcatheter valve implantation for patients with aortic stenosis: a position statement from the European Association of Cardio-Thoracic Surgery (EACTS) and the European Society of Cardiology (ESC), in collaboration with the European Association of Percutaneous Cardiovascular Interventions (EAPCI). *Eur Heart J* 2008;29:1463-70.

[31] Chukwuemeka A, Borger MA, Ivanov J, Armstrong S, Feindel CM, David TE. Valve surgery in octogenarians: a safe option with good medium-term results. *J Heart Valve Dis* 2006;15:191-6; discussion 196.

[32] Kolh P, Kerzmann A, Lahaye L, Gerard P, Limet R. Cardiac surgery in octogenarians; peri-operative outcome and long-term results. *Eur Heart J* 2001;22:1235-43.

[33] Unic D, Leacche M, Paul S, et al. Early and late results of isolated and combined heart valve surgery in patients > or =80 years of age. *Am J Cardiol* 2005;95:1500-3.

[34] Varadarajan P, Kapoor N, Bansal RC, Pai RG. Survival in elderly patients with severe aortic stenosis is dramatically improved by aortic valve replacement: Results from a cohort of 277 patients aged > or =80 years. *Eur J Cardiothorac Surg* 2006;30:722-7.

[35] Mihaljevic T, Cohn LH, Unic D, Aranki SF, Couper GS, Byrne JG. One thousand minimally invasive valve operations: early and late results. *Ann Surg* 2004;240:529-34; discussion 534.

[36] Attias D, Himbert D, Hvass U, Vahanian A. "Valve-in-valve" implantation in a patient with stentless bioprosthesis and severe intraprosthetic aortic regurgitation. *J Thorac Cardiovasc Surg* 2009;138:1020-2.

[37] Attias D, Himbert D, Brochet E, Laborde JC, Vahanian A. 'Valve-in-valve' implantation in a patient with degenerated aortic bioprosthesis and severe regurgitation. *Eur Heart J* 2009;30:1852.

[38] Napodano M, Cutolo A, Fraccaro C, et al. Totally percutaneous valve replacement for severe aortic regurgitation in a degenerating bioprosthesis. *J Thorac Cardiovasc Surg* 2009;138:1027-8.

[39] Wenaweser P, Buellesfeld L, Gerckens U, Grube E. Percutaneous aortic valve replacement for severe aortic regurgitation in degenerated bioprosthesis: the first valve in valve procedure using the Corevalve Revalving system. *Catheter Cardiovasc Interv* 2007;70:760-4.

[40] Krumsdorf U, Bekeredjian R, Korosoglou G, et al. Images and case reports in interventional cardiology. Percutaneous aortic "valve in valve" implantation for severe aortic regurgitation in a degenerated bioprosthesis. *Circ Cardiovasc Interv* 2010;3:e6-7.

[41] Ng AC, van der Kley F, Delgado V, et al. Percutaneous valve-in-valve procedure for severe paravalvular regurgitation in aortic bioprosthesis. *JACC Cardiovasc Imaging* 2009;2:522-3.

[42] Presbitero P, Mennuni MG, Pagnotta P, Gasparini GL, Ramondo A. Percutaneous aortic valve in severe valvular regurgitation caused by infective endocarditis. *Int J Cardiol* 2010.

[43] Messika-Zeitoun D, Serfaty JM, Brochet E, et al. Multimodal assessment of the aortic annulus diameter: implications for transcatheter aortic valve implantation. *J Am Coll Cardiol* 2010;55:186-94.

In: Percutaneous Valve Technology: Present and Future
Editors: Jose Luis Navia and Sharif Al-Ruzzeh
ISBN: 978-1-61942-577-4

Chapter IX

Surgical Perspective of Aortic Valve Disease: The Potential Role of Transcatheter Valve Technology

S. Chris Malaisrie, Virna L. Sales, John Kubasiak and Patrick M. McCarthy

Introduction

Transcatheter aortic valve implantation (TAVI) is a revolutionary therapy for patients with aortic valve disease, in particular aortic stenosis (AS). Treatment options for patients with AS have traditionally included aortic valve replacement (AVR), balloon aortic valvuloplasty (BAV), and medical therapy. A recent randomized trial has established TAVI as superior to medical management in patients considered not suitable for standard AVR (by both the cardiac surgeon and cardiologist);[1] and non-inferior to standard AVR in patients considered high-risk (Society of Thoracic Surgeons (STS) predicted risk of mortality greater than 10%).[2]

Future treatment groups may include intermediate-risk patients. However, an appropriate risk threshold remains to be determined, and will depend on the safety of the TAVI procedure, the durability of the stent-valve, and the need for concomitant procedures such as coronary artery bypass, other valve surgery, and atrial fibrillation surgery. The potential roles for transcatheter heart valves are several. A valve-in-valve procedure has impacts beyond a future treatment alternative for patients with failed prosthesis. The potential of a valve-in-valve option influences valve choice and valve size in patients requiring AVR today. Finally, by extending treatment options, TAVI has the potential of reducing the undertreatment of patients with AS.

Current Outcomes after Aortic Valve Replacement

The average age of the United States population is steadily increasing, with currently more than 11 million people with ages of 80 years or more, and an estimated 32 million by 2050.[3] The prevalence of senile, calcific AS in people over 65 years of age is 2-3% and will continue to increase.[4] Standard AVR with cardiopulmonary bypass was performed in 48,614 patients with AS in 2010 in the United States.[5] However, isolated AVR comprised only 44% of operations performed for AS. Of the remaining cases, 34% of patients also underwent concomitant CABG, 8% MV surgery, 2% TV repair, and 6% AF ablation.[5] The safety (operative mortality) and patient survival differs by procedure, however co-existing conditions such as obstructive coronary artery disease, or significant MR should not be left untreated. The benefit of the addition of tricuspid valve repair, and AF ablation to AVR is less clear, but nevertheless is important in the surgical decision-making process.

Isolated Aortic Valve Replacement

Data from the STS indicates that the operative mortality for patients 70 years of age or older who underwent isolated AVR or AVR with CABG between 1994 and 2003 has fallen from 10% to less than 6%[6] In the most recent analysis using the STS database on 108,687 patients from 1997 to 2006 with a mean age of 68 years undergoing isolated AVR, the in-hospital mortality was 2.6% with an observed stroke rate of 1.3% and length of stay of 7.8 days for the year 2006.[7] Among patients 80 to 85 years of age, 30-day mortality was less than 5% with an observed stroke rate less than 2.5%.[7]

Our experience at Northwestern shows that isolated AVR can be performed with <1% operative mortality.[8] Other similar single-center studies within the last 5 years have demonstrated significantly improved operative mortality after AVR even in higher-risk patients[9-12] (Table I). The incidence of peri-operative stroke ranged from 0 to 1.9% and the length of stay in these contemporary series was as low as 5 days.[8] Di Eusanio and colleagues[12] reported a 3-year survival comparable to the life-expectancy of an age- and gender-matched 2006 population (82% vs. 81%, p=.157). Overall, the reported patient survival at 1 and 3 years in these series were 94-97% and 88-94%, respectively.

In a recent prospective, randomized, multicenter Placement of Aortic Transcatheter Valves (PARTNER) trial[2] comparing high-risk patients (mean STS score 11.8%) receiving TAVI or AVR for AS, outcomes for both procedures in this trial were excellent. Patients undergoing either AVR (n= 351, mean age 85 years) or TAVI (n =348, mean age 84 years) revealed comparable mortalities at 30 days and 1 year (6.5% vs. 3.4%, p= 0.07; 26.8% vs. 24.2%, p =0.44, respectively), confirming that TAVI is non-inferior to AVR in a high-risk cohort. Early and late strokes and transient ischemic attacks were significantly lower in the AVR group than TAVI (30 days, 2.4% vs.5.5%, p =0.04; 1 year, 4.3% vs. 8.3%, p=0.04). Symptomatic improvement was observed in both cohorts at 1 year.

Table I. Summary of contemporary outcomes after isolated AVR for Aortic Stenosis

Authors 2007-2010	Study Period	n	Age, y (mean)	NYHA III/IV, %	Angina, %	STS score (mean)	Euro SCORE (mean)	30-day Mortality %	In-Hospital Mortality %	Peri-OP MI, %	Stroke, %	RF, %	Dialysis required, %	Post-op LOS, mean , d	Survival, % 1yr	Survival, % 3 yr	Survival, % 5 yr
Malaisrie et al., 2010	2004-2008	190	68	34	17	3.6		0	0.5	0	0	2.1	0.5	5 (3) median (IQR)	97	94	
Di Eusanio et al., 2010	2003-2007	2256	70	50			7.2		2.2	0.2	1.3	2.3	0.8		94	89	
Bakaeen et al., 2010	1991-2007	459	63	56				3.3		0.4	1.3		2				
Thourani et al., 2008	1996-2006	206	64	13	22				3.4	1.9	1.5	3.4	1.9	7.7± 9	94	89	84
Filsoufi et al., 2008	1998-2005	1077	61	34			13		4.4	0.4	2		1.9	7 (6-10) median (IQR)	96	88	
Brown et al, 2009 (STS Database)	2006	15,397	68	49	29				2.6		1.3			7.8			

YHA, New York Heart Association; OP, operative; MI, myocardial infarct; RF, renal failure; LOS, length of stay.

Minimally-invasive AVR (mini-AVR) as an alternative to AVR with full sternotomy has been shown to be safe and effective, while offering a cosmetically-appealing skin incision (Figure 1). In a meta-analysis of 26 studies comparing AVR through a partial sternotomy (n = 2054) and full sternotomy (n = 2532), no significant difference in operative mortality was found between groups [odds ratio 0.71, 95% confidence interval 0.49–1.02] despite a longer mean cross-clamp time [8-minute longer in partial sternotomy] and cardiopulmonary bypass time [12-minute longer in partial sternotomy].[13] Benefits of the mini-AVR included a shorter in-hospital stay (weighted mean difference [WMD] 0.9 days), less ventilator time (WMD 2.1 hours) and less blood loss within 24 hours (WMD 79 ml).

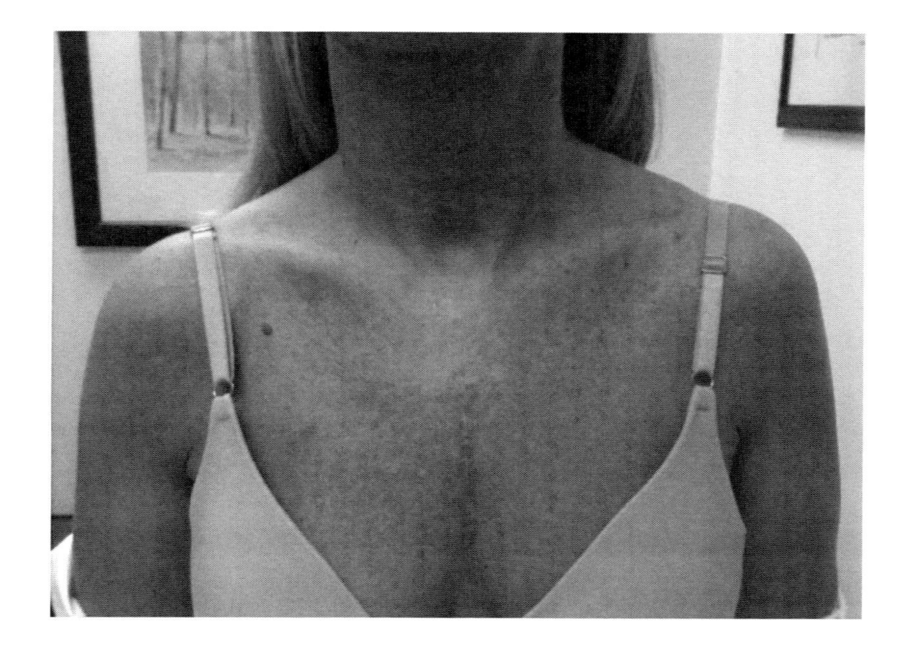

Figure 1. Minimally-invasive AVR.

Single-center retrospective studies published from 2004-2011 at experienced centers involving higher-risk patients (with advanced age and reoperations) have consistently shown that mini-AVR was associated with similar operative mortality (1.9-5.6% vs.3-11%)[14-17] and possibly better long-term survival (95% vs.89%, $p = 0.006$, median follow-up 39 months)[14] when compared with the full sternotomy.

In addition, shorter hospital stay (median 6-7 vs. 7-8 days, $p<0.01$)[14,15] and lower incidence of sternal complications (0% vs. 2.4%, $p< 0.08$)[15]were observed in patients undergoing mini-AVR.

Long-term follow-up of commonly-used bioprosthetic valves for the aortic position show good durability to over 15 years in several recent large series. Freedom from structural valve deterioration (SVD) for stented bovine pericardial valves has been reported to be 82.3% at 15 years for the Carpentier-Edwards Pericardial valve[18] and 62.3% at 20-years for the Sorin Mitroflow.[19] For stented porcine valves, the freedom form SVD has been reported to be 63.4% at 20 years for the Medtronic Hancock II valve[20] and the freedom from reoperation for SVD to be 61.1% for the Biocor valve.[21] Because age is the major determinant of durability, all of these series stratified their results by age and found that 20-year freedom from reoperation for SVD in patients 70 years and older to be between 84.8% (Mitroflow)[19] and 100% (Hancock II)[19]

In summary, the safety of AVR continues to improve with less than 1% operative mortality in specialized valve-centers. Low stroke rates, short length of stays and excellent patient survival is the standard against which TAVI should be compared. Despite increasing age and comorbidities in patients requiring isolated AVR, minimally-invasive AVR has been shown to have equivalent if not improved perioperative outcomes. Finally, AVR has been shown to maintain long-term patient survival using prosthetic valves of known durability.

AVR with Coronary Artery Bypass

Coronary bypass grafting (CABG) carries a class I recommendation for patients undergoing AVR with significant coronary arterial stenosis.[22] The STS database reported that unadjusted operative mortality in 2009 was 3% for the isolated AVR and 4.8% for AVR with CABG.[23] However, this difference reflected CAD as a strong risk factor for operative mortality as well as long-term survival rather than the actual risk of the CABG procedure itself.[24] Indeed, the addition of CABG to AVR has been shown to have no adverse effect on operative mortality in patients with AS and coexisting CAD.[25] The risks of omitting CABG, on the other hand, in patients with significant CAD include increased perioperative myocardial infarction,[26] postoperative systolic function,[27] and reduced long-term survival.[28] The strategy of "hybrid procedures" involving percutaneous coronary intervention for significant CAD followed by AVR has been untested. A single center series of 18 patients who underwent PCI followed by mini-AVR in high-risk elderly patients (mean age 75 years) with moderate CAD, demonstrated feasibility with 1 operative death (non-cardiac due to colonic perforation) with no late deaths at 19 months follow-up.[29] Such hybrid procedures have been used in selected, high-risk patients but have not been demonstrated to be equivalent to the widely-accepted strategy of AVR with CABG.

AVR with Mitral Valve Surgery

Patients with functional MR may improve after AVR alone and therefore not require concomitant MV surgery. In these patients, the degree of MR was found to decrease an average of 1.3 grades after AVR alone. [30-32] Other studies indicate that the persistence of significant MR (≥ 2+MR) after AVR alone was at 11-22% in up to 2 years of follow-up. [33,34] For patients with abnormal MV morphology, current 2008 ACC/AHA guidelines state that patients with severe AS and severe MR with symptoms, LV dysfunction, or pulmonary hypertension should undergo combined AVR and MV surgery.[22] The benefits of the addition of MV surgery to AVR include freedom from MV reoperation (91-100%,[35-37] 82-92%[35,38,39] and 75-80% [35] at 5, 10, and 15 years, respectively) and improvement in NYHA functional class.[36,38,40,41]

The STS database over the period of 1994-2003 analyzed 409,904 valve operations with and without CABG to determine operative mortality in single and multiple valve operations.[6] In this early study, the odds ratio (OR) for operative mortality for AVR/MVR compared to AVR alone was 2.02 (unadjusted mortality of 11.5% for AVR/MVR versus 5.7% for AVR alone)[6] In a more recent analysis of the STS database over the period of 2003-2007, the OR was found to be 2.31 (unadjusted mortality of 10.2% for AVR/MVR versus 4.4% for AVR alone).[42] The unadjusted operative mortalities in these studies reflect a broad group of patients including aortic regurgitation, infective endocarditis, and non-elective cases. In many single-center series including AS patients only, the operative mortality of combined AVR and MV surgery is reported to be 1-8% (Table 2).

AVR with Tricuspid Valve Repair

Results after AVR with tricuspid valve annuloplasty (TVA) have been under reported.[43-46] In a recent retrospective study, patients who underwent concomitant tricuspid repair (rigid ring annuloplasty) and left-sided valve procedures (AVR comprising 25% of the total 103 procedures), operative mortality was 1%.[45] At 15-month follow-up, significant TR was seen in 3% of patients.[45] Moreover, in patients undergoing left-sided valve procedures (AVR comprising 35% of the total 116 procedures) with known factors for recurrent TR such as preoperative pacemaker leads, the redevelopment of late TR was seen in less than 5% of patients by 19 months.[46] Mid-term outcomes of 789 patients undergoing left-sided valve surgery (AVR comprising 25%) and concomitant tricuspid repairs, overall significant TR was 31% after 8 years (17% for ring annuloplasty versus 33% for suture annuloplasty).[43] Similarly, long-term outcomes of concomitant ring annuloplasty (AVR comprising 33% of the total 209 procedures) showed redevelopment of late TR in 17% of patients at 15 years and an overall survival of 82% at 15 years.[44]

AVR with AF Ablation

Current ACC/AHA guidelines recommend the use of mechanical valves for AVR patients with preoperative AF with chronic anticoagulation.[22] Recent studies showed that surgical AF ablation can restore normal sinus rhythm (NSR) in AF patients[47-55] and may decrease the need for anticoagulation in this subgroup. AF ablation surgery has increased from 4,000 procedures in 2004 to 16,000 procedures in 2009 according to the most recent STS database report.23 Gammie and colleagues[56] using the STS database showed a 28% (2,965 of 10,590) prevalence of concomitant surgical AF ablation in patients undergoing AVR with or without CABG. However, nearly two thirds of AVR patients with preoperative AF are left untreated.[56]

Although older series with small patient numbers have shown an in-hospital mortality at 12%,[57] more recent series have demonstrated that the addition of AF ablation to AVR can be associated with zero in-hospital mortality.[58] These series have reported a freedom from AF of 68 - 85% with a follow-up of 6-12 months in AVR patients undergoing AF ablation (Table III).[47,49,50,59,60] Overall survival was reported to be 82% and 75% at 2 and 3 years, respectively.[48,57] Most importantly, our experience at Northwestern shows that up to 70% of patients after AVR with AF ablation were found to be free from warfarin, therefore making bioprosthetic valves an acceptable choice for an elderly group of patients (average age 74 years) while reducing the risks of long-term anticoagulation.[60]

Aortic Stenosis in High-Risk and Inoperable Patients

The important and often challenging preoperative determinants of outcomes in the high-risk AVR patient include both patient comorbidities and anatomic factors. Commonly cited comorbidities that contribute to surgical risk are advanced age, frailty, advanced heart failure, renal failure, and cirrhosis. Common anatomic considerations contributing to inoperability include porcelain aorta and reoperative surgery.

Advanced Age

Increased life expectancy has led to the growing elderly population frequently presenting with AS.[61] Age has been perceived as a major deterrent to AVR, despite well-published reports on the success of elderly patients undergoing isolated AVR (Table IV).[8-10,62,63] Because of excellent results with AVR in patients with advanced age, the 2008 AHA/ACC guidelines state that age itself is not a contraindication to AVR.[22] Operative mortality in previous single-center series have ranged from 2.4 to 11.6% in the octogenarian group. In the largest sample of patients involving 2945 octogenarians, the 2006 STS database reported a 4.7% mortality risk in patients 80-90 years of age after isolated AVR.7 Recent results from the PARTNER trial have established a benchmark for AVR in elderly patients.[2] In the group randomized to AVR, 351 patients had an average age of 84 years with an STS PROM of 12%. Observed 30-day mortality was 6.5% giving an impressive observed-to-expected (O:E) ratio of 0.54. Recovery is an equally important factor for patients with advanced age. Despite improvement in patient survival, patients with advanced age undergoing cardiac surgery are at greater risk for prolonged recovery, and poor functional outcome. Compared to patients less than 80 years, octogenarians are more likely to have a prolonged hospital stay after cardiac surgery, and approximately 50% of octogenarian are discharged to home directly from the hospital.[8,64] Functional outcome and quality of life in patients with advanced age after cardiac surgery has not been well-studied. Frailty scoring may emerge as a tool to predict poor functional outcome for octogenarians.[65] The identification of frail patients may allow better patient selection for less-invasive procedures.

Advanced Heart Failure

Patients with depressed EF but with ventricles capable of generating severe gradients across the aortic valve have afterload mismatch and have favorable outcomes after AVR. However, patients with low-gradient AS (LGAS) but with valve area consistent with severe AS have increased risk after AVR secondary to advanced heart failure. Aortic valve replacement for patients with LGAS was previously associated with poor operative outcomes with mortality as high as 21%.[66] Nevertheless, reduced operative mortality and increased long-term survival can be achieved as compared to dismal outcomes associated with medical therapy.

Table II. Summary of outcomes after AVR with Mitral Valve Surgery

Authors 1998-2010	Study Period	Age, y (mean)	n	MVr: MVR %	NYHA III/IV, %	MV etiology:	AF, %	AS	EF (mean), %	Preop MR, %	CABG, %	In-hospital Mortality, %	Freedom from MV reoperation, %
Kuwaki et al., 2007	1981-2003	51	128	37/63	14	IIIa				7		6	MVr: 84 (4 yr)
McGonigle et al., 2007	1977-1997	56 (median)	316	14/86	57	II (19-21%) IIIa (72-77%)		26		26	12	5.4	98 (6 yr)
Talwar et al., 2007	1995-2005	31	369	21/79	73	IIIa	41		56	44	0	8	93-100 (5 yr)
Ho Hq T. et al., 2004	1992-2001	36	609	33/67	17	IIIa	53	9	62	21	0	1	92-92 (9yr)
Hamamoto et al., 2003	1977-2000	54	379	21/79	47	II (5-25%) IIIa (54-61%)	70			22	0	4.5	92 (5 yr)
Gillinov et al., 2003	1975-1998	61 (mean)	813	36/64	39	II (20%) IIIa (71%)	38	27			29	6.4	98-99(1 yr) 91-97(5 yr) 88-89 (10 yr) 75-86(15 yr)
Turina et al., 1999	1975-1989	51	170	33/67	76	IIIa (41%)			55		4	4	
Mueller et al., 1998	1981-1996	56	200	19/81	86	II (41%) IIIa (55%)	62				9	5	

AVR, aortic valve replacement; MV, mitral valve ; MVr, MV repair; MVR, MV replacement; NYHA, New York Heart Association; AF, atrial fibrillation; AS, aortic stenosis; EF, ejection fraction; MR, mitral regurgitation; CABG, coronary artery bypass graft; DVR: MV replacement + AVR.

Table III. Summary of outcomes after AVR with AF Ablation

Authors 2003-2010	Study Period	Age, y (mean)	n	CABG,%	Predominant AF type, %	Predominant Ablation Procedure, %	Energy Source	In-Hospital Mortality, %	Rhythm F/U (mon)	Freedom from AF/Ablation, %	Survival %
Malaisrie, in press	2004-2009	74	80	49	Paroxysmal: 64	PVI :69	Bipolar RF Cryothermy	2.5	9	85	
Schopka et al., 2010	2007-2008	71	42	29	Long-standing persistent: 40	PVI :100	HIFU		12	68	
Deneke et al., 2009	2007-2008	68	13	100	Permanent: 100	LA Maze:61	Cryothermy		48	62	
Geidel et al., 2008	2003-2007	72	30	12	Permanent: 100	PVI :100	Bipolar RF	0			
Deneke et al., 2007	1997-2005	68	29	100	Permanent : 100	LA Maze: 72	Cryothermy		12	82	
Sie et al., 2004	1995-2001	68	20	40	Long-standing persistent: 100	Biatrial Maze: 100	Unipolar RF		40	85	75 (3 yr)
Knaut et al., 2004		68	53	0	Permanent: 100	PVI :55; LA Maze :45	Microwave		6	82	
Khargi et al., 2003	1997-2002		17	100	Permanent : 91	Biatrial :55 LA Maze: 44	Unipolar RF	12			82 (< 2 yr)

CABG, coronary artery bypass graft, LA, left atrium; AF, atrial fibrillation; AFL, atrial flutter; PVI, Pulmonary Vein Isolation; RF, Radiofrequency, F/U, follow-up; mon, months;

Table IV. Summary of outcomes after isolated AVR for Aortic Stenosis in patients ≥ 80 years

Authors 2007-2010	Study Period	n	Age ± SD,y (mean)	NYHA III/IV, %	Angina, %	STS score (mean)	Euro SCORE (mean)	Op Mortality, %	In-Hospital Mortality, %	Peri-OP MI, %	Stroke, %	RF, %	Dialysis required, %	Post-op LOS, d (mean)	Survival, % 1 yr	Survival, % 3 yr	Survival, % 5 yr
Smith et .al, 2011	2007-2009	351	84±6	94.0		12.0	29.0		6.5	0.6	2.4	1.2	3.0		73.0		
Malaisrie et. al, 2010	2004-2008	41	83±3	44.0	15.0	6.0		0.0	2.4	0	0	7.3	2.4	7 (2) median (IQR)			
Soltesz et al, 2007	2007	157	84 ≥ 80 (n= 34)					1.9 0 (≥ 80)									
Di Eusanio et al., 2010	2003-2007	430	≥ 80	58			13		3.7		2	3.7	2.6	16±8	91	82	
Bakaeen et. al, 2010	1991-2007	459	82±2	54				5.2		1.3	2.6		2.6				
Thourani et al. , 2008	1996-2006	88	83±2	21	31	6			5.7	0	3.4	4.6	1.1	10±11	87	68	61
Filsoufi et.al., 2008	1998-2005	231	83±3	49			23		6		<2.4						
Ferrari et al, 2010	1990-2005	124	82±2	48	10		13		6		0.7	11	2	15±6			88
STS, 2009	2006	2945	80-90						>5						89 (LR)		63 (LR)
Florath et al, 2010	1996-2006	156	83±2	57		7(LR)	18(LR)		5.1 (LR)						69 (HR)		35 (HR)
Florath et.al, 2010	1996-2006	95	83±2			9(HR)	24 (HR)		11.6(HR)					14±6	94	94	75
Huber et. al, 2007	1999-2003	34	82±1.8	62					3								

SD, Standard deviation, STS, Society of Thoracic Surgeons, OP, operative; NYHA, New York Heart Association; MI, myocardial infarct; RF, renal failure; LOS, length of stay; LR, Low-risk group; HR, High-Risk group.

In an effort to identify which patients with LGAS would benefit from AVR, a multicenter European study stratified patients with and without contractile reserve of the left ventricle as measured by dobutamine stress echocardiography.[67]

In patients with contractile reserve (defined as left ventricular stroke volume augmented with dobutamine infusion), operative mortality was as low as 5%. In contrast, patients without contractile reserve whose stroke volume were unable to be augmented with dobutamine infusion had a poor operative mortality of up to 31%. Despite this poor operative mortality, these patients with no contractile reserve that survived surgery demonstrated recovery of LV function similar to patients with contractile reserve.[68]

The AHA/ACC guidelines have no particular recommendation for AVR in patients with advanced heart failure. However, the European guidelines state that patients with LGAS with contractile reserve have a class IIa indication for AVR and patients with LGAS without contractile reserve have a class IIb indication.[69] Therefore, stratification of patients with DSE can help to differentiate patients who would benefit most from AVR versus those with advanced heart failure who are at high-risk for AVR.

Endstage Renal Failure

In a 30-year literature review on 615 patients with end-stage renal failure undergoing cardiac surgery with cardiopulmonary bypass, operative mortality was 19.3% in patients undergoing valve replacement and 39.5% in patients undergoing valve replacement and CABG.[70] In a more recent series of 1512 patients, in-hospital mortality for dialysis patients after AVR with or without CABG was 14.3%; 1-, 3-, 5-, and 10-year survival for the same cohort of patients was 59, 43, 29, and 12% respectively.[71] Moreover, non-dialysis dependent renal dysfunction has been shown to be a predictor of operative mortality (Figure 2). Using glomerular filtration rate (GFR) estimated using the Modification of Diet Renal Disease equation, preoperative GFR < 60 mL/min/1.73m^2 has been shown to be predictive of both mortality[72] and morbidity.[73] Considering the poor outcomes in these patients after valve replacement, the previous class IIa recommendation for the use of mechanical valves in dialysis patients has been removed from the current AHA/ACC guidelines.[22]

Cirrhosis

Liver cirrhosis is associated with increased risk after cardiac surgery with cardiopulmonary bypass. Commonly used models for preoperative risk assessment (STS PROM, log Euroscore, Ambler score) do not account for liver cirrhosis. The Child-Pugh classification for liver cirrhosis stratifies patients with liver cirrhosis and has been found to be predictive of outcomes after cardiac surgery. In a summary of 9 clinical studies involving 210 patients, Modi and colleagues reported an operative mortality for Child-Pugh A, B, and C of 5%, 32%, and 66%, respectively.[74] Similarly, patient survival has been reported to be poor with 1-year survival for Child-Pugh A, B, and C of 80%, 45%, and 16%.[75] Recent studies have excluded patient with Child-Pugh C due to prohibitive mortality.[76,77] The data support the safety of cardiac surgery in patients with Child-Pugh A; however, surgery should probably not be offered to patients with Child-Pugh B.[74] Additional factors including

MELD score,[75] platelet count,[76] and serum cholinesterase[77] may be useful in predicting risks for patient with Child-Pugh A.

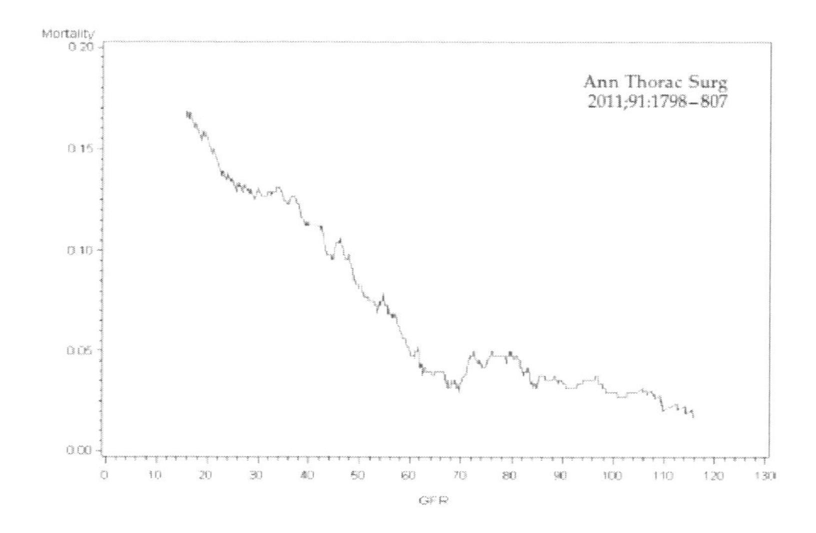

Figure 2. In-hospital mortality by preop GFR. Thourani, V. H., W. B. Keeling, et al. (2011). "Impact of preoperative renal dysfunction on long-term survival for patients undergoing aortic valve replacement." Ann Thorac Surg 91(6): 1798-1806; discussion 1806-1797.

Porcelain Aorta

Porcelain aorta is defined as extensive calcification and atherosclerotic plaque formation of the ascending aorta (Figure 3). Manipulation of an atherosclerotic aorta particularly during cannulation and cross-clamping can result in atheroemboli, greatly increasing the risk of stroke. Moreover, a heavily calcified aorta may increase the difficulty of aortotomy closure. Multiple strategies to manage the atherosclerotic aorta have been reported, all of which involve hypothermic circulatory arrest (Table V).

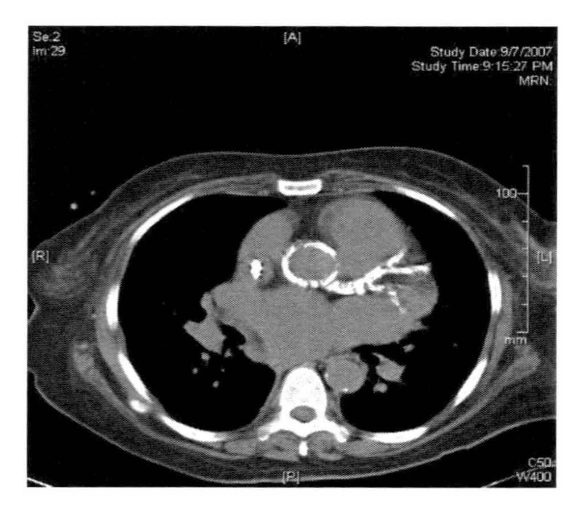

Figure 3. Porcelain Aorta.

Whether concomitant aortic endarterectomy or aortic replacement is superior to performing AVR under hypothermic circulatory arrest (leaving the aorta untouched) cannot be concluded.[78] However, AVR under circulatory arrest is associated with a prolonged period of cerebral ischemia compared to AVR with aortic replacement.[79] Overall, operative mortality ranges from 4% to 14% and stroke rates from 10-11%.[78-80]

Table V. Results of AVR with HCA for the atherosclerotic aorta

	Method (n)	Stroke, %	Mortality,%
Gillinov et al., 2000	Inspect and cross clamp (n=6)	0	0
	AVR, HCA (n=24)	17	12
	AVR, aortic endarterectomy, HCA (n=16)	12	19
	AVR, aortic replacement, HCA (n=12)	0	25
Aranki et al., 2005	AVR, HCA (n=13)	15	0
	AVR, aortic endarterectomy, HCA (n=13)	7.6	0
	AVR, aortic replacement, HCA (n=44)	11.3	6.8

AVR, aortic valve replacement; HCA, hypothermic circulatory arrest.

Reoperative Surgery

Reoperative cardiac surgery can be complicated by injury to bypass grafts, the heart, and great vessels.[81] Aortic valve replacement after previous cardiac surgery, in particular after previous CABG, was previously associated with operative mortality as high as 14%.[82]

Current series, however, show that operative mortality can be as low as 5% even in patients with patent bypass grafts.[83]

The presence of a patent IMA graft is associated with improved survival after reoperation; however, injury to the IMA graft during reoperation is associated with increased operative mortality.[84] When injury to the IMA does occur, operative mortality is associated with an operative mortality as high as 50%.[85] This has led to some surgeons to consider the presence of an IMA graft crossing midline and directly adherent to the posterior table of the sternum to be an indicator of inoperability.

Routine preoperative high-resolution CT may be particularly helpful in identifying patients with cardiovascular structures at risk for injury.[86] Exposure of peripheral vessels for cardiopulmonary bypass and institution of cardiopulmonary bypass prior to reentry are useful strategies when injury is imminent.[87] With improved operative techniques, operative mortality associated with injury to the IMA graft has more recently been reported to be 12% to 17.9% in two large series.[81,86]

Myocardial protection is another challenge in reoperative cardiac surgery. Identification and clamping of the patent LIMA graft during aortic cross-clamping must be weighed against the risk of injury to the LIMA during dissection. The strategy of leaving the LIMA unclamped has been shown to have an acceptable operative mortality compared to clamping the LIMA during cardioplegic arrest.[88,89] Components of successful myocardial protection in this strategy include systemic hypothermia and reliance on retrograde cardioplegia.[90]

Future Applications of TAVI

Lower Risk Patients with AS

Current US trials have randomized patients with an STS PROM of 10% or greater to TAVI versus AVR. Whether lower-risk patients would be acceptable candidates for TAVI is unknown. The lowest reported 30-day mortality after TAVI is 3.4%,[2] so it is reasonable that a lower-risk group of patients could be treated with TAVI.

In lower risk patients, however, valve durability becomes an important factor. The current ACC/AHA guidelines recommend mechanical valves for AVR in patients younger than 65 years if there is no contraindication for warfarin therapy.[22] This Class IIa is supported by long-term clinical outcomes performed 30 years ago. There are only two randomized studies (the Edinburgh Heart Valve Trials[91,92] and the Veterans Affairs Cooperative Studies on Valvular Heart Disease[93,94]) comparing patients receiving mechanical and bioprosthetic valves in the aortic position. These studies analyzed survival rates of patients enrolled in the late 1970s, receiving prostheses that are no longer implanted today (Bjork-Shiley single tilting-disk valve and first-generation porcine valve). In the VA trial,[94] 15-year survival was greater with mechanical valves (79% vs. 66%, $p<0.02$) compared to bioprosthetic valves. However, in the Edinburgh trial, the 12-year survival advantage favoring mechanical valves (51.5% versus 44.4%) was not statistically significant ($p=0.08$).[91] In addition, near-identical survival rate were observed in the same trial at 20-year follow-up (25.0% versus 22.6%, $p=0.39$).[92]

A meta-analysis published in 2006 reviewed 32 studies conducted between 1989 and 2004,[95] comparing 8,578 patients in the mechanical valve series (mean age 58) and 8,861 patients in the bioprosthetic valve series (mean age 69). Although unadjusted mortality favored mechanical valves (3.99% versus 6.33%/patient-year, $p<0.001$), no significant difference in mortality was observed after adjusting for age, NYHA class III/IV, aortic regurgitation, and concomitant CABG. The durability of transcatheter valves, however, is unknown; whether TAVI is good long-term option for patients who would otherwise receive a mechanical valve with proven durability or even third-generation bioprosthetic remains to be determined.

Valve-in-Valve Implantation for Failed Bioprosthetic Valves

The valve-in-valve procedure can be performed either on an emergency basis during initial TAVI to rescue a malfunctioning transcatheter valve, or on an elective basis for failed bioprosthetic valves. Increasing experience with elective valve-in-valve procedure using both the Edwards Sapien valve and Medtronic CoreValve has shown feasibility in high-risk patients.[96-99] These limited series show that both feasibility in both transapical and transfemoral approaches, applicability to variety of bioprosthetic valves both stented and stentless (although easier in stented valves with radiopaque metal frames), and no incidents of postoperative heart block. With current transcatheter heart valves, the smallest treatable bioprosthetic valve size is 21mm. The transapical approach offers the additional advantage of treating concomitant aortic and mitral pathologies (Figure 4).[98] Importance of exclusion criteria for valve-in-valve include acute or subacute endocarditis and presence of a paravalvular leak associated with the failed bioprosthetic.[97] Because calcification is the primary mode of failure in both bovine pericardial and porcine valves, some authors have advocated omitting the use of balloon aortic valvuloplasty prior to implantation of the transcatheter valve.[97]

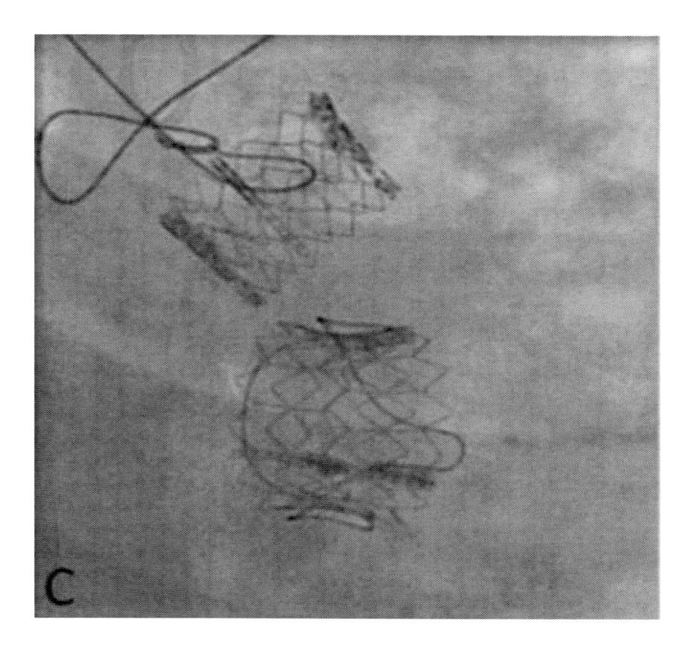

Figure 4. Transapical TAVI for stenotic native AV and failed mitral bioprosthesis. Webb, J. G., D. A. Wood, et al. (2010). "Transcatheter valve-in-valve implantation for failed bioprosthetic heart valves." Circulation 121(16): 1848-1857.

Valve Choice in AVR Patients

In recent years, the development of third-generation bioprosthetic valves with improved hemodynamic performance and purported increased durability has led to its increased use in AVR patients. From 1997 to 2006, the use of bioprosthetic valves increased to 78% of total valves with a corresponding decline in mechanical valve use to 20.5%.[7] In 2006, the life expectancy for people in the United States at age 65 was 18.5 years (17 years for men and 20 years for women).[100] Therefore, reoperative surgery for failed bioprosthetic valves will likely be commonplace. Fortunately, reoperative AVR carries a low operative mortality not significantly worse than primary AVR (reported to be as low as 3% in patients requiring elective reoperative AVR).[101] The option of TAVI for failed bioprosthetic valves ("valve in valve") has three potential impacts. The first impact is that patients with failed bioprosthetic valves may have TAVI as an alternative to repeat AVR as mentioned above.

The second is to reduce the age threshold where bioprosthetic valves are chosen (from the recommended 65 years). Finally, the third impact is the choice of valve size in patients undergoing AVR. Current transcatheter heart valves are limited to 2 sizes but with larger valves planned. However, small stented valves such as 19mm and possibly 21mm may be too small for valve-in-valve.[98]

Undertreatment of Aortic Stenosis

The natural history of aortic stenosis (AS) has been well characterized and largely unchanged since the condition was described by Frank and Braunwald in 1968.[102] The risk of sudden cardiac death has been shown to be ~1% / year in asymptomatic patients,[103] but with the onset of symptoms average survival is 2-3 years.[104] Despite being an AHA/ACC Class I recommendation for surgery, approximately one third of patients with symptomatic, severe AS do not receive AVR.[105,106]

Commonly cited patient-related reasons include advanced age, comorbidities, symptoms not from AS, and refusal of surgery.[105-109] Physician-related reasons include overestimation of operative risks, type of practice setting (academic, private practice, or VA), and under-referral to cardiac surgery.[105] Finally, the underutilization of stress tests to evaluate equivocal symptoms has been reported with rates below 10%[106,107] In our experience at Northwestern, we have shown that introduction of TAVI was associated with a decrease in the undertreatment of AS.[110] Increased evaluation by the cardiac surgeon as a part of a multidisciplinary heart team was a major factor in decreasing the rate of unoperated AS. These heart teams are mandatory in the preoperative evaluation, joint procedural performance, and postoperative management of these potentially complex patients.[111]

Conclusion

Transcatheter heart valve therapy represents a transformational technology in the treatment of patients with AS. Already a proven therapy for inoperable patients, next generation devices may allow TAVI to be a viable therapeutic option for lower-risk patients with isolated AS in addition to those high-risk patients with an estimated operative risk greater than 10%. Therapeutic options for patients with concomitant cardiac disease remain to be determined. The future impact of TAVI includes potential valve-in-valve option for failed bioprosthetic valves, increased enthusiasm for bioprosthetic valves during primary AVR, and a reduction in the undertreatment of AS

References

[1] Leon MB, Smith CR, Mack M, et al. Transcatheter aortic-valve implantation for aortic stenosis in patients who cannot undergo surgery. *The New England journal of medicine.* Oct 21 2010;363(17):1597-1607.

[2] Smith CR, Leon MB, Mack MJ, et al. Transcatheter versus surgical aortic-valve replacement in high-risk patients. *N Engl J Med.* Jun 9 2011;364(23):2187-2198.

[3] Population Division, U.S. Census Bureau 2008. Table 12. Projections of the Population by Age and Sex for the United States: 2010 to 2050 (NP2008-T12). *http://www.census.gov/population/www/projections/summarytables.html.*

[4] Nkomo VT, Gardin JM, Skelton TN, Gottdiener JS, Scott CG, Enriquez-Sarano M. Burden of valvular heart diseases: a population-based study. *Lancet.* Sep 16 2006;368(9540):1005-1011.

[5] Year 2010, The Adult Cardiac Surgery Database, *The Society of Thoracic Surgery,* Chicago, IL.

[6] Rankin JS, Hammill BG, Ferguson TB, Jr., et al. Determinants of operative mortality in valvular heart surgery. *J Thorac Cardiovasc Surg.* Mar 2006;131(3):547-557.

[7] Brown JM, O'Brien SM, Wu C, Sikora JA, Griffith BP, Gammie JS. Isolated aortic valve replacement in North America comprising 108,687 patients in 10 years: changes in risks, valve types, and outcomes in the Society of Thoracic Surgeons National Database. *J Thorac Cardiovasc Surg.* Jan 2009;137(1):82-90.

[8] Malaisrie SC, McCarthy PM, McGee EC, et al. Contemporary perioperative results of isolated aortic valve replacement for aortic stenosis. *The Annals of thoracic surgery.* Mar 2010;89(3):751-756.

[9] Filsoufi F, Rahmanian PB, Castillo JG, Chikwe J, Silvay G, Adams DH. Excellent early and late outcomes of aortic valve replacement in people aged 80 and older. *J Am Geriatr Soc.* Feb 2008;56(2):255-261.

[10] Thourani VH, Myung R, Kilgo P, et al. Long-term outcomes after isolated aortic valve replacement in octogenarians: a modern perspective. *The Annals of thoracic surgery.* Nov 2008;86(5):1458-1464; discussion 1464-1455.

[11] Bakaeen FG, Chu D, Huh J, Carabello BA. Is an age of 80 years or greater an important predictor of short-term outcomes of isolated aortic valve replacement in veterans? *The Annals of thoracic surgery.* Sep 2010;90(3):769-774.

[12] Di Eusanio M, Fortuna D, De Palma R, et al. Aortic valve replacement: Results and predictors of mortality from a contemporary series of 2256 patients. *J Thorac Cardiovasc Surg.* Jul 2 2010.

[13] Brown ML, McKellar SH, Sundt TM, Schaff HV. Ministernotomy versus conventional sternotomy for aortic valve replacement: a systematic review and meta-analysis. *J Thorac Cardiovasc Surg.* Mar 2009;137(3):670-679 e675.

[14] Mihaljevic T, Cohn LH, Unic D, Aranki SF, Couper GS, Byrne JG. One thousand minimally invasive valve operations: early and late results. *Ann Surg.* Sep 2004;240(3):529-534; discussion 534.

[15] Sharony R, Grossi EA, Saunders PC, et al. Minimally invasive aortic valve surgery in the elderly: a case-control study. *Circulation.* Sep 9 2003;108 Suppl 1:II43-47.

[16] Soltesz EG, Cohn LH. Minimally invasive valve surgery. *Cardiol Rev.* May-Jun 2007;15(3):109-115.

[17] ElBardissi AW, Shekar P, Couper GS, Cohn LH. Minimally invasive aortic valve replacement in octogenarian, high-risk, transcatheter aortic valve implantation candidates. *J Thorac Cardiovasc Surg.* Feb;141(2):328-335.

[18] McClure RS, Narayanasamy N, Wiegerinck E, et al. Late outcomes for aortic valve replacement with the Carpentier-Edwards pericardial bioprosthesis: up to 17-year

follow-up in 1,000 patients. *The Annals of thoracic surgery.* May 2010;89(5):1410-1416.

[19] Yankah CA, Pasic M, Musci M, et al. Aortic valve replacement with the Mitroflow pericardial bioprosthesis: durability results up to 21 years. *The Journal of thoracic and cardiovascular surgery.* Sep 2008;136(3):688-696.

[20] David TE, Armstrong S, Maganti M. Hancock II bioprosthesis for aortic valve replacement: the gold standard of bioprosthetic valves durability? *The Annals of thoracic surgery.* Sep 2010;90(3):775-781.

[21] Myken PS, Bech-Hansen O. A 20-year experience of 1712 patients with the Biocor porcine bioprosthesis. *The Journal of thoracic and cardiovascular surgery.* Jan 2009;137(1):76-81.

[22] Bonow RO, Carabello BA, Chatterjee K, et al. 2008 Focused update incorporated into the ACC/AHA 2006 guidelines for the management of patients with valvular heart disease: a report of the American College of Cardiology/American Heart Association Task Force on Practice Guidelines (Writing Committee to Revise the 1998 Guidelines for the Management of Patients With Valvular Heart Disease): endorsed by the Society of Cardiovascular Anesthesiologists, Society for Cardiovascular Angiography and Interventions, and Society of Thoracic Surgeons. *Circulation.* Oct 7 2008;118(15):e523-661.

[23] The Society of Thoracic Surgeons Adult Cardiac Surgery Database Spring 2010 Report. Available at *http://www.sts.org/documents/pdf/ndb2010/1stHarvestExecutiveSummary%5B1%5D.pdf.* Accessed August 14, 2010.

[24] Mullany CJ, Elveback LR, Frye RL, et al. Coronary artery disease and its management: influence on survival in patients undergoing aortic valve replacement. *J Am Coll Cardiol.* Jul 1987;10(1):66-72.

[25] Lund O, Nielsen TT, Pilegaard HK, Magnussen K, Knudsen MA. The influence of coronary artery disease and bypass grafting on early and late survival after valve replacement for aortic stenosis. *J Thorac Cardiovasc Surg.* Sep 1990;100(3):327-337.

[26] Iung B, Drissi MF, Michel PL, et al. Prognosis of valve replacement for aortic stenosis with or without coexisting coronary heart disease: a comparative study. *J Heart Valve Dis.* Jul 1993;2(4):430-439.

[27] Hwang MH, Hammermeister KE, Oprian C, et al. Preoperative identification of patients likely to have left ventricular dysfunction after aortic valve replacement. Participants in the Veterans Administration Cooperative Study on Valvular Heart Disease. *Circulation.* Sep 1989;80(3 Pt 1):I65-76.

[28] Czer LS, Gray RJ, Stewart ME, De Robertis M, Chaux A, Matloff JM. Reduction in sudden late death by concomitant revascularization with aortic valve replacement. *J Thorac Cardiovasc Surg.* Mar 1988;95(3):390-401.

[29] Brinster DR, Byrne M, Rogers CD, et al. Effectiveness of same day percutaneous coronary intervention followed by minimally invasive aortic valve replacement for aortic stenosis and moderate coronary disease ("hybrid approach"). *Am J Cardiol.* Dec 1 2006;98(11):1501-1503.

[30] Harris KM, Malenka DJ, Haney MF, et al. Improvement in mitral regurgitation after aortic valve replacement. *Am J Cardiol.* Sep 15 1997;80(6):741-745.

[31] Vanden Eynden F, Bouchard D, El-Hamamsy I, et al. Effect of aortic valve replacement for aortic stenosis on severity of mitral regurgitation. *The Annals of thoracic surgery.* Apr 2007;83(4):1279-1284.

[32] Wan CK, Suri RM, Li Z, et al. Management of moderate functional mitral regurgitation at the time of aortic valve replacement: is concomitant mitral valve repair necessary? *J Thorac Cardiovasc Surg.* Mar 2009;137(3):635-640 e631.

[33] Ruel M, Kapila V, Price J, Kulik A, Burwash IG, Mesana TG. Natural history and predictors of outcome in patients with concomitant functional mitral regurgitation at the time of aortic valve replacement. *Circulation.* Jul 4 2006;114(1 Suppl):I541-546.

[34] Waisbren EC, Stevens LM, Avery EG, Picard MH, Vlahakes GJ, Agnihotri AK. Changes in mitral regurgitation after replacement of the stenotic aortic valve. *The Annals of thoracic surgery.* Jul 2008;86(1):56-62.

[35] Gillinov AM, Blackstone EH, Cosgrove DM, 3rd, et al. Mitral valve repair with aortic valve replacement is superior to double valve replacement. *J Thorac Cardiovasc Surg.* Jun 2003;125(6):1372-1387.

[36] Talwar S, Mathur A, Choudhary SK, Singh R, Kumar AS. Aortic valve replacement with mitral valve repair compared with combined aortic and mitral valve replacement. *The Annals of thoracic surgery.* Oct 2007;84(4):1219-1225.

[37] Hamamoto M, Bando K, Kobayashi J, et al. Durability and outcome of aortic valve replacement with mitral valve repair versus double valve replacement. *The Annals of thoracic surgery.* Jan 2003;75(1):28-33; discussion 33-24.

[38] Ho HQ, Nguyen VP, Phan KP, Pham NV. Mitral valve repair with aortic valve replacement in rheumatic heart disease. *Asian Cardiovasc Thorac Ann.* Dec 2004;12(4):341-345.

[39] McGonigle NC, Jones JM, Sidhu P, Macgowan SW. Concomitant mitral valve surgery with aortic valve replacement: a 21-year experience with a single mechanical prosthesis. *J Cardiothorac Surg.* 2007;2:24.

[40] Mueller XM, Tevaearai HT, Stumpe F, et al. Long-term results of mitral-aortic valve operations. *J Thorac Cardiovasc Surg.* Jun 1998;115(6):1298-1309.

[41] Turina J, Stark T, Seifert B, Turina M. Predictors of the long-term outcome after combined aortic and mitral valve surgery. *Circulation.* Nov 9 1999;100(19 Suppl):II48-53.

[42] Lee R, Li S, Rankin JS, et al. Fifteen-year outcome trends for valve surgery in North America. *The Annals of thoracic surgery.* Mar 2011;91(3):677-684; discussion p 684.

[43] McCarthy PM, Bhudia SK, Rajeswaran J, et al. Tricuspid valve repair: durability and risk factors for failure. *J Thorac Cardiovasc Surg.* Mar 2004;127(3):674-685.

[44] Tang GH, David TE, Singh SK, Maganti MD, Armstrong S, Borger MA. Tricuspid valve repair with an annuloplasty ring results in improved long-term outcomes. *Circulation.* Jul 4 2006;114(1 Suppl):I577-581.

[45] Jeong DS, Kim KH. Tricuspid annuloplasty using the MC3 ring for functional tricuspid regurgitation. *Circ J.* 2010;74(2):278-283.

[46] Pfannmueller B, Hirnle G, Seeburger J, et al. Tricuspid valve repair in the presence of a permanent ventricular pacemaker lead. *Eur J Cardiothorac Surg.* May;39(5):657-661.

[47] Knaut M, Tugtekin SM, Jung F, Matschke K. Microwave ablation for the surgical treatment of permanent atrial fibrillation--a single centre experience. *Eur J Cardiothorac Surg.* Oct 2004;26(4):742-746.

[48] Sie HT, Beukema WP, Elvan A, Ramdat Misier AR. Long-term results of irrigated radiofrequency modified maze procedure in 200 patients with concomitant cardiac surgery: six years experience. *The Annals of thoracic surgery*. Feb 2004;77(2):512-516; discussion 516-517.

[49] Deneke T, Khargi K, Voss D, et al. Long-term sinus rhythm stability after intraoperative ablation of permanent atrial fibrillation. *Pacing Clin Electrophysiol*. May 2009;32(5):653-659.

[50] Schopka S, Schmid C, Keyser A, et al. Ablation of atrial fibrillation with the Epicor system: a prospective observational trial to evaluate safety and efficacy and predictors of success. *J Cardiothorac Surg*. 2010;5:34.

[51] Beyer E, Lee R, Lam BK. Point: Minimally invasive bipolar radiofrequency ablation of lone atrial fibrillation: early multicenter results. *J Thorac Cardiovasc Surg*. Mar 2009;137(3):521-526.

[52] Edgerton JR, McClelland JH, Duke D, et al. Minimally invasive surgical ablation of atrial fibrillation: six-month results. *J Thorac Cardiovasc Surg*. Jul 2009;138(1):109-113; discussion 114.

[53] Rodriguez E, Cook RC, Chu MWA, and Chitwood, WR. Minimally Invasive Bi-atrial CryoMaze operation for Atrial Fibrillation. *Operative Technique in Thoracic and Cardiovascular Surgery*. 2009;14(3):208-223.

[54] Edgerton JR, Brinkman WT, Weaver T, et al. Pulmonary vein isolation and autonomic denervation for the management of paroxysmal atrial fibrillation by a minimally invasive surgical approach. *J Thorac Cardiovasc Surg*. Mar 16.

[55] McCarthy PM, Kruse J, Shalli S, et al. Where does atrial fibrillation surgery fail? Implications for increasing effectiveness of ablation. *J Thorac Cardiovasc Surg*. Apr 2010;139(4):860-867.

[56] Gammie JS, Haddad M, Milford-Beland S, et al. Atrial fibrillation correction surgery: lessons from the Society of Thoracic Surgeons National Cardiac Database. *The Annals of thoracic surgery*. Mar 2008;85(3):909-914.

[57] Khargi K, Deneke T, Lemke B, Laczkovics A. Irrigated radiofrequency ablation is a safe and effective technique to treat chronic atrial fibrillation. *Interact Cardiovasc Thorac Surg*. Sep 2003;2(3):241-245.

[58] Geidel S, Lass M, Ostermeyer J. A 5-year clinical experience with bipolar radiofrequency ablation for permanent atrial fibrillation concomitant to coronary artery bypass grafting and aortic valve surgery. *Interact Cardiovasc Thorac Surg*. Oct 2008;7(5):777-780.

[59] Deneke T, Khargi K, Lemke B, et al. Intra-operative cooled-tip radiofrequency linear atrial ablation to treat permanent atrial fibrillation. *Eur Heart J*. Dec 2007;28(23):2909-2914.

[60] Malaisrie SC, Lee R, Kruse J, et al. Atrial Fibrillation Ablation in Patients Undergoing Aortic Valve Replacement. *J Heart Valve Dis*. In Press.

[61] Cohn LH, Narayanasamy N. Aortic valve replacement in elderly patients: what are the limits? *Curr Opin Cardiol*. Mar 2007;22(2):92-95.

[62] Di Eusanio M, Fortuna D, De Palma R, et al. Aortic valve replacement: Results and predictors of mortality from a contemporary series of 2256 patients. *The Journal of thoracic and cardiovascular surgery*. Jul 2.

[63] Huber CH, Goeber V, Berdat P, Carrel T, Eckstein F. Benefits of cardiac surgery in octogenarians--a postoperative quality of life assessment. *Eur J Cardiothorac Surg.* Jun 2007;31(6):1099-1105.

[64] Bardakci H, Cheema FH, Topkara VK, et al. Discharge to home rates are significantly lower for octogenarians undergoing coronary artery bypass graft surgery. *The Annals of thoracic surgery.* Feb 2007;83(2):483-489.

[65] Freiheit EA, Hogan DB, Eliasziw M, et al. Development of a frailty index for patients with coronary artery disease. *J Am Geriatr Soc.* Aug 2010;58(8):1526-1531.

[66] Carabello BA, Green LH, Grossman W, Cohn LH, Koster JK, Collins JJ, Jr. Hemodynamic determinants of prognosis of aortic valve replacement in critical aortic stenosis and advanced congestive heart failure. *Circulation.* Jul 1980;62(1):42-48.

[67] Monin JL, Quere JP, Monchi M, et al. Low-gradient aortic stenosis: operative risk stratification and predictors for long-term outcome: a multicenter study using dobutamine stress hemodynamics. *Circulation.* Jul 22 2003;108(3):319-324.

[68] Quere JP, Monin JL, Levy F, et al. Influence of preoperative left ventricular contractile reserve on postoperative ejection fraction in low-gradient aortic stenosis. *Circulation.* Apr 11 2006;113(14):1738-1744.

[69] Vahanian A, Baumgartner H, Bax J, et al. Guidelines on the management of valvular heart disease: The Task Force on the Management of Valvular Heart Disease of the European Society of Cardiology. *Eur Heart J.* Jan 2007;28(2):230-268.

[70] Horst M, Mehlhorn U, Hoerstrup SP, Suedkamp M, de Vivie ER. Cardiac surgery in patients with end-stage renal disease: 10-year experience. *The Annals of thoracic surgery.* Jan 2000;69(1):96-101.

[71] Thourani VH, Keeling WB, Sarin EL, et al. Impact of preoperative renal dysfunction on long-term survival for patients undergoing aortic valve replacement. *The Annals of thoracic surgery.* Jun 2011;91(6):1798-1806; discussion 1806-1797.

[72] Gibson PH, Croal BL, Cuthbertson BH, et al. The relationship between renal function and outcome from heart valve surgery. *Am Heart J.* Nov 2008;156(5):893-899.

[73] Ibanez J, Riera M, Saez de Ibarra JI, et al. Effect of preoperative mild renal dysfunction on mortality and morbidity following valve cardiac surgery. *Interact Cardiovasc Thorac Surg.* Dec 2007;6(6):748-752.

[74] Modi A, Vohra HA, Barlow CW. Do patients with liver cirrhosis undergoing cardiac surgery have acceptable outcomes? *Interact Cardiovasc Thorac Surg.* Nov;11(5):630-634.

[75] Filsoufi F, Salzberg SP, Rahmanian PB, et al. Early and late outcome of cardiac surgery in patients with liver cirrhosis. *Liver Transpl.* Jul 2007;13(7):990-995.

[76] Morisaki A, Hosono M, Sasaki Y, et al. Risk factor analysis in patients with liver cirrhosis undergoing cardiovascular operations. *The Annals of thoracic surgery.* Mar 2010;89(3):811-817.

[77] Murashita T, Komiya T, Tamura N, et al. Preoperative evaluation of patients with liver cirrhosis undergoing open heart surgery. *Gen Thorac Cardiovasc Surg.* Jun 2009;57(6):293-297.

[78] Aranki SF, Nathan M, Shekar P, Couper G, Rizzo R, Cohn LH. Hypothermic circulatory arrest enables aortic valve replacement in patients with unclampable aorta. *The Annals of thoracic surgery.* Nov 2005;80(5):1679-1686; discussion 1686-1677.

[79] Gillinov AM, Lytle BW, Hoang V, et al. The atherosclerotic aorta at aortic valve replacement: surgical strategies and results. *J Thorac Cardiovasc Surg.* Nov 2000;120(5):957-963.

[80] Vogt PR, Hauser M, Schwarz U, et al. Complete thromboendarterectomy of the calcified ascending aorta and aortic arch. *The Annals of thoracic surgery.* Feb 1999;67(2):457-461.

[81] Roselli EE, Pettersson GB, Blackstone EH, et al. Adverse events during reoperative cardiac surgery: frequency, characterization, and rescue. *J Thorac Cardiovasc Surg.* Feb 2008;135(2):316-323, 323 e311-316.

[82] Fighali SF, Avendano A, Elayda MA, et al. Early and late mortality of patients undergoing aortic valve replacement after previous coronary artery bypass graft surgery. *Circulation.* Nov 1 1995;92(9 Suppl):II163-168.

[83] Khaladj N, Shrestha M, Peterss S, et al. Isolated surgical aortic valve replacement after previous coronary artery bypass grafting with patent grafts: is this old-fashioned technique obsolete? *Eur J Cardiothorac Surg.* Feb 2009;35(2):260-264; discussion 264.

[84] Gillinov AM, Casselman FP, Lytle BW, et al. Injury to a patent left internal thoracic artery graft at coronary reoperation. *The Annals of thoracic surgery.* Feb 1999;67(2):382-386.

[85] Elami A, Laks H, Merin G. Technique for reoperative median sternotomy in the presence of a patent left internal mammary artery graft. *J Card Surg.* Mar 1994;9(2):123-127.

[86] Park CB, Suri RM, Burkhart HM, et al. Identifying patients at particular risk of injury during repeat sternotomy: analysis of 2555 cardiac reoperations. *J Thorac Cardiovasc Surg.* Nov 2010;140(5):1028-1035.

[87] Cohn LH. Myocardial protection for reoperative cardiac surgery in acquired heart disease. *Semin Thorac Cardiovasc Surg.* Apr 1993;5(2):162-167.

[88] Smith RL, Ellman PI, Thompson PW, et al. Do you need to clamp a patent left internal thoracic artery-left anterior descending graft in reoperative cardiac surgery? *The Annals of thoracic surgery.* Mar 2009;87(3):742-747.

[89] Park CB, Suri RM, Burkhart HM, et al. What is the optimal myocardial preservation strategy at re-operation for aortic valve replacement in the presence of a patent internal thoracic artery? *Eur J Cardiothorac Surg.* Jun 2011;39(6):861-865.

[90] Battellini R, Rastan AJ, Fabricius A, Moscoso-Luduena M, Lachmann N, Mohr FW. Beating heart aortic valve replacement after previous coronary artery bypass surgery with a patent internal mammary artery graft. *The Annals of thoracic surgery.* Mar 2007;83(3):1206-1209.

[91] Bloomfield P, Wheatley DJ, Prescott RJ, Miller HC. Twelve-year comparison of a Bjork-Shiley mechanical heart valve with porcine bioprostheses. *N Engl J Med.* Feb 28 1991;324(9):573-579.

[92] Oxenham H, Bloomfield P, Wheatley DJ, et al. Twenty year comparison of a Bjork-Shiley mechanical heart valve with porcine bioprostheses. *Heart.* Jul 2003;89(7):715-721.

[93] Hammermeister KE, Sethi GK, Henderson WG, Oprian C, Kim T, Rahimtoola S. A comparison of outcomes in men 11 years after heart-valve replacement with a mechanical valve or bioprosthesis. Veterans Affairs Cooperative Study on Valvular Heart Disease. *N Engl J Med.* May 6 1993;328(18):1289-1296.

[94] Hammermeister K, Sethi GK, Henderson WG, Grover FL, Oprian C, Rahimtoola SH. Outcomes 15 years after valve replacement with a mechanical versus a bioprosthetic valve: final report of the Veterans Affairs randomized trial. *J Am Coll Cardiol.* Oct 2000;36(4):1152-1158.

[95] Lund O, Bland M. Risk-corrected impact of mechanical versus bioprosthetic valves on long-term mortality after aortic valve replacement. *J Thorac Cardiovasc Surg.* Jul 2006;132(1):20-26.

[96] Kempfert J, Van Linden A, Linke A, et al. Transapical off-pump valve-in-valve implantation in patients with degenerated aortic xenografts. *The Annals of thoracic surgery.* Jun 2010;89(6):1934-1941.

[97] Pasic M, Unbehaun A, Dreysse S, et al. Transapical aortic valve implantation after previous aortic valve replacement: clinical proof of the "valve-in-valve" concept. *J Thorac Cardiovasc Surg.* Aug 2011;142(2):270-277.

[98] Webb JG, Wood DA, Ye J, et al. Transcatheter valve-in-valve implantation for failed bioprosthetic heart valves. *Circulation.* Apr 27 2010;121(16):1848-1857.

[99] Khawaja MZ, Haworth P, Ghuran A, et al. Transcatheter aortic valve implantation for stenosed and regurgitant aortic valve bioprostheses CoreValve for failed bioprosthetic aortic valve replacements. *J Am Coll Cardiol.* Jan 12 2010;55(2):97-101.

[100] U.S National Center for Health Statistics. National Vital Statistics Reports, U.S.Decennial Life Tables for 1999-2001, United States Life Tables, Vol.57, No.1, August 5,2008 and unpublished data.

[101] Potter DD, Sundt TM, 3rd, Zehr KJ, et al. Operative risk of reoperative aortic valve replacement. *J Thorac Cardiovasc Surg.* Jan 2005;129(1):94-103.

[102] Frank S, Braunwald E. Idiopathic hypertrophic subaortic stenosis. Clinical analysis of 126 patients with emphasis on the natural history. *Circulation.* May 1968;37(5):759-788.

[103] Pellikka PA, Sarano ME, Nishimura RA, et al. Outcome of 622 adults with asymptomatic, hemodynamically significant aortic stenosis during prolonged follow-up. *Circulation.* Jun 21 2005;111(24):3290-3295.

[104] Bonow RO, Carabello BA, Chatterjee K, et al. 2008 focused update incorporated into the ACC/AHA 2006 guidelines for the management of patients with valvular heart disease: a report of the American College of Cardiology/American Heart Association Task Force on Practice Guidelines (Writing Committee to revise the 1998 guidelines for the management of patients with valvular heart disease). Endorsed by the Society of Cardiovascular Anesthesiologists, Society for Cardiovascular Angiography and Interventions, and Society of Thoracic Surgeons. *J Am Coll Cardiol.* Sep 23 2008;52(13):e1-142.

[105] Bach DS, Siao D, Girard SE, Duvernoy C, McCallister BD, Jr., Gualano SK. Evaluation of patients with severe symptomatic aortic stenosis who do not undergo aortic valve replacement: the potential role of subjectively overestimated operative risk. *Circulation.* Nov 2009;2(6):533-539.

[106] Iung B, Baron G, Butchart EG, et al. A prospective survey of patients with valvular heart disease in Europe: The Euro Heart Survey on Valvular Heart Disease. *Eur Heart J.* Jul 2003;24(13):1231-1243.

[107] Freed BH, Sugeng L, Furlong K, et al. Reasons for nonadherence to guidelines for aortic valve replacement in patients with severe aortic stenosis and potential solutions. *Am J Cardiol.* May 1 2010;105(9):1339-1342.

[108] Iung B, Cachier A, Baron G, et al. Decision-making in elderly patients with severe aortic stenosis: why are so many denied surgery? *Eur Heart J.* Dec 2005;26(24):2714-2720.

[109] Varadarajan P, Kapoor N, Bansal RC, Pai RG. Survival in elderly patients with severe aortic stenosis is dramatically improved by aortic valve replacement: Results from a cohort of 277 patients aged > or =80 years. *Eur J Cardiothorac Surg.* Nov 2006;30(5):722-727.

[110] Malaisrie SC, Tuday E, Lapin B, et al. Transcatheter aortic valve implantation decreases the rate of unoperated aortic stenosis. *Eur J Cardiothorac Surg.* Jan 11 2011.

[111] Holmes DR, Jr., Mack MJ. Transcatheter valve therapy a professional society overview from the american college of cardiology foundation and the society of thoracic surgeons. *J Am Coll Cardiol.* Jul 19 2011;58(4):445-455.

In: Percutaneous Valve Technology: Present and Future ISBN: 978-1-61942-577-4
Editors: Jose Luis Navia and Sharif Al-Ruzzeh

Chapter X

Percutaneous Aortic Valve Implant – The US Experience – The Partner Trial

Imran N. Ahmad, E. Murat Tuzcu and Samir R. Kapadia

Introduction

Calcific aortic stenosis (AS) is the most common cause of aortic stenosis in adults with a prevalence of 2% in patients 65 years of age or older.[1, 2] Although patients may remain asymptomatic for many years, the onset of symptoms predicts rapid disease progression with an almost 50% mortality rate at 2 years.[3]

The gold standard therapy is surgical aortic valve replacement (AVR), however, in excess of 30% of patients may be denied surgery due to advanced age, significant left ventricular dysfunction, previous chest surgery or radiation, or other co-morbidities.[4-6] For this group of patients, until recently with the advent of transcatheter aortic valve implantation (TAVI) there were no therapies available that could provide either a mortality benefit or lasting symptom relief.[7]

In this chapter, we review the Edwards SAPIEN™ transcatheter aortic heart valve system (Edwards Lifesciences, Irvine, CA) in the context of the U.S. randomized Placement of Aortic Transcatheter Valves (PARTNER) trial including design, patient selection, role of imaging, and complications.

Edwards Sapien™ Transcatheter Heart Valve Technology Overview

Device

The Edwards SAPIEN™ valve is a catheter delivered aortic valve that combines a radiopaque, stainless steel balloon expandable stent with bioprosthetic valve technology (Figure 1). The trileaflet valve tissue is made from glutaraldehyde preserved bovine pericardium. Available in two sizes of 23 mm and 26 mm diameter, the valve is designed to fit through a 22-F or a 24-F inner diameter sheath, respectively.

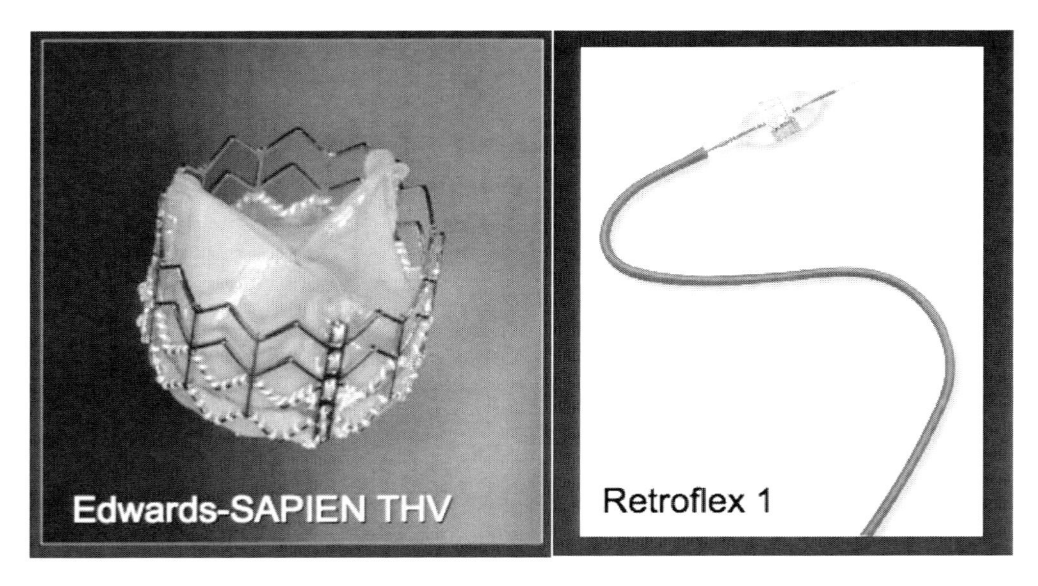

Figure 1. First generation Edwards SAPIEN™ transcatheter heart valve (THV) and RetroFlex™ balloon delivery catheter. The valve is made from bovine pericardium mounted on a radiopaque stainless steel balloon expandable stent.

Prior to implantation of the bioprosthesis, percutaneous balloon aortic valvuloplasty (BAV) is performed to facilitate passage of the delivery system and position the prosthetic valve within the native anulus. Contrast aortography at the time of balloon inflation aids in the assessment of anulur size as well as the risk of left coronary impeachment by native leaflets during prosthetic valve deployment. Prior to delivery, a crimping device is used to mount the valve onto the RetroFlex™ balloon delivery catheter system for the transfemoral retrograde approach or the Ascendra™ balloon delivery catheter system for the transapical antegrade approach. After careful delivery and positioning of the Edwards SAPIEN™ valve, rapid right ventricular pacing is employed to reduce stroke volume and thereby the risk of significant valve movement during deployment. The valve is then deployed through complete balloon expansion followed by balloon catheter delivery system removal and assessment for paravalvular regurgitation (Figure 2). In the context of the PARTNER trial, these procedures are performed under local and general anesthesia with intraprocedural imaging guidance by fluoroscopy and echocardiography.

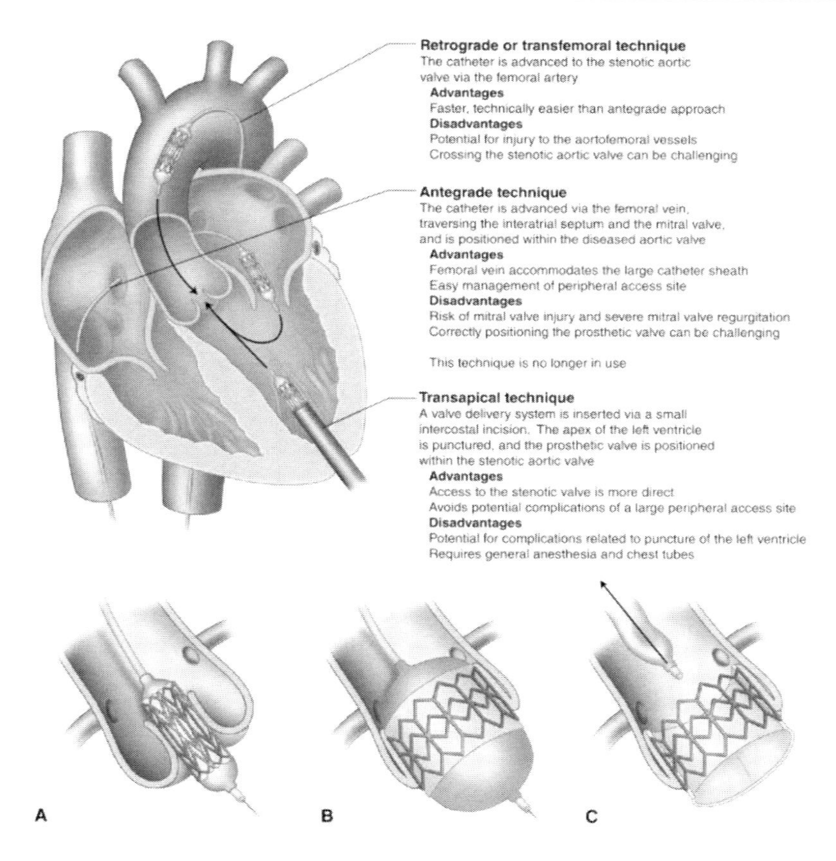

Figure 2. Overview of TAVI implantation via a retrograde, antegrade, or transapical approach. In all three approaches, the positioning of the prosthetic valve is determined by the patient's native valvular structure and anatomy and is guided by fluoroscopic imaging, supra-aortic angiography, and transesophageal echocardiography. The insets at the bottom show the position of the aortic valve prosthesis; it is placed at mid-position in the patient's aortic valve so as not to impinge on the coronary ostia or to impede the motion of the anterior mitral leaflet (a). The prosthesis is deployed by inflating (b), rapidly deflating, and quickly withdrawing the delivery balloon (c). (Adapted from Singh et al. []; with permission).

Non-Randomized Data Prior to PARTNER Trial

Dr. Alain Cribier in Rouen, France performed the first balloon expandable transcatheter aortic valve implantation in 2002.[8] He performed this procedure via the transseptal approach and in the Registry of Endovascular Critical Aortic Stenosis Treatment (RECAST) demonstrated an 82% procedural success rate.[9] Improving on the transfemoral approach Dr. John Webb in Vancouver, Canada described a technique using a steerable and deflectable guiding catheter in 18 patients.[10] His group reported a procedural success rate of 86% in their first 50 patients.[11] Based upon these and other reports, feasibility studies were organized through the development of multicenter registries from the United States [Transcatheter Endovascular Implantation of Valves II (REVIVAL-II)], the European Union [Registry of Endovascular Implantation of Valves in Europe II (REVIVE-II)], and Canada (Canadian Special Access). These included patients with a valve area ≤ 0.8 cm^2 and high predicted operative mortality. The REVIVAL-II registry included four centers: Cleveland Clinic in Ohio, William Beaumont Hospital in Michigan, Medical City in Dallas, Texas and Columbia University in New York. In the REVIVAL-II and REVIVE-II registries, the transfemoral implantation success rates were 88% and 87% while the 30-day mortality rates were 13.2% and 7.3% respectively. Advancements in transapical delivery during this time made it possible to include this approach under the REVIVAL-II registry. The 30-day mortality rate in the transapical cohort was 18.2%. The Canadian experience with 345 procedures (168 transfemoral and 177 transapical) at 6 centers between 2005 and 2009 in patients with severe AS and at high or prohibitive risk for surgery was recently published.[12] The overall procedural success rate was 93.3% and the 30-day mortality rate was 10.4% (9.5% transfemoral and 11.3% transapical).

With the approval of the Edwards SAPIEN™ valve in Europe under CE mark in 2007, the number of valve implants rapidly increased. Postmarketing studies including the Placement of Aortic Transcatheter Valve (PARTNER EU) registry and the Edwards Sapien Aortic Bioprosthesis European Outcome (SOURCE) registry allow for the continued review of TAVI procedures. In the SOURCE registry, the short-term procedural success rate was 93.8% with low rates of coronary obstruction (0.6%) and valve embolization (0.3%).[13, 14] Thirty day and one-year mortality rates were 8.5% and 23.9% respectively. Close to half of the deaths at one-year were non-cardiac in origin while about a quarter were classified as cardiac in origin. The 30-day and one-year stroke rates were 2.5% and 4.5% respectively. The incidence of vascular complications and permanent pacemaker implantation at 30-days was 12.8% and 7% respectively. As compared with transfemoral TAVI, transapical patients were a higher risk group with more co-morbid illnesses and a higher average logistic EuroSCORE. Although the outcome data for death is reliable, other unadjudicated endpoints such as stroke, paravalvular leak, and vascular complications may not be robust as this was a voluntary registry without core laboratory oversight.

Rationale for the PARTNER Trial

For TAVI to be clinically applicable and approved in the United States, two important questions have to be answered. First, does TAVI benefit patients with severe symptomatic aortic stenosis that do not have any surgical option? Second, does TAVI benefit patients with severe symptomatic aortic stenosis that may undergo surgical AVR albeit with high surgical risk? The PARTNER trial was designed to answer these very questions and in doing so, specific definitions were developed.

In reference to the first question, the definition of an inoperable patient is a very difficult task because in clinical practice many factors are weighed. In fact, some would argue that it is such an individualized decision that a universal definition of such a group for trial purposes remains elusive. Nonetheless, this definition had to be developed for the trial and was defined as patients who are likely to have a greater than 50% chance of mortality or serious irreversible morbidities if they underwent surgical AVR. In order for such a definition to work, each case had to be analyzed by unbiased expert cardiologists and cardiac surgeons.

Similarly, for the second question a definition for "high risk" surgical patient was developed. There are several available risk models for cardiac surgery each with significant limitations. The Logistic EuroSCORE is based on a 1995 European voluntary registry of 19,030 patients of whom less than 20% had any valve surgery. Because it is formulated on both older data and data from mostly non-valvular patients, it has significant limitations when applied to PARTNER trial patients in the current era.[15] It is clear that this algorithm overestimates mortality prediction in patients undergoing surgical AVR.[16] An alternative risk model is the Society of Thoracic Surgeons (STS) score developed from the voluntary registry of the STS National Adult Cardiac Surgery Database that included 67,292 patients undergoing isolated AVR from 2002 to 2006. This risk assessment algorithm can be found online and is updated every few years from more recent registry data. The main limitations of this score are selection and reporting bias as well as failure to weigh many common co-morbid illnesses. Despite underestimation of mortality in high risk patients, in the U.S. it is recognized as one of the more robust risk scoring systems and was chosen as the risk estimator when defining high risk patients in the PARTNER trial. The definition of high surgical risk was an STS score of at least 10% or coexisting conditions associated with a predicted 30-day risk of mortality ≥15%.

In addition to the definitions of inoperable and high risk groups, questions related to appropriate endpoints were considered. For example, the effect on mortality is a traditional and objective endpoint that is considered superior in many trials. However, in the PARTNER trial inoperable octogenarians and nonagenarians, improvement in quality of life may be the more relevant clinical endpoint. On the other hand, in younger high risk patients with different expectations improvement in survival likely takes precedence.

Study Design

The PARTNER trial is a multicenter randomized controlled prospective trial evaluating the safety and effectiveness of the Edwards SAPIEN™ valve in symptomatic patients with severe aortic stenosis at high or prohibitive risk for surgical AVR. Patients are initially stratified based on risk status and operability for aortic valve replacement surgery. Imaging studies are then used to determine feasibility of transfemoral approach based on vascular access criteria. Those not meeting criteria may be candidates for transapical delivery (Figure 3). The trial is designed such that it is essentially two parallel trials – high-risk patients in Cohort A and inoperable patients in Cohort B – each with an 85% power to detect a difference in all-cause mortality at one year. Out of 3,105 patients screened a total of 1,058 patients were entered into the study. Cohort A randomized approximately 700 patients to transfemoral TAVI or surgical AVR. Those not eligible for transfemoral delivery are randomized to transapical TAVI or surgical AVR. Cohort B randomized 358 patients to transfemoral TAVI or standard therapy including BAV. Patients ineligible for transfemoral TAVI were not randomized.

Patients were followed post-procedure at 1 week, 1 month, 3 months, 6 months, and then annually thereafter for a minimum of 5 years post-procedure. The complete trial analysis will focus on treatment arm versus control arm without any pooling of the data between cohorts. The primary endpoint in Cohort A is a non-inferiority endpoint for all cause mortality at one year, while the primary endpoint in Cohort B is a superiority endpoint for all cause mortality over the length of the trial.

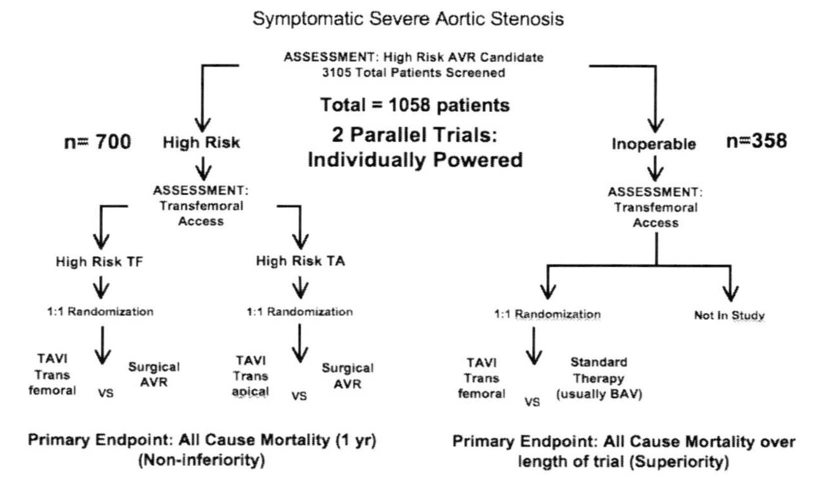

Figure 3. Overview of the PARTNER trial. Cohort B inoperable patients (n=358) were randomized to transfemoral TAVI versus standard therapy typically with BAV. Patients unsuitable for transfemoral TAVI in Cohort B were not included in the study.

There are a various secondary safety and efficacy endpoints including freedom from major adverse cardiovascular and cerebral events, echo assessments of valve function, quality of life and cost-effectiveness assessments, and functional improvement (Table 1 and 2).

Table 1. PARTNER trial secondary endpoints. VARC=Valve Academic Research Consortium, NYHA=New York Heart Association, QOL=Quality of Life, EOA=Effective orifice area

Secondary Endpoints
Cardiovascular Mortality
Repeat Hospitalization (after the index procedure)
Due to valve or procedure-related clinical deterioration
Mortality and repeat hospitalization (Kaplan-Meier analysis)
Major strokes (modified Rankin Score ≥ 2 at ≥ 30 days)
Mortality and major strokes (Kaplan-Meier analysis)
Major vascular complications (VARC definition)
NYHA symptom classification
QOL and cost-effectiveness assessments
Six-minute walk tests
Echo assessments of valve function (core lab)
EOA, mean gradient, aortic regurgitation

Table 2. Definitions of safety endpoints in the PARTNER Trial

Major Vascular Complications	Any thoracic aortic dissection
	Access site or access-related vascular injury leading to either: death, blood transfusions > 3 units, unplanned intervention (percutaneous or surgical), irreversible end-organ damage
	Distal embolization (non-cerebral) from a vascular source requiring surgery or resulting in amputation or irreversible end-organ damage
	Left ventricular perforation
Major Bleeding Complications	Clear site of bleeding resulting in:
	Death
	Hospitalization or hospitalization prolonged ≥ 24 hours
	Pericardiocentesis or open or endovascular procedure for hemostasis
	Permanent disability (e.g. blindness, paralysis, hearing loss)
	Transfusion > 3 units within a 24 hour period
Neurologic Events	
TIA	Focal neurologic event that was fully reversible in < 24 hours in the absence of any new imaging findings of infarction or other primary medical cause (hypoglycemia, hypoxia, etc.)
Stroke	Focal neurologic deficit lasting ≥ 24 hours
	Focal neurologic deficit lasing < 24 hours with imaging findings acute infarction or hemorrhage
Major Stroke	Stroke associated with a modified Rankin Scale of ≥ 2 at 30 days or longer after the event
	NIH Stroke Scale incorporated if available

Study Execution

Patient Selection

Patients are screened for severe symptomatic aortic stenosis as demonstrated by NYHA functional class II or greater and echocardiographic criteria: mean aortic valve gradient >40 mmHg or peak jet velocity greater than 4.0 m/s or an initial aortic valve area (AVA) of < 0.8 cm2 (indexed EOA < 0.5 cm2/m2).

As discussed above, the STS score is the risk assessment model selected for the PARTNER trial to aid in identifying patients who are at high risk for surgical AVR and therefore candidates for Cohort A. Patients with coexisting conditions associated with a predicted 30-day risk of ≥ 50% for death or serious irreversible morbidity were considered candidates for Cohort B. Such inoperable patients typically had conditions not captured by STS risk assessment such as severe calcification (porcelain) of the ascending aorta, chest wall deformity or radiation, multiple prior interventions, or severe respiratory insufficiency.

Although there are a number of exclusion criteria for the PARTNER trial, some of the most pertinent criteria relate to the feasibility of a transfemoral approach. Pre-procedural imaging of the aorta and ileofemoral arteries with aortography, multislice computed tomography (MSCT), magnetic resonance angiography, and peripheral intravascular ultrasound (IVUS) were all used in various combinations to evaluate for aneurysms, tortuosity, atheroma, severe calcifications, and vessel size that preclude transfemoral delivery of the large arterial sheath and RetroFlex™ catheter system. As experience has accumulated, MSCT with 3D reconstruction has taken on an invaluable role in the non-invasive screening process for TAVI.

Uniform Imaging Requirements

Echocardiography

As stated above only patients with severe symptomatic aortic stenosis diagnosed by transthoracic echocardiography (TTE) were eligible for the PARTNER trial. The whole echocardiogram study was reviewed not just the aortic anular size and gradient. In fact, TTE was invaluable in identifying patients who met exclusion criteria such as a congenital unicuspid or bicuspid valve, mixed aortic valve disease with predominant aortic regurgitation, severe mitral anular calcification, severe mitral insufficiency, hypertrophic cardiomyopathy, severe left ventricular (LV) dysfunction (ejection fraction < 20%), or evidence of intracardiac mass, thrombus, or vegetation. At the time of the procedure transesophageal echocardiography (TEE) is used to measure the native aortic valve anulus. The Edwards SAPIEN™ first generation valve comes in 23 mm and 26 mm diameter sizes and generally, anular diameter sizes of 16 mm to 21 mm would receive a 23 mm valve while anular diameter sizes of 22 mm to 24 mm would accommodate the 26 mm valve. Because of the available valve at the time of the study, patients with anular sizes less than 18 mm or greater than 25 mm were excluded from the trial. In many patients TEE was done prior to the procedure if TTE was inadequate to insure the anular diameter met study criteria. TEE during the procedure also characterized the degree of paravalvular regurgitation after deployment of the bioprosthetic valve.

Computed Tomography

As a comprehensive noninvasive imaging modality, MSCT with 3D reconstruction allows accurate assessment of the aortic valve structures and peripheral arteries. When making a decision between transfemoral or transapical approach, these images were reviewed for evidence of calcifications, tortuosity, and ileofemoral vessel size. Severe calcification, vessel size less than 7 mm, and extremely tortuous vessels excluded patients from the transfemoral approach. In these cases a transapical approach was used if patients were surgical candidates (only cohort A). While patients considered inoperable in cohort B were excluded from the study as there was no transapical arm in that group.

Fluoroscopy

Prior to implantation, aortography of the aortic root was used to define the optimal aortic valve plane such that all three sinuses are aligned (Figure 4).

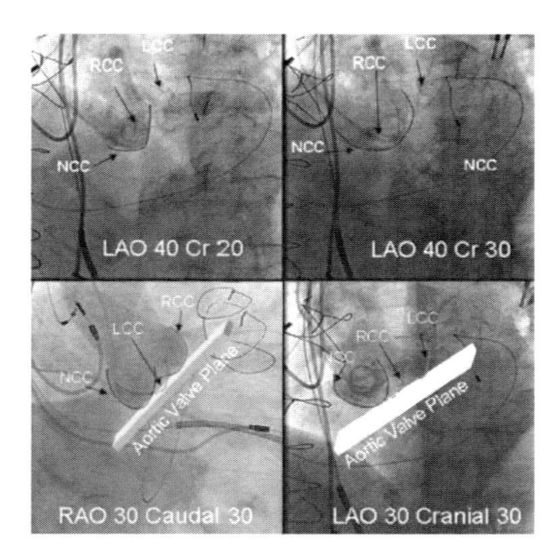

Figure 4. LAO and RAO views of the aortic root injection to demonstrate the coronary cusps. Note that the NCC is typically lower in this view. When the aortogram is performed in the cranial angulation, one can align the leaflets to properly visualize aortic valve plane. RAO caudal view is another common view for aortic plane. Abbreviations: LCC, left coronary cusp; RCC, right coronary cusp; NCC, noncoronary cusp.

Once defined TAVI positioning and deployment was performed under this fluoroscopic plane.

A descending aortogram was also performed to further assess the feasibility of transfemoral access. If vessel tortuosity was identified, then straightening of the vessel with a stiff wire could be attempted. As with any sheath, the large diameters sheaths used during TAVI traverse tortuous iliac vessels easier if they straightened first with a stiff wire.

Core Laboratory

The Duke Clinical Research Institute core laboratory was used for all electrocardiogram and echocardiogram studies to provide quality, uniformity, and reproducibility in both data acquisition and analysis. Echocardiographic efficacy endpoints included aortic valve area and mean gradient as well as LV ejection fraction (EF). Safety endpoints included prosthetic valve dysfunction, migration, thrombosis, paravalvular leak, LV injury, and mitral valve compromise. An economics and quality of life study headed by the Harvard Clinical Research Institute was included in the PARTNER trial to assess health-related quality of life and resource utilization. Neurological screening with the NIH Stroke Scale assessment was performed before and after each procedure by certified practitioners.

Case Screening and Site Education

Cases were reviewed twice a week and more often for expedited reviews via webcast presentations and conference calls. Screenings included review of clinical evaluations, echocardiographic and catheterization findings, and vascular access assessments. At these case reviews, cohort assignment and treatment strategies were discussed. All site operators and personnel completed a comprehensive training program including simulation training and proctoring. Sites were gradually enrolled approximately 1-2 per month to guarantee a personalized training experience for each site.

Trial Results

At this time only the results of Cohort B inoperable patients have been published and are discussed below.[17-25] Cohort A results are eagerly awaited and most likely to be presented at the 2011 American College of Cardiology meeting in March.

Baseline Characteristics

The two groups of patients TAVI and standard therapy were well balanced with respect to baseline characteristics (Table 3).

Table 3. Baseline characteristics of the PARTNER trial inoperable cohort B patients. CAD=coronary artery disease, MI=myocardial infarction, CABG=coronary artery bypass grafting, PCI=percutaneous coronary intervention, CVD=cerebral vascular disease, PVD=peripheral vascular disease, COPD=chronic obstructed pulmonary disease, HTN=hypertension

Characteristic	TAVI n=179	Standard Therapy n=179	P-value
Age - yr	83.1 ± 8.6	83.2 ± 8.3	0.95
Male sex (%)	45.8	46.9	0.92
STS Score	11.2 ± 5.8	12.1 ± 6.1	0.14
Logistic EuroSCORE	26.4 ± 17.2	30.4 ± 19.1	0.04
NYHA			
I or II (%)	7.8	6.1	0.68
III or IV (%)	92.2	93.9	0.68
CAD (%)	67.6	74.3	0.20
Prior MI (%)	18.6	26.4	0.10
Prior CABG (%)	37.4	45.6	0.17
Prior PCI (%)	30.5	24.8	0.31
Prior BAV (%)	16.2	24.4	0.09
CVD (%)	27.4	27.5	1.00
PVD (%)	30.3	25.1	0.29
COPD			
Any (%)	41.3	52.5	0.04
oxygen dependent (%)	21.2	25.7	0.38
Creatinine >2mg/dL (%)	5.6	9.6	0.23
Atrial fibrillation (%)	32.9	48.8	0.04
Permanent pacemaker (%)	22.9	19.5	0.49
Pulmonary HTN (%)	42.4	43.8	0.90
Frailty (%)	18.1	28.0	0.09
Porcelain aorta (%)	19.0	11.2	0.05
Chest wall radiation (%)	8.9	8.4	1.00
Chest wall deformity (%)	8.4	5.0	0.29
Liver disease (%)	3.4	3.4	1.00

The overall patient population was elderly with an elevated STS score of 11.6 ± 6% consistent with a high risk status. As shown in the table a number of patients had co-existing conditions such as porcelain aorta, COPD, chest wall deformity or radiation, or were very frail that added to their risk.

Outcomes

Death/Repeat Hospitalization

The results from Cohort B comparing transfemoral TAVI to best medical therapy, including BAV, showed a marked survival advantage of TAVI in non-surgical candidates.[17] Patients treated with standard therapy had a mortality rate (primary endpoint) by Kaplan-Meier analysis of 50.7% at one year compared with a rate of 30.7% with TAVI (hazard ratio with TAVI, 0.55; 95% confidence interval [CI], 0.40 to 0.74; $P<0.001$) (Figure 5). Specific causes of death (Table 4) revealed that there were more cardiovascular deaths in the standard therapy group but more non-cardiovascular deaths in the TAVI group.

Table 4. Specific causes of death in Cohort B inoperable patients

Cause of Death	TAVI n=179	Standard Rx n=179
All	71 (39.7%)	108 (60.3%)
Cardiovascular	27 (15.1%)	60 (33.5%)
Central nervous system	4 (2.2%)	4 (2.2%)
Vascular complication	3 (1.7%)	0
Sudden, unexpected	4 (2.2%)	18 (10.0%)
CHF	10 (5.6%)	32 (17.9%)
Endocarditis	2 (1.2%)	0
Myocardial infarction	1 (0.6%)	0
Arrhythmia	0	3 (1.7%)
Non-cerebral hemorrhage	0	3 (1.7%)
Other	3 (1.7%)	1 (0.6%)
Non-cardiovascular	27 (15.1%)	15 (8.4%)
Infection	9 (5.0%)	7 (3.9%)
Malignancy	4 (2.2%)	4 (2.2%)
Renal disease	3 (1.7%)	1 (0.6%)
Respiratory failure	3 (1.7%)	2 (1.2%)
Accidental	2 (1.2%)	0
Bleeding (GI, Intracerebral, Peritoneal)	2 (1.2%)	1 (0.6%)
Other	4 (2.2%)	0
Unknown	17 (9.5%)	33 (18.4%)

The composite endpoint of death or repeat hospitalization was also lower with TAVI at 42.5% compared with 71.6% in the standard therapy group (Figure 6). Therefore, in order to prevent one death at one year, five patients needed to be treated with TAVI and to prevent either one death or repeat hospitalization only three patients needed to be treated with TAVI. In the standard therapy group, approximately 84% of patients underwent BAV and initially event rates were lower in this group compared to patients who did not have BAV. However, after 3 months this benefit was reduced and by one year there was no clinically appreciable benefit of BAV in the standard therapy group (Figure 7). In essence, BAV did not alter the natural history of severe symptomatic aortic stenosis.

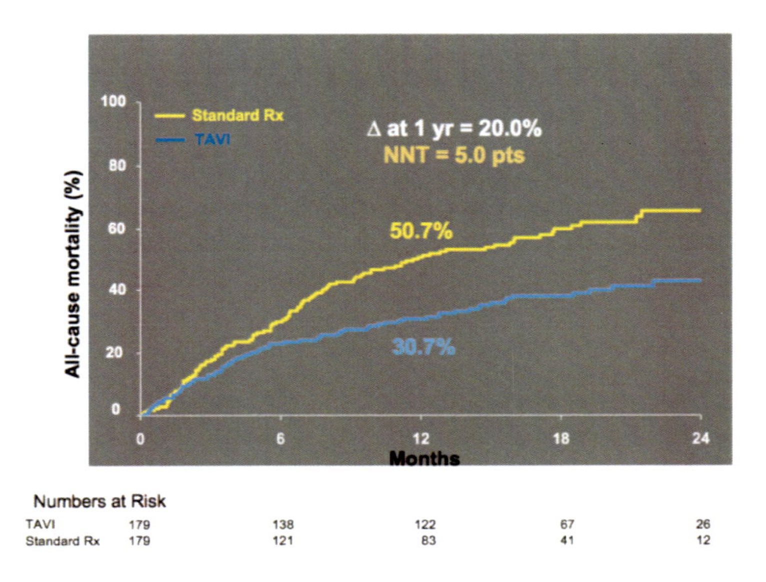

Figure 5. PARTNER Trial Cohort B results: death at one year. Patients treated with standard therapy had a mortality rate by Kaplan-Meier analysis of 50.7% at one year compared with a rate of 30.7% with TAVI (hazard ratio with TAVI, 0.55; 95% confidence interval [CI], 0.40 to 0.74; P<0.001). The number needed to treat to prevent one death with TAVI was only 5 patients.

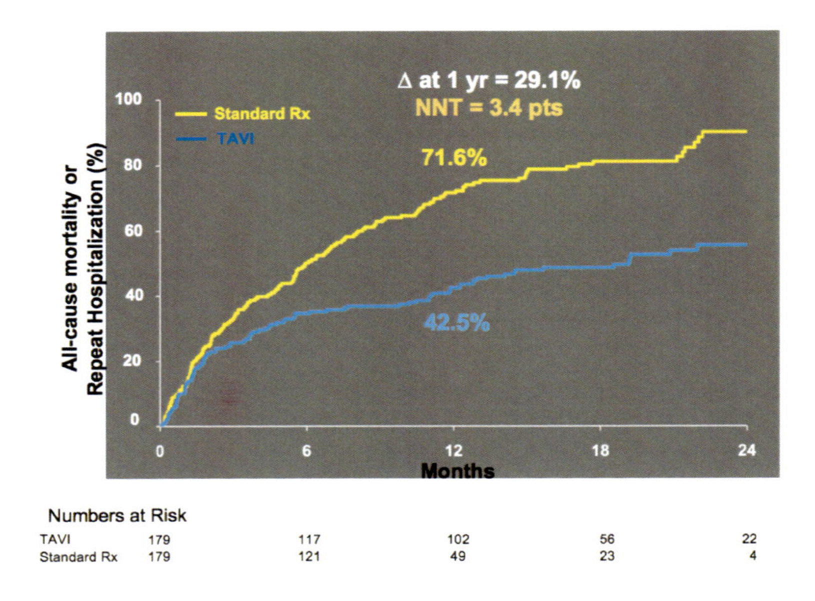

Figure 6. PARTNER Trial Cohort B results: death and repeat hospitalization at one year. The composite endpoint of death or repeat hospitalization was lower with TAVI at 42.5% compared with 71.6% in the standard therapy group (hazard ratio with TAVI, 0.46; 95% confidence interval [CI] 0.35 to 0.59; P (log rank) < 0.0001).

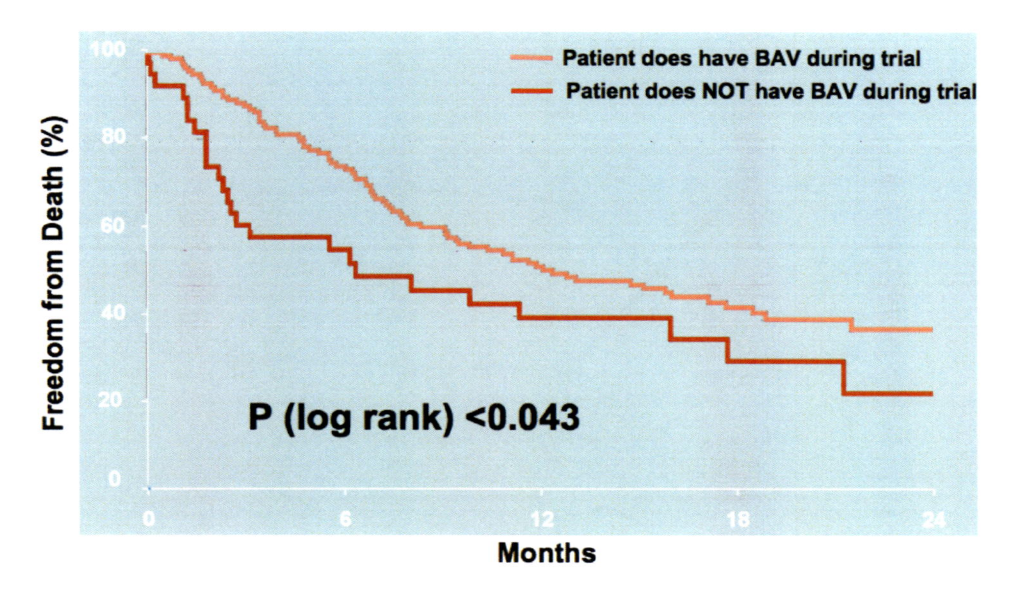

Figure 7. PARTNER Trial Cohort B outcomes: freedom from death in standard therapy with and without BAV. Patients treated with BAV demonstrate a catch-up effect so that by 12 months there is no appreciable benefit in mortality.

Hemodynamics

Echocardiograms were performed at baseline, discharge or day 7, 30 days, 6 months, and at one year. At baseline there was no difference between TAVI and standard therapy with respect to measures of aortic stenosis, systolic function, or mitral regurgitation (Table 5). Patients who underwent TAVI experienced marked and sustained improvements out to one year in aortic valve peak/mean gradients and valve area with rare prosthetic valve dysfunction (Figure 8). The safety analysis did not reveal any evidence of structural or nonstructural valve dysfunction, migration, thrombosis, LV injury, or mitral valve compromise. Although paravalvular AR was frequent, it was usually trace or mild, remained stable out to one year, and rarely required further therapy (Figure 9). Furthermore, there was no increase in total aortic regurgitation or total LV volume load.

Table 5. PARTNER Trial inoperable Cohort B baseline echocardiographic parameters. AV=aortic valve, LVEF=left ventricular ejection fraction, MR=mitral regurgitation

Parameter	TAVI n=179	Standard Rx n=179	P value
Aortic valve area (cm2)	0.6 ± 0.2	0.6 ± 0.2	0.96
Mean AV gradient (mm Hg)	44.5 ± 15.7	43.0 ± 15.3	0.39
Mean LVEF (%)	53.9 ± 13.1	51.1 ± 14.3	0.06
Mod-Severe MR (%) (≥ 3+)	22.2	23.0	0.90

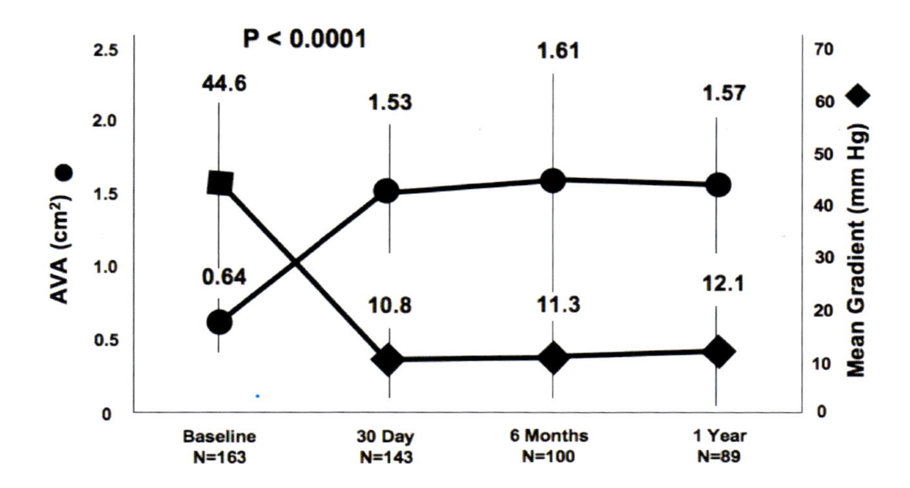

Figure 8. PARTNER Trial Cohort B results: echocardiographic measures in TAVI group. Patients treated with TAVI experienced a marked improvement in both aortic valve area (AVA) and mean gradients that was sustained out to one year.

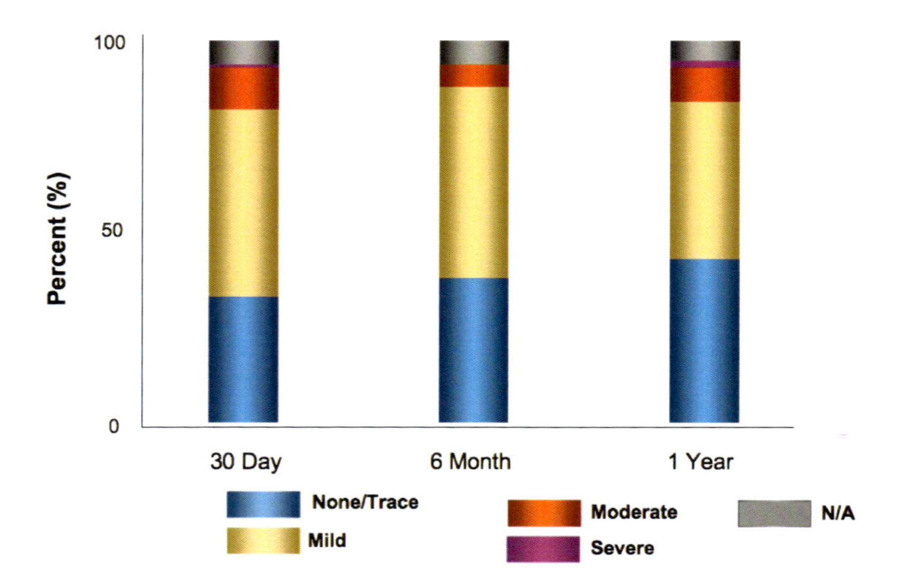

Figure 9. PARTNER Trial Cohort B outcomes: paravalvular regurgitation. Out of 179 TAVI treated patients, the most frequent grade of paravalvular regurgitation was trace or mild and remained stable out to one year. N/A=not applicable.

Complications

Vascular

With respect to safety endpoints more major vascular complications (16.8% vs. 2.2%, P<0.0001), more major bleeding (22.3% vs. 11.2%, P=0.007) (Figure 10), and more stroke or

TIA (10.6% vs. 4.5%, P=0.04) occurred in the TAVI treatment arm despite approximately 84% of patients in the standard treatment arm receiving a BAV procedure. The Edwards **SAPIEN™ valve** system used in the PARTNER trial is a first generation delivery system utilizing large size sheaths 22F (8mm outer diameter) or 24F (9mm outer diameter). Candidates for transfemoral TAVI were generally accepted only if the minimum access artery diameter was no more than 1mm less than the outer diameter of the sheath. Transfemoral TAVI complicated by a major vascular complication was associated with survival rate of 52.8% at one year compared with 72.3% in those without a major vascular complication (P log rank = 0.069) (Figure 11).

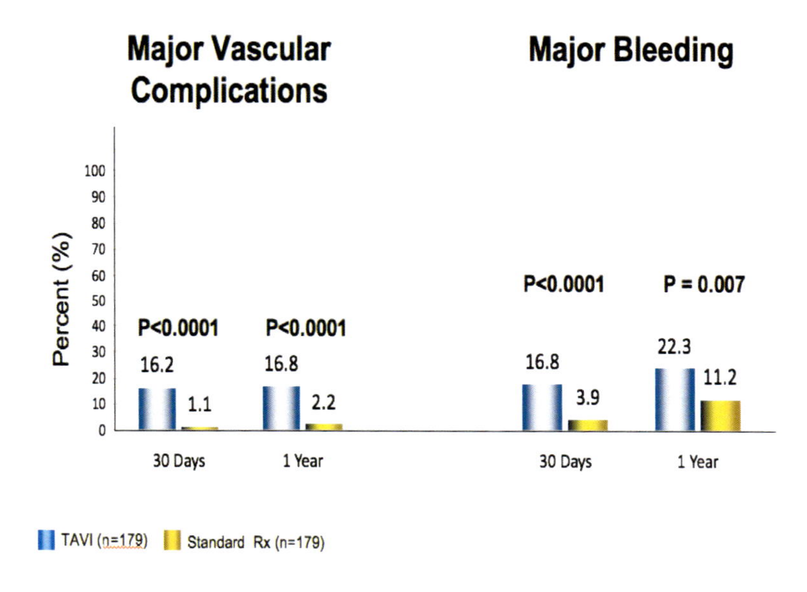

Figure 10. PARTNER Trial Cohort B outcomes: major vascular complications and major bleeding. At both 30-days and one year, TAVI patients experienced higher rates of major vascular complications and bleeding.

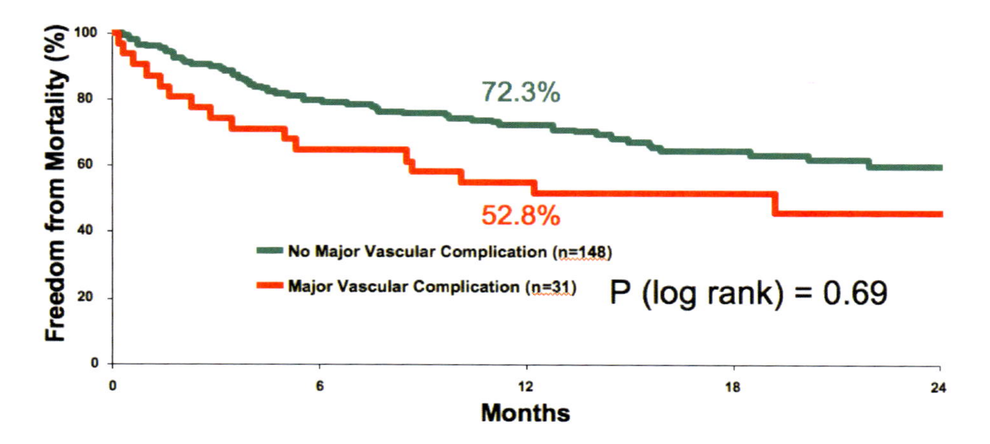

Figure 11. PARTNER Trial Cohort B outcomes: survival in TAVI with and without a major vascular complication. TAVI treated patients with major vascular complications experienced lower rates of survival than those without major vascular complications.

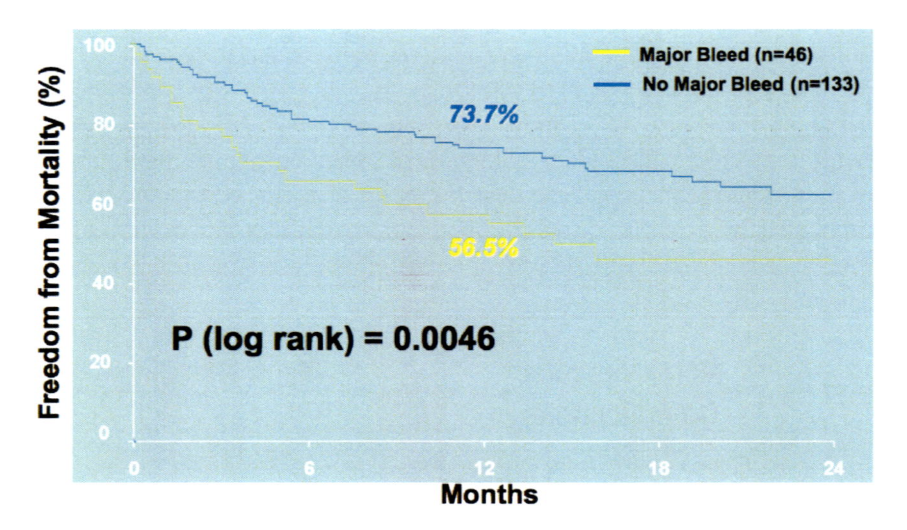

Figure 12. PARTNER Trial Cohort B outcomes: survival in TAVI with and without a major bleeding event. TAVI treated patients with major bleeding lower rates of survival than those without major bleeding events.

A major bleeding event was associated with a one-year survival rate of 56.5% compared with 73.7% in transfemoral TAVI patients without a major bleeding event (P log rank = 0.0046) (Figure 12). Therefore, vascular injury and bleeding are both associated with increased morbidity and mortality in patients undergoing transfemoral TAVI. However, with the introduction of the Edwards SAPIEN XT™ valve system that utilizes a new cobalt-chromium frame with a lower profile as well as the smaller 18F NovaFlex™ balloon delivery catheter, most operators believe that the rates of vascular complications and bleeding can be reduced (Figure 13).

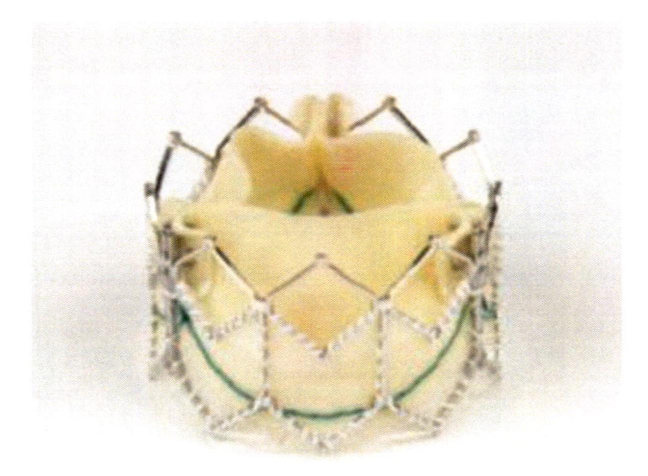

Figure 13. Edwards SAPIENT XT™ valve. This next generation valve is mounted on a cobalt-chromium frame with a lower profile and delivered via the smaller18F NovaFlex™ balloon delivery catheter.

Stroke

At one year TAVI was associated with a higher rate of stroke or TIA as well as major strokes (7.8% vs. 3.9%, P=0.18) (Figure 14). The survival rate in patients with a major stroke was 33.3% versus 72.3% in those without a major stroke (P log rank < 0.001) (Figure 15). Despite the stroke risk associated with TAVI, the combined endpoint of death or major stroke still favored TAVI (33% vs. 50.3%, P=0.001) over standard therapy at one year (Figure 16). Out of twenty-three neurologic events in the TAVI arm, five procedure related strokes occurred in the first three days and eight strokes occurred in patients while in atrial fibrillation. Out of eight neurologic events in the standard therapy arm, none occurred with BAV and four strokes occurred in patients while in atrial fibrillation. Given that the majority of strokes did not occur in the immediate peri-procedural period, it remains to be determined how stroke rates will be influenced by the use of embolic protection devices in conjunction with next generation delivery systems.

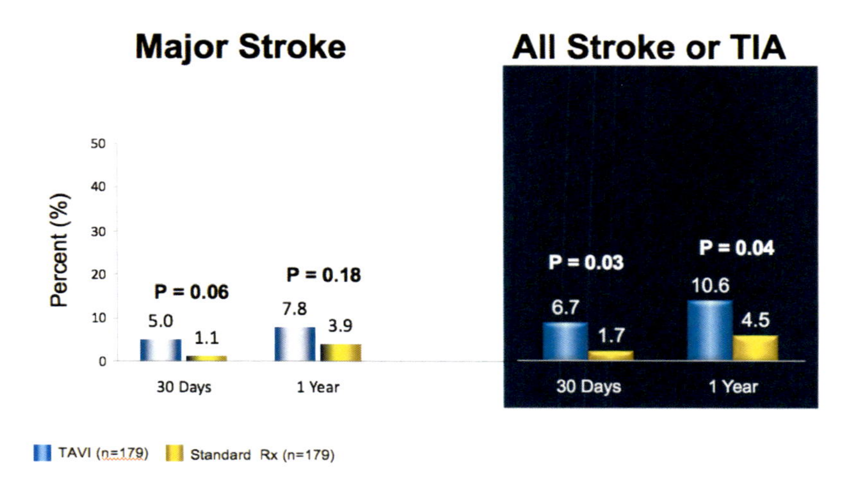

Figure 14. PARTNER Trial Cohort B outcomes: major stroke and all stroke or TIA. At 30-days and one year, major strokes trended higher in TAVI treated patients with the composite endpoint of all stroke or TIA significantly higher in the TAVI group.

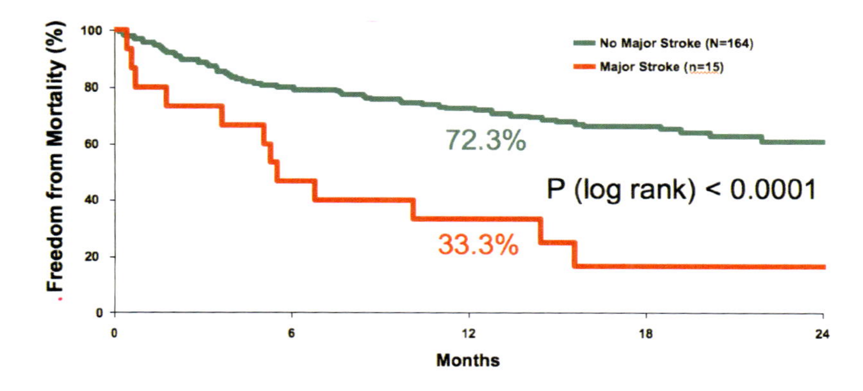

Figure 15. PARTNER Trial Cohort B outcomes: mortality rates in TAVI with and without a major stroke. TAVI treated patients with major strokes experienced higher rates of mortality than those without a major stroke.

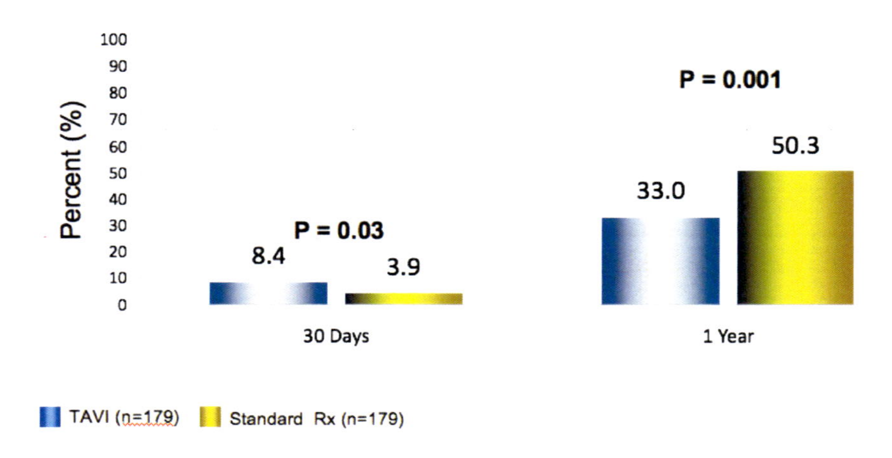

Figure 16. PARTNER Trial Cohort B outcomes: death or major stroke. At 30-days and one year, despite higher rates of stroke, TAVI treated patients experienced lower rates of the composite endpoint death or major stroke than standard therapy.

An analysis of TAVI risk in the PARTNER trial inoperable patients revealed several findings. First, the EuroSCORE and STS risk scoring models demonstrated weak correlation. This has been demonstrated before based on data from REVIAL II and PARTNER EU and may reflect the inherent differences in the original patient populations. Furthermore, the STS score predicted mortality better than the EuroSCORE in both the TAVI and control arm. Second, in subgroup analysis of all-cause mortality by STS score there was a significant risk reduction in the TAVI arm regardless of age above or below 85, LV ejection fraction above or below 55%, prior CABG or PCI, or STS score above or below 11. Therefore, TAVI appears to mitigate risk in certain subgroups. Third, in addition to all-cause mortality, the cardiovascular mortality at one year was lower with TAVI at 11.2% compared with 31.3% (P=0.000005) while non-cardiovascular causes were higher in the TAVI arm (14.5% vs. 7.3%). It may be the case that in a high-risk elderly population with multiple co-morbidities, survival after TAVI is ultimately limited by non-cardiac disease. Finally, a TAVI specific risk model that incorporates patient frailty and non-cardiac disease states is needed to more accurately predict candidates that would best benefit from this procedure.

Conclusion

Severe AS is the most common indication for surgical AVR. However, in the elderly population deemed inoperable due to frailty, multiple co-morbidities, or issues making surgery technically prohibitive, TAVI should be the new standard of care over medical therapy in conjunction with balloon aortic valvuloplasty. The PARTNER trial cohort B results highlight a significant survival advantage despite increased rates of vascular complications, strokes, and bleeding. Improvements in the Edwards SAPIEN™ valve related to lower valve profile, smaller size sheaths, as well as newer embolic protection devices hopefully will lower the rates of these adverse events. Results of the PARTNER trial cohort A will provide greater insight into how this new and exciting technology compares with surgical AVR in patients with high but acceptable surgical risk.

References

[1] Nkomo VT, Gardin JM, Skelton TN, Gottdiener JS, Scott CG, Enriquez-Sarano M. Burden of valvular heart diseases: a population-based study. *Lancet.* 2006;368 (9540):1005-1011.

[2] Otto CM. Timing of aortic valve surgery. *Heart.* 2000;84(2):211-218.

[3] Bonow RO, Carabello BA, Chatterjee K, de Leon AC, Jr., Faxon DP, Freed MD, Gaasch WH, Lytle BW, Nishimura RA, O'Gara PT, O'Rourke RA, Otto CM, Shah PM, Shanewise JS. 2008 Focused update incorporated into the ACC/AHA 2006 guidelines for the management of patients with valvular heart disease: a report of the American College of Cardiology/American Heart Association Task Force on Practice Guidelines (Writing Committee to Revise the 1998 Guidelines for the Management of Patients With Valvular Heart Disease): endorsed by the Society of Cardiovascular Anesthesiologists, Society for Cardiovascular Angiography and Interventions, and Society of Thoracic Surgeons. *Circulation.* 2008;118(15):e523-661.

[4] Bouma BJ, van Den Brink RB, van Der Meulen JH, Verheul HA, Cheriex EC, Hamer HP, Dekker E, Lie KI, Tijssen JG. To operate or not on elderly patients with aortic stenosis: the decision and its consequences. *Heart.* 1999;82(2):143-148.

[5] Iung B, Cachier A, Baron G, Messika-Zeitoun D, Delahaye F, Tornos P, Gohlke-Barwolf C, Boersma E, Ravaud P, Vahanian A. Decision-making in elderly patients with severe aortic stenosis: why are so many denied surgery? *Eur Heart J.* 2005;26(24):2714-2720.

[6] Pellikka PA, Sarano ME, Nishimura RA, Malouf JF, Bailey KR, Scott CG, Barnes ME, Tajik AJ. Outcome of 622 adults with asymptomatic, hemodynamically significant aortic stenosis during prolonged follow-up. *Circulation.* 2005;111(24):3290-3295.

[7] Krishnaswamy A, Tuzcu E, Kapadia S. Update on Transcatheter Aortic Valve Implantation. *Current Cardiology Reports.*1-11.

[8] Cribier A, Eltchaninoff H, Bash A, Borenstein N, Tron C, Bauer F, Derumeaux G, Anselme F, Laborde F, Leon MB. Percutaneous transcatheter implantation of an aortic valve prosthesis for calcific aortic stenosis: first human case description. *Circulation.* 2002;106(24):3006-3008.

[9] Cribier A, Eltchaninoff H, Tron C, Bauer F, Agatiello C, Nercolini D, Tapiero S, Litzler PY, Bessou JP, Babaliaros V. Treatment of calcific aortic stenosis with the percutaneous heart valve: mid-term follow-up from the initial feasibility studies: the French experience. *J Am Coll Cardiol.* 2006;47(6):1214-1223.

[10] Webb JG, Chandavimol M, Thompson CR, Ricci DR, Carere RG, Munt BI, Buller CE, Pasupati S, Lichtenstein S. Percutaneous aortic valve implantation retrograde from the femoral artery. *Circulation.* 2006;113(6):842-850.

[11] Webb JG, Pasupati S, Humphries K, Thompson C, Altwegg L, Moss R, Sinhal A, Carere RG, Munt B, Ricci D, Ye J, Cheung A, Lichtenstein SV. Percutaneous transarterial aortic valve replacement in selected high-risk patients with aortic stenosis. *Circulation.* 2007;116(7):755-763.

[12] Rodes-Cabau J, Webb JG, Cheung A, Ye J, Dumont E, Feindel CM, Osten M, Natarajan MK, Velianou JL, Martucci G, DeVarennes B, Chisholm R, Peterson MD, Lichtenstein SV, Nietlispach F, Doyle D, DeLarochelliere R, Teoh K, Chu V, Dancea

A, Lachapelle K, Cheema A, Latter D, Horlick E. Transcatheter aortic valve implantation for the treatment of severe symptomatic aortic stenosis in patients at very high or prohibitive surgical risk: acute and late outcomes of the multicenter Canadian experience. *J Am Coll Cardiol.* 2010;55(11):1080-1090.

[13] Thomas M, Schymik G, Walther T, Himbert D, Lefevre T, Treede H, Eggebrecht H, Rubino P, Michev I, Lange R, Anderson WN, Wendler O. Thirty-Day Results of the SAPIEN Aortic Bioprosthesis European Outcome (SOURCE) Registry: A European Registry of Transcatheter Aortic Valve Implantation Using the Edwards SAPIEN Valve. *Circulation.*122(1):62.

[14] Tuzcu EM, Kapadia S, Svensson LG. "SOURCE" of enthusiasm for transcatheter aortic valve implantation. *Circulation.*122(1):8-10.

[15] Brown ML, Schaff HV, Sarano ME, Li Z, Sundt TM, Dearani JA, Mullany CJ, Orszulak TA. Is the European System for Cardiac Operative Risk Evaluation model valid for estimating the operative risk of patients considered for percutaneous aortic valve replacement? *J Thorac Cardiovasc Surg.* 2008;136(3):566-571.

[16] Osswald BR, Gegouskov V, Badowski-Zyla D, Tochtermann U, Thomas G, Hagl S, Blackstone EH. Overestimation of aortic valve replacement risk by EuroSCORE: implications for percutaneous valve replacement. *Eur Heart J.* 2009;30(1):74-80.

[17] Leon MB, Smith CR, Mack M, Miller DC, Moses JW, Svensson LG, Tuzcu EM, Webb JG, Fontana GP, Makkar RR, Brown DL, Block PC, Guyton RA, Pichard AD, Bavaria JE, Herrmann HC, Douglas PC, Petersen JL, Akin JJ, Anderson WN, Wang D, Pocock S. Transcatheter Aortic-Valve Implantation for Aortic Stenosis in Patients Who Cannot Undergo Surgery. *NEJM.* 2010:1-11.

[18] Mack M. Neurologic Events in the PARTNER Inoperable Patients; Frequency, Timing, Causes, and Severity - on Behalf of the PARTNER Trial Investigators. *22nd Annual Transcatheter Cardiovascular Therapeutics (TCT).* Washington, DC; 2010.

[19] Webb J. Vascular Complications in the PARTNER Inoperable Patients: Frequency, Timing, Causes, and Impact on Short- and Long-term Outcome - for the PARTNER Investigators. *22nd Annual Transcatheter Cardiovascular Therapeutics (TCT).* Washington, DC; 2010.

[20] Svensson L. A Comprehensive Analysis of Causes of Death in the PARTNER Inoperable Patients - on Behalf of PARTNER Investigators. *22nd Annual Transcatheter Cardiovascular Therapeutics.* Washington, DC; 2010.

[21] Tuzcu EM. Clinical Outcomes from Standard Therapy in the PARTNER Inoperable Patients - on Behalf of PARTNER Investigators. *22nd Annual Transcatheter Cardiovascular Therapeutics.* Washingtion, DC; 2010.

[22] Douglas PS. Echocardiography in the PARTNER Trial: Methodology and Findings. *22nd Annual Transcatheter Cardiovascular Therapeutics.* Washington, DC; 2010.

[23] Leon MB. Study Design and Baseline Patient Characteristics - on Behalf of the PARTNER Investigators. *22nd Annual Transcatheter Cardiovascular Therapeutics.* Washington, DC; 2010.

[24] Smith CR. PARTNER Trial: Study Outcomes, Conclusions, and Implications - On Behalf of PARTNER Trial Investigators. *22nd Annual Transcatheter Cardiovascular Therapeutics.* Washington, DC; 2010.

[25] Martin B Leon CRS, Michael Mack, D Craig Miller, Jeffrey W Moses, Lars G Svensson, E Murat Tuzcu, John G Webb, Gregory P Fontana, Raj R Makkar, David L

Brown, Peter C Block, Robert A Guyton, Augusto D Pichard, Joseph E Bavaria, Howard C Herrmann, Pamela S Douglas, John L Petersen, Jodi J Akin, William N Anderson, Duolao Wang, Stuart Pocock, PARTNER Trial Investigators. Supplementary Appendix: Transcatheter aortic-valve implantation for aortic stenosis in patients who cannot undergo surgery. *N Engl J Med.* 2010;363(17):1597-1607.

In: Percutaneous Valve Technology: Present and Future ISBN: 978-1-61942-577-4
Editors: Jose Luis Navia and Sharif Al-Ruzzeh

Chapter XI

Transapical Aortic Valve Implantation and the User Experience

Lars Svensson

Abstract

The field of percutaneous aortic valves has advanced rapidly and the PARTNER A and B trials have shown promising results with the second generation devices. We review our method for the transapical approach and some of the results from our research.

Introduction

The field of management of critical aortic valve stenosis has expanded rapidly, particularly with percutaneous aortic valves [1-23]. Aortic valve stenosis in the general population in the United States is increasing and indeed 2.2% of patients over the age of 75 have severe aortic valve stenosis as defined as $0.8cm^2$ or smaller aortic orifice. Cardiac surgeons are increasingly operating on older patients and the number of patients that are not undergoing surgery appears to vary across the country. Data from Southern California shows that approximately two-thirds of patients with severe aortic valve stenosis do not undergo aortic valve replacement despite the fact that aortic valve replacement is one of the most successful cardiovascular procedures there is as far as improving quality of life and also longevity. In Europe, a similar high rate of not operating on severe aortic valve stenosis also has been reported. Part of the reason for these patients not undergoing surgery are because of comorbidity, patients being elderly and frail, and patients or their families not wishing to proceed with a procedure. This is despite the fact that in patients with symptomatic aortic valve stenosis only approximately 40% will be alive within a year of developing symptoms associated with severe aortic valve stenosis. Of interest the classic Ross-Braunwald curve of survival after development of symptoms still holds true based on an analysis on patients with severe aortic valve stenosis in the Medicare population. Indeed in the PARTNER B transcatheter Aortic Valve Replacement (TAVR) trial, only 50% of medically treated patients were alive at 1 year. [16]

In the late 1980s, H. R. Andersen from Denmark did some experimental work in animals with a tri-leaflet stented valve that was inserted in the aortic valve position. This he patented and the patent was bought subsequently by the PVT Company. This was further developed and resulted in the insertion in humans by Cribier of a percutaneous aortic valve in April 2002. The initial approach was through the femoral vein and transeptal puncture and then snaking the valve through the left ventricle into the aortic valve position and deploying the valve there with a balloon inflatable system. Some earlier attempts were made in the United States with this technique but the technique was quickly abandoned because of the complications. [6-17]

In late 2004 and 2005 the transapical approach of insertion of the valve (TA-TAVR) was studied in the animal model by Dewey and Mack and Svensson in sheep and pigs. It became clear that the transapical approach was a good approach for inserting the valves and this resulted in further animal studies in Leipzig with a plan to insert the first transapical aortic valve in Leipzig. This subsequently happened and lead to the expansion and development of the transapical approach. At the same time John Webb and colleagues in Vancouver were also working on the transfemoral (TF-TAVR) arterial approach with a retrograde catheter that was flexible to approach the aortic valve after passing through the aortic arch. The early success of the Vancouver group lead by Webb with both the insertion of the transfemoral and the transapical approach led to further research in the United States on the two new techniques. [6-17]

Initial United States Experience

In July 2008, after presentation at the Society of Thoracic Surgery Meeting in January of 2008, the complete results of the United States feasibility study was reported in the Annals of Thoracic Surgery. [17] Between December 2006 and February 2008 forty patients underwent a transcatheter insertion of a balloon expandable stainless steel stent with an internally mounted three leaflet pericardial valve developed by Edwards Lifesciences called the Sapien valve. This was deployed into the aortic annulus using a transapical left ventricle insertion approach with rapid pacing of the left ventricle during deployment of the balloon expandable stent. For entry into the study the patients had to be inoperable by conventional surgical methods or had to have an STS score calculated risk of death exceeding 15% or other documented risk factors which made surgery prohibitive, such as radiation heart disease or cirrhosis. Indeed 50% of the patients had previously had coronary artery bypass surgery or a large portion had peripheral vascular disease or had undergone previous coronary artery stent insertion or had in addition severe lung disease. This resulted in one of the highest risk group of patients of who have been studied for cardiovascular device procedures.

Of the forty patients in the study all the valves were successfully delivered and in thirty-five patients the valve was also successfully seated in the aortic annulus. Two patients had valves that embolized soon after insertion and required open aortic valve replacement and subsequently one patient who had severe aortic valve regurgitation around the prosthesis required an open aortic valve replacement. In two patients the hemodynamics instability required the patients to be placed on cardio-pulmonary bypass and in one of these patients the valve embolized and the other the valve migrated. There were seven deaths within thirty days for a mortality rate of 17.5% and a further two patients died before discharge at forty-two days and the other at seventy-two days after surgery, for a total of nine deaths. There were no immediate post-operative strokes in this series of patients with successful valve seating, however, one patient developed a stroke a few days after surgery related to atrial fibrillation that could not adequately be treated with anti-coagulants and one patient who had a porcelain aorta had to have an open replacement of the aortic valve and had a severe post-operative stroke. Hemodynamic performance in these patients showed marked improvement. The cross sectional area of the aortic valve improved from a mean of .62 cm^2 (standard deviation of 0.13) to 1.61 cm^2 (standard deviation of .37). This was highly significant at a P value of less than 0.0001. The mean perivalvular degree of regurgitation was 1.19 with a standard deviation of 0.8. The mean follow up in this series of patients was 143 days with standard deviation of 166. There were six further deaths related to comorbid disease and none of them were related to valvular or cardiac factors. The Kaplan-Meier survival curve at one month was 81.8% +/- 6.2% and 71.7% +/- 7.7% after three months. This trial clearly showed that the transapical approach was a feasible method of insertion of percutaneous aortic valves and that justified continuing with a prospective randomized trial called the PARTNER trial (Placement of Aortic Transcatheter Valve).

Subsequent studies in Leipzig showed that with reduction in the preoperative risk profile of the patients undergoing transapical valve insertion, the long term survival was improved since fewer patients were dying from their comorbid disease. Indeed the mortality rate at Leipzig with some three hundred patients has stabilized at approximately at 4%.

The United States feasibility study, while it showed the transapical approach could be used, it was hampered by the requirement that only twenty patients initially could be done before the FDA first reviewed the study and assessed the outcome. Thereafter the protocols had to be resubmitted to IRB for another twenty patients. This meant that there was a six month hiatus in between the two phases that clearly effected outcomes because teams had to re-learn the procedure. In addition the patients were extremely high risk for a surgical procedure including mini-thoracotomy.

During the same approximate time interval the feasibility trial in the United States was also undertaken with the transfemoral arterial approach. In this study 55 patients were enrolled in the feasibility trial at three centers. [17] The risk profile was not quite as high as the transapical approach and in addition the patients did not have severe peripheral vascular disease since they had to have access through the femoral arteries. In the 55 patients studied for the transfemoral retrograde approach the mortality was 7%, stroke 9% and 13% developed concurrent vascular injuries. [17] Nevertheless, once again, the trial showed that the transfemoral approach was feasible and that the results were probably improved with further experience.

Both the Edwards Sapein valve and the Medtronic Core valve were successful in very early obtaining European CE certification which allowed for the rapid expansion and sale of the devices in Europe. The price was approximately 20,000 euros per valve ($30,000 US dollar). This lead to the rapid deployment of the valve across Europe and the development of much more experience of the procedures although the collection of data and the follow up of patients was not as accurate as the FDA approved trials in the United States.

Partner Trial

The PARTNER trial was structured with two sub groups namely Group B, in which the patients who were inoperable by conventional means, or had a calculated risk of death or severe comorbidity exceeding 50%. [16] The other group was Group A, which were the patients who were high risk for surgery with a STS score exceeding 10 and a surgeon's estimate of mortality rate exceeding 15%. These patients were further divided according to whether they had access via the groins to either a transfemoral or transapical approach depending on whether the patient had peripheral access or not. The control group in the Group A arm were the patients who had conventional open surgery. In the PARTNER trial 690 patients were assigned to Group A and 350 patients to Group B. Entry criteria included that the patients had to have a valve area of less then 0.8cm^2 and symptoms related to their disease. There were also various entry and exclusion criteria. The Group B arm of the PARTNER trial was completed in mid March of 2009 and with one year plus thirty days of follow up the trial was completed in April of 2010. After completion of the trial the FDA allowed patients who were randomized to the control medical treatment arm to cross over into the device arm. Thus, those patients who survived over a year were allowed to cross over in treatment with a transfemoral approach. The PARTNER B trial showed the superiority of TAVR to medical treatment as far as survival and hospital readmission. Indeed 2 year survival was 67% better (delta) than medical treatment. [16] The Group A arm of the study was completed on the 18th of August of 2009 for enrollment in the trial. Follow up was completed at the end of 2010. The PARTNER A trial was a non-inferiority Trial and showed that in these high risk (average age 83 years, STS score 11%) patients, both TF-TAVR and TA-TAVR were non-inferior to the open control arms. [19] For the TA-TAVR group, the risk of stroke/TIA was also non-inferior, however, in the TF-TAVR group, the risk of stroke/TIA was three times higher (4.6% versus 1.4%, p=0.05).

Transapical Surgical Technique

Clearly the transapical approach for insertion has evolved over time but some common features have been developed by us at the Cleveland Clinic, Medical City in Dallas, Columbia in New York, and Leipzig. [17] At the same time Vancouver also developed a transapical approach that is very similar to the techniques used in most centers nowadays.

At the Cleveland Clinic there are some differences in the way we do the procedure that we believe have contributed to our success with the approach. Preoperative testing of all our patients is extensive prior to their procedure and includes cardiac catherization with pelvic vessel imaging and if needed by IVUS; CT scan of chest/abdomen and pelvis including careful examination of the aortic valve leaflets and the potential for them including the coronary artery and groin access; extensive pulmonary function testing with arterial blood gases; echocardiography to meet entry criteria; STS scoring; blood work with particular emphasis on the creatinine level; and the careful examination and evaluation in particularly for frailty and biological age prior to the procedures.

Currently the criteria require that the patients have a valve area of less than 0.8cm^2, a peak gradient exceeding 64 mm Hg or mean gradient of exceeding 40 mm Hg or a velocity exceeding 4 m/s. Patients require 2 of these 3 for entry into the continued access part of the trial. Patients must also have a STS score of approximately 10 but certainly more than 8 which is somewhat mitigated by the comorbid disease. Patients who are in Group B who have severe contraindications to cardiac surgery such as for example radiation heart disease or cirrhosis will be considered for the inoperable arm even though the STS score may not be as high as in the patients who are enrolled in the high risk surgical arm (Group A). Patients also cannot have severe renal dysfunctional namely dialysis or have a creatinine exceeding 3.0. The patients must also have no ongoing sepsis within 30 days of surgery and must not have undergone a coronary artery PCI procedure within 30 days of the procedure if a bare metal stent was used. If a drug eluting stent was used, then the period is 6 months. Patients also have to have a qualifying echo within two weeks of the procedure and the procedure has to be carried out within two weeks of presenting the patient to the national panel. Thus, most patients are over the age of 85 with comorbid disease and have frequently had coronary bypass surgery prior to being accepted into the study. Indeed a healthy 90 year old that has no comorbid disease but has undergone artery bypass surgery will often not be eligible for this study.

Operative Procedure

During the operation we position two towels under the pelvis and the shoulders and another one under the length of the vertebral column and drape the patient so they are somewhat elevated from the table but horizontal on the table. Some of the centers place the patient in a thoracotomy position but we have not done so since prior to the procedure, since we obtain the best angles of the aortic root that show the nadir of each sinus in the same position so that the valve can be accurately positioned prior to inflation of the balloon. This is checked both on CT scan and on angiography. Prior to cleaning and draping the patient, the patient is palpated for the left ventricular apex heave, if it is present. In addition, if needed, a transthoracic echo is performed to identify the best site for approaching apex of the left ventricle. A decision is then made on which intercostal space to use for entry. Once the patient is draped the intercostal space is entered and the apex of the left ventricle palpated. Based on the experience with MID-CAB operations we will often resect a piece of rib over the left ventricle apex to get the best possible exposure without having to stretch the intercostal muscles and thus produce later post operative chest pain.

The apex of the left ventricle is then identified and the pericardium opened and retracted. We then place three purse string sutures, two of them circumferentially and one as a horizontal mattress in the left ventricle apex using multiple pledgets with the purse string approximately one inch in diameter. At the same time a cutdown is made on the best femoral artery for potentially putting the patient on pump, with wires placed in the artery and the femoral vein. If the femoral artery is so heavily diseased and flow from below would be impossible in the case of trying to rescue the patient, a side graft is sewn onto the left subclavian artery for arterial in flow after heparinization. In addition, a percutaneous catheter is inserted into the femoral vein for the percutaneous transfemoral pacing wire that is fed into the right ventricle. A pig tail arterial catheter is placed in the other femoral artery and positioned in the aortic root.

The patient is then heparinized. The apex of the left ventricle is tapped with a finger prior to placing the purse string sutures to make sure the apex is identified and that the alignment with the aortic valve is on axis. This is often confirmed again after placing the purse string sutures.

A needle is then placed into the left ventricle apex and checked for arterial blood ejection. A short guide wire is then inserted into the left ventricle followed by a Cook size-14 dilator and sheath. The dilator is then withdrawn and with echo guidance a Berman catheter is then placed in the left ventricle cavity after withdrawing the wire, the balloon inflated, and then fed across the aortic valve into the ascending aorta and floated around the aortic arch down to the descending aorta. An extra stiff wire is then fed through this balloon catheter sheath down to approximately the renal arteries and then the balloon deflated and the catheter removed.

There is some variability as to when the large bore sheath is inserted but more recently we have gone to inserting the large bore delivery sheath at this point with the dilator over the guide wire into the left ventricle using the fluoroscopy for screening. This allows for quicker valve insertion if the patient becomes unstable after ballooning. The dilator is then withdrawn and the balloon for dilation of the stenotic aortic valve is then inserted. We have used balloons of various lengths but mostly use a 4cm 20mm diameter balloon for cracking the calcium in the aortic valve. This is done with breath holding and rapid pacing of the heart typically at 180 bpms and with either fluoroscopy or cine during the procedure. In patients who do not have elevated creatinine we will often also inject contrast in the aortic root with a pigtail to make sure that the left main coronary artery is not also occluded during inflation of the balloon. Typically only one inflation is required and the balloon is then withdrawn. The pacing is stopped and the patient is ventilated again. The stented valve device at this point is being crimped on the back table and is checked for correct orientation in the loader. This is then loaded onto the end of the sheath and pushed into the left ventricle. Prior to doing this, the sheath is de-aired as is the sheath for pushing the valve into position. The valve is then pushed out of the large bore sheath to the aortic valve and the aortic valve crossed and the so called "pusher" then withdrawn into the large bore sheath.

In most patients the large bore sheath is aimed at approximately the right shoulder to get the correct alignment on axis with the aortic valve. We typically do a dry run to make sure everything is checked and there is not much movement during breath holding and during rapid pacing. The sequence is holding a patients breath and rapid pacing the heart, turning on the cine and seeing if the position of the valve device changes in relation to the hinge points of the native aortic valve. Echocardiography is very important during a procedure to also check positioning of the new valve device. A root aortogram is also done at this time. The pacing is then stopped and the patient allowed to breathe again.

Once again positioning of the device is carefully performed to make sure both on the echo and the fluoroscopy it is in the correct position. We previously placed the valve 60% ventricle but we have more recently placed the valve 50/50 as far as the hinge points of leaflets for the transapical approach. With the transfemoral approach we tend to still use approximately 60% ventricle. The sequence is then repeated after withdrawing the pigtail to approximately to sinotubular junction and the balloon inflated. We previously inflated the balloon rapidly but have found it useful, as others have noted, that slower inflation allows for repositioning of the valve as expansion of the balloon occurs to make sure that the hinge points are correctly positioned in relation to the new stent valve. In addition if the balloon inflates on the aortic side first and the sinotubular junction is somewhat reduced this can so call "watermelon seed" the balloon and valve into the left ventricle and with a slower inflation of the balloon this can be corrected during the period of inflation. Immediately after deployment the balloon is withdrawn into the left ventricle, the pacing is stopped and the patient is allowed to breath. Attention is then turned to the echocardiogram to make sure that there is no severe aortic valve regurgitation. If there is severe peri-valve regurgitation we will sometimes do a repeat balloon inflation or insert another valve in valve. Indeed we have done eight valve in valve in patients who have had, typically, leaflets that do not function correctly or the valve height position is not quiet correct. An aortic root aortogram is then performed with the pigtail catheter and the device removed. We like to slip the Berman catheter back in over the wire and into the ascending aorta during wire removal so that the risk of the wires catching the struts of the percutaneous valves during withdrawal are reduced. In most patients we will leave the percutaneous femoral pacing wire in position over night and remove it the following day. Hemostasis is then obtained in the usual manner with one of the two chest tubes in the pleural cavity. The patients are placed on Plavix and returned to intensive care unit and extubated as soon as possible.

With this approach we have seen improved results with the transapical approach over time. Indeed as also with the transfemoral approach, we have been very satisfied with our results but continue to work towards improved results.

Future Partner Trials

The development of a new valve and delivery system has resulted in the FDA requiring a further PARTNER II trial for evaluation of the new device and delivery system. Hence, a new PARTNER Group B II protocol will become available with the entry criteria somewhat similar to the first PARTNER Group B protocol. The PARTNER II Group A protocol will probably become available towards the end 2011 and will likely include patients at lower risk for entry into the study.

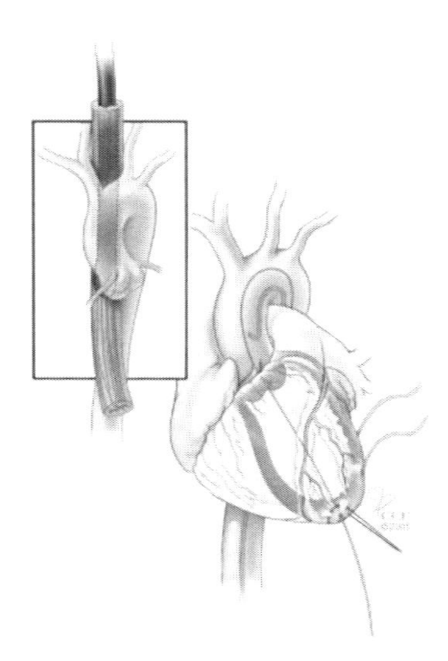

Figure 1. Placement of apical purse strings, guide wire, and transesophageal echocardiogram probe.

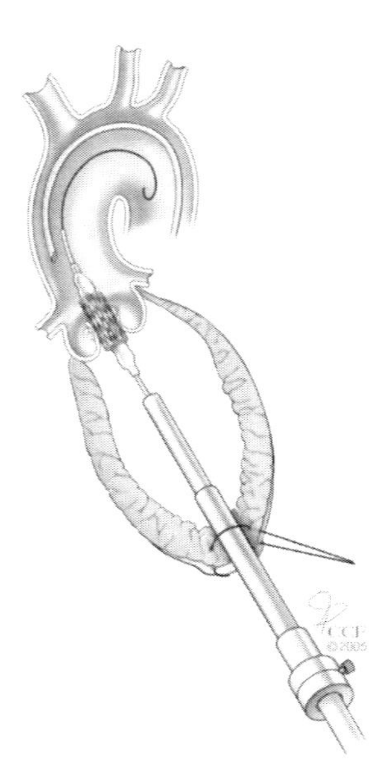

Figure 2. Insertion of delivery sheath and valve positioning.

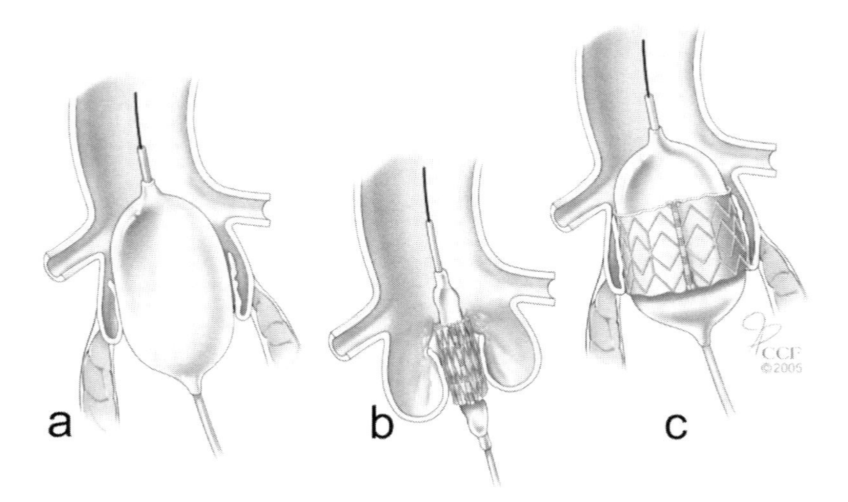

Figure 3. Steps for valve deployment a) Balloon valvuloplasty b) Device positioning, c) Balloon inflation and device deployment.

Conclusion

The rapid development of the percutaneous valve technologies both for transfemoral and transapical approach has been much more rapid than what would have been expected and more so than the initial animal studies would have suggested. Approximately 40,000 patients have had the procedure done. The unanswered questions will be the long term durability of the device and whether health insurance systems and governments will be able to afford the costs of the procedures. In PARTNER B the cost of the procedure was $78,000.00. Clearly the percutaneous valves meet the criteria for a successful aortic valve procedure namely ease of insertion, safety of insertion, and excellent effective orifice area. The criteria of durability will likely be not that different from the current pericardial valves since the stented Sapien Edwards device is made with the same leaflet material. Furthermore, a repeat valve in valve insertion is not difficult. The additional years of life and quality of life that this new device has brought to patients and will continue to contribute to the well being of the general population with congestive heart failure and the results after the initial animal studies have been gratifying to see.

References

[1] Svensson LG, Blackstone EH, Cosgrove DM 3rd. Surgical options in young adults with aortic valve disease. *Curr Probl Cardiol*. 2003; 417-80.

[2] Feldman T, Kar S, Rinaldi M, Fail P, Hermiller J, Smalling R, Whitlow PL, Gray W, Low R, Herrmann HC, Lim S, Foster E, Glower D; EVEREST Investigators. Percutaneous mitral repair with the MitraClip system: safety and midterm durability in the initial EVEREST (Endovascular Valve Edge-to-Edge Repair Study) cohort. *J Am Coll Cardiol*. 2009; 686-94.

[3] Mihaljevic T, Jarrett CM, Gillinov AM, Williams SJ, DeVilliers PA, Stewart WJ, Svensson LG, Sabik JF 3rd, Blackstone EH. Robotic repair of posterior mitral valve prolapse versus conventional approaches: potential realized. *J thorac Cardiovasc Surg*. 2011; 141(1):72-80

[4] Svensson LG, Atik FA, Cosgrove Dm, Blackstone EH, Rajeswaran J, Krishnaswamy G, Jin U, Gillinov AM, Griffin B, Navia JL, Mihaljevic T, Lytle BW. Minimally invasive versus conventional mitral valve surgery: a propensity-matched comparison; *J Thorac Cardiovasc Surg*. 2010; 139(4):926-32

[5] Mauri L, Garg P, Massaro JM, Foster E, Glower D, Mehoudar P, Powell F, Komtebedde J, McDermott E, Fledman T. The EVEREST II Trial: design and rationale for a randomized study of the evalve mitraclip system compared with mitral valve surgery for mitral regurgitation. *Am Heart J* 2010; 160(1):23-9

[6] Bleiziffer S, Ruge H, Mazzitelli D et al. Survival after transapical and transfemoral aortic valve implantation: talking about two different patient populations. *J Thorac Cardiovasc Surg* 2009;138:1073-80.

[7] Himbert D, Descoutures F, Al-Attar N et al. Results of transfemoral or transapical aortic valve implantation following a uniform assessment in high-risk patients with aortic stenosis. *J Am Coll Cardiol* 2009;54:303-11.

[8] Webb JG, Altwegg L, Boone RH et al. Transcatheter aortic valve implantation: impact on clinical and valve-related outcomes. *Circulation* 2009;119:3009-16.

[9] Thielmann M, Wendt D, Eggebrecht H, Kahlert P, Massoudy P, Kamler M, et al. Transcatheter aortic valve implantation in patients with very high risk for conventional aortic valve replacement. *Ann Thorac Surg* 2009;88:1468-74

[10] Rodes-Cabau J, Webb JG, Cheung A et al. Transcatheter aortic valve implantation for the treatment of severe symptomatic aortic stenosis in patients at very high or prohibitive surgical risk: acute and late outcomes of the multicenter Canadian experience. *J Am Coll Cardiol* 2010;55:1080-90

[11] Osten MK, Feindel C, Greutmann M, Chamberlain K, Meineri M, Rubin B, Mezodi M, Ivanov J, Butany J, Horlick EM. Transcatheter aortic valve implantation for high risk patients with severe aortic stenosis using the Edwards Sapien balloon-expandable bioprosthesis. A single centre study with immediate and medium-term outcomes. *Cath Cardiovasc Interv* 2010; 75:475–485

[12] Eltchaninoff H, Prat A, Gilard M, Leguerrier A, Blanchard D, Fournial G, Iung B, Donzeau-Gouge P, Tribouilloy C, Debrux JL, Pavie A, Gueret P. Transcatheter aortic valve implantation: Early results of the FRANCE (FRench Aortic National CoreValve and Edwards) registry. *Eur Heart J* 2010. Published online ahead of print 15 September 2010; doi:10.1093/eurheartj/ehq261.

[13] Thomas M, Schymik G, Walther T, et al. Thirty-Day Results of the SAPIEN aortic bioprosthesis European Outcome (SOURCE) Registry. A European Registry of transcatheter aortic valve implantation using the Edwards SAPIEN valve. *Circulation* 2010;122:62 9.

[14] Johansson M, Nozohoor S, Kimblad PO, Harnek J, Göran K, Olivecrona GK and Johan Sjögren J. Transapical Versus Transfemoral Aortic Valve Implantation: A Comparison of Survival and Safety. *Ann Thorac Surg* 2011;91:57–63

[15] Kodali SK, O'Neill WW, Moses JW, Williams M, Smith CR, Tuzcu M, Svensson LG, Kapadia S, Hanzel G, Kirtane AJ, Leon MB. Early and Late (One Year) Outcomes Following Transcatheter Aortic Valve Implantation in Patients With Severe Aortic Stenosis (from the United States REVIVAL Trial). *Am J Cardiol.* 2011 Apr 1;107(7):1058-64.

[16] Leon MB, Smith CR, Mack M, Miller DC, Moses JW, Svensson LG, Tuzcu EM, Webb JG, Fontana GP, Makkar RR, Brown DL, Block PC, Guyton RA, Pichard AD, Bavaria JE, Herrmann HC, Douglas PS, Petersen JL, Akin JJ, Anderson WN, Wang D, Pocock S; PARTNER Trial Investigators. Transcatheter aortic-valve implantation for aortic stenosis in patients who cannot undergo surgery. *N Engl J Med.* 2010 Oct 21;363(17):1597-607.

[17] Svensson LG, Dewey T, Kapadia S, Roselli EE, Stewart A, Williams M, Anderson WN, Brown D, Leon M, Lytle B, Moses J, Mack M, Tuzcu M, Smith C. United States feasibility study of transcatheter insertion of a stented aortic valve by the left ventricular apex. *Ann Thorac Surg.* 2008 Jul;86(1):46-54; discussion 54-5.

[18] Ewe SH, Delgado V, Ng AC, Antoni ML, van der Kley F, Marsan NA, de Weger A, Tavilla G, Holman ER, Schalij MJ, Bax JJ. Outcomes After Transcatheter Aortic Valve Implantation: Transfemoral Versus Transapical Approach. Ann Thorac Surg. 2011 Mar 19. [Epub ahead of print] Ewe etal; *Ann Thorac Surg*

[19] http://my.americanheart.org/idc/groups/ahamah-public/@wcm/@sop/@scon/documents/downloadable/ucm 425332.pdf/

[20] Svensson LG; Evolution and results of aortic valve surgery, and a 'disruptive' technology; *Cleveland Clin J Med*; 2008; Nov 75(11)802,804.

[21] O'Brien Sm, Shahian DM, Filardo G, Ferraris VA, Haan Ck, Rich JB, Normand SL, DeLong ER, Shewan CM, Dokholyan RS, Peterson ED, Edwards FH, Anderson RP;

Society of Thoracic Surgeons Quality Measurement Task Force. The Society of Thoracic Surgeons 2008 Cardiac surgery risk models: part 2—isolated valve surgery. *Ann Thorac Surg* 2009; Jul; 88(1 Suppl):S23-42.

[22] Bapat V, Thomas M, Hancock J, Wilson K; First Successful trans-catheter aortic valve implantation through ascending aorta using Edwards SAPIEN THV system. *Eur J Cardiothorac Surg* 2010; Dec;38(6):811-3.

[23] Kapadia SR, Goel SS, Svensson L, Roselli E, Savage RM, Wallace L, Sola S, Schoenhagen P, Shishenhbor MH, Christofferson R, Halley C, Rodriguez LL, Stewart W, Kalahasti V, Tuzcu EM. Characterization and outcome of patients with severe symptomatic aortic stenosis referred for percutaneous aortic valve replacement. *J Thorac Cardiovasc Surg* 2009 Jun;137(6):1430-5.

In: Percutaneous Valve Technology: Present and Future ISBN: 978-1-61942-577-4
Editors: Jose Luis Navia and Sharif Al-Ruzzeh

Chapter XII

Percutaneous Aortic Valve – The Canadian Experience: Present and Future Perspectives

Gilbert H. L. Tang, Mark Osten, Eric Horlick and Christopher M. Feindel

Abstract

Canada has been at the forefront of transcatheter aortic valve intervention (TAVI) since its initial inception. Both Edwards' balloon expandable valve and Medtronic's self expanding Corevalve have been used in different Canadian centers. Experience in transfemoral and transapical approaches, as well as valve-in-valve procedures have been reported. Combined multi-center experience with the Edwards valve demonstrates favorable short- and mid-term outcomes similar to those reported in Europe and the Placement of AoRTic TraNscathetER Valve B (PARTNER B) trial. In a publicly funded health care system, access to transcatheter valves has been restricted to the Special Access Program and requires case by case approval by Health Canada. Funding of most Canadian TAVI programs is currently through non-governmental sources and remains a significant challenge. Nonetheless, this emerging therapy will remain an important option for high risk inoperable patients and Canada will continue to play a leading role in the innovation and adoption of transcatheter valve technologies.

Introduction

Canadians were among the first groups in the world to report their experience with TAVI, with the Cribier-Edwards valve first implanted in January 2005 [1] and the Medtronic CoreValve first implanted in March 2005 [2].

Table 1. A summary of approximate case numbers among Canadian centers on transcatheter aortic valve intervention (as of December 2011, unless stated otherwise)

Institution	Edwards (Transfemoral)	Edwards (Transapical)	Medtronic CoreValve
Alberta Heart Institute, Edmonton	7	37	0
Centre Hopitalier d'Universite de Montreal	27	14	0
Hamilton General Hospital, Hamilton, Ontario (9/2010)	24	17	0
London Health Sciences Centre, London, Ontario	0	2	11
Montreal Heart Institute, Montreal, Quebec	12	30	155
New Brunswick Heart Centre, Saint John, New Brunswick	14	20	0
Ottawa Heart Institute, Ottawa, Ontario	12	20	140
Quebec Heart and Lung Institute, Laval, Quebec	86	154	0
Royal Victoria Hospital, Montreal, Quebec (9/2010)	10	18	8
St. Michael's Hospital, Toronto, Ontario (9/2010)	16	16	0
St. Paul's Hospital, Vancouver, British Columbia	321	175	13
Sunnybrook Health Sciences Centre, Toronto, Ontario	9	0	85
Toronto General Hospital, Toronto, Ontario	33	86	25

In Canada, both valves require special approval by the Department of Health and Welfare from the Federal government (Health Canada), for compassionate clinical use in patients deemed not suitable for surgery. Thus far, over 1100 Edwards valves and over 400 Medtronic Corevalves have been implanted in this country (Table 1). This chapter will review the pan-Canadian experience of TAVI, including techniques and outcomes from selected centres. We will discuss the regulatory process of how the transcatheter valves are approved for clinical use, and how the TAVI programs are funded at individual institutions. Finally, we will present a Canadian perspective of the future directions of TAVI.

A Brief History of Transcatheter Valves in Canada

Canada is known for a number of notable firsts in transcatheter valve intervention in North America. The first transcatheter Melody pulmonic valve implantation was performed in November 2005 at the Hospital for Sick Children by Benson, Horlick, and colleagues. The first Evalve Mitraclip was performed in September 2006 via a transseptal approach at Toronto General Hospital.

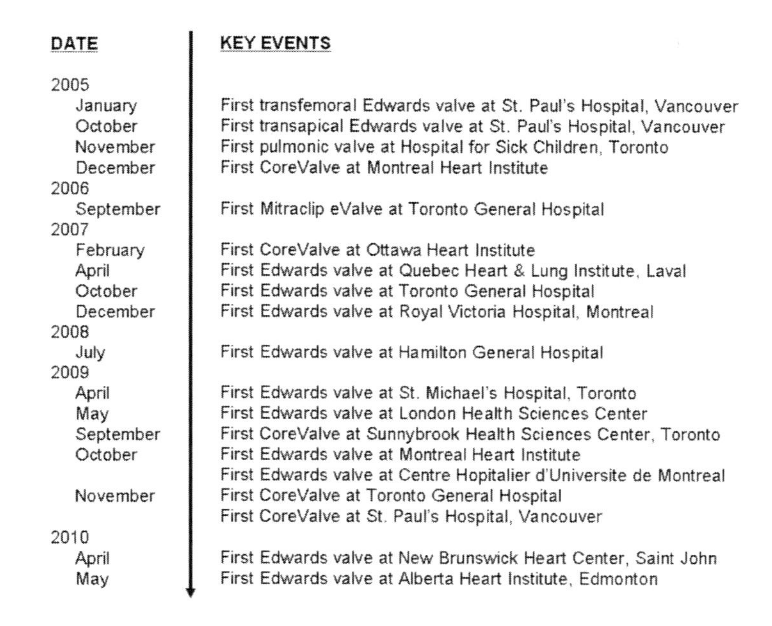

DATE	KEY EVENTS
2005	
January	First transfemoral Edwards valve at St. Paul's Hospital, Vancouver
October	First transapical Edwards valve at St. Paul's Hospital, Vancouver
November	First pulmonic valve at Hospital for Sick Children, Toronto
December	First CoreValve at Montreal Heart Institute
2006	
September	First Mitraclip eValve at Toronto General Hospital
2007	
February	First CoreValve at Ottawa Heart Institute
April	First Edwards valve at Quebec Heart & Lung Institute, Laval
October	First Edwards valve at Toronto General Hospital
December	First Edwards valve at Royal Victoria Hospital, Montreal
2008	
July	First Edwards valve at Hamilton General Hospital
2009	
April	First Edwards valve at St. Michael's Hospital, Toronto
May	First Edwards valve at London Health Sciences Center
September	First CoreValve at Sunnybrook Health Sciences Center, Toronto
October	First Edwards valve at Montreal Heart Institute
	First Edwards valve at Centre Hopitalier d'Universite de Montreal
November	First CoreValve at Toronto General Hospital
	First CoreValve at St. Paul's Hospital, Vancouver
2010	
April	First Edwards valve at New Brunswick Heart Center, Saint John
May	First Edwards valve at Alberta Heart Institute, Edmonton

Figure 1. A chronology of transcatheter valve implantation in Canadian centers.

Prior to the development of the Edwards Sapien valve, the Cribier-Edwards aortic valve was first implanted in North America via a transfemoral approach by Webb and colleagues in January 2005 at St. Paul's Hospital in Vancouver [1]. Later that year in October, Ye and colleagues from Vancouver reported the first transapical implantation of the Cribier-Edwards aortic valve [3]. In the meantime, the first North American implant of the Medtronic CoreValve was performed in December 2005 by Bonan and colleagues at the Montreal Heart Institute [4]. A timeline of the Canadian clinical development of transcatheter valves is outlined in Figure 1.

Transcatheter Aortic Valve by Edwards Lifesciences

Experience at the St. Paul's Hospital, Vancouver

Transfemoral Approach

The first Canadian transfemoral AVI series was reported by Webb and colleagues at St. Paul's Hospital using the transfemoral approach [1]. The rationale to use a retrograde, transfemoral approach was based on the limitations associated with the antegrade, transvenous approach originally described by Cribier and colleagues [5]. Beginning in January 2005, the TAVI option was considered for Canadian patients with symptomatic severe aortic stenosis who had multiple co-morbidities and excessive surgical risks. A team of cardiologists, cardiac surgeons and multidisciplinary staff discuss each patient to agree that surgery is not an option. In addition, patient's preference alone toward TAVI is not considered sufficient for the procedure, if the patient is deemed a surgical candidate. Patients are excluded if they are considered eligible for open aortic valve replacement, if anatomic criteria are not met (aortic annulus diameter needs to be between 18 and 25 mm), or if limited life expectancy or quality of life is expected [6].

Pre-procedural investigations include transthoracic echocardiography, iliofemoral contrast angiography and coronary angiography. Computed tomographic (CT) angiography is considered if the patient has borderline arterial access. The procedure is performed in a catheterization laboratory or a multipurpose operating room (Figure 2). The femoral artery is accessed percutaneously and patients receive systemic heparin at 100U/kg. After balloon valvuloplasty and valve deployment, valve positioning is assessed both by aortic root angiography and echocardiography. Aortoiliac angiography is performed at the end of the procedure to check for vascular injury. In the early series, the femoral access site was closed surgically. Later, percutaneous closure with the Prostar XL device or ProGlide device (Abbott Inc, Chicago, IL) was used instead.

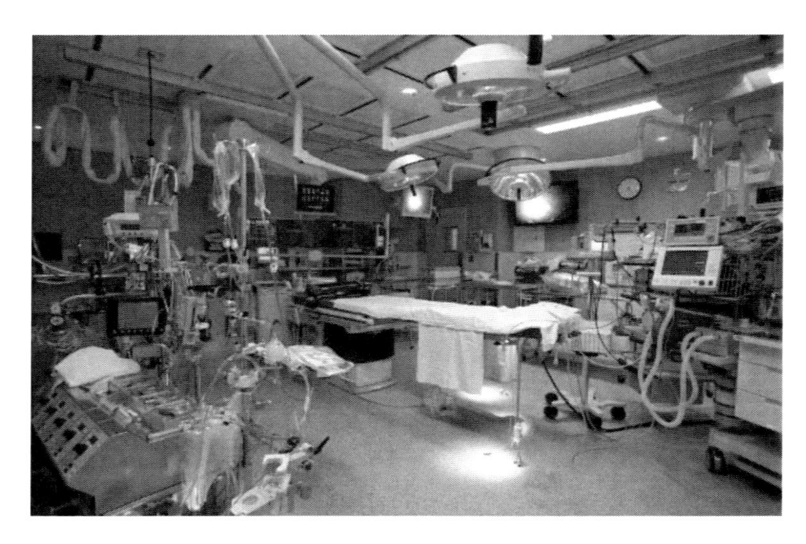

Figure 2. Photo of the hybrid operating room at St. Paul's Hospital, Vancouver (ceiling mounted C-arm imaging system not shown).

The Vancouver transfemoral AVI series were first reported for the initial 18 patients in 2006 [1] and the one-year follow-up of the first 50 patients was reported in 2007 [7]. Among the 50 patients, the mean Logistic European System for Cardiac Operative Risk Evaluation (EuroSCORE) risk score for procedural mortality was 28%[Comment: no STS score available in this paper]. Procedural success increased from 76% in the first 25 patients to 96% in the second 25, and 30-day mortality decreased from 16% to 8%. At one year, 17/43 patients who had a successful implant remained alive. Two patients sustained a stroke and two had sustained heart block requiring a permanent pacemaker. Three patients required reintervention for residual, ongoing symptomatic aortic stenosis: one had transapical AVI, one had transfemoral AVI and one had open aortic valve replacement.

Transapical Approach

The initial Vancouver experience on transapical AVI was reported on 7 patients who had the Cribier-Edwards valve [8]. Pre-procedural workup is performed similarly to that for the transfemoral AVI. A team of cardiologists and surgeons initially performed the transapical procedure in an operating room equipped with fluoroscopy, and subsequently in a hybrid multipurpose operating room (Figure 2). The procedure is done on a beating heart without cardiopulmonary bypass. Systemic heparinization is made with a target activated clotting time (ACT) of >250 seconds. A 5-8 cm left anterolateral thoracotomy is made via the sixth intercostal space and two pairs of orthogonally placed U-shaped pledgeted prolene purse string sutures are placed at the ventricular apex [9]. Temprorary rapid ventricular pacing is achieved with temporary epicardial pacer wires. After balloon valvuloplasty and valve deployment, the valve position was confirmed by both aortic root angiography and echocardiography. The purse string sutures are secured to close the ventricular apex access site.

The one and three-year transapical AVI experience in Vancouver were reported by Ye and colleagues [10, 11]. Thus far, approximately two-thirds of patients in Vancouver who were accepted for TAVI had their implant performed via the transfemoral approach, while one-third had transapical AVI. Of the 71 patients who received transapical TAVI, the mean EuroSCORE for procedural mortality was 35% and 12% by Society of Thoracic Surgeons (STS) Risk Calculator [11]. Twenty-eight patients received a 23 mm valve and 43 patients received a 26 mm valve. Procedural success was 100%. However, significant complications remain in this group of high risk patients. Two patients required a second valve-in-valve TAVI due to significant paravalular leak. One patient died in the operating room immediately after the procedure, probably due to occlusion of the left main coronary artery. One patient had a periprocedural cardiac arrest and was placed on cardiopulmonary bypass. While the valve was successfully deployed, that patient died of subsequent heart failure. Another patient had a perforation of the severely calcified aorta requiring emergency open surgery.

Overall, 12/71 patients died within the first 30 days, and 10 patients died subsequently of non-valve-related complications. The overall survival rate at 36 months was 58%. There were no valve-related complications, including structural deterioration. 78% of patients had paravalvular leak at follow-up, of which 5% were moderate. The degree of aortic insufficiency was unchanged and not clinically significant. Aortic valve area and mean gradients remained stable at 24 months. Despite an early learning curve, the mid-term outcomes were comparable to other reported transapical AVI series.

Combined Experience

Webb and colleagues recently compared their own institutional transfemoral and transapical AVI series [6]. Among the168 patients who had TAVI between January 2005 and April 2008, 113 were done transfemorally and 55 were done transapically. Patients in the transapical series had a significantly higher mean logistic EuroSCORE risk score (35% vs 25%, p=0.01) and STS risk score (10.3% vs 8.7%, p=0.02), previous myocardial infarction (84% vs 68%, p=0.03), and peripheral vascular disease (76% vs 16%, p<0.0001). After the procedure, transapical AVI patients had more new-onset atrial fibrillation (13% vs 0%, p<0.001), need for temporary hemodialysis (5.5% vs 0%, p=0.03) and longer median length of stay (7 vs 5 days, p<0.0001). In this series, the 30-day mortality between transapical and transfemoral AVI patients were not significantly different (18% vs 8%, p=0.07). Kaplan-Meier analyses show no significant differences in survival, valve-related events and hospital readmission rates at a maximum of >3 years between the two approaches.

Experience at the Laval Hospital, Quebec City

Rodes-Cabau and colleagues published their institutional experience on TAVI in 2008 [12]. The group devised selection criteria to determine if the patient will undergo transfemoral or transapical AVI (Table 2).

Table 2. The Quebec Heart and Lung Institute criteria for transfemoral vs transapical AVI*. A transapical approach is used if the patient has at least one of the following criteria

Criteria
Diameter of the femoral or iliac arteries <7 mm (23 mm valve) or <8 mm (26 mm valve) as determined by angiography
Significant stenosis or occlusion of both ilio-femoral arteries, or previous vascular bypass surgery
Severe calcification of both ilio-femoral arteries as determined by CT
Porcelain aorta
Horizontal ascending aorta

*Modified from [12].

Prospective TAVI candidates undergo systematic evaluation by a team of cardiologists, surgeons, anesthesiologists and internists. Imaging investigations consist of echocardiography, dobutamine stress echocardiography in stable patients with low left ventricular ejection fraction, coronary angiography, aortoiliofemoral angiography to evaluate femoral arterial diameters and CT to assess the degree of calcification of the aorta and vascular assess sites.

The transfemoral approach is performed in a similar fashion to other centers in the catheterization laboratory.

The femoral access site is surgically exposed at the beginning and closed at the end of the procedure. Valve positioning is confirmed under fluoroscopic, aortographic and echocardiographic guidance. In the transapical approach, the procedure is performed in the operating room under fluoroscopic and echocardiographic guidance. A Swan-Ganz pacing catheter is used for temporary rapid ventricular pacing. After valve deployment, the apex is closed with pledgeted Ethibond purse string sutures during rapid pacing.

From April 2007 to January 2008, 24 patients were found to be eligible for TAVI, of which 10 patients ultimately had a transfemoral AVI, while 12 patients underwent transapical AVI. Mean logistic EuroSCORE risk score for procedural mortality was 26%. Twelve patients received a 23 mm valve and 10 patients received a 26 mm valve. There was one intraprocedural death unrelated to valve positioning.

One patient received a second valve-in-valve due to severe aortic insufficiency after the initial implant. One patient had a tear in the ventricular apex after sheath removal, necessitating surgical repair under femoral-femoral cardiopulmonary bypass. In this series, there was one death due to pneumonia within the first 30 days. After a mean follow-up period of 6 months, there were no additional deaths or major complications. No strokes occurred in this series.

Experience at the Toronto General Hospital

We performed our first TAVI in January 2007. As of September 2010, we have implanted over 90 Edwards valves, 75 of which were via the transapical route. All patients who are assessed for TAVI at our institution are deemed to have a high surgical risk for open aortic valve replacement (estimated operative mortality >15%) by an experienced cardiac surgeon and a cardiologist. Prospective patients undergo the following imaging investigations to determine candidacy: aortoiliofemoral angiography, iliofemoral Doppler ultrasonography to determine the diameter of iliac and femoral arteries, coronary angiography, and transthoracic (TTE) and transesophageal (TEE) echocardiograms. All patients must have severe aortic stenosis as defined by the American Heart Association guidelines and at least NHYA Class III symptoms. In addition, the annular diameter is estimated from the parasternal long-axis view at the level of leaflet attachments on TTE, and a TEE annuluar measurement of <25 mm is considered the gold standard for approval for the procedure. In terms of exclusion from the transfemoral approach, patients would have at least either mobile aortic arch atheroma >5 mm or iliofemoral access precluding insertion of an 18 French sheath.

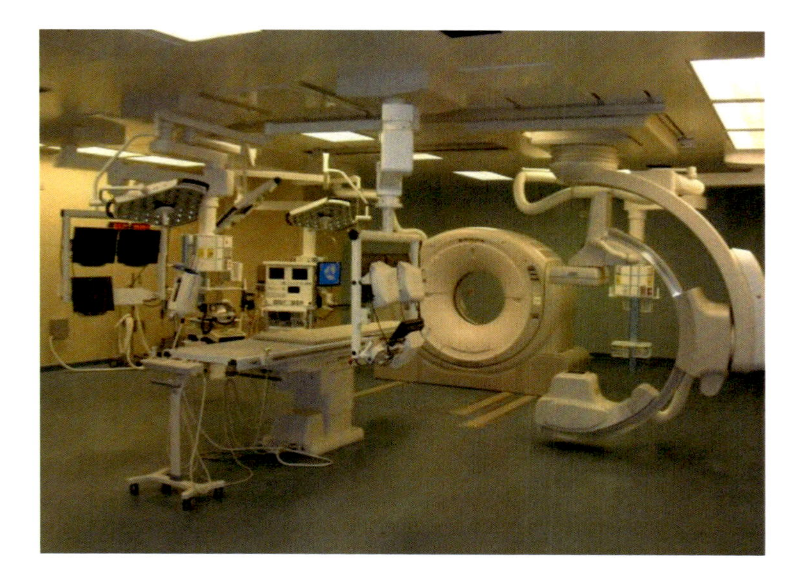

Figure 3. Photograph of the hybrid operating room at the Toronto General Hospital.

The transfemoral procedure was initially performed in the catheterization laboratory and the transapical procedure was performed in operating room. Subsequently all cases have been done in the hybrid multipurpose operating room (Figure 3). For the transfemoral approach, initially the femoral access site is closed surgically by our vascular surgical team. More recently, femoral access is made percutaneously and percutaneous devices (ProGlide, Abbott Inc, Chicago, IL) are used for vascular closure at the end of the procedure. Routine exit angiography is used to ensure the vasculature and access sites are not compromised. Our transapical approach is similar to that performed in Vancouver, except we use a high output pacing unit (Medtronic Inc model 2380) to ensure ventricular capture via temporary epicardial pacing wires during rapid pacing. In both approaches our target ACT after systemic heparinization is >300 seconds. In transapical AVI, we close the ventricular apex with pledgeted purse string sutures under temporary rapid pacing to minimize tension on the apex and ensure surgical hemostasis (Figure 4). To prevent acute severe mitral regurgitation from damage to the mitral valve from the valvuloplasty balloon, we routinely assess the mitral valve using TEE at baseline, after the wire crosses the aortic valve, after balloon introduction and before valve deployment – carefully noting changes in MR.

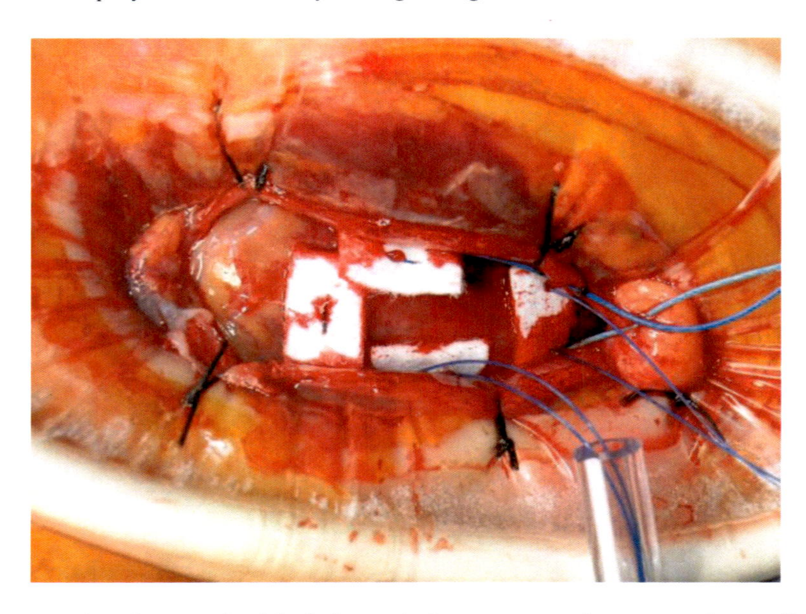

Figure 4. Intraoperative photograph of the left ventricular apex area where two orthogonally placed purse string sutures are placed. Temporary epicardial pacing wires (light blue) can be seen on the right side of the photo.

We recently reported the early- and mid-term results of our transfemoral and transapical series [13]. Until April 2009, 46 patients underwent TAVI procedures at our institution. 16 transfemoral AVI and 30 transapical AVI were performed. Our patient demographics between the two groups are similar. However, transfemoral AVI patients had more significant pulmonary hypertension (>60 mmHg), while transapical AVI patients had significantly higher incidence of chronic obstructive pulmonary disease and porcelain aorta. Mean logistic EuroSCORE and STS risk scores were comparable between the two groups (24% transfemoral vs 26% transapical, 7.2% vs 9.5% respectively).

Our procedural success in this series was 91% (88% transfemoral, 93% transapical). In our transfemoral procedures, one patient had difficulty crossing the native valve on a retroflex 1 delivery system due to the horizontal orientation of the aortic root. Another patient had a calcified obstruction of the external iliac artery precluding access, and so only a balloon valvuloplasty was performed. Subsequently, both patients underwent successful transapical AVI. In terms of transapical procedures, one valve (the first in the series) embolized to the aortic arch prior to deployment due to a faulty inflation device. This inflation device was later subject to a large scale recall by the company. The patient underwent emergency open aortic valve and hemiarch replacement, but subsequently died in the intensive care unit from a massive gastrointestinal bleed several weeks later from underlying cirrhosis. The second patient died of cardiac failure prior to valve deployment secondary to acute severe mitral regurgitation, likely from mitral subvalvular chordal entrapment during balloon valvuloplasty.

There were 4 in-hospital deaths, including one from an unrecognized iliac artery rupture. Access complications requiring reintervention occurred in 4 patients, including one patient who developed a ventricular pseudoaneurysm at the apical access site. Open surgical repair on cardiopulmonary bypass was required twice. Another patient from the transfemoral group required repair of a femoral pseudoaneurysm. Three patients from the transapical group and one from the transfemoral group required a permanent pacemaker. There were no myocardial infarctions, and 2/46 patients suffered a stroke.

39 patients (93%) survived during a mean follow-up of 7.4 months. The 3 late deaths were not cardiac or valve related. Both approaches had similar in-hospital and 30-day mortality rates. No other significant valve or access related complications were found. Only one patient had moderate paravalvular leak at 24 months follow-up. Most patients had a significant improvement in NYHA class, and aortic valve area and transvalvular mean gradient remained stable at 12 months.

Combined Experience in Canadian Centers

The multi-center Canadian experience of TAVI using the Cribier-Edwards and Edwards Sapien valves was recently published [14]. In addition to the above 3 centers, experience in St. Michael's Hospital in Toronto, Hamilton General Hospital and Royal Victorial Hospital in Montreal were included. The six centers reported their cases performed between January 2005 and June 2009, totaling 345 procedures performed in 339 patients. The 52 patients involved in the PARTNER trial were excluded. 168 transfemoral AVIs (1 repeat intervention) and 177 transapical AVIs (5 repeat interventions after transfemoral AVIs) were done. In addition to the aforementioned evaluation criteria for TAVI, frailty was used as a criterion for inoperability, after examination by the medical team and agreed upon by at least two cardiac surgeons.

In terms of valve selection, a 23 mm valve was implanted if the TEE measurement of the aortic annulus was between 17 and 21 mm, and a 26 mm valve was used if the annulus measured between 22 and 25 mm. The techniques for transfemoral and transapical AVIs were similar across institutions, and were detailed above and in published reports [1, 3, 8, 12, 13].

Early Outcomes

Procedural success among the 6 institutions was 93%. Procedural, post-procedural and 30-day mortality were 1.7% (N=6), 8.7% (N=30) and 10% (N=36), respectively. Aortic valve area and mean transvalvular gradient significantly increased (0.6 ± 0.2 cm2 to 1.6 ± 0.4 cm2, $p<0.0001$) and decreased (46 ± 17 mmHg to 10 ± 4 mmHg, $p<0.0001$), respectively. In the 61 patients with porcelain aorta, approximately half underwent transfemoral AVIs. The stroke and 30-day mortality rates (1.6% and 12% respectively) were similar to those without a porcelain aorta. Frailty was present in 85 patients, many of whom were women, older, and had a higher STS risk score. The procedural and 30-day mortality rates in this subgroup (2.4% and 8.2% respectively) were similar to those in the rest of the study population, but frail patients more frequently develop postoperative acute renal failure requiring temporary hemodialysis. Multivariate predictors of the cumulative 30-day mortality consisted of pulmonary hypertension, severe mitral regurgitation and the need for periprocedural hemodynamic support.

Mid-Term Outcomes

A median follow-up of 8 months was available in all patients. 39 patients (12%) died during follow-up, at a median period of 162 days after the procedure. There were no cases of structural valve deterioration, and 1 patient required reoperative open aortic valve replacement due to endocarditis of the transcatheter valve. Survival rates at one and two years were 76% and 64% respectively for the entire cohort, without significant difference between the transfemoral and transapical groups. There were no significant differences in survival rates between these two respective comorbidities and the rest of the study cohort. Predictors of cumulative mid-term mortality are listed in Table 3.

Table 3. Predictors of cumulative mid-term mortality in TAVI in 6 Canadian centers

Risk Factor	Hazard Ratio (95% Confidence Interval)
Periprocedural hemodynamic support	2.6 (1.1-6.0)
Pulmonary hypertension	1.9 (1.2-3.0)
Chronic kidney disease	2.3 (1.4-3.8)
Chronic obstructive pulmonary disease	1.8 (1.1-2.8)

Since the study was published, additional Canadian centres have also started implanting the Edwards Sapien valves (Table 1). Procedures take place in a mixture of catheterization laboratories and operating suites with a portable fluoroscopic imaging system. The Canadian multicenter study demonstrates favorable short- and mid-term outcomes of TAVI using the Edwards valve in both transfemoral and transapical groups. Transapical AVIs will continue to play an important role in the treatment of inoperable severe aortic stenosis in Canada. More importantly, we were the first group to report the favorable outcomes among those with a porcelain aorta or frailty as a high-risk co-morbidity.

CoreValve by Medtronic

With over 10,000 CoreValves implanted worldwide, Canada is one of the first countries to have piloted the device in high-risk, inoperable patients. Canadians were also the first in North America to report their clinical experience on the CoreValve, before the US pivotal trial that began in 2011.

Experience at the Montreal Heart Institute

The first CoreValve implant in Canada and North America took place in December 2005 at the Montreal Heart Institute. Bonan and colleagues reported their initial series of 11 patients in North America who received a CoreValve between December 2005 and August 2006 [2, 4]. Inclusion criteria consist of severe aortic stenosis (aortic valve area index ≤0.6 cm^2/m^2), aortic annulus diameter 20-26 mm, sinotubular junction diameter of ≤45 mm, and either age ≥80 years with a logistic EuroSCORE ≥20% mortality, or age ≥65 years plus at least one major comorbidity (e.g. previous cardiac surgery, pulmonary hypertension >60 mmHg). Exclusion criteria consist of a lack of peripheral arterial access with a femoral artery internal lumen diameter ≤7 mm or significant iliofemoral tortuosity. In this series, the first 4 patients were part of a local feasibility study, while the next 9 patients were part of a multicenter pilot study. Two patients had peripheral access limitations and could not undergo a CoreValve procedure. Preoperative assessment consists of TTE, iliofemoral contrast angiography and coronary angiography.

The CoreValve procedure was initially performed in the catheterization laboratory under femoral-femoral cardiopulmonary bypass but was subsequently changed to percutaneous ventricular assist support using the TandemHeart (PVAD Cardiac Assist, Pittsburgh, PA). Femoral arterial access was achieved via surgical cutdown. The CoreValve was deployed under fluoroscopic guidance, with its distal third adjacent to the calcified native valve leaflets. No rapid ventricular pacing was used during valve deployment. Valve position was confirmed with both aortography and TEE. More recently, the procedure has been performed without cardiopulmonary support.

Among the 13 patients, the median logistic EuroSCORE was 36% (5-48%) [4]. One patient had concomitant angioplasty and stent implantation of the left anterior descending artery. Another two patients required percutaneous angioplasty of the common iliac artery to enable advancement of the sheath. There were 2 in-hospital deaths (18%), both of which were not valve related. The 30-day mortality remained unchanged. There were 2 strokes. Three patients had vascular site complications, and 3 patients had persistent new onset heart block requiring permanent pacemaker implantation. Median follow-up was 305 days with 3 further deaths unrelated to prosthetic valve function. One patient survived up to the duration of the last follow-up of over 16 months [2]. All patients had a significant increase in aortic valve area and decrease in transvalvular mean gradient, with a majority having a significant improvement in NYHA class status. Since 2005, the Montreal Heart Institute have performed approximately 190 TAVI procedures, with 140 transfemoral CoreValves, 15 trans-subclavian CoreValves, 12 transfemoral Edwards Sapien valves, and 30 transapical Edwards Sapien valves.

Experience at the Ottawa Heart Institute

The first CoreValve was implanted in Ottawa in February 2007 (Dr. Marc Ruel, personal communication). Since then, 53 cases have been performed with an in-hospital mortality rate of 8% (4 deaths). The procedure is performed in the catheterization laboratory. No clinical follow-up has been published.

Experience at the Sunnybrook Health Sciences Center, Toronto

Sunnybrook had its first CoreValve implant in September 2009. All cases are performed in the catheterization laboratory without cardiopulmonary support. Recently, several cases have been performed under sedation and local anesthesia without mechanical ventilation. Femoral access is done via surgical cutdown and repair. CoreValve deployment is performed under fluoroscopic guidance, with only the initial section deployed under rapid ventricular pacing. Valve position is confirmed with fluoroscopy, aortography and TEE. In the case of patients being done under local anesthesia, fluoroscopy and aortography are used to confirm valve position.

Of the cases up to September 2010, there was one death secondary to multiorgan failure. One patient had severe paravalvular leak requiring multiple balloon valvuloplasty. One patient had a 26 mm CoreValve resheathed and a 29 mm valve implanted instead. One patient had only a balloon valvuloplasty due to hemodynamic instability from iliac artery dissection. One patient had a wire-induced ventricular perforation and cardiac tamponade, requiring emergency transfer to the operating room and open surgical repair. One patient had new onset sustained heart block requiring a permanent pacemaker. There were no other significant in-hospital complications. Significant improvement in NYHA class was observed among all surviving patients at 30 days after the CoreValve procedure.

Experience at the Toronto General Hospital

The first CoreValve was implanted in November 2009. So far, 25 cases have been performed without procedural death or complications. One patient died late in the postoperative course while in hospital. The patient had to be brought back to the hybrid OR 2 days after the initial implantation to reposition the valve due to severe aortic insufficiency. Unfortunately, the patient had a fall in hospital late after the procedure and developed a significant subdural hematoma that was ultimately fatal.

Experience at the St. Paul's Hospital, Vancouver

The first CoreValve was implanted in November 2009. So far, 13 cases have been performed, including one via the subclavian artery.

Canadian Experience in Valve-in-Valve

Transcatheter treatment of failing bioprostheses is emerging as a viable alternative to surgical reintervention, particularly in patients with significant comorbidities or risk factors for repeat surgery. Webb and colleagues at three Canadian centers (Vancouver, Toronto, Quebec City) were one of the first groups to present their experience in transcatheter valve-in-valve intervention for failing bioprostheses in aortic, mitral, tricuspid and pulmonic positions among 24 patients [15]. The patient group consists of 10 failing aortic, 7 mitral, 1 tricuspid and 6 pulmonic prostheses. No procedural deaths were observed and the 30-day mortality rate was 4.2%. 88% of patients had a significant improvement of NYHA class from III or IV to I or II. At a median follow-up of 135 days and a maximum follow-up of almost 3 years, survival rate was 92% with satisfactory valve function. The topic of transcatheter valve-in-valve intervention will be discussed in detail in another chapter.

Regulatory Process for Trancatheter Valves in Canada

In Canada, all transcatheter aortic valve procedures require approval by the Therapeutic Products Directorate, Department of Health and Welfare in Ottawa (Health Canada).

Health Canada / Santé Canada

PROTECTED WHEN COMPLETED

APPLICATION FORM FOR CUSTOM MADE DEVICES AND MEDICAL DEVICES FOR SPECIAL ACCESS

Return by Facsimile to: 1-613-957-1596
or e-Mail to: sap_devices_mdb@hc-sc.gc.ca

Please note that all fields must be completed or the application cannot be processed.

Health Care Professional Information: (Note: One Application per Health Care Professional)
Name and Title
Provincial Licence Number
Address: Number and Street
City, Province/Territory Postal Code
Telephone Facsimile E-Mail

Health Care Facility Information
Health Care Facility Name
Address: Number and Street
City, Province/Territory Postal Code
Date of Procedure (YYYY-MM-DD)

Device Information
Name of Device, Components and Accessories
Device Identifier (catalogue/model number) Quantity of each Catalogue/Model Number Required
Custom Made Device

Manufacturer Information
Manufacturer's Name
Contact Name and Title
Address: Number and Street
City, Province/Territory/State Postal Code or ZIP Code
Telephone Facsimile E-Mail

Importer or Distributor Information
Name of Importer or Distributor
Contact Name and Title
Address: Number and Street
City, Province/Territory Postal Code
Telephone Facsimile E-mail

Ver. 2009 Page 1 of 3

Canada

Application Form for Custom-Made Devices and Medical Devices for Special Access

Medical Rationale
1. Provide the diagnosis, treatment or prevention for which the device is required.
2. Provide the reasons why this unlicensed device was chosen over a licensed device or conventional therapies for this particular patient.
3. Identify and list the risks and benefits associated with the use of the device and indicate how the benefits obtained would outweigh the risks.
4. Compare the risks of the unlicensed device with conventional therapies.
5. In the case of a batch release request describe the emergency condition requiring treatment, and the number of devices required for one month.

Undertaking
Pursuant to Section 71(2)(f) of the Medical Devices Regulations, health care professionals are required to make an undertaking that they will inform the patient for whom the device is intended of the risks and benefits associated with its use.

I, the Health Care Professional, undertake to inform the patient ______ (Patient's Initials or Identifier)
who is to be treated with the device of the risks and benefits associated with the use of this unlicensed medical device.
(Electronic Signature or Signature Stamps can not be accepted.)

Health Care Professional's Signature and Date: ______ Signature Date (YYYY-MM-DD)

Please indicate if you have already informed the patient of the risks and benefits associated with its use.

I, the Health Care Professional, confirm that I have informed the patient, ______ (Patient's Initials or Identifier)
who is to be diagnosed or treated with the device of the risks and benefits associated with the use of this unlicensed medical device.

Notes
1. In the case of a Batch Release, it is the manufacturer or importer's responsibility to maintain a distribution record in respect of the device in accordance with Sections 52 to 56 of the *Medical Devices Regulations*.
2. Health care professionals are requested to return any unused devices to the manufacturers or importers. The distribution of the device(s) to patients or uses other than as authorized is not permitted.

Application Form for Custom-Made Devices and Medical Devices for Special Access

Declaration
I, the Health Care Professional, certify that the information given is true, correct and complete to the best of my knowledge. (Electronic Signature or Signature Stamps can not be accepted.)

Health Care Professional's Signature and Date: ______ Signature Date (YYYY-MM-DD)

Health Care Professional's Name : ______

Return the completed application form with any supporting documentation to the following address by fax or e-mail to:

Special Access Program
Device Evaluation Division
Medical Devices Bureau
Therapeutic Products Directorate
Health Canada
Room 1605, Main Building
150 Tunney's Pasture Driveway
Address Locator 0301H1
Ottawa, Ontario
K1A 0K9

Telephone: 1-613-946-8711
Facsimile: 1-613-957-1596
e-mail: sap_devices_mdb@hc-sc.gc.ca

Figure 5. A sample Health Canada application form to request special access approval for a transcatheter aortic valve in Canada. Ver. 2009.

The Medical Devices Special Access Program is "responsible for administering the Medical Devices Regulations, as part of the Special Access Provisions under the Canada Food and Drugs Act. This part of the Regulations permits health care professionals to access custom-made and unlicensed medical devices for emergency use or when conventional therapies have failed, are unavailable or are unsuitable to provide a diagnosis, treatment or prevention for patients under their care."[16] Applications are submitted individually for each patient. The

Medical Devices Bureau (MDB) is responsible for assessing the application and makes the decision.

Condition for approval consists of compassionate clinical use in patients with symptomatic severe aortic stenosis deemed to be inoperable or very high risk surgical candidates for open aortic valve replacement.

To get approval for an individual patient, a physician must complete a Special Access Program form (Figure 5). Criteria for approval include the patient's clinical background, the type of device requested, benefits and risks of the proposed device, and comparison of the proposed device with conventional treatment (in this case open aortic valve replacement). Approval is usually granted in 48-72 hours. Urgent submissions can be reviewed and approved within 24 hours.

Funding for Transcatheter Valve Programs in Canada

The Canadian Health Care System at a Glance

The Canadian health care system is a publicly funded system based on the Canada Health Act, which encompasses the following five principles [17]:

1) Universality: all insured persons are entitled to health coverage in uniform terms and conditions
2) Accessibility: all insured persons must be provided reasonable access to medical services without financial or other barriers
3) Portability: all insured persons must be provided health coverage when they move across Canada and travel abroad. Limitations may exist on coverage for services provided outside Canada
4) Comprehensiveness: all medically necessary services must be insured
5) Public administration: health plans must be operated on a non-profit basis by a public authority held accountable to the provincial and territorial governments

The federal government allocates a portion of health care funding to each province or territorial jurisdiction. Each province or territory allocates a specific amount of funding to individual hospitals. Each hospital is then responsible for allocating its funds to individual programs and services. Given hospitals are non-profit entities, they are responsible and held accountable to meeting their budgetary requirements.

Current Funding Models of Canadian Transcatheter Valve Programs

Because neither TAVI system is approved in Canada, indivdiaul cases must be approved through the Special Access program. As these devices are still considerd experimental, there has been no funding available through provincial governments to the hospitals to support

TAVI programs. Financial support for the programs varies from institution to institution, but has generally been provided through hospital foundations, individual donations, research funds, or in rare cases, hospitals' operational budgets. The exception is at St. Paul's Hospital in Vancouver, where the British Columbia government is able to provide funding for 150 TAVI cases per year.

At the Toronto General Hospital, our TAVI program is funded entirely by the hospital foundation. We have been able to continue offering this therapy to our patients through our institution's commitment to this program. Currently, patient and outcomes data on TAVI are collected in Ontario through the Cardiac Care Network (CCN). CCN is a network of 18 hospitals providing cardiac services in Ontario which advises the Ontario government in helping plan, coordinate, implement and evaluate cardiovascular care in Ontario. The CCN TAVI Registry includes variables pertaining to referral, wait times and procedural information for all TAVI patients in Ontario. The CCN data may be used in the future as part of a field analysis conducted by the Ontario Health Technology Advisory Committee (OHTAC), once Health Canada approval is received. OHTAC will then make recommendations to the Ontario Ministry of Health and Long-Term Care with respect to funding of TAVI procedures.

Challenges and Opportunities in Funding Canadian Transcatheter Valve Programs

Without direct government funding to most transcatheter valve programs in Canada, it has been a significant challenge for individual institutions to sustain their service offerings. Compared to an open aortic valve replacement, the procedural cost for a TAVI is higher. This is due to the increase in resources and personnel required for the TAVI procedure, as well as the higher cost of the prosthesis. Many programs across Canada, including ours, have been totally dependent on non-government sources for financing. Procedural volumes have been limited to the availability of funding to pay for the cost of the procedure and postoperative recovery.

As a result, the waiting list for TAVI is growing among centers across Canada. An increasing number of patients are found to benefit from this new therapy, and we have seen a growing number of referrals for TAVI at individual institutions, including our own. Yet, limited funding has restricted physicians' ability to manage the rising demand. For example, at the Toronto General Hospital, we have only been able to perform 4 TAVI procedures per month. London Health Sciences Center had to discontinue its program after completing only two procedures, because of a lack of funding.

In fact, across Canada, the obstacle in securing financial support for new technologies has not been limited to transcatheter valves. Broader adoption of procedures that utilize new technologies, such as ventricular assist device implantation, minimally invasive valve surgery and robotic cardiac surgery, have met with varying degrees of challenges to secure hospital funding. As a result, only a limited number of patients have been able to benefit from these new therapies. Canadians, born with a "birthright" to universal medical coverage, are well supplied with care but often suffer from late adoption of expensive new technologies, which need to fit within a preexisting funding envelope. The pace of increasing health care spending has also brought increasing scrutiny to dissemination of new technologies.

Future Directions in Transcatheter Valve Intervention in Canada and Beyond

Advances in Imaging

Fluoroscopy and TEE have remained as mainstay imaging modalities for TAVI and other transcatheter valve procedures. Three-dimensional rotational angiography (e.g. Siemen's DynaCT) and accompanying navigation software provide accurate anatomical landmarks and overlay of the reconstructed image over real-time fluoroscopy. Such enhancements in imaging technology may enable clinicians to improve accuracy in valve and device positioning and deployment. As imaging and navigation technologies continue to advance, various endocscopic and transcatheter approaches to the treatment of valvular heart disease will become possible.

Advances in Valve Technology

Canada will continue to be at the forefront of trialing and implementing new transcatheter valve technologies. Vancouver, Montreal and Toronto have respectively been pioneering centers in implanting transcatheter aortic, mitral and pulmonic valve devices. Various individuals have also been instrumental in developing new transcatheter valve technology through collaboration with industry partners. Canadian centers together have one of the largest transcatheter valve-in-valve series in the world. Our health care system and regulatory policies offer a favorable environment for industry partners to pilot new transcatheter valve devices in preclinical and clinical settings. In the future, we will see improvement in various components of transcatheter valve technology, including newer designs of valve prostheses, smaller delivery systems, more features on valve repositioning and retrieval, and apical closure devices. Although Europe may remain at the cutting edge in new technology adoption because of its regulatory environment, Canadians will certainly play an important role in developing and disseminating these innovations in North America.

Patient Selection and Preprocedural Planning

Currently, patient screening and selection for TAVI are done on an individual basis via multidisciplinary conferences at each institution. However, as indications for this procedure expands and the number of eligible patients increases, it would be important to develop a systematic approach to determine patient selection and the procedural approach. The Quebec Heart and Lung Institute has already devised selection criteria for transfemoral and transapical AVI. Developing a national consensus on a patient screening and selection algorithm would be a big step forward in devising a referral and care pathway for this patient population. This algorithm may become a model for other international centers to emulate. As the Canadian centers move forward with TAVI programs, we look forward to taking a leading role in making TAVI a safe and accessible treatment option to appropriate patients.

Finding a Sustainable Funding Model

Perhaps the most pressing issue that Canadian institutions need to address in the immediate future is finding a sustainable funding source for TAVI programs. The CCN data will be important to help centers in Ontario to present to the Ministry of Health for a recommendation to provide funding for this therapy. In addition, as the volume of TAVI expands, hospitals as a collective will need to negotiate with industry partners the pricing model of the new devices, so as to make the therapy financially feasible and accessible to eligible patients.

Conclusion

Canada has established itself as an innovator and early adopter in transcatheter aortic valve intervention. Experiences in Edwards and Medtronic devices have been reported and become important benchmarks for others in terms of early- and mid-term outcomes. Ongoing challenges include finding sustainable funding for institutions to continue this important therapy in high risk inoperable patients with symptomatic severe aortic stenosis. As indications for TAVI expand, it will be paramount for Canadian centers to create a common care pathway and national registry to ensure appropriate patient selection and follow-up in this high risk population.

Acknowledgments

We would like to thank the following individuals for kindly providing assistance to this book chapter: Kristeen Chamberlain, Ronen Gurvitch, Kori Kingsbury, Donna Riley, Dr. Anita Asgar, Dr. Gideon Cohen, Dr. Michael Chu, Dr. Benoit De Varennes, Dr. Ansar Hassan, Dr. Yoan Lamarche, Dr.David Latter, Dr. Jean-Bernard Masson, Dr. Giuseppe Matucci, Dr. Steven Meyer, Dr. Marc Pelletier, Dr. Sam Radhakrishnan, Dr. Josep Rodes-Cabau, Dr. Marc Ruel, Dr. Kevin Teoh, and Dr. John Webb.

References

[1] Webb JG, Chandavimol M, Thompson CR, et al. Percutaneous aortic valve implantation retrograde from the femoral artery. *Circulation* 2006;113:842-50.

[2] Marcheix B, Lamarche Y, Berry C, et al. Surgical aspects of endovascular retrograde implantation of the aortic CoreValve bioprosthesis in high-risk older patients with severe symptomatic aortic stenosis. *J Thorac Cardiovasc Surg* 2007;134:1150-6.

[3] Ye J, Cheung A, Lichtenstein SV, et al. Transapical aortic valve implantation in humans. *J Thorac Cardiovasc Surg* 2006;131:1194-6.

[4] Berry C, Asgar A, Lamarche Y, et al. Novel therapeutic aspects of percutaneous aortic valve replacement with the 21F CoreValve revalving system. *Catheter Cardiovasc Interv* 2007;70:610-6.

[5] Cribier A, Eltchaninoff H, Bash A, et al. Percutaneous transcatheter implantation of an aortic valve prosthesis for calcific aortic stenosis: First human case description. *Circulation* 2002;106:3006-8.

[6] Webb JG, Altwegg L, Boone RH, et al. Transcatheter aortic valve implantation: Impact on clinical and valve-related outcomes. *Circulation* 2009;119:3009-16.

[7] Webb JG, Pasupati S, Humphries K, et al. Percutaneous transarterial aortic valve replacement in selected high-risk patients with aortic stenosis. *Circulation* 2007;116:755-63.

[8] Lichtenstein SV, Cheung A, Ye J, et al. Transapical transcatheter aortic valve implantation in humans: Initial clinical experience. *Circulation* 2006;114:591-6.

[9] Wong DR, Ye J, Cheung A, Webb JG, Carere RG, Lichtenstein SV. Technical considerations to avoid pitfalls during transapical aortic valve implantation. *J Thorac Cardiovasc Surg* 2010;140:196-202.

[10] Ye J, Cheung A, Lichtenstein SV, et al. Transapical transcatheter aortic valve implantation: 1-year outcome in 26 patients. *J Thorac Cardiovasc Surg* 2009;137:167-73.

[11] Ye J, Cheung A, Lichtenstein SV, et al. Transapical transcatheter aortic valve implantation: Follow-up to 3 years. *J Thorac Cardiovasc Surg* 2010;139:1107,13, 1113.e1.

[12] Rodes-Cabau J, Dumont E, De LaRochelliere R, et al. Feasibility and initial results of percutaneous aortic valve implantation including selection of the transfemoral or transapical approach in patients with severe aortic stenosis. *Am J Cardiol* 2008;102:1240-6.

[13] Osten MD, Feindel C, Greutmann M, et al. Transcatheter aortic valve implantation for high risk patients with severe aortic stenosis using the edwards sapien balloon-expandable bioprosthesis: A single centre study with immediate and medium-term outcomes. *Catheter Cardiovasc Interv* 2010;75:475-85.

[14] Rodes-Cabau J, Webb JG, Cheung A, et al. Transcatheter aortic valve implantation for the treatment of severe symptomatic aortic stenosis in patients at very high or prohibitive surgical risk: Acute and late outcomes of the multicenter canadian experience. *J Am Coll Cardiol* 2010;55:1080-90.

[15] Webb JG, Wood DA, Ye J, et al. Transcatheter valve-in-valve implantation for failed bioprosthetic heart valves. *Circulation* 2010;121:1848-57.

[16] Health Canada. *The medical devices special access program* 2007:1-3.

[17] Health Canada. *Canada's health care system* 2005:2-26.

In: Percutaneous Valve Technology: Present and Future ISBN: 978-1-61942-577-4
Editors: Jose Luis Navia and Sharif Al-Ruzzeh

Chapter XIII

Sutureless Aortic Heart Valve Technology - Present and Future Perspectives

Eric Manasse

Abstract

Perceval™ S is a super-elastic, self-expanding, self-anchoring, sutureless surgical prosthetic aortic heart valve. It is designed to be a highly versatile and deployable prosthesis using a variety of techniques, including classic surgical aortic valve replacement (AVR) and minimally invasive surgery.

Several advantages can be expected from sutureless placement: avoidance of stitches through the annulus, improved haemodynamic performance, a substantially shorter cross-clamping time and faster recovery due to improved clinical outcome. Clinical experiences indicate that the valve has advantages over other 'sutureless' valves as well as over valves currently used with a transapical approach in TAVI.

Reports from the use of Perceval™ S in the open transaortic approach from cardiac surgery centres throughout Europe confirm the markedly reduced cardiopulmonary bypass and cross-clamping times compared with conventional surgical AVR, both in patients needing bypass grafting and in those with isolated AVR.

Available initial experiences with the deployment of Perceval S™ in minimally invasive valve replacement are also very promising. In selected patients, the intervention could be completed under epidural anaesthesia, awakening patients in the operating theatre.

The average skin-to-skin time for the entire procedure was 75 min. Thus, the sutureless valve is a further step towards the aspiration for the surgeon to minimise surgical time and patient discomfort in valve replacement.

Introduction

Aortic stenosis is the most common valvular heart disease in adults, with a dismal prognosis in symptomatic untreated patients. Approximately three quarters of patients with untreated symptomatic aortic stenosis die within 3 years [1, 2].

The gold standard, surgical aortic valve replacement (SAVR), through median sternotomy using classic cardioplegic cardiac arrest under cardiopulmonary bypass (CPB) produces high rates of excellent results in elderly patients. However, for high-risk patients in-hospital mortality is a relevant issue, ranging from 3% to 8% [3, 4]. Important independent predictors of survival after SAVR are the duration of aortic cross-clamping and CPB [5]. Improved technologies that reduce the times needed would bring significant reductions in the associated risks.

Transcatheter aortic valve implantation (TAVI) is a therapeutic option for high-risk patients, typically elderly and presenting with multiple and complex comorbidities, that are not considered to be suitable candidates for surgery. The randomised PARTNER trial recently showed prolonged survival with percutaneous transarterial TAVI with a 20% absolute increase in survival at 1 year in patients with severe aortic stenosis considered at too high risk for surgery [6]. Nevertheless TAVI remains a high-risk procedure: six-month mortality rates can be 48%, and it is associated with considerable complications. Rates of major adverse cardiovascular event rates at 30 days are up to 35%, driven by vascular complications, stroke, myocardial infarction, aortic dissection, wall fracture, major ventricular tachyarrhythmias, and implant failure [7, 8]. The incidence of complete AV block alone is up to 25% [7,9]. Most of these complications are not relevant issues with SAVR.

Importantly, in TAVI the diseased valve is not removed but dilated with angioplasty. Thus, the dilated calcified aortic root may generate debris which if dislodged increases the risk for peripheral and central embolism [10]. Paravalvular leakage and aortic regurgitation are further major causes for concern. While short-term clinical consequences of mild-to-moderate regurgitation are seen as relatively insignificant, the potential long-term complications from leakage and reduced valve performance are a barrier to wider adoption of the technologies [8, 11, 12].

Thus, for all valve replacements, there is a need to reduce the associated risks, improve survival chances and increase access to care.

Sorin Group has directed developmental efforts towards delivering a collapsible, stent-mounted aortic valve prosthesis that can be placed in a sutureless fashion either with median sternotomy or with a minimally invasive surgical technique through a right minithoracotomy [13]. The first clinical experiences with the valve were gathered in SAVR using CPB and aortic cross-clamping. In this setting, several advantages can be expected from the sutureless placement: avoidance of stitches through the annulus, improved haemodynamic performance, a substantially shorter cross-clamping time and faster recovery due to improved clinical oucome.

The surgical deployments of the valve provide experience with implanting sutureless valves under visual control and furnishes evidence on the safety and efficacy of sutureless aortic valve prostheses.

The Perceval S Sutureless Bioprosthesis

After extensive investigational clinical use with several cardiac surgeons and medical centers since 2007, the Perceval™ S super-elastic, self-expanding, self-anchoring, sutureless surgical prosthetic aortic heart valve (Figure 1) received European CE Mark in early 2011. The valve is currently commercially available in Europe and several countries throughout the world.

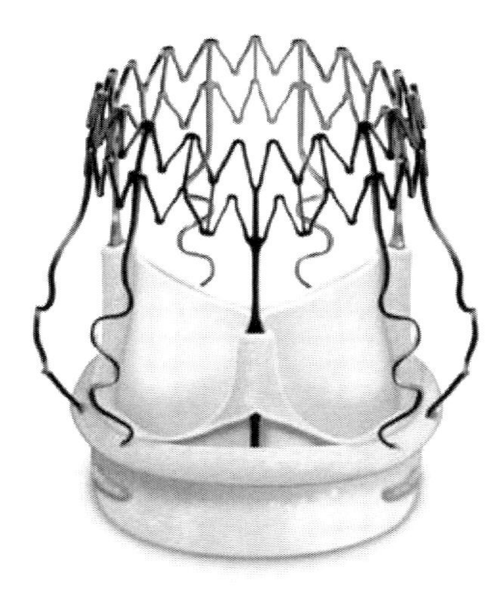

Figure 1. The Perceval™ S sutureless prosthetic aortic heart valve.

The Perceval™ S valve was designed to be easy to use with highly reproducible procedures leaving minimal opportunity for human error. The valve has a substantially smaller stent volume than other stented valves, while the expanded valve is of similar size to stentless valves.

The Perceval™ S valve design allows deployment of the prosthesis within a circular orifice, and ensures optimal adaptation to the native aortic sinus anatomy. Three valve sizes are commercially available at present; they cover annulus diameters ranging from 19 to 21 mm (size S), 21 to 23 mm (size M) and 23 to 25 mm (size L), respectively. One further valve, (size XL) for annulus 25-27 is expected to enter soon in clinical investigation.

The Perceval™ S valve is based on the Pericarbon bovine pericardium double-sheet valve platform (Sorin Biomedica Cardio Srl), that has been used in over 10,000 patients since 1985 with clinically proven durability [14], optimal haemodynamics [15,16] and excellent long-term results [17, 18]. A unique anchoring system was developed using a superelastic alloy able to endure significant deformation and then return to its original shape after the valve has been released from the proprietary prosthesis delivery system . Hence, the stent-mounted valve is collapsible within the valve delivery system and after implantation the anchoring device will expand upon release and develop an optimal fit within the patient aortic root anatomy.

A combination of straight commissural struts and sinusoidal struts is used to enable self-anchoring (Figure 2). The straight commissural struts provide valve support. The sinusoidal struts are necessary for the anchoring and good fitting within different Valsalva anatomies without interference with coronary ostia, and to prevent migration. All non-biological surfaces are coated with Carbofilm™, a highly biocompatible carbon coating that has been shown to reduce inflammatory tissue response[19].

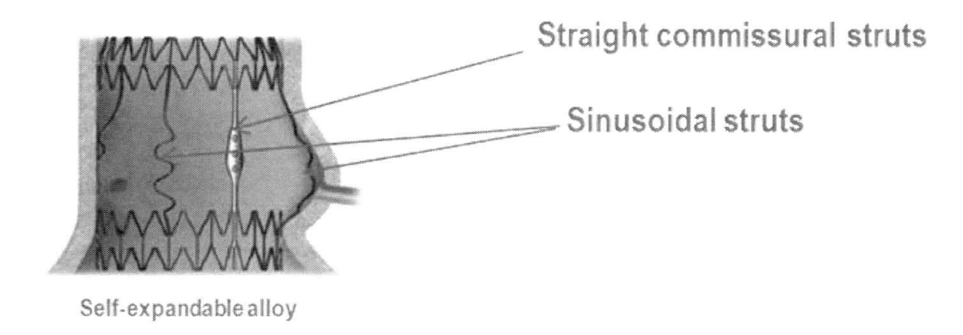

Figure 2. Self-anchoring strut design of the Perceval™ S supporting frame.

A dual-collar design with an intra-annular and a supra-annular sealing collar was developed to maximise the fit and prevent paravalvular leakage (Figure 3). Button holes were introduced into the intra-annular sealing collar for an accurate axial-rotational positioning in the native aortic root, using three guiding 3/0 Prolene sutures. These temporary sutures ensure the valve is aligned correctly with the native commissures and prevent the valve from being placed too low into the left ventricular outflow tract and after valve placement, the sutures are removed. In contrast to other so called 'fast deployment' valves, that require one or more permanent sutures [20], Perceval™ S is truly a sutureless prosthesis. This significantly reduces cross-clamping and CPB times [21, 22].

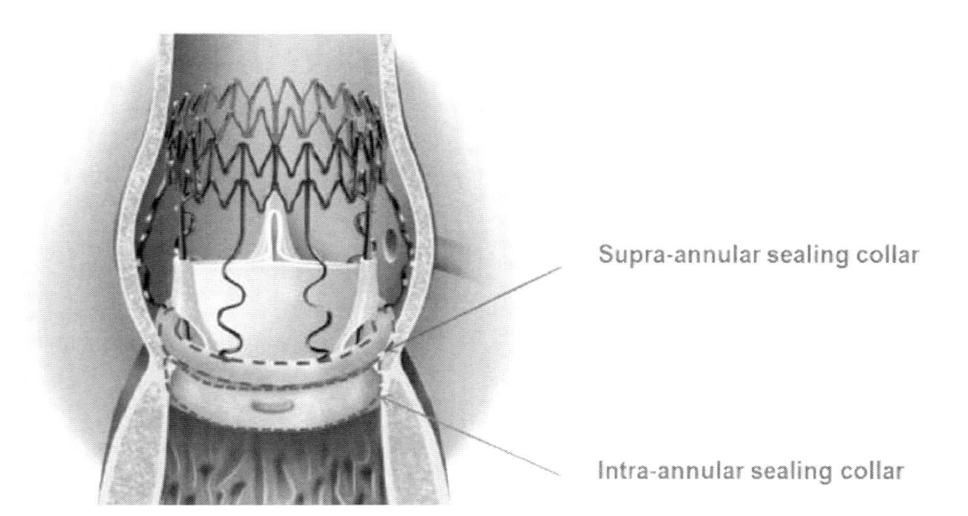

Figure 3. Perceval™ S dual-collar design to prevent paravalvular leakage.

Prior to implantation the prosthesis diameter is reduced to a suitable size and loaded on the delivery system (Figure 4). The collapsing system is designed to ensure an atraumatic device compression; importantly, the valve leaflets themselves are not affected by the collapse. This is in contrast to crimped TAVI valves on the market, where crimping involves valve leaflets and may put the long-term durability of the prosthesis at risk.

The low profile of the collapsed Perceval™ S (diameter down to 12 mm) allows for use in small aortic roots and will fit small aortic annuli without requiring long and technically demanding aortic enlargement plasty.

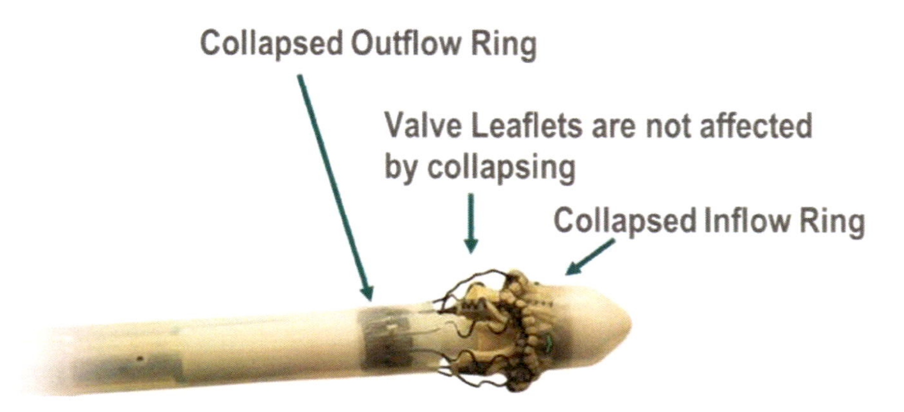

Figure 4. The Perceval™ S collapsing system.

The delivery system loaded with the collapsed stent-mounted valve is guided to its correct position by sliding it over the 3 guiding sutures, positioned at the nadir level of each resected cusp (the lowest part of the native leaflet insertion line for each valve sinus).

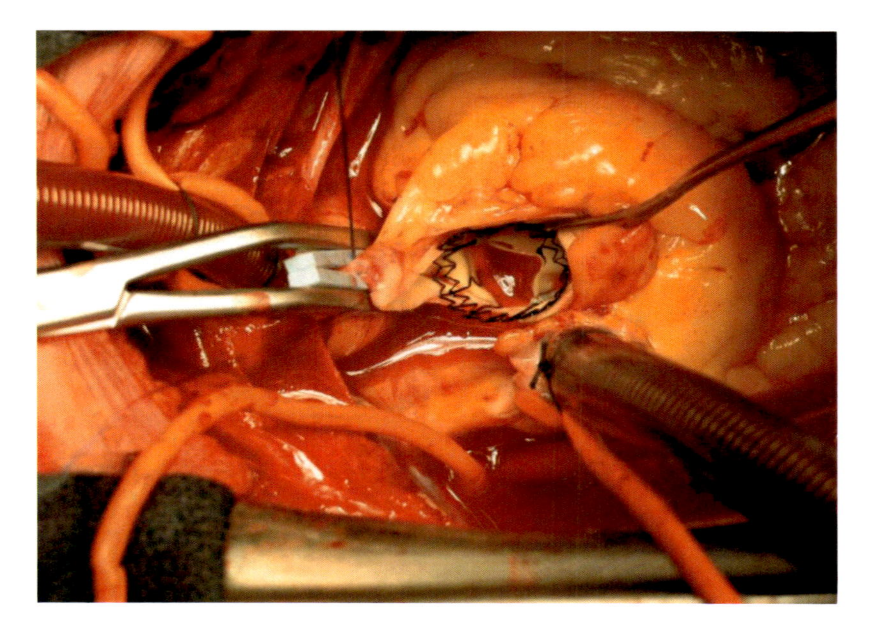

Figure 5. Perceval™ S during implantation after deployment.

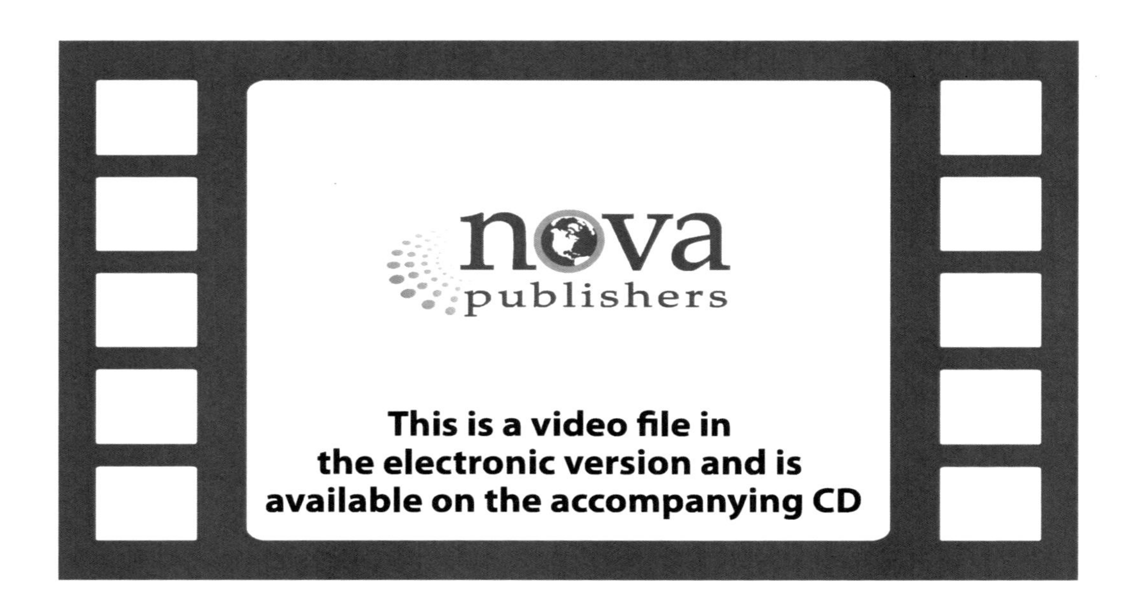

A video of an implant procedure is provided in the electronic version of this article. [http://www.symbols.it/sorin/videos/1.zip / http://www.symbols.it/sorin/videos/2.zip].

Once the delivery system is in position, the prosthesis is deployed by turning the release screw, pulling the transparent sheet and leaving the valve in place.

To optimise the area of contact between the prosthetic valve and the aortic annulus, post-dilation is performed. A specifically designed balloon is inserted in the valve and expanded for 30 seconds at a pressure of approximately 4 atm while instilling the aortic root with saline at physiological temperature. After visual inspection of the valve position, the aorta is closed by a 5-0 polypropylene suture.

The procedure is easy to implement and leaves little scope for human errors. In the initial experiences of surgeons, an impressively swift learning curve of typically 3-4 procedures has been reported that ensures rapid familiarisation and high reproducibility of the procedures.

Perceval S through Full or Partial Sternotomy Approach

At the time of writing (end-2011) there are clinical experiences from more than 45 cardiac surgery centres throughout Europe that have implanted the Perceval™ S prosthesis in approximately 900 patients using a staged approach with CPB and cross-clamping. The first systematically presented results, published in 2008 [23], reported short mean CPB and cross-clamping times and very little paravalvular leakage.

Table 1. CPB and cross-clamping times with Perceval™ S in SAVR. Data from two separate publications (21 22) and from an STS Database query August 2010

Multicentre study (21). N=30			Single-centre study (22) N=32			STS Database		
	Concomitant CABG n=14	Isolated AVR n=16		Concomitant CABG n=16	Isolated AVR n=16		Concomitant CABG	Isolated AVR
CPB time min (mean ±SD; range)	73.4 ±21.8 (41-130)	46.4 ±6.7 (34-60)	CPB time min (median; range)	62 (40-120)	35 (24-54)	CPB time mean	172	116
Cross-clamping time min (mean ±SD; range)	40 ±19 (16-79)	29 ±8 (23-55)	Cross-clamping time min (median; range)	22 (17-51)	17 (12-34)	Cross-clamping time mean	112	72

The results were included together with data from two further centres in a multicentre publication on 30 patients with 12 months' follow-up [21]. The mean age in the patients group was 81 (76-88) years and the logistic Euroscore 13%±7 (5-39). All patients were standard surgical intervention candidates at high risk for aortic valve stenosis. Fourteen patients needed concomitant coronary artery bypass grafting (CABG), as the location and/or extension of the stenosis precluded interventional therapy. The 21 mm (S) and 23 mm (M) valves were used in 11 and 19 patients, respectively.

Use of the Perceval™ S valve reduced CPB and cross-clamping times markedly compared with conventional surgical AVR, both in patients needing CABG and in those with isolated AVR (Table 1). Postoperative complications included 1 case of each of cardiac tamponade due to mediastinal bleeding, AV conduction block, wound infection, and gastrointestinal bleeding. There was 1 case of peripheral thromboembolism.

During 12 months' follow-up there were 3 deaths but none was related to the performance of the valve. The low rates of paravalvular leakage were confirmed over the follow-up period: there were 2 mild paravalvular leakages and 2 mild intravalvular regurgitation which remained stable over time. No migration nor dislodgement of the prosthesis occurred.

Gradients were low at discharge (10±5 mm Hg). Importantly, gradients remained low over the 12-month follow-up (9.1 mmHg for valve sizes S and M at 12 months follow up) [24]. All patients with complete follow-up (n=23) improved their NYHA functional class by ≥1 class [24].

More follow-up data were provided by Flameng et al [22] from a single-centre experience in 32 patients (median age 78 years; median logistic EuroScore 10) requiring aortic valve replacement with or without concomitant CABG. Median follow-up duration was 15.8 months.

The times needed for CPB and cross-clamping were comparable to those reported by the other centres, even somewhat shorter (Table 1). For isolated AVR without CABG, the mean cross-clamping time was as little as 17 ±6.2 min. Including the intermittent phases needed for distal CABG anastomoses, mean cross-clamping time was 23.4 ±10.4 min and mean CPB time was 54.2 ±25.4 min. Median intensive care unit stay was 2 days and mean hospital stay 15 days (4–30 days). The data on valve haemodynamic performances were consistent with those from the other groups (Table 2). Paravalvular regurgitations were absent to trivial in 27 patients and valvular regurgitations were absent to trivial in 25 patients. As in the multicentre report, gradients and effective orifice area values remained stable during follow-up.

Table 2. Haemodynamic parameters and leakages with Perceval™ S at 1-year follow-up after SAVR. Data from two separate publications [21 22].

	Multicentre study (21). N=30	Single-centre study (22). N=32
Peak gradient (mmHg)	18 (4-42)	19 (5–36)
Mean gradient (mmHg)	8 (2-21)	9 (3–21)
Orifice area (cm^2)	1.6 (1-2.3)	1.3 (0.8–2.4)
Paravalvular leakage	2 mild, paravalvular leakages (6.7%) 2 mild, stable intravalvular regurgitation	7 mild valvular regurgitation (23.3%) 1 endocarditis + severe valvular and paravalvular regurgitation (3.3%)

Regurgitation scores tended to shift from mild to absent/trivial. One patient underwent re-operation, as endocarditis and severe valvular and paravalvular regurgitation developed.

Clinical outcomes were favourable over the follow-up period. Three patients died, none of device-related causes. Only 1 patient developed AV block and received a permanent pacemaker implantation. There were no thromboembolic or bleeding events reported in any of the patients during follow-up.

The overall results of the clinical investigation conducted with the Perceval™ S valve have been recently presented (25th EACTS Annual Meeting). The cohort analyzed was made by 659 patients implanted in 25 investigational European centers. The mean age was 79 (63-92) years and the logistic Euroscore 11.3%±8.4. In the 33% of the cases the AVR was associated with CABG or other concomitant procedures. The maximum follow-up reached was 4.2 years; no valve thrombosis, no structural valve deterioration, and no post-operative migrations have occurred during the entire follow-up period. The early cardiac mortality was 1.6%, while major stroke occurred in 1.9% of the patients. The evaluation of the hemodynamic parameters showed good and stable performance with mean pressure gradient of 10.3±4.6 mmHg, 9.1±5.2 mmHg and 8.2±2.6 mmHg at discharge, 12 and 36 months respectively.

Perceval™ S Implanted by Minimally Invasive Surgery

Minimally-invasive valve replacement techniques represent an alternative to the conventional median sternotomy approach. Access through a right minithoracotomy offers the benefits of open heart operations with less pain and surgical trauma, less bleeding, earlier functional recovery, shorter hospital stay and greater patient satisfaction [25, 26, 27, 28]. Good experiences have been reported with the use of a 6-8 cm long right straight incision in the third intercostal space [13]. This approach gives a very good exposure of the aortic root, the aortic valve, the right atrium and the right superior pulmonary vein, and an appropriate working field to replace the aortic valve. The intervention is performed under general or epidural anaesthesia.

Concern has been raised that the minimally invasive approach may require longer perfusion and cross-clamp times than conventional surgery [29] with associated negative implications for long-term outcomes. One of the objectives when developing Perceval™ S was that the stent-mounted sutureless valve design would significantly shorten perfusion and cross-clamp times in minimally invasive surgical procedures for aortic valve replacement. This development promises to reduce mortality risk and complications.

Currently the deployment of Perceval™ S in minimally invasive valve replacement is at its early stages and there are less data available than for other applications of the valve. However, initial experiences are very promising. In selected patients (n=15), the intervention could be conducted under epidural anaesthesia, awakening patients in the operating theatre. The average skin-to-skin time for the entire procedure was an impressive 75 min. If these experiences are representative of the times achievable with the Perceval S™ valve in general use, the minimally invasive technique may finally come of age as a less traumatic and risky alternative to conventional surgery.

Conclusion

Perceval™ S represents a highly versatile prosthesis that can be deployed using a variety of techniques, including SAVR and minimally invasive surgery. The option of simultaneous CABG with the sutureless valve broadens the spectrum of indications for its use. The experiences gathered so far indicate that the valve has advantages over other so called 'fast-deployment' valves as well as over valves currently used in TAVI.

SAVR remains the gold standard procedure and the experiences with Perceval™ S outlined above are highly promising. Published data from different centres are impressively consistent with regards to procedural time, haemodynamic performance, success rates and safety, both short and mid-term. In particular, the reductions in aortic cross-clamp and CPB times and reduction in hospital stay are remarkable. The learning curve is short and it is reasonable to expect less than 20 minutes of aortic cross-clamping in routine procedures. Cross-clamping times with other so called 'sutureless' valves on the market range from 39 to 74 minutes[20, 30, 31]. With a truly sutureless valve such as Perceval™ S, only the native diseased leaflets are removed and the annulus does not need to be decalcified, shortening this phase as well and preventing possible tears on the aortic annulus. The positive impact on patient mortality as a result of these improvements will become apparent with time and increased patient numbers.

Much the same advantages are observed when Perceval™ S is deployed with minimally invasive surgery using the right minithoracotomy approach. While reducing surgical trauma and convalescence times, the procedure has hitherto been hampered by a reputation for needing longer perfusion and cross-clamp times than conventional surgery. The availability of a valve that reduces clamping time taking off the scene the most demanding part of a MIS procedure (ie. the suturing and tying) is thus a major achievement allowing the same clamping times regardless of the surgical approach (M Glauber presentation at Dallas-Leipzig meeting December 2011).

The low rates of perivalvular leaks, known risk-factor for worse prognosis and rate of rehospitalization, are very low in contrast to the experience with clinically available transcatheter valve procedures [30]. One may speculate that the collapsible design, which does not affect the valve leaflets, contributes to this advantage over crimped valves, thus probably allowing for a longer durability. Moreover, rates of pacemaker implantation with Perceval™ S have been low and consistent with surgical standards.

TAVI will remain the preferred strategy for inoperable patients. For operable and medium high risk patients, the sutureless valve should be preferred. In particular, the very low rates of paravalvular and valvular regurgitation are clear evidence of major advances in sutureless valve design. Gradients are low post-implant and remain low over time for at least 12 months.

The risk profile that defines a patient as suitable for SAVR or other valve replacement procedures is a moving target. Developments to technologies and procedures, both for SAVR and TAVI, force physicians continually to re-assess the most suitable procedure for each patient type. Risk stratification estimates have their use in predicting risk of medium-term survival, but are imprecise tools to predict perioperative survival [4] and may overpredict mortality for SAVR [32, 33] Thus, it is difficult to define "high surgical risk". There are reports indicating that patients with aortic stenosis who are considered at high risk for conventional AVR may be at greater mortality risk from TAVI than when treated surgically [7, 34]. Both surgical approaches have the added advantage over TAVI that there is no need to inject contrast fluid. This reduces the risk for renal complications, which should be taken into consideration when making decisions on the suitable procedure for individual patients.

The sutureless valve has brought us closer to the Surgeon goal of near 'zero impact' for the surgical AVR patient.[35,36]. But until we are there, developments in technologies need to be accompanied by developments in risk assessments.

References

[1] Iung B, Baron G, Butchart EG, et al. A prospective survey of patients with valvular heart disease in Europe: The Euro Heart Survey on Valvular Heart Disease. *Eur. Heart J.* 2003;24:1231-1243.

[2] Carabello BA, Paulus WJ. Aortic stenosis. *Lancet.* 2009;373:956-966.

[3] O'Brien SM, Shahian DM, Filardo G, et al. The Society of Thoracic Surgeons 2008 cardiac surgery risk models: part 2--isolated valve surgery. *Ann. Thorac. Surg.* 2009;88:S23-42.

[4] Leontyev S, Walther T, Borger MA, et al. Aortic valve replacement in octogenarians: utility of risk stratification with EuroSCORE. *Ann. Thorac. Surg.* 2009;87:1440-1445.

[5] Flameng WJ, Herijgers P, Szécsi J, et al. Determinants of early and late results of combined valve operations and coronary artery bypass grafting. *Ann. Thorac. Surg.* 1996;61:621-628.

[6] Leon MB, Smith CR, Mack M, et al. Transcatheter aortic-valve implantation for aortic stenosis in patients who cannot undergo surgery. *N. Engl. J. Med.* 2010;363:1597-1607.

[7] Yan TD, Cao C, Martens-Nielsen J, et al. Transcatheter aortic valve implantation for high-risk patients with severe aortic stenosis: A systematic review. *J. Thorac. Cardiovasc. Surg.* 2010;139:1519-1528.

[8] Vahanian A, Alfieri OR, Al-Attar N, et al. Transcatheter valve implantation for patients with aortic stenosis: a position statement from the European Association of Cardio-Thoracic Surgery (EACTS) and the European Society of Cardiology (ESC), in collaboration with the European Association of Percutaneous Cardiovascular Interventions (EAPCI). *Eur J Cardiothorac Surg.* 2008;34:1-8.

[9] Kallenbach K, Karck M. [Percutaneous aortic valve implantation - contra]. *Herz.* 2009;34:130-139.

[10] Webb JG, Pasupati S, Humphries K, et al. Percutaneous transarterial aortic valve replacement in selected high-risk patients with aortic stenosis. *Circulation.* 2007;116:755-763.

[11] Walther T, Falk V. Hemodynamic evaluation of heart valve prostheses paradigm shift for transcatheter valves? *J. Am. Coll. Cardiol.* 2009;53:1892-1893.

[12] Clavel M-A, Webb JG, Pibarot P, et al. Comparison of the hemodynamic performance of percutaneous and surgical bioprostheses for the treatment of severe aortic stenosis. *J. Am. Coll. Cardiol.* 2009;53:1883-1891.

[13] Glauber M, Farneti A, Solinas M, Karimov J. Aortic valve replacement through a right minithoracotomy. *Multimedia Manual of Cardiothoracic Surgery.* 2006;10:1826-1830.

[14] Seguin JR, Grandmougin D, Folliguet T, et al. Long-term results with the Sorin Pericarbon valve in the aortic position: a multicenter study. *J. Heart Valve Dis*. 1998;7:278-282.

[15] Gegouskov VA, Eckstein FS, Kipfer B, et al. [The Sorin pericardial bioprosthesis--a stentless aortic valve with very good hemodynamic performance]. *Swiss Surg*. 2003;9:247-252.

[16] García-Bengochea J, Sierra J, González-Juanatey JR, et al. Left ventricular mass regression after aortic valve replacement with the new Mitroflow 12A pericardial bioprosthesis. *J. Heart Valve Dis*. 2006;15:446-451.

[17] D'Onofrio A, Auriemma S, Magagna P, et al. Aortic valve replacement with the Sorin Pericarbon Freedom stentless prosthesis: 7 years' experience in 130 patients. *J. Thorac. Cardiovasc. Surg*. 2007;134:491-495.

[18] Nyawo B, Graham R, Hunter S. Aortic valve replacement with the Sorin Pericarbon Freedom stentless valve: five-year follow up. *J. Heart Valve Dis*. 2007;16:42-48.

[19] Vallana F, Pasquino E, Rinaldi S, et al. Carbofilm ^{TM}: Present and future applications in biomedical devices. *Ceramics International*. 1993;19:169-179.

[20] Martens S, Ploss A, Sirat S, et al. Sutureless aortic valve replacement with the 3f Enable aortic bioprosthesis. *Ann. Thorac. Surg*. 2009;87:1914-1917.

[21] Shrestha M, Folliguet T, Meuris B, et al. Sutureless Perceval S aortic valve replacement: a multicenter, prospective pilot trial. *J. Heart Valve Dis*. 2009;18:698-702.

[22] Flameng W, Herregods M-C, Hermans H, et al. Effect of sutureless implantation of the Perceval S aortic valve bioprosthesis on intraoperative and early postoperative outcomes. *J Thorac Cardiovasc Surg*. 2011; 1-5.

[23] Shrestha M, Khaladj N, Bara C, et al. A Staged Approach towards Interventional Aortic Valve Implantation with a Sutureless Valve: Initial Human Implants. *Thorac cardiovasc Surg*. 2008;56:398-400.

[24] Folliguet T, Dibie A, Laborde F. Future of cardiac surgery: minimally invasive techniques in sutureless valve resection. *Future Cardiol*. 2009;5:443-452.

[25] Bonacchi M, Prifti E, Giunti G, Frati G, Sani G. Does ministernotomy improve postoperative outcome in aortic valve operation? A prospective randomized study. *Ann. Thorac. Surg*. 2002;73:460-465.

[26] Doll N, Borger MA, Hain J, et al. Minimal access aortic valve replacement: effects on morbidity and resource utilization. *Ann. Thorac. Surg*. 2002;74:S1318-1322.

[27] Soltesz EG, Cohn LH. Minimally invasive valve surgery. *Cardiol Rev*. 2007;15:109-115.

[28] McClure RS, Cohn LH, Wiegerinck E, et al. Early and late outcomes in minimally invasive mitral valve repair: an eleven-year experience in 707 patients. *J. Thorac. Cardiovasc. Surg*. 2009;137:70-75.

[29] Mihaljevic T, Cohn LH, Unic D, et al. One thousand minimally invasive valve operations: early and late results. *Ann. Surg*. 2004;240:529-534.

[30] Breitenbach I, Wimmer-Greinecker G, Bockeria LA, et al. Sutureless aortic valve replacement with the Trilogy Aortic Valve System: multicenter experience. *J. Thorac. Cardiovasc. Surg*. 2010;140:878-884.

[31] Aymard T, Kadner A, Walpoth N, et al. Clinical experience with the second-generation 3f Enable sutureless aortic valve prosthesis. *J. Thorac. Cardiovasc. Surg*. 2010;140:313-316.

[32] Grossi EA, Schwartz CF, Yu P-J, et al. High-risk aortic valve replacement: are the outcomes as bad as predicted? *Ann. Thorac. Surg*. 2008;85:102-106.

[33] Ranucci M, Castelvecchio S, Menicanti LA, et al. An adjusted EuroSCORE model for high-risk cardiac patients. *Eur J Cardiothorac Surg*. 2009;36:791-797.

[34] Grube E, Schuler G, Buellesfeld L, et al. Percutaneous aortic valve replacement for severe aortic stenosis in high-risk patients using the second- and current third-generation self-expanding CoreValve prosthesis: device success and 30-day clinical outcome. *J. Am. Coll. Cardiol*. 2007;50:69-76.

[35] Nowicki ER. What is the future of mortality prediction models in heart valve surgery? *Ann. Thorac. Surg*. 2005;80:396-398.

[36] Manasse E. Cooks and recipes. *Eur J Cardiothorac Surg*. 2009;36:787-790.

In: Percutaneous Valve Technology: Present and Future ISBN: 978-1-61942-577-4
Editors: Jose Luis Navia and Sharif Al-Ruzzeh

Chapter XIV

Transcatheter Valve-in-valve for Failed Bioprosthetic Valves

R. Gurvitch, J. Je, A. Cheung and J.G. Webb

Introduction

All bioprosthetic heart valves, if given sufficient time, can be expected to eventually fail. Despite this, such valves are often favored over mechanical versions to avoid anticoagulation and the associated increased risk of bleeding[1] [2]. When bioprosthetic valves degenerate, repeat cardiac surgery is often at an increased risk given the nature of re-do cardiac surgery and the frequently advanced age of patients requiring such operations [3]. Certain co-morbidities such as advanced age, reduced ejection fraction, pulmonary disease and length of cardiopulmonary bypass time have been identified as independent predictive factors of poor outcomes following re-do surgery for failed aortic and mitral bioprostheses [4] [5].

In recent years, transcatheter heart valve (THV) implantation for stenosed native aortic valves has evolved as a viable alternative to open heart surgery particularly in high-risk surgical patients[6-8] [9] [10] [11] [12] [13]. As experience with the procedure widened and clinical outcomes improved, the concept of treating surgically degenerated valves using similar transcatheter techniques became a possibility. Such treatment is often referred to as "valve-in-valve" (VIV) implantation, as the new THV is implanted inside the degenerated bioprosthesis. In this chapter, we will review the techniques, outcomes and challenges of VIV therapy for failed surgical bioprostheses in the aortic, mitral, tricuspid and pulmonary positions.

Preclinical Animal Studies

Boudjemline et al. evaluated the concept of mitral VIV therapy by implanting Medtronic Mosaic (Medtronic Inc, Minneapolis, MN) valves with an added radiopaque ring in 6 sheep [14]. A bovine jugular valve mounted into a stent was then inserted off-pump via an atrial approach, with all but one procedure being successful. Walther et al. evaluated the feasibility of transcatheter implantation of an Edwards (Edwards Lifesciences, Irvine, CA) THV into Carpentier Edwards xenografts in the aortic and mitral position in 7 pigs [15]. The VIV procedure was performed transapically on the beating heart, with ventricular unloading via cardiopulmonary bypass and rapid ventricular pacing. Valve implantation was successful with reasonable hemodynamic function in all cases, and the authors noted that radiopaque markings on the surgical valves aided in valve positioning.

Current Transcatheter Systems

While a full review of current transcatheter systems is beyond the scope of this chapter, three main devices have been utilized in VIV therapy.

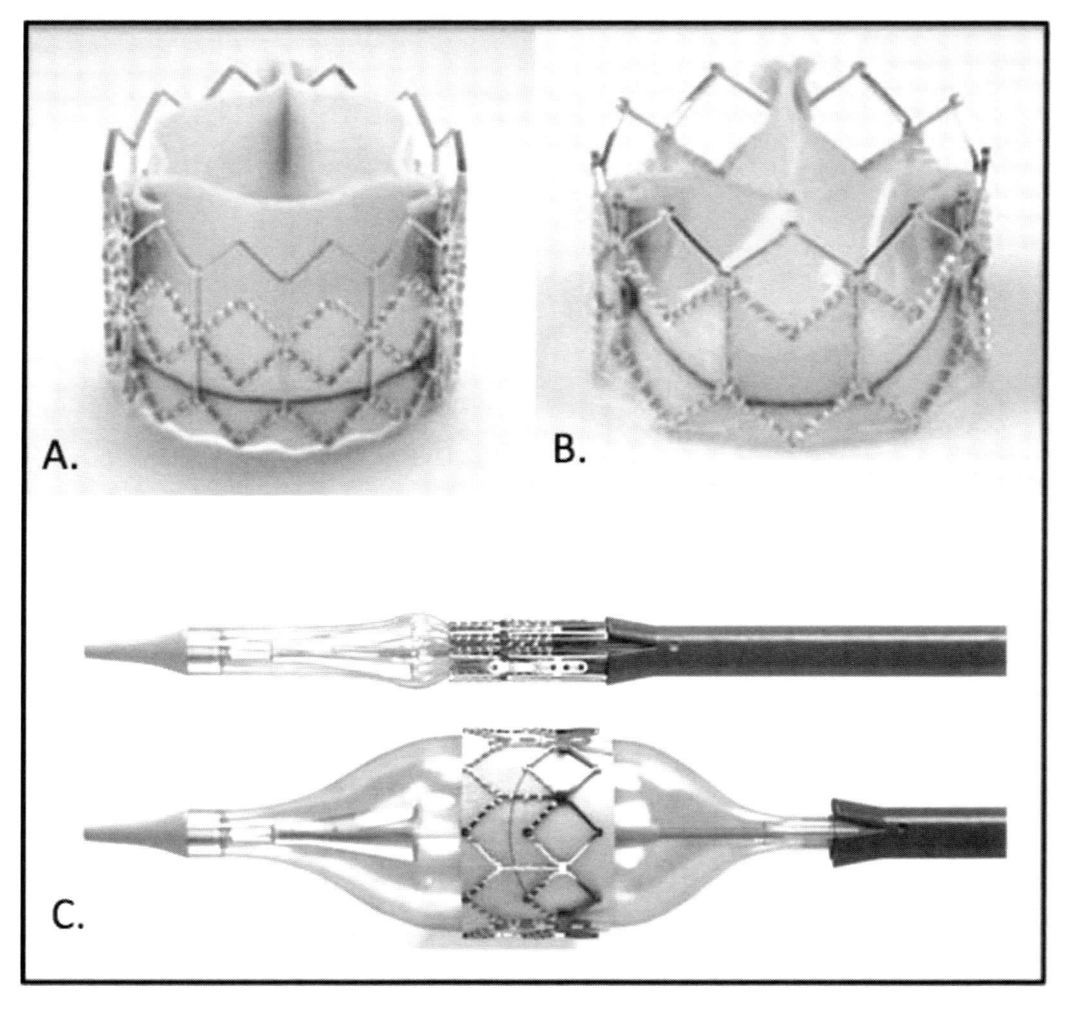

Figure 1. Edwards SAPIEN valve and delivery system. A. Edwards SAPIEN valve, B. Edwards SAPIEN XT valve, C. Edwards SAPIEN XT mounted on the Novaflex delivery system.

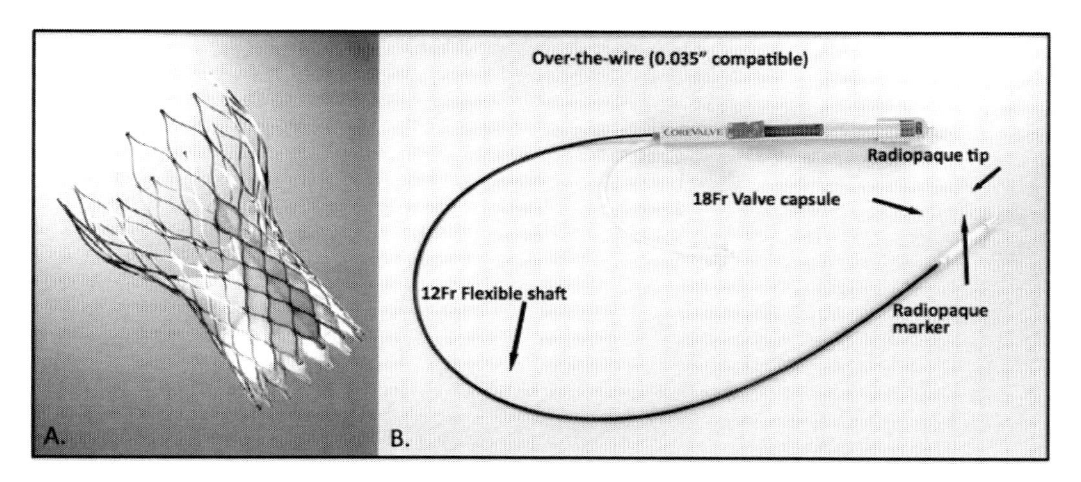

Figure 2. A. Medtronic CoreValve and, B. Medtronic CoreValve delivery system.

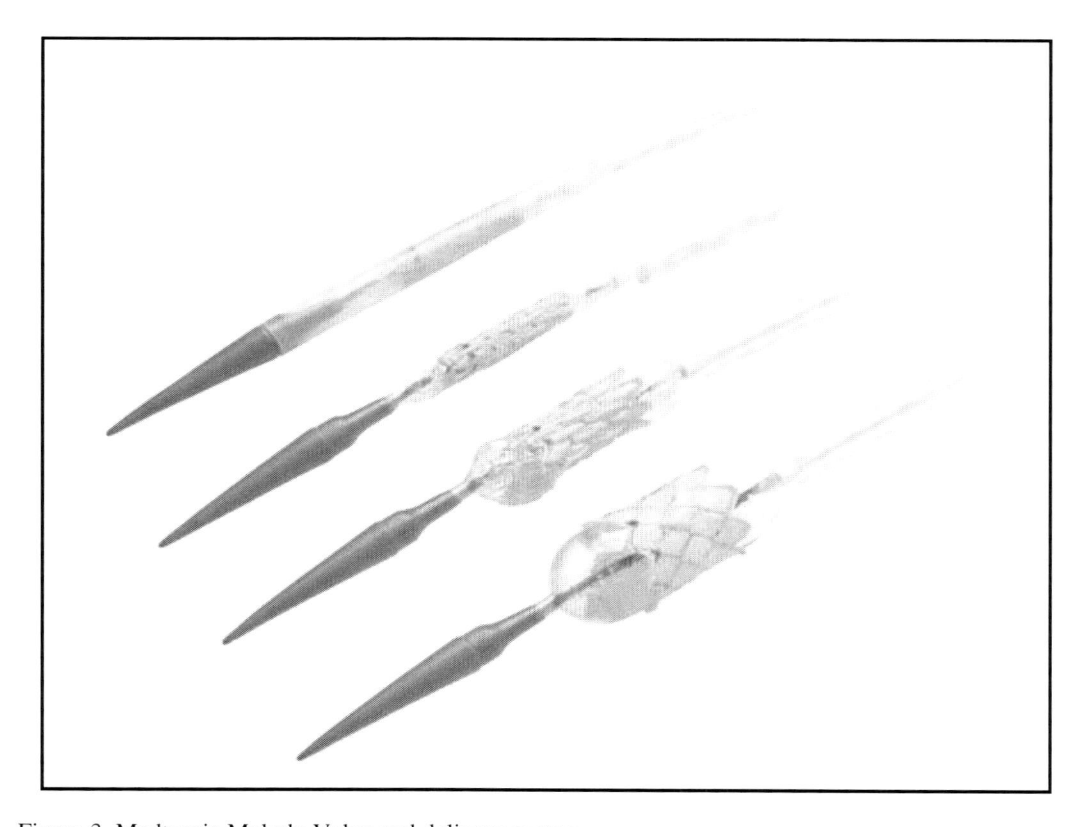

Figure 3. Medtronic Melody Valve and delivery system.

The Edwards SAPIEN system (Edwards Lifesciences, Irvine, California) is balloon expandable, consisting of a metal stent frame with valve leaflets crimped onto a balloon and deployed at high pressure [8, 9] (Figure 1). Early models were composed of stainless steel frames with equine leaflets, while more contemporary versions are cobalt chromium with bovine pericardial leaflets[16]. The valve is currently commercially available in two sizes, with expanded external diameters of 23mm and 26mm (20 and 29 mm diameter valves are undergoing evaluation). It is generally delivered via a transfemoral or transapical route and deployed under rapid ventricular pacing to decrease movement and prevent embolization while the balloon is inflated [17].

The CoreValve system (Medtronic Inc, Minneapolis, MN) is made of a self-expandable nitinol multilevel frame with porcine pericardial leaflets (Image 2). This valve is also available in two sizes: with inflow diameters of 26mm and 29mm. As the device is self-expanding and deployed by retraction of a sheath, rapid pacing is generally not required. The valve is generally delivered via a transfemoral or subclavian approach.

The Melody transcatheter valve (Medtronic Inc, Minneapolis, MN) is composed of bovine jugular venous valve leaflets in a platinum iridium stent scaffold delivered using a balloon-in-balloon system to facilitate positioning during expansion (Image 3). The valve is designed for use in the venous circulation, mostly to treat dysfunctional right ventricular outflow tract conduits or other pulmonary bioprostheses in patients with congenital heart disease.

Access Modes

Depending on the anatomical valve treated and the delivery system used, a number of approaches may be available for VIV therapy, with various advantages/disadvantages for each.

Aortic – The most frequently utilized approaches are transapical or transfemoral (Figures 4 and 5). The transapical approach offers the advantages of greater control given the shorter distance to the valve, more coaxial alignment and also easier crossing of the surgical valve as this is performed in an antegrade fashion. To date, only the Edwards system has been used via a transapical route for VIV therapy. The Medtronic CoreValve system has been generally delivered via the transfemoral approach. Both systems can also be delivered via a transaxillary/subclavian approach [18,19].

Mitral valve – Our initial attempts at first-in-human mitral VIV implantation using transvenous access with transeptal puncture and using a minithoracotomy with transatrial puncture were unsuccessful as we were unable to achieve coaxial alignment of the THV within the bioprosthetic valve [20]. All other attempts have been successfully performed transapically. To our knowledge, all successful mitral VIV procedures in humans have been via a transapical route utilizing the Edwards SAPIEN system.

Tricuspid valve – Small numbers of transcatheter tricuspid VIV procedures have been performed [20, 21]. We have performed two cases using a transatrial approach via a right mini-thoracotomy, and are aware of other successful cases via a similar route. In the only other published report to our knowledge, a percutaneous transjugular approach was used to implant a 22mm Medtronic Melody valve.

Pulmonary valve – The majority of cases have used the Melody valve, implanted via a femoral, right internal jugular or left subclavian venous approach [22]. Implants using the Edwards SAPIEN system have similarly been via a transvenous approach. While successful transapical pulmonary valve implantation has been described in animal models, there are not published cases of this access route in humans [23].

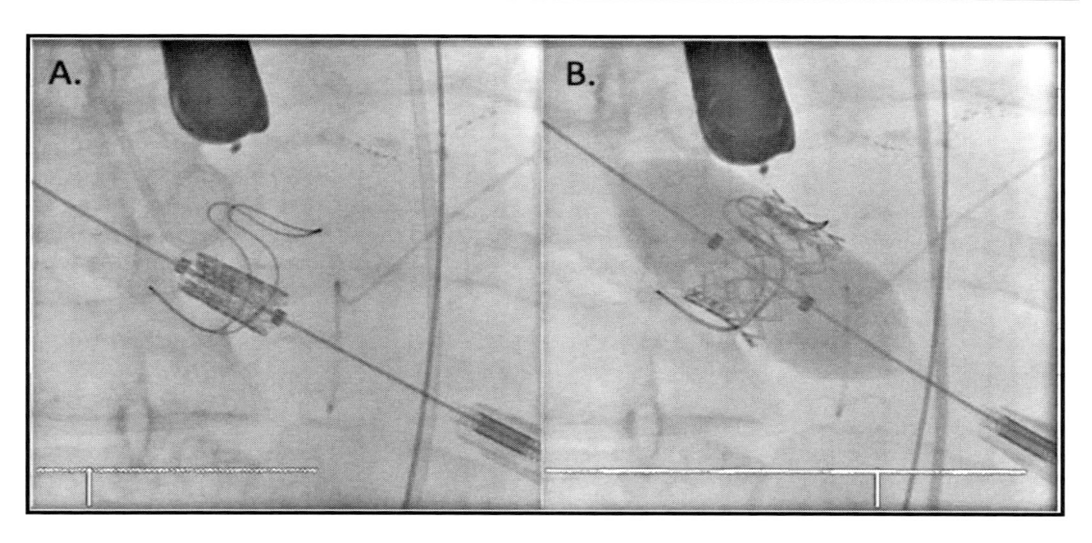

Figure 4. Transapical aortic VIV implantation. A. Positioning an Edwards SAPIEN 23mm valve within a Carpentier Edwards 25mm valve. B. Valve deployment under rapid ventricular pacing at 180 beats/minute.

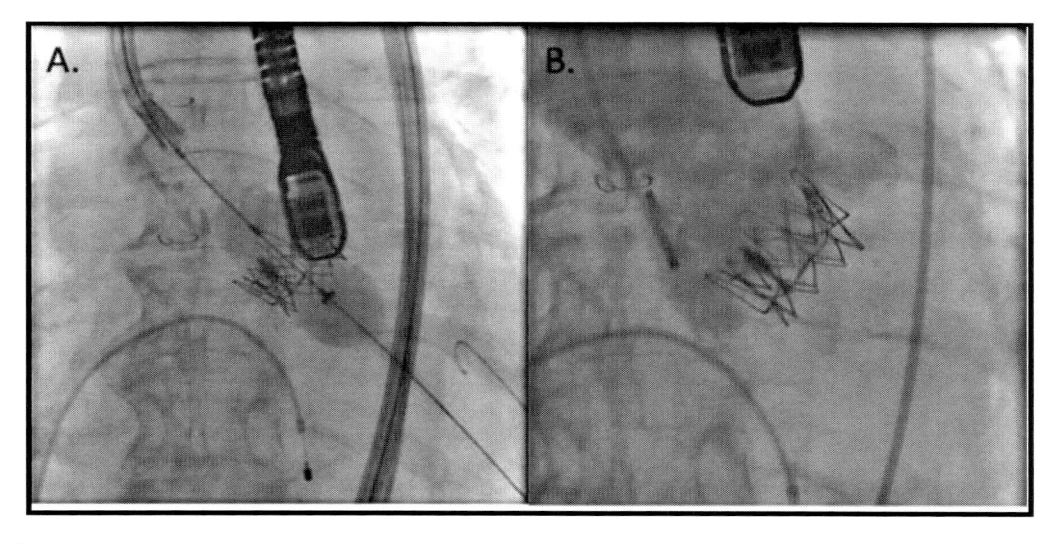

Figure 5. Transfemoral aortic VIV implantation. A. An Edwards SAPIEN XT 23mm valve is deployed within a Carpentier Edwards 23mm valve under rapid ventricular pacing at 180 beats/minute. B. Aortogram demonstrating the final result.

Positioning

Early bench models and animal studies suggested the THV should be positioned in the outflow portion of the surgical valve. At our first attempt of aortic VIV using the Edwards SAPIEN system, the THV was positioned in the outflow portions of the surgical bioprosthesis without overlapping the sewing ring. Balloon inflation splayed the surgical valve struts and resulted in embolization. Since then, we have adopted positioning the THV such that it overlaps within the annular sewing ring for improved fixation, without any further embolizations (image 6).

The operator must appreciate the angiographic landmarks and their corresponding anatomical correlates depending on the valve type being treated. Specifically, the location of the surgical sewing ring must be known in relation to radiopaque markers on the surgical valve. The location of radiopaque markers on different valves varies considerably, and familiarity with these appearances and the underlying structural elements relating to these markers is paramount prior to embarking on treating a particular valve. For example, some valves may have radiopaque markers very close to the sewing ring, while in others the markers may be close to the tip of the stent posts, or there may be no radiopaque markers at all (Image 7).

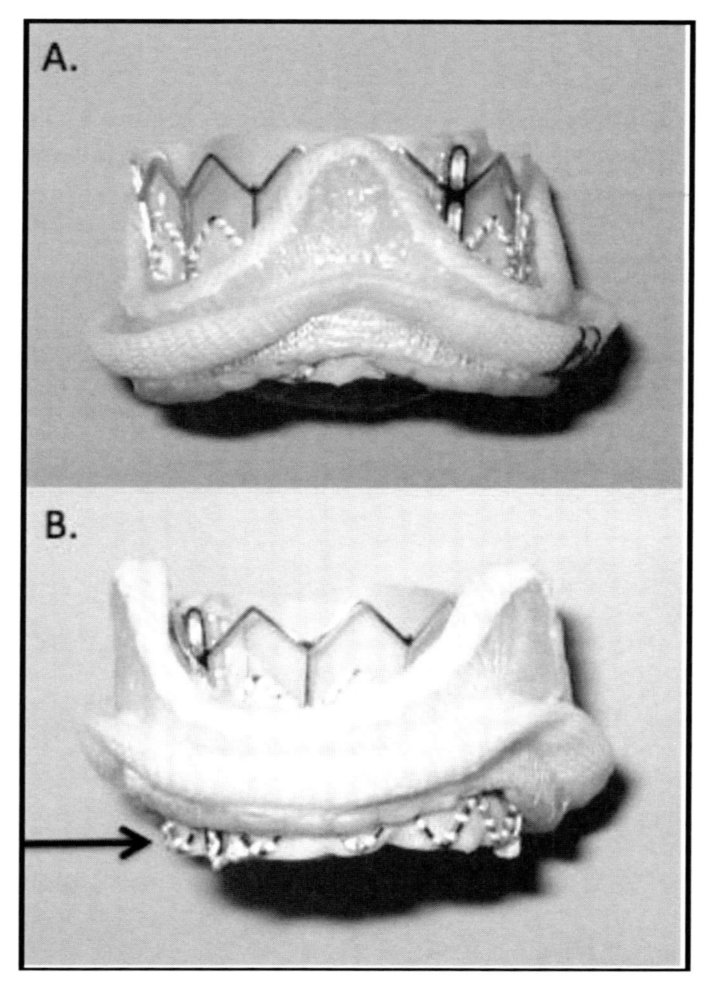

Figure 6. In vitro demonstration of a transcatheter valve (Edwards SAPIEN) implanted within a surgical valve (Carpentier Edwards). A. Incorrect Positioning: the transcatheter valve is implanted “too high”, within the outflow tract of the surgical valve. This may result in splaying of the surgical valve posts and transcatheter valve embolization. B. Correct valve positioning: The transcatheter valve (black arrow) is implanted such that it overlaps the surgical sewing ring, allowing better anchoring and a more secure position.

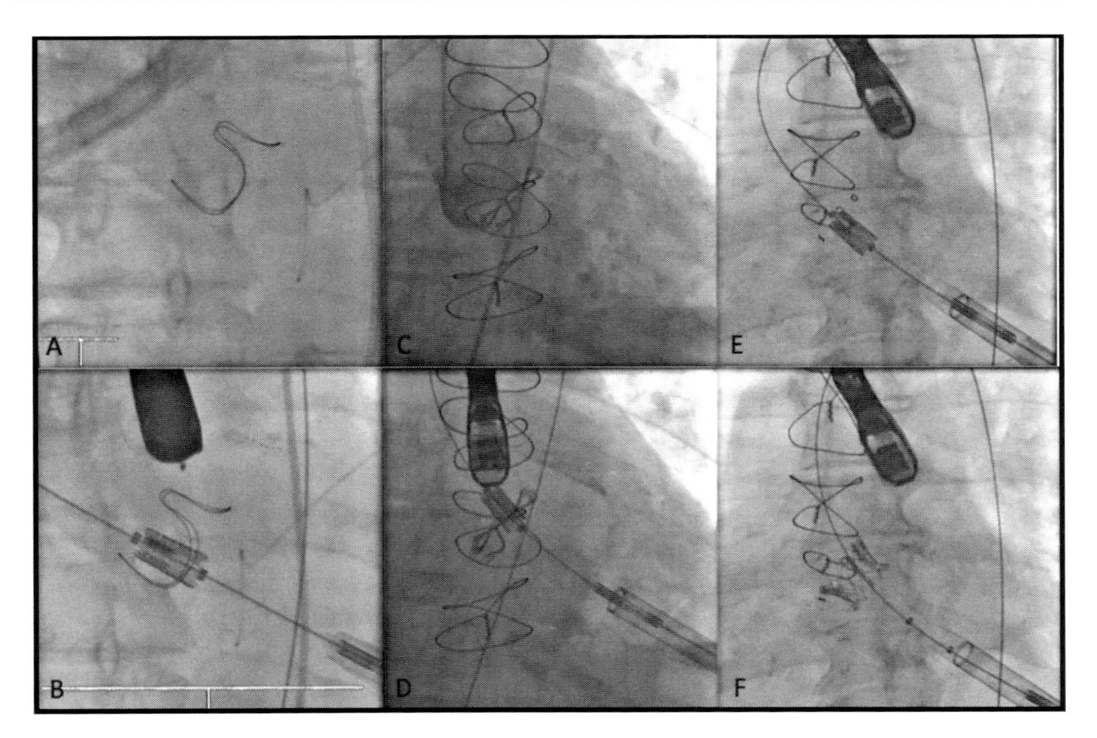

Figure 7. Fluroscopic Positioning: Importance of knowing the radiological appearance of the surgical valve treated. A. Carpentier Edwards Valve, B. Positioning of the Edwards SAPIEN just below the lowest radiopaque portion. C. Sorin Mitroflow Valve, D. Positioning the Edwards SAPIEN just below the lowest radiopaque portion. E. Medtronic Mosaic valve – the radiopaque markers are near the **top** of the surgical stent posts, hence the valve is positioned completely below these markers, F. Deployed Edwards SAPIEN valve. The "waist" at the lower part of the implanted valve demonstrates the narrowest location of the surgical valve.

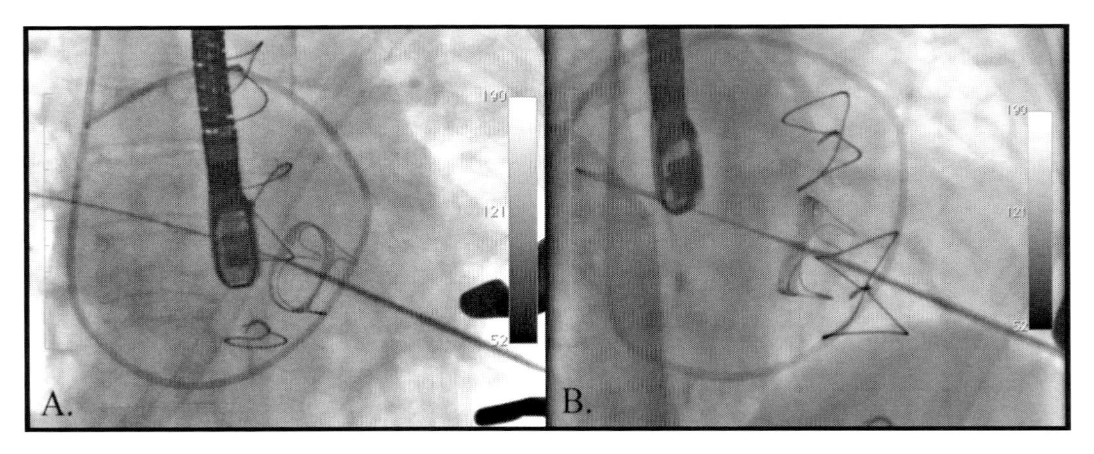

Figure 8. Perpendicular alignment for implantation. Flouroscopic images of a Carpentier Edwards Perimount valve in the mitral position. A. In the PA-straight projection, the valve is not perpendicular/orthogonal to the image intensifier, and is likely to lead to foreshortening. B. In the 25° right anterior oblique projection, the valve is now perpendicular/orthogonal to the image intensifier, allowing more accurate positioning of a transcatheter valve.

Co-axial positioning within the surgical valve is important to achieve prior to deployment. Angiographic C-arm angles which allow perpendicularity to the valve plane need to be determined. While these angles may sometimes be difficult to determine during transcatheter treatment of native aortic stenosis [24], the presence of angiographic markers on the surgical valve generally makes this easier during VIV therapy. For example, if the radiographic marker is a basal ring, rotating the C-arm until the ring is side on suggests appropriate perpendicularity to the valve plane (Figure 8), and this should form the implant view. Further manipulation may then be required to achieve co-axial alignment by techniques similar to those during native valve therapy, such as wire manipulation and tension, or device flexion/extension.

Procedural Consideration and Results

Aortic –VIV therapy for failed aortic bioprostheses has been the most frequently reported VIV procedure to date. As both the Edwards SAPIEN and Medtronic CoreValve systems are suitable for treating failed bioprostheses in this position, the majority of technical details are familiar to those already treating native aortic valve stenosis using transcatheter techniques.

Once the surgical valve is crossed with a guidewire, predilation to facilitate crossing with the THV may or may not be performed. The main risks of predilation are embolization of material from a bulky valve or structural damage causing disintegration. Using the transapical approach may reduce the need for predilation as the surgical valve is easier to cross antegrade. However, if the THV is advanced too far such that it needs to be pulled back through the valve, failure to predilate may make this more difficult. Rapid ventricular pacing is needed using the Edwards SAPIEN valve, but may be omitted for the Medtronic CoreValve device.

A variety of failed surgical bioprostheses have been successfully treated, both stented and stentless models [25] [26]. Our own group has performed 11 such cases (Table 1), with encouraging results overall. While the very first attempt resulted in embolization due to error in valve positioning, all subsequent transapical and transfemoral attempts resulted in THV implantation in the correct anatomical position.

Procedural outcomes have been encouraging, with satisfactory clinical outcomes especially given the high-risk nature of these patients. From our cohort of 11 patients, there was 1 procedural death due to acute coronary obstruction following treatment of a failed Mitroflow bioproshthesis, discussed in more detail below. All other patients were alive at 30-days.

Post-procedural gradients have been generally higher when compared to transcatheter treatment of native aortic stenosis. The average post-procedural mean transvalvular gradient in our cohort was 22mmHg. Similary, Seiffert reported an average transvalvular mean gradient of 19mmHg using the Edwards SAPIEN valve in 4 patients, and Khawaha an average transvalvular peak gradient of 33.5 mmHg using the Medtronic CoreValve [26, 27].

The degree of post-procedural regurgitation has been encouraging. As assessed by transesophageal echocardiography, we have not observed greater than trivial post-procedural regurgitation. Similarly, other published reports have generally noted less than 1+ aortic regugitation [26, 27].

Table 1. Mitral valve-in-valve implantations

Patient #	Age	Failed Surgical Valve	Type of Surgical Valve	Size of SAPIEN THV	Post MG	Post AI	Postop Paravalvular Leak	F/U (days)	Preop NYHA	Postop NYHA
1[*]	85	Regurgitation	Carpentier Edwards 29mm	N/A	N/A	N/A	N/A	1	4	N/A
2[τ]	80	Stenosis	Baxter Edwards 25mm	26	6	0	0	45	4	N/A
3	78	Stenosis	Edwards SAV 27mm	26	9	0	0	645	3	1
4	80	Regurgitation	Edwards SAV 27mm	26	9	0	0	485	4	1
5	84	Stenosis	Medtronic Mosaic 25mm	26	9	0	1	423	3	1
6	73	Regurgitation	Carpantier-Edwards 27mm	23	8	1	1	365	4	1
7	77	Stenosis/ regurgitation	Medtronic Intact 27mm	23	7	0	0	350	3	1
8	84	Regurgitation	Medtronic Mosaic 25mm	23	6	0	1	280	4	2
9	89	Regurgitation	Edwards Porcine 29mm	26	5	0	1	120	4	N/A
10	73	Regurgitation	Medtronic Mosaic 27mm	26	5	0	1	90	4	1
11	76	Stenosis/ regurgitation	Edwards Perimount 25mm	23	8	0	0	90	4	2
12	80	Stenosis	Medtronic Mosaic 29mm	23	7	1	1	18	3	2

All approaches were primary transapical, apart from: [*]Transvenous/transeptal approach, [τ] Transatrial then converted to transapical.

THV = Transcatheter Heart Valve, MG = Mean Gradient, AI = Aortic Incompetence, F/U = Follow-up, NYHA = New York Heart Association, SAV = Supra-annular valve.

Table 2. Aortic valve-in-valve implantation

Patient #	Age	Failed Surgical Valve	Type of Surgical Valve	Approach	Size of SAPIEN THV	MG Post	AI Post	Paravalvular Leak Post	F/U (days)	NYHA Pre	NYHA Post
1	87	Stenosis/ regurgitation	Carpentier-Edwards porcine 25mm	TF/TA*	23	11	0	0	1212	3	1
2	83	Stenosis	Edwards porcine 23mm	TA	23	24	0	0	610	4	1
3	85	Stenosis	EC Porcine 23mm	TA	23	27	0	0	540	4	1
4	86	Stenosis	Lonescu Shiley 21mm	TA	23	23	0	0	535	3	1
5	86	Stenosis	Edwards 25mm	TA	26	13	0	0	390	3	2
6	83	Stenosis	EC porcine 21mm	TA	23	24	1	1	380	4	N/A
7	82	Stenosis/ regurgitation	Medtronic Mosaic 21mm	TA	23	30	1	1	340	4	2
8	67	Regurgitation/ stenosis	EC porcine 23mm	TF	23	20	1	1	330	4	1
9	86	Stenosis	Sorin Mitroflow 21mm	TA	23	N/A	0	0	1	4	N/A
10	82	Regurgitation	Sorin Mitroflow 23mm	TA	23	32	0	1	120	4	1
11	80	Stenosis	Baxter Edwards 23mm	TF	23	20	0	1	14	3	2

* Initial approach was transfemoral but the valve embolized. Procedure converted to transapical which was successful.

THV = Transcatheter Heart Valve, MG = Mean Gradient, AI = Aortic Incompetence, F/U = Follow-up, NYHA = New York Heart Association, TA = Transapical, TF = Transfemoral.

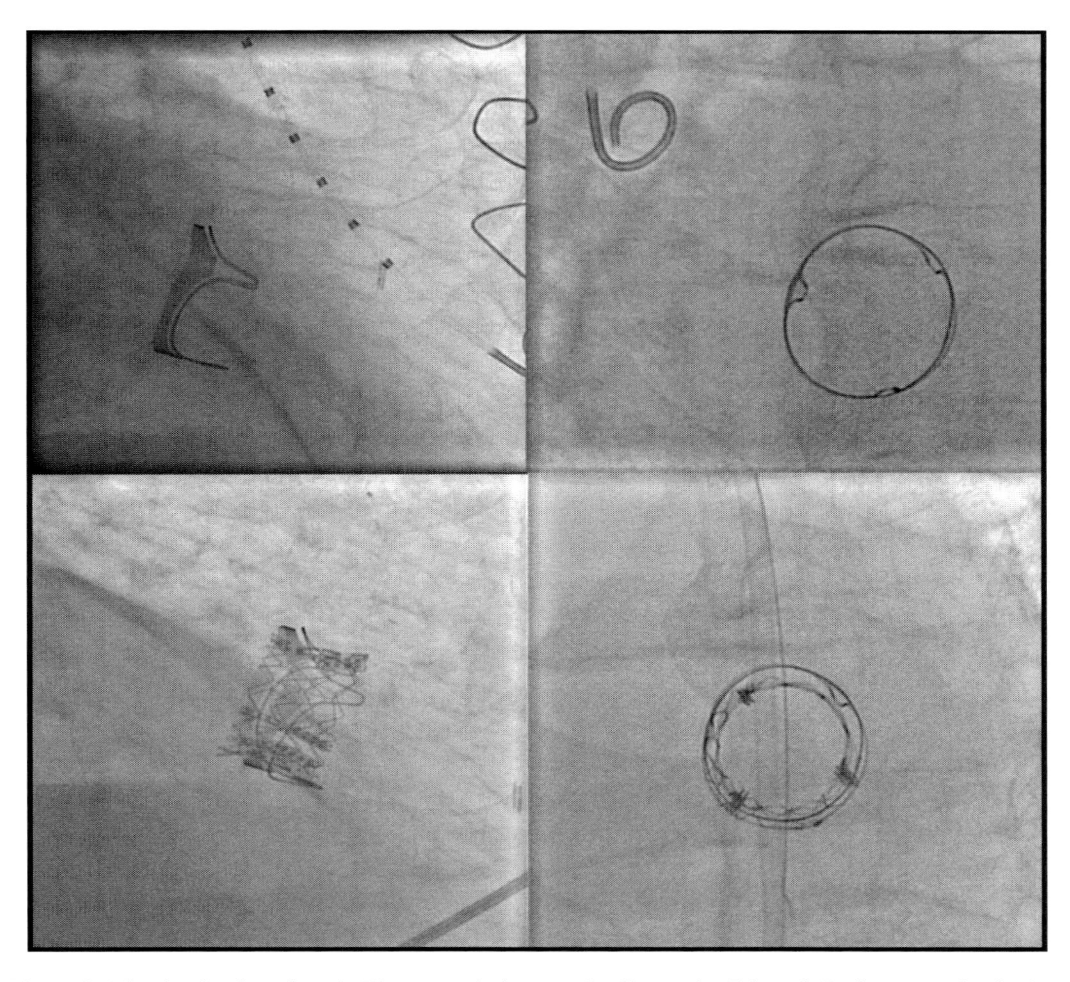

Figure 9. Mitral valve in valve. A. Flouroscopic image of a Carpentier Edwards Perimount valve in the mitral position. The valve is perpendicular to the image intensifier. B. Same valve is shown "down the barrel". This would be a poor angiographic projection in which to position a transcatheter valve. C. Perpendicular projection following implantation of an Edwards SAPIEN valve. D. "Down the barrel" projection following implantation of an Edwards SAPIEN valve. The new valve can be seen inside the surgical valve.

While long-term data is lacking, our first patient was in NYHA class I at 1212 days post procedure, with a transvalvular gradient of 18mmHg. Our overall survival at a median follow-up of 380 days (IQR 226 – 538 days) is 82%. Seiffert et al. reported on 1 patient with 12-month follow-up, in NYHA class 3 and a with transvalvular gradient of 34mmHg.

Mitral – Our first 2 transvenous and transatrial attempts were unsuccessful largely due to difficulties in co-axial positioning. The transatrial case was converted to a transapical procedure and was successful. All subsequent 11 procedures were performed transapically and were successful (Figure 9, Table 2).

Following transapical puncture, the valve is crossed with a stiff guidewire positioned in the left atrium. Predilation may or may not be performed, but is generally not required especially for regurgitant valves. Positioning principles are similar to aortic implants, with the aim of overlapping the surgical sewing ring. The Edwards SAPIEN valve should be deployed under rapid ventricular pacing. Great attention must be paid to mounting the valve in the correct direction on the balloon, as staff are generally accustomed to transapical native aortic valve implants which require the opposite valve orientation.

To our knowledge, only the Edwards SAPIEN valve has been implanted in this position in humans. Sizing is an important consideration given the tendency of mitral bioprostheses to be of larger diameter than aortic. While aortic bioprostheses are generally ≤27mm, for which the 26mm Edwards SAPIEN may be well suited, mitral bioprostheses are commonly >30mm and may be difficult to treat using currently available systems. Recently, a 29mm Edwards SAPIEN valve has become available and we have successfully used it in a patient with a 31mm diameter Medtronic Mosaic valve.

Clinical outcomes in our cohort have been very encouraging, with no procedural or 30-day mortality in the 11 primarily transapical procedures. The median transvalvular gradient post procedure was 7mmHg. Similarly to the aortic procedure, no greater than trivial post-procedural regurgitation was observed, even in patients treated for primary severe mitral regurgitation. In our series, the overall survival of primarily transapical procedures at a median follow-up of 315 days (IQR 101-408 days) was 90%.

Tricuspid – Tricuspid valve replacement is a relatively uncommon procedure, with the majority of surgical intervention aimed towards treating annular dilatation using annuloplasty rings. Likewise, limited experience exists with VIV procedures for failed tricuspid bioprostheses in humans. We have successfully performed two such cases, one other case has been published, and we are aware a small number of other cases successfully performed (Figure 10) [20, 21].

Utilizing a transatrial approach via a right mini thoracotomy, a stiff guidewire is positioned in the right ventricle or pulmonary artery. Again, valvuloplasty may or may not be required, although this can also be used to aid in valve sizing [21]. We have deployed the Edwards SAPIEN valve under rapid pacing. The Medtronic Melody valve is generally deployed without rapid pacing in the more commonly treated pulmonary position. Although rapid pacing may not be required to reduce transvalvular flow or gradients we have found it helpful in reducing cardiac motion during positioning. This may be particularly helpful when positioning the relatively short Edwards SAPIEN valve where the margin for error is small.

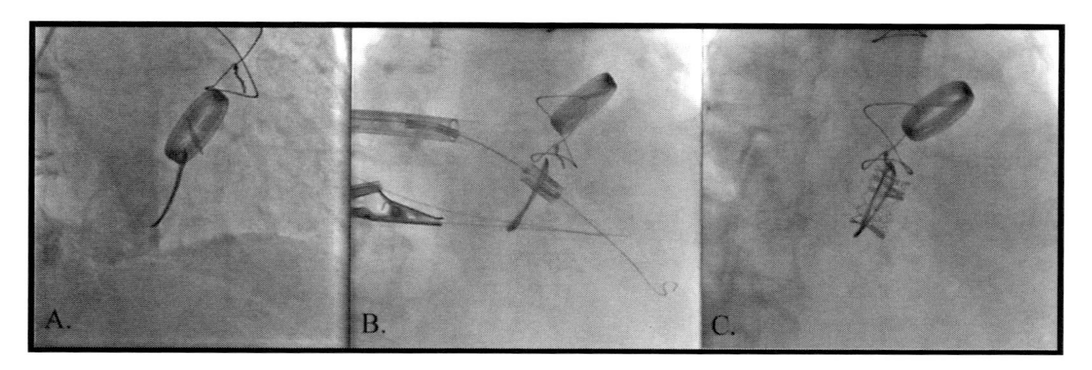

Figure 10. Tricuspid valve in valve. A. A tricuspid Mitroflow Synergy 27mm valve is seen perpendicular to the image intensifier (a bileaflet mechanical valve in the mitral position is also seen above it). B. A sheath is introduced via the right atrium through a mini right thoracotomy. An Edwards SAPIEN 26mm valve is being positioned. C. Final image following implantation.

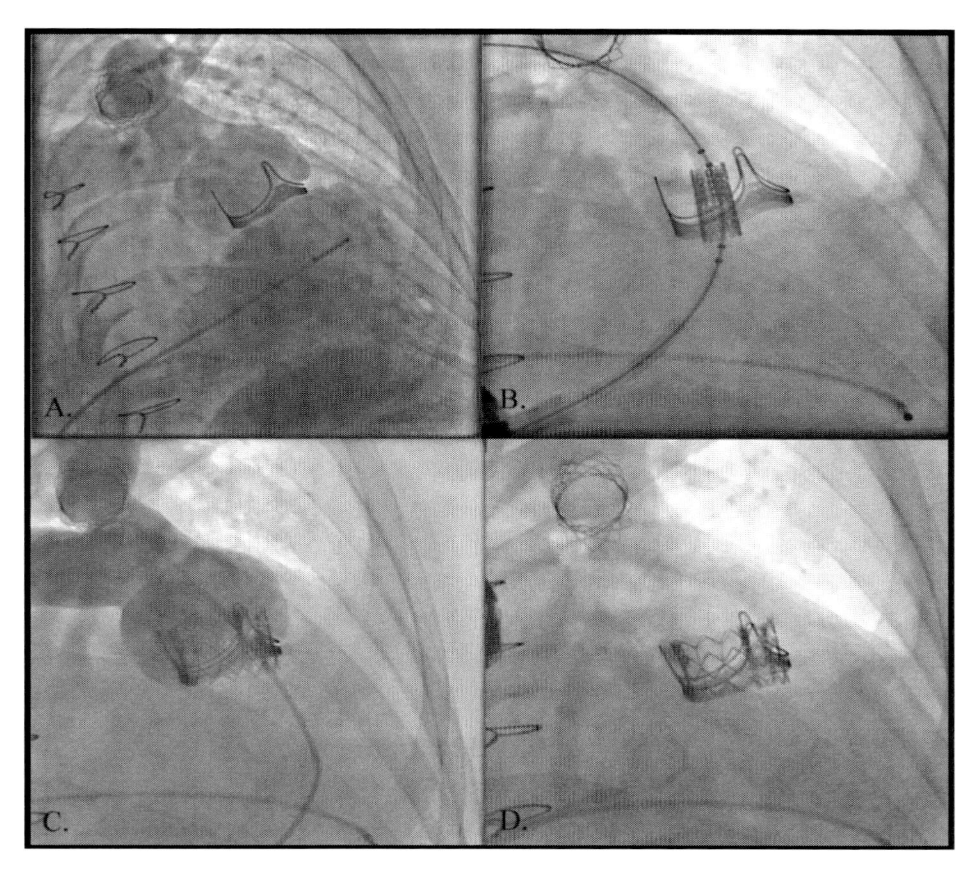

Figure 11. Pulmonary valve in valve. A. A Carpentier Edwards Perimount 27mm valve (a left pulmonary artery stent is also seen) in a 21 year old man with repaired tetralogy of fallot. The valve was severely regurgitant with moderate to severe stenosis B. An Edwards SAPIEN 26mm valve is being positioned. C. Post-deployment pulmonary angiogram demonstrating no residual pulmonary regurgitation. D. Final image post implantation.

Pulmonary - The implantation and creation of valved conduits in the right ventricular outflow tract has been an integral aspect of treating many congenital heart defects. Pulmonary conduits are low-pressure mostly tubular systems, often in patients who have undergone multiple previous procedures and hence ideally suited to THV implantation. Pulmonary valve disease outside of conditions involving more complex congenital structural heart disease is rare. Subsequently, these form a unique group of conditions, patients, and technical considerations, which are largely outside the scope of this chapter.

Bonhoeffer and his colleagues first described percutaneous implantation of a bovine jugular valve in a right ventricular to pulmonary artery conduit of a 12-year-old boy in 2000, and reported on their experience with 59 such patients in 2005 [28] [29]. This formed the platform for the Medtronic-Melody valve, the first transcatheter valve to be approved by the US FDA for therapy of dysfunctional right ventricular outflow tract conduits in pediatric or adult patients. Over 100 patients were treated as part of the Expanded Multicentre US Melody Valve Trial [30] [22]. Thus far short-term results have been very encouraging with high success rates and relatively low procedural complications. Rapid ventricular pacing is generally not required given the lower pressures in the right-sided circulation and longer stent length. While the majority of conduits treated have been homografts, a significant proportion of bioprosthetic valves have also been treated [22].

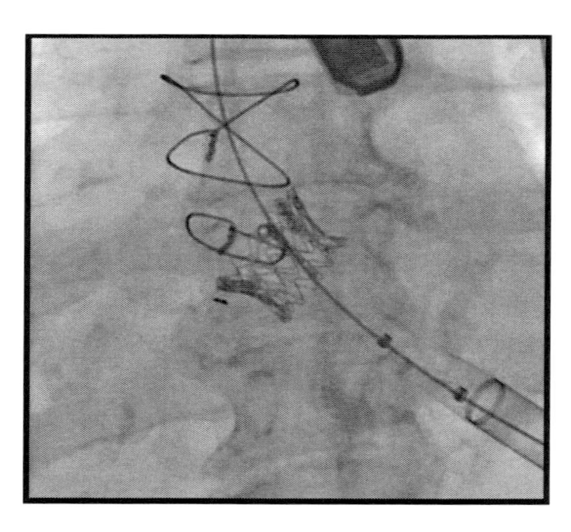

Figure 12. Underexpanded transcatheter valve in the aortic position. An Edward SAPIEN 23mm valve implanted within a Medtronic Mosaic 21mm valve for treatment of severe aortic regurgitation and moderately severe stenosis. The residual transaortic gradient was 30mmHg (with no residual regurgitation).

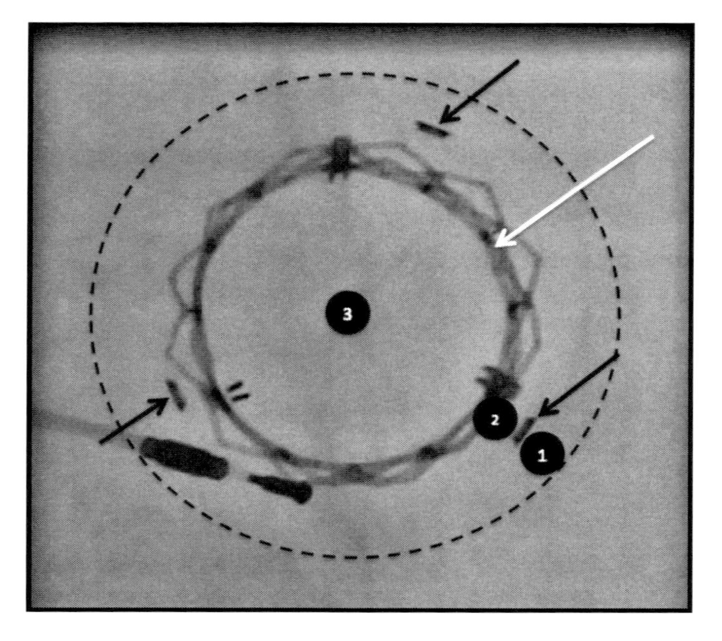

Figure 13. Possible sources of regurgitation following valve in valve implantation. "Down the barrel/end on" image of an Edwards SAPIEN valve (white arrow) implanted within a Medtronic Mosaic valve (black arrows showing the radiopaque markers). The large surrounding circle represents surrounding native tissue. Regurgitation may arise from 3 areas depicted schematically by the 3 black circles: (1) paravalvular, arising between the native tissue and the original failed bioprosthetic valve, (2) intervalvular – arising from the area *between* the old "outer" surgical valve and the new "inner" transcatheter valve, and (3) valvular – arising from within the transcatheter valve.

The Edwards SAPIEN system can also be used to treat failed homografts/conduits or bioprosthetic valves in the pulmonary position (Figure 11) [31]. Given the shorter length of the valve, a two-step procedure is often performed where the conduit is initially stented with a bare metal stent, allowing a greater margin of safety during positioning and increasing the chance of maintaining device circularity. When treating failed surgical bioprostheses, such "pre-stenting" can be omitted.

Valve function following VIV implants – Unlike in transcatheter valve therapy for native aortic valve disease, where relatively full expansion can be expected within the annulus, PHV expansion during VIV therapy can be constrained by the internal dimensions of the surgical bioprosthesis, particularly so by the relatively un-dilatable sewing ring (Figure 12).

Valve under-expansion appears to be relatively common during VIV therapy, and it may be expected that this would affect transvalvular gradients, effective orifice areas and possibly long-term durability. The average post procedural transaortic gradient in our series was 22mmHg and Kwaja et al. reported an average peak transaortic gradient 33.5 mmHg using the Medtronic-CoreValve. In comparison, mean gradients following trascatheter therapy for native aortic stenosis are generally around 10mmHg [32][33]. While elevated gradients may be acceptable in some patients who cannot undergo open-heart surgery, they may be inadequate in others with longer expected survival.

A report by Azadani et al. evaluated the hemodynamic performance of 23mm THVs within degenerated surgical bioprostheses ranging in size from 19mm to 23mm, hypothesizing that inadequate resolution of stenosis would be achieved in small valves [34]. They demonstrated in an in-vitro model that incomplete stent expansion resulted in leaflet distortion and central regurgitation when implanted in 19 and 21 mm bioprostheses. In a subsequent report, the same group used a custom designed supravalvular THV consisting of a stainless steel stent covered with Dacron (DuPont, Wilmington, DE), with a valve within an open stent positioned above the bioprosthetic posts [35]. More favorable hemodynamics were obtained using this design, with transvalvular gradients comparable to standard surgical valve replacement even in valves as small as 19mm. Such studies raise the possibility that future developments may result in transcatheter systems more ideally suited to VIV therapy with improved hemodynamics even when used in small valves.

There is currently insufficient long-term outcome data to understand the clinical sequela of such residual gradients. From our own experience, we have yet to see patients fail to improve or return for further intervention because of elevated gradients. For example, two patients from our cohort had transaortic gradients of 24mmHg and 27mmHg. At a follow-up of 610 and 540 days respectively, both remain asymptomatic in NYHA class I. However, it is conceivable that some patients may fail to obtain adequate symptomatic improvement is sufficiently low transvalvular gradients are not obtained.

Regurgitation appears to be less of an issue, and generally appears to be less than mild in published reports. We suggest reporting 3 sources of regurgitation post-procedure (Image 13):

1. Paravalvular – arising between the native valve and the original failed bioprosthetic valve.
2. Intervalvular – arising from the area *between* the old "outer" surgical valve and the new "inner" transcatheter valve.
3. Valvular – arising through the newly implanted valve,

If there is paravalular regurgitation around a surgical valve prior to VIV implantation, THV implantation is generally unlikely to ameliorate it given that no significant expansion of the surgical valve occurs during VIV therapy at the annular/sewing ring level.

Sizing Considerations

While current surgical bioprostheses are described according to their external diameters, the internal dimensions are more relevant for VIV therapy. However, the internal diameters vary significantly between manufacturer, valve model and size. While manufacturers generally provide internal diameters, these can sometimes be misleading [36] [37]. Also, VIV therapy need not necessarily be for valvular stenosis. Regurgitant valves may have less pannus and not be as bulky, making sizing considerations more complicated. A larger valve may need to be considered in order to achieve adherence to surrounding structures in such circumstances.

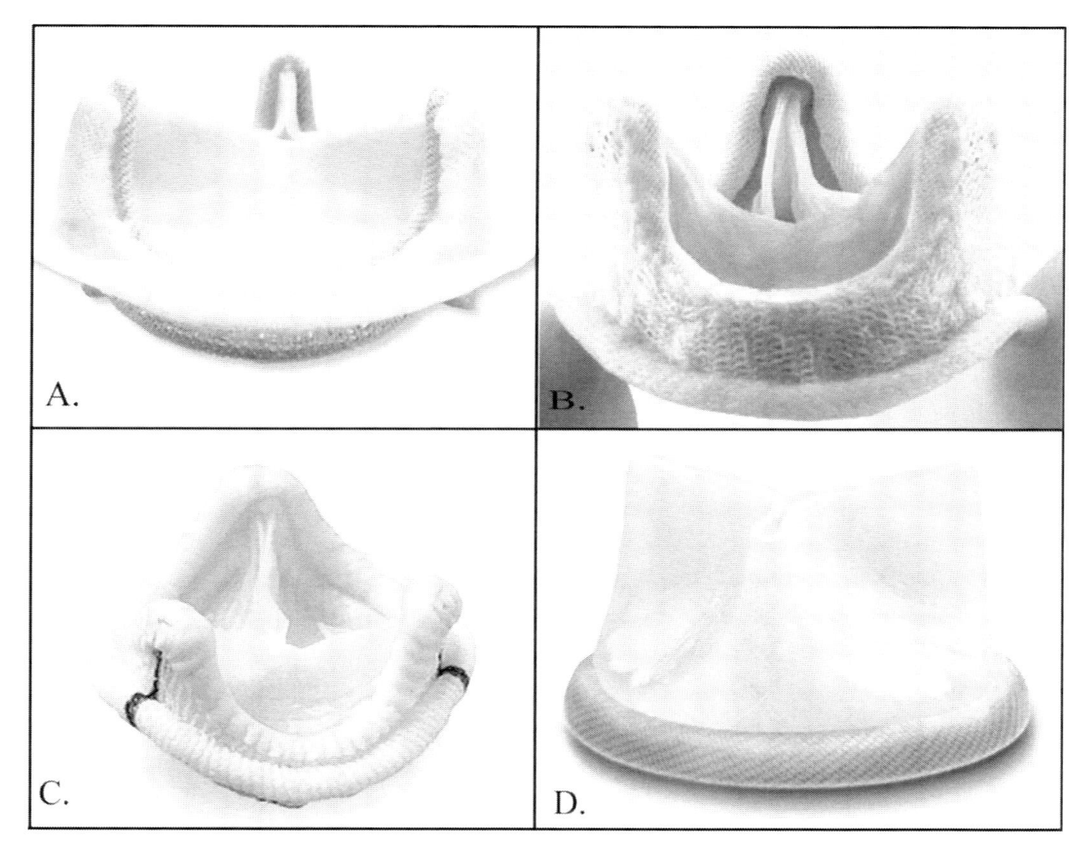

Figure 14. Different surgical bioprosthetic valves demonstrating the relative locations of the valve leaflets to the stent frame. (A) Carpentier Edwards PERIMOUNT, (B) Medtronic Mosaic, (C) St. Jude Medical EPIC, and (D) Sorin Medical Mitroflow valves. In A-C, the leaflets can be seen to be on the *inside* of valve stent frame. In D, the pericardial leaflets are seen on the *outside* of the valve stent frame (stent frame cannot be seen).

Oversizing which causes underexpansion of a large valve may result in compromised hemodynamics, while undersizing may result in embolization or patient prosthesis mismatch. Sizing needs to be considered carefully in each patient, taking into consideration the reported internal diameter, patient size, bulkiness of the degenerated valve, nature of the valve failure and the location of calcification or pannus.

Considerations Relating to Specific Valve Types

Thus far we have treated a range of failed surgical valves without particular preference for one over the other in the great majority (Tables 1 and 2). As previously discussed, operators need to be familiar with the unique radiological appearance of each valve and determine the internal diameter in each case. However, we have found that two valves types do deserve a special consideration:

- The Mitroflow valve (Sorin group, Vancouver, BC, Canada) is unique in that the leaflet tissue is mounted *externally over* the stent as opposed to *internally*, as is generally the case with other commercially available surgical prostheses (Image 14). During treatment of such a failed valve in the aortic position, one patient suffered acute coronary obstruction and died despite conversion to open thoracotomy. Leaflet tissue mounted outside the valve stent may pose a unique problem during transcatheter valve-in-valve therapy. When a new valve is positioned inside a failed bioprosthetic one, having the leaflets on the inside of the original valve frame ensures to some degree that sufficient space remains for blood to track down to the coronary vessels. However, with externally mounted leaflets especially in a supra-annular position, the transcatheter valve-in-valve may push externally mounted leaflets directly onto the aortic wall and impede coronary blood flow.
- The Medtronic Intact Porcine valve (model 705) appears not to have a significant radiopaque component to aid in angiographic positioning. We have successfully treated one such failed mitral valve with positioning performed utilizing transesophageal echocardiography guidance.

Conclusion

Transcatheter VIV implantation is a promising alternative for treatment of failed surgical valves especially for patients at high surgical risk. All four cardiac valves can be treated, with encouraging early to mid-term results in multiples series. A number of currently available transcatheter systems can be used, and future technological advances may continue to improve both hemodynamic and clinical outcomes.

References

[1] Gummert JF, Funkat A, Beckmann A et al. Cardiac surgery in Germany during 2008. A report on behalf of the German Society for Thoracic and Cardiovascular Surgery. *Thorac. Cardiovasc. Surg*. 2009;57:315–23.

[2] Ruel M, Chan V, Bedard P et al. Very long-term survival implications of heart valve replacement with tissue versus mechanical prostheses in adults <60 years of age. *Circulation*. 2007;116:I294–300.

[3] Jones JM, O'kane H, Gladstone DJ et al. Repeat heart valve surgery: risk factors for operative mortality. J. *Thorac. Cardiovasc. Surg*. 2001;122:913–18.

[4] Akins CW, Buckley MJ, Daggett WM et al. Risk of reoperative valve replacement for failed mitral and aortic bioprostheses. *Ann. Thorac. Surg*. 1998;65:1545–51; discussion 1551-2.

[5] Maganti M, Rao V, Armstrong S, Feindel CM, Scully HE, David TE. Redo valvular surgery in elderly patients. *Ann. Thorac. Surg*. 2009;87:521–25.

[6] Cribier A, Eltchaninoff H, Bash A et al. Percutaneous transcatheter implantation of an aortic valve prosthesis for calcific aortic stenosis: first human case description. *Circulation*. 2002;106:3006–08.

[7] Webb JG, Altwegg L, Masson JB, Al Bugami S, Al Ali A, Boone RA. A new transcatheter aortic valve and percutaneous valve delivery system. *J. Am. Coll. Cardiol*. 2009;53:1855–58.

[8] Webb JG, Chandavimol M, Thompson CR et al. Percutaneous aortic valve implantation retrograde from the femoral artery. *Circulation*. 2006;113:842–50.

[9] Lichtenstein SV, Cheung A, Ye J et al. Transapical transcatheter aortic valve implantation in humans: initial clinical experience. *Circulation*. 2006;114:591–96.

[10] Walther T, Dewey T, Borger MA et al. Transapical aortic valve implantation: step by step. *Ann. Thorac. Surg*. 2009;87:276–83.

[11] Webb JG. Percutaneous aortic valve replacement will become a common treatment for aortic valve disease. *JACC Cardiovasc. Interv*. 2008;1:122–26.

[12] Piazza N, Grube E, Gerckens U et al. Procedural and 30-day outcomes following transcatheter aortic valve implantation using the third generation (18 Fr) corevalve revalving system: results from the multicentre, expanded evaluation registry 1-year following CE mark approval. *EuroIntervention*. 2008;4:242–49.

[13] Tamburino C, Capodanno D, Mule M et al. Procedural success and 30-day clinical outcomes after percutaneous aortic valve replacement using current third-generation self-expanding CoreValve prosthesis. *J. Invasive Cardiol*. 2009;21:93–98.

[14] Boudjemline Y, Pineau E, Borenstein N, Behr L, Bonhoeffer P. New insights in minimally invasive valve replacement: description of a cooperative approach for the off-pump replacement of mitral valves. *Eur. Heart J*. 2005;26:2013–17.

[15] Walther T, Falk V, Dewey T et al. Valve-in-a-valve concept for transcatheter minimally invasive repeat xenograft implantation. *J. Am. Coll. Cardiol*. 2007;50:56–60.

[16] Nietlispach F, Wijesinghe N, Wood D, Carere RG, Webb JG. Current balloon-expandable transcatheter heart valve and delivery systems. *Catheter Cardiovasc. Interv*. 2010;75:295–300.

[17] Webb JG, Pasupati S, Achtem L, Thompson CR. Rapid pacing to facilitate transcatheter prosthetic heart valve implantation. *Catheter Cardiovasc. Interv.* 2006;68:199–204.

[18] Sharp AS, Michev I, Colombo A. First trans-axillary implantation of Edwards Sapien valve to treat an incompetent aortic bioprosthesis. *Catheter Cardiovasc. Interv.* 2010;75:507–10.

[19] Khawaja, MZ, Haworth, P Ghuran et al. Transcatheter aortic valve implantation for stenosed and regurgitant aortic valve bioprosthesis: corevalve for failed bioprosthetic aortic valve replacements. *Journal of the American College of Cardiology*. 2010;55, No 2:97–101.

[20] Webb JG, Wood DA, Ye J et al. Transcatheter valve-in-valve implantation for failed bioprosthetic heart valves. *Circulation*. 2010;121:1848–57.

[21] Roberts P, Spina R, Vallely M, Wilson M, Bailey B, Celermajer DS. Percutaneous tricuspid valve replacement for a stenosed bioprosthesis. *Circ. Cardiovasc. Interv.* 2010;3:e14–5.

[22] McElhinney DB, Hellenbrand WE, Zahn EM et al. Short- and medium-term outcomes after transcatheter pulmonary valve placement in the expanded multicenter US melody valve trial. *Circulation*. 2010;122:507–16.

[23] Huber CH, Hurni M, Tsang V, von Segesser LK. Valved stents for transapical pulmonary valve replacement. *J. Thorac. Cardiovasc. Surg*. 2009;137:914–18.

[24] Gurvitch R WDA, Leipsic J, Tay E, Johnson M, Ye J, Nietlispach F, Wijesinghe N, Cheung A, Webb JG. Multislice Computed Tomography for Prediction of Optimal Angiographic Deployment Projections During Transcatheter Aortic Valve Implantation. JACC: Cardiovas Interv. In Press

[25] Rodes-Cabau J, Dumont E, Doyle D, Lemieux J. Transcatheter valve-in-valve implantation for the treatment of stentless aortic valve dysfunction. *J. Thorac. Cardiovasc. Surg*. 2010;140:246–48.

[26] Khawaja MZ, Haworth P, Ghuran A et al. Transcatheter aortic valve implantation for stenosed and regurgitant aortic valve bioprostheses CoreValve for failed bioprosthetic aortic valve replacements. *J. Am. Coll. Cardiol*. 2010;55:97–101.

[27] Seiffert M, Franzen O, Conradi L et al. Series of transcatheter valve-in-valve implantations in high-risk patients with degenerated bioprostheses in aortic and mitral position. *Catheter Cardiovasc. Interv*. 2010

[28] Bonhoeffer P, Boudjemline Y, Saliba Z et al. Percutaneous replacement of pulmonary valve in a right-ventricle to pulmonary-artery prosthetic conduit with valve dysfunction. *Lancet*. 2000;356:1403–05.

[29] Khambadkone S, Coats L, Taylor A et al. Percutaneous pulmonary valve implantation in humans: results in 59 consecutive patients. *Circulation*. 2005;112:1189–97.

[30] Zahn EM, Hellenbrand WE, Lock JE, McElhinney DB. Implantation of the melody transcatheter pulmonary valve in patients with a dysfunctional right ventricular outflow tract conduit early results from the u.s. Clinical trial. *J. Am. Coll. Cardiol*. 2009;54:1722–29.

[31] Boone RH, Webb JG, Horlick E et al. Transcatheter pulmonary valve implantation using the edwards SAPIEN transcatheter heart valve. *Catheter Cardiovasc. Interv*. 2010;75:286–94.

[32] Grube E, Buellesfeld L, Mueller R et al. Progress and current status of percutaneous aortic valve replacement: results of three device generations of the CoreValve Revalving system. *Circ. Cardiovasc. Interv.* 2008;1:167–75.

[33] Webb JG, Altwegg L, Boone RH et al. Transcatheter aortic valve implantation: impact on clinical and valve-related outcomes. *Circulation.* 2009;119:3009–16.

[34] Azadani AN, Jaussaud N, Matthews PB, Ge L, Chuter TA, Tseng EE. Transcatheter aortic valves inadequately relieve stenosis in small degenerated bioprostheses. *Interact. Cardiovasc. Thorac. Surg.* 2010;11:70–77.

[35] Azadani AN, Jaussaud N, Matthews PB et al. Valve-in-valve implantation using a novel supravalvular transcatheter aortic valve: proof of concept. *Ann. Thorac. Surg.* 2009;88:1864–69.

[36] Christakis GT, Buth KJ, Goldman BS et al. Inaccurate and misleading valve sizing: a proposed standard for valve size nomenclature. *Ann. Thorac. Surg.* 1998;66:1198–203.

[37] Shibata T, Inoue K, Ikuta T, Bito Y, Yoshioka Y, Mizoguchi H. Which valve and which size should we use in the valve-on-valve technique for re-do mitral valve surgery? *Interact. Cardiovasc. Thorac. Surg.* 2009;8:206–10.

In: Percutaneous Valve Technology: Present and Future ISBN: 978-1-61942-577-4
Editors: Jose Luis Navia and Sharif Al-Ruzzeh

Chapter XV

Complications of Transcatheter Aortic Valve Implantation

Roberto Lorusso, Sandro Gelsomino, Giuseppe De Cicco, Cesare Beghi, Domenico Corradi, Pompilio Faggiano, Enrico Vizzardi, Antonio D'Aloia, Salvatore Curello, Claudia Fiorina, Giuliano Chizzola, Mario Frontini and Federica Ettori

Transcatheter aortic valve implantation (TAVI) is emerging as a valuable procedure to treat patients with severe aortic valve stenosis at high risk or not candidate for conventional aortic valve replacement. Besides obvious shortcomings related to the learning curve, adverse events do occur because of the inherent features of TAVI strictly linked to the application of the procedure as well as of the preoperative patient clinical profiles and comorbidities. These complications may profoundly affect procedural success rate as well as patient outcome at early and mid-term. Despite recent improvements due to advances in technological components as well as in transcatheter procedural management, several complications are still critical issues, and some may not be reduced by better device design or improved procedural strategies. Thorough awareness, therefore, of the prevalence and type of adverse events, potential predisposing factors or determinants, and management strategies to treat them once occurred, might be crucial to allow further improvement in patient outcome and reduce negative results, either in hospital or post discharge. This chapter will provide an overview about prevalence and features of TAVI complications, with particular emphasis on the impact on patient outcome and some insights about management as well as preventing strategies.

Since the first clinical procedure performed by Cribier in 2002 [1], an overwhelming number of clinical series of trans-catheter aortic valve implantation (TAVI) has been recorded (table). In a few years, remarkable advances in valve design and procedural management have been achieved, with substantial improvements in TAVI success rate. However, TAVI accounts for several technical and clinical challenges which may expose the patient at high risk for the occurrence of variable adverse events, some of them being potentially lethal. Complications in TAVI may account for several factors [2] which are inherently linked to the procedure itself, namely advanced patient age, poor clinical conditions at treatment, and numerous and severe comorbidities to be faced intra or peri-procedurally, access and site of intervention, procedural management, last, but not least, type and extent of cardiovascular involvement. All these factors variably contribute to the occurrence and prognosis of TAVI complications, together with the kind of treatment applied to counteract such adverse events. Technical advances in instrument design and size, growing expertise, and refinement in patient selection and intra-procedural imaging, as well as careful peri-procedural management, are all factors supporting the ongoing progressive reduction in complication rate, enhancement in management, and increase in procedural success. Several misadventures, however, still occur during the procedure and appropriate recognition and treatment might lead to more favourable patient outcome, although careful planning and technical skill are paramount to prevent immediate or early untoward events. A comprehensive awareness and knowledge of complication profiles, therefore, are critical to prevent or limit untoward events.

The different types and prevalence of TAVI adverse events will be herein reviewed, the potential determinants or predisposing factors discussed, and the reported strategies to manage them described.

Access-Related Complications (Vascular or Cardiac/Apex)

The first TAVI cases [1] were performed through an atrial transeptal approach, adopting the technique applied for mitral valvuloplasty. It came evident, however, that advancing a bulky device such as the first ones available for TAVI at that time, could lead to unsatisfactory procedural success rate. A trans-arterial approach was then proposed by Webb and associates obviously limited by the arterial access in relation to device size initially available [3]. First trans-arterial experiences with TAVI were characterized by complex procedural preparation (patient intubated and mechanically ventilated, groin vessel cut-down) and performance (large-size and stiff introducer, mechanical cardiocirculatory assistance). Progressive enhancement of TAVI instruments and prosthesis, experience in patient and procedural management gradually simplified the percutaneous access and reduced the related complications. Furthermore, a true percutaneous approach thanks to the low-profile prosthesis, the adoption of a trans-subclavian artery or the cardiac apex, certainly reduced procedural complexity and misadventures.

Regarding the trans-arterial approach, the reduction in size of TAVI delivery catheter and sheath (from 25/22-Fr. sheaths to 18-Fr sheath) as well as the selection of alternative approach with regards to the arterial routes, have enhanced the insertion and deployment of the prosthetic valve inside the diseased aortic valve, overcoming initial obstacles, like restricted, tortuous or occluded femoral or iliac vessels, aneurysmatic or severely calcified abdominal aorta, or severely atheromatous descending thoracic aorta or aortic arch. Nonetheless, despite enhanced TAVI access and pre-procedural vascular screening, vascular or cardiac access still represent a frequent site of unfavourable and sometimes dreadful events [2]. Approach-related complications have been reported to occur in up to 32% of patients submitted to trans-femoral approach, with a 23% of major vascular complication [4]. Limited vascular injury, vessel perforation or dissection, vessel avulsion, distal embolism, or retroperitoneal hemorrhage have been all reported, sometimes requiring massive blood transfusions, endovascular or surgical repair, with obvious negative impact on patient morbidity and ultimate patient outcome [2,4,5].

Predisposing factors for such potentially lethal complications are represented by bulky aortic atheroma, marked vessel tortuosity, and reduced lumen calibre of the vascular access [2]. Current device design and size, and careful observation of a vessel 1 or 2 mm greater than the chosen device sheath may be helpful to prevent catastrophic events [2]. Pre-interventional screening of vessel anatomy have certainly improved procedural planning and management, with reduced incidence of mishaps. It is self-explanatory that appropriate procedural environment and personnel are highly recommended in order to appropriately and quickly provide successful management of potentially lethal complications involving the arterial vascular system [6-8].

With regards of the trans-arterial access, the percutaneous trans-femoral approach is usually the preferred entry-site due to enhanced patient management. The previous use of large-bore balloon-expandable device has shown to increase the risk of vascular injury, dissection, or bleeding. Once a vascular injury is suspected or diagnosed, however, conservative treatment may be still successful, and, in most instances of major vascular damage, endovascular interventions with stent might be applied. In case of complex injury surgical repair may be mandatory. As far as endovascular intervention is concerned, reinsertion of an occlusive sheath over the guidewire or inflating a soft balloon upstream to the area of injury or bleeding may prevent progression of the vascular damage or limit bleeding at the entry site of extravascular hemorrhage (retroperitoneal hemorrhage). The puncture of the femoral vessel above the bifurcation is also recommended since it enhances the deployment of a suture-mediated closure device or allow any endovascular procedure if necessary [6].

The trans-apical access has been proposed to overcome the risk of atheromatous embolism from the aortic arch or ascending aorta intimately linked to a retrograde TAVI approach, and also to prevent major vascular injuries [2,4, 9]. Furthermore, the antegrade approach might allow a better device-alignement through the outflow tract and, theoretically, the implantation of a larger prosthetic size. Nonetheless, a few cases of left ventricular bleeding, rupture, or pseudoaneurysm at the cardiac apex have been reported [10-19]. Age-related frailty of cardiac tissue, complicated or long-lasting procedure, presence of infarcted apex or dilated and thinned left ventricle, may predispose to such negative events. Additional damages to the near structure (lung) are also possible (particularly in patients with chronic obstructive pulmonary disease), but rare [2, 4]. Data from the SOURCE Registry [12], including 575 patients from 32 centres, showed that major approach-related complications, using the trans-apical access, occurred only in 2,4% (14 patients) of the registry, obviously mainly related to left ventricular apex. Of note, this adverse event was significantly correlated to high mortality rate (7 over 14 patients, 50% mortality), as compared to patients not experiencing any major vascular/access-related complication. No case of bleeding in patients submitted to TAVI through a transapical approach has been also reported [20] underlying that although cardiac tissue may be prone to tear or rupture in elderly patients, safety and effective control of access site is possible. Bleiziffer and associates have described in details access-related complications in patients submitted to trans-apical TAVI [7]. In this series, 11 patients over 50 experienced adverse events related to the site of approach, namely bleeding (10%), left ventricular aneurysm (1%), new hypokinesia or akinesia at the apex at 6-month echocardiography (8%). Only one patient died, with the majority of complications solved without any further event. In another clinical series of 60 patients submitted to trans-apical TAVI, left ventricular apical hemorrhage occurred in 3 patients (5%), and apical pseudoaneurysm in 4 (6.6%), making the hemostatic control of the access site, therefore, the most critical aspect of this experience [10]. The use of pledget-reinforced purse-string or a box-type suture have been proposed as advisable options to control bleeding at the apical entry-site. Several other technical aspects have been suggested to accomplish a safe trans-apical access : a clear view of the apex must be obtained, temptatively avoiding fatty tissue area if possible, to ensure accurate recognition of the apical puncture site (avoiding the left ventricular free wall) and of the placement of the para-apical sutures. Large needle with deep bites are also advisable together with a large purse-string suture to allow an unrestricted passage of the transcatheter sheath. Undue sheath manipulation should be also avoided to prevent myocardial tearing or excessive puncture-site enlargement. Finally, pericardial tissue should not be incorporated in the suture, and in case of any difficulty in controlling apical bleeding, temporary LV unloading with a femoro-femoral extracorporeal circulation or a transient rapid ventricular pacing might be helpful to reduce tissue tension and allow effective repair and hemostasis [10]. Avoidance of postoperative anticoagulation (use aspirin and clopidogrel instead) and hypertension may prevent or reduce bleeding complications as well as pseudoaneurysm formation [10, 11].

A word of caution has been raised also by the observation of impairment of cardiac contractility induced by the ventricular-related damage induce by apical access [7], but such an aspect deserves further confirmation, particularly at medium and long term.

Infection at the surgical incision (minithoracotomy) may also represent a potential complication although with low incidence rate [7, 10, 19, 20].

Obviously, further studies and larger numbers of treated patients will be necessary to conclusively elucidate whether cardiac apex represents an alternative access for TAVI or should be exclusively considered as complementary once trans-femoral or trans-subclavian approach are contraindicated.

Coronary Artery-Related Complications

Due to the pre-procedural profile of the current "usual" TAVI candidates (elderly, advanced comorbidities, severely calcified aortic stenosis, concomitant atherosclerosis-related risk factors) coronary artery disease (CAD) is frequently encountered during pre-TAVI investigations. Besides the impact of coexisting CAD, however, the coronary system may be jeopardized, particularly at the level of the coronary ostia, by several mishaps induced or related to the transcatheter biological prosthesis.

Regarding the prevalence of CAD in TAVI patients, a recent international series [21] showed that CAD was found in almost 50% of treated patients, being more common in patients undergoing trans-apical implantation (74% of the patient cohort) and, as expected by the current enrolment criteria for such a transcatheter approach, with higher EUROScore and prevalence of atherosclerosis-related risk factors as compared to patients undergoing trans-femoral procedure. In this experience, overall mortality was significantly higher in patients with CAD (35.7%) as compared to non-CAD patients (18.4%), with a 2.3 higher risk of dying as compared to non-CAD subjects, and this unfavourable impact was also confirmed at long-term survival. This finding has been recently confirmed by the SOURCE Registry [12], which included almost equal number of patients submitted to the two TAVI approaches (trans-femoral and trans-apical). In this registry there was a slight, although significant, predominance of CAD in the transapical group, with relevant prevalence of pre-TAVI CABG (17.6% in the trans-femoral group, and 26.9% in the trans-apical group, respectively). Overall, myocardial ischemia-related events related to impaired coronary flow vary a great deal, ranging from 0 to 17,5% of the treated patients (table). These events encompass myocardial infarction due to coronary flow supply/demand imbalance, but can be induced by direct coronary vascular damage, occlusion, or emboli [15, 22]. Other indirect cause of impaired coronary perfusion may arise, during TAVI, in patients with previous CABG, particularly in case of internal thoracic artery anastomosed to the LAD and of trans-subclavian access for TAVI [23]. In this condition, vascular damage may jeopardize a critical source of myocardial perfusion and further complicate the already ongoing vascular injury by generating substantial myocardial ischemia.

Iatrogenic injury to the coronary system may be generated by catheters floating in the aortic root, by valve ballooning, by valve implantation, and by valve frame positioning or by the sealing cuff placed over the coronary ostia. Calcified debris may certainly be ejected or direct into the coronary system, either during preparatory valvuloplasty or during prosthetic valve deployment. An in vitro study has shown that coronary occlusion or embolization by small or large particulate material (larger than 1 mm) may indeed occur after valvuloplasty of a calcified aortic valve [24]. Predisposing factors to coronary obstruction during TAVI, are rare, but usually related to bulky native valve leaflets [13, 25, 26] or short distance (between 8 and 14 mm) of the coronary ostia from the valve annulus [2, 14], and narrowed sinuses of Valsava [2]. It is therefore paramount to carefully define the take-off position and distance of the coronary ostia in relation to the valvular ring or leaflet attachment, and the height or bulkiness of the leaflets themselves in order to predict coronary obstruction or closure during native leaflet crashing against the aortic wall. As mentioned, also the prosthetic skirt, designed to reduce or prevent paravalvular leak, if improperly positioned too high may impinge the coronary ostia thereby variably reducing blood flow.

Acute coronary or aortic dissection may be also part of the vascular complication seen in a few TAVI cases (figure 1). Too high positioning of the transcatheter valve may also jeopardize both coronary ostia [26, 27], and patient symptoms or signs of ongoing myocardial ischemia may also appear in the subacute_phase of TAVI [27]. Indeed, refractory cardiogenic shock may represent a sequeale of an otherwise apparently successful TAVI procedure. Echocardiographic and angiographic evaluations, if sudden cardiocirculatory impairment occurs, should immediately documents if different cause of hypotension or TAVI-related cardiocirculatory dysfunction are present. Valve repositioning or immediate direct main stem stenting [28] are usually sufficient to solve proximal coronary obstruction. However, a few cases of failure to restore proximal patency have been reported, with some fatal events or with the need of immediate surgical revascularization. Cardiocirculatory assistance with femoro-femoral access or through a transeptal-femoral approach [28] may provide proper support to address the coronary complication and enhance heart and organ recovery. It has been suggested to measure the distance between the coronary ostia and the hinge point of the native valve. In case of high risk for such a coronary ostia occlusion or severe stenosis, an additional "safety wire" positioned in the LAD through a guiding catheter from another arterial access might be advanced at the time of the valve deployment to provide immediate access to the obstructed coronary ostium in case of necessity [28].

Impaired flow to the coronary territory because of occlusion or stenosis of previously implanted arterial or vein grafts are, as mentioned, possible, albeit extremely rare. Occlusion of the internal thoracic artery due to subclavian artery dissection, or of CABG grafts by prosthetic valve frame or aortic dissection, have been reported and successfully managed [23].

Finally, there are evidences of post-implant embolization of calcified particles. Such an event might be acute or, by micro and repetitive coronary embolization, chronic and may represent the underlying cause of unexplained sudden death or quick clinical deterioration observed in the post-procedural period, along with aortic wall or annular rupture or coronary occlusion or cerebral embolization, or malignant cardiac arrhythmia.

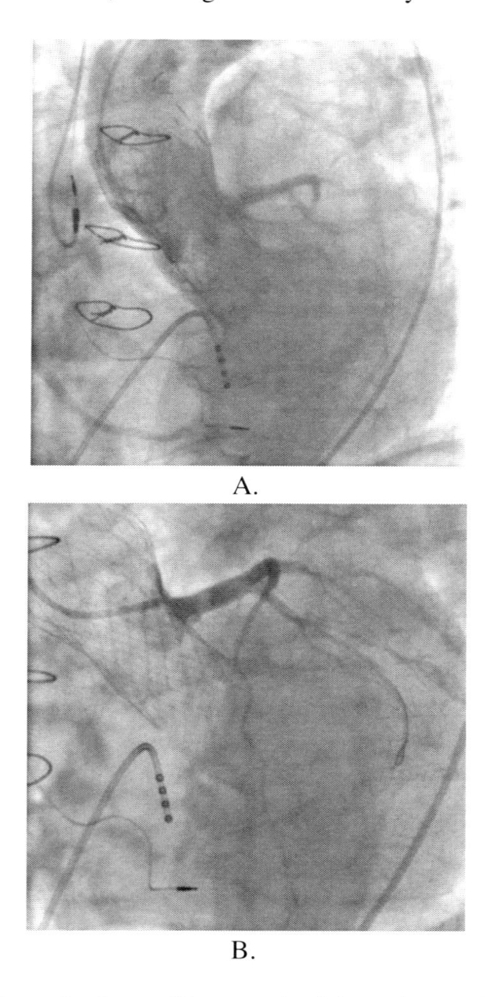

A.

B.

Figure 1. Fluoroscopy showing a diaphragm-like stenosis of the main stem (A) which was normal before the TAVI procedure. Main stem stenting performed with complete resolution of the vessel injury (B).

Prosthesis Migration

Prosthesis embolization does represents a likely misadventure of TAVI, either backward in the left ventricle or forward into the ascending aorta or more distally. The event rate varies a great deal (table), ranging from 0% to almost 14% [7, 12-21, 29-39]. Obviously, management of prosthetic migration depends on the type of device chosen for the procedure. Indeed, the CoreValve Revalving System does not allow repositioning in case of significant improper deployment, although very little adjustments of the prosthetic net may still be obtained using the wire loop or with an additional ballooning. The Edwards Sapien device can still allow slight repositioning. Currently available prostheses, however, do not allow recapturing and repositioning after full deployment, although development of devices with these characteristics is ongoing and maybe soon available.

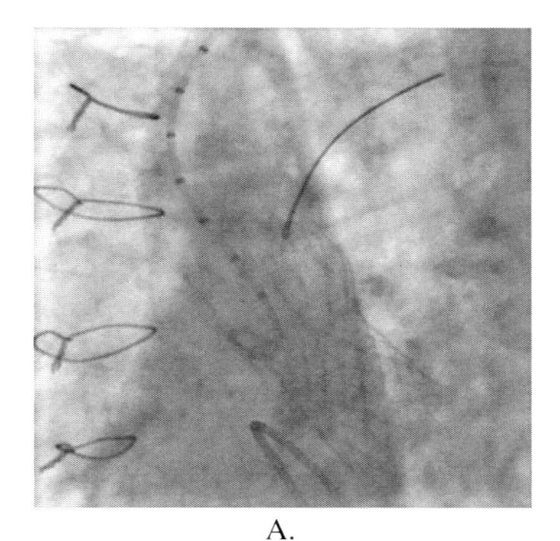

A.

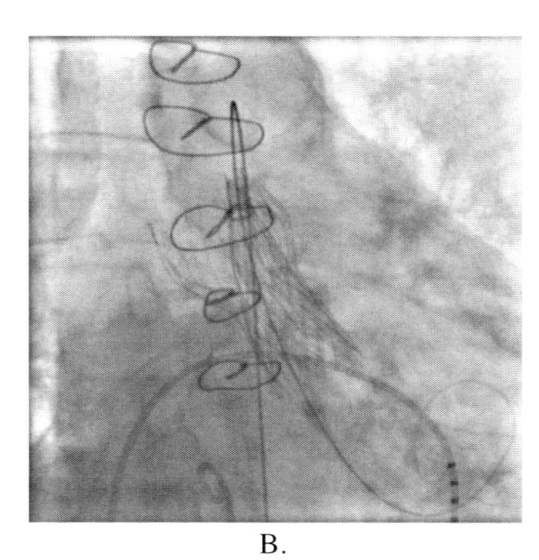

B.

Figure 2. Malposition of a transcatheter valve (too low) which was firstly managed with a prosthetic hook to attempt valve pulling and repositioning (A). Due to failure of the prosthetic pulling, a second CoreValve was deployed within the first one (B) with adequate positioning.

Prosthetic displacement usually occurs once effective ventricular ejection reappears after cessation of rapid ventricular pacing. Malpositioning (figure 2) obviously predisposes to prosthetic migration. In case of distal migration of the implanted device, surgery can still be avoided by adjusting the device landing in a safe portion of the distal part of the ascending aorta, followed by implantation of another transcatheter valve (figure 3). Prosthetic migration in the aortic arch are also likely [2]. In these cases, usually no major complications occur being the supra-aortic vessels adequately perfused thanks to the device frame which allows unrestricted flow. Any malpositioning, if not substantial, might be managed with attempts to correct the landing of the prosthesis with a catheter-based technique, particularly if the prosthesis is not totally released. In this case a valve repositioning is still feasible [40].

Impingement of the superior edge of the prosthetic frame into the aortic intima, with a progressive erosion of the aortic wall potentially leading to aortic dissection or rupture, may also occur and mandates surgical removal.

Prosthetic migration in the left ventricle may occur, and require prompt surgical intervention, particularly for the potential deleterious effect on the mitral valvular apparatus, with high risk of infringing the mitral chordae leading to de novo or increased mitral regurgitation. Furthermore, as it will be described later on in this chapter, migration of the prosthesis towards the left ventricular outflow tract may cause further complications to the anterior mitral leaflet due to the presence of the mitro-aortic continuity [41, 42].

Surgical conversion of TAVI does pertain, as it might be expected, a high mortality rate, particularly in case of emergent procedure and usually represent a negative determinant of patient outcome either in terms of mortality or morbidity [2].

The availability of a hybrid room and a surgical stand-by may allow a more expeditious and effective management, particularly in the emergent situations, but it is obviously the type of complication to be treated which confers the prognosis to the treated case.

Prompt access to peripheral-based mechanical circulatory support, presence or absence of cardiac arrest, presence or absence of severe comorbidities, are all critical factors which may allow also successful surgical management.

Post-procedural migration (after one day) have been rarely observed, although two cases of valve embolization 2 days and 55 days, respectively, after the TAVI procedure have been reported [10, 43].

Aortic Dissection/Perforation/Aortic Annular Rupture

As seen for the other untoward events, also aortic vessel-related complications vary a great deal, ranging from 0% to almost 4% [2, 4-39] of TAVI series. These conditions, however, occur infrequently, and progressively increasing experience, better device-related systems and instruments, or also alternative accesses for native valve approach, all contributed to the decline of such frightening events.

The use of antegrade (trans-apical) approach was suggested as an effective mean to avoid such complications, particularly in relation to a reduced incidence of vascular-related injury or relatively safer route for catheter-based valve insertion. However, most of the reported aortic dissection or rupture are usually localized near the native valve area (annular rupture or intimal tear above the annular plane), mechanism shared among all the applied routes of prosthetic implantations. Additional factor potentially linked to aortic injury might have been related to the need of balloon-expandable prosthetic devices, in contrast to self-expandable prosthetic systems which do not required operator-mediated ballooning for deployment. Data from published literature [2, 4-39] do not support this hypothesis, being more consistent with inherent and individual characteristics of the ballooned native valve and of the patient aortic wall features (bulky and ulcerated atheroma, thickness, tissue frailty, and so forth).

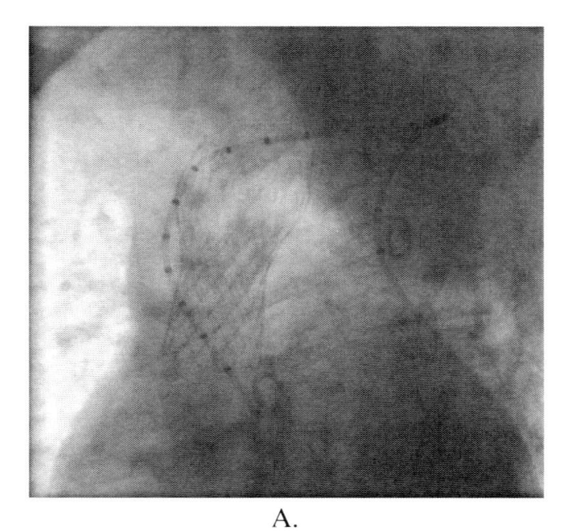

A.

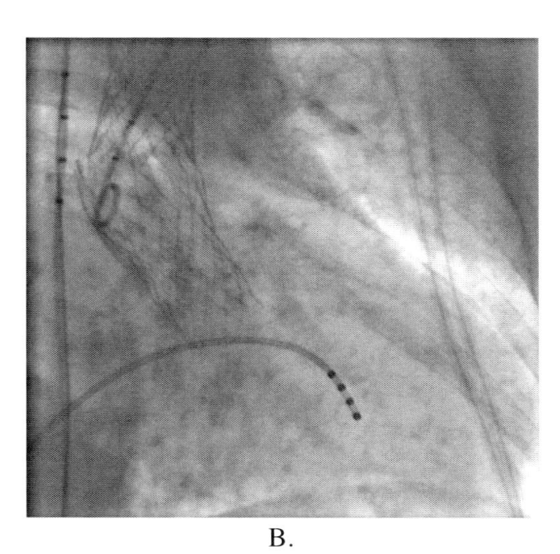

B.

Figure 3. Prosthetic valve migration in the ascending aorta (A) immediately after the cessation of rapid pacing with prosthetic ejection from the annular site. A second transcatheter valve was then deployed in the proper position (B) with the first prosthesis lining in the distal ascending aorta and initial portion of the aortic arch with no flow impairment of the supra-aortic vessels.

In some circumstances, the aortic wall involvement may start after native valve ballooning and progress just after TAVI (figure 4). Once occurred, aortic vessel involvement may be life threatening and require immediate surgical treatment, but it may also lead to sudden patient death. Sudden atrio-ventricular (AV) block, severe hypotension, cardiac tamponade, severe chest pain, or ischemic-like changes of the ECG due to coronary involvement may represent signs and symptoms announcing major aortic vessel compromise. In most of the cases, surgical treatment, if feasible, should be taken into account. However, the presence of absolute contraindications for previous surgical treatment, or the impact of a demanding surgery in usual TAVI candidates (aortic root replacement) should be considered and weighted. In a few cases, immediate relief of cardiac tamponade and absence of progression of the tearing process may not lethally compromise the immediate patient outcome. A conservative and limited treatment (controlled systemic arterial pressure) might be an option for patients with absolute contraindications for surgery although prognosis of untreated acute aortic dissection is notoriously dismal.

Aortic dissection may also develop a few days after surgery [44] and usually linked to intimal injury by the prosthetic frame or by the device-related introducer or sheath. Therefore, post-procedural echocardiographic as well as chest-x ray should be carried out during the first days after TAVI in order to disclose any sign of such a dreadful complication, although its incidence at variable time from the intervention appears low. In case of type B dissection [44], a conservative approach might be undertaken, or, in case of further complication, an endovascular procedure might be considered. In the presence of the dissection of the ascending aorta, surgery must be obviously considered immediately, unless hopeless for the patient comorbidities and status, or alternative techniques (hybrid approach) may represent another extreme option.

Conversion to Surgical Aortic Valve Replacement

Despite the inherent features and risks of TAVI, the rate of surgical conversion has been low in the published clinical series, ranging from 0 to 8% (table). It must be taken into account, however, that some patients have absolute contraindications to surgical procedure or have been treated, particularly in the initial TAVI experience, for compassionate reasons. Therefore, in a few cases, either because of no possibility linked to the kind of adverse event, lack of hybrid room, or no chance to survive the surgical intervention, despite dreadful complications, patients have not been treated surgically, and hence the true rate of surgical conversion might have been underestimated. The most common indications for surgical revision are cardiac tamponade due to ventricular rupture and valve migration (either in the left ventricle or in the ascending aorta or arch). Additional events requiring surgical intervention have been aortic valve annular rupture or aortic dissection, ventricular septal defect (VSD), mitral valve-related complications, coronary-related adverse events (coronary occlusion not amenable of PCI, coronary or previously implanted coronary arterial or vein grafts).

Indications for surgical procedure during the TAVI procedure account for immediate danger for the patient life, and, hence, emergent surgical treatment must be carried out to treat above mentioned complications. This condition, obviously, affects patient mortality and morbidity, although successful surgical procedures have been repetitively reported. Unfortunately, sepsis or multi-organ failure may intervene after successful bail-out surgical treatment, and poor preoperative patient condition does greatly influence postoperative course and outcome.

As mentioned, the presence of a multi-disciplinary team and approach, with ready-to use ECC and cardiocirculatory support may play a critical role in this scenario.

Atrio/Ventricular Conduction Defects

Permanent AV conduction abnormalities are frequent after conventional aortic valve replacement requiring permanent pacemaker (PM) implantation up to 7% of the surgical patients [45]. Presence of aortic insufficiency, advanced age and preoperative bundle-branch block are negative determinant of definitive PM implantation in surgical series [45, 46]. The incidence of AV block or abnormalities to require permanent pacemaker implantation in TAVI experiences has been shown to range from 4% to 32%, although no case of AV conduction defect and no need of PM implantation has been reported in a clinical experience of trans-apical TAVI with Sapien prosthesis [37].

The presence of pre-procedural right bundle branch block [47, 48], or of a narrow left ventricular outflow tract and severe mitral annular calcification were strong predictors for the need of permanent PM [48].

The potential mechanisms underlying this complications are variable, accounting for hematoma of the periannular tissue, with compression and damage of the adjacent conduction system tissue and fibers [49]. Compression of the His bundle by an interventricular septum hematoma secondary to TAVI was described in a patient submitted to necroscopy study following a TAVI procedure [50] and this might represent the most frequent cause of AV conduction disorders in this setting. Obviously, aging-related abnormalities and pre-procedural AV conduction abnormalities might be exacerbated by traumatic injury (valve ballooning or prosthetic deployment) ultimately lead to irreversible AV conduction disorders.

Interestingly, clues about a difference in the incidence of permanent PM dependence according to the type of prosthesis implanted has been underlined, with an apparent higher rate in the CoreValve series as opposed to the Edwards Sapien-related experience [13, 50, 51], and the findings in the most numerous clinical series show a PM need ranging from 9% to 32% in CoreValve patients, and from 0% to 22% in Sapien patients, respectively (table).

As far as the access-site is concerned, besides anecdotal data, there is still no evidence that the TAVI approach may play a role in the incidence of post-procedural AV conduction defects, although trans-femoral access appear to be linked to higher incidence of conduction disorders.

A slightly higher deployment of the prosthesis within the LV outflow tract, by sparing the delicate spot where the bundle of His, just below the membranous septum and along the crest of the ventricular septum, splits into the left and right bundles, appear to reduce the incidence of PM implantation [41]. The superficial course, particularly of the left bundle, may therefore explain the high incidence of such complications, with little hope, thus far based on the current prosthetic design, to significantly reduce their occurrence.

Paravalvular Leak

Transcatheter valve deployment is frequently characterized by paravalvular leak occurrence at the end of the procedure due to the intimate features of the technique itself. Indeed, the leaflet and annular squeezing induced by the valve deployment leads to irregular tissue-related folds and fragments, often leading to imperfect fitting of the valve frame along the native valve annulus [52]. Prevalence of mild (2 plus) or greater paravalvular leak following TAVI ranges from 1.4% to almost 50% of the treated cases (table), making paravalvular leak the most frequent complication after TAVI [53]. Usually, paravalvular leak are trivial or mild [54]. Apparently, patients with greater height, large annulus and smaller cover index, given by 100 X (prosthesis diameter-transesophageal echocardiography annulus diameter)/prosthesis diameter, are more prone to develop paravalvular leak with a regurgitation >2/4, whereas patients with an aortic annulus smaller than 22 mm or a cover index >8% may be free from such a complication [53].

The effects of paravalvular leak at mid or long term are unknown, although data from studies assessing late results in the presence of paravalvular leak after conventional aortic valve replacement are well established [55]. In contrast, no information are obviously available regarding the influence of such a functional and anatomical defect in TAVI patients. Recently, an in vivo study adopting the pulse duplicator technique has analysed the hemodynamic and mechanical features related to paravalvular leak and has shown that there is a substantial energy loss in the presence of mild paravalvular leak during diastole following a TAVI procedure [56]. This volume regurgitation, moreover, generates a higher workload of the left ventricle as compared to similar leakage in the presence of a conventionally (sutured) implanted bioprosthetic valve. These findings indicate that additional and/or more detailed information will be necessary to elucidate the actual effects of paravalvular leak in TAVI patients, although upcoming technical advance in prosthetic design and implantation may reduce the incidence of such an event.

Angiography tends to overestimate the actual extent of aortic regurgitation and, therefore, transesophageal echocardiography is highly recommended to consistently evaluate the hemodynamically impact and degree of such a complication. Usually, paravalvular leak is related to underexpansion of the prosthesis, and, therefore, frequently solved with repeated intravalvular balloon dilatation. Additional cause of hemodinamically significant paravalvular leaks is a too low or too high valve deployment. In the first case, a forward valve retrieval with a goose-neck snare might be sufficient to reallocate appropriately the transcatheter valve. Unfortunately, as mentioned, such a condition may also lead to mitral valve dysfunction or damage, namely mitral regurgitation due to impingement of the prosthetic frame against the inferior surface of the anterior mitral leaflet. The second condition, in contrast, may be counteracted by sight prosthetic retrieval or by a second prosthetic deployment (valve-in-valve).

Another important aspect to be considered relates to the morphology of the diseased valve to be treated: the presence of a calcified and severely stenotic bicuspid valve appears an unfavourable setting for a TAVI procedure. The peculiar anatomical features of these valves may not enhance annular/prosthetic frame contact, leading to improper fitting along the annulus, generating structural distortion, and, hence, leaflet dysfunction [57, 58]. Of note, an anatomical study performed in patients submitted to valved stent implantation showed that valve misdeployment, a critical determinant of paravalvular leak, was constant in patients with bicuspid calcified aortic valve, whereas, in the presence of tricuspid aortic valve, adequate valve deployment was achieved in the majority of the cases [58]. Furthermore, the usual elliptical morphology of the bicuspid valve may be also not favourable in terms of native tissue compression towards the aortic wall, with uneven distribution of the native calcified tissue, with valve-related calcium protruding towards the prosthetic frame and representing a potential cause for prosthetic leaflet injury and degeneration at long term [58].

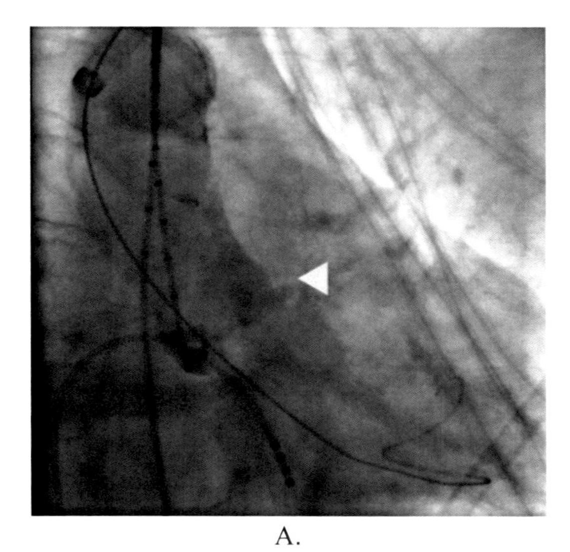

A.

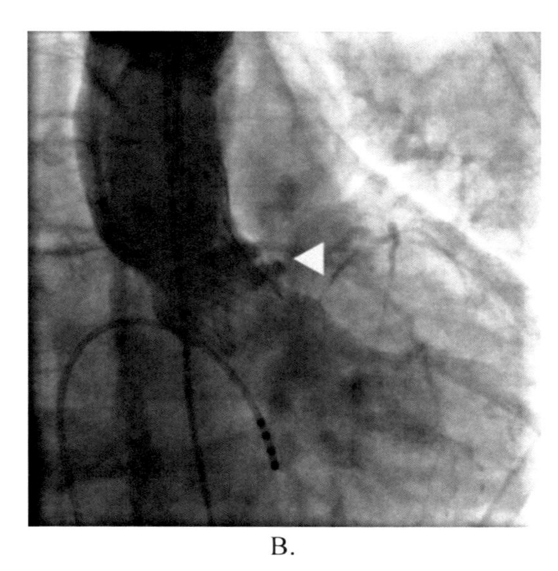

B.

Figure 4. Aortic annular rupture. The first sign of aortic annular rupture is shown just after balloon valvuloplasty and before TAVI (A - white arrowhead). Sign of aortic annulus rupture is also evident in the angiography following valve deployment (B - white arrowhead).

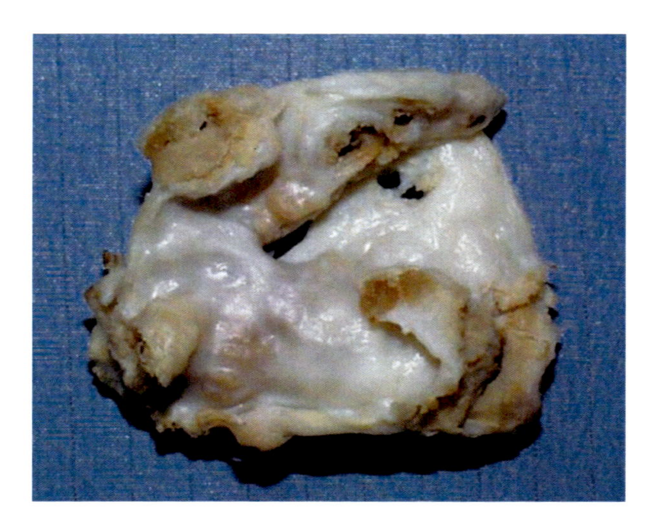

Figure 5. Macroscopic view of a severely calcified bicuspid aortic valve. The marked derangement and the extensive calcification of the aortic valve underline the risk either of transcatheter valve misdeployment and high risk of paravalvular leak and prosthetic deformation, the danger of coronary occlusion and calcific material embolization.

The different behaviour of tricuspid versus bicuspid native stenotic aortic valve has shown that "circular" (that is, more appropriate) deployment is strictly dependent on valve morphology, being the prosthetic adaptation more effective in the presence of a tricuspid valve (77% of the cases, versus 19% of patients with bicuspid valves, respectively) and that a better prosthetic adaptation along the native annulus was observed with an increased radial force applied by a prosthetic frame (stiffer stent) again in tricuspid valves, whereas no beneficial effects was shown in bicuspid valves [59]. Furthermore, it is well known that patients with stenotic bicuspid aortic valve often present with severe calcification of the valve leaflet and annulus, and sometimes with a remarkable derangement of the original valve morphology (figure 5) making adequate deployment extremely difficult, and perhaps increasing the rate of related complications (paravalvular leak, migration or particulate emboli). Nonetheless, successful valve deployment in the presence of a bicuspid aortic valve have been anecdotally reported using an Edwards Sapien prosthesis [60, 61].

It is therefore rather evident that with the current devices a severely calcified bicuspid aortic valve does represent a relative contraindication to TAVI. In this setting high rate of paravalvular leak, prosthetic deformation and valve tissue-related abnormalities due to unfavourable geometry and transvalvular flow features, and valve dysfunction due to altered leaflet coaptation or prolapse, may occur and should be seriously taken into consideration if any other alternative treatments (valvuloplasty) are unfeasible in the process of TAVI decision making by performing an accurate evaluation of valve anatomy.

Mitral Valve-Related Complications

Mitral insufficiency (MI) in the presence of severe aortic stenosis has been a matter of debate in the surgical community regarding the actual need of combined intervention. Indeed, it has been shown that, provided that the mitral dysfunction be not secondary to primitive organic disease and not of severe degree, the correction of the aortic barrage to forward blood flow usually leads to substantial improvement of the mitral function with significant reduction of regurgitation [62-64]. Although percutaneous procedures to treat mitral valve insufficiency are ongoing [65], combined transcatheter mitral and aortic dysfunction have not been simultaneously addressed yet and, therefore, severe involvement of the mitral valve still represents a contraindication fro TAVI. Less than severe MI, however, does not preclude TAVI and the actual impact of MI on TAVI outcome has been poorly elucidated. Tzikas and associates have analysed the data of 79 patients treated with transfemoral valve implantation and found that MI improved in 17% of the patients, was unchanged in 61%, and worsened in 22%, respectively [66]. Furthermore, by analysing preoperative patient features, it has been shown that patients with lower pre-TAVI procedure left ventricular ejection fraction experienced a greater improvement. These findings have been confirmed by Gotzmann who showed that TAVI did not significantly influence overall mitral function at early and mid term, with no change of the degree of MI either at 30-day or at 6-month follow-up [67].

The effects of TAVI on mitral valve function deserve further investigations and may rely on the actual impact of the TAVI on intra-ventricular hemodynamics and geometrical changes induced by the device deployment. The implantation and presence of frame-based prosthesis, indeed, has been shown to be potentially dangerous particularly_to the anterior mitral leaflet based on the close anatomically relationship with the aortic annulus. Cases of anterior leaflet perforation and aneurysm formation has been described [68]. Mitral valve insufficiency due to traction of the subvalvular apparatus induced by an entangled guidewire has been also reported [69].

The close anatomical as well as functional relationship between the aortic and mitral valves is well known [41] and, therefore, such adverse events are possible and any unexplained hypotension or new-onset MI should alert the operator during any TAVI procedure, particularly in case of a "too low" implant, although apparently satisfactory results from a prosthetic valve function standpoint.

Patient-Prosthesis Mismatch

Patient-prosthesis mismatch (PPM) has been claimed to be related to early and long-term adverse outcome following conventional AVR [70, 71], although robust clinical series appear to disagree upon this concept [72, 73]. Jilaihawi and co-workers have addressed the prevalence of PPM following TAVI in 50 patients who received a CoreValve bioprosthesis [74]. In their experience, such a condition was present in 16 patients (32%) and was strictly related to the prosthetic valve positioning. Indeed, in patients who had an "optimal positioning" (defined in their series as a prosthetic deployment between 5 mm. to 10 mm. below the native aortic annulus measured with fluoroscopy) there was an inverse correlation with the incidence of PPM, achieving such a favourable results in 50% of the cases. Interestingly, PPM occurrence was unrelated to the aortic valve annulus or body surface area. The authors suggested that a suboptimal valve positioning may induce an incomplete stent expansion which, in turn, may generate a restricted forward flow. Additionally, small aortic annuli did no represent per se, in this series, a predisposing factor for PPM development. As mentioned, the impact of PPM on postoperative patient outcome, however, is still controversial [72, 73] and, hence, may not represent a major determinant of early or mid-term prognosis of the currently TAVI population. Furthermore, it must be emphasized that current patient selection for TAVI enrol patients with a native aortic annuli ranging from 20 and 27 mm, thereby excluding those with smaller valve dimensions and markedly limiting de facto PPM occurrence. Further studies, therefore, are required to provide additional insights on this particular anatomical and hemodynamic situation

Cardiogenic Shock

Detailed information about incidence of cardiogenic shock in TAVI patients are somehow lacking, but a few published series have described such a complication occurring between 0% and 43% (table) of treated subjects, underlining that such a condition is certainly not usually reported.

Episodes of severe cardiac contractile impairment or cardiac arrest may account for several causes, either directly related to myocardial dysfunction (acute myocardial ischemia, arrhythmias, ventricular hematoma or septal defect) or indirectly evoked by adverse events (tamponade, aortic dissection). Usually, depressed myocardial function after TAVI, if not directly linked to a precise complication, has a limited time span, with almost full recovery of contractility within a few hours. Mechanical circulatory support to temporarily assist the dysfunctional heart has been variably reported, and usually by adopting a femoro-femoral extracorporeal circulation or ECMO in case of concomitant refractory lung dysfunction. Vrancks and associates have described the use of a transeptal approach of the left atrium to decompress the impaired and dilated left ventricle in 10 patients undergoing elective TAVI with successful weaning in all patients, and vascular access-related complications occurring in 2 patients [75].

The prompt availability of a mechanical circulatory support is highly advisable and recommended. The presence of guidewires in the femoral vessels may be also used to introduce the ECC cannulae using the Seldinger technique. Rarely, in the presence of severely depressed left ventricle or for other high risk conditions, a prophylactic ECC may be used while performing the TAVI. This situation was predominantly seen in the initial experience of TAVI and currently used only as a temporarily support or in case of catastrophic complications as a bail-out manoeuvre.

Cerebral Emboli

In principle, any intervention, either surgical or catheter-based, acting in the left cardiac compartments or at the supra-aortic arterial vessels and in patients with atherosclerotic-related complications (that is, atheroma, dissection, stenosis, vegetations, calcifications) may be subjected to dislocation of particled or gasseous emboli and generate cerebral ischemic events and related injury [76]. These potentially catastrophic events are sometimes fortunately subclinical with no apparent neurologic functional impairment. Stolz and associates has shown, using a diffusion-weighted imaging (DWI), that new perioperative DWI lesions occurred in 38% of the study patients submitted to conventional AVR, of whom only 3 patients (6,6%) developed overt neurological deficit [77]. This finding was confirmed by other studies [78, 79] which have shown that a significant number of patients experienced new focal brain lesions which were variably clinically relevant, and almost all affecting the neurocognitive function in the immediate postoperative phase. The neurocognitive decline, however, disappeared in all affected patients a few months after surgery. It is well known that also simple aortic catheterization may generate cerebral emboli. Indeed, Omran and colleagues has shown, in a randomized-case control study, the passage of the catheter through the stenotic aortic valve induced new focal lesions, as assessed by DWI, in the brain in 22% of the patients (with 3 clinically relevant neurologic events), versus no event in the patients who had no valve crossing with the angiographic catheter [80].

The inherent features of TAVI, namely retrograde passage of the guidewires and catheters along the atherosclerotic thoracic aorta and aortic arch, as well as the native valve ballooning and prosthetic valve deployment with subsequent annular squeezing and leaflet pushed aside, pose the patient at consistent risk for emboli. Despite the apparent high risk for such an adverse event, the actual prevalence of stroke or other kind of neurological events following TAVI have ranged from 0% to 10% (table). Obviously, in case of such a dreadful complication, patient prognosis is dismal, particularly in the presence of previous neurologic events. Silent cerebral embolic events, however, are not strictly linked to the intra-procedural phase, they do also occur in the immediate hours or days after TAVI [81-83]. Current limited long-term data suggest that significant neurologic event potentially attributable to the native valve or to aortic calcific emboli are not common.

Ghanem and associates have prospectively investigated 22 patients undergoing TAVI, and preoperatively as well postoperatively (3 days, and 3 months, respectively) submitted to diffuse-weighted MRI to disclose correlation between silent or apparent embolism and cerebral MRI-related changes [81]. In 16 patients (72%) a total of 75 new lesions were shown, with the great majority [75] of such an ischemic injury located at the supratentorial region. Notwithstanding, only 3 patients suffered from overt neurological deficit (one had transient cerebellar ataxia, one transient dysarthria, and one persistent left-sided hemiparesis, respectively). This experience also showed that all patients undergone to valve frame dilatation (nr. 4) had embolic events, and the presence of cerebrovascular and peripheral vascular disease were slightly more prevalent in these subjects. Khalert analysed data obtained in 32 patients undergoing balloon-expanded or self-expandable retrograde TAVI : also in this experience many new foci suggestive of embolic-based ischemic cerebral injury were shown in 27 (84%) patients and significantly more frequent as compared to conventional valve replacement. However, in this series, no overt neurological deficit could be shown, and 80% of these new lesions were completely solved after 3 months from TAVI [82].

Post-discharge incidence of neurologic event likely due to cerebral emboli is not widely available, also due to the limited post-procedural follow-up carried out. Nonetheless, Gurvitch and associates has recently reported about the 3-year follow-up of 70 patients submitted to TAVI and who survived more than 30 days, showing an overall rate of 8.6% of new neurological events at 3 years from TAVI [83]. This complication occurred more than months from TAVI in more than two thirds of cases, indicating that this risk may indeed persist, although no information was provided about the actual source (and maybe impossible to disclose) of the neurological injury.

Table. Overview of complication data and rates of clinical series (published and personal unpublished) including more than 20 patients

Series	Pts	Logistic Euro score (mean, %)	30-day Mortality (%)	Late (> 6 months) Mortality (%)	Coronary Complications / AMI (%)	Access-related Complications /Bleeding (%)	Aortic Complications (dissection/ perforation) (%)
Thomas	1.038	25,7	88 (8,5%)	na	6 (0,6%)	106 (9,3%)	14 (1,3%)
Ussia	110	26,7	13 (12)%	nr	nr	nr	nr
Grube	25	11*	5 (20%)	nr	0	6 (24%)	0
Dewey	171	30,9	12 (7%)	nr	21 (12,2%)	10 (11,7%)	nr
Dworakowski	151	21,6	15 (9,9%)	na	0	13 (8,6%)	nr
Petronio	514	20,1	28 (5,4%)	51 (15,2%)	3 (0,6%)	14 (2,7%)	nr
Webb	50	28	6 (12%)	0	1 (2%)	6 (12%)	1 (2%)
Grube	86	23,4	10 (12%)	nr	1 (1%)	nr	0
Piazza	646	23,1	52 (8%)	na	3 (0,5%)	12 (1,9%)	4 (0,6%)
De Jaegere	33	20,3	1 (3)%	1 (3%)	nr	nr	nr
Webb	168	28,6	19 (11,3%)	nr	nr	11 (6,6%)	nr
Kahlert	60	21,6	7 (12%)	nr	0	19 (32%)	nr
Leon	179	26,4	11 (6,4%)	55 (30,7%)§	0	29 (16,2%)	nr
Eltchaninoff	244	25,6	31 (12,7%)	na	3 (1,2%)	14 (5,6%)	2 (0,8%)
Svensson	40	nr	15	6	7 (17,5%)	nr	1
Bleiziffer	203	22	21 (10,4%)	15 (7,4%)	nr	29 (14,2%)	nr
Walther	59	27	8 (13,6%)	13 (22%)	0	8	0
Zierer	26	36,5	4 (15,3%)	na	2 (7,7%)	2 (7,7%)	1 (3,8%)
Walther	50	27,6	4 (8%)	nr	2 (4%)	0	1 (2%)
Ye	26	37	6 (23%)	3 (12%)	1 (4%)	3 (12%)	0
Rodés-Cabau	22	26	2 (8,7%)	na	0	1 (4,1%)	0
Tchetche	45	25,2	2 (4,4%)	na	5 (11,1%)	4 (8,9%)	0
Wendler	575	29,1	59 (10,3%)	na	4 (0,7%)	12 (2,1%)	6 (0,2%)
Pasic	175	38,3	9 (5,1%)	25 (14,5%)	2 (1,1%)	6 (3,4%)	0
Personal Exp. (unpublished)	105	21	6 (5,7%)	12 (11,4%)	1 (0,9%)	2 (1,9%)	2 (1,9%)

Post-Implant Shock (%)	Valve Migration/ Malposition (%)	Cerebro-vascular Events (%)	Other Major Complication (Ventr. Rupture)	PVL (mild or >) (%)	Transfusio n > 2 Units (%)	ARF (dyalisis) (%)	PM Implant (%)	Conversion to surgery (%)
nr	3 (0,3%)	27 (2,5%)	13 (1.2%)	20 (1,9%)	97 (9,3%)	47 (4,3%)	73 (7%)	28 (2,7%)
nr	1 (0,9%)	2 (1,8%)	1 (0,9%)	8 (7,2%)	nr	nr	nr	1 (0,9%)
nr	0	1 (4%)	1 (4%)	1 (4%)	nr	nr	nr	2 (8%)
1 (1,1%)	nr	12 (7%)	17 (9,9%)	nr	nr	nr	nr	2 (2,3%)

Post-Implant Shock (%)	Valve Migration/ Malposition (%)	Cerebro-vascular Events (%)	Other Major Complication (Ventr. Rupture)	PVL (mild or >) (%)	Transfusion > 2 Units (%)	ARF (dyalisis) (%)	PM Implant (%)	Conversion to surgery (%)
nr	nr	9 (6%)	nr	6 (3,9%)	nr	nr	8 (5,3%)	nr
nr	71 (13,8%)	9 (1,8%)	nr	90 (17,5 %)	53 (10,3%)	15 (2,9%)	84 (16,3%)	5 (1%)
2 (4%)	2 (4%)	2 (4%)	nr	3 (6%)	9 (18%)	nr	2 (4%)	0
nr	nr	9 (10%)	8 (9,3%)	nr	nr	nr	nr	6 (12%)
nr	nr	4 (0,6%)	11 (1,7%)	nr	nr	nr	60 (9,3%)	3 (0,5%)
nr	0	nr	nr	18 (54,5 %)	nr	nr	nr	0
4 (2,4%)	nr	7 (4,2%)	10 (6%)	nr	19 (11,5%)^	3 (1,8%)	9 (5,4%)	1 (0,6%)
13 (22%)	1 (2%)	0	2 (3%)	nr	nr	nr	13 (22%)	0
nr	1 (0,6%)	12 (6,7%)	nr	20 (11,8 %)	nr	2 (1,1%)	6 (3,4%)	0
nr	2 (0,8%)	9 (3,6%)	5 (2,0%)	23 (9,5%)	nr	4 (1,6%)	29 (11,8%)	nr
1	3	2	nr	5	nr	nr	nr	2
41 (46%)	nr	11 (7%)	5 (2,4%)	nr	nr	17 (8,3%)	nr	2 (1%)
nr	0	2	6	15	nr	8	nr	4
3 (12%)	1 (3,8%)	0	1 (3,8%)	nr	nr	3 (12%)	nr	2 (7,7%)
1 (2%)	1 (2%)	0	0	nr	nr	7 (14%)	2 (4%)	3 (6%)
nr	0	1 (4%)	1 (4%)	9 (34,6 %)	3 (12%)	0	3 (12%)	0
0	0	0	1 (4,1%)	nr	nr	nr	0	0
1 (2,2%)	nr	0	1 (2,2%)	4 (9,5%)	18 (40%)	10 (22,2%)	7 (15,6%)	0
nr	3 (0,5%)	16 (2,6%)	11 (??%)	13 (2,3%)	nr	41 (7,1%)	42 (7,3%)	20 (3,5%)
2 (1,1%)	0	1 (0,5%)	1 (0,5%)	nr	nr	nr	10 (5,7%)	0
1 (0,9%)	1 (0,9%)	3 (2,8%)	0	16 (15,2 %)	na	0	34 (32,3%)	1 (0,9%)

Valve Type	Procedural Approach (Pts)	Study	Procedural Success (%)	Overall 30-day Pts with MACE events (%)	Reference
Edwards Sapien	Trans-apical (575)/ Trans-femoral (463)	Multi-Centre	956 (93,8%)	nr	[12]
Medtronic CoreValve	Trans-femoral (107) Trans-subclavian (3)	Single-Centre	102 (93,6%)	nr	[29]
Medtronic CoreValve	Trans-femoral (13)/ Trans-subclavian (3)/Trans-iliac (9)	Single-Centre	22 (88%)	8 (32%)	[30]

(Continued)

Valve Type	Procedural Approach (Pts)	Study	Procedural Success (%)	Overall 30-day Pts with MACE events (%)	Reference
Edwards Sapien	Trans-apical (35) / Trans-femoral (136)	Multi-Centre	nr	nr	[21]
Edwards Sapien	Trans-apical (84)/ Trans-femoral (67)	Single-Centre	148 (98%)	nr	[31]
Medtronic CoreValve	Trans-femoral (460) /Trans-subclavian (54)	Multi-Centre	507 (98,6%)	39 (7,6%)	[32]
Edwards Sapien	Trans-femoral	Single-Centre	43 (86%)	nr	[14]
Medtronic CoreValve	Trans-femoral (nr)/ Trans-subclavian (nr)/Trans-iliac (nr)	Multi-Centre	(74%)	19 (22%)	[34]
Medtronic CoreValve	Trans-femoral (nr)/ Trans-subclavian (nr)/Trans-iliac (nr)	Multi-Centre	626 (97%)	60 (9,3%)	[35]
Medtronic CoreValve	Trans-femoral	Single-Centre	33 (100%)	nr	[36]
Edwards Sapien	Trans-apical (55) / Trans-femoral (113)	Single-Centre	150 (94,1%)	25 (14,9%)	[33]
Sapien / CoreValve	Trans-femoral	Single-Centre	59 (98%)	nr	[6]
Edwards Sapien	Trans-femoral	Multi-Centre	173 (97,7%)	nr	[5]
CoreValve (78) / Edwards Sapien (166)	Trans-apical (71)/ Trans-femoral (161) / Trans-subclavian (12)	Multi-Centre	240 (98,3%)	nr	[13]
Edwards Sapien	Transpapical	Multi-Centre	36 (90%)	21 (52%)	[15]
CoreValve (154) / Sapien (49)	Trans-apical (50)/ Trans-femoral (153)	Single-Centre	203 (100%)	nr	[7]
Edwards Sapien	Trans-apical	Multi-Centre	100%	nr	[16]
Edwards Sapien	Trans-apical	Single-Centre	25 (96%)	nr	[17]
Edwards Sapien	Transapical	Single-Centre	49 (98%)	nr	[20]
Edwards Sapien	Trans-apical	Single-Centre	26 (100%)	9 (34,6%)	[18]
Edwards Sapien	Trans-apical (11) / Trans-femoral (11)	Single-Centre	22 (91%)	nr	[37]
CoreValve (21) / Sapien (24)	Trans-femoral / Trans-subclavian	Single-Centre	44 (97,8%)	4 (8,9%)	[38]
Edwards Sapien	Trans-apical	Multi-Centre	533 (92,7%)	nr	[39]
Edwards Sapien	Trans-apical	Single-Centre	175 (100%)	nr	[19]
Medtronic CoreValve	Trans-femoral (101) Trans-subclavian (4)	Single-Centre	105 (100%)	39 (36,1%)	na

Pts : patients; AMI : Acute myocardial infarction; PVL : Paravalvular Leak; ARF : Acute Renal Failure; PM : Pacemaker; nr : not reported; na : not applicable; * : median; ^: > than 5 Units of packed cells; §:data at 1 year post-implant.

External or intravascular device designed to block or deviate far from the supra-aortic vessel dislodged particles are under investigation or development, and, therefore, such misadventures will probably further decrease.

Acute Aortic Insufficiency and Structural Prosthetic Dysfunction

Aortic valve insufficiency following TAVI is usually related to trivial or mild paravalvular leak. Sudden aortic valve insufficiency may occur just after native valve ballooning and lead to acute left ventricular dysfunction with cardiogenic shock and pulmonary edema. This event is rare and immediate prosthetic deployment may solve the ongoing left ventricular impairment. Rarely, temporary cardiocirculatory support may be required to let the heart recover from stunning and transient myocardial ischemia related to sudden rise in left ventricular end-diastolic pressure.

Intra-prosthetic regurgitation may occur at time. This complication may be generated by an improper function of an otherwise well positioned prosthesis. Immobile valve leaflet have been described [84] requiring an immediate valve-in-valve procedure to solve the adverse event. The mechanisms underlying such a structural defect may account for incomplete valve deployment [69], by guidewire impingement onto a bioprosthetic cusp [69], by leaflet or valve frame damage during deployment, by a severe PPM (valve deformation) or by excessive calcified vegetation inducing frame deformation [85].

Prosthetic valve crimping, as performed to prepare the bioprosthesis for trans-catheter implantation, has been claimed to induce damage of the prosthetic leaflet tissue and to some extent also to the valve frame.

Regarding specific prosthesis-related behaviour following deployment it should be mentioned that Zegdi and coworkers analysed the geometrical and morphological changes of the Edwards Sapien bioprostheses in 19 patients submitted to trans-femoral TAVI [86]. In this limited observational study the authors found that rather constant deformation of the prosthetic stent, particularly at the level of the distal portion of the frame (the one supporting the free edges of the leaflets) induced a stent-to-leaflet mismatch and, hence, a likely site of mechanical stress. Since it is well known that increased mechanical stress is the prerequisite for subsequent biological tissue performance and durability, further studies are certainly mandatory to thoroughly investigate such an aspect.

Another aspects which was variably claimed to be dangerous for the leaflet mechanics and, hence, for the prosthetic performance and hemodynamics, was the biological and_tissue-related processes generated by the presence of the stent in the aortic root, particularly in terms of pannus formation over the nitinol frame. Noble and co-workers has shown in 4 cases of explanted CoreValve that the biological reactions induced by the presence of the prosthetic components vary according to the time elapsed from the implantation [87]. Indeed, an initial inflammatory reaction has been observed in the leaflet tissue early after implantation, specifically characterized by fibrin deposition associated with an inflammatory reaction and slight foreign body response. At 3 months from implantation fibrin deposition is substituted by smooth muscle and endothelial cells, with a final appearance of neointimal tissue featured predominantly by fibrosis and fewer cells. Neointimal tissue covered almost entirely the nitinol portions in contact with the native aortic wall, and no sign of nitinol fracture or leaflet tissue degeneration was observed in this post-mortem study, thereby providing encouraging inputs regarding postoperative tissue valve durability and performance. Interestingly, a patient with amyloidosis showed a more pronounced neointimal formation, indicating that this condition (senile amyloidosis) may predispose to excessive inflammatory reaction and potential danger to the prosthetic integration at the aortic root level [87]. Regarding the valve-in-valve condition, the pathological examination showed an optimal integration between the two artificial valves with proper fibrin coverage along both luminal surfaces, again indicating that this peculiar condition may not represent a risk factor for uncontrolled or enhanced inflammatory reaction ultimately leading to neointima overgrowth.

No case of structural or non-structural valve deterioration, and postprocedural prosthetic valve insufficiency unchanged over time from discharge, with only slight increase in trans-valvular gradient (from 10 at discharge to 12 mmHg at follow-up, respectively), has been shown by Gurvitch and co-workers in 70 patients at 3 years from TAVI procedure [83], thereby providing encouraging information about long-term performance of implanted prostheses, although additional data are warranted to draw any further conclusion in this respect.

Other Potential Complications

The occurrence of *acute renal failure* after TAVI varies a great deal, as all the other complications, and may occur up to 22% of treated patients [36]. The cause of such an adverse event may account for embolism, decreased renal perfusion or dye-related kidney dysfunction. The presence of hypertension, chronic obstructive pulmonary disease, and blood cell transfusion have been shown to be independently related to increase rate of acute kidney dysfunction in TAVI patients [88]. Notably, the incidence of acute renal failure was 11.7% in a series of 117 patients without preoperative chronic renal failure [88]. Furthermore, the occurrence of acute renal failure was significantly correlated with in-hospital mortality, underlying the importance of prevention and appropriate management in this respect, although TAVI in high risk patients appeared to reduce two to three folds the incidence of acute kidney impairment as compared to conventional aortic valve replacement [88].

Perforation of cardiac structures by direct injury of catheters or as consequence of prosthetic deployment is likely although fortunately rather uncommon. Rupture of the aortic wall or aortic valve-related structures have been previously discussed, but perforation of the membranous interventricular septum [89], of the left ventricular wall by the TAVI catheter, or of the right ventricular wall by the pacing lead, are all possible adverse events and variably reported in the literature. Ventricular or septal hematoma are also possible and may lead to delayed complications, particularly tamponade, often requiring surgical intervention, but minimal treatment (percutaneous pericardiocentesis) may also allow resolution without any further action.

Ventricular fibrillation or other kind of sustained and clinically relevant arrhythmia are again likely, particularly during rapid ventricular pacing. Usually, these arrhythmias are self-limiting and extinguish rather quickly. In the presence of severe left ventricular dysfunction or decompensated patients or markedly hypertrophic hearts rapid pacing may induce a sort of "myocardial stunning" involving also the conduction system, with persistent left ventricular hypocontractility and extreme bradicardia. If appropriate ventricular pacing rate will not be sufficient to restore adequate cardio-circulatory conditions, IABP or peripheral-based ECC may be required for a transient mechanical circulatory support.

Thrombosis of the implanted TAVI prosthesis has been reported a few months following trans-apical aortic valve implantation [90].

Perspectives

Despite being a rather invasive procedure in a very critical site of the cardiovascular system, complication rate does not appear to be unacceptably high, particularly taking into account the candidate profile and comorbidities usually characterizing TAVI candidates. Obviously the learning curve does play a critical role, but results of the latest series indicate that this issue might be mitigated. Several events (see pacemaker implantation) might be difficult to decline, but device-related technical advances either in terms of system design or operational access may enhance early outcome and reduce drastically the complication rate. Additionally, new device (internal or external) might be helpful to reduce cerebral embolization of calcified material during TAVI [24], most likely deviating the emboli from the supra-aortic vessels to the lower thoracic or abdominal aorta. Other devices, however, are under development and investigation to act as filters and barrier to dislodged valve-related calcium to prevent or markedly limit such an adverse event.

It is clear, however, that full and comprehensive awareness and knowledge of type, extent, prognosis, and kind of management of adverse events during TAVI represent a mandatory background for the operator to be involved in TAVI. It is self-explanatory that further reduction or prevention of any misadventure will be critical for any further extension of TAVI indications, besides the important clues about prosthetic performance and related complications at long term.

Finally, this overview of the existing literature about TAVI experiences underlines how heterogeneous has been the reporting of complication-related information. It would be, therefore, extremely advisable to use a common language and a uniform attitude, as already existing in relation to surgically implanted valvular prosthesis [91], and maybe modifying such guidelines of reporting mortality and morbidity taking into account TAVI procedures. By using a standard and common language relevant and comprehensive data will be available for analysis and interpretation, particularly in view of early and long-term assessment of TAVI results.

Finally, it is also extremely evident that the wide range of type and complexity of complications during TAVI procedures calls for a well integrated team approach, which may also not be limited to cardiologist and cardiac surgeon, but maybe involving also interventional radiologist and vascular surgeon, underlining the need of a well equipped and organised centre as a pre-requisite for starting a TAVI program [10, 92].

References

[1] Cribier A, Eltchaninoff H, Bash A, Borestein N, Tron C, Bauer F, Derumaux G, Anselme F, Laborde F, Leon M. Percutaneous transcatheter implantation of an aortic valve prosthesis for calcifid aortci stenosis : first human case description: *Circulation* 2002;106:3006-8.

[2] Masson JB, Kovac J, Schuler G, Ye J, Cheung A, Kapadia S, Tuzcu ME, Kodali S, Leon MB, Webb JG. Transcatheter aortic valve implantation : review of the nature, management, and avoidance of procedural complications. *J. Am. Coll. Cardiol. Intv.* 2009;2:811-20.

[3] Webb JG, Chandavimol M, Thompson CR, Ricci DR, Carere RG, Munt BI, Buller CE, Pasupati S, Lichtestein S. Percutaneous aortic valve implantation retrograde from the femoral artery. *Circulation* 2006;113:842-50.

[4] Yan TD, Cao C, Martens-Nielsen J, Padang R, Ng M, Vallely MP, Bannon PG. Transcatheter aortic valve implantation for high-risk patients with severe aortic stenosis: a systematic review. *J. Thorac. Cardiovasc. Surg.* 2009;139;1519-28.

[5] Leon MB, Smith CR, Mack M, Miller CE, Moses JW, Svensson LG, Tuscu EM, Webb JG, Fontana GP, Makkar RR, Brown DL, Block PC, Guyton RA, Pichard AD, Bavaria JE, Herrmann HC, Douglas PC, Petersen JL, Akin JJ, Anderson WN, Wang D, Pocock S. PARTNER Trial. Transcatheter aortic-valve implantation for aortic stenosis in patients who cannot undergo surgery. *N. Eng. J. Med.* 2010 (electronic publication; ahead of print).

[6] Kahlert P, Al-Rashid F, Weber M, Wendt D, Heine T, Kottenberg E, Thielmann M, Kuhl H, Peters J, Jakob HG, Sack S, Erbel R, Eggebrecht H. Vascular access site complications after percutaneous transfemoral aortic valve implantation. *Herz* 2009;34:398-408.

[7] Bleiziffer S, Ruge H, Mazzitelli D, Hutter A, Opitz A, Bauernshmitt R, Lange R. Survival after transapical and transfemoral aortic valve implantation : talking about two different patient populations. *J. Thorac. Cardiovasc. Surg.* 2009;138:1073-80.

[8] Marcheix B, Lamarche Y, Berry C, Asgar A, Laborde JC, Basmadijan A, Ducharme A, Denault A, Bonan R, Cartier R. Surgical aspects of endovascular retrograde implantation of the aortic CoreValve bioprosthesis in high-rik older patients with severe symptomatic aortic stenosis. *J. Thorac. Cardiovasc. Surg.* 2007;134:1150-6.

[9] Ye J, Cheung A, Lichtestein SV, Carere RG, Thompson CR, Pasupati S, Transapical aortic valve implantation in humans. *J. Thorac. Cardiovasc. Surg.* 2006;131:1194-6.

[10] Wong DR, Ye J, Cheung A, Webb JG, Carere RG, Lichtenstein SV. Technical considerations to avoid pitfalls during trans-apical valve implantation. *J. Thorac. Cardiovacs. Surg.* 2010;140:196-202.

[11] Al-Attar N, Raffoul R, Himbert D, Brochet E, Vahanian A, Nataf P. Lase aneurysm after transapical aortic valve implantation. *J. Thorac. Cardiovasc. Surg.* 2009;137:e21-2.

[12] Thomas M, Schymik G, Walther T, Himbert D, Lefevre T, Treede H, Eggebrecht H, Rubino P, Michev I, Lange R, Anderson WN, Wendler O. Thirty-day results of the SAPIEN aortic bioprosthesis European Outcome (SOURCE) Registry. *Circulation* 2010;122:62-9.

[13] Eltchaninoff H, Prat A, Gilard M, Leguerrier A, Blanchard D, Fournial G, Iung B, Donzeau-Gouge P, Tribouilloy C, Debrux JL, Pavie A, Gueret P. France Registry Investigators. Transcatheter aortic valve implantation : early results of the FRANCE (FRench Aortic National CoreValve and Edwards) registry. *Eur. Heart J.* 2010 (electronic publication; ahead of print).

[14] Webb JG, Altwegg L, Boone RH, Cheung A, Ye J, Lichtestein S, Lee M, Masson JB, Thompson C, Moss R, Carere R, Munt B, Nietlispach F, Humphries K. Transcatheter aortic valve implantation : impact on clinical and valve-related outcomes. *Circulation* 2009;119:3009-16.

[15] Svensson LG, Dewey T, Kapadia S, Roselli EE, Stewart A, Williams M, Anderson WN, Brown D, Leon M, Lytle B, Moses J, Mack M, Tuzcu M, Smith C. United States

feasibility study of transcatheter insertion of a stented aortic valve by the left ventricular apex. *Ann. Thorac. Surg.* 2008;86:46-55.

[16] Walther T, Simon P, Dewey T, Wimmer-Greinecker G, Falk V, Kasimir MT, Doss M, Borger MA, Schuler G, Glogar D, Fehske W, Wolner E, Mohr FW, Mack M. Transapical minimally invasive aortic valve implantation : multicenter experience. *Circulation* 2007;116(Suppl I):I-240--I-245.

[17] Zierer A, Wimmer-Greinecker G, Martens S, Moritz A, Doss M. The transapical approach for aortic valve implantation. *J. Thorac. Cardiovasc. Surg.* 2008;136:948-53.

[18] Ye J, Cheung A, Lichtestein SV, Altwegg LA, Wong DR, Carere RG, Thompson CR, Moss RR, Munt B, Pasupati S, Boone RH, Masson JB, Ali AA, Webb JG. Transapical transcatheter aortic valve implantation: 1-year outcome in 26 patients. *J. Thorac. Cardiovasc. Surg.* 2009;137:167-73.

[19] Pasic M, Unbehaun A, Dreysse S, Drews T, Buz S, Kukucka M, Mladenow A, Gromann T, Hetzer R. Transapical aortic valve implantation in 175 consecutive patients. *J. Am. Coll. Cardiol.* 2010;56:813-20.

[20] Walther T, Falk V, Kempfert J, Borger MA, Fassl J, Chu MWA, Schuler G, Mohr FW. Transapical minimally invasive aortic valve implantation : the initial 50 patients. *Eur. J. Cardio-Thorac. Surg.* 2008;33:983-8.

[21] Dewey TM, Brown DL, Herbert MA, Culica D, Smith CR, Leon MB, Svensson LG, Tuzcu M, Webb JG, Cribier A, Mack MJ. Effect of concomitant coronary artery disease on procedural and late outcomes of transcatheter aortic valve implantation. *Ann. Thorac. Surg.* 2010;89:758-67.

[22] Moss RR, Ivens E, Pasupati S, Humphries K, Thompson C, Munt B, Sinhal A, Webb JG. Echocardiography and percutaneous aortic valve implantation. *J. Am. Coll. Cardiol. Imaging* 2008;1:15-24.

[23] Gerckens U, Latsios G, Mueller R, Buellesfeld L, Sauren B, Iversen S, Felderhof T, Grube E. Left main PCI after trans-subclavian CoreValve implantation : successful outcome of a combined procedure for management of a rare complication. *Clin. Res. Cardiol.* 2009;98:687-90.

[24] Haberthur D, Lutter G, Appel M, Attman T, Schramm R, Schmitz C, Bombien Quaden R. Percutaneous aortic valve replacement : valvuloplasty studies in vitro. *Eur. J. Cardio-Thorac. Surg.* 2010 (electronic publication; ahead of print)

[25] Webb JG. Coronary obstruction due to transcatheter valve implantation. *Cath. Cardiovasc. Intv.* 2009;73:973.

[26] Tops LF, Wood DA, Delgado V, Schuijf JD, van der Wall EE, Schalij MJ, Webb JG, Bax JJ. Noninvasive evaluation of the aortic root with multislice computed tomography: implications for transcatheter aortic valve replacement. *J. Am. Coll. Cardiol. Imaging* 2008;1:321-30.

[27] Bagur R, Dumont E, Doyle D, Larose E, Lemieux J, Bergeron S, Bilodeau S, Bertrand OF, De Larochellerière R, Rodés-Cabau J. Coronary ostia stenosis after transcatheter aortic valve implantation. *JACC Cardiovasc. Interv.* 2010;3:253-5.

[28] Kapadia SR, Svensson L, Tuzcu EM. Successful percutaneous management of left main trunk occlusion during percutaneous aortic valve replacement. *Catheter Cardiovasc. Interv.* 2009;73:966 –72.

[29] Ussia GP, Barbanti M, Immè S, Scarabelli M, Mulè M, Cammalleri V, Aruta P, Pistritto AM, Capodanno D, Deste W, Di Pasqua MC, Tamburino C. Management of implant

failure during trancatheter aortic valve implantation. *Cathet. Cardiovasc. Intv.* 2010 (electronic publication; ahead of print).

[30] Grube E, Laborde JC, Gerckens U, Felderhoff T, Sauren B, Buellesfeld L, Mueller R, Menichelli M, Schimdt T, Zickmann B, Iversen S, Stone GW. Percutaneous implantation of the CoreValve self-expanding valve prosthesis in high-risk patients with aortic valve disease: the Siegburg first-in-man study. *Circulation* 2006;114:1616-24.

[31] Dworakowski R, Maccarthy PA, Monaghan M, Redwood S, El-Ganel A, Young C, Bapat V, Hancock J, Wilson K, Brickham B, Wendler O, Thomas MR. Transcatheter aortic valve implantation for severe aortic stenosis: a new paradigm for multidisciplinary intervention. A prospective cohort study. *Am. Heart J.* 2010;160:237-43.

[32] Petronio AS, De Carlo M, Bedogni F, Marzocchi A, Klugmann S, Maisano F, Raimondo A, Ussia GP, Ettori F, Poli A, Brambilla N, Sala F, De Marco F, Colombo A. Safety and efficacy of the subclavian approach for transcatheter aortic valve implnantation with the CoreValve Revalving System. *Circ. Cardiovasc. Interv.* 2010 (electronic publication; ahead of print).

[33] Webb JG, Pasupati S, Humphries K, Thompson C, Altwegg L, Moss R, Sinhal A, Carere RG, Munt B, Ricci D, Ye J, Cheung A, Lichtestein SV. Percutaneous transarterial aortic valve replacement in selected high-risk patients with aortic stenosis. *Circulation* 2007;116:755-63.

[34] Grube E, Schuler G, Buellesfeld L, Gerckens U, Linke A, Wenaweser P, Sauren B, Mohr FW, Walther T, Zickmann B, Iversen S, Felderhoff T, Cartier R, Bonan R. Percutaneous aortic valve replacement for severe aortic stenosis in high-risk patients using the second and current third-generation slef-expanding Corevalve prosthesis. *J. Am. Coll. Cardiol.* 2007;50:69-76.

[35] Piazza N, Grube E, Gerkens U, den Heijer P, Linke A, Luha O, Ramondo A, Ussia G, Wenaweser P, Windecker S, Laborde JC, de Jaegere PP, Serruys PW. Procedural and 30-day outcomes following transcatheter aortic valve implantation using the third generation (18 Fr) CoreValve revalving system : results from the multicentre, expanded evaluation registry 1-year following CE mark approval. *Eurointervention* 2008;4:242-9.

[36] de Jaegere PP, Piazza N, Galema TW, Otten A, Soliman OI, Van Dalen BM, Geleijnse ML, Kappetein AP, Garcia HM, Van Es GA, Serruys PW. Early echocardiographic evaluation following percutaneous implantation with the self-expanding CoreValve Revalving System aortic valve bioprosthesis. *Eurointervention* 2008;4:351-7.

[37] Rodés-Cabau J, Dumont E, De LaRochellière R, Doyle D, Lemieux J, Bergeron S, Clavel MA, Villeneuve J, Raby K, Bertrand OF, Pibarot P. Feasibility and initial results of percutaneous aortic valve implantation including selection of transfemoral or transapical approach in patients with severe aortic stenosis. *Am. J. Cardiol.* 2008;102: 1240-6.

[38] Tchetche D, Dumonteil N, Sauguet A, Descoutures F, Garcia O, Soula P, Gabiache Y, Fournial G, Marcheix B, Carrie D, Fajadet J. Thirty-day outcome and vascular complications after trans-arterial aortic valve implantation using both Edwards Sapien and Medtronic CoreValve bioprostheses in a mixed population. *Eurointervention* 2010;5:659-65 32.

[39] Wendler O, Thomas W, Nataf P, Rubino P, Schroefel H, Thielmann M, Treede H, Thomas M. Transapical aortic valve implantation : univariate and multivariate analysis of the early results from the SOURCE Registry. *Eur. J. Cardio-Thorac. Surg.* 2010;38: 119-27.

[40] Vavouranakis M, Vrachatis DA, Toutouzas KP, Chrysohoou C, Stafanidis C. "Bail out" procedures for malpositioning of aortic valve prostheses. *Int. J. Cardiol.* (electronic publication; ahead of print).

[41] Piazza N, de Jaegere P, Schultz C, Becker AE, Serruys PW, Anderson RH. Anatomy of the aortic valvar complex and its implications for transcatheter implantation of the aortic valve. *Circ. Cardiovasc. Intervent.* 2008;2008;1:74-81.

[42] Akhtar M, Tuzcu EM, Kapadia SR, et al. Aortic root morphology in patients undergoing percutaneous aortic valve replacement. *J. Thorac. Cardiovasc. Surg.* 2009; 137:950–6.

[43] Clavel MA, Dumont E, Pibarot P, Doyle D, De Larochellière R, Villenueve J, Bergeron S, Couture C, Rodés-Cabau J. Severe valvular regurgitation and late prosthesis embolization after percutaneous aortic valve implantation. *Ann. Thorac. Surg.* 2009;87: 618-21.

[44] Zahn R, Schiele R, Kilkowski C, Klein B, Zeymer U, Werling C, Lehmann A, Layer G, Saggau W. There are two sides to everything : two cases reports on sequelae of rescue interventions to treat complications of trancatheter aortic valve implantation of Medtronic CoreValve prosthesis. *Clin. Res. Cardiol.* 2010 (electronic publication; ahead of print).

[45] Dawkins S, Hobson AR, Kalra PR, Tang ATM, Monro JL, Dawkins KD. Permanent pacemaker implantation after isolated aortic valve replacement : incidence, indications, and predictors. *Ann. Thorac. Surg.* 2008;85:108-12.

[46] Koplan BA, Stevensomn WG, Epstein LM, Aranki SF, Maisel WH. Development and validation of a simple risk score to predict the need for permanent pacing after cardiac valve surgery. *J. Am. Coll. Cardiol.* 2003;41:795-801.

[47] Piazza N, Onuma Y, Jesserun E, Kint PP, Maugenest AM, Anderson RH, de Jaegere PPY, Serruys PW. Early and persistent intraventricular conduction abnormalities and requirements for pacemaking after percutaneous replacement of the aortic valve. *J. Am. Coll. Intv.* 2008;1:310-6.

[48] Baan J, Yong ZY, Koch KT, Henriques JPS, Bouma BJ, Vis MM, Cocchieri R, Piek JJ, de Mol BAJM. Factors associated with cardiac conduction disorders and permanent pacemaker implantation after percutaneous aortic valve implantation with the Corevalve prosthesis. *Am. Heart J.* 2010;159:497-503.

[49] Sinhal A, Altwegg L, Pasupati S, Humphries KH, Allard M, Martin P, Cheung A, Ye J, Kerr C, Lichtenstein SV, Webb JG. Atrioventricular block after transcatheter balloon expandable aortic valve implantation. *J. Am. Coll. Cardiol. Intv.* 2008;1:305-9.

[50] Moreno R, Dobarro D, Lopez de Sà E, Prieto M, Morales C, Orbe LC, Moreno-Gomez I, Filguerias D, Sanchez-Recalde A, Galeote G, Jimenez-Valero S, Lopez-Sendon JL. Cause of complete atrioventricular block after percutaneous aortic valve implantation. *Circulation* 2009;120:e29-e30.

[51] Godin M, Eltchaninoff H, Furuta A, Tron C, Anselme F, Bejar K, Sanchez-Giron C, Bauer F, Litzler PY, Bessou JP, Cribier A. Frequency of conduction disturbances after

trancatheter implantation of an Edwards Sapien aortic valve prosthesis. *Am. J. Cardiol.* 2010;106:707-12.

[52] Bombien R, Humme T, Schunke M, Lutter G. Percutaneous aortic valve replacement : computed tomography scan after valved stent implantation in human cadaver hearts. *Eur. J. Cardio-Thorac. Surg.* 2009;36:592-4.

[53] Ussia GP, Barbanti M, Immè S, Scarabelli M, Mulè M, Cammalleri V, Aruta P, Pistritto AM, Capodanno D, Deste W, Di Pasqua MC, Tamburino C. Management of implant failure during transcatheter aortic valve implantation. *Cath. Cardiovasc. Intv.* 2010 (electronic publication; ahead of print).

[54] Détaint D, Lepage L, Himberg D, Brochet E, Messika-Zeitoun D, Iung B, Vahanian A. Determinants of significant paravalvular regurgitation after transcatheter artic valve implantation. *J. Am. Coll. Cardiol. Intv.* 2009;2:821-7.

[55] Ionescu A, Fraser AG, Bruchart EG. Prevalence and clinical significance of incidental paraprosthetic valvar regurgitation : a prospective study using transesophageal echocardiography. *Heart* 2003;89:1316-21.

[56] Azadani AN, Jaussaud N, Matthews PB, Ge L, Guy S, Chuter TAM, Tseng EE. Energy loss due to paravalvular leak with transcatheter aortic valve implantation. *Ann. Thorac. Surg.* 2009;88:1857-63.

[57] Zegdi R, Khabbaz Z, Ciobataru V, Noghin M, Deloche A, Fabiani JN. Calcific bicuspid aortic stenosis : a questionable indication for endovascular valve implantation ? *Ann. Thorac. Surg.* 2008;85:342.

[58] Zegdi R, Ciobataru V, Noghin M, Sleilaty G, Lafint A, Latremouille C, Deloche A, JN Fabiani. Is it reasonable to treat all calcified stenotic aortic valves with a valved stent ? *J. Am. Coll. Cardiol.* 2008;51:579-84.

[59] Zegdi R, Lecuyer L, Achouh P, Blanchard D, Lafont A, Latremouille C, Fabiani JN. Increased radial force improves stent deployment in tricuspid, but not in bicuspid stenotic native aortic valves. *Ann. Thorac. Surg.* 2010;89:768-72.

[60] Chiam PTL, Chao VTT, Tan SY, Koh TH, Lee CY, Tho VYS, Sin YK, Chua YL. Percutaneous transcatheter heart valve implantation in a bicuspid aortic valve. *J. Am. Coll. Cardiol. Cardiovasc. Interv.* 2010;3:559-61.

[61] Wijesinghe N, Ye J, Rodas-Cabau J, Cheung A, Velianou J, Natarajan M, Dumont E, Nietlispach F, Gurvitch R, Wood D, Tai E, Webb J. Transcatheter aortic valve implantation in bicuspid aortic valve stenosis. *Heart Lung Circ.* 2010;19S:S156.

[62] Vanden Eynden F, Bouchard D, El-Hamamsy I, Butnaru A, Demers P, Carrier M, Perrault LP, Tardif JC, Pellerin M. Effect of aortic valve replacement for aortic stenosis on severity of mitral regurgitation. *Ann. Thorac. Surg.* 2007;83:1279-84.

[63] Waisbren EC, Stevens LM, Avery EG, Picard MH, Vlahakes GJ, Agnihotri AK. Changes in mitral regurgitation after replacement of the stenotic aortic valve. *Ann. Thorac. Surg.* 2008;86:56-62.

[64] Wan CKN, Suri RM, Li Z, Orszulak TA, Daly RC, Schaff HV, Sundt TM. Management of moderate functional mitral regurgitation at the time of aortic valve replacement : is concomitant valve repair necessary ?- *J. Thorac. Cardiovasc. Surg.* 2009;137:635-40.

[65] Feldman T, Kar S, Rinaldi M, Fail P, Hermiller J, Smalling R, Whitlow PL, Gray W, Low R, Hermann HC, Lim S, Foster E, Glower D. EVEREST Investigators. Percutaneous mitral repair with the MitraClip system : safety and midtterm durability in the initial EVEREST cohort. *J. Am. Coll. Cardiol.* 2009;54:686-94.

[66] Tzikas A, Piaza N, van Dalen BM, Schultz C, Geleijnse ML, van Geuns RJ, Galema TW, Nuis RJ, Otten A, Gutierrez-Chico JL, Serruys PW, de Jaegere PP. Changes in mitral regurgitation after transcatheter aortic valve implantation. *Catheter Cardiovasc. Intv.* 2010;75:43-49.

[67] Gotzmann M, Lindstaedt M, Bojara W, Mugger A, Germing A. Hemodynamic results and changes in myocardial function after transcatheter aortic vave implantation. *Am. Heart J.* 2010;159:926-32.

[68] Piazza N, Marra S, Webb J, D'Amico M, Rinaldi M, Boffini M, Comoglio C, Scacciatella P, Kappetein AP, de Jaegere P, Serruys PW. Two cases of aneurysm of the anterior mitral valve leaflet associated with transcatheter aorti valve endocarditis : a mere coincidence ? *J. Thorac. Cardiovasc. Surg.* 2010;140:e36-8.

[69] Al-Attar N, Ghodbane W, Himbert D, Rau C, Raffoul R, Messika-Zeitun D, Bochet E, Vahanian A, Nataf P. Unexpected complications of transapical aortic valve implantation. *Ann. Thorac. Surg.* 2009;88:90-4.

[70] Walther T, Rastan A, Falck V, Lehmann S, Garbade J, Funkat AK, Mohr FW, Gummert JF. Patient prosthesis mismatch affects short- and long-term outcomes after aortic valve replacement. *Eur. J. Cardio-Thorac. Surg.* 2006;30:15-9.

[71] Mohty D, Dumesnil JG, Echahidi N, Mathieu P, Dagenais F, Voisine P, Pibarot P. Impact of prosthesis-patient mismatch on long-term survival after aortic valve replacement : influence of age, obesity, and left ventricular dysfunction. *J. Am. Coll. Cardiol.* 2009;53:39-47.

[72] Blackstone EH, Cosgrove DM, Jamieson EWR, Birkmeyer NJ, Lemmer JH, Miller CG, Butchart EG, Rizzoli G, Yacoub M, Chai A. Prosthesis size and long-term survival after aortic vave replacement. *J. Thorac. Cardiovasc. Surg.* 2003;126:783-96.

[73] Moon MR, Lawton JS, Moazami N, Munfakk NA, Pasque MK, Damiano RJ. POINT : Prosthesis-patient mismatch does not affect suvival for patients greater than 70 years of age undergoing bioprosthetic aortic valve replacement. *J. Thorac. Cardiovasc. Surg.* 2009137:278-83.

[74] .Jilaihawi H, Chin D, Spyt T, Jeilan M, Vasa-Nicotera M, Bence J, Logtens E, Kovac J. Prosthesis-patient mismatch after transcatheter aortic valve implantation with the Medtronic Corevalve bioprosthesis. *Eur. Heart J.* 2010;31:857-64.

[75] Vranckx P, Otten A, Schultz C, Van Domburg R, de Jaegere P, Seruys PW. Assisted circulation using the Tandemheart, percutaneous traseptal left ventricular assist device, during percutaneous aortic valve implantation : the Rotterdam experience. *Eurointervention* 2009;5:465-9.

[76] Adams HP. Ischemic cerebrovascular complications of cardiac procedures. *Circulation* 2010;121:846-7.

[77] Stolz E, Gerriets T, Kluge A, Klovekorn WP, Kaps M, Bachmann G. Diffusion-weighted magnetic resonance imaging and neurobiochemical markers after aortic valve replacement. *Stroke* 2004;35:888-92.

[78] Knipp SC, Matatko N, Schlamann M, Wilhelm H, Thielmann M, Forsting M, Diener HC, Jakob H. Small ischemic brain lesions after cardiac valve replacement detected by diffusion-weighted magnetic resonance imaging : relation to neurocognitive function. *Eur. J. Cardio-Thorac. Surg.* 2005;28:88-96.

[79] Floyd TF, Shah PN, Price CC, Harris F, Ratcliffe SJ, Acker MA, Bavaria JE, Rahmouni H, Kuersten B, Wiegers S, McGarvey ML, Woo JY, Pochettino AA, Melhem ER.

Clinically silent cerebral ischemic events after cardiac surgery : their incidence, regional vascular occurrence, and procedural dependence. *Ann. Thorac. Surg.* 2006;81: 2160-6.

[80] Omran H, Schmidt H, Hackenbroch M, Illien S, Bernhardt P, von der Recke G, Fimmers R, Flacke S, Layer G, Pohl C, Luderitz B, Schild H, Sommer T. Silent and apparent cerebral embolism after retrograde catheterisation of the aortic valve in valvular stenosis : a prospective, randomised study. *Lancet* 2003;361:1241-46.

[81] Ghanem A, Muller A, Nahle CP, Kocurek J, Werner N, Hammerstingl C, Schild HH, Schwab JO, Mellert F, Fimmers R, Nickenig G, Thomas D. Risk and fate of cerebral embolism after transfemoral aortic valve implantation. *J. Am. Coll. Cardiol.* 2010;55: 1427-32.

[82] Kahlert P, Knipp SC Schlamann M, Thielmann M, Al-Rashid F, Weber M, Johansson U, Wendt D, Jakob HG, Forsting M, Sack S, Erbel R, Eggebrecht H. Silent and apparent cerebral ischemia after percutaneous transfemoral aortic valve implantation. *Circulation* 2010;121:870-8.

[83] Gurvitch R, Wood DA, Tay EL, Leipsic J, Ye J, Lichtestein SV, Thompson CR, Carere RG, Wijesinghe N, Nietlispach F, Boone RH, Lauck S, Cheung A, Webb JG. Transcatheter aortic valve implantation. Durability of clinical and hemodynamic outcomes beyond 3 years in a large patient cohort. *Circulation* 2010;122;1319-27.

[84] Pasupati S, Puri A, Devlin G, Fisher R. Trancatheter aortic valve implantation complicated by acute structural valve failure requiring immediate valve-in-valve implantation. *Heart Lung Circulation* 2010 (electronic publication; ahead of print).

[85] Zahn R, Schiele R, Kilwoski C, Zeymer U. Severe aortic regurgitation after percutaneous transcatheter aortic valve implantation : on th eimportance to clarify the underlyig pathology. *Clin. Res. Cardiol.* 2010;99:193-7.

[86] Zegdi R, Blanchard D, Achouh P, Lafont A, Berrebi A, Cholley B, Fabiani JN. Deployed Edwards Sapien prosthesis is always deformed. *J. Thorac. Cardiovasc. Surg.* 2010;140:e54-6.

[87] Noble S, Asgar A, Cartier R, Virmani R, Bonan R. Anatomo-pathological analysis after Corevalve Revalving sytem implantation. *Eurointervention* 2009;5:78-85.

[88] Bagur R, Webb JG, Nietlispach F, Durmont E, De Larochelliere R, Doyle D, Masson JB, Gutiérrez MJ, Clavel MA, Bertrand OF, Pibarot P, Rodés-Cabau J. Acute kidney injury following transcatheter valve implantation : predictive factors, prognostic value, and comparison with surgical aortica valve replacement. *Eur. Heart J.* 2010;31:865-74.

[89] Tzikas A, Schultz C, Piazza N, van Geuns RJ, Serruys PW, de Jaegere PP. Perforation of the membranous interventircular septum after trancatheter aortic valve implantation. *Circ. Cardiovasc. Interv.* 2009;2:582-3.

[90] Trepels T, Martens S, Doss M, Fichtlescherer S, Schachinger V. Thrombotic restenosis after minimally invasive implantation of aprtic valve stent. *Circulation* 2009;120:e23-e24.

[91] Akins CW, Miller CD, Turina MI, Kouchoukos NT, Blackstone EH, Grunkemeier GL, Takkenberg JJM, David TE, Butchart EG, Adams DH, Shahian DM, Hagl S, Mayer JE, Lytle BW. Guidelines for reporting mortality and morbidity after cardiac valve interventions. *Eur. J. Cardio-Thorac. Surg.* 2008;33:523-8.

[92] Vassiliades TA, Block PC, Cohn LH, Adams DH, Borer JS, Feldman T, Holmes DR, Laskey WK, Lytle BW, Mack MJ, Williams DO. The clinical development of

percutaneous heart valve technology : a position statement of the STS, AATS and SCAI. *J. Thorac. Cardiovasc*. 2005;129:970-6.

Mitral Valve

In: Percutaneous Valve Technology: Present and Future ISBN: 978-1-61942-577-4
Editors: Jose Luis Navia and Sharif Al-Ruzzeh

Chapter XVI

Cardiology Perspective of Mitral Valve Disease - The Potential Role of Percutaneous Treatment

Amar Krishnaswamy and Brian P. Griffin

Introduction

The characteristic shape of the mitral valve (MV) was first described by Andre Vesalius in 1543. Our understanding of the valve has grown considerably since that time with regard to normal valve function and the anatomic and histopathologic mechanisms of disease. Furthermore, the imaging modalities for diagnosis and percutaneous strategies for treatment are continually evolving, and represent a paradigm shift in our approach to mitral valve disease. In this chapter, we will provide an overview of normal mitral valve anatomy, the etiology and mechanisms of mitral stenosis and mitral regurgitation, as well as the available medical and percutaneous options for treatment.

Normal Mitral Valve Anatomy

The mitral valve (MV) is a complex structure composed of multiple components that together provide a non-regurgitant valvular structure with minimal obstruction to forward flow and also maintain the structure and function of the left ventricle (LV). The MV complex consists of the mitral annulus (MA), leaflets, chordae, and papillary muscles (PM), all within the context of the left atrium (LA) and ventricle (Figure 1).

The MA is a thin membrane described as having a characteristic “saddle shape” with its most basal portions anteriorly and posteriorly and its most apical portions at the level of the commisures. It is attached anteriorly to the aortic annulus, composing the region known as the intervalvular fibrosa, and the posterior annulus separates the musculature of the LA and LV.

Due to its continuity with the muscular walls of the cardiac chambers, the annulus also contracts during atrial and ventricular systole [1].

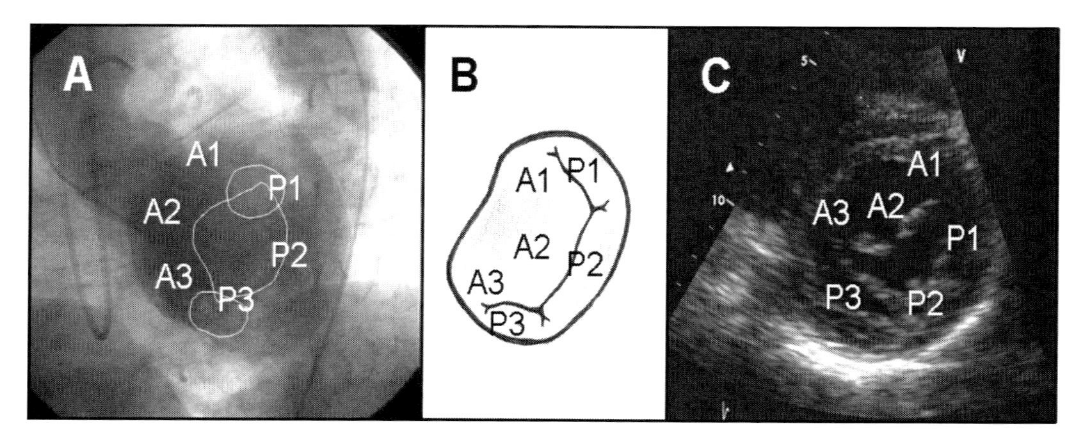

Figure 1. Normal mitral valve anatomy. A) left ventriculogram in the left anterior oblique projection showing the mitral valve in short axis; B) a schematic of the mitral valve in short axis; C) a transthoracic echocardiographic image of the mitral valve in the parasternal short axis projection. This figure was originally published in Topol & Teirstein's Textbook of Interventional Cardiology (6th edition); Krishnaswamy and Kapadia; Percutaneous Mitral Valve Repair (Chapter 49); Copyright Elsevier 2011.

The mitral leaflets are divided into 3 apposing parts on the basis of the 3 "scallops" of the posterior leaflet: from lateral to medial, A1/P1, A2/P2, and A3/P3, respectively. The free, coapting edges of the leaflets are referred to as the "rough zones;" the remaining portion of the leaflets are the "clear" zones. The zone of coaptation extends along the valve line and to a depth of about 1 cm. This coaptation depth provides a degree of redundancy which counterbalances the tethering forces of the chordae and ensures a barrier to regurgitation during ventricular systole.

There are more than 100 chordae that attach to the MV leaflets. Primary chords are thin, attach to the free leaflet margins, and function to maintain apposition. Secondary chords are thicker, attach to the ventricular surface of the leaflets, and serve to maintain LV structure and function. A subset of the secondary chords, termed "strut chords," are thicker and longer than the rest and attach exclusively to the anterior MV leaflet. They provide a continuous relationship between the MA, leaflets, and LV [2]. Severing the strut chords results in a perturbation of LV geometry and systolic function [3,4]. Both primary and secondary chords originate from the papillary muscles, and each PM contributes chordae to each leaflet. The tertiary chords, on the other hand, originate directly from the LV and attach only to the posterior MV leaflet. Their function is not known.

The anterolateral and posteromedial papillary muscles usually attach to the mid-portion of the LV. Blood supply to the anterolateral PM is from the left anterior descending (LAD) and left circumflex coronary arteries; the posteromedial PM receives blood from the right coronary artery (RCA) [5]. Contraction of the PMs reflects a coordinated action along with the rest of the left ventricle, and results in MV closure and apical displacement of the same. The thickening and rotational movement of the PMs also results in the creation of a "pathway" for blood to the left ventricular outflow tract (LVOT) [6].

Histologically, the MV is composed of 3 distinct layers. The atrialis, on the atrial side of the leaflets, is a later of collagen and elastic tissue. The spongiosa is the middle layer, and contains proteoglycans and structural proteins. The ventricularis, composed primarily of collagen, is also referred to as the fibrosa and is on the ventricular aspect of the leaflets [7].

Mitral Stenosis

Mitral stenosis (MS) was first described in the early 18th century, and was the first valvular lesion to be diagnosed by echocardiography and treated successfully with surgery [8]. Worldwide, the leading cause of MS is rheumatic heart disease (RHD), with a [likely underestimed] prevalence in some developing nations of 6 per 1000 children (compared with 0.5 per 1000 in the United States) [9]. In developed countries, other etiologies such as severe mitral annular calcification due to end-stage renal disease (ESRD), endocarditis, inflammatory disorders (ie lupus and rheumatoid arthritis), radiation therapy, and LA myxoma causing MV obstruction are more often considered.

Left untreated, MS is a slowly progressive disease that results in atrial fibrillation (AFib), pulmonary hypertension, decreased cardiac outpt, and the morbidities and mortalities associated therein. The increased loading conditions of pregnancy also present a particular challenge in patients with MS. Once symptoms develop, patients face a dismal prognosis, with at least 70% dead at 10 years [10]. Medical therapy is aimed at treating acute rheumatic fever and preventing its recurrence, avoiding systemic embolization in patients with atrial fibrillation, and maintaining optimal hemodynamics across the stenotic valve by controlling the heart rate. Percutaneous balloon mitral valvuloplasty (PBMV) has evolved as the 1st line of therapy in appropriately selected patients [11]. Surgical valve repair or replacement is reserved for those patients who are not good candidates for the percutaneous method based on anatomic characteristics or concomitant significant mitral regurgitation.

Etiology and Pathology of Mitral Stenosis

Acute rheumatic fever is the result of Group A streptococcal pharyngitis, and may affect up to 4% of patients with untreated infection. It has a number of manifestations including polyarthritis, chorea, and carditis. The inflammatory process affecting the MV begins with nodule formation at the leaflet edges, followed by leaflet thickening, commissural fusion, and chordal thickening and shortening. Eventually, fibrosis, scarring, and calcifications develop. This slowly progressive condition is likely the result of both smoldering inflammation and turbulent flow across the deformed mitral apparatus [15].

Patients with rheumatic MV disease may present with MS, MR, or combined disease. The mean time to symptom presentation is 16 years [16]. In a study of more than 700 patients in South Africa operated on for rheumatic MV disease between 1983 and 1986, Marcus and colleagues demonstrated an almost equal distribution of patients with MS (275 patients, 38%), MR (219 patients, 31%), and combined MS and MR (220 patients, 31%) [17]. Of note, almost all patients with pure MR required surgery before age 30 years (89%), and more often presented with ongoing inflammation than their counterparts with pure MS (47% vs 2%, $p <$

0.001). Furthermore, surgical examination revealed that the valvular lesions of pure MS and pure MR differed significantly. In patients with pure MS, only a minority had annular dilation (30%), most of which was mild (22%); almost all had shortened chords (90%); and almost half had rigid or scarred valves (38%). Patients with pure MR usually had some degree of annular dilation (95), elongated (92%) or ruptured chords (25%). Most patients with mixed disease had annular dilation (83%), and approximately half had shortened chords (49%) and rigid leaflets (56%).

Patients with end-stage kidney disease on hemodialysis are known to have disordered calcium metabolism. Mitral annular calcification (MAC) occurs in the majority of patients on dialysis, and increasing duration of dialysis and higher calcium*phosphate product are both associated with greater degree of valvular calcification [18,19]. With progressive calcification of the annulus and involvement of the leaflets, clinically meaningful gradients may present due to a smaller mitral orifice, especially with concomitant restricted leaflet motion [20]. MR may also be present as a result of MAC.

Other causes of MS include systemic inflammatory disorders (ie systemic lupus erythematosis (SLE) and rheumatoid arthritis), radiation heart disease, carcinoid disease, infiltrative disease (ie mucopolysaccharidosis), and MV obstruction by left atrial myxoma or valvular vegetation [16]. In contrast to rheumatic MS, in which the smallest valve area is at the leaflet tips, obstruction in non-rheumatic MS is predominantly at the annular level.

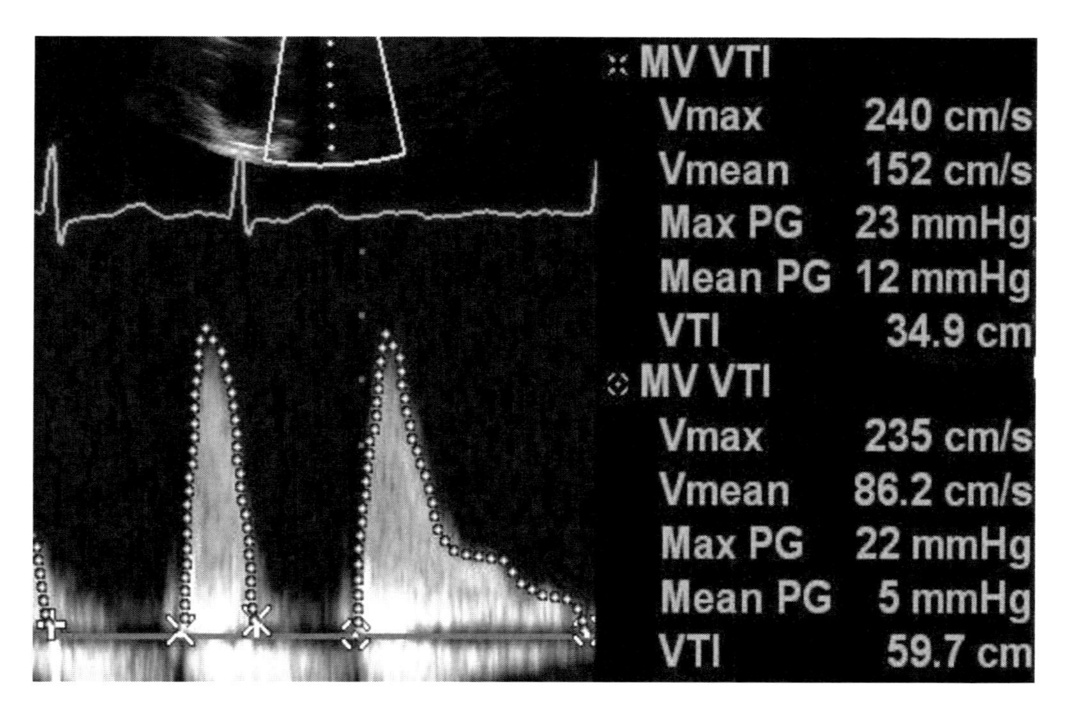

Figure 2. Patient with moderate MS and atrial fibrillation. The mean gradient across the mitral valve is significantly increased in the setting of decreased diastolic filling time (beat 1; 12 mmHg) compared with a longer R-R interval (beat 2; 5 mmHg).

Pathophysiology of Mitral Stenosis

Normal flow across the mitral valve is driven by the minimal pressure difference that exists between the LA and LV at the start of diastole, as well as the contribution of atrial systole. With the development of mitral stenosis, however, the increased impedence to flow caused by the valve gradient required a higher LA pressure and increases the significance of the diastolic filling time (the R-R interval) and atrial systole. Generally, a shorter R-R interval produces an increase in the MV gradient (Figure 2) [8]. The increased gradient results in elevated LA pressure, eventually causing atrial fibrillation and pulmonary venous congestion.

Table 1. Grading of mitral stenosis severity. Reproduced from Baumgartner et al; Echocardiographic assessment of valve stenosis: EAE/ASE recommendations for clinical practice; Eur Heart J 2009;1:1-25 by permission of Oxford University Press

	Mild	Moderate	Severe
Specific findings			
Alve area (cm^2)	>1.5	1.0-1.5	<1.0
Supportive findings			
Mean gradient (mmHg)[a]	<5	5-10	>10
Pulmonary artery pressure (mmHg)	<30	30-50	>50

[a] At heart rates between 60 – 80 bpm and in sinus rhythm.

Table 2. Echocardiographic scoring system for mitral valve stenosis. Reproduced from Wilkins et al; Percutaneous balloon dilatation of the mitral valve: an analysis of echocardiographic variables related to outcome and the mechanism of dilatation; Heart 1988;60:299-308 with permission from BMJ Publishing Group Ltd

Grade	Mobility	Subvalvar thickening	Thickening	Calcification
1	Highly mobile valve with only leaflet tips restricted	Minimal thickening just below the mitral leaflets	Leaflets near normal in thickness (4-5mm)	A single area of increased echo brightness
2	Leaflet mid and base portions have normal mobility	Thickening of chordal structures extending up to one third of the chordal length	Mid-leaflets normal, considerable thickening of margins (5-8mm)	Scattered areas of brightness confined to leaflet margins
3	Valve continues to move forward in diastole, mainly from the base	Thickening extending to the distal third of the chords	Thickening extending through the entire leaflet (5-8mm)	Brightness extending into the mid-portion of the leaflets
4	No or minimal forward movement of the leaflets in diastole	Extensive thickening and shortening of all chordal structures extending down to the papillary muscles	Considerable thickeningof all leaflet tissue (>8-10mm)	Extensive brightness throughout much of the leaflet tissue

The total echocardiographic score was derived from an analysis of mitral leaflet mobility, valvar and subvalvar thickening, and calcification which were graded from 0 to 4 according to the above criteria. This gave a total score of 0 to 16.

The normal mitral valve is > 4.0 cm^2 in diameter, and patients may remain asymptomatic with a decrease up to 2.0 cm^2. When the valve area decreases to < 1.5 cm^2, patients may experience mild symptoms or symptoms with exertion, and severe symptoms usually present with valve area < 1.0 cm^2. As a general rule, conditions that increase flow (ie pregnancy), raise heart rate, or diminish atrial function (ie atrial fibrillation) cause an increase in the transmitral gradient at a given valve area.

Imaging in Mitral Stenosis

Transthoracic Echocardiography

Echocardiography, as in other valvular heart diseases, is instrumental in defining the extent of disease and planning the treatment approach. A thorough assessment of MS requires an evaluation of the anatomy and calcification of the valvular apparatus, definition of valve area using planimetry and the pressure half-time (derived from Doppler data), a measurement of gradients across the valve, and estimation of pulmonary artery pressures (Table 1) [24].

The initial subjective evaluation considers leaflet mobility and thickness (usually revealing "doming" of the anterior leaflet and restriction of the posterior leaflet), and should also include an assessment of the commisures, subvalvular fusion, and associated calcification. A more thorough scoring system of leaflet mobility and calcification was provided by Wilkens and colleagues, and is useful in assessing the feasibility of percutaneous balloon mitral valvotomy (Table 2) [25]. The percutaneous approach is generally favorable in patients with relatively mobile leaflets, little commissural fusion, and minimal calcification of the valvular apparatus. This is discussed further below.

Calculation of mitral valve area (MVA) can be accomplished using multiple methods, and it is recommended that all of them be interpreted to appropriately determine MVA. Planimetry of the valve in the parasternal short-axis projection has shown the best correlation surgically obtained measurements [26]. However, accurate assessment relies on proper positioning of the ultrasound slice perpendicular to the valve at the leaflet tips.

The pressure half-time (PHT) method relies on the Doppler signal across the mitral valve, and measures the time required for the maximal MV gradient to decrease by half. The MVA is calculated using the following equation: MVA = 220/PHT. Of note, the PHT method is unreliable in patients with aortic regurgitation, decreased LA compliance, and LV diastolic dysfunction. This method is therefore not recommended in patients with severe calcific MS, as they tend to be elderly and have abnormalities in diastolic function.

Measurement of gradients across the MV also utilize the Doppler signal (Figure 2). The mean gradient, which is the clinically relevant hemodynamic measurement, is obtained by tracing the mitral inflow. The gradient can be significantly altered by changes in the R-R interval, so assessment in patients with atrial fibrillation should use an average of 5 cardiac cycles for greatest accuracy. Additionally, changes in cardiac output and MR can affect the measured gradients and should be considered.

Chronic left-sided volume overload from MS can cause pulmonary venous congestion and pulmonary hypertension. The right ventricular systolic pressure (RVSP) is estimated from the tricuspid regurgitation velocity, and is used as a proxy for the pulmonary artery (PA) pressure. A PA pressure of > 50 mmHg at rest is considered an indication for intervention, even in patients without symptoms [11]

Three-Dimensional Echocardiography

Three-dimensional echocardiography (3DE) acquires an entire 3D volume of the mitral valve apparatus, thereby allowing the echocardiographer to 'slice' the image in any plane, reducing the risk of incorrectly measuring the valve area. The technology holds great promise, and has been shown to improve the accuracy of MVA assessment [27]. Furthermore, visualization of the valve in 3 dimensions allows a more thorough appreciation of valve morphology.

Transesophageal Echocardiography

Transesophageal echocardiography (TEE) is useful in patients for whom standard surface imaging provides suboptimal data. The same measurements obtained in the transthoracic exam are evaluated. TEE may also be helpful to characterize the degree of MR in patients for whom the TTE is suspected to underestimate regurgitation. Furthermore, assessment of the LA and LA appendage for thrombus prior to percutaneous balloon valvotomy is imperative, as the presence of clot is an absolute contraindication to the procedure.

Stress Echocardiography

Some patients with mild or moderate MS on rest TTE provide a clinical history that is indicative of greater stenosis. In these patients, the physiologic changes of activity (increased heart rate, higher loading conditions) may cause an increase in the transvalvular gradient that is not appreciated on the routine exam. When this is clinically suspected, exercise echocardiography may be considered. An increase in the mean MV gradient to $\geq$ 15 mmHg or pulmonary artery pressure to > 60 mmHg provides an indication for intervention if the valve morphology is amenable to percutaneous treatment [11].

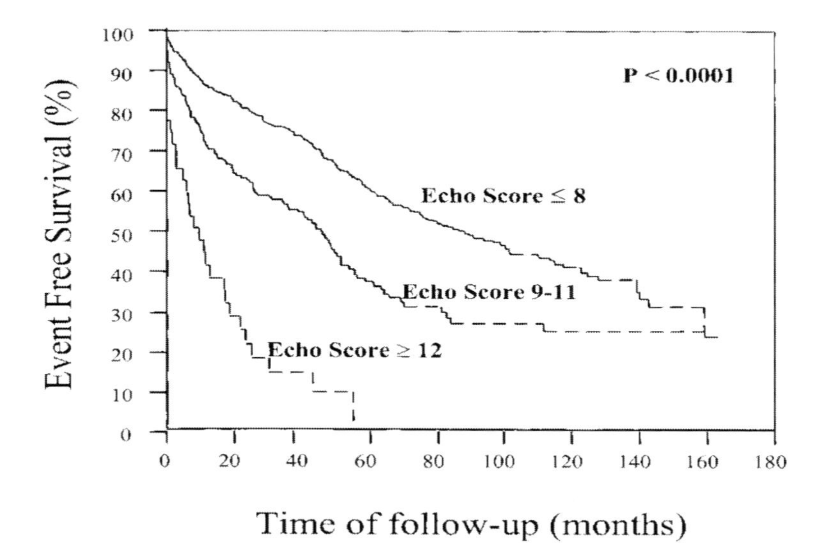

Figure 3. Survival of patients undergoing PMBV based upon pre-procedural Wilkens echocardiographic score. Reproduced with permission from Palacios et al; Which patients benefit from percutaneous mitral balloon valvuloplasty?: Prevalvuloplasty and postvalvuloplasty variables that predict long-term outcome; Circulation 2002;105:1465-71.

Medical Management of Mitral Stenosis

The vigilant diagnosis and treatment of streptococcal pharyngitis is of paramount importance in minimizing the risk of developing ARF and subsequently RHD. Large public health campaigns have been launched in developing nations to increase awareness of the disease, especially in light of the fact that treatment within 9 days of symptom onset with 1 dose of intramuscular penicillin is sufficient to prevent ARF [30]. Once rheumatic fever has developed, however, treatment with penicillin, salicylates, NSAIDs, or corticosteroids (all aimed at decreasing inflammation) has not been shown to decrease the incidence of RHD [8]. In patients with a history of ARF of RHD, however, antibiotic prophylaxis is recommended by the World Health Organization (WHO) to reduce the recurrence of infection [31]. This may be accomplished by daily oral administration of penicillin, erythromycin, or sulfonamide, or monthly administration of intramuscular penicillin. Duration of treatment varies: 5 years for patients without proven carditis (or until age 18 years, whichever is longer), 10 years for patients with mild or healed carditis (or until age 25 years, whichever is longer), and lifelong for patients with more severe valvular heart disease or requiring surgery.

Likely catalyzed by LA enlargement and/or pulmonary venous dilation, atrial fibrillation occurs up to 50% of patients with symptomatic MS [8]. Loss of concerted atrial contraction and decrease in diastolic filling time (if the ventricular rate is not well controlled) both contribute to increased gradients across the mitral valve, and results in the development, or exacerbation, of symptomatic MS (Figure 2). Aggressive rate control of AFib with beta-blockers, calcium channel blockers, and/or digoxin is therefore imperative. In patients for whom rate control is not adequate, cardioversion to sinus rhythm is recommended. A small study of patients with rheumatic atrial fibrillation found an increased exercise time, functional class, and mortality for patients treated with a rhythm control strategy compared with rate control [32].

Systemic embolization presents a further challenge, presenting in up to 20% of patients with MS [33]. The American College of Cardiology/American Heart Association (ACC/AHA) Guidelines therefore recommend anticoagulation with warfarin (goal INR 2.5 – 3.5) for all patients with MS and atrial fibrillation, irrespective of the CHADS2 score [11]. Anticoagulation is also recommended for patients with history of embolism or LA thrombus (even with sinus rhythm), and is suggested for patients with very enlarged LA (> 5.5cm). The risks and benefits of anticoagulation in individual patients must of course be considered. For patients not amenable to (or not desiring of) anticoagulation, full dose aspirin may also be considered.

Percutaneous Mitral Balloon Valvuloplasty

Percutaneous mitral balloon valvuloplasty (PMBV) was first reported in 1984 by Inoue and colleagues [34]. Since that time, it has evolved to become the first-line treatment for patients with MS and favorable valve morphology. In patients with favorable morphology for PMBV, the ACC/AHA recommends intervention for symptomatic patients with moderate or severe stenosis (Class I. Intervention may be considered for symptomatic patients with mild stenosis and elevated gradient (> 15 mmHg) or PA pressure (> 60 mmHg) with exercise (Class IIb). PMBV is also recommended for asymptomatic patients with moderate or severe

MS and elevated PA pressures (> 50 mmHg at rest or > 60 mmHg with exercise), and may be considered in asymptomatic patients with moderate or severe MS and new-onset atrial fibrillation.

As noted previously, assessment of the Wilkin's echocardiographic score is imperative for appropriate patient selection. Multiple investigators have shown that patients with a score of 8 or less have the greatest freedom from death and valve surgery, and the largest improvement in MVA with PMBV (Figure 3) [35-37]. Early event-free survival can range from > 95% in patients with favorable anatomy to less than 60% with a high echocardiographic score [38]. Generally, the procedure is most effective in patients with rheumatic MS; patients with non-rheumatic disease and severe, diffuse calcification fare less well and are often not candidates for percutaneous treatment.

Palacios and colleagues provided their center's experience with 879 patients followed for a mean of 4.2 years [38]. Average MVA for the entire group increased from 0.9 to 1.9 cm^2 (p <_0.0001). Six-hundred and one patients (68%) with an echo score < 8 enjoyed a greater degree of procedural success (defined as post-PMBV MVA > 1.5 cm^2 or > 50% increase in MVA, and MR $\leq$ 2+) (86.5% versus 76.6%, P_0.0002). Those with a score > 8 had more heavily calcified valves and more often presented with NYHA class IV symptoms (25.2% *vs.* 7.5%, $p < 0.0001$). Independent pre-procedural predictors of PMBV success included greater MVA, less MR, and lack of prior surgical commissurotomy. In the overall group, 27.7% required MVR and 6.4% required re-do PMBV at long-term follow-up.

Complications of PMBV are highly variable and largely depend on center experience [39]. In the series above, in-hospital mortality rate was 1.9%, and is generally reported at 0 – 3%, comparable to surgical risk [8]. Systemic embolization can also occur, and underscores the need for TEE evaluation of the LA and LA appendage prior to the procedure, as well as adequate anticoagulation during the intervention. Severe MR is the most dreaded complication, and can result in acute hemodynamic collapse and refractory pulmonary edema requiring emergent open-heart surgery. MR > 3+ may be seen in up to 10% of patients, though < 1% of patients require urgent surgical intervention [40]. This complication is most often seen in patients with unfavorable valve anatomy, or with overzealous balloon dilation.

The threshold to intervene in MS is higher when PMBV is not an appropriate option. Surgical correction includes commisurotomy, which may also be feasible in patients with mixed MS/MR who receive a valve ring annuloplasty as well. Mitral valve surgery (repair preferred over replacement) is indicated in patients with moderate or severe MS and NYHA III-IV symptoms when PMBV is unavailable, or is contraindicated due to Wilkin's store or concomitant severe MR. Surgical treatment is considered reasonable for patients with severe MS and NYHA I-II symptoms and concomitant severe pulmonary hypertension (PASP > 60 mmHg), or patients with moderate or severe MS and recurrent embolic events despite therapeutic anticoagulation.

Mitral Regurgitation

More than 2 million people in the United States alone are affected by mitral regurgitation (MR) [41]. While medical therapy may provide some relief from symptoms, and is imperative in treating patients with concomitant ischemic heart disease or heart failure, there is no proven benefit of medications on the MR itself. Left untreated, chronic MR leads to left atrial enlargement, atrial fibrillation, pulmonary hypertension, and progressive left ventricular (LV) dilation and dysfunction. Surgery is therefore recommended in symptomatic patients with severe MR, or asymptomatic patients with severe MR and LV cavity dilation or systolic dysfunction [11]. Surgery is also considered reasonable in asymptomatic patients with pulmonary hypertension or atrial fibrillation at centers where repair is considered likely and low-risk. Unfortunately, due to significant comorbidities up to 50% of patients, usually those who are elderly or have significant left ventricular (LV) dysfunction, are deemed to be unfit for surgery [42]. Percutaneous therapies may provide an important alternative treatment modality in patients with chronic MR.

Classification and Pathophysiology of Mitral Regurgitation

In order to understand mitral valve repair, one must first understand the disease process. This allows a more critical appraisal of the feasibility of each of the devices being studied, as well as an insight into appropriate patient selection for each of these evolving percutaneous procedures.

Mitral regurgitation is broadly divided into 2 groups: primary and secondary. Primary MR is the result of problems with the valve itself, and in the developed world is usually due to myxomatous or degenerative disease, or mitral valve prolapse (MVP; Barlow's Disease). In developing nations, MR is often the result of rheumatic heart disease, and as discussed above usually presents at a younger age than those patients with MS or mixed MR and MS.

Myxomatous mitral valve disease is defined by thickening of the leaflets and chordae. Histologically, there is an accumulation of proteoglycans and glycosaminoglycans in the spongiosa that extends into the chords, and decreased collagen in the fibrosa [43]. The resultant redundancy of valve tissue and/or chordal elongation can result in mitral valve prolapse [44,45]. MVP may be associated with genetic connective tissue disorders such as Marfan's Syndrome or the Ehlers-Danlos Syndrome, but most cases are idiopathic in nature.

Secondary MR is usually referred to as 'functional' or 'ischemic' MR, and is the result of problems with the left ventricle. It may seen in the setting of previous myocardial infarction, or in patients with non-ischemic causes of LV cavity dilation and dysfunction. In either case, the mitral valve (MV) is dysfunctional due to a disordered geometry within the LV, but not due to a problem with the MV itself.

Disorders of the MV causing regurgitation may also be classified using the Carpentier system which specifies the anatomic lesion(s): Type I is the result of annular dilation with normal leaflet motion; Type II is due to leaflet prolapse; and Type III is caused by restricted leaflet motion [46]. Primary MR most commonly falls into the 'Type II' category. As discussed previously, however, rheumatic MR may be the result of 'Type I, II, or III' pathophysiology [17].

Ischemic or functional MR may manifest all 3 Carpentier types. For instance, there could be MV annular dilation due to LV cavity dilation, apical leaflet tethering due to cavity dilation with papillary muscle displacement or due to papillary muscle dysfunction after infarction, excessive leaflet motion due to chordal avulsion or papillary muscle rupture, or some combination of all of these [47,48].

Table 3. Echocardiographic determination of MR severity. Reproduced with permission from Krishnaswamy et al; Ischemic mitral regurgitation: pathophysiology, diagnosis, and treatment; Coron Art Dis 2011;22:359-70

	Degree of Mitral Regurgitation		
	Mild	Moderate	Severe
Color Flow Mapping			
RJA/LAA	< 20%	20 - 40%	> 40%
VC (cm)	< 0.40	0.40 - 0.69	> 0.70
ERO (cm2)	< 0.20	0.20 - 0.40	> 0.40
RV (ml/beat)	< 30	30 - 60	> 60
Pulsed Wave Doppler			
Mitral E-wave velocity			> 1.2 m/sec
PV flow pattern			Systolic blunting or reversal

* RJA: regurgitant jet area, LAA: left atrial area, VC: vena contracta, ERO: effective regurtitant orifice, RV: regurgitant volume, PV: pulmonary vein.

Imaging in Mitral Regurgitation

Imaging is used for diagnosis, pre-procedural planning, procedural guidance, and surveillance after repair. Transthoracic (TTE) and transesophageal echocardiography (TEE) are the traditional mainstays of imaging, but computed tomography (CT) and three-dimensional (3D) echocardiography are increasingly important in contemporary practice.

Echocardiography

In evaluating patients with mitral regurgitation, TTE is used for quantifying the degree of MR, evaluating LV function, and defining the anatomic characteristics of the MV. The degree of MR is determined using a combination of parameters including color Doppler, continuous and pulsed wave Doppler, and pulmonary venous flow pattern (Table 3) [49]. LV size and function are important in determining the causes and effects of chronic MR, and also provide prognostic information regarding surgical outcome. In planning open surgery or percutaneous repair, TTE is used to precisely characterize the MV leaflets, annulus, and MV:LV geometry to determine what procedure(s) or device will be most effective. Another important assessment is of MR jet origin in the parasternal short-axis view, as certain treatments such as edge-to-edge repair are much more effective in central-origin lesions.

In situations where the surface echocardiogram is not sufficient, more information can be gleaned from a TEE. The transesophageal exam may also be more sensitive in detecting papillary muscle rupture or suspected severe regurgitation in the setting of acute myocardial infarction.

Three-dimensional (3D) echocardiography, now available in "real time" during transesophageal examinations, is a developing technology that has the ability to more precisely define the mechanism(s) of MR [50]. In light of the complexity of MV anatomy, and the fact that ischemic MR is the result of disruptions in multiple aspects of valvulo-ventricular function, 3D echocardiography holds great promise for a better understanding of the disease, and has the possibility to provide information to more appropriately choose a treatment strategy. For instance, 3D echocardiography has shown that in many cases of ischemic MR there is restricted motion on the medial side of the valve which gives rise to one regurgitant jet; and on the lateral side of the valve there is excess motion which gives rise to a more severe MR jet.

Computed Tomography

Percutaneous MV repair devices that exploit the proximity of the coronary sinus (CS) with the mitral annulus (MA) are under various stages of development. The use of these devices requires a detailed anatomic understanding of the relationship between the CS and MA, as well as an awareness of the course of the CS with respect to the left circumflex coronary artery (LCx). A seminal paper by Choure and colleagues demonstrated significant variability in the CS:MA distance, and that compared to normal controls patients with severe MR have a greater distance between the CS and MA [51]. Furthermore, they found that the CS crosses the LCx in more than 80% of patients, though the region of crossing is highly variable (Figure 4). These anatomic considerations have important implications for the efficacy and safety of percutaneous CS-based annuloplasty devices. Imaging with cardiac CT should therefore be an essential part of pre-procedural planning in these cases.

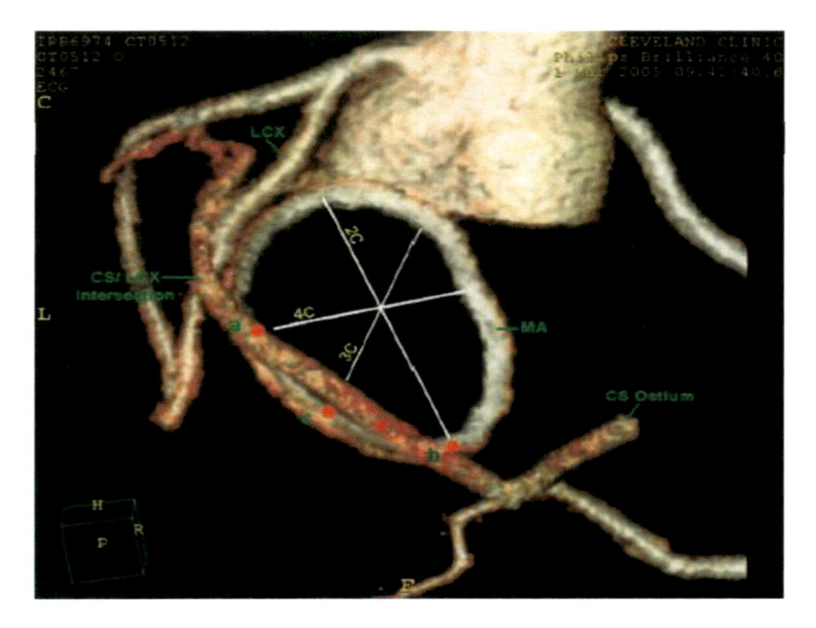

Figure 4. Reconstructed 3-dimensional image of mitral annulus (MA), coronary sinus (CS), coronary arteries, and aorta. (Point a) Mitral annulus diameter in 4-chamber view (4C). (Point b) Mitral annulus diameter in 2-chamber view (2C); and (point c) Mitral annulus diameter in 3-chamber view (3C). All MA to CS measurements obtained in 2-demensional images. LCX = left circumflex coronary artery. Reprinted from Choure et al; In Vivo Analysis of the Anatomical Relationship of Coronary Sinus to Mitral Annulus and Left Circumflex Coronary Artery Using Cardiac Multidetector Computed Tomography: Implications for Percutaneous Coronary Sinus Mitral Annuloplasty; J Am Coll Cardiol;48:1938-45 with permission from Elsevier.

Medical Therapy for Mitral Regurgitation

Medical treatment in patients with MR may be beneficial in stabilizing patients acutely, in treating underlying heart failure, or in mitigating some symptoms. Medications are also useful in patients for whom surgery is not an option. There is no established role, however, for its use to alter the natural course of the disease [11].

Acute MR is most often due to MI or infective endocarditis, though sometimes patients with MV prolapse may suddenly develop a flail leaflet. It may be poorly tolerated with regard to both symptoms and hemodynamics. Medical management with intravenous afterload reduction (ie sodium nitroprusside) or inotropic therapy (ie dobutamine) is used to decrease the regurgitant fraction and pulmonary congestion, and to improve forward cardiac output and hemodynamics [52]. Intra-aortic balloon counterpulsation (IABP) may be required in those patients with significant hypotension. In any case, each or all of these therapies are used almost exclusively to stabilize the patient for definitive surgical treatment.

For chronic primary MR, studies of angiotensin converting enzyme (ACE) inhibitors in very small numbers of patients with severe MR and normal EF have suggested an improvement in regurgitant fraction and beneficial effects on LV size [53,54]. However, there are no large clinical trials providing evidence for clinical benefit. Similarly, studies of angiotensin receptor blockers (ARBs) have failed to showed a meaningful benefit [55].

Patients with functional MR present a different substrate for medical treatment than those with primary disease. Due to underlying coronary artery disease and/or heart failure, medical therapy is the staple of treatment. Studies of beta blockers in patients with chronic MR show a decrease in regurgitant fraction and improvements in aortic outflow [56]. Afterload-reducing agents such as ACE inhibitors and ARBs also have proven merit in this group of patients [57]. As such, medical therapy plays a role in secondary MR to improve symptoms and possibly the prognosis of heart failure, and may be a reasonable choice for patients who are either unwilling to undergo valve surgery or who present prohibitive operative risk. For the rest, however, valve repair or replacement is ultimately necessary, though the outcomes of repair or replacement are far from ideal.

Percutaneous Mitral Valve Repair

Percutaneous procedures are likely to first find a place in the treatment of patients who are high-risk candidates for surgical mitral replacement or repair. The application of these technologies to low- or intermediate- risk patients with primary MR will require a demonstration of safety and efficacy similar to current surgical techniques which have a proven track record of success [58]. In patients with secondary MR, though, current surgical techniques have proven to be both ineffective and carry a significant surgical risk [59]. In fact, due to the clinical equipoise that exists in patients with moderate functional MR, an NIH-sponsored study is currently randomizing patients with functional MR undergoing CABG to MV repair vs CABG alone. As such, percutaneous repair may have a greater role in treating this difficult group of patients.

The percutaneous therapies for mitral repair include devices designed to perform indirect CS-based annuloplasty, direct annuloplasty, cardiac chamber remodeling, and edge-to-edge repair. Of these strategies, edge-to-edge repair with the MitraClip™ system (Evalve Inc,

Menlo Park, CA) is the best studied thus far with results of the pivotal stage II randomized trial recently reported, and has received CE Mark approval for use in Europe. The CARILLON™ Mitral Contour system (Cardiac Dimensions, Kirkland, WA), a CS-based annuloplasty device, has also received CE Mark approval and clinical trials are ongoing. Numerous other devices are in development across the spectrum from preclinical to clinical stages (Table 4).

Table 4. Phase of development of the percutaneous mitral valve repair technologies

Method	Device	Trials
Indirect Coronary-Sinus Based Annuloplasty	Carillon™ Mitral Contour System (Cardiac Dimensions, Kirkland, WA)	Phase II trial underway CE Mark approval
	Percutaneous Transvenous Mitral Annuloplasty (Viacor Inc, Wilmington, MA)	Phase II trial underway
	Monarc™ system (Edwards Lifesciences Inc., Irvine, CA)	Phase I trial completed
	Percutaneous Mitral Valve Repair (PMVR) Device (St. Jude Medical, St. Paul, MN)	Preclinical testing
Direct Retrograde Annuloplasty	Mitralign Direct Annuloplasty System (Mitralign, Tewksbury, MA)	First-in-man implants
	GDS Accucinch Annuloplasty System (Guided Delivery Systems, Santa Clara, CA)	Preclinical testing
Radiofrequency Annuloplasty	QuantumCor corporation (Lake Forest, CA)	Preclinical testing
Dynamic Annuloplasty	Dynaplasty (MiCardia Corporation, Irvine, CA)	Phase I trial enrolling
Cardiac Chamber Remodeling	Coapsys™ (Myocor, Maple Grove, MN)	Phase I trial completed No longer in development
	iCoapsys™ (Myocor, Maple Grove, MN)	Preclinical testing No longer in development
	Percutaneous Septal Sinus Shortening (PS^3) System (Ample Medical Inc, Foster City, CA)	First-in-man implants No longer in development
Edge-to-edge Repair	MitraClip™ (Evalve Inc, Menlo Park, CA)	Phase II trial completed CE Mark approval
	Mobius™ Leaflet Repair System (Edwards Lifesciences, Inc.; Irvine, CA).	Phase I trial completed No longer in development
Percutaneous Mitral Valve Replacement	CardiAQ Valve Technologies (Winchester, MA)	Preclinical testing

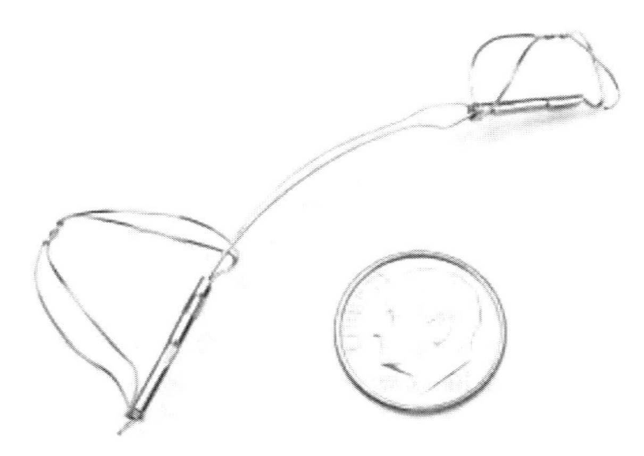

Figure 5. Carillon mitral contour system (Cardiac Dimensions, Kirkland, WA). Reprinted from http://www.cardiacdimensions.com/PhysicianResources/technology .

Indirect Coronary-Sinus-Based Annuloplasty Devices

Surgical annuloplasty is the current mainstay of treatment in functional MR, and usually achieves a reduction of 25% in the diameter of the mitral annulus (MA). Remodeling the MA percutaneously requires an exploitation of the CS:MA relationship. The CS parallels almost 80% of the posterior intertrigonal distance 50% of the MA perimeter, and a number of devices have been developed that take advantage of this relationship [60]. As previously mentioned, however, the proximity of the LCx coronary artery and variability in the relationship of the CS and MA to each other are significant barriers to widespread use and efficacy of these procedures [51].

Carillon™ Mitral Contour System

The Carillon™ Mitral Contour System (Cardiac Dimensions, Kirkland, WA) is delivered percutaneously through the internal jugular vein, and consists of 2 anchors bridged by a fixed-length nitinol tensioning rod (Figure 5). The distal anchor is deployed in the CS and locked, followed by passage of the nitinol rod into the CS. Tension is applied which results in tissue plication, reduction in MA diameter, and thereby MR. Procedural results are verified by real-time echocardiography prior to deployment of the proximal anchor. If there is any concern for safety of positioning or efficacy, the device can be collapsed and removed or adjusted prior to final deployment.

Ovine and canine models used in preclinical testing of the Carillon system were promising, and paved the way for clinical feasibility evaluation in the prospective AMADEUS (Carillon Mitral Annuloplasty Device European Union Study) trial of 48 patients with functional MR and LV systolic dysfunction [61]. The predicted 1-year mortality of the group was 10%. Successful implantation was achieved in 30 patients, and at 6-months follow-up there was a 23% reduction in MR, 10% decrease in MA diameter (4.2 to 3.78cm), and improvement in NYHA class (2.9 to 1.8). Quality-of-life scores and 6-minute walk testing was also improved.

An analysis of patients who did not have procedural success revealed a CS-related complication in 3 and failure of the catheterization laboratory imaging equipment in 2 patients. Thirteen patients had retrieval of the device due to coronary complication or inadequate reduction in MR as assessed by echocardiogram. A total of 7 complications were noted in 6 patients (13%), and included multi-organ failure leading to death (n = 1), MI without need for PCI (n=3), and CS dissection or perforation (n = 3).

As a result of these encouraging results, the Carillon system was granted CE Mark approval in Europe. Enrollment in the follow-up TITAN (Tighten the Annulus Now) study was completed in late 2008, and included 53 patients in 8 centers across Europe [62]. Successful implantation was achieved in 68%; coronary obstruction requiring device removal occurred in 15%. Major adverse events occurred in 1 patients who died of contrast-related complications; notably, the patient had not had a device implanted. At 6-months, there was a sustained 1 class reduction in NYHA class and 35% decrease I MR.

Percutaneous Transvenous Mitral Annuloplasty System

The Percutaneous Transvenous Mitral Annuloplasty (PTMA) device (Viacor Inc, Wilmington, MA) is composed of nitinol and stainless steel rods 35 to 85 mm in length. The distal portion is advanced to the anterior interventricular branch of the great cardiac vein via an internal jugular approach, and rods of varying length are introduced until the optimal reduction in MA diameter has been achieved. If necessary, up to 3 rods may be delivered. The procedure is initially conducted using a 'diagnostic' system to determine the optimal combination of rods, and is then exchanged for the therapeutic device. If necessary, the number and stiffness of rods can be subsequently modified.

Initial trials in sheep demonstrated significant reductions in MR and led to human feasibility studies [63,64]. Results in the first 27 patients, all of whom had moderate or severe functional MR, have been reported [65]. Procedural success was achieved in 70% (n = 19) of patients and reduced MR by at least 1 grade in 48% (n = 13). The diagnostic device was exchanged for the therapeutic device in 33% (n = 9). Five patients had evaluation at between 3 months and 1 year, and demonstrated sustained reduction in MA diameter, though the reduction in MR was described as only "modest."

With regard to complications, 1 patient experienced pericardial effusion (without cardiac tamponade) and 1 patient had LCx impingement. One patient died of progressive heart failure at 6 months, 3 patients required subsequent surgical annuloplasty (at 84 days, 197 days, and 216 days), and 1 patient had fracture of the device at day 7.

Use of the Viacor PTMA system has been encouraging, though long-term efficacy is not yet clear. The multicenter, international PTOLEMY (Percutaneous TransvenOus Mitral AnnuloplastY) safety and efficacy trial is currently enrolling patients. The results of this trial will be integral to the future development of this device.

Monarc™ System

The Monarc™ system (Edwards Lifesciences Inc., Irvine, CA) consists of distal and proximal anchors and a unique bridging segment composed of nitinol and biodegradable "spacers" (Figure 6). These spacers dissolve over 3-6 weeks, resulting in a slow conformational change in the coronary sinus and further reducing any residual MR that may be present immediately post-procedure. The device cannot be retrieved after implantation, and like the others is delivered via the internal jugular vein.

A multicenter feasibility and safety trial, EVOLUTION (clinical EValuation of the Edwards Lifesciences PercUTaneous mItral annulOplasty system for the treatment of mitral regurgitation) has been completed. Enrolled patients had 2-4+ functional MR; severe LV dysfunction (EF < 25%), CS leads, primary MV disease, and severe mitral annular calcification were notable exclusions. While the results have not yet been formally published, interim follow-up on 72 patients at 2 years has been presented [66].

Device implantation was achieved in 59 of the 72 patients (82%); 13 patients were not implanted due either to significant venous tortuosity or unfavorable size. Degree of MR at 2 years was available in 21 patients who demonstrated a non-significant decrease from 2.3 to 1.9 ($p = 0.11$). There were also trends toward sustained decrease in MA diameter and LV volume over this period. NYHA class was available at 2-years follow-up in 24 patients who demonstrated an average decrease from 2.7 to 2.0 ($p = 0.002$). With regard to safety, freedom from the cumulative secondary endpoint (device migration, MI, tamponade, CS thrombosis, or pulmonary embolism) was realized in 83% at 6 months, 81% at 1 year, and 72% at 2 years.

The investigators also noted interesting differences among subgroups in their analysis. At 90-days, patients with 2+ MR had no change in MR, but patients with 3-4+ MR had a significant reduction from 3.3 to 1.9 ($p = 0.001$). Similarly, patients with worse NYHA class demonstrated greater efficacy with the device. Among patients with NYHA class III-IV, 75% had a decrease in MR grade of ≥ 1, compared with 44% of patients with NYHA class II.

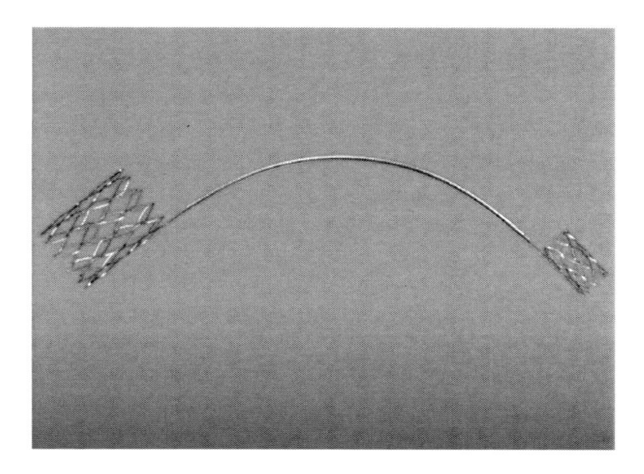

Figure 6. Monarc system (Edwards Lifesciences Inc, Irvine, CA). Reprinted from Chiam and Ruiz; Percutaneous Transcatheter Mitral Valve Repair: A Classification of the Technology; J Am Coll Cardiol Intv 2011;4:1-13 with permission from Elsevier.

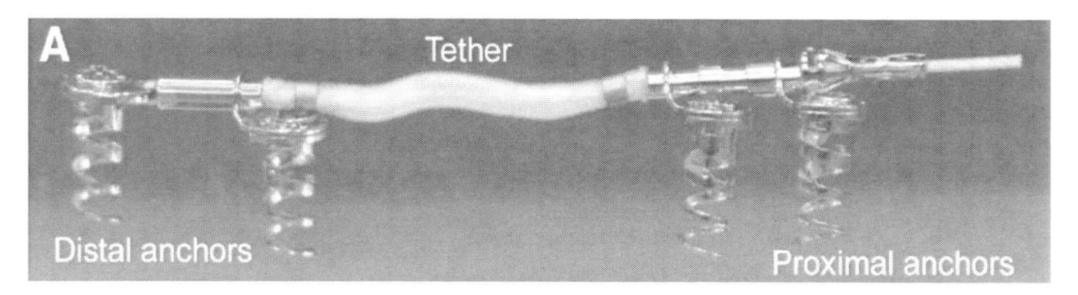

Figure 7. Percutaneous Mitral Valve Repair (PMVR) device (St. Jude Medical, St. Paul, MN). Reprinted from Sorajja et al; A Novel Method of Percutaneous Mitral Valve Repair for Ischemic Mitral Regurgitation; J Am Coll Cardiol Intv 2008;1:663-72 with permission from Elsevier.

For the time being, the device seems to be most effective in patients with moderate or severe MR. However, while report of the 2-year results provides some insight into use of the Monarc device, formal publication of the results is eagerly awaited, as is completion of the follow-up EVOLUTION II study.

Percutaneous Mitral Valve Repair Device

The Percutaneous Mitral Valve Repair (PMVR) device (St. Jude Medical, St. Paul, MN), is currently under preclinical development, but presents a unique approach among the CS-based devices (Figure 7). As described above, ischemic MR often originates at the medial segment of the mitral valve due to preferential involvement of the posteromedial papillary muscle. With this in mind, the PMVR is designed to preferentially affect the medial annulus. The device is passed via the jugular vein into the CS, but the distal anchors are actually screwed into the LV myocardium through the CS at the area of the P2 segment and the proximal anchors are screwed in near the posteromedial trigone. The nitinol bridging segment thereby provides tension on the annulus and shortening of the MA diameter. This device can be repositioned prior to final deployment.

The PMVR was evaluated by Sorajja and colleagues in 8 pigs [67]. They achieved a decrease in MA diameter of 20%, a reduction that is similar to surgical annuloplasty. Echocardiography was not performed. The authors comment that due to the device's medial placement, complications involving the laterally coursing LCx are unlikely and the CS is also more directly apposed to the MA in its medial portion.

Direct Retrograde Annuloplasty

Given the concerns of LCx coronary artery proximity to the CS, variability in the CS:MA relationship, and inconsistent results from the indirect CS-based devices, percutaneous approaches to direct annuloplasty are being actively pursued.

Mitralign Direct Annuloplasty System

While surgical annuloplasty is usually performed with implantation of a ring, suture annuloplasty has been performed with salutary results and allows preservation of annular contraction [68,69]. The Mitralign Direct Annuloplasty System (Mitralign, Tewksbury, MA) employs a similar strategy. The device is placed through a retrograde, arterial approach, and consists of 3 anchors that are deployed into the ventricular aspect of the annulus (one at each posterior leaflet scallop). These anchors are connected by suture material which is subsequently cinched and results in annular plication. Subsequent to initial preclinical animal trials, 3 devices have been successfully implanted in patients as part of the pilot clinical study [70].

GDS AccuCinch Annuloplasty System

The GDS Accucinch Annuloplasty System (Guided Delivery Systems, Santa Clara, CA) is similar to the Mitralign system, and also consists of anchors placed in the ventricular aspect of the mitral annulus. Initial animal models were promising, and 3 patients have been implanted thus far in Europe as part of a first-in-man study.

Other Annuloplasty Devices

The QuantumCor corporation (Lake Forest, CA) is currently developing a device to scar and shrink the mitral annulus through the direct application of subablative levels of radio frequency (RF) energy. The device is intended for percutaneous treatment through a trans-septal approach as well as surgical use. Preclinical study in 16 sheep (via left thoracotomy) was encouraging, with a reduction in the antero-posterior dimension of the MA by 23.8% immediately and sustained at 21.4% at 30-days in the 7 surviving sheep [71].

A unique device under early development is the Dynaplasty (MiCardia Corporation, Irvine, CA) which consists of an annuloplasty ring implanted during open heart surgery that can change configuration in response to electrical stimulation. The ring can be reshaped during surgery, or percutaneously thereafter using a trans-septal approach. The ring is designed for use in both the mitral and tricuspid positions. Enrollment in the phase I DYANA (Dynamic Annuloplasty Activation) study was recently completed in Europe and results are eagerly awaited [72].

Cardiac Chamber Remodeling Devices

Functional MR is a disorder not of the mitral valve itself, but is due to geometric alterations in the left ventricle and left atrium and their relationship with the mitral annulus. Surgical and percutaneous devices have been designed to address this disordered perivalvular geometry, and have provided encouraging initial results. However, due to financial concerns, further study is not currently ongoing.

Coapsys™ and iCoapsys™

The Coapsys™ (Myocor, Maple Grove, MN) annuloplasty system consists of pericardial implants that are placed on the epicardial surface of the heart. A cord connecting the 2 pads crosses the left ventricle internally and is cinched to correct the disordered LV geometry, decrease MA diameter, and ultimately reduce MR (Figure 8). The device is placed off-pump, providing the potential for combined coronary revascularization and mitral valve repair without the need for cardiopulmonary bypass.

The Coapsys was implanted in 34 patients with functional MR at the time of CABG in the initial feasibility trial. Mishra and colleagues provided results on the first 11 patients completing 1-year follow-up [73]. There was impressive reduction in MR (grade 2.9 to 1.1; jet area 7.4 cm^2 to 3.0 cm^2) and improvement in NYHA class (2.5 to 1.2). The randomized RESTORE-MV (Randomized Evaluation of a Surgical Treatment for Off-pump Repair of the Mitral Valve) trial was designed to compare traditional CABG and MV repair to CABG with Coapsys placement. The trial was prematurely terminated due to funding constraints after randomization of 165 patients. To date, the only published report from this trial is of intraoperative results from the first 19 Coapsys implants [74]. The patients achieved a considerable reduction in MR (2.7 ± 0.8 to 0.4 ± 0.7, $p < 0.0001$) acutely.

A percutaneous version of the system, the iCoapsys™, is implanted through a pericardial access sheath. While a preclinical study in 12 sheep was successful, the VIVID (Valvular and Ventricular Improvement Via iCoapsys Delivery) clinical trial, designed to demonstrate feasibility, was prematurely discontinued due to financial considerations [75].

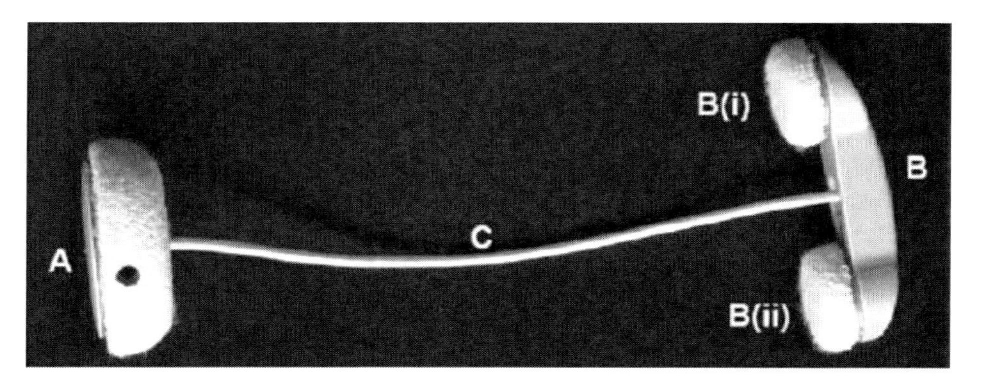

Figure 8. Coapsys device (Myocor, Maple Grove, MN). (A) Anterior epicardial pad; (B) Posterior epicardial pad with superior (B(i)) and inferior (B(ii)) heads; (C) Ventricular cord. Reprinted with permission from Mishra et al; Coapsys mitral annuloplasty for chronic functional ischemic mitral regurgitation: 1-year results. Ann Thorac Surg 2006;81:42-6 with permission from Elsevier.

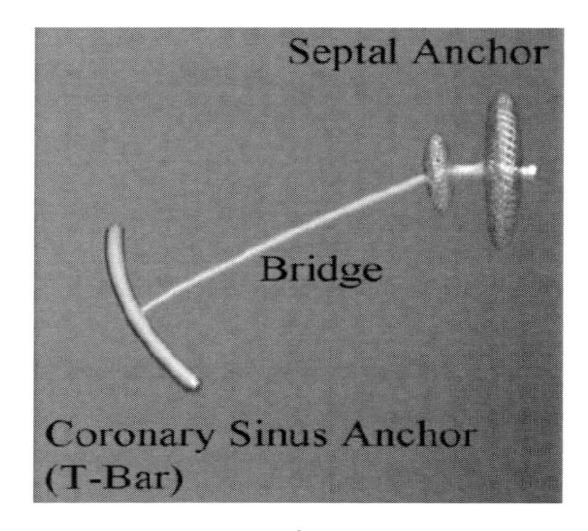

Figure 9. Percutaneous Septal Sinus Shortening (PS^3) system (Ample Medical Inc, Foster City, CA). Reprinted with permission from Palacios et al; Safety and feasibility of acute percutaneous septal sinus shortening: First-in-human experience Catheter Cardiovasc Interv 2007:69:513-18 with permission from John Wiley and Sons.

Percutaneous Septal Sinus Shortening (PS^3) System

As opposed to the Coapsys, which creates a transventricular bridge, the percutaneous septal sinus shortening (PS^3) system (Ample Medical Inc, Foster City, CA) creates a transatrial bridge (Figure 9). A distal "T-bar" device is anchored in the coronary sinus and attached to an atrial septal anchor device via a bridging cord. Tension applied to this bridge reshapes the annulus and left atrium as a result of traction between the interatrial septum and the CS at the P2 mitral valve segment. MV leaflet coaptation is improved and MR is reduced.

Initial preclinical testing was conducted in sheep with tachycardia-induced cardiomyopathy, 19 of which were evaluated immediately after implantation and 4 of which were evaluated at 30-days [76]. Post-procedurally, a 24% reduction in septal-lateral diameter was achieved (32.5mm to 24.6mm, $p < 0.001$) with a correspondingly significant reduction in MR grade (2.1 to 0.4, $p < 0.001$). The reductions in MA dimension and MR were maintained in the animals designated for 30-day follow-up. No animals had LCx coronary artery complications and CS patency was maintained.

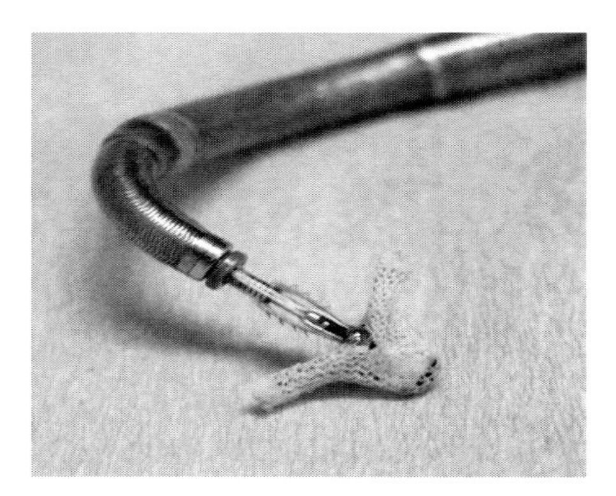

Figure 10. MitraClip (Evalve, Menlo Park, CA). Reprinted with permission from Feldman et al; Percutaneous Mitral Repair With the MitraClip System: Safety and Midterm Durability in the Initial EVEREST (Endovascular Valve Edge-to-Edge REpair Study) Cohort; J Am Coll Cardiol 2009;54:686-94 with permission from Elsevier.

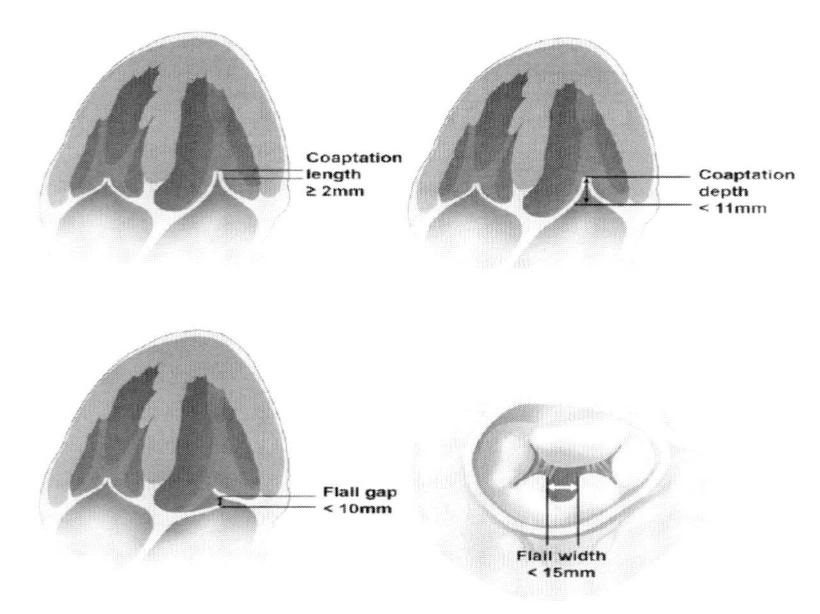

Figure 11. Anatomic characteristics required for MitraClip placement. The coaptation length must be at least 2 mm. Coaptation depth must be <11 mm. If a flail leaflet exists, the flail gap must be $\leq$ 10 mm, and the flail width must be $\leq$ 15mm. These anatomic characteristics are necessary for sufficient leaflet tissue for mechanical coaptation when the MitraClip device is used. Reprinted with permission from Feldman et al; Percutaneous Mitral Repair With the MitraClip System: Safety and Midterm Durability in the Initial EVEREST (Endovascular Valve Edge-to-Edge REpair Study) Cohort; J Am Coll Cardiol 2009;54:686-94 with permission from Elsevier.

The same investigators also studied another group of 12 healthy sheep for up to 12-months after implantation [77]. At follow-up, the PS^3 device demonstrated almost complete tissue ingrowth without evidence of erosion or migration. Furthermore, the reduction in MA diameter were sustained.

Clinical work with the PS^3 system is currently on hold due to financial considerations. However, results of implantation in 2 patients (prior to undergoing planned open-heart surgery) has been published as part of the first-in-man experience [78]. The 2 patients experienced a reduction in MR grade of 2 to 1 and 3 to 1, respectively. MA diameter was reduced by 31% in one and 29% in the other, a result which is substantially better than that achieved by the indirect CS-based annuloplasty devices. Given these initial findings, future trials are eagerly awaited.

Edge-to-edge (Double-Orifice) Leaflet Repair

Surgical edge-to-edge repair, otherwise known as the "Alfieri Stitch," consists of placing a suture to connect the anterior and posterior mitral leaflets and creating a double-orifice mitral valve [79]. The procedure is effective when combined with annuloplasty, but has shown reasonable long-term results even without concomitant placement of a ring [80]. Two devices have been tested which mimic the surgical procedure using a percutaneous approach.

MitraClip™ System

The MitraClip™ system (Evalve Inc, Menlo Park, CA) has undergone the most extensive clinical study of any percutaneous mitral valve repair device (Figure 10). It consists of a clip which is advanced to the mitral valve via a trans-septal approach. The clip grasps the anterior and posterior mitral leaflets and is then locked into position, effectively creating a double-orifice repair. The device can be unlocked and repositioned if necessary. Furthermore, multiple clips can be placed if one does not sufficiently reduce the degree of MR. The clip is covered in a polyester fabric to facilitate tissue ingrowth , and as with the surgical repair fibrosis and scarring eventually occurs at the anterior-posterior bridging segment [81]. Key anatomic features necessary for MitraClip placement are shown in Figure 11.

Long-term follow-up (12-months) on the 55 patients enrolled in the prospective, multi-center feasibility EVEREST I (Endovascular Valve Edge-to-Edge Repair Study) trial and the first 52 patients enrolled in the pivotal EVEREST II phase II trial have been published [82]. The majority of patients (79%) had primary MR, and 21% had functional disease. Acute procedural success (APS; defined as clip implantation with MR $\leq$ 2+) was achieved in 79 patients (74%), some of whom required 2 clips. In patients with APS, 77% were discharged with MR $\leq$ 2+, and 50 of 76 patients (66%) had $\leq$ 2+ MR at 12-months. Of the patients who did not achieve APS, 17 (16%) had severe residual MR even after clip placement and 11 did not have a clip placed. The primary efficacy endpoint (MR $\leq$ 2+, freedom from MV surgery, and freedom from death) was achieved in 66% of patients at 12-months. The first human implant has been in place for over 2 years and the patients remains with only mild MR and has undergone positive LV remodeling [83].

Of the group above, a total of 32 patients have undergone surgery, 23 of whom had MitraClip placement and 9 of whom did not. Of the patients who had undergone clip placement, 10 required surgery for partial clip detachment, 9 for MR > 2+, 2 for atrial septal defect, 1 for device malfunction, and 1 for suspected mitral stenosis (incorrectly diagnosed).

Twenty-one patients had successful mitral valve repair, providing evidence that surgical repair after MitraClip placement is feasible, even up to 18-months later [84].

The phase II EVEREST II trial is a multi-center trial which was designed to randomize patients in a 2:1 fashion to MitraClip *vs.* standard surgical repair, the results of which were recently reported [85]. A total of 279 patients, 73% with degenerative MR and 27% with functional MR, were randomized (184 to MitraClip and 85 to surgery). Of the 184 patients assigned to MitraClip, 178 underwent treatment and APS was achieved in 137 (77%).

The trial was designed with 2 primary endpoints, one for safety and one for efficacy. The safety endpoint was defined as the occurrence of major adverse events (death, stroke, MI, re-operation, transfusion, and others), and was designed to show superiority of the endovascular strategy. The endpoint was experienced by 9.6% of the percutaneous group and 57% of the "control" surgical group at 30-days. It should be noted, however, that the great majority of this difference can be accounted for by the need for > 2 units of blood transfusion in the surgical group (53.2% vs 8.8%). Also notable was the freedom from death, major stroke, urgent/emergent surgery, or MV reoperation in all of the 136 patients who achieved APS with MitraClip placement.

The efficacy endpoint was designed to show non-inferiority to cardiac surgery, and was designed as a composite of freedom from surgery for valve dysfunction, death, and MR ≥ 2+. The device achieved non-inferiority compared with surgery with Analysis of clinical effectiveness showed the MitraClip to be "non-inferior" to surgery (72.4% vs 87.8%, pre-specified margin for non-inferiority 31%). At 12-months of follow-up there was also a significant decrease in LV dimension noted in both groups. Of the 137 patients with APS, echocardiogram was available in 119 patients at 12 months: 81.5% remained with ≤ 2+ MR. NYHA class I or II symptoms were noted in 97.6% of the MitraClip group compated with 87.9% of the surgical group.

While clinical trials of the MitraClip system have been encouraging in both primary and secondary MR, it should be mentioned that the device is likely to be most effective in MR that has a more central origin as clip placement close to the commissures is not technically feasible. The device has garnered CE Mark approval, and to date more than 1,000 patients have received the clip. Its use in Europe, as well as the ongoing REALISM (Real World ExpAnded MuLtIcenter Study of the MitraClip System) continued access registry of high-risk and non-high risk patients in the US, will provide more experience and insight into its applications and appropriate patient selection.

Mobius™ Leaflet Repair System

The Mobius™ Leaflet Repair System (Edwards Lifesciences, Inc, Irvine, CA). uses vacuum suction to engage the mitral leaflets, followed by suturing of the 2 leaflets together. Encouraging animal studies led to a clinical trial in 15 patients. Acute procedural success was achieved in 9 (60%), but at 30-days only 6 of the patients (40%) had a successful stitch in place [40]. Development of the device is currently suspended.

Percutaneous Mitral Valve Replacement

Percutaneous mitral valve replacement, also known as transcatheter mitral valve implantation, is a challenging area of research. Unlike transcatheter aortic valve prostheses, radial force cannot be used to secure mitral prosthetics, and this has presented a significant impediment to evolution of the field. A transcatheter valve being developed by CardiAQ Valve Technologies (Winchester, MA) holds some promise. Initial studies in an animal model have demonstrated secure implantation, unobstructed LV outflow, and freedom from perivalvular MR.

Patient Selection

Surgery for primary mitral regurgitation in low-risk surgical candidates can be performed quite safely effectively with durable long-term results. While percutaneous edge-to-edge repair with the MitraClip device has provided encouraging results, it is still a procedure in development and in the United States can only be performed under the auspices of a clinical trial. As such, with rare exceptions, surgical repair is likely to remain the mainstay of treatment for primary MR for some time to come. Another possibility to consider would be the use of percutaneous edge-to-edge repair as an initial therapy as patients can still undergo successful surgical repair thereafter.

Conversely, mitral valve repair for functional regurgitation has poor long-term results in a group of patients that is also usually of moderate- or high- surgical risk. Surgical outcomes have been so variable, in fact, that trials are still being conducted randomizing patients with moderate functional MR to CABG with or without mitral valve repair. Percutaneous approaches to mitral repair may therefore present a good alternative to surgery (or medical therapy) in this group of patients.

Appropriate patient selection for these procedures consists not only of an estimation of surgical risk and candidacy, but also a thorough evaluation of the pathophysiologic basis of each patients' MR. Using the imaging modalities discussed above will provide insight into whether the best approach would be percutaneous edge-to-edge repair or annuloplasty via direct or indirect methods. In patients undergoing CS-based repair, a proper assessment of the CS:MA and CS:LCx relationships is imperative. In addition to progress in device design, the evolution of imaging technology and our understanding of the mechanisms of disease should provide further insights into the factors that dictate patient selection and improve procedural success.

References

[1] Ormiston JA, Shah PM, Tei C, Wong M. Size and motion of the mitral valve annulus in man. I. A two-dimensional echocardiographic method and findings in normal subjects. *Circulation* 1981;64(1):113-20.

[2] David TE. Papillary muscle-annular continuity: is it important? *J. Card. Surg.* 1994;9(2 Suppl):252-4.

[3] Rodriguez F, Langer F, Harrington KB, Tibayan FA, Zasio MK, Cheng A, Liang D, Daughters GT, Covell JW, Criscione JC and others. Importance of mitral valve second-order chordae for left ventricular geometry, wall thickening mechanics, and global systolic function. *Circulation* 2004;110(11 Suppl 1):II115-22.

[4] Obadia JF, Casali C, Chassignolle JF, Janier M. Mitral subvalvular apparatus: different functions of primary and secondary chordae. *Circulation* 1997;96(9):3124-8.

[5] James TN. Anatomy of the coronary arteries in health and disease. *Circulation* 1965;32(6):1020-33.

[6] Armour JA, Randall WC. Structural basis for cardiac function. *Am. J. Physiol.* 1970; 218(6):1517-23.

[7] Olsen EG, Al-Rufaie HK. The floppy mitral valve. Study on pathogenesis. *Br. Heart J.* 1980;44(6):674-83.

[8] Chandrashekhar Y, Westaby S, Narula J. Mitral stenosis. *Lancet* 2009;374(9697):1271-83.

[9] Padmavati S. Rheumatic fever and rheumatic heart disease in India at the turn of the century. *Indian Heart J.* 2001;53(1):35-7.

[10] Selzer A, Cohn KE. Natural history of mitral stenosis: a review. *Circulation* 1972; 45(4):878-90.

[11] Bonow RO, Carabello BA, Chatterjee K, de Leon AC, Jr., Faxon DP, Freed MD, Gaasch WH, Lytle BW, Nishimura RA, O'Gara PT and others. ACC/AHA 2006 guidelines for the management of patients with valvular heart disease: a report of the American College of Cardiology/American Heart Association Task Force on Practice Guidelines (writing Committee to Revise the 1998 guidelines for the management of patients with valvular heart disease) developed in collaboration with the Society of Cardiovascular Anesthesiologists endorsed by the Society for Cardiovascular Angiography and Interventions and the Society of Thoracic Surgeons. *J. Am. Coll. Cardiol.* 2006;48(3):e1-148.

[12] Guidelines for the diagnosis of rheumatic fever. Jones Criteria, 1992 update. Special Writing Group of the Committee on Rheumatic Fever, Endocarditis, and Kawasaki Disease of the Council on Cardiovascular Disease in the Young of the American Heart Association. *JAMA* 1992;268(15):2069-73.

[13] Kemeny E, Husby G, Williams RC, Jr., Zabriskie JB. Tissue distribution of antigen(s) defined by monoclonal antibody D8/17 reacting with B lymphocytes of patients with rheumatic heart disease. *Clin. Immunol. Immunopathol.* 1994;72(1):35-43.

[14] Gibofsky A, Khanna A, Suh E, Zabriskie JB. The genetics of rheumatic fever: relationship to streptococcal infection and autoimmune disease. *J. Rheumatol. Suppl.* 1991;30:1-5.

[15] Braunwald E, editor. 2005. Robert O Bonow and Eugene Braunwald. Chapter 57: Valvular Heart Disease. 7th Edition. ed. Philadelphia, PA: Elsevier Saunders.

[16] Horstkotte D, Niehues R, Strauer BE. Pathomorphological aspects, aetiology and natural history of acquired mitral valve stenosis. *Eur. Heart J.* 1991;12 Suppl B:55-60.

[17] Marcus RH, Sareli P, Pocock WA, Barlow JB. The spectrum of severe rheumatic mitral valve disease in a developing country. Correlations among clinical presentation, surgical pathologic findings, and hemodynamic sequelae. *Ann. Intern. Med.* 1994; 120(3):177-83.

[18] Torun D, Sezer S, Baltali M, Adam FU, Erdem A, Ozdemir FN, Haberal M. Association of cardiac valve calcification and inflammation in patients on hemodialysis. *Ren. Fail* 2005;27(2):221-6.

[19] Braun J, Oldendorf M, Moshage W, Heidler R, Zeitler E, Luft FC. Electron beam computed tomography in the evaluation of cardiac calcification in chronic dialysis patients. *Am. J. Kidney Dis.* 1996;27(3):394-401.

[20] Muddassir SM, Pressman GS. Mitral annular calcification as a cause of mitral valve gradients. *Int. J. Cardiol.* 2007;123(1):58-62.

[21] Heidenreich PA, Kapoor JR. Radiation induced heart disease: systemic disorders in heart disease. *Heart* 2009;95(3):252-8.

[22] Carlson RG, Mayfield WR, Normann S, Alexander JA. Radiation-associated valvular disease. *Chest* 1991;99(3):538-45.

[23] Heidenreich PA, Hancock SL, Lee BK, Mariscal CS, Schnittger I. Asymptomatic cardiac disease following mediastinal irradiation. *J. Am. Coll. Cardiol.* 2003;42(4):743-9.

[24] Baumgartner H, Hung J, Bermejo J, Chambers JB, Evangelista A, Griffin BP, Iung B, Otto CM, Pellikka PA, Quinones M. Echocardiographic assessment of valve stenosis: EAE/ASE recommendations for clinical practice. *Eur. J. Echocardiogr.* 2009;10(1):1-25.

[25] Wilkins GT, Weyman AE, Abascal VM, Block PC, Palacios IF. Percutaneous balloon dilatation of the mitral valve: an analysis of echocardiographic variables related to outcome and the mechanism of dilatation. *Br. Heart J.* 1988;60(4):299-308.

[26] Faletra F, Pezzano A, Jr., Fusco R, Mantero A, Corno R, Crivellaro W, De Chiara F, Vitali E, Gordini V, Magnani P and others. Measurement of mitral valve area in mitral stenosis: four echocardiographic methods compared with direct measurement of anatomic orifices. *J. Am. Coll. Cardiol.* 1996;28(5):1190-7.

[27] Messika-Zeitoun D, Brochet E, Holmin C, Rosenbaum D, Cormier B, Serfaty JM, Iung B, Vahanian A. Three-dimensional evaluation of the mitral valve area and commissural opening before and after percutaneous mitral commissurotomy in patients with mitral stenosis. *Eur. Heart J.* 2007;28(1):72-9.

[28] Messika-Zeitoun D, Serfaty JM, Laissy JP, Berhili M, Brochet E, Iung B, Vahanian A. Assessment of the mitral valve area in patients with mitral stenosis by multislice computed tomography. *J. Am. Coll. Cardiol.* 2006;48(2):411-3.

[29] Meille L, Paul JF. Multislice computed tomography in mitral and aortic stenosis. *Arch. Cardiovasc. Dis.* 2008;101(10):681-2.

[30] Robertson KA, Volmink JA, Mayosi BM. Antibiotics for the primary prevention of acute rheumatic fever: a meta-analysis. *BMC Cardiovasc. Disord.* 2005;5(1):11.

[31] WHO Technical Report Series. Rheumatic Fever and Rheumatic Heart Disease. 2004. www.who.int/cardiovascular_diseases/resources/trs923/en/. Accessed May 27, 2010.

[32] Vora A, Karnad D, Goyal V, Naik A, Gupta A, Lokhandwala Y, Kulkarni H, Singh B. Control of rate versus rhythm in rheumatic atrial fibrillation: a randomized study. *Indian Heart J.* 2004;56(2):110-6.

[33] Hwang JJ, Kuan P, Chen JJ, Ko YL, Cheng JJ, Lin JL, Tseng YZ, Lien WP. Significance of left atrial spontaneous echo contrast in rheumatic mitral valve disease as a predictor of systemic arterial embolization: a transesophageal echocardiographic study. *Am. Heart J.* 1994;127(4 Pt 1):880-5.

[34] Inoue K, Owaki T, Nakamura T, Kitamura F, Miyamoto N. Clinical application of transvenous mitral commissurotomy by a new balloon catheter. *J. Thorac. Cardiovasc. Surg.* 1984;87(3):394-402.

[35] Abascal VM, Wilkins GT, O'Shea JP, Choong CY, Palacios IF, Thomas JD, Rosas E, Newell JB, Block PC, Weyman AE. Prediction of successful outcome in 130 patients undergoing percutaneous balloon mitral valvotomy. *Circulation* 1990;82(2):448-56.

[36] Palacios IF. Percutaneous mitral balloon valvotomy for patients with mitral stenosis. *Curr. Opin. Cardiol.* 1994;9(2):164-75.

[37] Herrmann HC, Wilkins GT, Abascal VM, Weyman AE, Block PC, Palacios IF. Percutaneous balloon mitral valvotomy for patients with mitral stenosis. Analysis of factors influencing early results. *J. Thorac. Cardiovasc. Surg.* 1988;96(1):33-8.

[38] Palacios IF, Sanchez PL, Harrell LC, Weyman AE, Block PC. Which patients benefit from percutaneous mitral balloon valvuloplasty? Prevalvuloplasty and postvalvuloplasty variables that predict long-term outcome. *Circulation* 2002;105(12): 1465-71.

[39] Multicenter experience with balloon mitral commissurotomy. NHLBI Balloon Valvuloplasty Registry Report on immediate and 30-day follow-up results. The National Heart, Lung, and Blood Institute Balloon Valvuloplasty Registry Participants. *Circulation* 1992;85(2):448-61.

[40] Cubeddu RJ, Palacios IF. Percutaneous techniques for mitral valve disease. *Cardiol. Clin;* 28(1):139-53.

[41] Enriquez-Sarano M, Akins CW, Vahanian A. Mitral regurgitation. *Lancet* 2009;373 (9672):1382-94.

[42] Mirabel M, Iung B, Baron G, Messika-Zeitoun D, Detaint D, Vanoverschelde JL, Butchart EG, Ravaud P, Vahanian A. What are the characteristics of patients with severe, symptomatic, mitral regurgitation who are denied surgery? *Eur. Heart J.* 2007; 28(11):1358-65.

[43] Baker PB, Bansal G, Boudoulas H, Kolibash AJ, Kilman J, Wooley CF. Floppy mitral valve chordae tendineae: histopathologic alterations. *Hum. Pathol.* 1988;19(5):507-12.

[44] Olson LJ, Subramanian R, Ackermann DM, Orszulak TA, Edwards WD. Surgical pathology of the mitral valve: a study of 712 cases spanning 21 years. *Mayo Clin. Proc.* 1987;62(1):22-34.

[45] Davies MJ, Moore BP, Braimbridge MV. The floppy mitral valve. Study of incidence, pathology, and complications in surgical, necropsy, and forensic material. *Br. Heart J.* 1978;40(5):468-81.

[46] Carpentier A, Chauvaud S, Fabiani JN, Deloche A, Relland J, Lessana A, D'Allaines C, Blondeau P, Piwnica A, Dubost C. Reconstructive surgery of mitral valve incompetence: ten-year appraisal. *J. Thorac. Cardiovasc. Surg.* 1980;79(3):338-48.

[47] Paparella D, Malvindi PG, Romito R, Fiore G, Tupputi Schinosa Lde L. Ischemic mitral regurgitation: pathophysiology, diagnosis and surgical treatment. *Expert Rev. Cardiovasc. Ther.* 2006;4(6):827-38.

[48] Timek TA, Lai DT, Tibayan F, Liang D, Rodriguez F, Daughters GT, Dagum P, Ingels NB, Jr., Miller C. Annular versus subvalvular approaches to acute ischemic mitral regurgitation. *Circulation* 2002;106(12 Suppl 1):I27-I32.

[49] Zoghbi WA, Enriquez-Sarano M, Foster E, Grayburn PA, Kraft CD, Levine RA, Nihoyannopoulos P, Otto CM, Quinones MA, Rakowski H and others. Recommendations for evaluation of the severity of native valvular regurgitation with two-dimensional and Doppler echocardiography. *J. Am. Soc. Echocardiogr.* 2003;16 (7):777-802.

[50] Daimon M, Saracino G, Gillinov AM, Koyama Y, Fukuda S, Kwan J, Song JM, Kongsaerepong V, Agler DA, Thomas JD and others. Local dysfunction and asymmetrical deformation of mitral annular geometry in ischemic mitral regurgitation: a novel computerized 3D echocardiographic analysis. *Echocardiography* 2008;25 (4):414-23.

[51] Choure AJ, Garcia MJ, Hesse B, Sevensma M, Maly G, Greenberg NL, Borzi L, Ellis S, Tuzcu EM, Kapadia SR. In vivo analysis of the anatomical relationship of coronary sinus to mitral annulus and left circumflex coronary artery using cardiac multidetector computed tomography: implications for percutaneous coronary sinus mitral annuloplasty. *J. Am. Coll. Cardiol.* 2006;48(10):1938-45.

[52] Yoran C, Yellin EL, Becker RM, Gabbay S, Frater RW, Sonnenblick EH. Mechanism of reduction of mitral regurgitation with vasodilator therapy. *Am. J. Cardiol.* 1979; 43(4):773-7.

[53] Host U, Kelbaek H, Hildebrandt P, Skagen K, Aldershvile J. Effect of ramipril on mitral regurgitation secondary to mitral valve prolapse. *Am. J. Cardiol.* 1997;80(5):655-8.

[54] Schon HR. Hemodynamic and morphologic changes after long-term angiotensin converting enzyme inhibition in patients with chronic valvular regurgitation. *J. Hypertens Suppl.* 1994;12(4):S95-104.

[55] Dujardin KS, Enriquez-Sarano M, Bailey KR, Seward JB, Tajik AJ. Effect of losartan on degree of mitral regurgitation quantified by echocardiography. *Am. J. Cardiol.* 2001; 87(5):570-6.

[56] Capomolla S, Febo O, Gnemmi M, Riccardi G, Opasich C, Caporotondi A, Mortara A, Pinna GD, Cobelli F. Beta-blockade therapy in chronic heart failure: diastolic function and mitral regurgitation improvement by carvedilol. *Am. Heart J.* 2000;139(4):596-608.

[57] Evangelista A, Tornos P, Sambola A, Permayer-Miralda G. Role of Vasodilators in Regurgitant Valve Disease. *Curr. Treat Options Cardiovasc. Med.* 2006;8(6):428-434.

[58] Braunberger E, Deloche A, Berrebi A, Abdallah F, Celestin JA, Meimoun P, Chatellier G, Chauvaud S, Fabiani JN, Carpentier A. Very long-term results (more than 20 years) of valve repair with carpentier's techniques in nonrheumatic mitral valve insufficiency. *Circulation* 2001;104(12 Suppl 1):I8-11.

[59] Mihaljevic T, Lam BK, Rajeswaran J, Takagaki M, Lauer MS, Gillinov AM, Blackstone EH, Lytle BW. Impact of mitral valve annuloplasty combined with revascularization in patients with functional ischemic mitral regurgitation. *J. Am. Coll. Cardiol.* 2007;49(22):2191-201.

[60] Iansac E, Di Centa I, Al Attar N, Baron F, Lali M, Detaint D, Bel A, Hvass U, Raffoul R, Nataf P. Percutaneous mitral annuloplasty through the coronary sinus: an anatomical point of view. *Circulation* 2006;114(suppl):II-565.

[61] Schofer J, Siminiak T, Haude M, Herrman JP, Vainer J, Wu JC, Levy WC, Mauri L, Feldman T, Kwong RY and others. Percutaneous mitral annuloplasty for functional mitral regurgitation: results of the CARILLON Mitral Annuloplasty Device European Union Study. *Circulation* 2009;120(4):326-33.

[62] http://www.medicalnewstoday.com/articles/136541.php. Accessed May 15, 2010.

[63] Liddicoat JR, Mac Neill BD, Gillinov AM, Cohn WE, Chin CH, Prado AD, Pandian NG, Oesterle SN. Percutaneous mitral valve repair: a feasibility study in an ovine

model of acute ischemic mitral regurgitation. *Catheter Cardiovasc. Interv.* 2003;60(3): 410-6.

[64] Daimon M, Fukuda S, Adams DH, McCarthy PM, Gillinov AM, Carpentier A, Filsoufi F, Abascal VM, Rigolin VH, Salzberg S and others. Mitral valve repair with Carpentier-McCarthy-Adams IMR ETlogix annuloplasty ring for ischemic mitral regurgitation: early echocardiographic results from a multi-center study. *Circulation* 2006;114(1 Suppl):I588-93.

[65] Sack S, Kahlert P, Bilodeau L, Pierard LA, Lancellotti P, Legrand V, Bartunek J, Vanderheyden M, Hoffmann R, Schauerte P and others. Percutaneous transvenous mitral annuloplasty: initial human experience with a novel coronary sinus implant device. *Circ. Cardiovasc. Interv.* 2009;2(4):277-84.

[66] Harnek J. 2-year Interim Results of the Percuataneous MONARC™ System for the Treatment of Functional Mitral Regurgitation. EuroPCR 2009.

[67] Sorajja P, Nishimura RA, Thompson J, Zehr K. A novel method of percutaneous mitral valve repair for ischemic mitral regurgitation. *JACC Cardiovasc. Interv.* 2008;1(6):663-72.

[68] Aybek T, Risteski P, Miskovic A, Simon A, Dogan S, Abdel-Rahman U, Moritz A. Seven years' experience with suture annuloplasty for mitral valve repair. *J. Thorac. Cardiovasc. Surg.* 2006;131(1):99-106.

[69] Nagy ZL, Bodi A, Vaszily M, Szerafin T, Horvath A, Peterffy A. Five-year experience with a suture annuloplasty for mitral valve repair. *Scand. Cardiovasc. J.* 2000;34(5): 528-32.

[70] Mitralign News and Information. www.mitralign.com/eurostudy.shtml. Accessed May 18, 2010.

[71] Heuser RR, Witzel T, Dickens D, Takeda PA. Percutaneous treatment for mitral regurgitation: the QuantumCor system. *J. Interv. Cardiol.* 2008;21(2):178-82.

[72] MiCardia News/Events: Press Releases. www.micardia.com/Mitral-valve-prolapse-and-regurgitation-news/Mitral-valve-repair-for-Mitral-valve-prolapse-PR.php. Accessed May 18, 2010.

[73] Mishra YK, Mittal S, Jaguri P, Trehan N. Coapsys mitral annuloplasty for chronic functional ischemic mitral regurgitation: 1-year results. *Ann. Thorac. Surg.* 2006;81(1): 42-6.

[74] Grossi EA, Saunders PC, Woo YJ, Gangahar DM, Laschinger JC, Kress DC, Caskey MP, Schwartz CF, Wudel J. Intraoperative effects of the coapsys annuloplasty system in a randomized evaluation (RESTOR-MV) of functional ischemic mitral regurgitation. *Ann. Thorac. Surg.* 2005;80(5):1706-11.

[75] Pedersen WR, Block P, Leon M, Kramer P, Kapadia S, Babaliaros V, Kodali S, Tuzcu EM, Feldman T. iCoapsys mitral valve repair system: Percutaneous implantation in an animal model. *Catheter Cardiovasc. Interv.* 2008;72(1):125-31.

[76] Rogers JH, Macoviak JA, Rahdert DA, Takeda PA, Palacios IF, Low RI. Percutaneous septal sinus shortening: a novel procedure for the treatment of functional mitral regurgitation. *Circulation* 2006;113(19):2329-34.

[77] Rogers JH, Rahdert DA, Caputo GR, Takeda PA, Palacios IF, Tio FO, Taylor EA, Low RI. Long-term safety and durability of percutaneous septal sinus shortening (The PS(3) System) in an ovine model. *Catheter Cardiovasc. Interv.* 2009;73(4):540-8.

[78] Palacios IF, Condado JA, Brandi S, Rodriguez V, Bosch F, Silva G, Low RI, Rogers JH. Safety and feasibility of acute percutaneous septal sinus shortening: first-in-human experience. *Catheter Cardiovasc. Interv.* 2007;69(4):513-8.

[79] Maisano F, Torracca L, Oppizzi M, Stefano PL, D'Addario G, La Canna G, Zogno M, Alfieri O. The edge-to-edge technique: a simplified method to correct mitral insufficiency. *Eur. J. Cardiothorac. Surg.* 1998;13(3):240-5; discussion 245-6.

[80] Maisano F, Vigano G, Blasio A, Colombo A, Calabrese C, Alfieri O. Surgical isolated edge-to-edge mitral valve repair without annuloplasty: clinical proof of the principle for an endovascular approach. *EuroIntervention* 2006;2:181-6.

[81] Fann JI, St Goar FG, Komtebedde J, Oz MC, Block PC, Foster E, Butany J, Feldman T, Burdon TA. Beating heart catheter-based edge-to-edge mitral valve procedure in a porcine model: efficacy and healing response. *Circulation* 2004;110(8):988-93.

[82] Feldman T, Kar S, Rinaldi M, Fail P, Hermiller J, Smalling R, Whitlow PL, Gray W, Low R, Herrmann HC and others. Percutaneous mitral repair with the MitraClip system: safety and midterm durability in the initial EVEREST (Endovascular Valve Edge-to-Edge REpair Study) cohort. *J. Am. Coll. Cardiol.* 2009;54(8):686-94.

[83] Condado JA, Acquatella H, Rodriguez L, Whitlow P, Velez-Gimo M, St Goar FG. Percutaneous edge-to-edge mitral valve repair: 2-year follow-up in the first human case. *Catheter Cardiovasc. Interv.* 2006;67(2):323-5.

[84] Argenziano M, Skipper E, Heimansohn D, Letsou GV, Woo YJ, Kron I, Alexander J, Cleveland J, Kong B, Davidson M and others. Surgical revision after percutaneous mitral repair with the MitraClip device. *Ann. Thorac. Surg;* 89(1):72-80; discussion p 80.

[85] Feldman T, on behalf of the EVEREST II investigators. Endovascular valve edge-to-edge repair study (EVEREST II) randomized clinical trial: primary safety and efficacy endpoints. American College of Cardiology/i2 Late Breaking Clinical Trials session. Atlanta, GA. March 14, 2010.

In: Percutaneous Valve Technology: Present and Future ISBN: 978-1-61942-577-4
Editors: Jose Luis Navia and Sharif Al-Ruzzeh

Chapter XVII

Functional Anatomy of the Mitral Valve: Surgical Perspective of Mitral Valve Disease. Setting the Field for Percutaneous Valve Repair

Joanna Chikwe and David H. Adams

Introduction

Mitral valve repair is the only treatment known to restore normal life expectancy to patients with severe mitral regurgitation[1], but despite repair rates of 90% at high volume centres [2-5], overall repair rates in Europe and the US average less than 50%[6-8]. The wide variation in successful repair primarily reflects the extremely heterogeneous morphology of regurgitant valves, which poses a particular challenge to percutaneous repair techniques. This chapter focuses on the functional anatomy and pathology of the mitral valve from a surgical perspective, providing an insight into the impact of valve morphology on the potential applications and limitations of percutaneous approaches to mitral regurgitation.

Definitions and Nomenclature

The mitral valvular apparatus is a complex assembly of interdependent anatomical structures consisting of the anterior and posterior valve leaflets and commissures (valve tissue), mitral annulus, the chordae tendinae and papillary muscles (subvalvular apparatus), and the left ventricle (Figure 1). Failure to identify the precise dysfunction of each of these components, any of which may reduce leaflet coaptation causing regurgitation, reduces the likelihood of successful repair. The first step in repair is to clearly identify the abnormal pathology causing regurgitation, which requires the different etiologies and resultant lesions to be differentiated, hampered by the use of imprecise nomenclature such as "billowing", "prolapse", "flail", "myxomatous disease", "floppy valve", and "Barlow's valve" [9]. A systematic method of describing mitral regurgitation was therefore introduced by the cardiac surgeon Alain Carpentier in the 1960's, in which the regurgitant valve is described first by disease aetiology (e.g. degenerative disease, endocarditis, rheumatic) then by the primary lesion (e.g. chordal rupture, annular dilatation); and finally by the resultant leaflet dysfunction (Table 1).

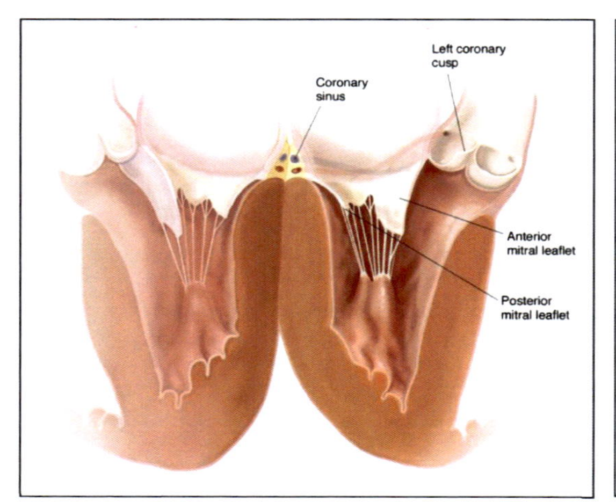

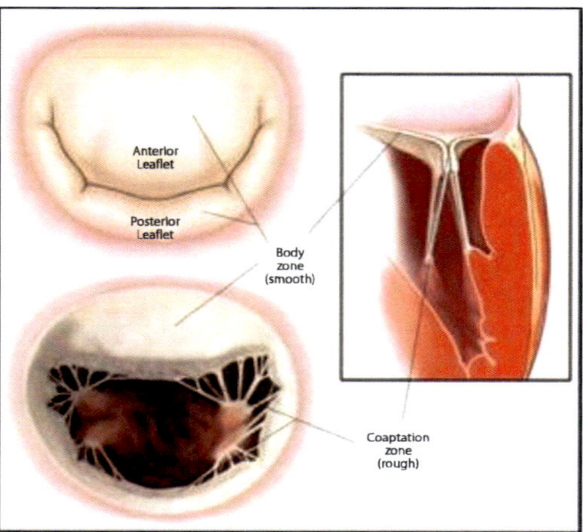

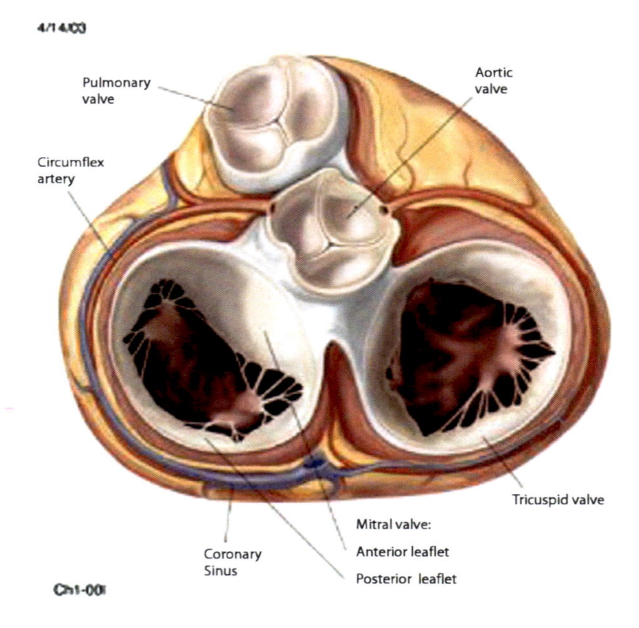

Figure 1. The mitral valvular apparatus is a complex assembly of interdependent anatomical structures consisting of the anterior and posterior valve leaflets and commissures (valve tissue), mitral annulus, the chordae tendineae and papillary muscles (subvalvular apparatus), and the left ventricle. Leaflet coaptation can be affected by changes in any of these components, resulting in regurgitation.

Table 1. Carpentier's pathophysiologic triad of mitral regurgitation, composed of etoilogy, valve lesions and leaflet dysfunction, with specific surgical repair techniques, and possible percutaneous equivalent

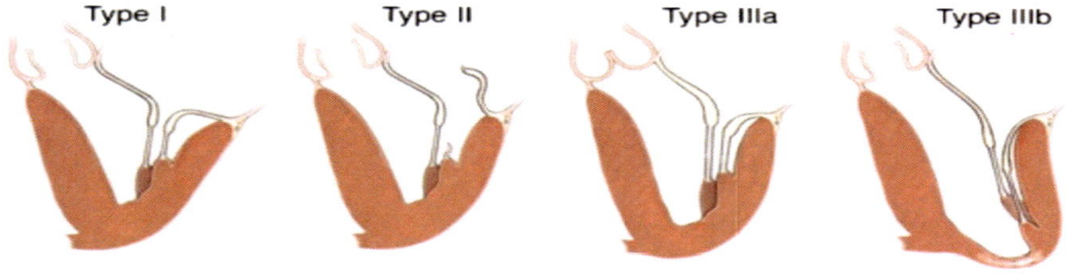

Leaflet Dysfunction	Type I	Type II	Type IIIa	Type IIIb
Lesions	Annular dilatation Annular deformation Leaflet perforation Leaflet cleft	Myxomatous degeneration Chordal elongation or rupture Papillary muscle elongation or rupture	Leaflet thickening or retraction Commissural fusion Chordal thickening or retraction Chordal fusion Calcification Ventricular endomyocardial fibrosis	Leaflet tethering Papillary muscle displacement Ventricular dilatation Ventricular aneurysm Endomyocardial fibrosis
Etiology	Ischemic cardiomyopathy Dilated cardiomyopathy Endocarditis Congenital	Degenerative disease (fibroelastic deficiency, Barlows, Marfans) Endocarditis Rheumatic disease Acute myocardial infarct (PM rupture) Ischemic cardiomyopathy Trauma	Rheumatic disease Carcinoid Radiation Lupus erythematosus Ergotamine use	Ischemic cardiomyopathy Dilated cardiomyopathy
Surgical Repair Technique	Downsized annuloplasty Primary or patch closure of perforations Cleft closure	Leaflet resection +/- chordal reconstruction + annuloplasty	Commissurotomy Chordal fenestration Pericardial patch leaflet augmentation	Downsized annuloplasty Chordal cutting
Percutaneous Repair Technique	Coronary sinus devices e.g. Viacor PTMA, Carillon, Edwards Monarc, Transventricular Mitral annuloplasty e.g. Mitralign Ample PS3 system Myocardial support e.g. Coapsys	Leaflet edge-toedge e.g. Mitraclip	Balloon valvotomy	Myocardial support e.g. Coapsys

Text in black represents lesions and surgical techniques for which there is currently no percutaneous equivalent.

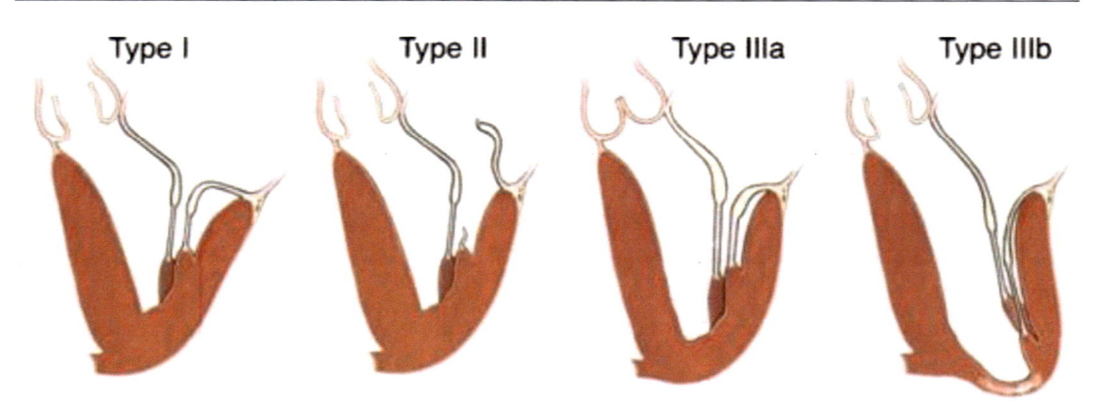

Figure 2. Carpentier originally classified leaflet dysfunction into three types: Type I or normal motion, Type II or excessive leaflet motion, and Type III or restricted leaflet motion. Type III is subdivided into restricted opening (IIIa) and restricted closure (IIIb).

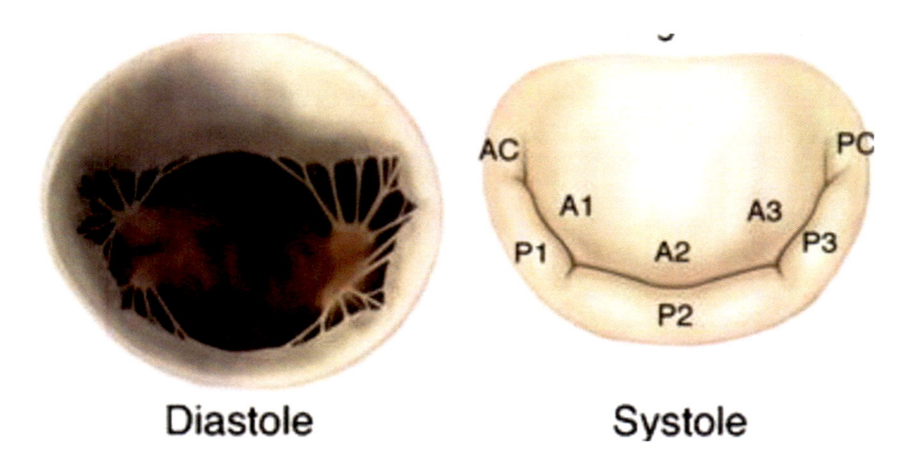

Figure 3. segmental valve anatomy.

Carpentier classified leaflet dysfunction into three types: Type I or normal motion, Type II or excessive leaflet motion, and Type III or restricted leaflet motion (Figure 2) [10, 11]. Type III mitral regurgitation is subdivided into Type IIIa resulting from restricted leaflet opening, most commonly due to rheumatic valve disease; and Type IIIb caused by restricted leaflet closure, and most commonly due to chordal restriction from lateral displacement of the posteromedial papillary muscle as a result of ischemic ventricular dysfunction and dilatation [12]. He combined this classification with segmental valve anatomy (Figure 3), to provide a system of nomenclature and valve analysis that is central to planning mitral valve repair. Taking each component of the mitral valve in turn, this chapter reviews the normal anatomy, common pathological changes resulting in mitral regurgitation, and the potential avenues in each case for valve repair. Table 1 summarises the main lesions by leaflet dysfunction, and lists the relevant surgical and potential percutaneous repair methods where available for each one.

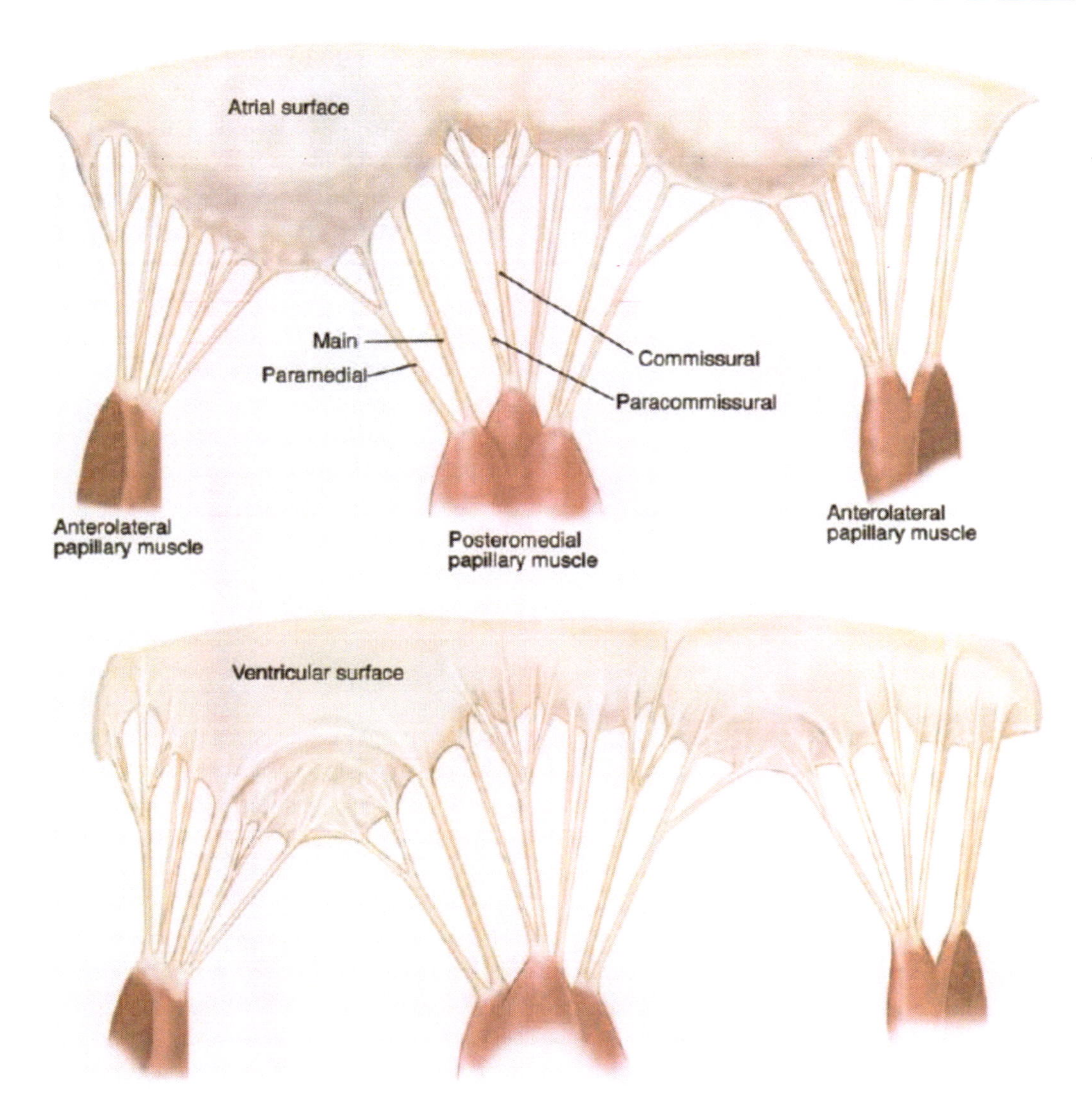

Figure 4. The atrial surface of the leaflets are further divided into two zones, one peripheral smooth zone and one central rough zone which corresponds to the coaptation area, and which is the insertion site of most of the chordae tendineae.

Leaflets

Leaflet Anatomy

The leaflet tissue consists of two leaflets - anterior and posterior, as well as two commissures (posteromedial and anterolateral) which define the area where the anterior and posterior leaflets meet at their insertion into the annulus (Figure 3). The leaflets insert onto the entire circumference of the mitral annulus, with fibrous continuity between the anterior leaflet of the mitral valve and the left and noncoronary cusps of the aortic valve. The anterior (aortic) leaflet has a semicircular shape, no indentations, is attached to two fifths of the annular circumference, and defines the boundary between the inflow and outflow tracts of the left ventricle. The posterior (mural) leaflet is attached to three fifths of the annular circumference, and has a quadrangular shape divided into three scallops by two deep indentations. The leaflets have similar surface areas although the anterior leaflet is taller than the posterior leaflet. The atrial surface of the leaflets is further divided into two zones, one peripheral smooth zone and one central rough zone which corresponds to the coaptation area, and which is the insertion site of most of the chordae tendinae (Figure 4). A curved line, called the coaptation line, separates these two areas.

The mitral valve is separated into eight segments (Figure 3). The three scallops of the posterior leaflet are identified as P1 (anterior scallop), P2 (middle scallop), and P3 (posterior scallop). The three corresponding segments of the anterior leaflet are A1 (anterior segment), A2 (middle segment), and A3 (posterior segment). The anterolateral and posteromedial commissures comprise the last two segments. This anatomical nomenclature is the basis of segmental valve analysis, and allows precise location of valve pathology which may occur anywhere in the leaflet tissue.

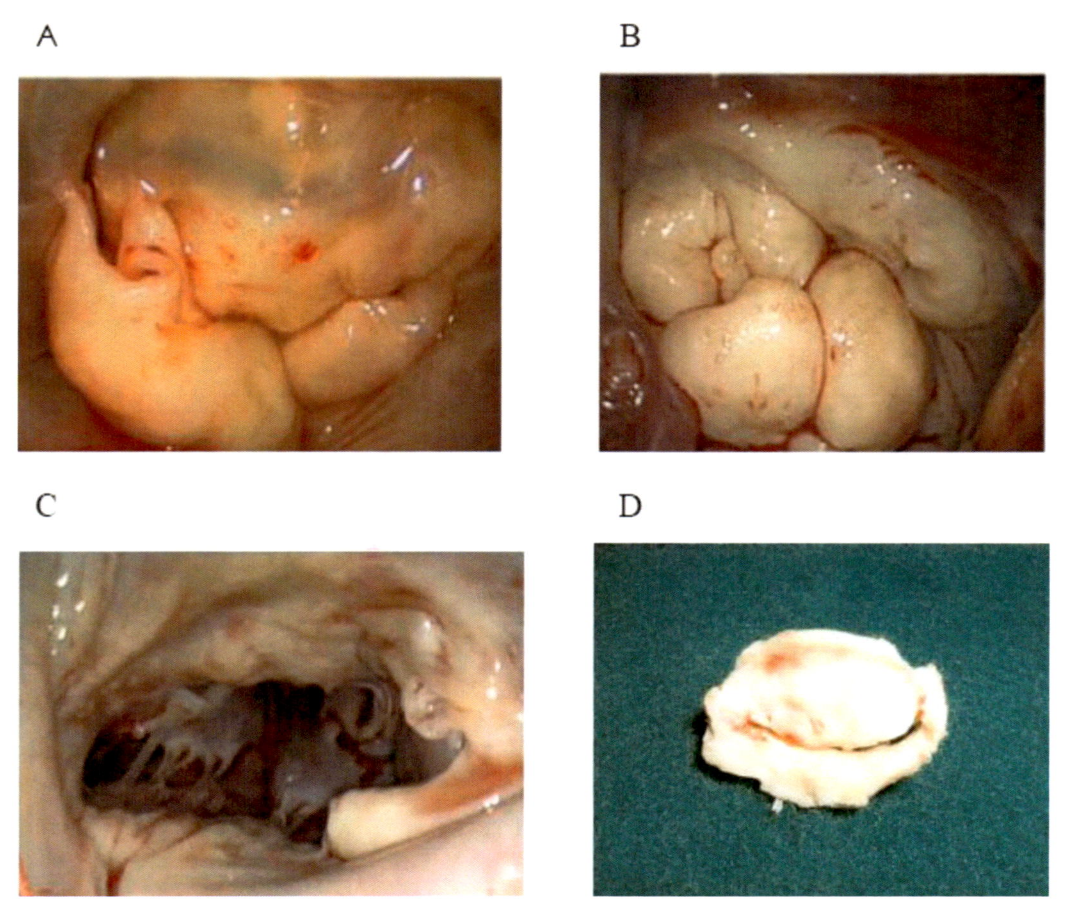

Figure 5. Examples of the more common etiologies of mitral regurgitation. A: fibroelastic deficiency. B: Barlow's disease. C: ischemic mitral regurgitation. D: rheumatic valve disease.

Leaflet Pathology

The commonest pathology to directly involve the mitral valve leaflets is degenerative mitral valve disease in the West, and rheumatic valve disease in undeveloped countries. Degenerative disease is defined as a spectrum of conditions in which infiltrative or dysplastic tissue changes cause elongation or rupture of the mitral valve chordae resulting in leaflet prolapse and / or annular dilatation[9] (Figure 5). At one end of the spectrum of degenerative mitral disease is fibroelastic deficiency (Figure 5A), characterised by insufficient tissue in a normal sized valve: leaflets are thin and translucent, and chordae are flimsy and elongated. Regurgitation is most frequently caused by rupture of a single chord associated with a single thickened, prolapsing segment, usually P2, resulting in Type II leaflet dysfunction. At the opposite end of the spectrum of degenerative mitral regurgitation is Barlow's disease, characterised by excess tissue in a very dilated valve (Figure 5B). Leaflet tissue is thickened and there is obvious redundancy in multiple segments, with thick, elongated, mesh-like chordae[13]. Regurgitation is due to the multiple areas of bileaflet prolapse (Type II leaflet dysfunction). Degenerative valve disease may occupy the range within this spectrum, and it is this diverse morphology that requires a tailored approach for successful mitral valve repair. Coronary artery disease is often present in patients with mitral valve regurgitation due to degenerative disease, and these patients may be incorrectly described as having ischemic mitral valve disease.

Leaflet involvement in rheumatic disease is characterized by thickening, stiffening, and eventually calcification, associated with fusion of the commissures and subvalvular apparatus (Figure 5C). These lesions reduce leaflet mobility throughout the cardiac cycle (type IIIa dysfunction), leading to mixed regurgitant and stenotic lesions. Occasionally chordal elongation of the anterior leaflet primary chordae results in a type II dysfunction; combined anterior leaflet prolapse and posterior leaflet restriction (type II anterior, type IIIa posterior) is one of the most common mechanisms of mitral regurgitation in young rheumatic patients.

The leaflets are not directly involved by the pathological changes found in ischemic mitral valve disease. The characteristic Carpentier Type IIIb leaflet dysfunction results from restricted closure of morphologically normal leaflets due to papillary muscle displacement posteriorly as a result of left ventricular dilatation in the setting of coronary artery disease (Figure 5D). Restricted leaflet motion results in poor coaptation and mitral regurgitation. These valves are usually small, as annular dilatation is not a feature until very late in the disease process.

Valve leaflets may be involved by any of several lesions in endocarditis, which is usually defined by the presence of a history of endocarditis or evidence of valvular vegetations (Figure 5E). Mitral valve endocarditis usually occurs in patients with a structurally leaflets (due to degenerative or rheumatic valve disease). Primary native mitral endocarditis may cause several types of lesions, including vegetations, chordal rupture, leaflet abscess or perforation, and annular abscess. Aortic valve endocarditis may also cause native mitral valve endocarditis by extension of the infective process. In some cases an aortic annular abscess can track to the fibrous body and involve the mitral annulus, and anterior leaflet of the mitral valve. Furthermore, the diastolic jet of aortic regurgitation resulting from aortic endocarditis may also cause secondary mitral endocarditis with vegetations or leaflet perforation on the ventricular surface of the anterior leaflet, known as "kissing lesions".

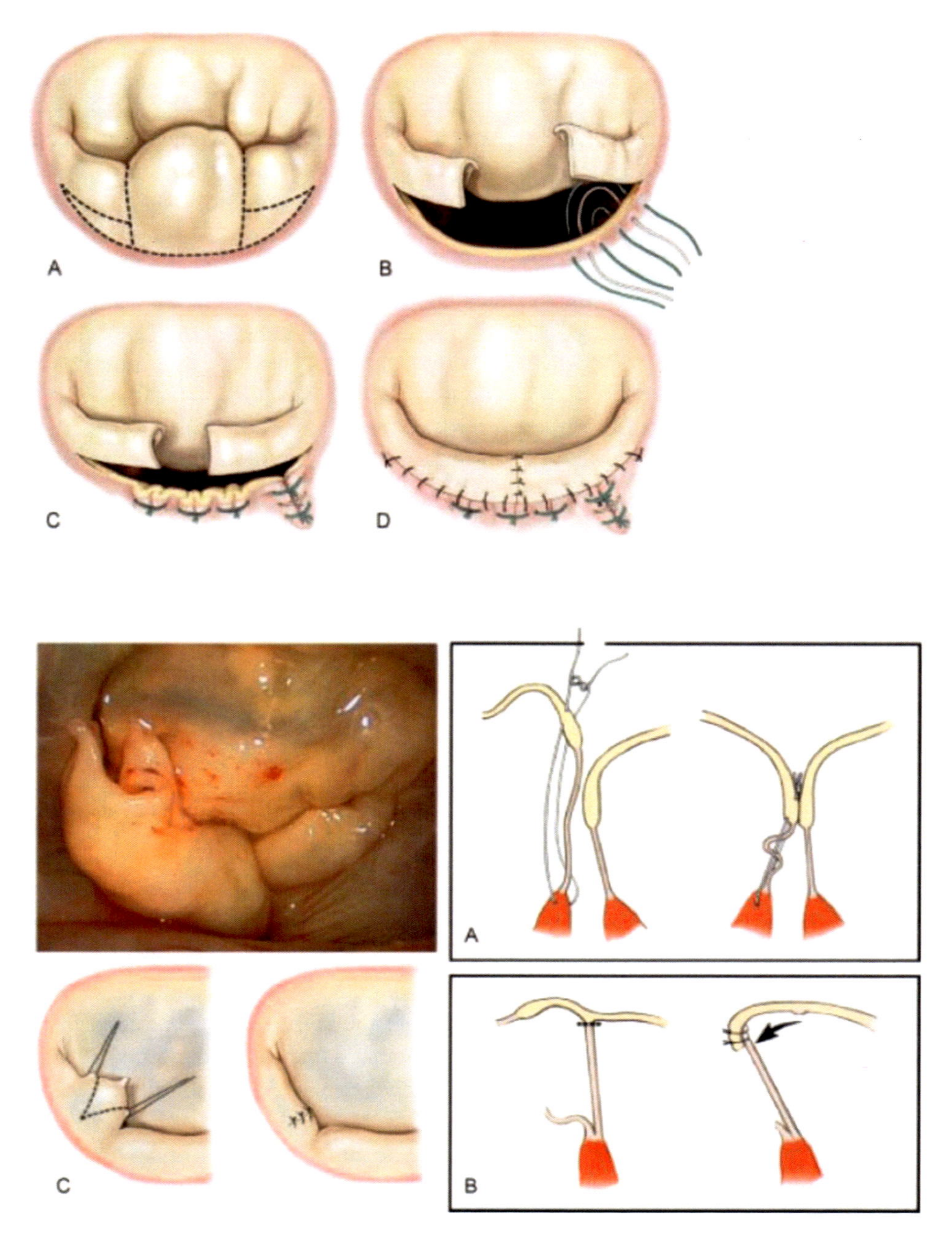

Figure 6. Examples of surgical repair techniques. A: triangular resection. **B" quadrangular resection and** sliding plasty. C: pericardial patch augmentation. D: asymmetric annuloplasty. E: Commisurotomy

Leaflet Repair Techniques

Surgical: It is crucial to distinguish between regurgitation due to type II (leaflet prolapse) and type III (leaflet restriction), as the techniques required to achieve a satisfactory repair for these different mechanisms are very different.

From a surgical perspective it is important to further differentiate between prolapse in the setting of excess leaflet tissue (e.g. Barlow's valves) versus that occurring in valves with limited leaflet tissue (e.g. fibroelastic deficiency or endocarditis) as the latter is best addressed with very conservative resection or chordal reconstruction (Figure 6A), rather than aggressive quadrangular resection and sliding plasty (Figure 6B) which has traditionally been the technique of choice for the former pathology. Tissue resection in valves with limited tissue must be approached with caution, as the surgeon runs the risk of leaving insufficient leaflet tissue to complete a successful repair, and edge-to-edge closure may produce a functional stenosis in what is usually a small valve.

The edge-to-edge (Alfieri suture) technique (Figure 6C) was developed to treat anterior leaflet prolapse, but can also be applied to ischemic mitral regurgitation [14]. The technique sutures the anterior and posterior leaflets with a single stitch, resulting in a double orifice if applied at the coaptation of A2 and P2, or a reduced orifice if applied towards the commissures. Proponents of this simple technique have reported good early and late results when it is used in conjunction with other repair methods, notably annuloplasty [15]. The edge to edge repair in isolation does not correct the primary lesions of ischemic mitral regurgitation (leaflet tethering and annular dilatation), and has little or no impact on the geometric valvular and subvalvular changes associated with chronic mitral regurgitation [16]. Aggressive tissue resection and / or chordal reconstruction (Figure A) are mainstays of surgical repair in these Barlow's valves, because edge-to-edge closure is unlikely to achieve a significant reduction in regurgitation which is usually due to multi-segment prolapse.

In ischemic mitral regurgitation, an isolated, asymmetrical annuloplasty addressing the characteristic type IIIb lesion which is usually most pronounced in the P2/3 area (Figure 6D), may be sufficient to reduce or eliminate mitral regurgitation, but frequently division of restrictive chordae is required to eliminate regurgitation in a durable fashion. An edge-to-edge repair on its own is unlikely to achieve a competent valve in type IIIb regurgitation, as the repair does not address the leaflet restriction and may result in a functional stenosis in what are usually small valves.

Rheumatic valves are particularly challenging to repair because of the widespread reduction in leaflet mobility. Edge-to-edge repair is likely to result in adding significant stenosis to residual regurgitation, whereas an isolated annuloplasty fails to address the leaflet prolapse or restriction. Commonly used surgical techniques for repairing regurgitant mitral valves include autologous glutaraldehyde fixed pericardial patch augmentation (Figure 6E). Commisurotomy if required is carried out stopping 3-4mm from the annulus to prevent extension of the incision and an incompetent valve (Figure 6F).

Patch augmentation is a useful technique to address leaflet perforations in endocarditis where a key part of surgical treatment is complete debridement of all infected and devitalized tissue to minimize the risk of recurrent infection. Several surgical repair techniques may be required including patch repair of augmentations, leaflet resection and resuspension and annuloplasty.

Percutaneous: Balloon valvuloplasty has been the mainstay of percutaneous approaches to the mitral valve for decade. This effects a blunt commisurotomy which can be used to reduce stenosis in the absence of severe leaflet calcification, but the presence of more than moderate regurgitation is a contraindication. The MitraClip device is designed to perform an edge-to-edge type repair in patients with severe mitral regurgitation. Up to a third of patients have moderate to severe recurrent mitral regurgitation within six months of treatment with the device[17], possibly reflecting the surgical literature outlined above that has demonstrated the importance of adjunctive annuloplasty in stabilizing this type of repair, as well as the difficulty of satisfactorily addressing any lesion other than single segment prolapse with this approach.

Commissures

Commissural Anatomy

The anterolateral and posteromedial commissures are identified using two anatomical landmarks: the axis of corresponding papillary muscles and the commissural chordae, which have a net like structure. The free edge of the commissures, which occasionally take the form of a clearly defined commissural leaflet, is usually several millimeters from the annulus.

Commisural Pathology

Commissural thickening and fusion are early features of rheumatic valve disease, where progressive loss of leaflet mobility and narrowing of the valve orifice eventually results in stenotic lesions. The commissures may be affected in degenerative disease, with prolapse in that area, although more commonly leaflet tissue is deficient there. Eccentric regurgitant commissural jets are often seen in endocarditis caused by commissural prolapse or perforations.

Commisural Repair Techniques

Surgical: Commisural prolapse or perforations may be the cause of severe mitral regurgitation, neither of which would be successfully addressed by percutaneous P2 to A2 edge-to-edge closure, or annuloplasty techniques, although a commissural edge-to-edge repair may achieve a satisfactory result in this setting. Commisurotomy (Figure 6E) may be performed for mitral stenosis due to commissural fusion, dividing the fused leaflet to around 5mm short of the annulus to avoid causing commissural regurgitation. Pericardial patch augmentation is a useful way of addressing commissural leaks due to perforations or inadequate leaflet tissue.

Mitral Annulus

Annular Anatomy

The mitral annulus is the saddle shaped fibrous junction between the left ventricle and atrium and is the site of insertion for the mitral valve leaflets and commissural tissue. It lies in the atrioventricular groove close to important anatomical structures including the noncoronary and right coronary aortic sinuses, the circumflex coronary artery and the coronary sinus (Figure 1). It incorporates the two fibrous trigones: the right fibrous trigone is where the fibrous annular tissue of the mitral, tricuspid, and noncoronary cusps of the aortic valve and the membranous septum coalesce, and the left fibrous trigone which is formed by the junction of both left fibrous borders of the aortic and the mitral valve. The mitral annulus is thinnest at the insertion of the posterior leaflet, and as this segment is not attached to any rigid structures, it is particularly prone to annular dilation, which can also occur to a moderate degree at the anterior portion of the mitral annulus between the trigones. The commissural areas move apically during systole, whereas the annular diameter narrows increasing the area of leaflet coaptation.

Annular Pathology

The normal ratio between the antero-posterior and transverse diameter of the mitral annulus is 3:4 in systole (Figure 7A). This ratio inverts as the annulus dilates in chronic mitral regurgitation, exacerbating poor leaflet coaptation and regurgitation. This progressive defect affects the anterior annulus to a lesser extent than the posterior annulus which is thinner and only supported by the left ventricular free wall.

Annuloplasty Techniques

Surgical: The objective of remodelling annuloplasty, which was introduced in the 1970's by Carpentier is to restore the mitral annulus to its systolic 3:4 ratio, preventing further annular dilatation, preserving leaflet mobility, relieving tension on the leaflets helping to stabilize the repair, and increasing the area of coaptation minimising mitral regurgitation [18].

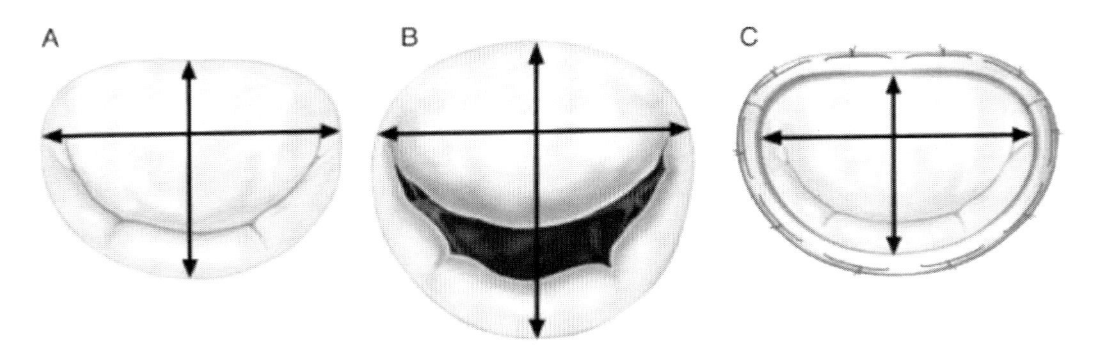

Figure 7A. The normal ratio between the anteroposterior and transverse diameter of the mitral annulus is 3:4 in systole. B: Annular dilatation occurs in a predictable fashion in primarily affecting the posterior annulus which is less supported by the fibrous skeleton of the heart than the anterior annulus which remains relatively fixed in the intertrigonal distance resulting in a change to a 4:3 systolic ratio and the valve becoming more circular. C: Remodelling annuloplasty improves coaptation not only by reducing annular circumference to that of the surface area of the anterior leaflet, but restores the normal 3: systolic ratio.

From a surgical standpoint annuloplasty may be achieved using suture techniques or rings, which may be rigid, semi-rigid or flexible, complete or incomplete. Most annuloplasty rings are semi-rigid two-dimensional rings that are designed to reduce the circumference (reduction annuloplasty) and restore the 3:4 systolic ratio (remodelling annuloplasty)(Figure 7B). Asymmetric rings, with a reduced diameter in the P3 region, have successfully been used to address the asymmetric leaflet tethering: these are most commonly used in ischemic mitral valve repair (Figure 7C)[19]. Several studies have suggested that ring annuloplasty offers superior long-term freedom from mitral regurgitation to repair techniques not using ring annuloplasty[20], and that chronic mitral regurgitation may be best treated by remodelling the annulus with a complete ring, rather than by using incomplete bands that do not prevent dilation of the anterior annulus, or address the change in annular proportions[21, 22], and that failure to correctly employ ring annuloplasty is the main predictor of residual and recurrent regurgitation.

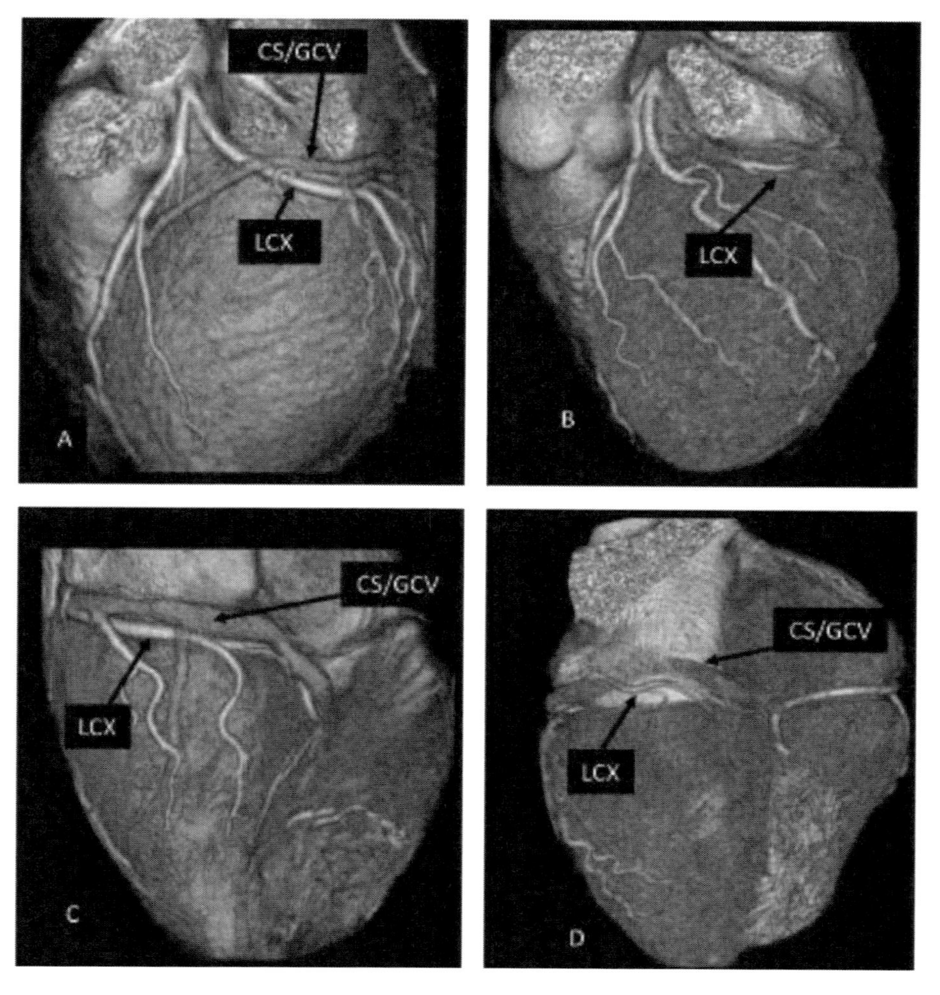

Figure 8. Volume-rendered images of the heart showing different projections. The circumflex (LCX), and occasionally the obtuse marginal and posterolateral coronary arteries lie between the coronary sinus and great cardiac vein (CS/GCV) and the mitral annulus for part of their course. Rreproduced from.

Percutaneous: The coronary sinus lies in close proximity to much of the annulus, and has been proposed as a potential route for percutaneous annuloplasty devices. The primary issue with coronary sinus based techniques is that the coronary sinus does not reach the anterior mitral annulus (Figure 1, so limited reduction can be achieved in the antero-posterio dimension (particular in the A1 P1 area), which is the primary type of annular dilatation in mitral regurgitation of most etiologies (Figure 7). Care must be taken to avoid excessive distortion of the posterior annulus and compromise of the circumflex artery with posterior annuloplasty techniques. Recent cross-sectional imaging studies suggest that circumferential compression type devices placed within the coronary sinus could compromise coronary blood flow as, in over 80% of subjects studied, the circumflex, and occasionally the obtuse marginal and posterolateral coronary arteries lie between the coronary sinus and the mitral annulus for part of their course [23-25] (Figure 8). In a porcine animal model of a percutaneous coronary sinus annuloplasty device, the circumflex coronary artery was entrapped by the device in all cases resulting in subtotal angiographic occlusion and 50% reduction in blood flow.

Chordae Tendineae

Chordal Anatomy

The chordae tendinae are thin fibrous structures connecting the papillary muscles to the leaflets. They are classified according to the site of insertion: marginal (primary) chordae insert on the free margin of the leaflets and limit leaflet prolapse, intermediate (secondary) chordae insert onto the ventricular surface of the leaflets and reduce tension on the leaflet and primary chordae, and basal (tertiary) chordae are attached to the posterior leaflet base connecting it to the mitral annulus (Figure 4).

Chordal Pathology

Mitral regurgitation is almost invariably associated with loss of normal chordal architecture or function. Degenerative valve disease and rheumatic valve disease are the two pathologies that most commonly directly affect the chordae tendinae resulting in mitral regurgitation.

In fibroelastic deficiency the chordae are often very thin, with a tendency to rupture most frequently in the marginal chordae of the P2 segment resulting in prolapse (Figure 5A).

In Barlow's disease the chordae are characteristically thickened and elongated, which also leads to prolapse, usually of multiple segments (Figure 5B). Rheumatic disease is characterized by chordal fusion, shortening and calcification resulting in a type IIIa leaflet dysfunction. Endocarditis is often associated with chordal rupture. Ischemic and dilated cardiomyopathy are not characterized by chordal pathology, but result in type IIIb leaflet restriction as the chordal attachments are displaced posteriorly (Figure 5C).

Chordal Repair Techniques

Surgical: Several repair techniques are useful to address chordal pathology (Figure 6F). Chordal techniques may be applied to prolapsing segments caused by elongated or ruptured chordae of either leaflet, particularly when there is insufficient tissue to permit leaflet resection; or to correct leaflet tethering caused by chordal shortening or ventricular dilatation[10, 18, 26]. Where there is a flail segment the two main options are chordal reconstruction with polytetrafluoroethylene (PTFE) [27] (Figure 11) or chordal transfer[26] (Figure 6H). Intermittently testing valve competency with normal saline as the neo-chord is tied down is one method of ensuring the correct neo chordal height is selected[9], an alternative is selecting pre-formed PTFE loops (Figure 13) based on measurement of distance between a reference leaflet margin point to the base of the nearest papillary muscle with callipers. Chordal transfer involves the selection of a normal looking nearby secondary chord, or adjacent chord from the opposite leaflet[28]. The cord is detached from its insertion on its leaflet, and reattached to the margin of the anterior leaflet with 5/0 prolene. Although this is a reliable repair method using normal tissue, the technique is limited by the number of normal chordae available in valves affected by extensive disease.

Chordal shortening, where the base of the chord is buried in a trench created in the papillary muscle, is an alternative method of treating flail leaflet segments caused by chordal elongation [10]. Failure rates over 30% have been reported with chordal shortening [29]. A alternative to chordal shortening, transfer and reconstruction is papillary muscle repositioning where the taller anterior head of the posterior papillary muscle is divided from its attachments, and fixed to the shorter posterior head, effectively shortening the chordae and correcting associated leaflet prolapse[30].

Leaflet restriction, which is most commonly a feature of ischemic mitral regurgitation, is addressed by resection of restrictive secondary chordae, and division of chordal meshes [18]. Selection of an appropriate asymmetric annuloplasty ring is a useful adjunct in the treatment of tethering in the P3 region (Figure 7C). Rheumatic chordal involvement can sometimes be addressed by chordal cutting and fenestration, but extensive involvement usually means that durable repair is challenging. Currently there are no percutaneous devices designed to emulate surgical chordal repair techniques, even through chordal lesions are amongst the commonest causes of mitral regurgitation.

Papillary Muscles and Left Ventricular Wall

Papillary Muscle Anatomy

There are two papillary muscles: the anterolateral which is usually composed of one body arises from the lateral ventricular wall between the mid third and apex, and the posteromedial which has two bodies arises from the middle third to apex of the posterior septal wall. Each papillary muscle provides chordae to both leaflets. The anterolateral papillary muscle has a dual blood supply from the left anterior descending and the diagonal or marginal branches of the circumflex coronary arteries. The blood supply to the posteromedial papillary muscle comes from either the right or the circumflex coronary artery depending on the coronary dominance.

Ventricular Pathology

The lack of a dual blood supply means that the posteromedial papillary muscle is most commonly affected in acute (papillary muscle rupture) and chronic ischemic cardiomyopathy (papillary muscle dysfunction or elongation). The relationship of the papillary muscle to the lateral ventricular wall and annular plane plays the most important role in the pathogenesis of mitral regurgitation in patients with ischemic cardiomyopathy, where chronic progressive ventricular dilatation results in posterior displacement of the posteromedial papillary muscle. As the chordae tendinae remain the same length, the mitral leaflets, particularly the P2/3 region which receives chordae from the posteromedial papillary muscle are prevented from achieving full coaptation (type IIIb dysfunction). Lack of coaptation results in mitral regurgitation which further contributes to the left ventricular dysfunction and dilatation. Occasionally acute ischemia will contribute to papillary muscle dysfunction. More commonly rupture of the posteromedial papillary muscle is seen 5-10 days after acute posterior myocardial infarction resulting in acute, severe mitral regurgitation.

Papillary Muscle and Ventricular Repair Techniques

Surgical: The most commonly used repair technique for ischemic mitral regurgitation is an annuloplasty – which focuses on the mitral leaflets and annulus in a bid to compensate for subvalvular pathology. The durability of this approach has been reported to be poor in several large series[31, 32], partly because of failure to appreciate the value of a rigid, down-sized remodelling ring over partial, flexible and true-sized annuloplasty rings, inadedquate use of techniques such as chordal cutting cutting to eliminate leaflet restriction, and failure to address the underlying ventricular pathology[33, 34]. Systematic use of downsized rigid remodelling rings to treat Type IIIb dysfunction due to ischemic cardiomyopathy has been associated with better outcomes[35]. Attempts to restore normal papillary muscle geometry, such as papillary muscle relocation, have not been demonstrated to enhance long-term freedom from ischemic mitral regurgitation compared to rigid, down-sized annuloplasty alone[36], although papillary muscle shortening techniques have a useful role in Type II degenerative disease. The standard approach to acute rupture of an infarcted papillary muscle is mitral valve replacement as the durability of repair of necrotic papillary muscle tissue is poor.

Percutaneous: The only percutaneous device designed to address papillary muscle geometry is the iCoapsys device, which aimed to reposition and stabilize the papillary muscles as well as decreasing the antero-posterior mitral annular dimension. The need to place the devices across the full thickness of the anterior left ventricle wall, potentially in close proximity to the left anterior descending coronary artery presents significant technical challenges. Percutaneous revascularisation for multi-vessel disease in the setting of ischemic mitral regurgitation has not been shown to impact papillary muscle geometry, degree of regurgitation or survival.

Conclusion

Carpentier described three basic tenets of mitral valve repair over thirty years ago, which remain fundamental to successful repair today: preserve leaflet mobility, restore a large coaptation surface, and remodel the annulus[10]. The nature and combination of surgical repair techniques can be tailored precisely to the etiology of the disease process and the resultant lesions, to achieve these aims and produce a durable, competent repair. A detailed understanding of the range of valve morphology seen in mitral regurgitation also helps define the uses and limitations of percutaneous approaches to mitral valve repair.

References

[1] Bonow, R.O., et al., ACC/AHA 2006 guidelines for the management of patients with valvular heart disease: a report of the American College of Cardiology/American Heart Association Task Force on Practice Guidelines (writing committee to revise the 1998 Guidelines for the Management of Patients With Valvular Heart Disease): developed in collaboration with the Society of Cardiovascular Anesthesiologists: endorsed by the Society for Cardiovascular Angiography and Interventions and the Society of Thoracic Surgeons. *Circulation*, 2006. 114(5): p. e84-231.

[2] Bonow, R.O., et al., ACC/AHA 2006 guidelines for the management of patients with valvular heart disease: a report of the American College of Cardiology/American Heart Association Task Force on Practice Guidelines (writing Committee to Revise the 1998 guidelines for the management of patients with valvular heart disease) developed in collaboration with the Society of Cardiovascular Anesthesiologists endorsed by the Society for Cardiovascular Angiography and Interventions and the Society of Thoracic Surgeons. *J. Am. Coll. Cardiol*, 2006. 48(3): p. e1-148.

[3] Sousa Uva, M., et al., Surgical treatment of asymptomatic and mildly symptomatic mitral regurgitation. *J. Thorac. Cardiovasc. Surg*, 1996. 112(5): p. 1240-8; discussion 1248-9.

[4] Seeburger, J., et al., Minimal invasive mitral valve repair for mitral regurgitation: results of 1339 consecutive patients. *Eur. J. Cardiothorac. Surg*, 2008.

[5] Enriquez-Sarano, M., et al., Quantitative determinants of the outcome of asymptomatic mitral regurgitation. *N. Engl. J. Med*, 2005. 352(9): p. 875-83.

[6] Executive Summary STS Spring 2006 Report, 2006, The Society of Thoracic Surgery.

[7] Keogh B, K.R., The Society of Cardiothoracic Surgeons of Great Britain and Ireland Fifth National Adult Cardiac Surgical Database Report 20032004, Henley-on-Thames: Dendrite Clinical Systems.

[8] Iung, B., et al., A prospective survey of patients with valvular heart disease in Europe: The Euro Heart Survey on Valvular Heart Disease. *Eur. Heart J*, 2003. 24(13): p. 1231-43.

[9] Adams, D.H., et al., Current concepts in mitral valve repair for degenerative disease. *Heart Fail Rev,* 2006. 11(3): p. 241-57.

[10] Carpentier, A., Cardiac valve surgery--the "French correction". *J. Thorac. Cardiovasc. Surg,* 1983. 86(3): p. 323-37.

[11] Carpentier, A., et al., Reconstructive surgery of mitral valve incompetence: ten-year appraisal. *J. Thorac. Cardiovasc. Surg*, 1980. 79(3): p. 338-48.

[12] Carpentier, A.F., et al., The "physio-ring": an advanced concept in mitral valve annuloplasty. *Ann. Thorac. Surg*, 1995. 60(5): p. 1177-85; discussion 1185-6.

[13] Anyanwu, A.C. and D.H. Adams, Etiologic classification of degenerative mitral valve disease: Barlow's disease and fibroelastic deficiency. *Semin. Thorac. Cardiovasc. Surg,* 2007. 19(2): p. 90-6.

[14] Fucci, C., et al., Improved results with mitral valve repair using new surgical techniques. *Eur. J. Cardiothorac. Surg*, 1995. 9(11): p. 621-6 discuss 626-7.

[15] De Bonis, M., et al., Mitral valve repair for functional mitral regurgitation in end-stage dilated cardiomyopathy: role of the "edge-to-edge" technique. *Circulation*, 2005. 112(9 Suppl): p. I402-8.

[16] Timek, T.A., et al., Edge-to-edge mitral valve repair without ring annuloplasty for acute ischemic mitral regurgitation. *Circulation*, 2003. 108 Suppl 1: p. II122-7.

[17] Feldman, T., et al., Percutaneous mitral repair with the MitraClip system: safety and midterm durability in the initial EVEREST (Endovascular Valve Edge-to-Edge REpair Study) cohort. *J. Am. Coll. Cardiol*, 2009. 54(8): p. 686-94.

[18] Carpentier, A.A., DH. Filsoufi, F., Carpentier's Techniques of Valve Reconstruction2006, Philadelphia: W.B.Saunders.

[19] Daimon, M., et al., Mitral valve repair with Carpentier-McCarthy-Adams IMR ETlogix annuloplasty ring for ischemic mitral regurgitation: early echocardiographic results from a multi-center study. *Circulation*, 2006. 114(1 Suppl): p. I588-93.

[20] Gillinov, A.M., et al., Durability of mitral valve repair for degenerative disease. *J. Thorac. Cardiovasc. Surg,* 1998. 116(5): p. 734-43.

[21] Kaji, S., et al., Annular geometry in patients with chronic ischemic mitral regurgitation: three-dimensional magnetic resonance imaging study. *Circulation*, 2005. 112(9 Suppl): p. I409-14.

[22] Ahmad, R.M., et al., Annular geometry and motion in human ischemic mitral regurgitation: novel assessment with three-dimensional echocardiography and computer reconstruction. *Ann. Thorac. Surg*, 2004. 78(6): p. 2063-8; discussion 2068.

[23] Choure, A.J., et al., In vivo analysis of the anatomical relationship of coronary sinus to mitral annulus and left circumflex coronary artery using cardiac multidetector computed tomography: implications for percutaneous coronary sinus mitral annuloplasty. *J. Am. Coll. Cardiol*, 2006. 48(10): p. 1938-45.

[24] Maselli, D., et al., Percutaneous mitral annuloplasty: an anatomic study of human coronary sinus and its relation with mitral valve annulus and coronary arteries. *Circulation*, 2006. 114(5): p. 377-80.

[25] Gopal, A., et al., The role of cardiovascular computed tomographic angiography for coronary sinus mitral annuloplasty. *J. Invasive Cardiol*, 2010. 22(2): p. 67-73.

[26] Sousa Uva, M., et al., Transposition of chordae in mitral valve repair. Mid-term results. *Circulation*, 1993. 88(5 Pt 2): p. II35-8.

[27] David, T.E., J. Bos, and H. Rakowski, Mitral valve repair by replacement of chordae tendineae with polytetrafluoroethylene sutures. *J. Thorac. Cardiovasc. Surg,* 1991. 101(3): p. 495-501.

[28] Uva, M.S., et al., Mitral valve repair in patients with endomyocardial fibrosis. *Ann. Thorac. Surg,* 1992. 54(1): p. 89-92.

[29] Smedira, N.G., et al., Repair of anterior leaflet prolapse: chordal transfer is superior to chordal shortening. *J. Thorac. Cardiovasc. Surg*, 1996. 112(2): p. 287-91; discussion 291-2.

[30] Dreyfus, G.D., O. Souza Neto, and S. Aubert, Papillary muscle repositioning for repair of anterior leaflet prolapse caused by chordal elongation. *J. Thorac. Cardiovasc. Surg,* 2006. 132(3): p. 578-84.

[31] Grossi, E.A., et al., Ischemic mitral valve reconstruction and replacement: comparison of long-term survival and complications. *J. Thorac. Cardiovasc. Surg*, 2001. 122(6): p. 1107-24.

[32] Gillinov, A.M., et al., Is repair preferable to replacement for ischemic mitral regurgitation? *J. Thorac. Cardiovasc. Surg*, 2001. 122(6): p. 1125-41.

[33] Anyanwu, A.C. and D.H. Adams, Ischemic mitral regurgitation: recent advances. *Curr. Treat Options Cardiovasc. Med*, 2008. 10(6): p. 529-37.

[34] Filsoufi, F., et al., Physiologic basis for the surgical treatment of ischemic mitral regurgitation. *Am. Heart Hosp. J,* 2006. 4(4): p. 261-8.

[35] Braun, J., et al., Restrictive mitral annuloplasty cures ischemic mitral regurgitation and heart failure. *Ann. Thorac. Surg*, 2008. 85(2): p. 430-6; discussion 436-7.

[36] Gazoni, L.M., et al., A change in perspective: results for ischemic mitral valve repair are similar to mitral valve repair for degenerative disease. *Ann. Thorac. Surg*, 2007. 84(3): p. 750-7; discussion 758.

In: Percutaneous Valve Technology: Present and Future ISBN: 978-1-61942-577-4
Editors: Jose Luis Navia and Sharif Al-Ruzzeh

Chapter XVIII

Current Concepts for Surgical Treatment of Mitral Valve Pathology

Jose Luis Navia, Nicolas Ariel Brozzi and Sharif Al-Ruzzeh

Introduction

Mitral valve pathology affects 2,4% of the population in the United Stated, mainly manifested as mitral valve insufficiency of degenerative etiology.[1] Around twenty thousand patients require surgical treatment every year. [2]

In developing countries, however, rheumatic etiology continues to be the most prevalent cause of mitral valve pathology, causing stenosis or mixed valvular lesions.

Surgical treatment of mitral valve disease has evolved in recent years with the introduction of minimally invasive approaches through limited incisions, robotic surgery, and the development of devices designed for trascatheter implantation.

This chapter will review the general indications for surgery in mitral valve pathology, describe alternative surgical approaches, and discuss the evolution of surgical techniques.

Mitral Valve Anatomy

The mitral valve apparatus regulates blood flow during the cardiac cycle between the left atrium to the left ventricle. It is formed by three components that present continuity with both chambers: annulus, leaflets, and subvalvular apparatus.

The mitral annulus is a thin, fibrous membrane in continuity with the fibrous skeleton of the heart, and presents two segments connected by the right and left fibrous trigones. (Figure 1) The anterior segment of the mitral annulus constitutes one third of the circumference and is anatomically related to the aortic annulus (aorto mitral curtain), while the posterior segment constitutes two thirds of the circumference. Actually, the shape of the mitral annulus is better described as a hyperbolic paraboloid, resembling a riding saddle, that undergoes conformational changes along the cardiac cycle as a result of extrinsic forces imposed by adjacent atrial and ventricular musculature. [3] These changes result in a reduction of the mechanical stress exerted on the valve leaflets. [4] A simultaneous translational movement along the left ventricular major axis results from the torsion of the base of the left ventricle, and has been correlated with stroke volume. [5,6]

The mitral valve leaflets are formed by a connective tissue core covered by a layer of endocardial cells. Both leaflets present continuity with the mitral annulus with a high anterior leaflet implanting in the anterior segment of the mitral annulus, and a shorter but longer posterior leaflet arising from the posterior segment of the annulus. Both leaflets are in continuity at the commissures.

The surface area of both leaflets taken together is 2,5 times the area of the valvular orifice. In systole, the leaflets coapt over a height of approximatelly 8 mm, providing an overlapping reserve in case of annular dilation. [7] The posterior mitral leaflet presents indentations called scallops, separated by slits, that allow the leaflet to accommodate to the curved shape of the line of valve closure. [8] Three regions are identified in the ventricular side of the leaflets. The rough zone is located towards the free edge where the primary chords attach, the clear zone is located below and receiving the implantation of secondary chords, and the basal zone in the posterior leaflet receives the tertiary chords directly from the postero-lateral ventricular wall or the trabeculae carnae. Both primary and secondary chords arise from the papillary muscle heads and present a fan type distribution to both leaflets. While primary chords maintain leaflet apposition and facilitate valve closure, secondary chords play a role in maintaining normal left ventricular size and geometry. [9] Two papillary muscles (anterolateral and posteromedial) arise most frequently form the middle third of the left ventricular wall avoiding the interventricular septum, and present variable number of heads that anchor the chordate tendinae. They present autonomic inervation and contract during systole contributing to the conformational changes that maintain the competency of the mitral valve apparatus.

Segmental description of mitral valve anatomy allow surgeons to perform a thorough assessment of mitral valve apparatus to determine the most appropriate repair technique for mitral valve disease. (Figure 1)

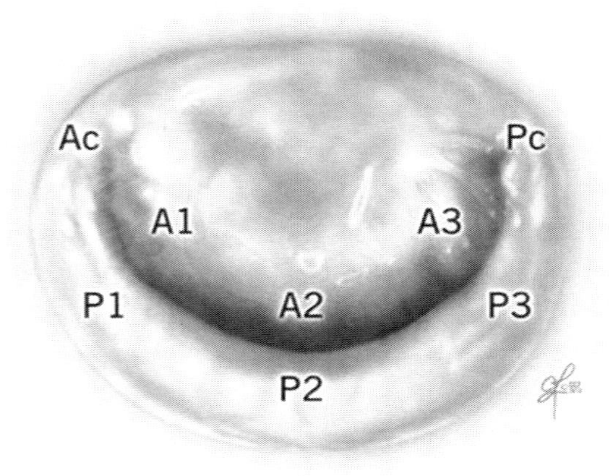

Figure 1. Segmental anatomy of the mitral leaflets.

Mitral Valve Stenosis

Mitral valve stenosis causes obstruction of the inflow tract of the left ventricle affecting left ventricular diastolic loading. Rheumatic disease is the most frequent cause of mitral stenosis, responsible for 99% of cases. Up to 40% of patients with rheumatic heart disease present isolated mitral stenosis, and 60% of patients with isolated mitral stenosis have a history of rheumatic fever. [10] Additional causes of mitral valve stenosis are rare, including congenital malformations, left atrial mixoma, mitral valve vegetations or thrombosis, carcinoid syndrome, mucopolisacaridosis, and severe annular calcification.

Women present twice the incidence of isolated mitral stenosis than men. [11] Rheumatic fever continues to be the main cause of acquired valvular disease in the world. It evolves with an acute phase characterized by a diffuse inflammatory reaction in the heart (pancarditis), most evident on the endocardium and cardiac valves, particularly the mitral valve. During this acute phase the left ventricle may become distended, with associated distention of the mitral annulus that can cause transient mitral insufficiency that resolves when the left ventricular function recovers. During the chronic stage of the disease, permanent changes occur in the heart with initial fusion of the commissures, followed by fibrosis and thickening of mitral leaflets. These structural changes of the leaflets produce turbulent blood flow that, along with the chronic inflammatory process, affect the subvalvular apparatus with thickening, shortening and fusion of chordae tendinae and papillary muscles, resulting in a funnel shape mitral apparatus with restricted motion, causing stenosis or mixed lesions including stenosis and regurgitation. [12] (Figure 2)

Normal mitral valve area is 4,0 to 5,0 cm^2. Symptoms like shortness of breath and dyspnea develop when the blood flow increases or diastolic period decreases during exercise, emotional stress, infection, pregnancy or atrial fibrillation with rapid ventricular response in patients with mitral valve area $\leq$2,5 cm^2, and are evident in a resting patient when the area is $\leq$ 1,5 cm^2. [13] Mitral stenosis associated to rheumatic disease shows a slow progression, so that patients may remain asymptomatic during 20 to 40 years, but may experience rapid deterioration when symptoms develop at advanced stages of disease. [14]

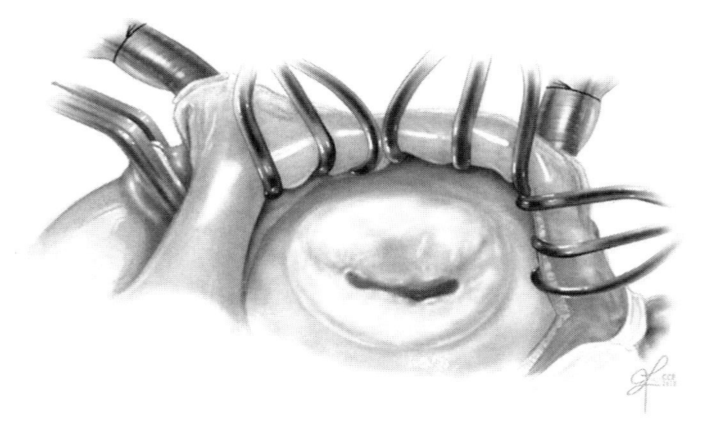

Figure 2. Intraoperative view shows changes related to mitral valve stenosis.

Table 1. Echocardiographic determinants of mitral stenosis

Severity	Mild	Moderate	Severe
Mean gradient † (mmHg)	<5	5 - 10	>10
PASP (mmHg)	<30	30 - 50	>50
Valve area (cm^2)	>1,5	1,0 – 1,5	<1,0

† Valve gradients are flow dependent and when used as estimates of severity of valve stenosis should be assessed with knowledge of cardiac output or forward flow across the valve.

* Modified from the Zoghbi WA, et al. Recommendations for evaluation of the severity of native valvular regurgitation with two-dimensional and Doppler echocardiography. *Journal of the American Society of Echocardiography* 2003;16:777–802.

Diagnosis of rheumatic mitral valve stenosis is most frequent in patients in their fifth or sixth decade of life. Long term survival is related to symptoms, so that 10 year survival is 80 % for patients asymptomatic at time of diagnosis, 50% to 60% for patients with symptoms, and 15% when severe symptoms are present. [9] Development of severe pulmonary hypertension is related to a median survival of 3 years. [15]

Diagnosis of mitral stenosis requires a complete medical history along with a thorough physical examination. Patients may be asymptomatic for many years, until they develop fatigue, exertional dyspnea, or pulmonary edema, although the initial presentation in some patients may be new onset atrial fibrillation or an embolic event. A high pitched S_1 with opening snap, and presystolic and medial systolic low pitched murmur are often present in the physical exam, although they can be absent in patients with severe pulmonary hypertension, low cardiac output or heavily calcified mitral valve.

Complimentary tests will contribute to the diagnosis, showing left atrial enlargement or pulmonary congestion on the chest X-ray; or large p waves or atrial fibrillation in the EKG. Transthoracic Doppler echocardiography is essential to evaluate cardiac dimensions and function, mitral valve morphology and presence of associated valve lesions, thrombus in the left atrial appendage, associated myocardial or pericardial pathology. [16] (Table 1) Transesophageal echocardiography should be considered when transthoracic echocardiography provides insufficient information to evaluate the morphology and severity of mitral valve disease. [17] A stress echocardiography may result usefull in sedentary patients, when a transvalvular gradient increase ≥15 mmHg or systolic pulmonary pressures ≥60 mmHg are documented, identifying patients with a clear limitation to exercise that may benefit from invasive therapy by percutaneous balloon valvulotomy or conventional surgery. When non-invasive tests results are inconclusive, or there is discrepancy between the clinical symptoms of the patient and the tests results, a left and right heart catheterization study will determine hemodynamic gradients across the valve and provide more accurate information about the severity of mitral valve stenosis and pulmonary pressures. [18] Gorlin's formula is used to estimate the mitral valve area. [19]

Surgical Treatment of Mitral Stenosis

Mitral valve commisurotomy was proposed by Brunton in 1902, but it was not until early 1950's that Harken and Bailey established the technique as a valid therapeutic alternative.

[20, 21] The original technique consisted of a thoracotomy approach to the left atrial appendage, where a purse string was sutured, and allowed the surgeon to introduce a finger or a Hegar dilator into the left atrium and through the mitral valve valve to produce mechanical dilatation of the stenotic annulus. Surgical commissurotomy can be perfomed blindly approaching the mitral valve with closed cardiac chambers through a transatrial or transventricular approach. Both techniques produce significant improvement in symptoms, and offer better long term survival than medical treatment alone. [22] Even though closed surgical commissurotomy continues to be the preferred technique in many developing countries, open commissurotomy is preferred in US and Europe, because it provides direct view of the mitral valve allowing for a more complete evaluation and treatment by dividing the commissures, separating fussed chordae tendinae and papillary muscles, and debriding deposits of calcium. [23] (Figure 3) When the compromise of the valve precludes a safe repair, mitral valve replacement should be considered. Additionally, most surgeons resect the left atrial appendage to decrease the risk of postoperative thrombo-embolic events. [24] Since most patients are referred for surgical treatment at advanced stages with extensive structural compromise of the mitral valve, only 25% of patients will benefit from a conservative surgical approach with commissurotomy, while 75% of patients will require mitral valve replacement.

The introduction of mitral balloon valvuloplasty in 1984 changed the initial approach to most patients with mitral stenosis becoming the initial therapeutic consideration for most patients with advanced mitral stenosis. [25] Surgery for moderate or severe mitral valve stenosis is indicated in symptomatic patients (NYHA III-IV) with acceptable operative risk when percutaneous ballon valvuloplasty is not possible, or is contraindicated by the presence of left atrial thrombus,moderate to severe mitral insufficiency, or unsuitable anatomy (indication class I, level of evidence B). Symptomatic patients with severe mitral stenosis and concomitant moderate to severe mitral insufficiency should receive valve replacement, unless mitral valve repair is possible at time of surgery (indication class I, level of evidence C). Mitral valve replacement is considered reasonable in patients with severe mitral stenosis and severe pulmonary hypertension (>60 mmHg) with NYHA I-II symptoms who are not candidates for ballon valvuloplasty or mitral valve repair (indication class IIa, level of evidence C).

Table 2. Echocardiographic grading system based on mitral valve characteristics *

Grade	Leaflet mobility	Subvalvular thickening	Leaflet Thickening	Calcification
1	High	Minimal	Near normal (4-5 mm)	Single area
2	Normal mid and basal leaflet motion	Proximal 1/3 of chordal structures	Thickened margins (5-8 mm)	Scattered marginal areas
3	Base of leaflets move forward in diastole	Down to distal 1/3 of the chords	Diffuse (5-8 mm)	Extends to mid portion of leaflets
4	No movement of leaflets in diastole	Extensive compromise down to papillary muscles	Diffuse (>8-10 mm)	Most areas of both leaflets

* Adapted from Wilkins G. et al. Percutaneous balloon dilatation of the mitral valve: an analysis of echocardiographic variables related to outcome and the mechanism of dilatation. *Br. Heart J.* 1988;60:299-308.

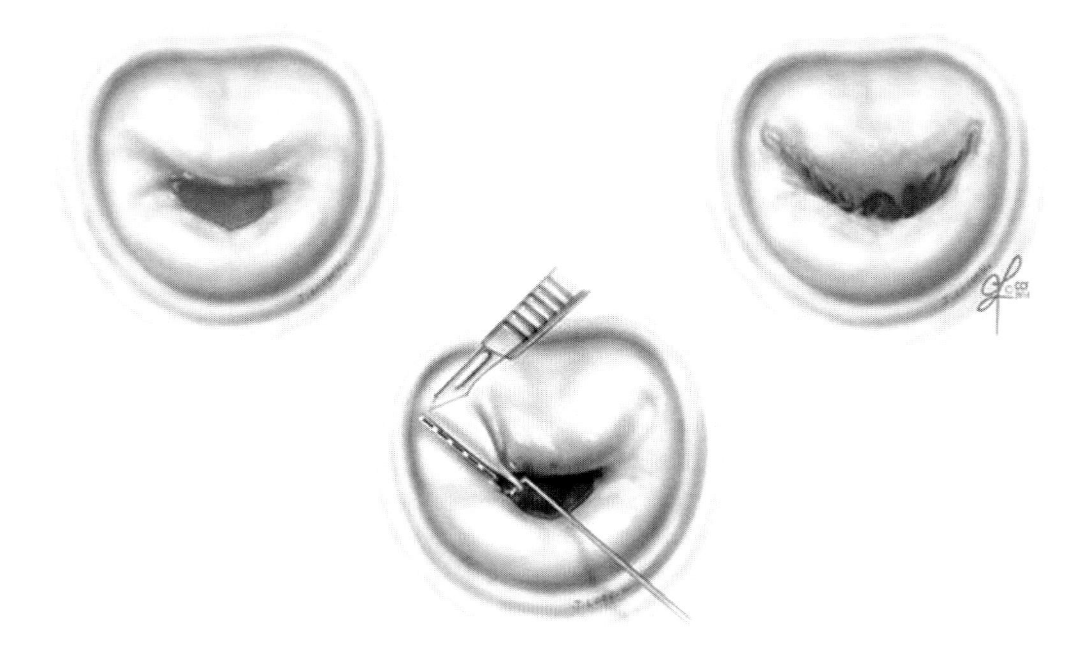

Figure 3. Surgical mitral commisurotomy.

Mitral valve repair can be considered in asymptomatic patients with moderate to severe mitrals stenosis and favorable anatomy for valvular repair that present recurrent embolic events while on adequate anticoagulation therapy (indication class IIb, level of evidence C).

Mitral valve replacement is a valid alternative in patients with severe mitral valve stenosis that are not candidates for percutaneous ballon valvuloplasty or surgical commissurotomy. Symptomatic patient with severe mitral stenosis and moderate to severe pulmonary hypertension (>50 mmHg) constitute a high risk group for hospital mortality after mitral valve replacement that has been reported between 5% and 20%. [26] Operative morality is particularly increased in patients with pulmonary hypertension in the range of systemic pressures, in patients with acute congestive heart failure, and severe left or right ventricular dysfunction. In patients with extensive compromise of the mitral valve requiring mitral valve replacement significant postoperative symptomatic improvement is observed with 5 and 10 years survival of 80 % and 64%, respectively.

Transcatheter Mitral Balloon Valvuloplasty

Transcatheter mitral baloon valvuloplasty was described by Inoue et al in 1984, and followed the same basic therapeutic principles of the original surgical techniques, but was performed by percutaneous placement of a balloon inside the mitral valve that could be insufflated to produce progressive dilatation of the mitral annulus. [25] By opening the commissures that were fussed by the rheumatic process, mitral valve area is increased and transvalvular gradients decrease. Patients with movile, non-calcified mitral valves, with minimal fussion of the subvalvular apparatus obtain the best therapeutic results. [27]

Wilkins' echocardiographic score estimates the possibility of performing a successful mitral valvuloplasty by assigning points (1-4 points) according to the compromise of the different components of the mitral valve apparatus. (Table 2) A score lower than 8 points indicates high chances of performing a successful percutaneous mitral valvuloplasty. [28]

The following indications have been described for percutaneous mitral balloon valvuloplasty: [27]

Class I: symptomatic patients (NYHA II-IV) with moderate to severe mitral stenosis and favorable valve anatomy, in patients without left atrial thrombus or moderate to severe mitral insufficiency (level of evidence A), and in patients with baseline pulmonary systolic arterial pressure greater than 50 mmHg or grater than 60 mmHg during exercise (level of evidence C).

Class II a: symptomatic patients (NYHA FC III-IV) with moderate or severe mitral stenosis and favorable anatomy that are considered high risk or not candidates for surgical treatment (level of evidence C).

Class II b: percutaneous mitral balloon valvuloplasty can be considered for asymptomatic patients with moderate or severe mitral stenosis and favorable anatomy that present recent onset atrial fibrillation, with no evidence of left atrial appendage thrombus or mitral insufficiency (level of evidence C), in symptomatic patients (NYHA II-IV) with mitral valve area greater than 1,5 cm^2 and hemodinamic findings of severe mitral stenosis (level of evidence C), and can be considered an alternative to surgery for symptomatic patients in NYHA III-IV functional class and favorable anatomy (level of evidence C).

Percutaneous mitral balloon valvuloplasty is contraindicated in patients with left atrial thrombus, moderate or severe mitral stenosis, severe calcification or the mitral valve or severe pathology of the subvalvular apparatus.

Similar early hemodynamic results and complication rates have been reported for both percutaneous balloon valvuloplasty and closed surgical commissurotomy techniques but valvuloplasty would offer more sustained symptomatic relief and improved long-term results. [29] Two studies comparing open surgical commissurotoy with percutaneous balloon valvuloplasty reported similar results with surgical open commissurotomy and percutaneous balloon valvuloplasty. [30, 31]

In the follow up to seven years mitral valve restenosis presented in 6,6% of patients after balloon valvuloplasty versus 33% in the closed commissurotomy technique; while 87%, and 90% of patients that had received balloon valvuloplasty or open commissurotmy remained in NYHA class I, versus only 33% of patients that received closed mitral commissurotomy.

The lower morbidity associated to the percutaneous nature of balloon valvuloplasty, which does not require thoracotomy or cardiopulmonary by-pass, has led some authors to propose it as the initial intervention for patients with symptomatic moderate to severe mitral valve stenosis. [30] However, some authors have argued that open mitral commissurotomy provides larger mitral valve areas, a better functional recovery, and a lower incidence of late mitral regurgitation after the procedure. [31] Current indications for open mitral commissurotomy include presence of left atrial thrombus, severe subvalvular disease, mitral valve calcification, associated disease of other valves, and failure or restenosis after closed or ballon mitral valvuloplasty. Excellent results with operative mortality below 1%, and 10 year freedom from mitral valve failure of 87% have been reported. [32]

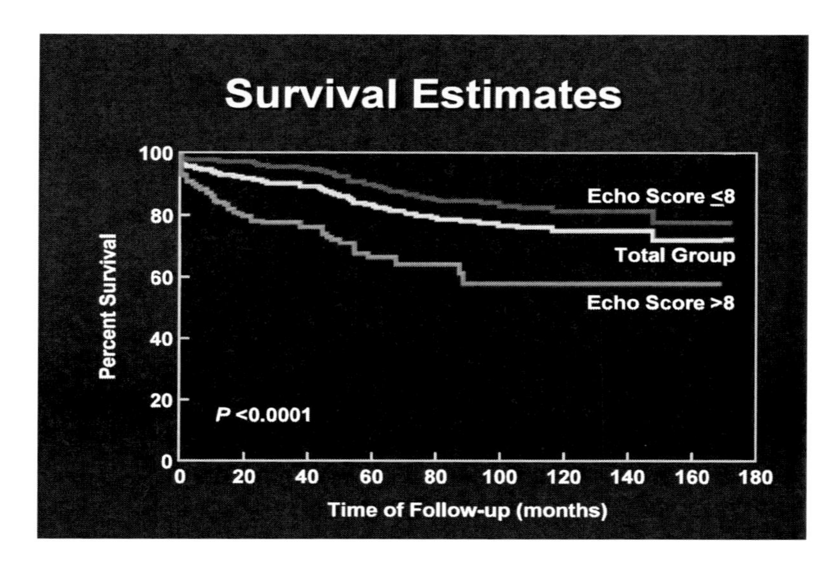

Figure 4. Survival curves after mitral balloon valvuloplasty.

Mitral valve morphology plays a major role in the outcome of percutaneous mitral valvuloplasty. Presence of fussed commissures and severe calcification are associated with higher rate of complications and symptoms recurrence, while patients with non-calcified movable leaflets, with mild subvalvular fussion, and no commissural calcium present high therapeutic success rate (>90%), with low complication rates (<3%), and sustained long-term symptomatic improvement in 80% to 90% of patients. [33] Independents predictors of combined events at long-term follow up and mortality after mitral ballon valvuloplasty include echocardiographic score ≥8, age, prior commissurotomy, NYHA IV, elevated pulmonary arterial pressures, and degree of mitral valve regurgitation particularly when ≥2 before the procedure, or ≥3 after the procedure (Figure 4). [34]

Patients older than 65 years of age have been reported to obtain less benefit from mitral valvuloplasty with success rates of 50%, more complications, and higher mortality associated to the procedure. This may reflect a population of sicker patients with more advanced disease at time of intervention. [35]

Symptomatic improvement after surgical commissurotomy or percutaneous baloon valvulotomy is almost immediate, with improvement in hemodynamic parameters manifested as a decrease in left atrial and pulmonary artery pressures, a decrease in pulmonary arteriolar resistance, and increase in cardiac output. These parameters can continue to improve for several months after the procedure. [36]

Mitral Valve Insufficiency

Etiology of Mitral Valve Insufficiency

Degenerative mitral insufficiency is the most frequent indication for surgical repair of the mitral valve in the United States, accounting for more than 50% of cases. [37, 38, 39, 40, 41] Rheumatic fever is still the most common cause of mitral valve disease in developing countries, frequently causing a combination of regurgitation and stenosis that requires surgical intervention in advanced stages. [11] Other causes of mitral regurgitation include ischemic disease, as up to 30% of patients evaluated for coronary surgery present with some degree of mitral valve insufficiency, infective endocarditis that results in pure mitral regurgitation in 2% to 8% of patients, connective tissue disease such as Marfan's Syndrome and Ehlers-Danlos Syndrome, and idipathic calcification of the mitral annulus. [42]

Most common pathologic changes related to degenerative mitral valve insufficiency include annular dilatation, leaflet thickening, mixomatous degeneration, elongation and rupture of chordae tendinae, and annular or leaflet calcification. [43, 44, 45]

Carpentier described three basic mechanisms of mitral insufficiency: [46] (Figure 5)

Type I: normal leaflet motion, related mainly to annular dilatation, or leaflet perforation.
Type II: excessive leaflet motion, including leaflet prolapse and chordal elongation or rupture.
Type III: restricted leaflet motion, subdivided into restricted opening (IIIa), and restricted closure (IIIb)

Mitral Valve Prolapse

Mitral valve prolapse is defined as the systolic protrusion of one or both mitral leaflets towards the left atrium with or without concomitant mitral insufficiency. Echocardiography definition includes mitral leaflet prolapse of more than 2 mm above the plane of the mitral annulus in the long parasternal axis view, that may be accompanied by leaflet thickening (>5 mm) with or without mitral regurgitation. [47] The incidence of mitral valve prolapse is about 1% to 2,5% of the general population. [48] Up to 5% of patients with mitral valve prolapse will develop moderate to severe mitral insufficiency that require surgical treatment. [49] Posterior leaflet prolapse is the most frequent cause of mitral insufficiency requiring surgical treatment. [53, 55] Surgical repair offers the best long-term results in spite of preserving and using pathologic leaflet tissue to perform the repair. [50]

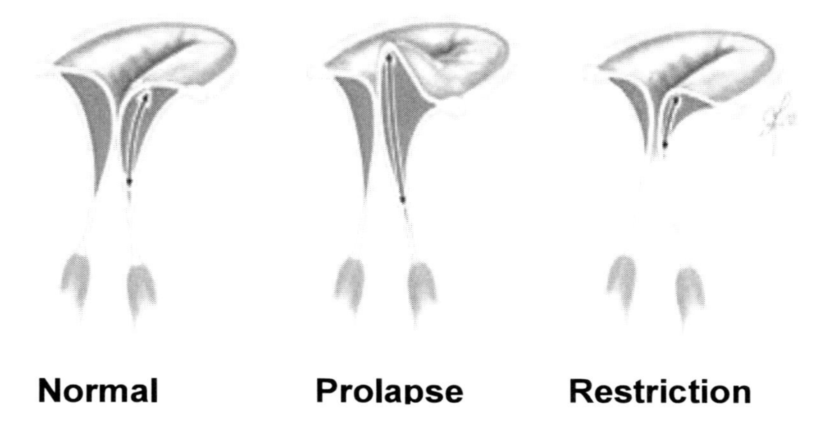

Figure 5. Carpentier's classification for mechansims of mitral valve insufficiency.

The natural history of patients with asymptomatic mitral valve prolapse is widely heterogeneous, with most patients presenting a benign evolution with normal life expectancy, to subsets with high morbidity or even excess mortality directly related to development of mitral regurgitation. [51] Patients with asymptomatic prolapse but moderate to severe mitral regurgitation and left ventricular dysfunction lower than 50% face a 10 year mortality of 45% that represents the strongest argument to offer them surgical treatment.

Progression of mitral insufficiency is variable and determined by progression of lesions or mitral annulus size. [52] Gradual progression of chronic mitral insufficiency results in progressive dilatation of left atrium and left ventricle. The resulting increase in left ventricular end-diastolic volume permits an increase in total stroke volume to compensate for the increasing regurgitant volume and to restore forward cardiac output. [53] During the compensated phase of mitral regurgitation, the increase in left ventricular and left atrial size allows accommodation of the regurgitant volume at lower filling pressures, deferring the development of symptoms. This compensated phase is variable and patients may remain asymptomatic for many years. The prolonged burden of volume overload will eventually overcome compensatory mechanisms resulting in left ventricular dysfunction with increase in left ventricular filling pressures and atrial fibrillation. [47] Increasing pressures in the pulmonary circulation can generate right ventricular dysfunction. These hemodynamic events result in reduced forward output and patients can enter a phase of rapid deterioration. [54] Development of complications associated to mitral valve prolapse is low, with spontaneous chord rupture being the most frequent complication, followed by infective endocarditis, fibrinous microembolization that has been related to transient visual symptoms and rarely, complex ventricular tachiarhythmias that can lead to sudden death.

Natural history of degenerative mitral disease with severe valve insufficiency presents an annual mortality of 6% - 7%. Over 10 years, 90% of symptomatic patients with severe mitral insufficiency will require surgical treatment or die. Patients at highest risk for death are those with ejection fraction below 60%, and those with NYHA functional class III-IV symptoms. [55]

Clinical improvement after surgery is more limited when preoperative symptoms have progressed to NYHA functional class III-IV. [56]

Diagnostic Evaluation of Patients with Mitral Valve Insufficiency

Clinical history along with a through physical examination are the mainstays of diagnosis for patients with mitral valve regurgitation. Displacement of left ventricular apical impulse indicates cardiac enlargement secondary to severe chronic mitral regurgitation. A third heart sound and early diastolic rumble are usually present, and findings consistent with pulmonary hypertension may also be present. Complimentary exams play a major role in the staging of patients and evaluation of their condition. An ECG will provide information about the rhythm while the chest X-ray will provide images of the cardiac silhouette, pulmonary vascularity and pulmonary congestion.

Transthoracic echocardiogram plays a major role to assess the severity of mitral regurgitation, morphology of heart chambers, and the underlaying mechanism of disease. Pulmonary pressure may be estimated, along with left ventricular size and function. It provides baseline parameters for follow up as well as parameters related to worse prognosis that may determine the indication of surgery even for asymptomatic patients (Table 3).

Left ventriculography and hemodynamic measurements are indicated when noninvasive tests are inconclusive regarding severity of mitral valve regurgitation, and left ventricular function, when pulmonary artery pressure is out of proportion to the severity of mitral regurgitation, and when there is a discrepancy between clinical and noninvasive findings regarding severity of mitral regurgitation. Coronary angiography is performed before mitral valve surgery in patients at risk for coronary artery disease. [47]

Indications for Surgery

Surgery is the most appropriate treatment for symptomatic patients with mitral valve insufficiency and normal left ventricular function. Mitral valve repair is the operation of choice when the valve is suitable for repair as it preserves native tissues without prosthesis, avoiding the risk of chronic anticoagulation or prosthetic valve failure late after surgery. Preserving the mitral apparatus leads to better postoperative left ventricular function and survival. [57] A Maze procedure or current alternatives should be performed at time of mitral valve surgery in patients presenting with atrial fibrillation because normal sinus rhythm can be obtained in most patients, avoiding the need for chronic anticoagulation, and reducing the risk of postoperative embolic stroke.

Current ACC/AHA guidelines for the management of patients with valvular heart disease consider the following indications for surgery of the mitral valve. [47]

Class I Indications:

- Symptomatic patients with acute severe mitral insufficiency (Level of Evidence B)
- Symptomatic patients with chronic severe mitral insufficiency with left ventricular function > 30% and end-dyastolic diameter < 55mm (Level of Evidence C)
- Asymptomatic patients with severe chronic mitral insufficiency and mild to moderate left ventricular dysfunction (LVEF 30% to 60% and end-systolic left ventricular diameter $\geq$0,40) (Level of Evidence B)

Mitral valve repair rather than replacement is recommended for most patients with severe chronic mitral insufficiency requiring surgery, and patients should be referred to centers experienced in mitral valve repair (Level of Evidence C).

Class II indications:

Mitral valve surgery is considered reasonable (Class IIa) in the following group of asymptomatic patients with chronic severe mitral insufficiency and normal left ventricular function:

- Surgery to be performed in a center of large experience and high indices on mitral valve repair without residual mitral insufficiency in more than 90% of patients (Level of Evidence B)
- New onset of atrial fibrillation (Level of Evidence C)
- Pulmonary arterial hypertension (> 50 mmHg at rest, or > 60 mmHg with exercise) (Level of Evidence C).

- Patients with severe chronic mitral insufficiency primarily related to anomalies of mitral valve apparatus presenting with symptoms in NYHA functional class III-IV, with severe left ventricular dysfunction (LVEF < 30% and left ventricular end-systolic diameter > 55mm) provided high chances of reparability (Level of Evidence C).

Mitral valve repair may also be considered for patients with chronic severe secondary mitral regurgitation due to severe left ventricular dysfunction who have persistent HYHA functional class III-IV symptoms despite optimal therapy for heart failure, including biventricular pacing. (Indication Class IIb, Level of Evidence C).

Table 3. Determinants of severity of mitral valve regurgitation

Degree of mitral regurgitation	Mild	Moderate	Severe
Qualitative			
Angiographic grade	1	2	3-4
Color Doppler jet area	Small, central jet (less than 4 cm2 or less than 20% LA area)	Signs of MR greater than mild present but no criteria for severe MR	Vena contracta width greater than 0.7 cm with large central MR jet (area greater than 40% of LA area) or with a wallimpinging jet of any size, swirling in LA
Doppler vena contracta width (cm)	< 0.3	0.3–0.69	≥ 0.70
Quantitative (cath or echo)			
Regurgitant volume (ml per beat)	<30	30–59	≥ 60
Regurgitant fraction (%)	< 30	30–49	≥ 50
Regurgitant orifice area (cm2)	< 0.20	0.2–0.39	≥ 0.40
Additional essential criteria			
Left atrial size			Enlarged
Left ventricular size			Enlarged

Valve gradients are flow dependent and when used as estimates of severity of valve stenosis should be assessed with knowledge of cardiac output or forward flow across the valve.

* Modified from the Zoghbi WA, et al. Recommendations for evaluation of the severity of native valvular regurgitation with two-dimensional and Doppler echocardiography. *Journal of the American Society of Echocardiography* 2003;16:777–802.

The type of procedure considered as well as the skill and experience of the surgical team may influence the optimal timing for surgery. Highly experienced teams with high mitral valve repair success rate may have a lower threshold to indicate surgery in asymptomatic or mildly symptomatic patients at the earliest echocardiographic development of signs of ventricular function deterioration.

Nonrheumatic posterior leaflet prolapse due to degenerative mitral valve disease or a ruptured chordae tendineae can usually be repaired by a limited leaflet resection and annuloplasty, while pathologic involvement of the anterior mitral leaflet or both leaflets make the repair more challenging and affect long term prognosis. [43] Rheumatic involvement and calcification of mitral annulus or leaflets decrease the chances of repair even in experienced hands. [58]

The STS cardiac surgery database shows that mitral valve repair has increased in the Unites States in the last decade. A report over 58.370 patients that received isolated mitral valve surgery in more than 900 US hospitals shows an increase in mitral valve repair from 51% in the year 2000 to 69% in the year 2007. Among patients receiving mitral valve replacement, the implantation of mechanical valves decreased in the same period from 68% to 37%. Hospital mortality for mitral valve replacement was 3,8% versus 1,4% global mortality for mitral valve repair, and 0,6% mortality for mitral repair in asymptomatic patients. [59]

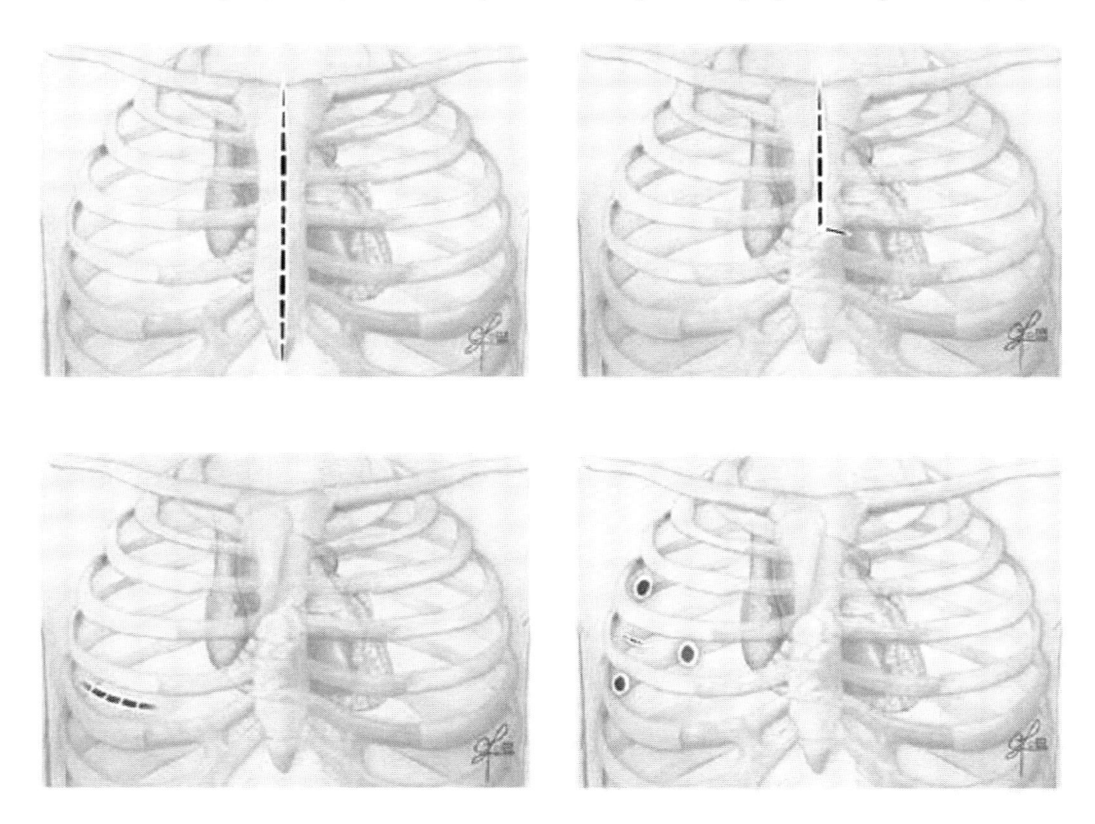

Figure 6. Approaches for mitral valve surgery include median sternotomy (A), limited upper hemisternotomy (B), limited right anterior thoracotomy (C), and port-access incisions for robotically assisted techniques (D).

The indication for surgical repair of the mitral valve in asymptomatic patients is controversial, but most authors agree that surgery should be considered when signs of left ventricular dysfunction are present in echocardiography, as surgery will likely prevent further deterioration of ventricular function and improve long-term survival.

Another dilemma arises when considering the indication for surgery in a symptomatic patient with mitral insufficiency and severe left ventricular dysfunction as it is often difficult to distinguish primary cardiomyopathy with secondary mitral regurgitation from primary mitral regurgitation with secondary myocardial dysfuntion. When the primary problem is mitral regurgitation, surgery should still be contemplated if mitral valve repair appears likely, as it will contribute to prevent further left ventricular function deterioration and improve symptoms. [60]

Mitral valve repair should always be considered as the initial surgical treatment for mitral insufficiency, as it preserves native valve leaflets and the chordal apparatus, preserves left ventricular function and is associated with improved long-term survival compared to mitral valve replacement with disruption of subvalvular apparatus. [61] If repair cannot be accoplished and replacement of the mitral valve is performed, every effort should be made to preserve the chordal apparatus in order to preserve left ventricular geometry, and prevent left ventricular dilatation and progressive dysfunction.

The long-term freedom from reoperation is similar for mitral valve repair and replacement, with 7% to 10% reoperation rate at 10 years in patients undergoing mitral valve repair, usually for severe recurrent mitral regurgitation. [62]

Surgical Procedures for Mitral Valve Pathology

Surgical Approach (Figure 6)

Multiple approaches have been described to expose the mitral valve, since the original descriptions through a left thoracotomy with a purse-string suture of the left atrial appendaje, allowing to blindly enter a dilator into the left atrium and through the mitral valve.

Median stenotomy has been the standard approach for many years and still remains the first choice when concomitant cardiac procedures are perfomed. (Figure 6 A) Alternativelly, an upper hemisternotomy followed by incision of the right atrium and the interatrial septum provides excellent exposure of the mitral and tricuspid valves using conventional intruments. (Figure 6 B)

Technological development over the last two decades has contributed to advance the field of minimally invasive mitral valve surgery, approaching the valve through a limited right thoracotomy (6-8 cm incision in the forth intercostal space); or endoscopically with incicions that are smaller than one inch by using robotic surgical techniques. (Figures 6 C, and 6 D) The visualization of the mitral valve with these techniques is excellent, particullarly with the robotic technology. However, both approaches require peripheral cannulation to establish cardiopulmonary by-pass, and their indication is limited by advanced peripheral vascular disease or in the presence of small femoral arteries.

In 1996 our group introduced less Invasive approaches for treating myxomatous mitral valve disease to reduce trauma while preserving the safety and quality achieved by surgery through complete sternotomy. [53, 54] Partial upper sternotomy. (Figure 7), and limited right mini-anterolateral thoracotomy (Figure 8) reduce incision size while still allowing surgery under direct visualization using conventional instruments. [55, 56, 57] Robotic mitral valve repair represents the latest development in less invasive surgery, and is the least invasive approach for mitral valve repair. [58] (Figure 9). A recent data from Cleveland Clinic Foundation compared the four alternative approaches for repair of posterior mitral valve prolapse including conventional median sternotomy, partial sternotomy, right mini-anterolateral thoracotomy, and robotic surgery, showing that robotic repair is as safe and effective as conventional approaches. Even though technical complexity of robotic approach was related to longer operative times, this is compensated for by lesser invasiveness and shorter hospital stay that is about 1 day lower than with any of the other three approaches. [68]

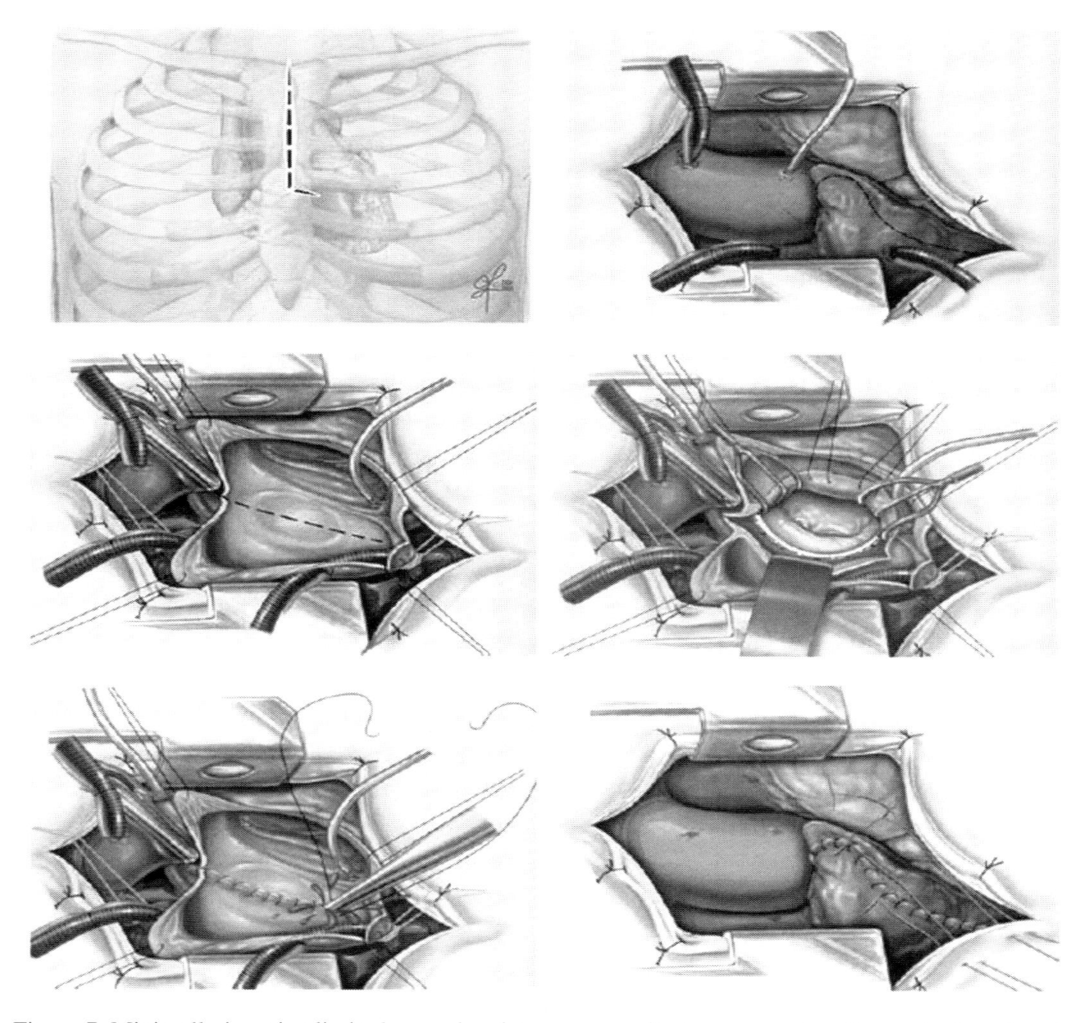

Figure 7. Minimally invasive limited upper hemisternotomy mitral valve repair with annuloplasty band.

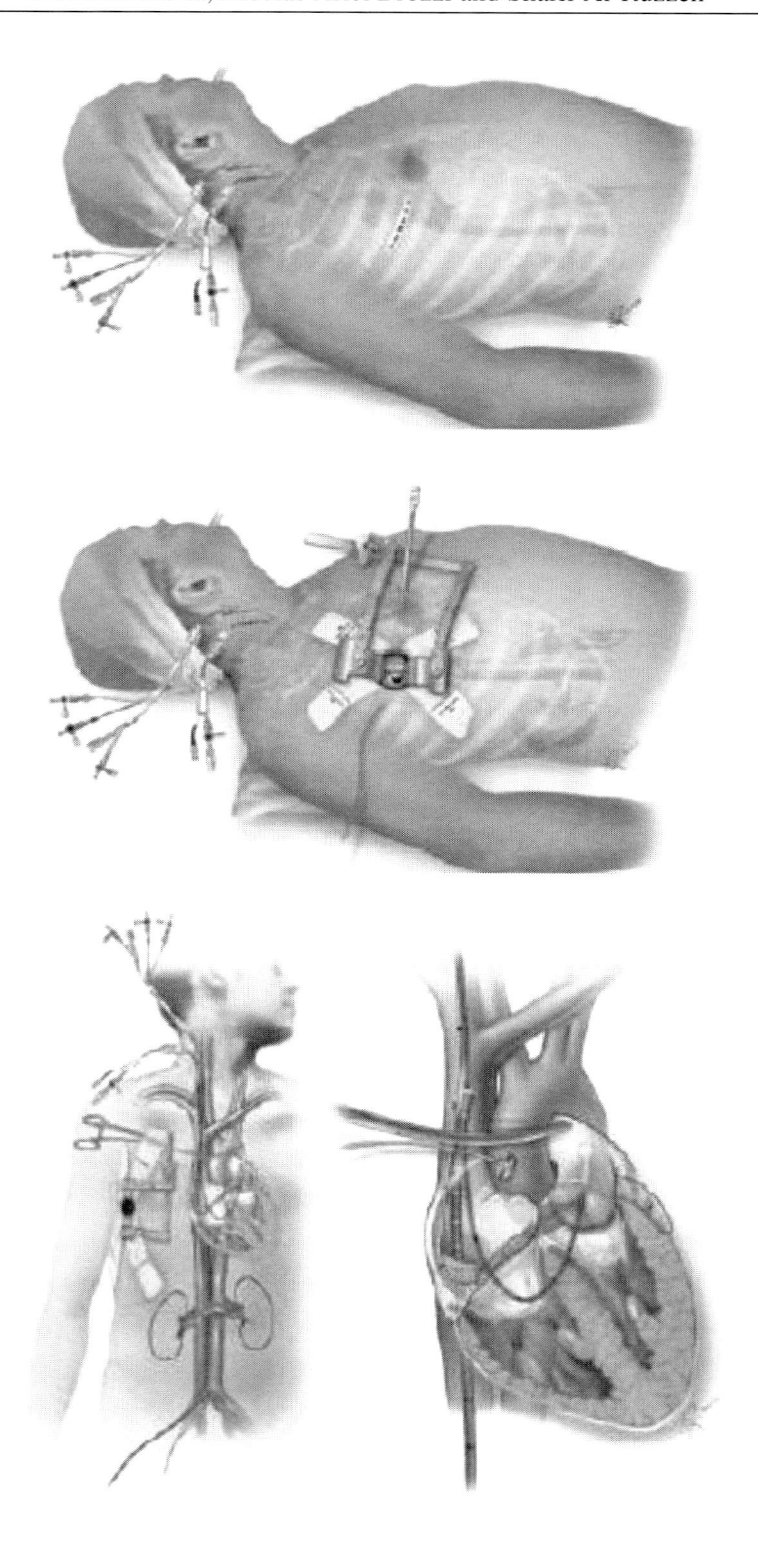

Figures 8. Right thoracotomy mitral valve surgery.

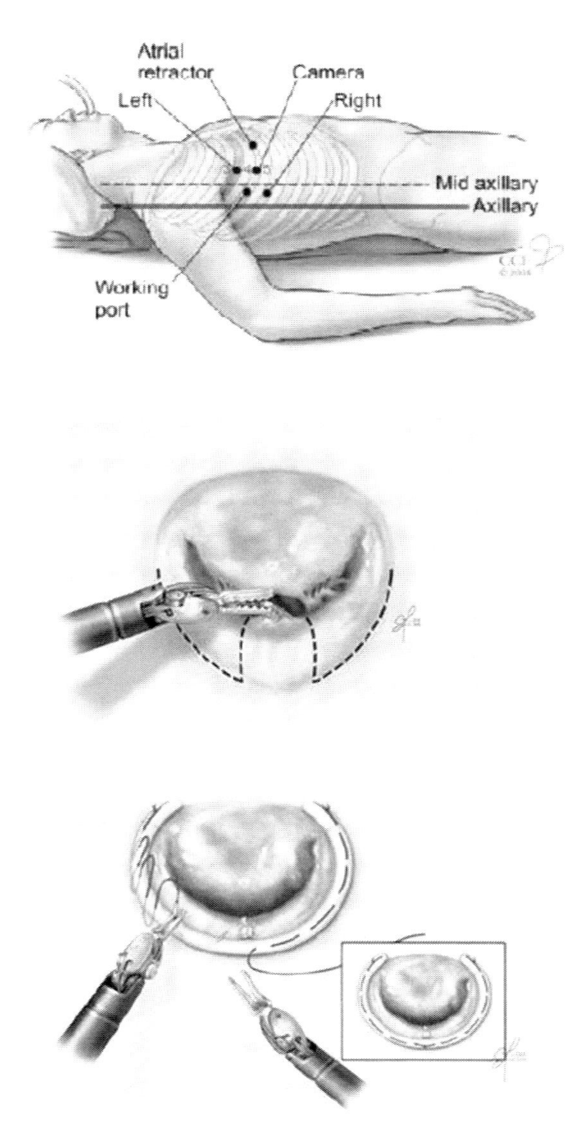

Figure 9. Robotic mitral valve repair employs videoscopic techniques and remote directed instruments to perform the repair.

Cannulation strategies for cardiopulmonary by-pass in the less invasive techniques of right mini-thoracotomy and robotic approaches require peripheral cannulation of both femoral artery and vein, and sometimes additional venous drainage through the internal yugular vein from the superior vena cava. Additionally, surgeons performing these techniques require specific trainning using long-shafted instruments for the right thoracotomy approach or specific training to work with the robot. In contrast, limited sternotomy approaches can be performed under direct vision with single lumen intubation, regular cannulation techniques and conventional instruments.

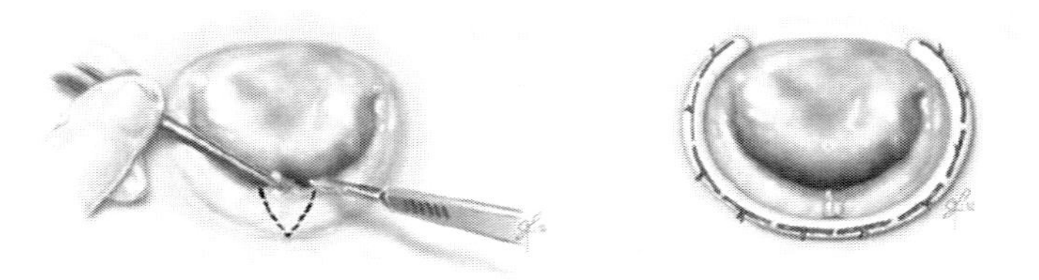

Figure 10 A. Limited resection with primary approximation of edges and band annuloplasty.

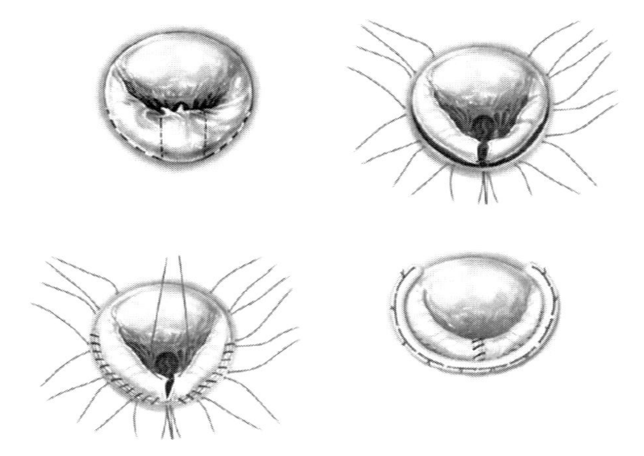

Figure 10 B. More complex repair involving resection of one segment, with additional sliding technique of adjacent segments, and band annuloplasty.

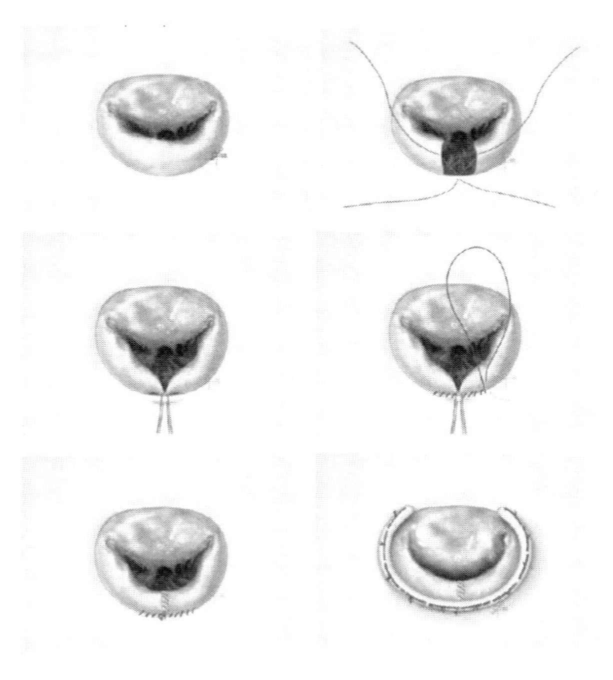

Figure 10 C. Folding repair, a less complex repair technique involving resection of one segment, without additional sliding technique of adjacent segments, and band annuloplasty.

The mitral valve can be exposed through different cardiac incisions, including direct left atriotomy through Sondergaard's groove with retraction of the interatrial septum, or right atriotomy and transeptal approach which is most frequently used when performing an upper median hemisternotomy, or when performing additional procedures on the tricuspid valve or Maze procedure.

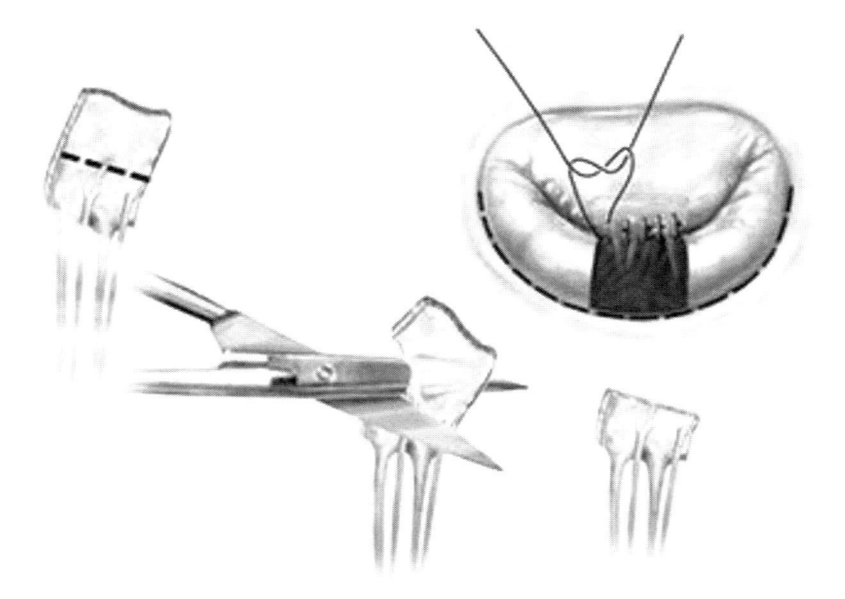

Figure 11. Chordal transfer from a segment of posterior leaflet to improve anterior leaflet diastolic apposition.

Interventions over the Mitral Valve

Three surgical interventions are used in the treatment of mitral valve insufficiency, including mitral valve repair, mitral valve replacement preserving the valve apparatus, and mitral valve replacement with resection of the mitral valve apparatus. Each procedure has specific indications, benefits and disadvantages. The type and severity of the valvular lesion, along with the surgical experience of the operating team will determine the technique that will be employed in any specific case, but mitral valve repair is the procedure of choice every time it can be accomplished because it preserves native valve tissues, mantains fluid dynamics within the left heart, avoids the risks related to chronic anticoagulation exept in those patients that require it for atrial fibrillation, and does not present risks related to prosthetic valve failure. Preserving the subvalvular apparatus mantains left ventricular geometry and is associated to better ventricular function and improved long-term survival. [69, 70, 71, 72, 73]

Mitral valve replacement preserving the subvalvular apparatus provides a competent mitral prosthesis, preserves left ventricular geometry contributing to preserve left ventricular function and improve long-term survival in comparison to mitral valve replacement with resection of the subvalvular apparatus. (Figures 12 A and B) Disadvantages related to prosthetic valve implantation include risk of paravalvular leak, hemolisis, infection, long-term prosthetic deterioration for tissue valves oscilating between 12% and 15% at 15 years, and mechanical valves carry additional risks related to chronic anticoagulation. [74, 75]

Mitral valve replacement with resection of the subvalvular apparatus is infrequent and should only be performed when there are no alternatives to preserve at least part ot it. Artificial chords have expanded the possibilities to reparir some mitral valves in patients with advanced rheumatic disease. [76]

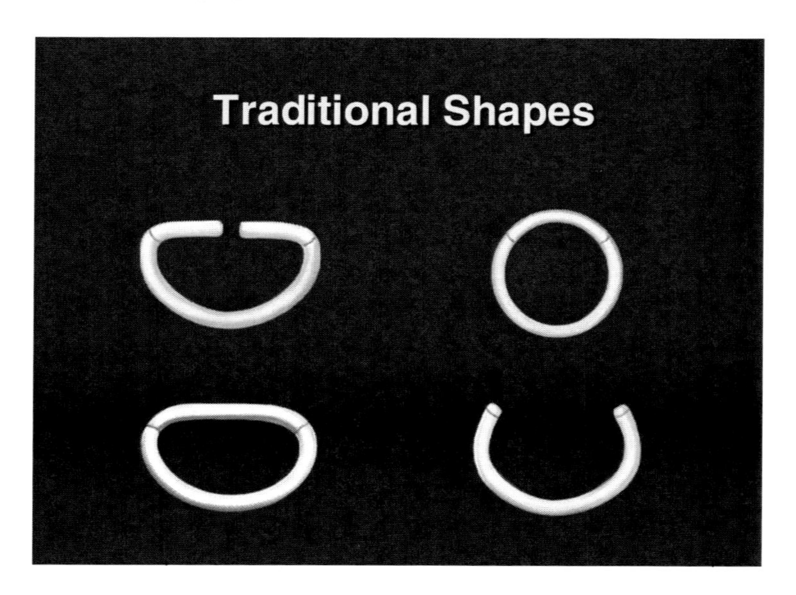

Figure 12 A. Mitral Annuloplasty Rings.

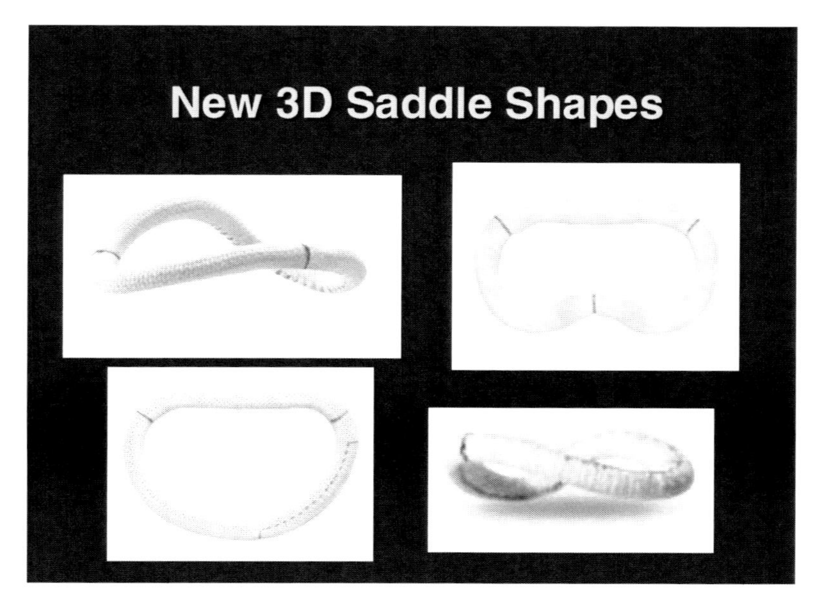

Figure 12 B. Mitral 3D Saddle Shape Annuloplasty Rings.

Repair of the Mitral Valve

Mitral valve repair offers benefit to a wide range of patients with mitral valve insufficiency. In asymptomatic patients with normal left ventricular function and severe mitral valve insufficiency, repairing the valve will prevent the deletereous effects of chronic volume overload; while in patients with advanced symptoms related to severe mitral insufficiency with left ventricular dysfunction, repairing the mitral valve and preserving the mitral apparatus mantains the ventricular geometry, and prevents further ventricular deterioration that could occur after replacement of the mitral valve. [77] The recurrence of severe mitral regurgitation is very low with only 7% to 10% of patients requiring reoperation over 10 years of follow up.[62, 43] The best results are achieved when only the posterior leaflet is repaired with 96% freedom from reoperation at 12 years, in comparison to 94% and 88% for both leaflets, or anterior leaflet repair respectively. [45]

Intraoperative echocardiography allows the surgeon to determine the underlying mechanism of mitral valve insufficiency to implement the best repair technique in each patient, and has become standard of practice when performing mitral valve repair as it has been related to the best long-term outcomes with over 98% freedom from reoperation at 10 years.

Mitral Valve Repair Techniques

Carpentier's clasification of functional mechanisms associated to mitral valve insufficiency standardized the intraoperative evaluation of mitral valve anatomy and the criteria for repair. Individual evaluation of each of the eight functional segments of the mitral valve (Figure 1) provides a systematic description of the mechanism of mitral insufficiency: Type I with normal leaflet movement; type II with leaflet prolapse; and type III with restricted leaflet movement during dyastole (IIIa) or systole (IIIb). (Figure 5). [46]

Mitral valve repair techniques are tailored to correct the mechanism responsible for the valve incompetence. Every attempt is made to repair the mitral valve with native tissue. Technical complexity can vary from a simple approximation of medial segments of both leaflets, to a procedure involving both leaflets with chordal transposition, or artificial chords implant, and ring annuloplasty. In cases requiring limited resections, leaflet edges can generally be reaproximated (Figures 10 A), while more extensive resections may require movilization of adjacent segments to be repositioned and approximated ("sliding technique") (Figure 10 B), or a folding repair, consisting on a limited resection without additional sliding of adjacent segments (Figure 10 C)

When chordal elongation or rupture cause segmental leaflet prolapse, chordal transfer from another redundant segment can be considered (Figure 11). Artificial chordaes offer an alternative solution with very high rate of success when utilized for repair of degenerative mitral valve disease and excellent long-term results and over 85% of patients free of recurrent mitral insufficiency at 15 years in recently published series. [78, 79] In all cases, an annuloplasty band is used to reinforce the repair , increase leaflet copatation when necessary, and optimize long-term valve competency.

Several types of mitral annuloplasty rings are used to complete the repair, depending on the mechanism of mitral insufficiency. Flexible bands are used in degenerative mitral valve disease with dilatation limited to the posterior segment of the mitral annulus (Figure 12 A), while more rigid and complete annuloplasty rings with 3D saddle shape are used when severe anular dilatation involving the anterior segment of the mitral annulus is present like in patients with congestive heart disease or ischemic myocardial pathology with associated mitral insufficiency (Figure 12 B).

Specific conditions

The following section describes several conditions that may require particular diagnostic and therapeutic considerations.

a) Ischemic Mitral Regurgitation

Ischemic cardiomyopathy is the most common cause of heart failure in the United States. This advanced form of coronary artery disease is marked by diffuse myocardial damage, left ventricular remodeling, and often functional ischemic mitral regurgitation (MR). [80] Ischemic mitral regurgitation is estimated to affect 2.8 million Americans and is associated with worse survival prognosis.

The MV itself is usually anatomically normal, and MR is secondary to papillary muscle displacement, annular dilatation, and tethering of the mitral leaflets. The mechanism of MR in chronic ischemic disease is local LV remodeling (apical and posterior displacement of papillary muscles) and annular dilatation, which lead to excess valvular tenting and loss of systolic annular contraction. [81, 82] The evolution of patients with ischemic MR is substantially worse than that for regurgitation from other causes. [83, 84]

With 1-year mortality rates as high as 40%, recent practice guidelines of professional societies recommend repair or replacement of the mitral valve in patients with severe MR, although there remains a lack of conclusive evidence supporting either intervention. The choice between therapeutic options is characterized by the trade-off between reduced operative morbidity and mortality with repair versus a better long-term correction of mitral insufficiency with replacement. The long-term benefits of repair versus replacement remain unknown, which has led to significant variation in surgical practice. [85] Chan and colleagues performed a propensity-based, case-matched analysis to examine whether patients who undergo mitral valve repair and those who undergo mitral valve replacement for IMR have similar long-term outcomes. Late survival was the similar in both groups, but recurrent mitral regurgitation (≥2+) at late follow-up was observed in 23% of patients after repair. Patients in both groups had similar freedom from valve-related complications and similar left ventricular function at follow-up. Mitral valve replacement remains a viable option for the treatment of ischemic MR. Although mitral valve repair effectively protects against persistent or recurrent moderate-to-severe MR, mitral valve replacement provides better freedom from mild-to-moderate MR in this population, with a low incidence of valve-related complications. Notably, there was no significant difference in left ventricular function between the valve-repair and valve-replacement groups at follow-up. [86]

Whether moderate functional ischemic MR in patients with ischemic cardiomyopathy should be addressed with mitral valve repair at the time of coronary artery bypass grafting (CABG) is still debated, and current prospective trials are being done to answer this question. Arguments against concomitant mitral valve repair are that CABG alone, by decreasing ischemia and improving left ventricular function, often decreases functional ischemic MR, and adding mitral valve repair to CABG increases operative complexity and risk. Arguments favoring concomitant mitral valve repair are that mitral valve repair consistently decreases functional ischemic MR, and CABG alone does not predictably improve postoperative MR. [80] Preoperative myocardial viability studies, including dobutamine stress echocardiography, single-photon emission computed tomography, positron emission tomography, or magnetic resonance imaging (MRI) can assist making the decision to add a mitral valve repair to coronary arteries revascularization in patients with moderate functional ischemic MR. Penicka and colleagues reported that the absence of preoperative papillary muscle dyssynchrony and presence of viability in myocardial segments adjacent to papillary muscles were associated with improvement in postoperative functional ischemic MR in >90% of patients. In contrast, the absence of myocardial viability and presence of significant papillary muscle dyssynchrony were associated with no improvement or worsening postoperative MR. The changes in postoperative MR are associated with clinical outcomes. Patients with improved postoperative functional ischemic MR had better functional status and survival compared with those whose MR remained the same or worsened after surgery. [87]

The proper way of revascularization remains controversial in patients with ischemic mitral regurgitation (IMR). Kang and colleagues compared the long-term results of percutaneous coronary intervention (PCI) and surgical revascularization in a group of 185 consecutive patients with IMR. The survival and cardiac mortality rates were not significantly different between the 2 groups, but the risk of cardiac events was significantly lower in the surgical group than in the PCI group. Compared with patients who underwent coronary artery bypass graft surgery alone, event-free survival rates were significantly higher in those who underwent additional mitral annuloplasty. They concluded that surgical revascularization is associated with an improved long-term event-free survival when compared with PCI, and concomitant mitral annuloplasty should be considered in patients with significant ischemic MR. [88]

b) Infective Endocarditis

Bacterial endocarditis can compromise normal valves, but a higher incidence occurs in patients with preexisting valve pathology (ie, degenerative mitral valve disease). Duke's criteria provide the most accurate variables for diagnosis. Depending on the organism involved and the patient's immune system, the infective process may manifest as an isolated small vegetation that resolves with antibiotic treatment, or compromise the anatomic structure of the valve with leaflet invasion and erosion of the mitral annulus. Progression of the infective process with leaflet perforation or rupture of chords may result in severe acute mitral insufficiency. Local extension of the infective process rarely involves the subvalvular apparatus or the aortic valve. The most appropriate time for surgical treatment will be determined by the patient's clinical evolution. While hemodynamic stability without evidence of peripheral embolism allows to treat patients conservativelly with antibiotics, those patients that do not improve with antibiotic treatment, present hemodynamic instability, progressive end-organ dysfunction, or evidence of peripheral embolism will require immediate surgical treatment.

Basic concepts related to any surgery for advanced infection are applied during surgical treatment of infective endocarditis with resection of all vegetations, extensive debridement of all necrotic tissue, and functional preservation of the affected structure. Several techniques can be employed to preserve mitral valve competency, including suture of pericardial patch to cover leaflet perforations, and chordal transposition to restablish leaflet coaptation.

When tissue necrosis is so extensive that a reconstruction cannot be accomplished, mitral valve replacement can be performed using either mechanical or biologic prosthesis. Some groups have recently advocated the implantation of homografts in the mitral position to replace part or all the mitral valve, although operative mortality for patients with endocarditis was 8,5%.

Partial homografts allow for a localized reconstruction of a segment of the mitral valve, and lower early failure (2,6%) have been reported as compared to complete homograft reconstruction of the mitral valve (early faliure of 6,2%), most frequently related to sizing missmatch. [89]

When the infective process compromises both aortic and mitral valves, the most common pattern includes a jet lesion on the anterior mitral leaflet, while continuous spread of infection, and involvelment of the fibrous skeleton of the heart are rare. The most common indication for surgery is congestive heart failure. A surgical strategy that involves repair of the mitral valve is recommended whenever feassible. Surgical treatment can be accomplished with good early results, late survival, and freedom from recurrent infection similar to those found in patients with infection of only one valve. [90] When the infective process compromises the fibrous trigone, disrupting both aortic and mitral valve annulus, a more extensive debridement should be performed, requiring pericardial patch reconstruction of the trigone ("commando operation") associated with increased mortality (up to 31%). As an alternative, some authors have advocated the implantation of aorto-mitral homograft that enables for the reconstruction of both valves. [91, 92] (Figure 13)

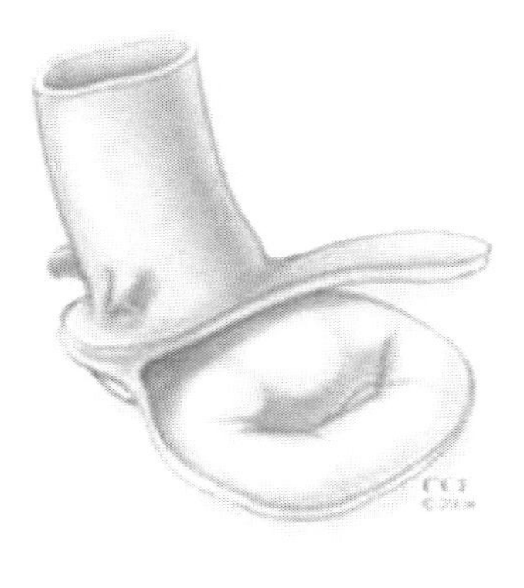

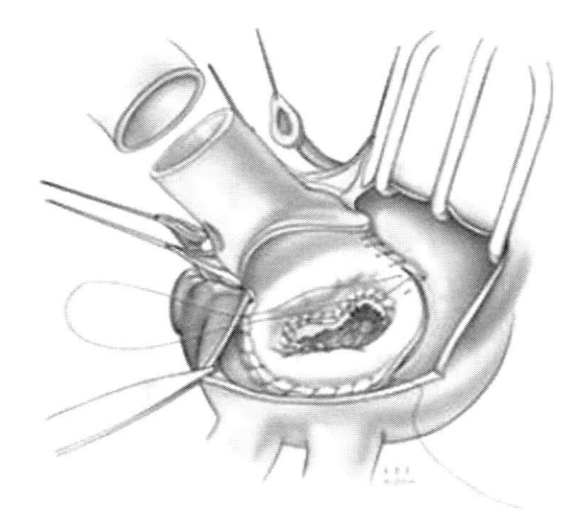

Figure 13. Recently introduced aorto-mitral monoblock for simultaneous treatment of aortic and mitral valve endocarditis presenting extensive tissue destruction. After complete tissue debridement, the combined homograft allows adequate reconstruction of both valves.

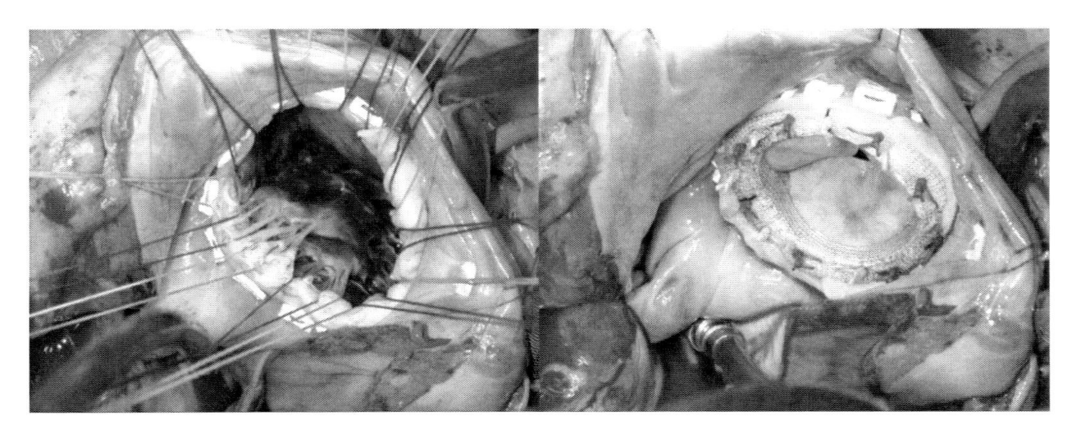

Figure 14. Mitral valve replacement with chordal preservation.

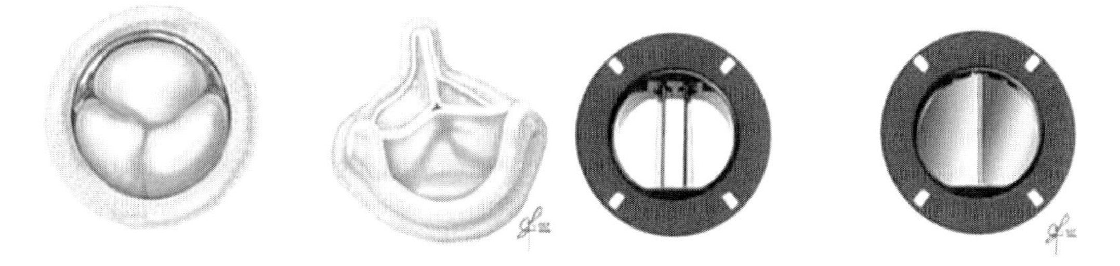

Figure 15. Bioprosthetic valves (A), and Mechanical valves (B).

During the last decade, operative mortality for infective endocarditis have decreased from 7,5% to < 2% in our institution, probably associated to an earlier indication of surgical treatment.

c) Mitral Valve Replacement

Repair has become the most frequent mitral valve procedure in the United States, performed in more than 70% of patients with degenerative disease. However, there is still a group of patients with combined pathology or mainly stenosis in whom the mitral valve will not be salvageable and will require valve replacement.

Ventricular physiology should always be considered when replacing the mitral valve, and every effort should be done to preserve native mitral valve apparatus, including the leaflets in continuity with the tendinous chords and papillary muscles in order to preserve left ventricular geometry and function (Figure 14). Selection of prosthesis type to be implanted will be determined by factors related to the patient, and the undelying pathology. Bioprosthesis offer the advantage of avoiding anticoagulation, particullarly in patients with regular rhythm, elderly patients, or young females considering pregnancy; but present elevated rate of structural deterioration, reported to be over 20% after 10 years of implantation (Figure 15 A). Structural deterioration is lower in patients older than 70 years of age. [93]

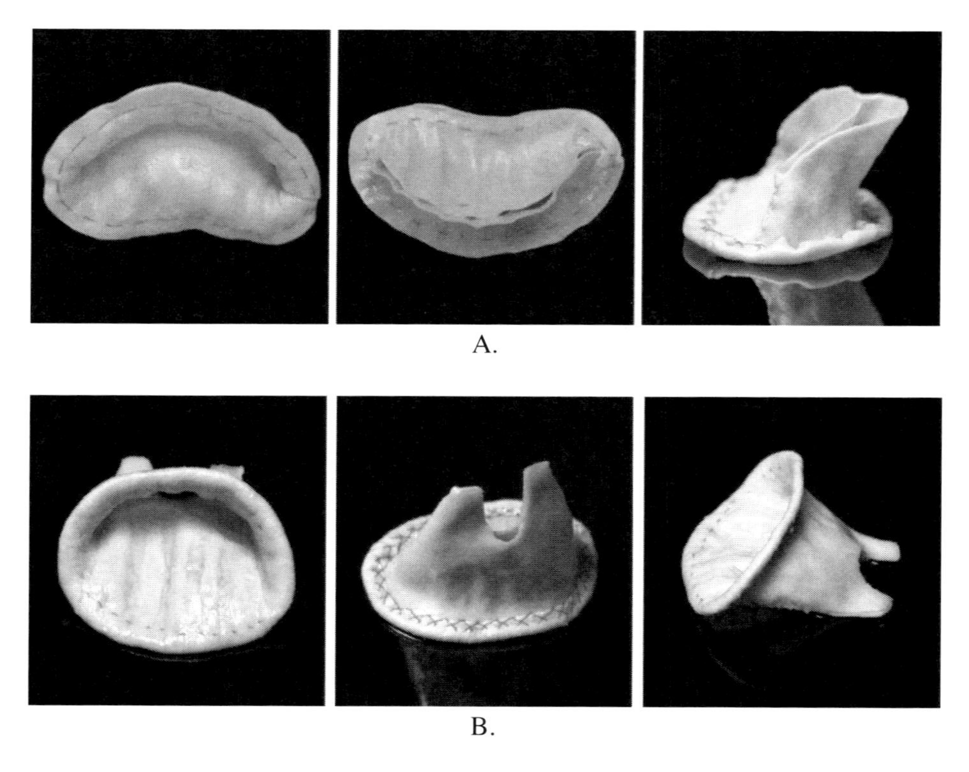

Figure 16. Stentless bioprosthetic mitral valves without chordae (A), and with chordae (B).

Mechanical valves do not present structural deterioration, but require anticoagulation usually on a higher therapeutic level than in the aortic position. Their long-term durability makes them particularly usefull in young patients, and patients requiring anticoagulation for associated pathology like atrial fibrillation. (Figure 15 B).

According to ACC/AHA guidelines, a bioprosthesis is indicated for mitral valve replacement in a patient who will not take warfarin, is incapable of taking warfarin, or has a clear contraindication to warfarin therapy (Indication Class I C), in patients older than 65 years of age (indication Class IIa C), or in patients younger than 65 years of age that request it in order to avoid chronic anticoagulation treatment provided they understand the long-term chances of requiring a reoperation for structural valve deterioration (indication Class IIa C). A mechanical prosthesis is reasonable in patients younger than 65 years of age with long-standing atrial fibrillation (indication Class IIa C).

d) Stentless Mitral Prosthesis

Alternative approaches have been reported when the valve cannot be repaired, including replacement with mitral homografts, or implantation of stentless bioprosthesis.

During the cardiac cycle, the fibrous mitral annulus undergoes complex conformational changes as a result of extrinsic forces imposed by adjacent atrial and ventricular musculature that determine a sphincteric contraction that reduces the annular area by approximately 25%, and a translational motion along the LV major axis as a consequence of the torsion of the base of the LV. [94, 95]

Recent studies have emphasized the importance of maintaining the native annulus shape when repairing the mitral valve to decrease the shear stress on the anterior mitral valve leaflet that may jeopardize long-term results. We have recently developed and described two alternative models of stentless bioprosthesis mitral valves that are actually sewn to the base of the native mitral leaflets. (Figure 16) The absence of a prosthetic ring allows the valve to accommodate and respect the saddle shape of the native mitral annulus. Implantation technique is simpler than implantation of mitral homografts, and early echocardiographic results in animal models have shown good hemodynamic performance. [96, 97] Presumably, valve geometry and function would be preserved on the chronic phase because of reverse ventricular remodeling that might occur after eliminating the diseased mitral valve, although further animal studies are under way to evaluate this hypothesis.

e) Transcatheter Mitral Valve Therapy

The field of percutaneous catheter-based treatment of valvular heart disease has expanded rapidly in the last decade. Percutaneous and transpical implantation of aortic and pulmonary valved stents have shown promising results, and are gaining acceptance in clinical practice. [98]

Several approaches have been explored to reproduce basic surgical principles of mitral valve repair with trancatheter therapies, but applying transcatheter techniques to the mital valve is not as simple as it may seem. The complex mitral valve anatomy, and the different etiologies and pathophysiology of mitral regurgitaion create a tremendous challenge for a successful treatment of these patients.

Current pecutaneous mitral valve repair technologies provide only half of what sugical repair techniques can do combining leaflet repair and anuloplasty rings; and doing only one or the other procedure results in an incomplete repair and imperfect outcomes, when compared against the gold standard surgical repair technique.

Research studies have reported that approximately 49% of patients with severe mitral regurgitation do not receive surgery. [99] Patients who are considered high risk for surgery include the elderly, patients with reduced left ventricular systolic function, or other comorbidities. [100] The interest to treat these high risk patients with functional MR has recently expanded inview of the resonable results demostrated in the percutaneous edge-to-edge tecnique device trial (MitraClip - EVEREST), which reported 1 year freedom from severe MR grade in 66% of the patients, and showed an initial reverse remodeling of the left ventricle. [101]

The application of catheter-delivery technologies in selected high risk patients is becoming more and more challenging, this is more specifically true for patients with mitral regurgitation who present a burgeoning clinical unmet need for therapeutic advances. A transcatheter implanted mitral valve may offer a very effective treatment alternative, and this begins with the sutureless implantation of such device that can completely eleminate the MR.

The next frontier for valve surgery is the development of a clinical sutureless transcatheter delivered MV prosthesis. Despite substantial technical progress in development of sutureless MVR designs, most of the emerging transcatheter mitral devices remain in their early developmental stages, and will ultimately need to be proven safe and effective when compared to surgical gold standards. [102, 103, 104] While technically and surgically demanding, this technology can become an important alternative in a selected group of patients with high operative risks and a low probability for successful MV repair. [105] The first description of sutureless mitral prosthetic implantation in animals with a self-expanding valved stent was reported by Segesser's group in 2005. [102] Use of a transapical approach for suturelss MV implantation in animals was reported by Lutter and his group. [106] Goetzenich and coworkers presented a novel collapsible hollow-body atrioventricular valve prosthesis tested in 8 pigs which does not require anchoring within the mitral annulus. [107] Berreklouw introduced a mitral bioprosthesis sutured to a fabric covered nitinol attachment ring which was successfully delivered through a left atriotomy in 9 pigs. 108] Designs reported to be closest to clinical use appear to be the following: Endovalve, Inc. (Princeton, New Jersey) which is developing an MVR system for insertion during a minimally invasive surgical procedure without the need for CPB, and is targeting 2012 for initial trials; and CardiAQ Valve Technologies, Inc. (Winchester, Massachussets) is in pre-clinical development phase of its transcatheter MV implantation system. [109]

At our institution, The Cleveland Clinic, we have developed a balloon-expandable tri-leaflet mitral bioprostheses that was designed for deployment within a catheter delivery system (Figures 17 A and B).

Device Description

The valve is fabricated from glutaraldehyde cross-linked bovine pericardial tissue leaflets sutured to a prefabricated expandable stent, laser cut from a Cobalt-Chromium tube 15 mm in diameter and 0.7 mm wall thickness. [110] Radially arranged anchoring wings are incorporated into the proximal and distal ends of the stent. The valve profile (height) is about 18 mm for both 30 mm and 42 mm prostheses. The trans-mitral delivery catheter was designed for direct valved stent dilation and consists of a 40 mm long inflatable balloon dilatation system on which the crimped prosthesis is mounted prior to deployment (Figure 17 C).

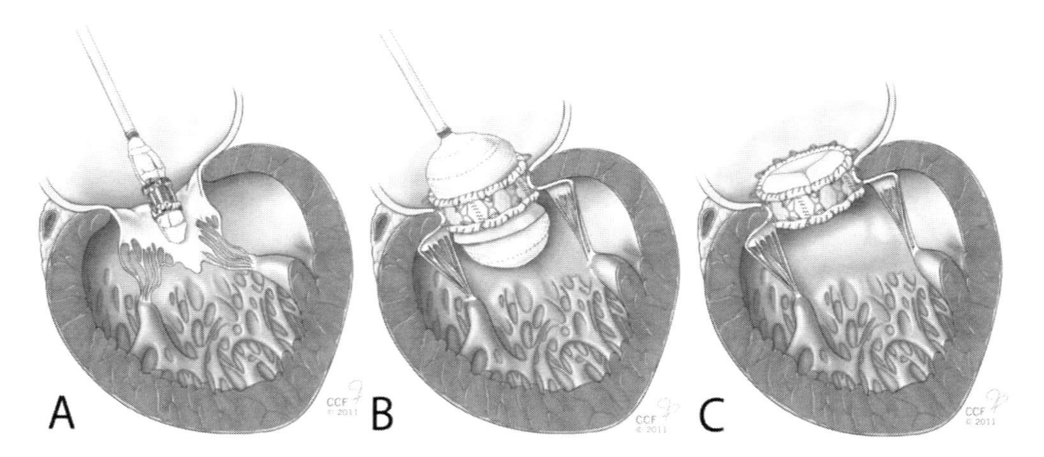

Figure 17. Evolving models for transcatheter mitral valve implantation.

A surgical transcatheter based delivery system of a metallic support frame incorporating a tissue derived valve puts considerable constraints on device specifications. Expansion to a large diameter from the catheter diameter without mechanical fracture involves advanced device design, and appropriate material processing and selection. Our newest frame concept incorporates wings that protrude during expansion to establish adequate fixation. Expansion characteristics of the design in relation to annulus fixation were quantified through finite element analysis predictions of the frame wing span and angles. Computational modeling and physical prototyping was used to identify many favorable design features for the transcatheter mitral valve frame and obtain desired expansion diameters (30-42mm), acceptable radial and axial stiffness (2.7N/mm), and ensure limited risk of failure based on predicted plastic deformations.

A large diameter frame is required for a mitral valve replacement device because the diseased annulus is larger than the healthy annulus. The engineered frame could be manufactured into a large diameter, yet still be delivered through a small catheter size and have acceptable plastic strains accumulated upon deployment. Uniform deployment of the stent and wings is an influential factor for overall fatigue performance, and the structures of the device need to be expanded homogeneously. The mitral valve design comprises a prosthetic valve secured within an expandable CoCr frame, knowing that CoCr material has been used successfully previously for heart valve applications. And lastly, because the annulus not only moves but also changes shape during the cardiac cycle, the distinctive wing fixation features act as a lock to secure the valve to the position on the tissue shelf, which is important for prevention of dislodgement. [111]

The acute *in vivo* animal studies of our balloon-expandable mitral bioprosthetic valve under thoracotomy and cardiopulmonary bypass in a beating heart, and with direct visualization of the native valve through an atriotomy were encouraging. The new design of contractible and expandable mitral valve prosthesis requires a minimal amount of surgical manipulation for implantation, and provides a secure engagement of the native annulus without compromising the subvalvular apparatus, showing a reliable valve performance. Further chronic studies are underway to verify these results, and evaluate reliability of implantation procedures, biocompatibility, and valve durability. Transition to a transcatheter valve delivery system without opening the heart or need of CPB may be eased by the attributes of this new device.

Conclusion

Surgical treatment of mitral valve pathology has benefited from the evolution of surgical concepts. Refinement of repair techniques allowed performing a successful repair in most patients with degenerative or ischemic mitral insufficiency in experienced centers. Mitral valve repair may be more difficult in patients with rheumatic disease or infective endocarditis. Technological development has enabled surgeons to perform mitral valve surgery through limited incisions including ministernotomy, right minithoracotomy, and robotic mitral valve repair. All these approaches allow the surgeon to reproduce conventional surgical techniques, but through limited incisions that are benefitial for patient recovery.

For patients undergoing mitral valve replacement, preservation of the chordal apparatus preserves left ventricular function, and enhances postoperative survival compared with mitral valve replacement with resection of the mitral apparatus.

Performing atrial fibrillation surgery at time of mitral valve surgery does not increase surgical risk, and provides additional benefits to patients that will recover normal sinus rhythm in 75% to 90% of cases, avoiding life-long medical therapy with antiarrhythmic and anticoagulant medication.

Minimally invasive and transcatheter approaches have become very popular particularly for aortic valve procedures. While the former continues to improve the operative technique, the application of catheter delivery technologies in selected high risk patients is becoming more and more challenging. This is particularly true for patients with mitral regurgitation who present a burgeoning clinical unmet need for therapeutic advances. A transcatheter implanted mitral valve may offer a very effective treatment alternative and this begins with the sutureless implantation of such device.

References

[1] Singh JP, vans JC, Levy D. Pevalence and clinical determinants of mitral, tricuspid and aortic regurgitation (the Framingham Study). *Am. J. Cardiol.* 1999;83:897-902.

[2] Executive Summary : 10 years STS Report. Presented at the 46th Annual Meeting of the Society of Thoracic Surgeons in Ft Lauderdale, Florida. January 27th, 2010.

[3] Levine RA, Handshumacher MD, Sanfilipo AJ, et al. Three-dimensional echocardiograpic reconstruction of the mitral valve, with implications for the diagnoss of mitral valve prolapsed. *Circulation* 1989;80:589-98.

[4] Salgo IS, Gorman JH, Gorman RC, et al. Effect of annular shape on leaflet curvature in reducing mitral leaflet stress. *Circulation* 2002;106:711-7.

[5] Burns AT, McDonald IG, Thomas JD, et al. Doin' the twist: new tools for an old concept of myocardial function. *Heart* 2008;94:978-83.

[6] Carlsson M, Ugander M, Mosen H, et al. Atrioventricular plane displacement is the major contributor to left ventricular pumping in healthy adults, athletes, and dilated cardiomyopathy. *Am. J. Heart Circ. Physiol.* 207;292:H1452-9.

[7] Van Mieghem NM, Piazza N, Anderson RH, et al. Anatomy of the mitral valvular complex and its implications for transcatheter interventions fo mitral regurgitation. *J. Am. Coll. Cardiol.* 2010;56:617-26.

[8] Silbiger JJ, Bazaz R. Contemporary insights into the functional anatomy of the mitral valve. *Am. Heart J.* 2009;158:887-95.

[9] Obadia JF, Casali C, Chassignolle F, et al. Mitral subvalvular apparatus: different functions of primary and secondary chordae. *Circulation* 1997;96:3124-8.

[10] Rowe JC, Bland EF, Sprangue HB, White PD. The course of mitral stenosis without surgery: ten- and twenty- year perspectives. *Ann. Intern. Med.* 1960;52:741-9.

[11] Olensen KH. The natural history of 271 patients with mitral stenosis under medical treatment. *Br. Heart J.* 1962;24:349-57.

[12] Roberts WC, Perloff JK. Mitral valvular disease: a clinicopathologic survey of the conditions causing the mitral valve to function abnormally. *Ann. Intern. Med.* 1972; 77: 939-75.

[13] Hugenholtz PG, Ryan TJ, Stein SW, Belmann WH. The spectrum of pure mitral stenosis: hemodynamic studies in relation to clinical disability. *Am. J. Cardiol.* 1962; 10: 773-84

[14] Wood P. An appreciation of mitral stenosis, I: clinical features. Br. Med. J. 1954;4870: 1051-63.

[15] Ward C, Hancock BW. Extreme pulmonary hypertension caused by mitral valve disease: natural history and results of surgery. *Br. Heart J.* 1975;37:74-8.

[16] Martin RP, Rakowski H, Kleiman JH, Beaver W, London E, Popp RL. Reliability andr eporducibility of two dimensional echocardiograph measurement of the stenotic mitral valve orifice area. *Am. J. Cardiol.* 1979;43:560-8.

[17] Bonow RO, Carabello BA, Chatterjee K, et al. ACC/AHA 2006 Guidelines for the management of patients with valvular heart disease: A report of the American College of Cardiology/American heart Association Task Force on practice guidelines. *JACC* 2006; 48(3):e1-148.

[18] Branwald E, Moscovits HL, Mram SS, et al. The hemodynamics of the left side of the heart as studied by simultaneous left atrial, left ventricular, and aortic pressures; particular reference to mitral stenosis. *Circulation* 1955;15:69-81.

[19] Gorlin R, Gorlin SG. Hydraulic formula for calculation of the area of the stenotic mitral valve, other cardiac valves, and central circulatory shunts. *Am. Heart J.* 1951;41:1-29.

[20] Harken DE, Ellis LB, Ware PF, Norman LR. The surgical treatment of mitral stenosis. *N. Engl. J. Med.* 1948;239:801-8.

[21] Bailey CP. The surgical treatment of mitral stenosis (mitral commissurtotomy). *Dis. Chest* 1949;15:377-84

[22] John S, Bashi VV, Jairaj PS, et al. Closed mitral valvulotomy: early results and long-term follow-up of 3724 consecutive patients. *Circulation* 1983;68:891-6.

[23] Gross RI, Cunningham JN Jr., Snively SL, et al. Long-term results of open radical mitral commissurotomy: ten year follow-up study of 202 patients. *Am. J. Cardiol.* 1981;47:821-5.

[24] Garcia-Fernandez MA, Perez DE, Quiles J, et al. Role of left atrial appendage obliteration in stroke reduction in patients with mitral valve prosthesis: a transesophageal echocardiographic study. *J. Am. Coll. Cardiol.* 2003;42:1253-8.

[25] Inoue K, Owaki T, Nakamura T, et al. Clinical application of transvenous mitral commissurotomy by a new balloon catheter. *J. Thorac. Cardiovasc. Surg.* 1984;87:394-402.

[26] Camara ML, Aris A, Padro J, Caralps JM. Long-term results of mitral valve surgery in patients with severy pulmonary hipertensión. *Ann. Thorac. Surg.* 1988;45:133-6.

[27] Lock JE, Khalilullah M, Shrivastava S, Bahl V, Keane JF. Percutaneous catheter commissurotomy in rheumatic mitral stenosis. *N. Engl. J. Med.* 1985;313(24):1515-8.

[28] Abascal VM, Wilkins GT, Choong CY, Thomas JD, Palacios IF, Block PC, Weyman AE. Echocardiographic evaluation of mitral valve structure and function in patients followed for at least 6 months after percutaneous balloon mitral valvuloplasty. *J. Am. Coll. Cardiol.* 1988;12(3):606-15.

[29] Reyes VP, Raju BS, Wynne J, et al. Percutaneous balloon valvuloplasty compared with open surgical commissurotomy for mitral stenosis. *N. Engl. J. Med.* 1994;331:961-7.

[30] Ben Farhat M, Ayari M, Maatouk F, et al. Percutaneous balloon versus surgical closed and open mitral commissurtotomy: seven-year follow-up results of a randomized trial. *Circulation* 1998;97:245-50.
[31] Cotrufo M, Renzulli A, Ismeno G, et al. Percutaneous mitral commissurotomy versus open mitral commmissurotomy: a comparison study. *Eur. J. Cardiothorac. Surg.* 1999; 15:646-51.
[32] Choudhary SK, Dhareshwar J, Govil A, Airan B, Kumar AS. Open mitral commissurotomy in the current era: indications, technique, and results. *Ann. Thorac. Surg.* 2003;75:41-6.
[33] Hernandez R, Banuelos C, Alfonso F, et al. Long-term clinical and echocardiographic follow-up after percutaneous mitral valvuloplasty with the Inowe balloon. *Circulation* 1999;99:1580-6.
[34] Palacios IF, Sanchez PL, Harrell LC, et al. Which Patients Benefit From Percutaneous Mitral Balloon Valvuloplasty?: Prevalvuloplasty and Postvalvuloplasty Variables That Predict Long-Term Outcome. *Circulation* 2002;105:1465-71.
[35] Tuzcu Em, Block PC, Griffin BP, Newell JB, Palacios IF. Immediate and long-term outcome of percutaneous mitral valvulotomy in patients 65 years and older. *Circulation* 1992;85:963-71.
[36] Braunwald E, Braunwald NS, Ross JJ, Morrow AG. Effects of mitral valve replacement on the pulmonary vascular dynamics of patients with pulmonary hypertension. *N. Engl. J. Med.* 1965;273:509.
[37] Cosgrove DM, mitral valve repair in patients with elongated chordae tendineae. *J. Card Surg.* 1989;4:247-53.
[38] Reul RM, Cohn LH. Mitral valve reconstruction for mitral insufficiency. *Prog. Cardiovasc. Dis.* 1997;39:567-99.
[39] David TE, Armstrong S, Sun Z, et al. Late results of mitral valve repair for mitral inregurgitation due to degenerarive disease. *Ann. Thorac. Surg.* 1993;56:7-14.
[40] Olson LJ, Subramanian R, Ackerman DM, et al. Surgical pathology of the mitral valve: a study of 712 cases spanningn 21 years. *Mayo Clin. Proc.* 1987;62:22-34.
[41] Gillinov AM, Coosgrove DM. Mitral valve repair. Oper Tech Thor Cardiovasc Surg 1998; 3:95-108.
[42] Fenster MS, Feldman MD. Mitral regurgitation: an overview. *Curr. Prob. Cardiol.* 1995; 20:193-228.
[43] Gillinov AM, Cosgrove DM, Blackstone EH, et al. Durability of mital valve repair for degenerative disease. *J. Thorac. Cardiovasc. Surg.* 1998;116:734-43.
[44] Suri RM, Schaff HV, Dearani JA, et al. Survival advantage and improved durability of mitral repair for leaflet prolapse subsets in the current era. *Ann. Thorac. Surg.* 2006;82: 819-26.
[45] David TE, Ivanov J, Armstrong S, et al. A comparison of outcomes of mitral valve repair for degenerative disease with posterior, anterior, and bileaflet prolapse. *J. Thorac. Cardiovasc. Surg.* 2005;130:1242-9.
[46] Carpentier A. Cardiac valve surgery – the "French" correction. *J. Thorac. Cardiovasc. Surg.* 1983;86:323-37.
[47] Freed LA, Benjamin EJ, Levy D, et al. Mitral valve prolapse in the general population: the benign nature of echocardiographic features in the Framingham Heart Study. *J. Am. Coll. Cardiol.* 2002;40:1298-304.

[48] Freed LA, Benjamin EJ, Levy D, et al. Prevalence and clinical outcome of mitral-valve prolapse. *N. Engl. J. Med.* 1999;341:1-7.

[49] Wilken DE, Hickey AJ. Lifetime risk for patients with mitral valve prolapse of developing severe valve regurgitation requiring surgery. *Circulation* 1988;78:10-4.

[50] Braunberger E, Deloche A, Berrebi A, et al. Very long-term results (more than 20 years) of mitral valve repair with Carpentier's techniques in nonrheumatic mitral valve insufficiency. *Circulation* 2001;104(Suppl):I-8-11.

[51] Avierinos JF, Gersh Bh, Melton LJ III, et al. Natural history of asymptomatic mitral valve prolapse in the community. *Circulation* 2002;106:1355-61.

[52] Enriquez-Sarano M, Basmadjian AJ, Rossi A, Bailey KR, Seward JB, Tajik AJ. Progression of mitral regurgitation: a prospective Doppler echocardiographic study. *J. Am. Coll. Cardiol.* 1999;34: 1137– 44.

[53] Zile MR, Gaasch WH, Carroll JD, Levine HJ. Chronic mitral regurgitation: predictive value of preoperative echocardiographic indexes of left ventricular function and wall stress. *J. Am. Coll. Cardiol.* 1984;3:235–42.

[54] Fontana ME, Sparks EA, Boudoulas H, Wooley CF. Mitral valve prolapsed and the mitral valve prolapsed syndrome. *Curr. Probl. Cardiol.* 1991;16:309-75.

[55] Ling LH, Enriquez-Sarano M, Seward JB, et al. Clinical outcome of mitral regurgitation due to flail leaflet. *N. Engl. J. Med.* 1996;335:1417-23.

[56] Tribouilloy CM, Enriquez-Sarano M, Schaff HV, et al. Impact of preoperative symptoms on survival after surgical correction of organic mitral regurgitation: rationale for optimizing surgical indications. *Circulation* 1999;99:400-5.

[57] Enriquez-Sarano M, Schaff HV, Orszulak TA, Tajik AJ, Bailey KR, Frye RL. Valve repair improves the outcome of surgery for mitral regurgitation: a multivariate analysis. *Circulation* 1995;91: 1022– 8.

[58] Feindel CM, Tufail Z, David TE, Ivanov J, Armstrong S. Mitral valve surgery in patients with extensive calcification of the mitral annulus. J Thorac Cardiovasc Surg 2003;126:777–82.

[59] Gammie JS, Sheng S, Griffith BP, Peterson ED, O'Brien SM, Brown JM. Trends in mitral valve surgery in the United States: results from the Society of Thoracic Surgeons Adult Cardiac surgery Database. *Ann. Thorac. Surg.* 2009;87(5):1431-7.

[60] Bonow RO, Nikas D, Elefteriades JA. Valve replacement for regurgitant lesions of the aortic or mitral valve in advanced left ventricular dysfunction. *Cardiol. Clin.* 1995; 13:73– 83, 85.

[61] David TE, Burns RJ, Bacchus CM, Druck MN. Mitral valve replacement for mitral regurgitation with and without preservation of chordae tendineae. *J. Thorac. Cardiovasc. Surg.* 1984;88:718–25.

[62] Gillinov AM, Cosgrove DM, Lytle BW, et al. Reoperation for failure of mitral valve repair. *J. Thorac. Cardiovasc. Surg.* 1997;113: 467–73.

[63] Chitwood WR Jr, Wixon CL, Elbeery JR, Moran JF, Chapman WH, Lust RM. Video-assisted minimally invasive mitral valve surgery. *J. Thorac. Cardiovasc. Surg.* 1997; 114:773-82.

[64] Mihaljevic T, Cohn LH, Unic D, Aranki SF, Couper GS, Byrne JG. One thousand minimally invasive valve operations: early and late results. *Ann. Surg.* 2004;240:529-34.

[65] Navia JL, Cosgrove DM, 3rd. Minimally invasive mitral valve operations. *Ann. Thorac. Surg*. 1996;62:1542-4.

[66] Cosgrove DM, 3rd, Sabik JF. Minimally invasive approach for aortic valve operations. *Ann. Thorac. Surg*. 1996;62:596-7.

[67] Cosgrove DM, 3rd, Sabik JF, Navia JL. Minimally invasive valve operations. *Ann. Thorac. Surg*. 1998; 65:1535-8; discussion 8-9.

[68] Mihaljevic T, Jarrett CM, Gillinov AM, et al. Robotic repair of posterior mitral valve prolapse versus conventional approaches: Potential realized. *J. Thorac. Cardiovasc. Surg*. 2011;141:72-80.

[69] Duran CG, Pomar JL, Revuelta JM, et al. Conservative operation for mitral insufficiency: critical analysis supported by postoperative hemodynamic studies of 72 patients. *J. Thorac. Cardiovasc. Surg*. 1980;79:326-37.

[70] Yacoub M, Halim M, Radley-Smith R, McKay R, Nijveld A, towers M. Surgical treatment of mitral regurgitation caused by floppy valves: repair versus replacement. *Circulation* 1981;64:II210-6.

[71] David TE, Uden DE, Strauss HD. The importance of the mitral apparatus in left ventricular function after correction of mitral regurgitation. *Circulation* 1983;68:II76-82.

[72] Goldman ME, Mora F, Guarino T, Fuster V, Mindich BP. Mitral valvuloplasty is superior to valve replacement for preservation of left ventricular function: an intraoperative two-dimensional echocardiographic study. *J. Am. Coll. Cardiol*. 1987; 10:568-75.

[73] Tischler MD, Cooper KA, Rowen M, Lewinter MM. Mitral valve replacement versus mitral valve repair: a Doppler and quantitative stress echocardiograpic study. *Circulation* 1994;89:132-7.

[74] Myken PS, Bech-Hansen O. A 20 year experience of 1712 patients with the Biocor procine bioprosthesis. *J. Thorac. Cardiovasc. Surg*. 2009;137:76-81.

[75] Kirali K, Güler M, Tuncer A, et al. Fifteen-year clinical experience with the Biocor porcine bioprostheses in the mitral position. *Ann. Thorac. Surg*. 2001;71:811-5.

[76] Privitera S, Butany J, Silversides C, Leask RL, David TE. Artificial chordate tendinae: long-term changes. *J. Card. Surg*. 2005;20:90-2.

[77] Ling LH, Enriquez-Sarano M, Seward JB, et al. Early surgery in patients with mitral regurgitation due to flail leaflets: a long-term outcome study. *Circulation* 1997; 96: 1819-25.

[78] Rankin JS, Orozco RE, Rodgers TL, et al. Adjustable artificial chordal replacement for repair of mitral valve prolapse. *Ann. Thorac. Surg*. 2006;81:1526-8.

[79] Salvador L, Mirone S, Bianchini R, et al. A 20-year experience with mitral valve repair with artificial chordae in 608 patients. *J. Thorac. Cardiovasc. surg*. 2008;135:1280-7.

[80] Mihaljevic T, Gillinov AM, Sabik JF III. Functional ischemic mitral regurgitation: Myocardial viability as a predictor of postoperative outcome after isolated coronary artery bypass grafting. *Circulation* 2009, 120:1459-61.

[81] Kwan J, Shiota T, Agler DA, et al. Geometric differences of the mitral apparatus between ischemic and dilated cardiomyopathy with significant mitral regurgitation: real-time three-dimensional echocardiography study. *Circulation* 2003;107:1135– 40.

[82] Levine RA, Schwammenthal E. Ischemic mitral regurgitation on the threshold of a solution: from paradoxes to unifying concepts. *Circulation* 2005;112:745–58.

[83] Akins CW, Hilgenberg AD, Buckley MJ, et al. Mitral valve reconstruction versus replacement for degenerative or ischemic mitral regurgitation. *Ann. Thorac. Surg*. 1994; 58:668 –75.

[84] Flemming MA, Oral H, Rothman ED, et al. Echocardiographic markers for mitral valve surgery to preserve left ventricular performance in mitral regurgitation. *Am. Heart J.* 2000;140:476–82.

[85] Perrault LP, Moskowitz AJ, Kron IL, et al. Optimal surgical management *J. Thorac. Cardiovasc. Surg*. 2011 Nov 3. [Epub ahead of print]

[86] Chan V, Ruel M, Mesana TG. Mitral valve *Ann. Thorac. Surg*. 2011 Oct;92(4):1358-65.

[87] Penicka M, Linkova H, Lang O, et al. Predictors of improvement of unrepaired moderate ischemic mitral regurgitation in patients undergoing elective isolated coroanary artery bypass graft surgery. *Circulation* 2009;120:1474-81.

[88] Kang DH, Sun, Kim DH, Yun SC, et al. Percutaneous versus surgical revascularization in patients with ischemic mitral regurgitation *Circulation*. 2011 Sep 13;124(11 Suppl):S156-62.

[89] Ali M, Lung B, Lansac E, et al. Homograft replacement of the mitral valve: eight-year results. *J. Thorac. Cardiovasc. Surg*. 2004;128:529-34.

[90] Gillinov AM, Diaz R, Blackstone EH, et al. Double valve endocarditis. *Ann. Thorac. Surg*. 2001;71:1874-9.

[91] Obadia JF, Raisky O, Sebbag L, et al. Monobloc aorto-mitral homograft as a treatment of complex cases of endocarditis. *J. Thorac. Cardiovasc. Surg*. 2001;121:584-6.

[92] Navia JL, Al-Ruzzeh S, Gordon S, et al. The incorporated aortomitral homograft: a new surgical option for double valve endocarditis. *J. Thorac. Cardiovasc. Surg*. 2010;139: 1077-81.

[93] Jamieson WRE, Gudas VM, Burr LH, et al. Mitral valve disease: if the mitral valve is not repairable/failed repair, is bioprosthesis suitable for replacement? *European Journal of Cardio-thoracic Surgery* 2009;35:104-110.

[94] Ryan LP, Jackson BM, Hamamoto H, *et al*: The influence of annuloplasty ring geometry on mitral leaflet curvature. *Ann. Thorac. Surg. 2008;*86: 749–760.

[95] Jimenez JH, Liou SW, Padala M, *et al*: A saddle shape annulus reduces systolic strain on the central region of the mitral valve anterior leaflet. *J. Thorac. Cardiovasc. Surg*. 2007;134: 1562–1568.

[96] Navia JL, Brozzi NA, Doi K, Garcia M, Al-Ruzzeh S, Atik FA, Fukamach K, Xu XF, Kamohara K, Gonzalez-Stawinski GV, Lytle B. Implantation Technique and Early Echocardiographic Performance of Newly Designed Stentless Mitral Bioprosthesis. *ASAIO Journal* 2010;56:497-503.

[97] Navia JL, Doi K, Atik FA, Fukamachi K,. Kopcak MW Jr., Dessoffy R, Ruda-Vega P, Garcia M, Martin M, Blackstone EH, McCarthy PM, Lytle B. Acute In Vivo Evaluation of a New Stentless Mitral Valve. *J. Thorac. Cardiovasc. Surgery* 2007, Volume 133,Number 4:986-994.

[98] Leon MB, Smith CR, Mack M, et al; PARTNER Trial Investigators. Transcatheter aortic-valve *N. Engl. J. Med.* 2010 Oct 21;363(17):1597-607. Epub 2010 Sep 22.

[99] Mirabel M., Lung B., Baron G. et al., 2007, "What are the characteristics of patients with severe symptomatic, mitral regurgitation who are denied surgery?" *Eur. Heart J,* 28, pp.1358-1365.

[100] Munt B., Webb J., 2006, "Percutaneous valve repair and replacement techniques". *Heart*, October; 92(10), pp.1369–1372.

[101] Feldman T, Kar, Rinaldi M, et al. for the EVEREST Investigators. Percutaneous Mitral Repair With the MitraClip System. Safety and Midterm Durability in the Initial EVEREST (Endovascular Valve Edge-to-Edge REpair Study) *Cohort Journal of the American College of Cardiology* Vol. 54, No. 8, 2009.

[102] Ma L, Tozzi P, Huber CH, et al. Double-crowned valved stents for off-pump mitral valve replacement. *Eur. J. Cardiothorac. Surg*. 2005;28:194-9.

[103] Lutter G, Quaden R, Osaki S, et al. Off-pump transapical mitral valve replacement. *Eur. J. Cardiothorac. Surg*. 2009;36:124-8.

[104] Cubeddu RJ, Palacios IF. Percutaneous techniques for mitral valve disease. *Cardiol. Clin*. 2010;28:139-53.

[105] Attmann T, Pokorny S, Lozonschi L, et al. Mitral valved stent implantation: an overview. *Minim. Invasive Ther. Allied Technol*. 2011;20:78-84.

[106] Lutter G, Cremer J. Off-pump mitral valve replacement: an attack on conventional heart surgery? *Eur. J. Cardiothorac. Surg*. 2005;28:198-9.

[107] Goetzenich A, Dohmen G, Hatam N, et al. A new approach to interventional atrioventricular valve therapy. *J. Thorac. Cardiovasc. Surg*. 2010;140:97-102.

[108] Berreklouw E, Leontyev S, Ossmann S, et al. Sutureless mitral valve replacement with bioprostheses and Nitinol attachment rings: Feasibility in acute pig experiments. *J. Thorac. Cardiovasc. Surg*. 2011;142:390-5.e1.

[109] Chiam PT, Ruiz CE. Percutaneous transcatheter mitral valve repair: a classification of the technology. *JACC Cardiovasc. Interv*. 2011;4:1-13.

[110] Fumoto H, Chen JF, Zhou Q, Navia JL, et al. Performance of Bioprosthetic Valves After Glycerol Dehydration, Ethylene Oxide Sterilization, and Rehydration. *Innovations* 2011;6:32-6.

[111] Ormiston JA, Shah PM, Tei C, et al "Size and motion of the mitral valve annulus in man. A two-dimensional echocardiographic method and findings in normal subjects," *Circulation* 1981;64:113–120.

In: Percutaneous Valve Technology: Present and Future
Editors: Jose Luis Navia and Sharif Al-Ruzzeh
ISBN: 978-1-61942-577-4

Chapter XIX

Percutaneous Mitral Valve Repair -E-Clip the US Experience- EVEREST Trial

Uygar C. Yuksel, Samir R. Kapadia and E. Murat Tuzcu

Abstract

Catheter based mitral valve repair systems offer a new option to those who have prohibitively high risk for conventional mitral valve surgery. MitraClip™ Mitral Valve Repair System (Evalve Inc., Menlo Park, California) is a multi-axial catheter system utilizing a clip to grasp and stitch the mitral leaflets percutaneously by a transvenous transseptal approach. Data from the EVEREST trials (Endovascular Valve Edge-to-Edge Repair Study) demonstrated the catheter based MitraClip™ system has clinical benefits and is safe and effective for selected patients with moderate to severe mitral regurgitation. In this chapter the therapeutic potential of the MitraClip™ system is discussed on the basis of available data from the EVEREST trials.

Introduction

Mitral regurgitation (MR) is a common valvular heart disease with a 60% 5 year mortality rate in severe symptomatic cases if left uncorrected [1, 2]. Epidemiological data show that moderate or severe MR is the most frequent valve disease in the USA [3]. The current standard of care for patients with severe MR is cardiac surgery. In general, mitral valve (MV) repair is preferred to MV replacement because of improved survival, better preservation of left ventricular function, increased freedom from thromboembolism and side effects of chronic anticoagulation [4, 5]. However, there is a large patient population suffering from MR that is currently not treated with heart surgery because of significant morbidity and mortality risks [6, 7]. Percutaneous techniques for MV repair are under development and several clinical trials reported encouraging clinical results in the recent years. In this monograph we will discuss the percutaneous edge to edge repair of the mitral valve with MitraClip™ device and the current clinical status of the procedure based on the available evidence.

Degenerative vs. Functional MR

A wide variety of disease conditions, including degenerative (myxomatous) disease, ischemic heart disease, cardiomyopathy, rheumatic disease and infective endocarditis can lead to MR by causing anatomical abnormalities in any of the components of MV apparatus. MR initiated as a consequence of a degenerative process is called "degenerative MR" [8]. Degenerative disease includes Barlow's disease (myxomatous degeneration) and fibroelastic deficiency, both of which can result in MV leaflet prolapse and mitral regurgitation. Fibroelastic deficiency is the most common etiology encountered among surgical mitral valve repair population in the US. MR in the absence of a degenerative cause is called "functional MR". Ischemic heart disease is the most common cause of functional MR. Ischemic cardiomyopathy causes anular dilation and ventricular remodeling with otherwise preserved normal leaflet anatomy causing functional MR. Regional left ventricular dysfunction may cause tethering of papillary muscles which in turn may also lead to functional MR. Selecting the appropriate treatment modality largely depends on the type and cause of the MR.

Major causes of mitral regurgitation treated by surgical intervention in western countries are degenerative (myxomatous disease, flail leaflets, anular calcification), representing 60–70% of cases, followed by ischemic mitral regurgitation (20%), endocarditis (2–5%), rheumatic (2–5%), and miscellaneous causes (cardiomyopathies, inflammatory diseases, drug-induced, traumatic, congenital) [9].

Basic Anatomy for the Procedure

Before undertaking surgical or percutaneous repair procedures, anatomy of the MV apparatus must be well understood. The mitral valve apparatus is a complex structure consisting of the anterior and posterior mitral leaflets, chordae tendinae, anterolateral and posteromedial papillary muscles, the annulus, and the left ventricular wall. All of these structures are essential for proper functioning of the mitral valve and play an important role in left ventricular performance. Failure of any component may initiate MR.

The mitral valve tissue is composed of two leaflets: anterior (or aortic) and posterior (or mural). The anterior leaflet has a roughly triangular shape and occupies one third of the anular circumference (approximately 3 cm). The posterior leaflet is longer but narrower than the anterior leaflet. It occupies the remaining two-third of the annulus. The overall orifice areas covered by each leaflet are similar in size.

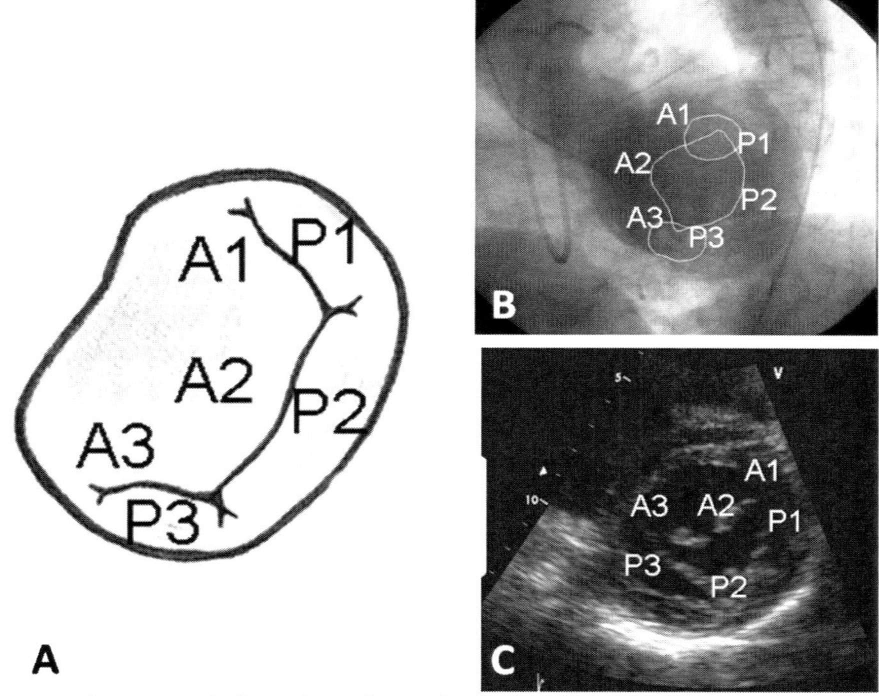

The valve tissue is composed of anterior and posterior leaflets (Panel A). The posterior leaflet is longer but narrower than the anterior leaflet. The overall orifice areas covered by each leaflet are almost identical. The leaflets are divided into three or more scallops by small indentations and are identified as A1, A2 and A3 from lateral to medial for the anterior leaflet and P1, P2 and P3 for the posterior leaflet. The middle scallop is generally larger than the other two. Leaflets and scallops as seen in aortography (Panel B) and echocardiography (Panel C).

Figure 1. Mitral valve leaflets and scallops.

The posterior leaflet is divided into three or more scallops by small indentations. These scallops are identified as P1, P2 and P3 from lateral to medial. The middle scallop (P2) is generally larger than the other two. The corresponding areas of the anterior leaflet are defined as A1, A2 and A3 (Figure 1). Dividing the mitral leaflets into scallops is important for repair surgery since regurgitation from different scallops require different approach. Anatomic partitions of mitral valve are also important for percutaneous edge to edge repair, since optimum placement of the MitraClip™ depends on the location of the regurgitant jet.

The mitral annulus is a saddle shaped structure composed of fibrous and muscular fibers. The annulus establishes fibrous continuity between the fibrous trigones. As the mitral annulus continues away from the fibrous trigone, it becomes thinner and is more prone to distortion and dilatation. The fibrous skeleton of the heart is fixed and its length doesn't change with mitral valve disease [10]. Mitral anular dysfunction generally occurs in the posteromedial region of the valve. The annulus is a dynamic structure and moves synchronously during the cardiac cycle. It undergoes substantial area changes throughout the cardiac cycle reaching maximum in diastole and minimum in systole. The posterior flexible portion of the annulus plays a major role in reduction of anular area. The anterior annulus is relatively fixed during the cycle. Anular dilatation, along with ventricular remodeling, plays a major role in the pathogenesis of functional MR. Annuloplasty procedures aim to limit the further dilatation of the annulus which causes mal-coaptation of mitral leaflets. Coronary sinus, due to its close proximity to posterior mitral annulus, provides a percutaneous access for percutaneous annuloplasty procedures.

Overview of Surgical Repair Techniques and the Alfieri Stitch

The subvalvular apparatus (chorda tendinea and papillary muscles) plays an important role in maintaining normal shape and function of the left ventricle. If the papillary muscles and their chordal attachments to the valve and valve annulus are severed during the surgery, the ventricle dilates, wall stress and afterload increase and contractile function deteriorates [11]. Preservation of subvalvular apparatus during MV replacement surgery results in significantly better outcomes. In mitral valve repair surgery the entire subvalvular apparatus is preserved.

The classic mitral valve repair technique developed by Carpentier primarily involved quadrangular leaflet resection for those with prolapse, transposition of normal chords to other areas of prolapsing leaflet tissue if needed, and a remodeling annuloplasty with a complete ring prosthesis [8]. Newer techniques have been introduced which are frequently used in combination.

A simple mitral valve repair method in which the leading edges of the mitral leaflets are attached to each other by a suture (Alfieri procedure or "bow-tie" repair), creating a double orifice mitral valve, was introduced by Alfieri and colleagues [12].

Double-orifice mitral valve is an uncommon but well defined congenital anomaly of mitral leaflets characterized by a mitral valve with a single fibrous annulus with two orifices opening into the left ventricle. Patients with this anomaly may suffer from mitral regurgitation or stenosis depending on the severity of the accompanying leaflet or chordal anomalies. The observation of completely healthy subjects despite having this anomaly inspired Ottavio Alfieri to approximate the free edges of mitral leaflets by a stitch at the site of regurgitation when other surgical repair approaches are ineffective. An annuloplasty is generally performed in conjunction with the surgical edge-to-edge technique.

The double-orifice repair is technically simple, but careful evaluation of the mitral valve is necessary in selecting the right site for the approximation of the leaflets and the appropriate extension of the suture. The aim of the procedure is to completely abandon the regurgitation while maintaining the largest possible mitral valve orifice area. Inadequate application of the technique may result either in residual MR or in mitral stenosis.

Percutaneous Edge to Edge Repair

The simplicity and elegance of Alfieri stitch with its potential percutaneous applicability quickly drew the attention of the interventional cardiologists. Goar et al. demonstrated the possibility of the edge to edge repair using an endovascular approach in a non-diseased porcine model [13]. After extensive testing in animals revealed considerable efficacy, a U.S. Food and Drug Administration Investigational Device Exemption - approved phase I safety feasibility trial (EVEREST: Endovascular Valve Edge-to-Edge Repair Study) was initiated for the percutaneous edge to edge repair device: The MitraClip™ Mitral Valve Repair System.

The Mitraclip™ Mitral Valve Repair System

MitraClip™ Mitral Valve Repair System (Evalve Inc., Menlo Park, California) is a multi-axial catheter system utilizing a clip to grasp and stitch the mitral leaflets percutaneously by a transvenous transseptal route. The system is composed of three main subsystems (Figure 2):

1) A steerable guide catheter,
2) A clip delivery system,
3) The MitraClip™ device (implant).

The guide catheter is steerable using a steering knob on the proximal end of the catheter which allows flexion and lateral movement of the distal tip. The 24 F guide catheter tapers to 22 F at the distal tip. After a transseptal puncture the distal tip of the guide catheter is advanced into the left atrium over a guidewire with a tapered dilator.

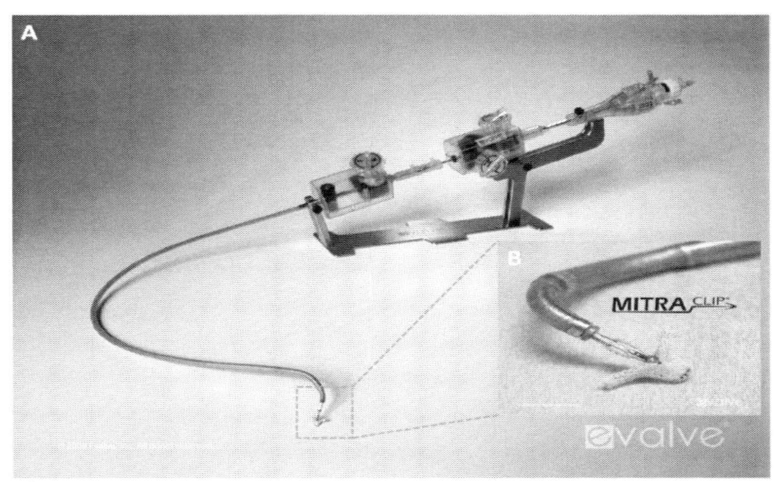

Panel A: MitraClip™ delivery system.
Panel B: The poly-ester covered cobalt/chromium MitraClip™ implant (arms opened).

Figure 2. The Evalve MitraClip™ Percutaneous Edge-to-Edge Repair System.

The clip delivery system is advanced through the guide catheter with the clip attached to its distal end. The clip delivery system is steerable using a two knob co-axial system that permits three dimensional positioning.

The clip is poly-ester covered cobalt/chromium implant with two arms that are opened and closed by control mechanisms on the clip delivery system. In the closed position the clip has an outside diameter of 15 F and in fully opened position the two arms have a span of 20 mm. The clip is designed to grasp a valve tissue of up to 8 mm of height and 4 mm of width in order to replicate the surgical Alfieri stitch [13]. U shaped gripping elements are placed in the inner portion of the clip. These grippers are small, flexible, multi-prolonged friction elements that appose and stabilize the leaflet tissue against the clip arms. When the clip is closed leaflet tissue is secured by clip arms on the ventricular side and by the grippers on the atrial side. The clip can be repositioned using echocardiographic and fluoroscopic guidance to attain the best possible result before final deployment.

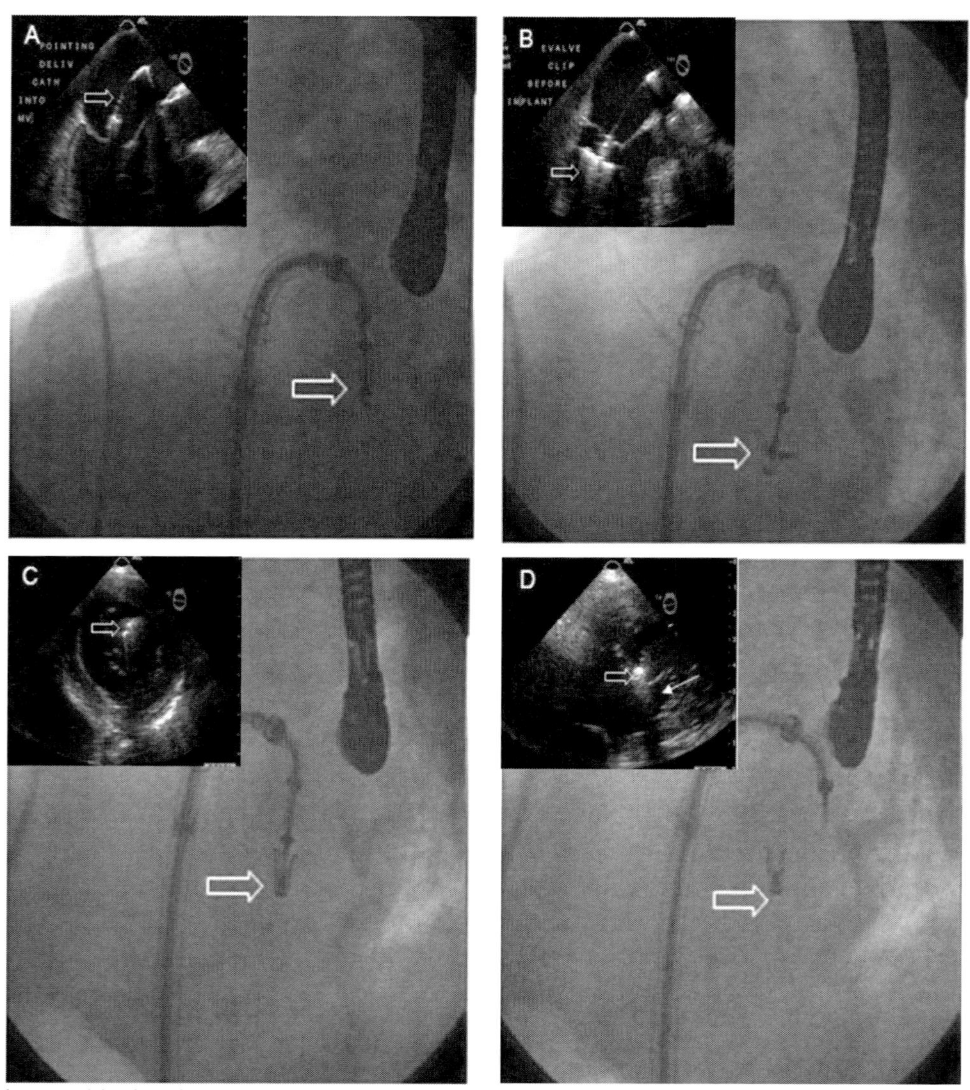

Panel A: Positioning the MitraClip™.
Panel B: The MitraClip™ advanced into the left ventricle with the arms extended.
Panel C: The mitral leaflets are grasped.
Panel D: Final deployment.
(Arrows are depicting the location of the clip).

Figure 3. Fluoroscopic and corresponding transesophageal echocardiographic views of the The MitraClip™ procedure.

Procedure Technique

The procedure is performed in the cardiac catheterization laboratory under general anesthesia using both fluoroscopic and transesophageal echocardiographic guidance. Real time transesophageal echocardiographic (TEE) guidance, in conjunction with fluoroscopy, is vital for procedural success [14]. Unlike standard transseptal puncture which primarily depends on fluoroscopic guidance and tactile feedback, TEE guidance is essential for transseptal puncture in this procedure since the MitraClip™ usually requires a higher and posterior puncture site. To facilitate positioning and maneuvering, adequate superior clearance must be achieved from the mitral anular plane. This is especially important in cases with highly prolapsing leaflets. Before the puncture, atrial septal tenting caused by the catheter tip should be assessed at various angles by TEE for establishing the ideal site. The mid esophageal 0° image shows a 4-chamber view including the mitral and tricuspid valves. This is one of the views used for locating the optimal interatrial septal puncture site. Many investigators prefer general anesthesia as esophageal intubation time may be prolonged.

After transseptal puncture, heparin is administered. A 0.035 inch guidewire is passed into the left atrium and the transseptal sheath is exchanged for guide catheter of the MitraClip™ system. The guide catheter is advanced with its tapered dilator over the supportive guidewire and the distal tip of the catheter is placed in the mid left atrium. The distal tip of the guide catheter is positioned over the mitral valve using manual torque and steering knob.

After the guiding catheter is carefully de-aired and flushed the clip delivery catheter with the clip attached in closed position to its tip is introduced into the guide catheter. After the delivery catheter is introduced into the left atrium the re-positionable clip is moved under fluoroscopic and echocardiographic guidance in multiple iterations until it is centered over the mitral orifice in three planes (Figure 3). At this stage TEE is used as the principal imaging modality to approach the mitral valve. A particular view, called inter-commissural view is obtained by rotating the transducer to 40-60°, when the probe is at the mid esophageal level. It shows A2 segment typically in the middle of the left ventricular inflow with P1 and P3 on either side. Aortic long axis view which is obtained at the mid esophagus level with 120° rotation visualizes anterior and posterior leaflets. Most frequently A2 and P2 segments are seen in this view. Together with inter-commissural view, long axis view provides the necessary orientation needed to optimize the clip angle to the mitral annulus plane.

The two arms of the clip are opened in the left atrium once the clip is aligned with the long axis of the heart near the origin of the MR jet. Under echocardiographic guidance the arms of the clip are oriented perpendicular to the long axis of the mitral leaflet edges. This orientation generally requires a transgastric short axis view. If satisfactory short axis views can not be obtained by transesophageal imaging, transthoracic echocardiography can be tried for better results.

After proper orientation the clip is advanced into the left ventricle just below the mitral leaflet tips and the vertical orientation to the leaflet edges is verified again by echocardiography. Then the clip is closed to 120° and pulled back until the mitral leaflets are captured in the arms of the clip. To facilitate grasping a midesophageal long axis left ventricular outflow tract (LVOT) view is used. The grippers are then lowered onto the atrial aspect of the leaflets. The clip is partially closed. If both leaflets have been grasped successfully, a double orifice is maintained by edge-to-edge approximation of mitral leaflets.

If successful grasping of the leaflets is verified by echocardiography with a double orifice, the clip is closed incrementally and the reduction in MR jet is assessed by Doppler echocardiography (Figure 4). An adequate grasp of both mitral leaflets does not ensure an adequate reduction in MR. Suboptimal positioning of the clip, capture of chords or just the leaflet edge in the clip arms may cause suboptimal results. Therefore a careful assessment of residual MR must be performed before the clip is fully deployed. If the location of the effectiveness of the clip is not acceptable then the grippers are raised and clip arms are opened to release the leaflet tips. In case that the clip must be withdrawn back into the left atrium, the clip arms are everted to prevent entangling the chordae tendinea. After repositioning, the procedure is repeated until a sufficient reduction in MR jet is obtained. When optimal result is achieved the clip is released from the delivery catheter and the delivery catheter and guide catheter are withdrawn (Figure 5, 6). More than one clip may be required to reduce the MR satisfactorily. After a clip is placed aspirin 325 mg daily for 6 months and clopidogrel 75 mg daily for 30 days are administered to the patients.

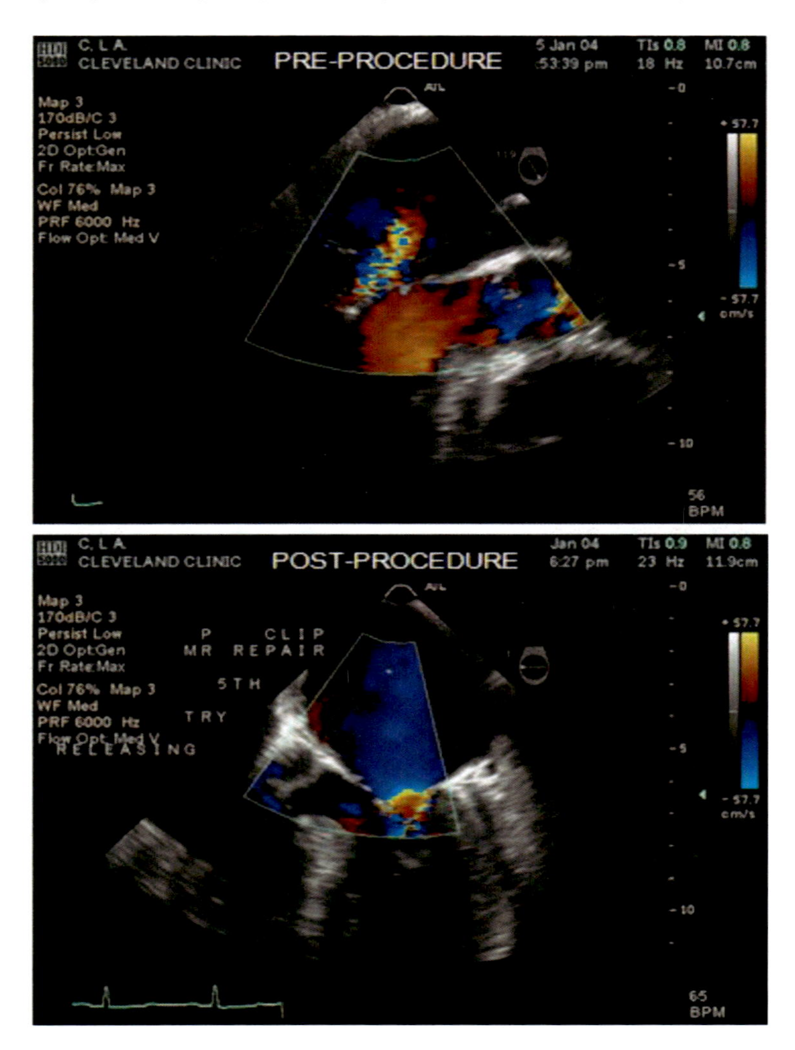

Figure 4. Pre and immediate post procedural mitral regurgitation.

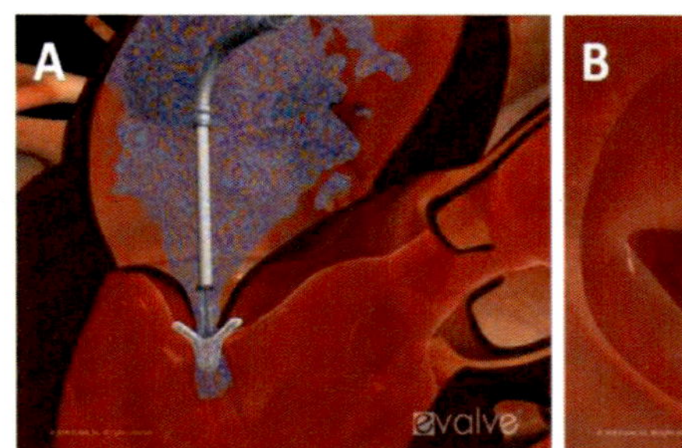

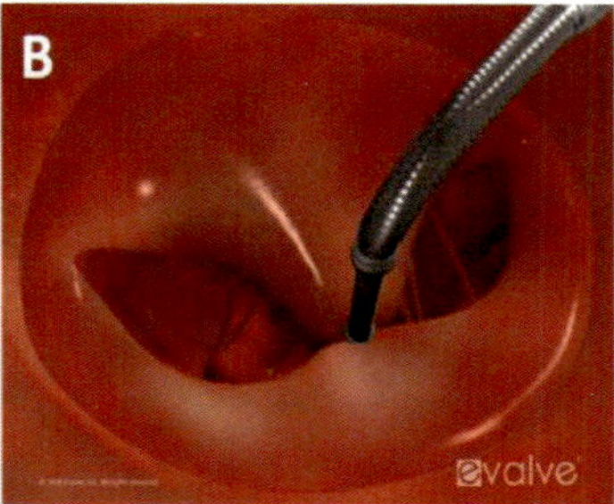

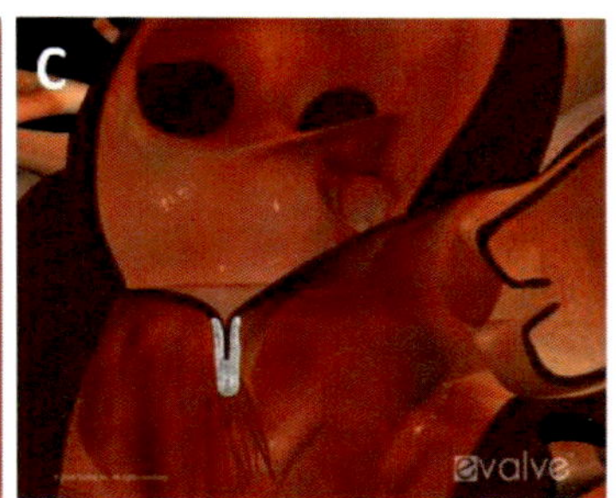

Panel A: The mitral leaflets are grasped by the MitraClip™ device.
Panel B: The double orifice mitral valve.
Panel C: Deployed MitraClip™.

Figure 5. Schematic representation of the procedure.

Table 1. Key eligibility and exclusion criteria for the EVEREST cohort

KEY ELIGIBILITY CRITERIA
Candidate for mitral valve repair or replacement surgery.
Moderate to severe (3+) or severe (4+) chronic mitral regurgitation and symptomatic with LVEF > 25 % and LVID-s ≤ 55 mm.
Asymptomatic moderate to severe (3+) or severe (4+) chronic mitral regurgitation with one of the followings: LVEF < 60 % (not less then 25 %) LVID-s ≥ 40 mm (not wider than 55 mm) New onset atrial fibrillation Pulmonary hypertension (Pulmonary artery systolic pressure > 50 mmHg at rest or > 60 mmHg with exercise)
KEY EXCLUSION CRITERIA*
Recent Myocardial Infarction
Any interventional or surgical procedure within 30 days of the index procedure
Mitral valve orifice area < 4 cm^2
Renal Insufficiency
Endocarditis
Rheumatic Heart Disease
Severe mitral anular calcification
If leaflet tethering is present, coaptation depth > 11 mm, vertical coaptation length < 2mm
Leaflet anatomy that may preclude clip implantation and proper clip positioning including evidence of calcification in the grasping area, presence of significant cleft, bileaflet flail or severe mitral valve prolapsus.

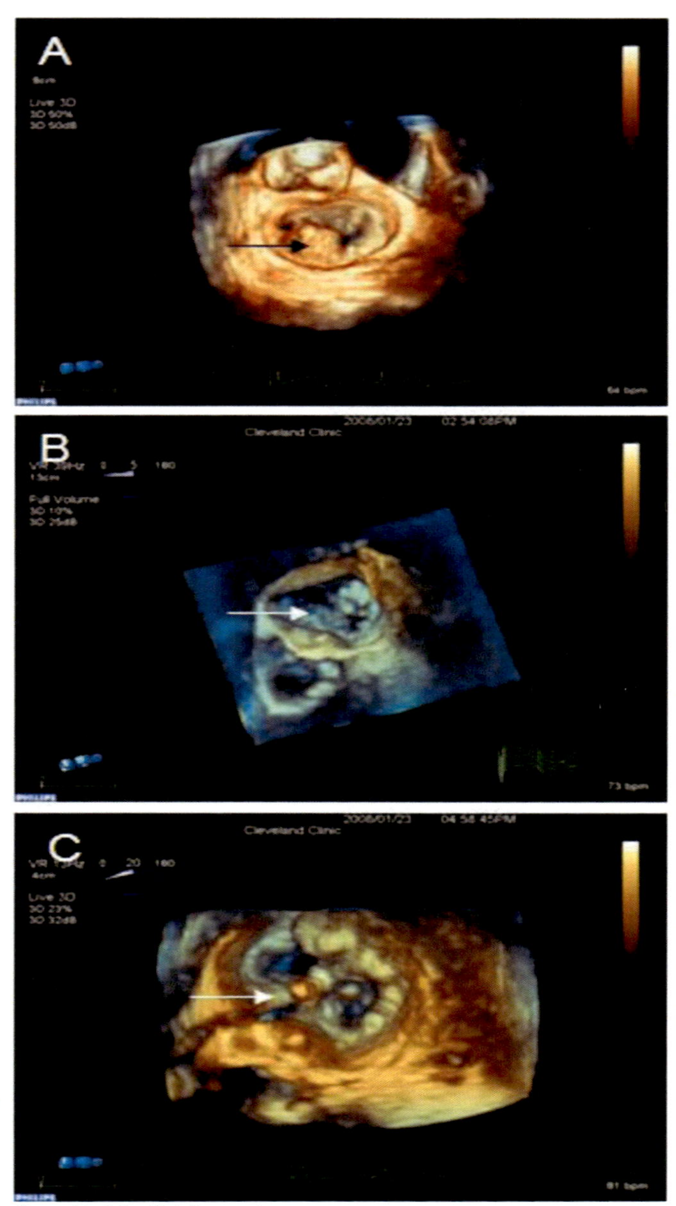

Panel A: Flail posterior mitral leaflet (arrow).
Panel B: The double orifice mitral valve.
Panel C: Deployed MitraClip™.

Figure 6. 3D Echocardiogram revealing the deployment of MitraClip™.

The U.S. Experience – Everest Trials

After the encouraging results in animal models a U.S. Food and Drug Administration Investigational Device Exemption-approved phase I safety feasibility trial (EVEREST: Endovascular Valve Edge-to-Edge Repair Study) was initiated. The initial phase I study included 55 patients which aimed to evaluate the safety and the feasibility of percutaneous edge-to-edge mitral valve repair technique [15]. The key eligibility and exclusion criteria for the EVEREST cohort is listed in table 1. The primary endpoint for the EVEREST I trial was safety at 30 days. Safety was defined as freedom from death, myocardial infarction, cardiac tamponade, cardiac surgery for failed clip or device, clip detachment, permanent stroke or septicemia. Secondary safety endpoints included in-hospital vascular complications, 30-day and 6-month bleeding, endocarditis, clip thrombosis, hemolysis and cardiac surgery for late device failure.

Initial phase I feasibility trial showed percutaneous edge-to-edge mitral valve repair can be performed safely and the degree of MR can be reduced significantly with the percutaneous approach and the trial proceeded to phase II (EVEREST II) in 2007 to evaluate the performance of endovascular mitral repair in comparison to open mitral valve surgery.

Recently, Feldman et al. reported the midterm durability and safety of the MitraClip™ device in the initial EVEREST cohort [16]. This report included the mid term results of the 107 patients of which 23 (21%) had pure functional MR and the rest had either pure degenerative MR or degenerative disease combined with functional MR. One clip was placed in 65 patients (61%) and 2 clips in 31 patients (29%). In 11 patients clipping can not be accomplished either due to complications or inability to achieve a significant reduction in MR before final deployment. There was a steep procedural learning curve, with rapid reduction in the procedure and device times throughout the study. In the overall cohort, device time, defined as time from guide catheter insertion to MitraClip™ delivery system retraction into the guide catheter, was 175 min. The device time decreased to 146 minutes in the last 30 patients in this cohort. There was no procedural mortality. Ten patients experienced a major adverse event at 30 days, including a single death in an 81-year-old patient with a Society of Thoracic Surgeons (STS) operative mortality risk score of 18.3% in whom no clip was placed and MR was not reduced, resulting in a composite primary safety end point of 9.1 % by intention to treat. One patient with a history of transient ischemic attack had a non-embolic stroke with a neurological deficit lasting >72 hours, which resolved within 30 days. Non-elective cardiac surgery was performed in 2 patients for transseptal complications. Bleeding requiring transfusion ≥2 U occurred in 4 patients. Of the ten patients meeting a major adverse event, the cause was transfusion ≥2 U in approximately one-half of the patients. There was no procedure related mortality. In-hospital mortality was <1%.

No clip embolization has occurred at any time point. Partial clip detachment, defined as detachment of a single leaflet from the clip, occurred in 10 patients (9%). None of the partial clip detachments were associated with urgent intervention.

Overall, acute procedural success was achieved in 79 patients (74 %). Of those 79 patients, 51 (64 %) were discharged with mild MR (1+) and 10 (13%) had MR graded as mild to moderate (1+ to 2+).

The composite primary efficacy end point (freedom from MR >2+, freedom from cardiac surgery for valve dysfunction, and freedom from death at 12 months) was 66%. In patients with acute procedural success Kaplan-Meier freedom from death was 95.9%, 94.0%, and 90.1% at 1, 2, and 3 years, and Kaplan-Meier freedom from surgery was 88.5%, 83.2%, and 76.3% at 1, 2, and 3 years, respectively. The 23 patients with functional MR showed similar acute results and durability compared with the overall population.

EVEREST II is a prospective, multicenter, randomized, non-blinded trial to evaluate the safety and effectiveness of the MitraClip™ system as a percutaneous approach to the repair of

MR compared with standard MV repair surgery under cardiopulmonary bypass [17]. The trial is conducted at 37 sites in the United States and Canada and enrolled 279 patients. 184 patients were randomized to MitraClip™ procedure (device group) and 95 patients were randomized to surgery (control group). After randomization, but before either treatment, patients are required to undergo a transesophageal echocardiogram within 3 days of the procedure to exclude the presence of intracardiac mass, thrombus, or vegetation. Clinical, laboratory, and echocardiographic follow-up was planned at predischarge and at 30 days, 6 months, 12 months, 18 months, 24 months, and annually to 5 years. The primary efficacy end point of the EVEREST II trial is freedom from the composite end point of death from any cause, surgery for valve dysfunction, and moderate-severe (3+) or severe (4+) MR at 12 months. The primary safety end point is the proportion of patients with major adverse events , a composite end point of all cause death, myocardial infarction and additional adverse events listed in table II.

Table 2. Primary safety endpoints for the EVEREST cohort

• Death (all cause)
• Myocardial infarction
• Reoperation for failed surgical repair or replacement
• Nonelective cardiovascular surgery for adverse events
• Stroke
• Renal failure
• Deep wound infection
• Ventilation for >48 hours
• Gastrointestinal complication requiring surgery
• New onset of permanent atrial fibrillation
• Septicemia
• Transfusion of 2 or more units of blood

EVEREST II is designed and powered with a pre-specified superiority safety margin and non-inferiority effectiveness margin to show the superiority of the device regarding to safety and show the non-inferiority of the device compared to control treatment [17].

It was reported that the primary safety end points were observed in 9.6% and 57% in the device and control group respectively which reveals a clear superiority for the MitraClip™ treatment regarding to safety (Pre-specified margin = 6%, Observed difference = 47.4%; P_{sup} <0.0001). Superiority in safety was mostly derived from the difference of need for transfusion ≥ 2 units between the groups.

Need for transfusion ≥2 units was 8.8% vs. 53.2% in the device and control group respectively (P<0.0001). When transfusions are excluded, MitraClip™ was still superior for safety endpoints (0.7% vs 16.5%; P<0.0001). In the two groups there was significant improvement in left ventricular function, NYHA functional class and quality of life.

In the EVEREST cohort 41 patients in the device group had unsuccessful initial procedures, 28 of those patients were referred to surgery.

Nine patients with an initially successful MitraClip™ procedure also required surgery for late onset device failure which makes a total of 37 cases who required surgery after the the

MitraClip™ procedure. In the 12 month follow-up, the outcomes of this patient sub-group was found to be as successful as the initial control group which shows surgery is still a safe and effective option after a failed MitraClip™ procedure.

Mitraclip™ in High Risk Patients

EVEREST researchers formed an additional cohort of 78 high risk patients who were not randomized in the EVEREST II trial. This registry, which is named EVEREST High Risk Registry (EVEREST HRR) included patients who have prohibitively high risk for surgery. Patients with 3+ or 4+ symptomatic MR (either functional or degenerative) and predicted procedural mortality risk > 12 % (STS calculated or surgeon estimated based on pre-specified co-morbidities) were included in this registry.

In September 2009, Dr. Patrick L. Whitlow from Cleveland Clinic presented the results of this registry at the Transcatheter Cardiovascular Therapeutics (TCT) meeting, San Francisco, CA [18]. In this registry, primary end point was 30 day mortality and secondary end point was major adverse events. Major effectiveness endpoints were MR reduction, freedom from death, NYHA class, left ventricular dimensions and re-hospitalization for congestive heart failure at 12 months. Patients with an LVEF ≤ 20 % and/or LVESD > 60 mm, unsuitable mitral leaflet anatomy for the procedure and mitral valve area < 4 cm^2 were not enrolled into this registry. Patients that were eligible for HRR but for some reason (e.g. institutional review board approval, patient refusal, insurance reasons etc) could not be treated with MitraClip served as a control population. Dr. Whitlow reported that the procedural success was 96% in the HRR. 46 patients required 1 clip, and 29 patients required 2 clips for procedural success.

In three patients procedure was unsuccessful and no clips were implanted. The predicted 30 day mortality -based on the STS scores- of the patient cohort was 18.2 %. The observed mortality in those patients were found to be 7.7% (P=0.006). Total number of patients who met a major adverse event was 20 (6 deaths, 1 renal failure, 1 permanent atrial fibrillation, 1 prolonged (>48 hours) ventilation and 11 blood transfusions (≥2 Units). There was no difference in 30 day mortalities between the HRR group and HRR control group. However, freedom from death at 12 months was 76.4 % and 55.3 % respectively in the HRR group and HRR control group (P=0.037).

There was a 45 % reduction in the rate of re-hospitalizations from congestive heart failure in the HRR group (P=0.02) compared to their pre-procedural re-hospitalization rates. Both end systolic and end diastolic diameters and ejection fractions were significantly improved in the HRR group compared to their baseline. The EVEREST HRR revealed that MitraClip™ device can be successfully implanted to high risk patients who are considered ineligible for surgery and clinical benefits are found to be superior to the conventional medical therapy. The improvement in mortality rate, NYHA class, ventricular functions and re-hospitalization rates were sustained at 12 months.

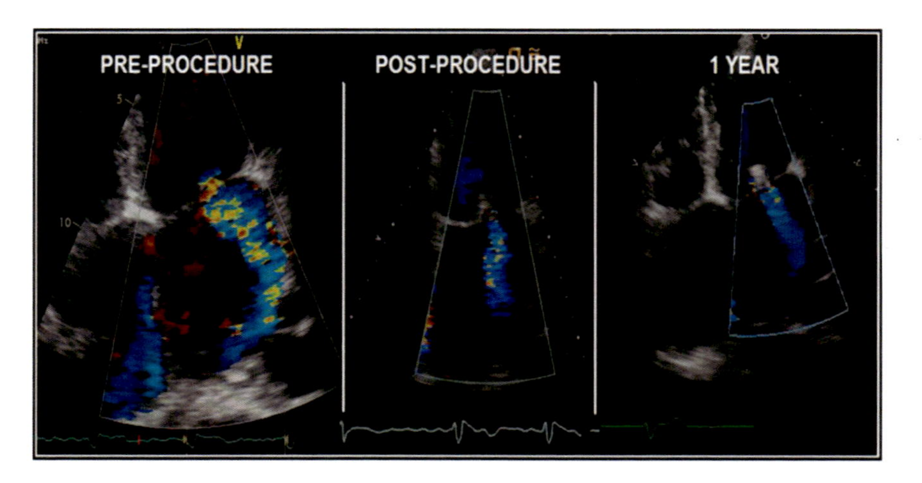

Figure 7. Pre-procedural, 30 day post-procedure and 12 months follow-up echocardiograms of a MitraClip™ patients.

Conclusion

The US experience with the MitraClip™ device yielded promising results. The EVEREST trials showed that the procedure was non-inferior to surgery with regards to effectiveness and superior with regards to complications. EVEREST HRR showed that patients who are considered ineligible for MV surgery because of their high surgical risk also benefited from the procedure. The procedure yielded similar results both in the functional and degenerative MR patients. Despite the absence of adjunctive annuloplasty the procedure remained effective at 12 months (Figure 7). Even though current evidence, based on relatively short term follow up, did not reveal a clear need for annuloplasty, there are still ongoing concerns about long term durability of the percutaneous procedure in functional MR patients without an annuloplasty. Percutaneous annuloplasty procedures are still under development and will provide additional durability to MitraClip™ procedure in the long run. However, long term follow-up data will be required to make robust conclusions about the durability of the procedure.

References

[1] Ling LH, Enriquez-Sarano M, Seward JB, Tajik AJ, Schaff HV, Bailey KR, et al. Clinical outcome of mitral regurgitation due to flail leaflet. *N. Engl. J. Med.* 1996 Nov 7;335(19):1417-23.

[2] Trichon BH, Felker GM, Shaw LK, Cabell CH, O'Connor CM. Relation of frequency and severity of mitral regurgitation to survival among patients with left ventricular systolic dysfunction and heart failure. *Am. J. Cardiol.* 2003 Mar 1;91(5):538-43.

[3] Nkomo VT, Gardin JM, Skelton TN, Gottdiener JS, Scott CG, Enriquez-Sarano M. Burden of valvular heart diseases: a population-based study. *Lancet.* 2006 Sep 16; 368(9540):1005-11.

[4] Lawrie GM. Mitral valve repair vs replacement. Current recommendations and long-term results. *Cardiol. Clin.* 1998 Aug;16(3): 437-48.

[5] Lee EM, Shapiro LM, Wells FC. Superiority of mitral valve repair in surgery for degenerative mitral regurgitation. *Eur. Heart J.* 1997 Apr; 18(4):655-63.

[6] Gillinov AM, Wierup PN, Blackstone EH, Bishay ES, Cosgrove DM, White J, et al. Is repair preferable to replacement for ischemic mitral regurgitation? J. *Thorac. Cardiovasc. Surg.* 2001 Dec;122(6):1125-41.

[7] Goodney PP, Stukel TA, Lucas FL, Finlayson EV, Birkmeyer JD. Hospital volume, length of stay, and readmission rates in high-risk surgery. *Ann. Surg.* 2003 Aug;238(2):161-7.

[8] Carpentier A, Chauvaud S, Fabiani JN, Deloche A, Relland J, Lessana A, et al. Reconstructive surgery of mitral valve incompetence: ten-year appraisal. *J. Thorac. Cardiovasc. Surg.* 1980 Mar;79(3):338-48.

[9] Enriquez-Sarano M, Akins CW, Vahanian A. Mitral regurgitation. *Lancet.* 2009 Apr 18;373(9672):1382-94.

[10] Lillehei CW, Levy MJ, Bonnabeau RC, Jr. Mitral Valve Replacement With Preservation Of Papillary Muscles And Chordae Tendineae. *J. Thorac. Cardiovasc. Surg.* 1964 Apr;47:532-43.

[11] Rozich JD, Carabello BA, Usher BW, Kratz JM, Bell AE, Zile MR. Mitral valve replacement with and without chordal preservation in patients with chronic mitral regurgitation. Mechanisms for differences in postoperative ejection performance. *Circulation.* 1992 Dec;86(6):1718-26.

[12] Alfieri O, Maisano F, De Bonis M, Stefano PL, Torracca L, Oppizzi M, et al. The double-orifice technique in mitral valve repair: a simple solution for complex problems. *J. Thorac. Cardiovasc. Surg.* 2001 Oct;122(4):674-81.

[13] St Goar FG, Fann JI, Komtebedde J, Foster E, Oz MC, Fogarty TJ, et al. Endovascular edge-to-edge mitral valve repair: short-term results in a porcine model. *Circulation.* 2003 Oct 21;108(16):1990-3.

[14] Silvestry FE, Rodriguez LL, Herrmann HC, Rohatgi S, Weiss SJ, Stewart WJ, et al. Echocardiographic guidance and assessment of percutaneous repair for mitral regurgitation with the Evalve MitraClip: lessons learned from EVEREST I. *J. Am. Soc. Echocardiogr.* 2007 Oct;20(10):1131-40.

[15] Feldman T, Wasserman HS, Herrmann HC, Gray W, Block PC, Whitlow P, et al. Percutaneous mitral valve repair using the edge-to-edge technique: six-month results of the EVEREST Phase I Clinical Trial. *J. Am. Coll. Cardiol.* 2005 Dec 6;46(11):2134-40.

[16] Feldman T, Kar S, Rinaldi M, Fail P, Hermiller J, Smalling R, et al. Percutaneous mitral repair with the MitraClip system: safety and midterm durability in the initial EVEREST (Endovascular Valve Edge-to-Edge REpair Study) cohort. *J. Am. Coll. Cardiol.* 2009 Aug 18;54(8):686-94.

[17] Mauri L, Garg P, Massaro JM, Foster E, Glower D, Mehoudar P, et al. The EVEREST II Trial: design and rationale for a randomized study of the evalve mitraclip system compared with mitral valve surgery for mitral regurgitation. *Am. Heart J.* 2010 Jul;160(1):23-9.

[18] Whitlow PL, editor. Percutaneous Edge-To-Edge Evalve Mitral Valve Repair in the US "High Risk" Registry. Transcatheter Cardiovascular Therapeutics (TCT) Meeting, 21-25 September 2009, San Francisco, CA.

In: Percutaneous Valve Technology: Present and Future ISBN: 978-1-61942-577-4
Editors: Jose Luis Navia and Sharif Al-Ruzzeh

Chapter XX

Current Percutaneous Coronary Sinus Mitral Annuloplasty Devices in Patients with Dilated Cardiomyopathy

Tohru Takaseya, Sharif Al-Ruzzeh and Kiyotaka Fukamachi

Introduction

Mitral regurgitation (MR) is an important clinical entity in which blood leaks from the left ventricle (LV) back into the left atrium during systole. Patients with significant MR may suffer from shortness of breath, symptoms of congestive heart failure, and atrial arrhythmias. MR is caused by a variety of different mechanisms and pathologies affecting various components of the mitral valve. The father of surgical mitral valve repair, Alain Carpentier, MD, PhD, described a three-tier classification system (types I, II, and III), which incorporates annular size, leaflet mobility, and coaptation, as well as LV and papillary muscle function in determining the structural changes causing MR. This classification remains relevant to the modern-day surgeon and in the new era of percutaneous mitral valve repair [1] (Figure 1).

The terms *functional* and *ischemic* MR are often used interchangeably in clinical medicine, but some relevant differences exist. Functional MR usually occurs when mitral leaflets fail to coapt despite normal leaflet motion (Carpentier type I dysfunction) and can be seen with increased LV sphericity [2,3], papillary muscle tethering from nonischemic LV enlargement [4], or mitral annular dilatation [5]. Myocardial infarction, often with regional involvement of the posterolateral LV wall and the posterior papillary muscle, can also result in LV/mitral annular enlargement and so-called ischemic MR. Ischemic MR arises from apical papillary muscle displacement with primarily posterior leaflet tethering and restricted motion during systole (Carpentier type IIIb dysfunction). Apical displacement of both leaflets with restricted motion in systole and diastole, often with associated rheumatic valve disease, results in type IIIa dysfunction. Almost half the patients with LV dysfunction have at least moderate MR [6, 7]. Due to its vicious downward cycle, the prognosis is poor in patients with functional MR [6, 8]. Chronic ischemic MR, also called "Functional" MR or "Secondary"

MR, is an independent predictor of higher mortality and higher risk of developing heart failure in the post myocardial infarction population [8, 9].

Ischemic MR occurs in 10-20% of the patients with coronary artery disease (CAD) [10], translating to an incidence of approximately 50,000 to 100,000 patients. Despite the increased mortality and risk of heart failure, there is currently no therapy that demonstrates a survival benefit for the ischemic MR population [10-13]. Prosthetic ring annuloplasty is a key in most cases of surgical valve repair because there is always some degree of annular dilation in severe chronic MR. Surgical mitral annuloplasty is widely used to treat chronic MR, either in isolation or, most often, in combination with other techniques. However, the operative procedure requires access to and manipulation of the valve annulus via a left atriotomy and stitching of the ring is a time-consuming process. Furthermore, the procedure currently requires the patient to be placed on cardiopulmonary bypass (CPB) to facilitate the treatment. Research indicates that CPB constitutes a greater risk to patient outcomes than does the access means associated with the procedure (sternotomy, thoracotomy). Longer CPB times have been suggested as a cause of minor neurological deficits following open-heart procedures, and the use of heparin during CPB results in an increased risk of stroke complications. Finally, the outcome of the annuloplasty ring placement cannot be adequately assessed until the patient is weaned from CPB. These complications result in added procedural and anesthetic times and are typical reasons for increased morbidity/mortality rates in treated patients. Surgery may be high risk or even contraindicated in a substantial group of patients due to the presence of severe comorbidities and/or very severe LV dysfunction.

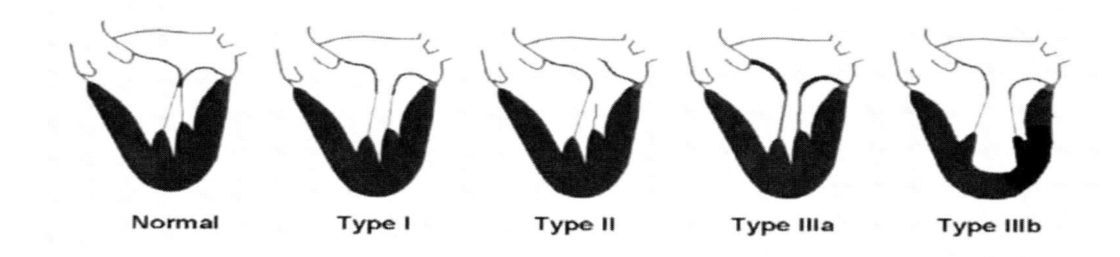

Figure 1. The Carpentier classification of mitral valve regurgitation encompasses the basic mechanistic etiologies for mitral regurgitation. In reality,more than one type can coexist in any given individual. Shown at left is the normal mitral valve apparatus. Type I indicates normal leaflet motion with annular dilation. Type II indicates increased leaflet motion (leaflet prolapse or flail). Type IIIa indicates restricted leaflet motion in systole and diastole, usually associated with leaflet and subvalvular thickening (rheumatic). Type IIIb indicates restricted leaflet motion in systole, often seen in ischemic cardiomyopathy with history of infarct (dark region in left ventricle). Reproduced with permission.

These findings set the stage for the new percutaneous techniques. There is a great variety of innovative therapies that have been proposed. Several of them have taken advantage of the close anatomical relationship of the coronary sinus (CS) / great cardiac vein (GCV) to the posterior mitral annulus. Blood that supplies the heart via the coronary arteries returns to the venous system by way of venous drainage, which coalesces into the GCV. This vein lies in the posterior atrioventricular groove between the left atrium and LV. The GCV becomes the CS, which drains into the right atrium. The GCV/CS is located slightly more on the atrial side of the atrioventricular groove, which is slightly superior to the mitral annulus. Although the distance between the CS and the mitral annulus is variable, it averages between 5 mm and 10 mm [14]. By taking advantage of this relationship, several devices are under development that can be placed within the CS. Through tensioning of these systems by various means, the circumference of the mitral annulus can be decreased, with attendant reduction in the septal-lateral dimension and reduction in MR. Several therapeutic approaches have proposed placing a device within the CS/GCV to place some force on the mitral annulus, reduce the septal-lateral diameter of the mitral annulus [15, 16], and/or cinch the mitral annulus. Several experimental studies have been performed in animals with acute and chronic models of moderate functional regurgitation and have shown potential to reduce the size of the mitral annulus and the degree of MR [17, 18]. To date, more than 100 cases of CS annuloplasty have been performed in man with three different devices: the Monarc device [19], the CARILLON Mitral Contour System [20], and the Viacor percutaneous mitral annuloplasty device (PTMA) [21].

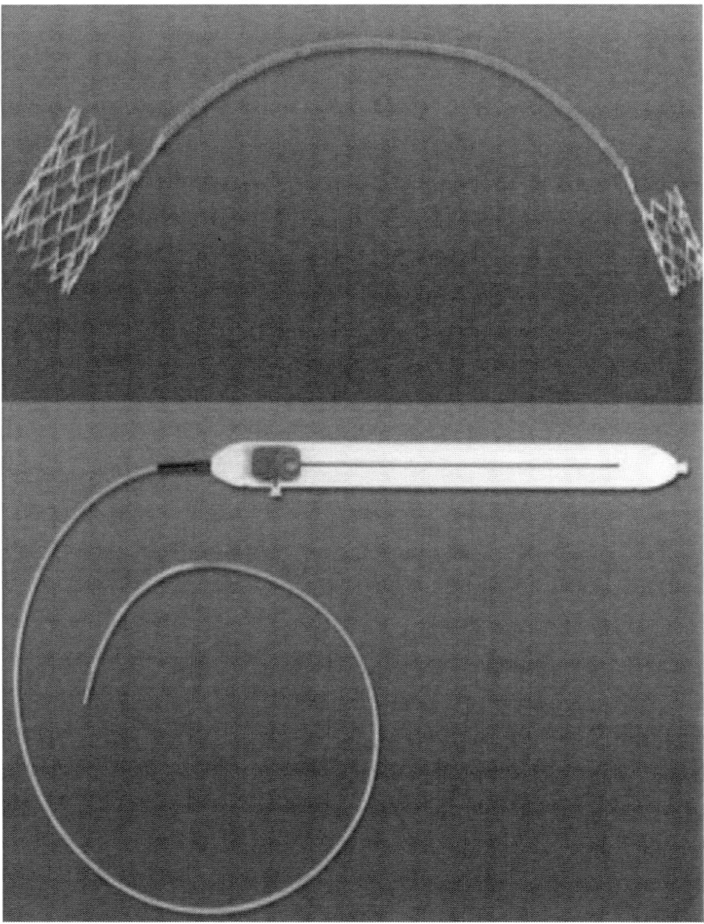

Figure 2. Top: The Monarc percutaneous mitral valve annuloplasty device (formery manufactures by Edwards Lefesciences, Inc.) was constructed of nitinol and consisted of a large proximal anchor, a flexible shortening bridge segment, and a small distal anchor. Bottom: The delivery system consisted of an over-the-wire inner catheter on which was mounted the compressed implant and an outer restraining sheath. The sheath was retracted with a thumb sliding mechanism that sequentially released the self-expanding distal and then the proximal anchor. Reproduced with permission.

Keywords: mitral valve annuloplasty, coronary sinus, minimally invasive surgery, off-pump surgery

Monarc*

Device Description

The Monarc Percutaneous Mitral Annuloplasty System (Edwards Lifesciences Inc; Figure 2)was composed of two self-expanding stents (one proximal, one distal) connected by a bridge element, which had a delayed foreshortening capacity (after 3 to 6 weeks) due to presence of absorbable material. The systemconsisted of a 12 F outer-diameter guide catheter and dilator, a 9 F delivery catheter, and a nickel-titanium alloy (nitinol) implant (Figure 2) [19]. The implant itself was made up of 3 sections: a distal self-expanding anchor, a springlike "bridge," and a proximal self-expanding anchor. The distal anchor was deployed in the GCV; the proximal anchor was deployed in the proximal CS. The bridge has shape-memory properties that result in shortening forces at body temperature. The distal stent is designed to be placed within the anterior interventricular vein, the tributary vessel of the GCV that is furthermost from the CS, running near the ventricular septum. The proximal stent was placed in the CS. Thus, as the spacers in the connecting bridge dissolve, a foreshortening force was created with the intention of cinching the mitral annulus. This device was not retrievable and did not allow for immediate assessment of efficacy and risk of compression of the circumflex artery.

Study Results

Clinical experience with second-generation devices has only been reported in five patients [19]. All patients in these preliminary studies had functional MR either of ischemic origin or in cardiomyopathy. Four of five patients had chronic ischemic MR $\geq$2+ and ejection fractions >30%. Device implantation was successful in 4 of 5 patients. In one patient (patient 2), the device could not be advanced fully into the CS because of difficulty in obtaining coaxial guide position. The one unsuccessful patient had perforation of the anterior interventricular vein. At the 3-month follow-up, all patients remained alive. There was one late death (day 148) caused by progressive heart failure. There was a reduction in MR grade from 3.0 ± 0.7 to 1.6 ± 1.1 at the last postimplantation visit in those with an intact device. Three patients experienced separation of the nitinol bridge segment, visualized on chest X ray, at days 22, 28, and 81. Coronary angiograms were obtained at 3 months in the other 3 patients who received implants. There was no evidence of compromise of the circumflex coronary artery as a result of the device implanted in the adjacent GCV. Patency of CS was documented in all patients.

The Monarc device was tested in the EVOLUTION I study, which was a feasibility study [19]. This study was not designed to formally address clinical efficacy endpoints, although some data are available in a subset of patients. In the 72 patients enrolled, 59 received implants, with anatomic reasons limiting implants in the rest. All the patients had cardiomyopathy with 2 to 4+ MR, with 57% symptomatic. Results from the first five patients were published to demonstrate proof of efficacy [19]. Four of these five patients received a device, and reduction in MR was seen in three of those four patients acutely. In those three patients, bridge separation occurred, with return of MR. Thus, this therapy demonstrated effectiveness when the device was intact, but showed a lack of efficacy with loss of integrity. The device has since been redesigned to avoid separations. Data have recently been presented on 2-year efficacy in a subset of patients with available data. In 21 patients, the MR grade was reduced from a mean of 2.3 to 1.9 at 2 years (P = .1), and in 24 patients, the New York Heart Association (NYHA) classification was reduced from 2.7 to 2 at 2 years (P = .002). Using quantitative assessments of MR, there appeared to be little deterioration from 1 to 2 years.

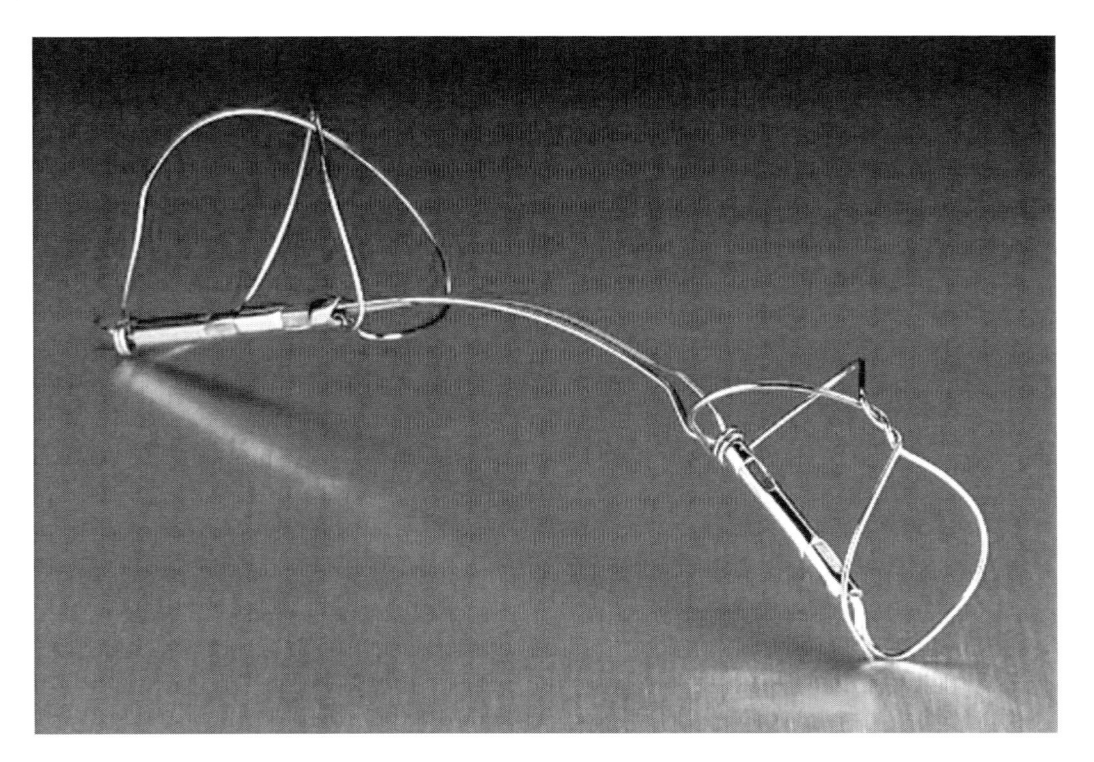

Figure 3. The CARILLON Mitral Contour System is a fixedlength, double-anchor, nitinol device designed to be positioned within the CS/GCV to reduce FMR. The arc of the nitinol ribbon, which connects the 2 anchors, serves to orient the device automatically during deployment. Reproduced with permission.

A larger clinical study, EVOLUTION II, has been initiated in Europe and Canada [22]. The EVOLUTION II study will commence in the near future and will be a nonrandomized multicenter prospective consecutive registry study. There will be 19 clinical sites, which expect to enroll 150 patients. Primary safety end-points will be 30-day freedom from major adverse cardiovascular cerebrovascular events, and the primary efficacy end-point will examine the 6-month reduction of at least 1 grade of MRion from baseline.

Carillon

Device Description

The Carillon Mitral Contour System (Cardiac Dimensions, Kirkland, WA; Figure 3) also has a proximal and a distal anchor, which are joined by a nitinol wire element. This latter device is retrievable and allows for immediate assessment of efficacy and risk of compression of the circumflex artery. The CARILLON Mitral Contour System device [20] uses the concept of mitral annular placation (i.e., cinching of the MA) to reduce MR. The device consists of two major components: (i) a distal anchor device intended for temporary placement in the GCV; (ii) a catheter-based delivery system through which the distal anchor device is deployed. The anchors are mirror-image double helices that have shape memory characteristics. The anchors may be deployed and subsequently recaptured within a titanium crimping tube. The distal anchor is available in diameters of 3.5–9.0 mm. After deployment of the distal anchor in the GCV, tension is applied by pulling on the system resulting in plication (i.e., cinching) of the mitral annulus. Traction is released if there is hemodynamic compromise, coronary artery compression, displacement of the distal anchor, adequate reduction in MR, or 8 cm translation of the proximal anchor marker. Once adequate tension has been applied, the proximal anchor is deployed and the device is uncoupled from the delivery catheter system. This device is recapturable and removable until it is released, which may be done if there is inadequate efficacy in reducing MR, or if there is coronary artery compromise.

Study Results

The CARILLON Mitral Contour System has been studied in the European AMADEUS study [23]. This study looked at symptomatic patients with dilated (ischemic and nonischemic) cardiomyopathy, depressed LV ejection fraction, and 2 to 4+ MR as assessed by an echocardiographic core lab. Implantation of the CARILLONdevice was attempted in 48 patients, with 29 receiving implants. Reasons for nonimplantation included distal anchor slipping of an early version of the device (resolved with minor redesign), inability to access the CS/GCV, insufficient reduction in MR, and/or coronary artery compromise. Although coronary arteries were crossed in 84% of cases, coronary artery compromise limited implantation in 15%. There were three non-ST-elevation myocardial infarctions in this study. In one, the event was clinically relevant, but no clear obstruction was observed. This patient developed worsening renal failure and died 3 weeks later; this was the only procedure-related (within 30 days) death of the study. The overall 30-day major adverse event rate was 13%, which appears to be acceptable because in this high-risk cohort, there is a > 20% predicted 1-year mortality rate, and half of the complications were related to vascular access. It is of note that a subsequent European study (TITAN) has completed enrollment, and there was only one 30-day complication in the 53 patients enrolled, providing a major adverse event rate of < 2%. In AMADEUS, efficacy was assessed using a variety of modalities. MR was assessed by a core lab using quantitative assessments. Overall, in AMADEUS, there was a 27% quantitative reduction in MR. Clinical parameters improved as well. At baseline, 88% of patients were in NYHA class III or IV, whereas at 6 months, only 12% of patients receiving an implant were in NYHA class III or IV. There were marked improvements in functional capacity, as assessed by 6-minute walk tests, as well as in quality-of-life tests.

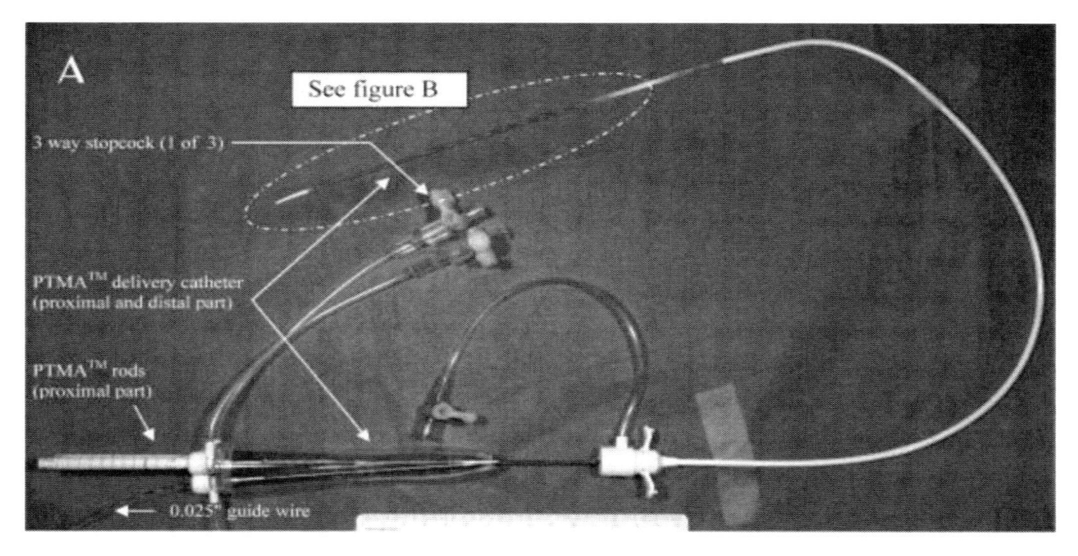

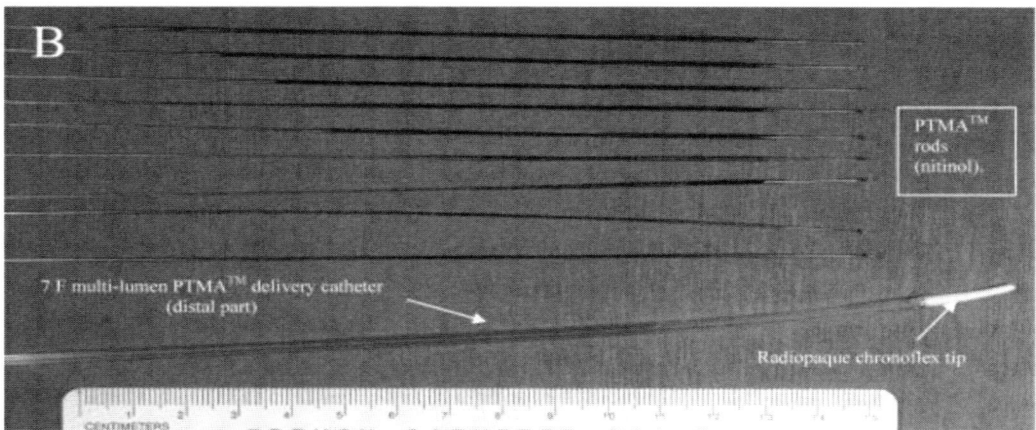

Figure 4. PTMA temporary implant. (A) PTMA device. (B) Distal part of the PTMA device placed in the CS. PTMA, percutaneous transvenous mitral annuloplasty. The device consists of straight and rigid nitinol rods that are inserted into a 7 F multilumen custom catheter with the atraumatic silicone distal tip seated into the anterior interventricular vein. Up to 3 rods may be inserted into the parallel lumens of the delivery catheter. Reproduced with permission.

PTMA

Device Description

The PTMA (Viacor, Inc., Wilmington, MA; Figure 4) is a device used for "percutaneous transvenous mitral annuloplasty" and consists of a polytetrafluoroethylene catheter in which rods of different stiffness are introduced, putting pressure on the posterior annulus at the P2 segment of the mitral valve. After testing to find the appropriate combination of rigid elements, permanent implantation is performed. Here again, the device is retrievable in cases of absence of efficacy or circumflex cinching. The Viacor PTMA consists of straight and rigid nitinol rods that are inserted into a 7 F multilumen custom catheter with the atraumatic silicone distal tip seated into the anterior interventricular vein [21]. Up to three rods may be inserted into the parallel lumens of the delivery catheter to obtain the desired tension and graded conformational change in the mitral annulus. The rods are available in two hinge stiffnesses (100 and 200 g/cm of pressure), six distal treatment lengths (70, 90, 110, 120, 130, and 140 mm), and three tapers (full, half, and quarter). The proximal and distal treatment barrels can be supplied in different lengths, resulting in a total of 15-rod configurations. As opposed to other mitral annuloplasty CS devices, the Viacor device exerts an outward force at its proximal and distal segments (i.e., commissural points) because of its straight and rigid element. This results in anterior displacement of the midportion of the posterior annulus toward the anterior annulus, thus decreasing the anterior-posterior diameter of the mitral annulus. This increases leaflet coaptation and reduces MR. By varying the number, stiffness, and treatment length of the rods, incremental changes in mitral annular geometry can be obtained.

Study Results

MR was assessed and the PTMA device adjusted to optimize efficacy. If MR reduction ($\geq$ 1 grade) was observed, placement of a PTMA implant was attempted. Implanted patients were evaluated with echocardiographic, quality of life, and exercise capacity metrics. Nineteen patients received a diagnostic PTMA study. Diagnostic PTMA was effective in 13 patients (MR grade 3.2 $\pm$ 0.6 reduced to 2.0 $\pm$ 1.0), and PTMA implants were placed in 9 patients. Four devices were removed uneventfully (at 7, 84, 197, and 216 days), and three for annuloplasty surgery due to observed PTMA device migration and/or diminished efficacy. No procedure- or device-related major adverse events with permanent sequelae were observed in any of the diagnostic or implant patients. Sustained reductions of mitral annulus septal-lateral dimension from 3D echo reconstruction dimensions were observed (4.0 $\pm$ 1.2 mm at 3 months) [24].

Temporary implants suggested efficacy, and the subsequent PTOLEMY trial found a reduction of MR by at least 1 grade was achieved in 13 of 19 patients with limited follow-up suggesting durability [25].

Comment

The proximity between the CS and the mitral annulus is exploited on the basis of the theory that a device with foreshortening capacities placed in the former may reduce the size of the latter and increase leaflet coaptation. However, several studies based on anatomy and/or imaging using multislice computed tomography or magnetic resonance imaging have shown several potential limitations of this approach.

First, several groups [19, 26-28] reported that the left circumflex artery was located between the CS and the mitral valvular annulus in 63% to 80% patients. This frequency increased up to 96% of cases when severe MR was present [28]. This anatomic reality is raising concern over the potential for coronary ischemia from devices located in the CS. The contraindication to implantation of the PTMA included the presence of a proximal coronary circumflex stent and a left dominant coronary circulation. Second, the anatomic proximity of the CS and mitral annulus is of great concern. Maselli *et al.* [14] examined the detailed anatomic relationship between the CS, coronary arteries, and mitral valve annulus in 61 excised cadaveric human hearts and reported that the maximal distance from the CS to the mitral annulus was up to 19 mm (mean: 9.7 ± 3.2 mm). Sorgente *et al.* [28] are consistent with Maselli *et al.* [14] and showed that *in vivo* and in a large group of patients with normal ventricular function CS always lies behind the posterior wall of the left atrium at a significant distance from the mitral annulus. In patients with normal dimensions of the left chambers, they also observed a large variability in the distance between the CS and the mitral annulus. This distance was quantified by the angle in axial section and by the area between the CS and mitral annulus.

The anatomic position of the CS behind the left atrial wall in patients with normal left chamber volume is not a rare finding. Indeed, the anatomic position of the CS behind the left atrial wall may be indicative of anatomical reserve of the CS. The plasticity of the CS they are hypothesizing is substantiated by the observed high correlation between elongation of the CS and volumetric changes of LV chambers. This novel observation is also concordant with remodeling of the mitral annulus area. Sorgente *et al.* [28] also demonstrated that a gradual but progressive shift of CS toward the mitral annulus occurred when left chambers enlarge, as evident by changes in both angular and planimetric measures. However, due to the strong mutually dependence of left atrial and ventricular sizes, it was not possible to discriminate the main determinant (atrial or ventricular dimension) of this relationship. The gradual and progressive shift of the CS toward the mitral annulus was equally evident in patients with coronary artery disease or idiopathic cardiomyopathy. Patients with moderate to severe MR frequently present with larger left atrial and ventricular volumes. These patients may particularly benefit from the percutaneous CS mitral annuloplasty due to the closer proximity of CS to the mitral annulus. However, Choure *et al.* [27] showed in a study of 36 patients that the CS-to-mitral annulus distance increases in patients with severe MR and annular dilation, mainly in the posterolateral location.

The third potential disadvantage to the use of annuloplasty devices that pass through the CS is that such devices are only applied along the posterior annulus, leaving the anterior annulus untreated. The ring inserted into the CS is necessarily incomplete and localized to the posterior half of the annulus covering only 120° or 140° of the circumference of the mitral annulus, leaving the commissures and the anterior half of the annulus unsupported. There is a possibility of dilatation of the trigone-to-trigone area [29], which may cause a potential recurrence of MR in the long term. Thus, efficacy is a concern in cases in which surgeons usually use undersized and complete rings. We need to evaluate all of the above risks before committing to CS treatment. Multislice computer tomography is an extremely valuable technique for precisely assessing morphological and anatomical changes of CS and its relation to coronary arteries in patients with heart failure undergoing nonpharmacological device-based therapies delivered via the CS.

Conclusion

The potential benefits of these percutaneous CS mitral annuloplasty devices still require considerable study, but the current results are encouraging. These devices are effective for high-risk patients who have ischemic or nonischemic functional, moderate or severe MR with LV dysfunction. These devices need preoperative screening for anatomic relationship among the CS, mitral annulus, and left circumflex from multislice computed tomography. There are a number of issues that still necessitate clarification; (1) the need for standardized measurements of mitral annular and CS dimensions; (2) the possibility of combining transcatheter mitral valve devices for additive effects (i.e., CS annuloplasty and mitral valve leaflet repair systems); and (3) the use of such devicesto limit the hemodynamic stress of MR and possibly reduce the need for or prolong the time to mitral valve surgery.

References

[1] Carpentier A. Cardiac valve surgery: the "French correction." *J. Thorac. Cardiovasc. Surg.* 1983;86:323-337.

[2] Kono T, Sabbah HN, Rosman H, et al. Left ventricular shape is the primary determinant of functional mitral regurgitation in heart failure. *J. Am. Coll. Cardiol.* 1992;20:1594-1598.

[3] Sabbah HN, Rosman H, Kono T, et al. On the mechanism of functional mitral regurgitation. *Am. J. Cardiol.* 1993;72:1074-1076.

[4] Otsuji Y, Handschumacher MD, Schwammenthal E, et al. Insights from three-dimensional echocardiography into the mechanism of functional mitral regurgitation: direct in vivo demonstration of altered leaflet tethering geometry. *Circulation.* 1997;96:1999-2008.

[5] Boltwood CM, Tei C, Wong M, et al. Quantitative echocardiography of the mitral complex n dilated cardiomyopathy: the mechanism of functional mitral regurgitation. *Circulation.* 1983;68:498-508.

[6] Koelling TM, Aaronson KD, Cody RJ, Bach DS, Armstrong WF. Prognostic significance of mitral regurgitation and tricuspid regurgitation in patients with left ventricular systolic dysfunction. *Am. Heart J.* 2002;144:524-9.

[7] Robbins JD, Maniar PB, Cotts W, Parker MA, Bonow RO, Gheorghiade M. Prevalence and severity of mitral regurgitation in chronic systolic heart failure. *Am. J. Cardiol.* 2003;91:360-2.

[8] Grigioni F, Enriquez-Sarano M, Zehr KJ, Bailey KR, Tajik AJ. Ischemic mitral regurgitation: long-term outcome and prognostic implications with quantitative Doppler assessment. *Circulation* 2001;103:1759-64.

[9] Lamas GA, Mitchell GF, Flaker GC, Smith SC, Jr., Gersh BJ, Basta L, Moye L, Braunwald E, Pfeffer MA. Clinical significance of mitral regurgitation after acute myocardial infarction. Survival and Ventricular Enlargement Investigators. *Circulation* 1997;96:827-33.

[10] Borger MA, Alam A, Murphy PM, Doenst T, David TE. Chronic ischemic mitral regurgitation: repair, replace or rethink? *Ann. Thorac. Surg.* 2006;81:1153-61.

[11] Harris KM, Sundt TM, 3rd, Aeppli D, Sharma R, Barzilai B. Can late survival of patients with moderate ischemic mitral regurgitation be impacted by intervention on the valve? *Ann. Thorac. Surg.* 2002;74:1468-75.

[12] McGee EC, Gillinov AM, Blackstone EH, Rajeswaran J, Cohen G, Najam F, Shiota T, Sabik JF, Lytle BW, McCarthy PM, Cosgrove DM. Recurrent mitral regurgitation after annuloplasty for functional ischemic mitral regurgitation. *J. Thorac. Cardiovasc. Surg.* 2004;128:916-24.

[13] Fukamachi K. Percutaneous and off-pump treatments for functional mitral regurgitation. *J. Artif. Organs* 2008; 11:12–18.

[14] Maselli D, Guarracino F, Chiaramonti F, Mangia F, Borelli G, Minzioni G. Percutaneous mitral annuloplasty: an anatomic study of human CS and its relation with mitral valve annulus and coronary arteries. *Circulation.* 2006 Aug 1;114(5):377-80. Epub 2006 Jul 24.

[15] Palacios IF, Condado JA, Brandi S, Rodriguez V, Bosch F, Silva G, Low RI, Rogers JH. Safety and feasibility of acute percutaneous septal sinus shortening: first-in-human experience. *Catheter Cardiovasc. Interv.* 2007;69(4):513-8.

[16] Sack S, Kahlert P, Erbel R. Percutaenous mitral valve *Minim. Invasive Ther. Allied Technol.* 2009;18(3):156-63.

[17] Kaye DM, Byrne M, Alferness C, Power J. Feasibility and short-term efficacy of percutaneous mitral annular reduction for the therapy of heart failure-induced mitral regurgitation. *Circulation.* 2003;14;108(15):1795-7.

[18] Byrne MJ, Kaye DM, Mathis M, Reuter DG, Alferness CA, Power JM. Percutaneous mitral annular reduction provides continued benefit in an ovine model of dilated cardiomyopathy. *Circulation.* 2004;110(19):3088-92.

[19] Webb JG, Harnek J, Munt BI, et al. Percutaneous transvenous mitral annuloplasty initial human experience with device implantation in the CS. *Circulation* 2006;113: 851–855.

[20] Schofer J, Siminiak T, Haude M, Herrman JP, Vainer J, Wu JC, Levy WC, Mauri L, Feldman T, Kwong RY, Kaye DM, Duffy SJ, Tübler T, Degen H, Brandt MC, Van Bibber R, Goldberg S, Reuter DG, Hoppe UC. Percutaneous mitral annuloplasty for functional mitral regurgitation: results of the CARILLON Mitral Annuloplasty Device European Union Study. *Circulation.* 2009 Jul 28;120(4):326-33. Epub 2009 Jul 13.

[21] Sack S, Kahlert P, Erbel R. Percutaenous mitral valve: A non-stented CS device for the treatment of functional mitral regurgitation in heart failure patients. *Minim. Invasive Ther. Allied Technol.* 2009;18(3):156-63.

[22] Edwards Lifesciences. MONARC system. http://www.edwards.com/eu/products/investigational/monarcclinical.htm?MONARC=1. Accessed June 08, 2010.

[23] Siminiak T, Hoppe UC, Schofer J, Haude M, Herrman JP, Vainer J, Firek L, Reuter DG, Goldberg SL, Van Bibber R. Effectiveness and safety of percutaneous CS-based mitral valve repair in patients with dilated cardiomyopathy (from the AMADEUS trial). *Am. J. Cardiol.* 2009 Aug 15;104(4):565-70. Epub 2009 May 29.

[24] Sack S, Kahlert P, Bilodeau L, Pièrard LA, Lancellotti P, Legrand V, Bartunek J, Vanderheyden M, Hoffmann R, Schauerte P, Shiota T, Marks DS, Erbel R, Ellis SG. Percutaneous transvenous mitral annuloplasty: initial human experience with a novel CS implant device. *Circ. Cardiovasc. Interv.* 2009 Aug;2(4):277-84. Epub 2009 Jun 23.

[25] Kahlert P, Al-Rashid F, Kottenberg-Assenmacher E, Peters J, Hoffmann R, Erbel R, Sack S. Percutaneous transvenous mitral annuloplasty (PTMA): initial human experiences with a CS implant device for the treatment of functional mitral regurgitation in patients with heart failure. *Eur. Heart J.* 2008;29(abstract supplement): 580.

[26] Tops LF, Van de Veire NR, Schuijf JD, de Roos A, van der Wall EE, Schalij MJ, Bax JJ. Noninvasive evaluation of CS anatomy and its relation to the mitral valve annulus: implications for percutaneous mitral annuloplasty. *Circulation.* 2007 Mar 20;115(11): 1426-32. Epub 2007 Mar 12.

[27] Choure AJ, Garcia MJ, Hesse B, Sevensma M, Maly G, Greenberg NL, Borzi L, Ellis S, Tuzcu EM, Kapadia SR. In vivo analysis of the anatomical relationship of CS to mitral annulus and left circumflex coronary artery using cardiac multidetector computed tomography: implications for percutaneous CS mitral annuloplasty. *J. Am. Coll. Cardiol.* 2006 Nov 21;48(10):1938-45. Epub 2006 Nov 1.

[28] Sorgente A, Truong QA, Conca C, Singh JP, Hoffmann U, Faletra FF, Klersy C, Bhatia R, Pedrazzini GB, Pasotti E, Moccetti T, Auricchio A. Influence of left atrial and ventricular volumes on the relation between mitral valve annulus and CS. *Am. J. Cardiol.* 2008 Oct 1;102(7):890-6. Epub 2008 Jul 10.

[29] Timek TA, Dagum P, Lai DT, Liang D, Daughters GT, Tibayan F, Ingels NB Jr, Miller DC. Tachycardia-induced cardiomyopathy in the ovine heart: mitral annular dynamic three-dimensional geometry. *J. Thorac. Cardiovasc. Surg.* 2003;125:315–324.

In: Percutaneous Valve Technology: Present and Future ISBN: 978-1-61942-577-4
Editors: Jose Luis Navia and Sharif Al-Ruzzeh

Chapter XXI

Percutaneous Valve Technology – University of Leipzig Experience – Present and Future Perspectives

David M. Holzhey, Martin Haensig, Friedrich W. Mohr and Ardawan J. Rastan

Introduction

Since the first transcatheter aortic valve implantation (TAVI) by Alain Cribier in the year 2002 a rapid evolution of the catheter-based therapy to treat severe symptomatic aortic valve stenosis in risk patients has taken place and transapical as well as transfemoral aortic valve implantation has become a routine procedure at many centers [1,16-20]. These new therapeutic approaches for formerly inoperable or very high risk patients have reduced the threshold for treating aortic valve disease far towards higher age and acceptance of significant comorbidities [10]. In parallel, transcatheter technologies have sensitized not only cardiologist but also internal and home doctors to offer these alternative techniques to their old patients with symptomatic aortic stenosis for whom they in former years would have accepted soon death as a natural course. This had led to a significant increase of TAVI procedures worldwide.

Recent studies showed a clear benefit of survival for patients receiving aortic valve implantation compared to optimal medical therapy including aortic valvuloplasty [10,14,21]. These results gave a further boost for both industry and treating physicians to get even more involved in this relatively young field. However, results of TAVI are far from perfect and several questions had to be answered to improve results in the future. One major issue is the right indication for a TAVI and if, whether it should be performed transapically or transfemorally [3]. Second is how to reduce present technical limitations like a high rate of atrioventricular block, a high rate of (minimal to severe) paravalvular leaks and a comparably high rate of at least minor strokes [10,14,21,22]. Whether these drawbacks will influence long term results and quality of life remains unclear at the present state. In this chapter we aim to summarize our five year experience with TAVI starting with our program in 2006 and to describe lessons we have learned and improvement that were made over the time. Finally we would give some perspectives for the future, especially on new devices which eventually overcome some of the current device limitations.

Hybrid Operation Room and Team Building – Optimal Preconditions for Catheter-Based Valve Implantation

The surge with catheter valves has led to a worldwide demand for hybrid operation suites. At our center we were lucky to have one of these facilities available from the early beginning. Since 2009 a second hybrid suite was opened [Figure 1]. The combination of a high quality fluoroscopic imaging system and the space, sterility, optimal anesthesiology and heart lung machine setup of an operation room is a highly recommendable precondition for both, transapical and transfemoral valve implantation. Having prerequisites for coronary interventions, cardiopulmonary bypass and standard heart surgery available is important, because a variety of complications can occur during implantation that needed early decision and potentially emergency intervention.

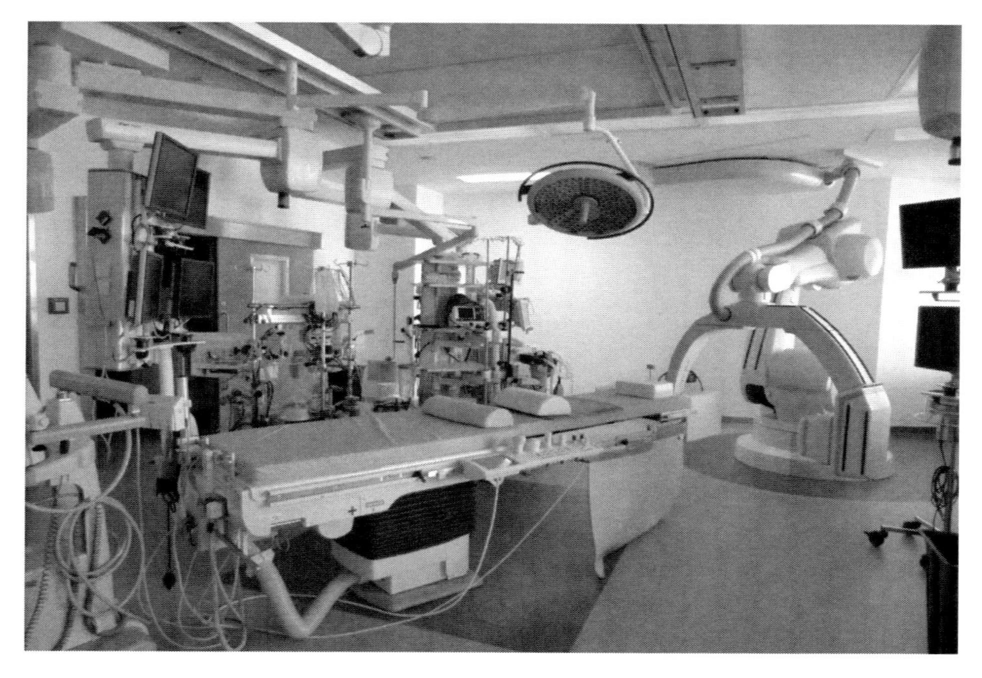

Figure 1. Newest hybrid suite at the Heart Center Leipzig with a floor-mounted C-arm system (Siemens Zeego). It combines all prerequisites of a cathlab like cardiac measuring unit, advanced imaging and contrast agent injector with surgical needs for sterility, table mobility and operating light. The availability of the heart lung machine, instruments and technology for conventional heart surgery and percutaneous coronary interventions as well as the team approach allow optimal implantation safety and to immediately address potential complications.

A second valuable precondition for the development of a smoothly running catheter valve program at our center was the team building between dedicated cardiologists and cardiac surgeons even before the first implantation. In a time when competition is fare more common than collaboration among cardiac surgeons and cardiologists, the TAVI program not only propelled the partnership in this field but eventually lead to better understanding in general. So far, virtually all procedures were done with at least one cardiologist and one surgeon at the table. Within the specialties, however, TAVI procedures were limited to few specialized doctors. So throughout the five years only three cardiologists and four cardiac surgeons were substantially involved in the actual implantation program. This way a substantial amount of practice and thus a high quality could be obtained.

The treating physicians were certainly the main driving force within the program. Patient selection, conduction of the procedure, postoperative care and research are chiefly in their hands. For the success of the actual operation, on the other hand, it is very important to integrate specialized scrub nurses, perfusionists and anesthesiologists into the team. Standardization of patient preparation, transesophageal echo protocols, operation room setup and management of emergency scenarios has lead to a high degree of safety during the implantation. It was also very helpful to maintain a comprehensive database of all patients from the beginning. This has made retrospective analyses easy and is the base for clinical research.

In summary the integrated team approach and an optimal stable environment of a hybrid operating suite are preconditions to ensure patient safety and procedural success, particularly during an ongoing development of new valve prostheses and delivery systems.

Oversizing, Rapid Pacing, Safety Net – Lessons Learned from the First Cases

The first two cases were planned at a time when hardly any implants worldwide had been performed. So two putatively “optimal” cases with an aortic annulus measured at exactly 23mm were selected for the implantation of a 23mm valve prosthesis. Both patients had to be converted to conventional surgery, one during and the other shortly after the operation, because both valves had migrated and caused severe cardiac problems. After a few more weeks in the laboratory, the concept of oversizing was evaluated and inaugurated into clinical practice since then. Based on an annulus measurement in systole and in the long axis of a transesophageal echocardiogram, the standard recommendation now is to have at least a 2 mm valve oversizing. This concept has been transferred to the recommendations of all recently launched new valve prostheses.

A serious concern in the beginning was the potentially high stroke rate which had was assigned to the balloon valvuloplasty. The friction of the balloon against the aortic wall and the break-up of the calcified cusps were accounted for the release of debris and potential harmful embolism. The danger of this effect was considered to be even worse under full cardiac output and when primarily using a balloon with a stent-mounted valve. Thus, the first transapical valve implants were done initially under cardiopulmonary bypass to reduce cardiac output and by making an initial balloon valvuloplasty using a reduced balloon volume. However, especially in hypertrophied left ventricles there was still some residual movement of the balloon. This could be overcome be using a short period of rapid ventricular pacing at a rate of 180 to 220 beats per minute. For this purpose epicardial pacing wires were placed on the left ventricle at the beginning of the transapical procedure or floating pacemaker leads were transfemorally forwarded into the right ventricle for transfemoral cases. The rapid pacing became the method of choice for all procedures on the aortic valve to reduce cardiac output whenever required.

As mentioned above the first procedures were done under protection of the heart lung machine [17-19]. This was true for transapical and transfemoral cases. Usually a ten minutes run of cardiopulmonary bypass (CPB) was sufficient to perform the valvuloplasty and valve implantation. With growing experience and considering the experience from other centers the application of CPB was reduced stepwise. At first the femoral vessels were still dissected and the cannulas inserted without starting CBP, then the tubes were only prepared but not actually connected to the patient. Eventually the so called safety net remained and has saved many a live together with the fact of having the heart lung machine ready in the operating room. The safety net basically consists of an arterial sheath which is also used for root angiography and a venous wire which is percutaneously advanced into the right atrium. The wire allows to forward a venous cannula very easily even under mechanical resuscitation. In case of the necessity of CPB the arterial sheath is exchanged by a standard wire which makes it easy to advance the arterial cannula percutaneously [17]. With these preparations and with the perfusionist being present in the room (usually he is crimping the valve) it takes some two minutes to go on-pump as it is necessary in about 2% of the cases.

All in all, after the first 20 patients the setup and all the procedural steps were clear and standardized and have hardly changed ever since [19].

Patient Selection

Patient selection today is one of the most crucial parts in the transcatheter valve business and is still controversial. With the inauguration of new valve technologies, operability of patients had to be redefined [3,7]. Today patients, referring physicians, cardiologists and cardiac surgeons are faced to three possible operative techniques – transfemoral, transapical and conventional valve replacement.

Because in the very beginning no valid data on implantation success and valve function were available, it was obvious that TAVI could only applied to old patients having a risk being prohibitively too high for conventional surgery. Of course, there was no clear definition what inoperability meant and definition varied between surgeons, cardiologists, institutions and countries. With a more widespread use of TAVI it is, however, an unwelcome danger that inoperability for conventional aortic valve replacement is exclusively ascertained by interventional cardiologist never having seen a single conventional operation. Thus, it is clearly defined in the current recommendations of our medical societies that inoperability of a particular patient should be assessed by both, cardiologist and cardiac surgeon as a team decision [15].

With more experience in the field and better scientific evaluation, TAVIs also became an option for operable patients. This development by nature was more driven by interventionalists, but surgeons also adapted to these developments and learned transcatheter technologies early during their training [12].

With growing experience in the field of catheter-based valve implantation, guidelines and recommendations were developed and published. They acknowledge the still somewhat experimental character of TAVI procedures, the lack of long-term results and take into consideration the very good results of conventional aortic valve surgery. Based on these recommendations TAVI was considered in patients older than 75 years of age having a high operative risk expressed by a logistic EUROScore >20% or an STS Score >10% [15]. However these rather formal criteria reflect only part of the truth. Thus the guidelines also mentioned several risk factors that are in better accordance with the daily clinical practice. Accordingly patients with porcelain aorta, history of CABG (especially with a patent LIMA to LAD graft), severely impaired respiratory function, liver failure, status post mediastinal radiation or mediastinitis as well as patients with a degenerated biologic valve prosthesis in aortic position are potential candidates for TAVI [8,9]. Aside from the guideline recommendations our clinical practice showed a few other comorbidities where TAVI might be an alternative approach. These include terminal renal insufficiency with long-term dialysis, long term cortisone or immunosuppressive therapy, systemic lupus erythematosus or other severe rheumatic diseases, severe osteoporosis or other malformations of the skeletal system.

Last but not least some aged patients present with a not-well defined status summarized as frailty. This is an important, but less clearly defined subset of patients. It summarizes the physical and mental impairment that usually occurs towards the end of a person's life. Often frailty can be judged quiet easily from clinical experience. There are also scoring systems to evaluate and quantify frailty, but most of them are too comprehensive and impractical for daily routine screening. So far the experienced physician has to judge whether a person is too frail to be eligible for conventional surgery or even too frail for any kind of intervention [13].

Because the direct vision of the aortic valve and the aortic root is not possible during a TAVI procedure, beside clinical aspects the Heart Team has also to consider important anatomical details before a final decision. For this preoperative diagnostic tools had to be adopted to answer these questions (see below). Not only the size and shape of the aortic annulus, the morphology of the aortic root including the distance of the coronary ostia, the distribution of the calcium within the leaflets, but also the calcification and character of the aorta and the pelvic vessels became of particular interest and need to be addressed accurately.

Another crucial step is to decide for the transfemoral versus the transpical TAVI approach. It is estimated the about 70% of all TAVI candidates are potentially amenable for both catheter-based approaches. The transfemoral approach should be preferred in patients with coincidence of severe obstructive pulmonary disease or severely impaired lung function (FEV_1 <60% of normal), while transapical approach is primarily indicated in patients with obstructive arterial disease at the level of the pelvic arteries and in severely diseased thoracic aorta including the aortic arch. Optimally the decision for either approach should be independent from a physician´s personal preference or skill and free from any financial interest.

In conclusion, the indication for TAVI is still based on a Heart team decision considering individual clinical and anatomical patient characteristics. Future studies might give us a clearer cut-off point for clinical parameters to choose the best treatment option for a particular patient.

Advanced Imaging Technology

Transoesophageal Echocardiogram (TOE)

With the development of TAVI several imaging methods moved into the center of interest and remained of utmost importance for the feasibility of the procedure and its final results. Different to conventional surgery where the valve size is determined under direct vision after having removed all calcified debris, in TAVI the valve size has to be chosen by indirect measurements.

The most important parameter for the selection of the right valve is the size of the aortic annulus. There are several imaging methods to obtain an exact measurement of the annulus. At our institution the most commonly used method is the transoesophageal echocardiography (TOE) where we measure the annulus in the long axis view with the widest possible view of the aortic root and always in systole. TOE is used as the screening method in all potential TAVI patients.

Apart from the annulus size it gives additional information about the calcium distribution, symmetry of the valve, anatomy of the entire artic root and other cardiac conditions of interest like concomitant mitral valve regurgitation, pulmonary hypertension and ventricular function. As this investigation is observer dependent, valve size is always reassessed by TOE when the patient is under general anesthesia to finally reconfirm the annular size.

Computed Tomography (CT)

Besides TOE other imaging modalities have developed and can contribute to complete the preoperative picture of the patient. Particularly, multi-slice ECG-triggered CT scanning can provide many a useful information. With appropriate protocols the annular shape and size as well as the distances to the coronary ostia can be determined very accurately. Optimal root imaging can only be achieved using contrast medium, thus all contraindications to the contrast agent application limit routine preoperative CT scan.

This is particularly true for impaired renal function which is unfortunately prevalent in many TAVI candidates. However, especially in cases where TOE measurement of the annulus is of borderline between two valve sizes, CT should be enforced to avoid intraoperative problems. The additional information about the optimal thoracic incision site is very precious. From the many CT scans we learnt that the annulus is almost always oval with a difference of 3-5 mm between the largest and the smallest diameter. By encircling the annulus an effective diameter can be calculated reflecting the size of the annulus as if it was pressed into a truly round shape.

This effective diameter is almost always 1-2mm larger than the annulus measured by TOE. This fact reconfirmed the concept of oversizing. In our preoperative routine a customized TAVI CT protocol using only 60 ml of contrast medium is performed in all transapical patients with normal renal function.

Intraoperative Dyna-CT

The so-called Dyna-CT is a software solution based on the Syngo DynaCT Cardiac imaging application that is integrated in Siemens high quality angiography systems. It provides a CT-like three-dimensional image of the thorax during a rotational angiography [4,5]. In practice the Dyna-CT is used in most transapical patients. During a short period of apnea and rapid ventricular pacing today 15 ml of contrast medium diluted to 75ml are injected into the aortic root via a pigtail catheter. After a short delay the C-arm of the system rotates around the thorax of the patient collecting radiographic data. This data is computed immediately into a three-dimensional picture of the aortic root. Furthermore, important landmarks like the hinge points of all aortic sinuses, the commissures and the coronary ostia are detected automatically [4,5,23]. The landmarks are depicted and additional center lines and measurements allow different 2D and 3D views of the entire aortic root [Figure 2]. In this virtual environment an optimal angulation of the C-arm for a perpendicular of the aortic root can be simulated without any additional application of contrast medium or radiation. The landmarks can later on be overlaid over the live image and be used as guidance. This is especially helpful for new generation valve technologies aiming an anatomically positioned TAVI valve position (see below).

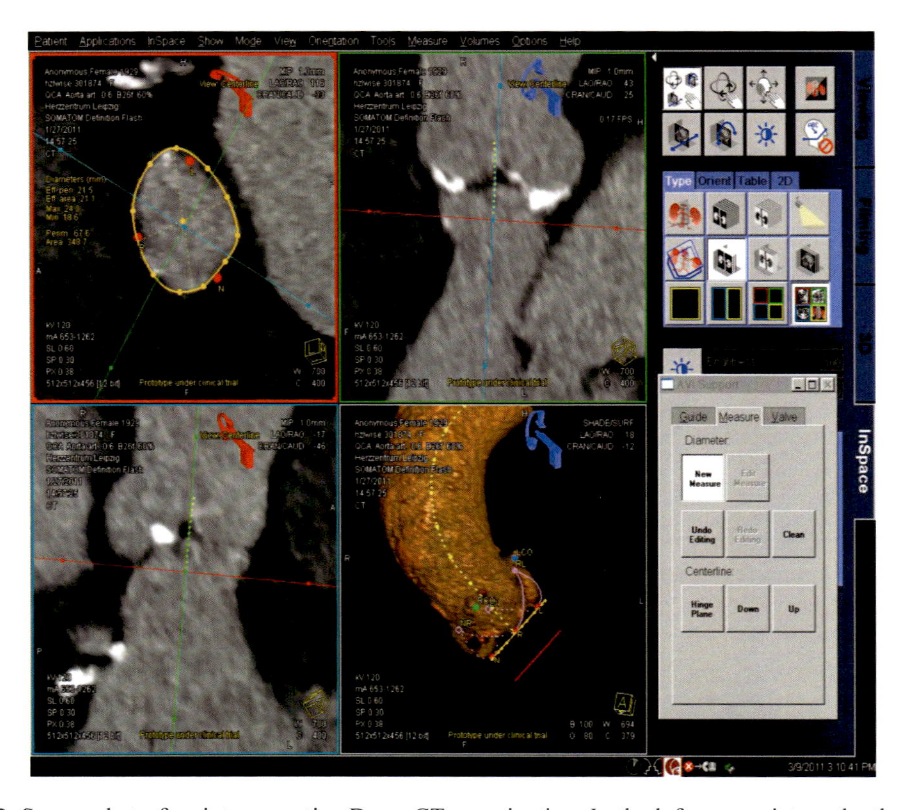

Figure 2. Screen shot of an intraoperative Dyna-CT examination. In the left upper picture the three hinge points of the aortic valve are automatically identified. The right lower picture depicts the automatically segmented ascending aorta, both coronary ostia (RCA and LCA) and an optimal perpendicular view to the aortic root.

High Quality Fluoroscopy

X-ray imaging in operation rooms in former decades used to be done with a mobile C-arm. This was sufficient for pacemaker and ICD applications. However, with the growing number of aortic stent implants and devices for cardiac resynchronization and even more with an increasing number of TAVIs, more and more hybrid suites are built to address the need of modern cardiovascular therapy. These rooms combine a high quality fluoroscopy unit with the sterile environment and the necessary equipment of an operating room. With respect to TAVI there are two other inferior options currently used in practice. First, the procedures is done with a mobile C-arm in an operating room. This maintains sterility (mandatory for transapical procedures), and conversion to sternotomy and/or cardiopulmonary bypass can usually be done within an appropriate time in an emergency situation. However, the quality of the fluoroscopic image might be acceptable for normal implants, but is inferior in the event of complications to evaluate coronary perfusion or aortic root perforation. Different angulations for an optimal perpendicular view are also difficult to attain as advanced techniques like the Dyna-CT are impossible.

The second option is to perform TAVI procedures in a cardiac catheterization lab. This allows for a good imaging and cardiologists work in a familiar environment. Conversely, there is barely enough space for the surgical equipment including a heart-lung-machine and the logistic prerequisites of an operative environment concerning material and manpower are also very limited in an emergency situation. As a consequence a hybrid operation room is one of the best investments towards ideal working conditions and eventually patient safety and thus recommended as the ideal solution in the current recommendations [15].

Pitfalls and Unfavorable Conditions

The following issues reflect a number of unfavorable situations or conditions that can occur during TAVI procedures. Additionally, possible solutions are given. A conversion to full sternotomy and cardiopulmonary bypass can become necessary at all times although mostly can be avoided. However, one lesson learnt is not to wait too long for the decision for cardiopulmonary bypass support or sternotomy in the case of intraoperative hemodynamic compromise. While a stable situations allows for several interventional solutions, a beginning hemodynamic instability or increasing inotropic support require early conversion, because of the very bad outcome known for patients developing cardiogenic shock during TAVI.

Very Low Ejection Fraction

Bad ventricular function (i.e. ejection fraction below 30%) is associated with an increasing perioperative risk of a patient and is found in TAVI candidates in up to 25% of cases. First of all the indication for a TAVI had to be very carefully reconsidered regarding whether or not the aortic stenosis is the primary and leading cardiac pathology or not. This is most important in patients presenting a so-called low-gradient stenosis. In case of bad LV function and severe aortic stenosis (i.e. highly calcified valve, orifice era <0.5 cm^2) the recovery of the ventricle is likely and almost all patients experience a fast clinical improvement after TAVI. If patients demonstrate a less severe valve pathology (less calcified aortic valve, orifice era 0.6-1.0 cm^2) a valvular cardiomyopathy is less likely and benefit of the procedure is more questionable, especially in concomitant coronary artery disease. These patients, however, are on a high risk of postoperative low output syndrome.

If TAVI is indicated one option is to reduce or completely avoid the number of rapid ventricular pacing episodes as reported by some teams. With the current balloon-expandable and Nitinol devices we do not prefer this approach because of the potentially increased risk of paravalvular leak (see below), valve dislocation and adverse embolic events. Alternatively, for those patients one option is to carry out the operation primarily under the protection of CBP. This is usually advisable if the LVEF is less than 15%. In all the other patients a few steps allow to be prepared if the patient remains unstable after rapid ventricular pacing. A series of treatment options are described in the following to manage this event successfully:

1. During the implantation and especially before induction of rapid ventricular pacing the mean arterial pressure should be kept >80 mmHg to avoid coronary ischemia.
2. A syringe of epinephrine 100µg/10ml should always be ready on the operative table. It can be fractionally applied directly in the aortic root via the pigtail catheter to bridge the circulation time of intravenous drug application. Very often this is sufficient.
3. If the reason for cardiac decompensation is the event of severe aortic regurgitation after valvuloplasty it might be advisable to go ahead with the valve implantation very quickly. For this reason it is essential that the valve preparation process is completed before starting the valvuloplasty or even any cardiac manipulation.
4. If all measures fail the connection of cardiopulmonary bypass through the femoral vessels is the last option. As mentioned, this should not be delayed for a too long time. For effective volume deloading of the heart the venous cannula needs to be placed in the right atrium. For this reason it is very important that the "safety net" venous wire had been placed correctly at the beginning of the procedure. From our experience the arterial sheath can be exchanged easily by an arterial cannula with the help of a superstiff wire. Further preconditions for a fast CPB support are the heart lung machine being ready in the room, the perfusionist being available and all necessary materials being stacked close to the operation table. With all this precautions and an experienced team it is possible to go on pump within two minutes.

Residual Leak after Valve Implantation

A mild paravalvular leak after TAVI a common finding. The decision whether or not a leak is hemodynamically relevant remains probably one of the most crucial decisions during the implantation. First of all angiographic and echocardiographic findings had to be used to locate and classify the degree of paravalvular leak and to distinguish it from an intravalvular regurgitation. Invasive hemodynamic measurements are helpful in these cases. We then use the diastolic pressure after implantation compared to that before implantation and the pressure difference between diastolic pressure and left ventricular end diastolic pressure. In general, patients with a good left ventricular ejection fraction tolerate a mild artic regurgitation well. In patients with a low ejection fraction, paravalvular leaks need to be addressed more aggressively.

The first step to address a paravalvular leak is to consider re-ballooning. Especially in self-expanding valve prostheses, but also in balloon-expandable valve concepts post-dilatation of the valve can reshape the annulus and rearrange the calcium in relation to the stent and thus seal off a paravalvular leak. Postdilatation should be more liberally performed in case of high-grade paravalvular leak, only moderate oversizing, in stable hemodynamics and normal coronary anatomy, while it should be more restrictively used in small root anatomy, severely calcified leaflets, oversizing of >3mm and less significant leaks. Of note, in central leaks a redilatation is contraindicated and useless.

In case of unsuccessful reballooning the next option is to place a second TAVI valve in the first one. This so-called bail out valve-in-valve procedure is a promising alternative if the position of the first valve is not optimal (too high, too low, oblique). It is also an option when annular complications like ventricular septal defects or small annular rupture occur. The covered part of the second TAVI valve can then be placed exactly where the lesion is. A second valve can also be helpful when it is realized that the choice of the first valve was too small for the annulus. If the second valve is dilated to its full extend the first (outer) valve will then be overextended adding some 1-2mm in diameter to the whole structure.

In case of a persisting severe leak a conversion to conventional surgery should be considered early. While patients are usually stable during and shortly after the procedure they tend to deteriorate during the following hours and days. Hemodynamics and lab values (e.g. lactate) should be monitored in short intervals to early recognize signs of cardiac decompensation.

Access Problems. Fragile Apex and Groin Complications

Very fragile tissue can be expected in patients with long-term cortisone or other immunosuppressive therapy. If one encounters a butter-like texture of the apex during a transapical procedure, conversion to a transfemoral implant should be considered if possible. This again supports the approach of a close collaboration between cardiologists and cardiac surgeons. Complications with the apical access are very rare (~1%), but difficult to handle. It can be controlled by using rapid ventricular pacing to reduce arterial pressure and using large Teflon-felted sutures (e.g. Prolene 2-0). In rare cases an apical bleeding might require CPB to deload the ventricle. In these cases a patch reconstruction might be helpful.

Vascular access problems during transfemoral TAVI are comparably more frequent but by nature less life-threatening [14]. In case of bleeding a cell-saver system should be used early. Open cut down of the vessels is the most commonly used technique. After bleeding control, direct vessel suturing or in case of severe vessel injury, a vascular prosthetic interponat might be indicated. Alternatively, in some patients we implanted a covered vascular stent delivered by a contralateral femoral artery approach with good results.

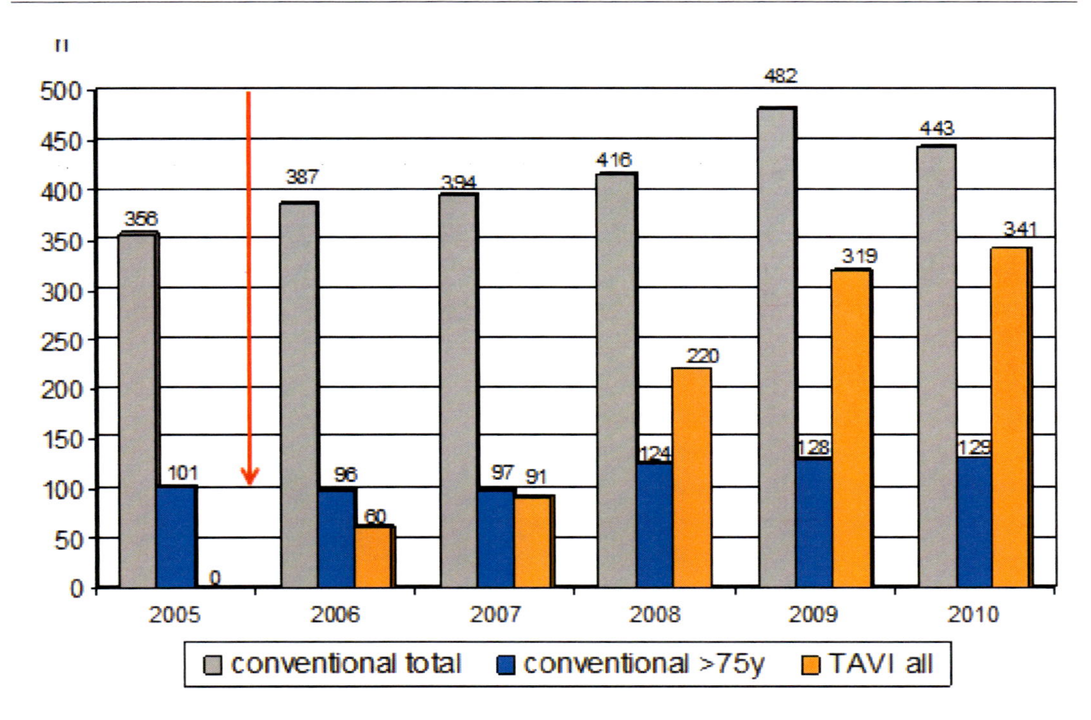

Figure 3. Isolated AV - Surgery (Leipzig): Conventional aortic valve surgery (overall and in patients >75 years of age) versus transcatheter (transfemoral and transapical) aortic valve implantation. Development over a 6-year period. The red arrow indicates the begin of our TAVI program.

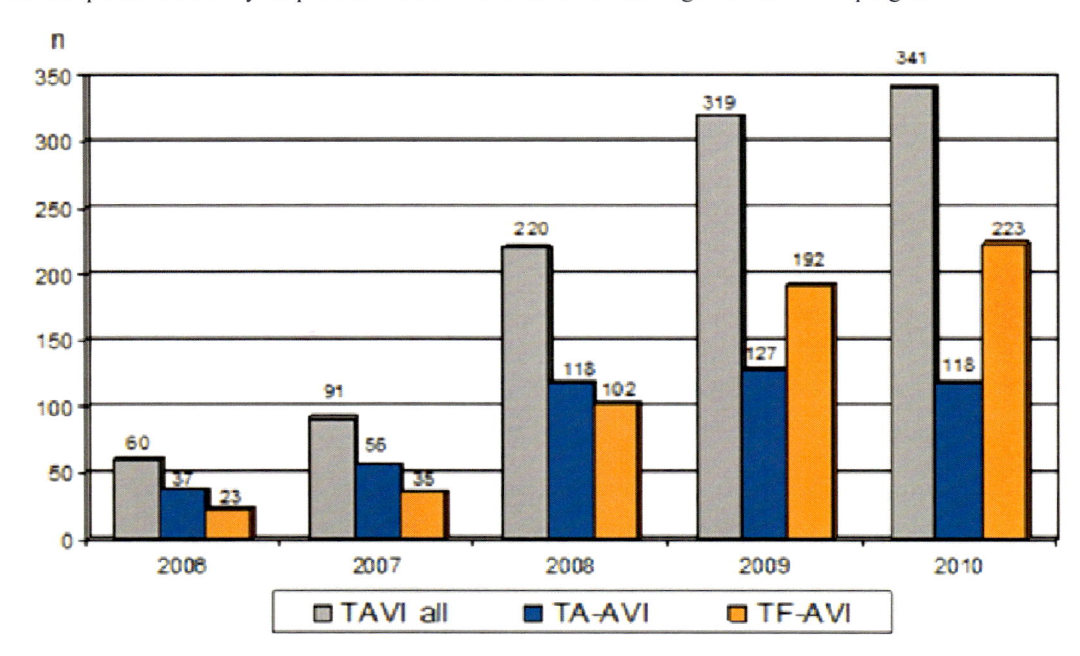

Figure 4. Case load development of transapical and transfemoral aortic valve implantations between 2006 and 2010.

Leipzig TAVI Experience

Between 01/2006 and 12/2010, 1.031 TAVI patients were treated in Leipzig (575 transfemoral, 456 transapical). During that time period, overall 2.122 patients received isolated aortic valve surgery through a conventional approach, of whom 574 patients were older than 75 years of age (Figure 3). Despite an increasing TAVI case volume, the number of conventional aortic valve surgery also increased. More interesting, even in the target group of patients >75 years of age the number of conventional surgery for isolated aortic valve disease grew. This demonstrate that even in the presence of a functioning TAVI program it is rather competitive than supplemental for conventional valve surgery. Having a constant countrywide data in mind these data also support the suggestion that a missing TAVI program potentially bears the risk to loose conventional aortic valve patients to centers having all options available [11,12].

Over the years there was a comparable increase of patients for transfemoral and transapical approach. However, during the last two years the increase in transfemoral implantations was more significant (Figure 4). Patients´ characteristics of TF and TA patients were given in Table 1 demonstrating a significantly higher operative risk score measured by the EuroSCORE for transapical patients, which is good comparable to data known from the literature [14,21]. As mentioned above, from our experience overall 70% of all TAVI candidates are eligible for both, TF and TA approach. However, all TAVI candidates were discussed by a common Heart Team consisting of Cardiac surgeons and interventional cardiologists who are actively implanting transcatheter valves. Echocardiographic and radiology data were assessed by specialized radiologists and echocardiographists. If TAVI is indicated, the choice of the TAVI delivery route is based on medical data and when both approaches are possible also on the primarily involved discipline. In addition to an informed consent all treatment options including conventional surgery were discussed with a particular patient and the family.

Table 1. Preoperative demographics of 1031 TAVI patients treated between 2006 and 2010

01/2006 - 12/2010	TA-AVI	TF-AVI
Number of patients, n	456	575
Age, years	82.0 ± 6.2	81.2 ± 6.4
Female gender, %	66.9%	55.2%
NYHA class	3.0 ± 0.6	2.9 ± 0.8
Body weight, kg	67.9 ± 15.4	73.8 ± 44.1
Additive EuroScore, points	10.1 ± 2.4	9.5 ± 2.4
Logstic EuroSCORE, %[a]	23.9 ± 14.6	20.3 ± 13.2
LVEF, %	52.7 ± 17.6	51.9 ± 17.4

TA-AVI;transapical aortic valve implantation. TF-AVI;transfemoral aortic valve implantation. NYHA;New York Heart Association. LVEF;left ventricular ejection fraction.
[a] estimated risk of mortality.

With the growing experience, the mortality of TAVI decreased significantly over time and recently ranged between 5% and 8%. The implant success today is more than 98%. Thus we have to consider that in an era of safe implantation techniques mortality can only be reduced by opening indication to less ill patients and by being more restrictive in very frail and comorbid patients at their end of life. This is probably one of the most important considerations that had to be done when discussing outcome data of TAVI patients comparing TF versus TA approach, randomized versus registry data and potentially also data from Europe versus North America. However, what we found as a side effect of picking the sick patients for TAVI, the mortality of conventional aortic valve surgery in patients >75 years of age decreased significantly to less than 2% compared to 4.6% in the pre-TAVI period.

Future Developments

Beside the above mentioned improvements in imaging technologies, two major developments have to be mentioned. First is an expected change in indication and second is an improvement in valve technologies.

One crucial disadvantage of TAVI remains the not well foreseeable risk of more than trivial degree of paravalvular leakage. This event had been observed in a significant number of patients and its clinical relevance on early and long term follow-up is unclear so far [10,14,22]. However, it is well accepted that this finding is not well tolerated in hypertrophied and stiff, but also in dilated left ventricles. Today paravalvular leak is one of the major limitations to liberate the indication for TAVI to younger, less ill patients [11]. The second major limitation of presently available CE-mark approved TAVI devices is a high rate of atrioventricular block and consecutive pacemaker implantation in up to 40%, of patients, which is significantly higher than reported for conventional aortic valve replacements [22]. These shortcomings had pushed the development of 2nd generation self-expandable Nitinol-based devices for subcoronary implantation which aim to reduce the degree of paravalvular leak and AV-block by anatomical orientated positioning of the valve into the aortic root. Three upcoming devices are shortly described which are currently under clinical evaluation by transapical delivery route (Figure 5).

One device is the Symetis ACURATE TA™ aortic stent valve (Symetis, Lausanne, Switzerland) consists of an aortic stentless porcine valve that is mounted and sutured on a self-expanding nitinol alloy stent with a Dacron interface. The stent assembly consists of a three stabilization arches, commissural totems, inflow-edge hooks, and an upper and lower anchoring crown.

The EngagerTM Aortic Valve Bioprosthesis (Medtronic, Inc., M-inneapolis, MN, USA) is a flexible heart valve prosthesis composed of three leaflets, cut from tissue-fixated bovine pericardium, sewn to a polyester sleeve, and mounted on a compressible and selfexpanding Nitinol frame [2]. The stent assembly consists of a main frame and a support frame, which are coupled together so as to form the commissural posts of the valve.

The JenaValveTM (JenaValve, Munich, Germany) device consists of a self-expandable Nitinol stent designed for subcoronary implantation [6]. Using three Nitinol 'feelers' meant to embrace the native calcified aortic valve leaflets the stent design relies on axial in addition to radial fixation. Inside the Nitinol stent a regular porcine tissue-valve (Elan, Vascutek Inc.) is mounted. A sheathless delivery system is used for antegrade transapical implantation. The stent assembly consists of three positioning arches with associated retaining arches, a distal and a proximal anchoring region.

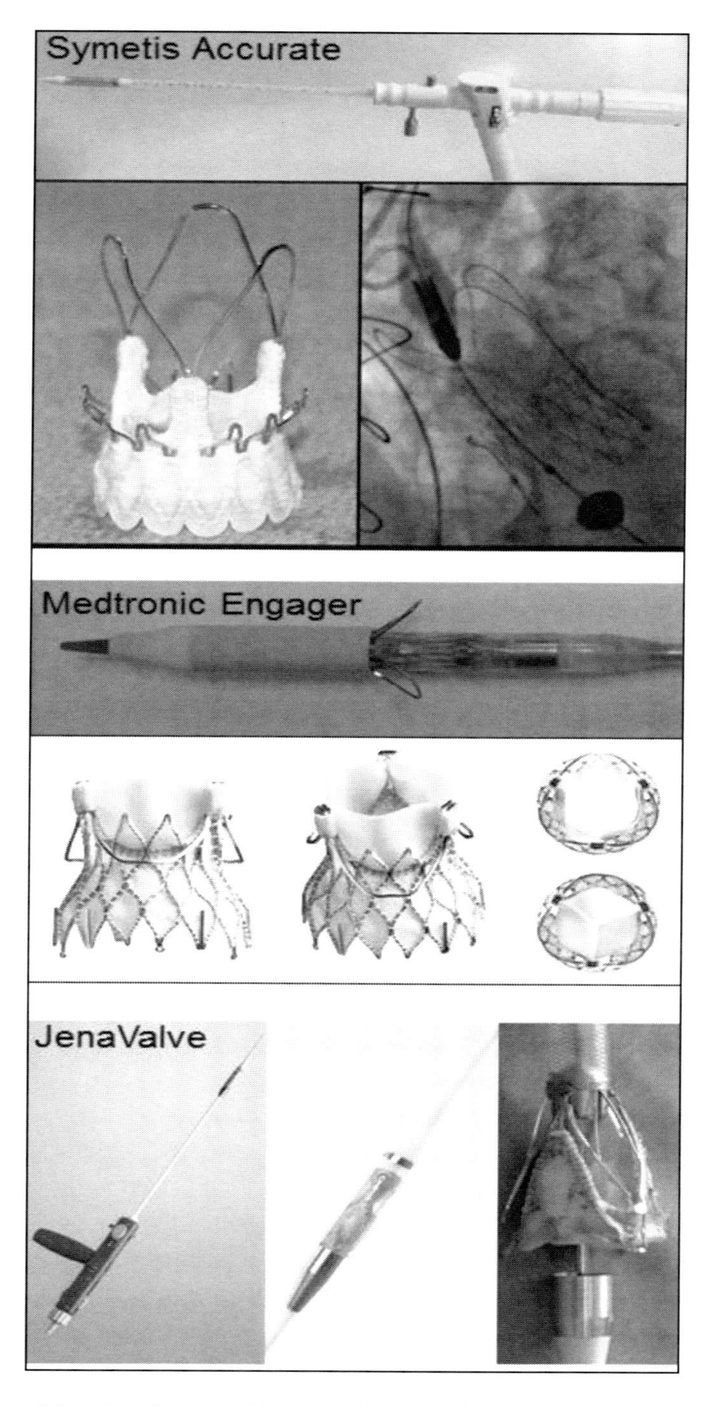

Figure 5. New Nitinol-based self-expandable transcatheter aortic valve systems for transapical approach, which are currently under clinical evaluation. Details see text.

Conclusion

TAVI today is a well-accepted alternative for high risk patients with symptomatic aortic valve stenosis. Surgeons should not fear, but keeping involved in the decision making of conventional surgery versus transcatheter valve implantation and had to adapt their surgical skills to all kinds of TAVI procedures as a primary surgical competence. Indication for treatment followed by the kind of procedure had to be done by a common Heart Team. If not, comparable to what we know from the experience in coronary artery disease a potential risk exists that without any heart team decision the gate keeper privilege to guide patients in the direction of TAVI will occur. At the moment this is not justified either by clinical outcome data, functional valve results nor economic considerations. Thus, a Heart team decision had to be the central element in TAVI programs. New TAVI devices are under clinical evaluation. However, there potential benefit over presently available TAVI systems remains to be seen.

The authors do not have any disclosures.

References

[1] Cribier A, Eltchaninoff H, Bash A, Borenstein N, Tron C, Bauer F, Derumeaux G, Anselme F, Laborde F, Leon MB. Percutaneous transcatheter implantation of an aortic valve prosthesis for calcific aortic stenosis: first human case description. *Circulation* 2002;106:3006-8.

[2] Falk V, Walther T, Schwammenthal E, Strauch J, Aicher D, Wahlers T, Schäfers J, Linke A, Mohr FW. Transapical aortic valve implantation with a self-expanding anatomically oriented valve. *Eur. Heart J.* 2011;32:878-87.

[3] Grant SW, Devbhandari MP, Grayson AD, Dimarakis I, Kadir I, Saravanan DM, Levy RD, Ray SG, Bridgewater B. What is the impact of providing a transcatheter aortic valve implantation service on conventional aortic valve surgical activity: patient risk factors and outcomes in the first 2 years. *Heart* 2010;96:1633-7.

[4] John M, Liao R, Zheng Y, Nöttling A, Boese J, Kirschstein U, Kempfert J, Walther T. System to guide transcatheter aortic valve implantations based on interventional C-arm CT imaging. *Med. Image Comput. Comput. Assist. Interv.* 2010;13:375-82.

[5] Karar ME, Merk DR, Chalopin C, Walther T, Falk V, Burgert O. Aortic valve prosthesis tracking for transapical aortic valve implantation. *Int. J. Comput. Assist. Radiol. Surg.* 2010; [Epub ahead of print].

[6] Kempfert J, Rastan AJ, Mohr FW, Walther T. A new self-expanding transcatheter aortic valve for transapical implantation - first in man implantation of the JenaValve™. *Eur. J. Cardiothorac. Surg.* 2011; [Epub ahead of print].

[7] Kempfert J, Van Linden A, Holzhey D, Rastan AJ, Blumenstein J, Mohr FW, Walther T. The evolution of transapical aortic valve implantation and new perspectives. *Minim. Invasive Ther. Allied Technol.* 2011;20:107-16.

[8] Kempfert J, Van Linden A, Linke A, Borger MA, Rastan A, Mukherjee C, Ender J, Schuler G, Mohr FW, Walther T. Transapical off-pump valve-in-valve implantation in patients with degenerated aortic xenografts. *Ann. Thorac. Surg.* 2010;89:1934-41.

[9] Kempfert J, Van Linden A, Linke A, Schuler G, Rastan AJ, Lehmann S, Lehmkuhl L, Mohr FW, Walther T. Transapical aortic valve implantation: therapy of choice for patients with aortic stenosis and porcelain aorta? *Ann. Thorac. Surg.* 2010;90:1457-61.

[10] Leon MB, Smith CR, Mack M, Miller DC, Moses JW, Svensson LG, Tuzcu EM, Webb JG, Fontana GP, Makkar RR, Brown DL, Block PC, Guyton RA, Pichard AD, Bavaria JE, Herrmann HC, Douglas PS, Petersen JL, Akin JJ, Anderson WN, Wang D, Pocock S; PARTNER Trial Investigators. Transcatheter aortic-valve implantation for aortic stenosis in patients who cannot undergo surgery. *N. Engl. J. Med.* 2010;363:1597-607.

[11] Linke A, Walther T, Schuler G. The utility of trans-catheter aortic valve replacement after commercialization: does the European experience provide a glimpse into the future use of this technology in the United States? *Catheter. Cardiovasc. Interv.* 2010; 75:511-8.

[12] Mack M.J. Does transcatheter aortic valve implantation mean the end of surgical aortic valve replacement? *Tex. Heart Inst. J.* 2010; 37:658-9.

[13] Sündermann S, Dademasch A, Praetorius J, Kempfert J, Dewey T, Falk V, Mohr FW, Walther T. Comprehensive assessment of frailty for elderly high-risk patients undergoing cardiac surgery. *Eur. J. Cardiothorac. Surg.* 2011;39:33-7.

[14] Thomas M, Schymik G, Walther T, Himbert D, Lefèvre T, Treede H, Eggebrecht H, Rubino P, Michev I, Lange R, Anderson WN, Wendler O. Thirty-day results of the SAPIEN aortic Bioprosthesis European Outcome (SOURCE) Registry: A European registry of transcatheter aortic valve implantation using the Edwards SAPIEN valve. *Circulation* 2010;122:62-9.

[15] Vahanian A, Alfieri O, Al-Attar N, Antunes M, Bax J, Cormier B, Cribier A, De Jaegere P, Fournial G, Kappetein AP, Kovac J, Ludgate S, Maisano F, Moat N, Mohr F, Nataf P, Piérard L, Pomar JL, Schofer J, Tornos P, Tuzcu M, van Hout B, Von Segesser LK, Walther T; European Association of Cardio-Thoracic Surgery; European Society of Cardiology; European Association of Percutaneous Cardiovascular Interventions. Transcatheter valve implantation for patients with aortic stenosis: a position statement from the European Association of Cardio-Thoracic Surgery (EACTS) and the European Society of Cardiology (ESC), in collaboration with the European Association of Percutaneous Cardiovascular Interventions (EAPCI). *Eur. Heart J.* 2008;29:1463-70.

[16] Vahanian A, Iung B, Himbert D, Nataf P. Changing demographics of valvular heart disease and impact on surgical and transcatheter valve therapies. *Int. J. Cardiovasc. Imaging* 2011; [Epub ahead of print].

[17] Walther T, Dewey T, Borger MA, Kempfert J, Linke A, Becht R, Falk V, Schuler G, Mohr FW, Mack M. Transapical aortic valve implantation: step by step. *Ann. Thorac. Surg.* 2009;87:276-83.

[18] Walther T, Falk V, Borger MA, Dewey T, Wimmer-Greinecker G, Schuler G, Mack M, Mohr FW. Minimally invasive transapical beating heart aortic valve implantation--proof of concept. *Eur. J. Cardiothorac. Surg.* 2007;31:9-15.

[19] Walther T, Falk V, Kempfert J, Borger MA, Fassl J, Chu MW, Schuler G, Mohr FW. Transapical minimally invasive aortic valve implantation; the initial 50 patients. *Eur. J. Cardiothorac. Surg.* 2008;33:983-8.

[20] Walther T, Kempfert J. Transcatheter aortic valve implantation: the right procedure for the right patient by the right team. *Eur. J. Cardiothorac. Surg.* 2011;39:623-4.

[21] Wendler O, Walther T, Schroefel H, Lange R, Treede H, Fusari M, Rubino P, Thomas M. The SOURCE Registry: what is the learning curve in trans-apical aortic valve implantation? *Eur. J. Cardiothorac. Surg*. 2011;39:853-60.

[22] Zahn R, Gerckens U, Grube E, Linke A, Sievert H, Eggebrecht H, Hambrecht R, Sack S, Hauptmann KE, Richardt G, Figulla HR, Senges J; German Transcatheter Aortic Valve Interventions-Registry Investigators. Transcatheter aortic valve implantation: first results from a multi-centre real-world registry. *Eur. Heart J*. 2011;32:198-204.

[23] Zheng Y, John M, Liao R, Boese J, Kirschstein U, Georgescu B, Zhou SK, Kempfert J, Walther T, Brockmann G, Comaniciu D. Automatic aorta segmentation and valve landmark detection in C-arm CT: application to aortic valve implantation. *Med. Image Comput. Comput. Assist. Interv*. 2010;13:476-83.

In: Percutaneous Valve Technology: Present and Future ISBN: 978-1-61942-577-4
Editors: Jose Luis Navia and Sharif Al-Ruzzeh

Chapter XXII

Percutaneous Valve Technology in China: Experience, Present and Future

Xin Chen and Fuhuang Huang

Abstract

Since its introduction 30 years ago by Andreas Gruntzig, interventional cardiology has expanded its scope from coronary disease to valve diseases gradually. And now, a variety of percutaneous methods to treat mitral regurgitation and to replace pulmonic and aortic valves have already been successfully employed in patients. In China, the first pulmonic balloon valvuloplasty was reported in 1985 and was rapidly followed by applications to the mitral valves and aortic valves. Moreover, percutaneous valve replacement has been developed in numerous studies in animal models recent years. In the future, these creative new transcatheter approaches may change the face of valve therapy in China.

Introduction

Thirty-two years after its introduction by Andreas Gruntzig, interventional cardiology has become a major player not only in the management of coronary artery disease, but also in both congenital and acquired valve diseases. Developmental efforts to achieve percutaneous catheter based therapies for cardiac valve repair and replacement have advanced rapidly over the past several years. Although the principal therapies for valvular heart disease are surgical, operative risk may be high due to age and comorbidities. More importantly, a certain proportion of patients are not referred for surgery because of higher expected mortality according to the risk scores. The risks of open heart surgery have prompted investigation of alternative therapies, including balloon valvuloplasty, transcatheter valve implantation, and other less invasive procedures. In this chapter, an overview of the past and current technology for percutaneous valve intervention in China is provided. In addition, the possible future improvements on transcatheter valve implantation is discussed.

Experience

Percutaneous balloon valvular commissurotomy (PBVC) was an important achievement of cardiology in 1980s. The technique involves positioning one or more balloon catheters across the stenotic valve, usually over an extra-stiff guide wire and inflating the balloons with diluted contrast material, thus producing valvotomy. Percutaneous treatment of valvular heart diseases is mostly made up of Percutaneous Balloon Pulmonary Valvuloplasty (PBPV), percutaneous mitral commissurotomy (PMC) and percutaneous aortic valvuloplasty (PAV). The procedure is effective; now has a 30-year track record with excellent success in patients with suitable valvular and subvalvular morphology. In the past, surgical valvotomy was the treatment of choice; however, more recently PVBC has gained acceptance as the first option in the management of valve stenosis.

Percutaneous Balloon Pulmonary Valvuloplasty (PBPV)

Since the first description of balloon pulmonary valvuloplasty in 1982 by Kan, the procedure has been extensively utilized by several groups of workers for relief of pulmonary valve stenosis. It is generally recommended that the procedure be performed for patients with peak gradients in excess of 50 mmHg. In China, the first pulmonic balloon valvuloplasty was reported in 1985.

In China, pulmonary stenosis is one of the common disorders, comprises of 8% of all congenital heart defects. It is also the most common cause of rightside heart failure in children. In the past, surgical repair was the only option. Since Chuan-Rong Chen et al. introduced the technique of balloon dilation of the stenotic pulmonary valve in 1985, percutaneous balloon pulmonary valvuloplasty (PBPV) had gained increasing acceptance in China as an alternative to surgical pulmonary commissurotomy. At first, he used traditional cylindrically shaped balloons. He started using the Inoue balloon catheter technique of PBPV in November 1985 and thus had accumulated over 15 years experience. Based on his experience and that of others, he recommended as follows: ①The diagnosis and assessment of pulmonary valve stenosis are made by the usual clinical, radiographic, electrocardiographic, and echo-Doppler data. ② the procedure be performed for peak to peak gradients in excess of 50 mm Hg. ③ Percutaneous femoral venous route is the most preferred entry site for balloon pulmonary valvuloplasty and should be used routinely. ④ The double-balloon procedure is not technically difficult but it does depend on high quality angiography for valve location and definition. ⑤The recommended balloon/annulus ratio is 1.2:1.35. ⑥ Severe and critical obstructions, irrespective of age and pulmonary valve dysplasia are amenable to balloon dilatation.

In 1986, Li huata and Dai ruping employed PBMV and applied to the mitral and aortic valves. Wang guanyi, from the PLA General Hospital conducted a study of 1,200 congenital patients who underwent PBMV 5–10 years earlier. Immediate reduction of peak-to-peak gradient across the pulmonary valve and right ventricular peak systolic pressure along with slight increase in pulmonary artery pressure occurs following balloon dilatation. The width of the jet of contrast material passing through the pulmonary valve increases. Pulmonary valve leaflets open more freely with less doming as observed on echocardiographic studies. 10 years Follow-up results, restenosis, defined as gradient >50 mm Hg, only has been observed in 3‰ patients, Pulmonary valve insufficiency is noted in 10% patients.

Long-term comparisons of balloon valvuloplasty versus surgery for pulmonary valve stenosis have also shown excellent outcomes. Although surgery generally yielded lower long-term gradients and results in longer freedom from reintervention initially, patients who underwent balloon dilation with a balloon 25-30% larger than the valve annulus, the recurrences were not found. As the result, balloon valvuloplasty seems the better choice of treatment, because they take the less risk from surgery and even have equal effect, especially when patients have adequate balloon dilation.

In summary, it appears that balloon pulmonary valvuloplasty is effective in neonates as well as in adults and is the first line therapeutic option for treatment of isolated pulmonary valvar stenosis.

Percutaneous Balloon Mitral Valvuloplasty (PBMV)

Although the incidence of rheumatic fever and the prevalence of rheumatic heart disease as a sequela are decreasing in most countries, an estimated 12 million people are currently affected by rheumatic fever and rheumatic heart disease worldwide. Several studies were conducted on the prevalence of rheumatic heart disease, reporting 1.86/1000 in China. Based on researches, rheumatic heart disease is the most prevalent pathological cause for mitral valve stenosis (MS). The treatment options for symptomatic MS at present are either surgical open mitral commissurotomy (OMC) or percutaneous balloon mitral valvuloplasty (PBMV).

Percutaneous balloon mitral valvuloplasty, first performed by Inoue in 1982, was a rational progression from 4 decades of experience with the blunt surgical dilatation technique of closed mitral commissurotomy. As with surgical commissurotomy, balloon valvuloplasty relieves mitral stenosis by the splitting of fused commissures. The initial objectives of the procedures are to increase the crosssectional valve area and simultaneously to reduce the transmitral pressure gradient, left atrial pressure, and mean pulmonary artery pressure. The ultimate objectives are to improve overall cardiac pump function, the ability to exercise, quality of life, and prognosis. The procedure is effective; over 88% of patients showed significant improvement in valve function with a final valve area over 1.5 cm^2 and no severe regurgitation. In experienced centers incidence of severe complications is low. In China, Guangdong Cardiovascular Institute reported the first clinical application of a Inoue balloon catheter in 1985. Since then, this method has been used extensively by Chinese interventional cardiologists as an alternative to surgical mitral commissurotomy.

In 1988, Chen et al. working in Guangdong Cardiovascular Institute used Inoue balloon catheter in 30 Chinese patients with rheumatic mitral stenosis (Figure 1.). PBMV with the Inoue balloon catheter was successfully performed in 27 patients without any significant complications. The mean left atrial pressure decreased from 20.15±6.75 to 7.06±4.54 mm Hg; mitral valve area increased from 1.27±0.31 to 2.13±0.43 cm^2. Results of follow-up examinations at 8 to 20 months showed that both subjective and objective improvement was well maintained. Subsequent to the report of Chen et al, Yip AS, et al in Grantham Hospital, Hong Kong introduced a doubleballoon technique for mitral valvuloplasty in China. Twenty-one patients with moderate to severe mitral stenosis were treated with percutaneous balloon mitral valvuloplasty using Inoue mitral double balloon catheters and proved to be a effective and safe nonsurgical method that can yield very good results in relieving symptomatic rheumatic mitral stenosis, with minimal morbidity and no mortality in this group.

The encouraging results obtained with PBMV in these early studies were soon confirmed in larger patient series. Between November 1985 and January 1994, 4832 patients with rheumatic mitral stenosis from 120 medical centers in China underwent PBMV by the Inoue technic. The procedure success rate was 99.30%. Major complications included death in 0.12%, mitral regurgitation in 1.41%, cardiac tamponade in 0.81%, and thromboembolism in 0.48%. After PBMV, the mean left atrial pressure decreased from 26.2±7.6 mm Hg to 11.4±6.1 mm Hg; pulmonary artery systolic pressure decreased from 51.2±14.8 mm Hg to 33.9±8.8 mm Hg; cardiac output increased from 3.8±1.3 L/min to 4.8±1.2 L/min; and mitral valve area expanded from 1.1±0.3 cm2 to 2.1±0.2 cm2. The rate of restenosis was 5.2% over a follow-up period of 32.2 months in the entire group and 4.6% over a follow-up period of 5.1 years in Guangdong Cardiovascular Institute, where PBMV was begun in China.

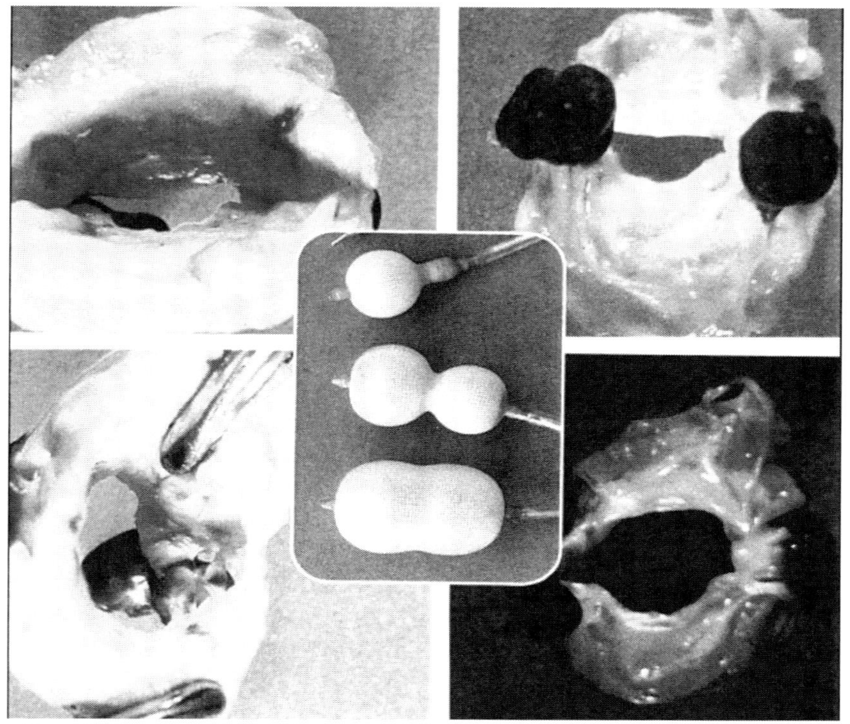

Form Chuan-Rong Chen, et al. Catheterization and Cardiovascular Diagnosis 1998;43:132–139.

Figure 1. A stenotic mitral valve before (top) and after (bottom) dilation with the Inoue balloon catheter (inset), viewed from the left atrium (left) and left ventricle (right). Inset: Progressive stages of inflation of the Inoue balloon.

There followed several reports of the efficacy of PBMV in the treatment of rheumatic mitral stenosis in complicated conditions such as advanced ages, the presence of severe tricuspid regurgitation , severe pulmonary hypertension (PH), and aortic regurgitation. Shu Maoqin et al, in Third Military Medical University, Chongqing, performed successful PBMV with 44 patients with MS complicated by severe PH (systolic pulmonary pressure >80 mm Hg, group S) and 67 patients with MS complicated by mild PH (systolic pulmonary pressure <50 mm Hg, group M) and compared their immediate and late results after a follow-up period of 24 months after PBMV.

The successful rate and the incidence of severe complications from the PBMV procedure were similar in both groups. There were more cases of post-PBMV mitral valve area 1.5 cm^2 in group M than in group S. After PBMV, NYHA class obviously improved in both groups, but there were more patients with NYHA class II in group M than in group S at discharge.

During the 24 months follow-up, 7 patients (10.5%) in groupM and 11 (25.0%) in group S developed cardiac events. Cumulative event-free survival was 89.6% in group M and 75.0% in group S. NYHA class I or II was present for 80.6% in group M and 59.1% in group S. The study has demonstrated that PBMV can significantly improve immediate and long-term clinical outcomes of patients with rheumatic MS complicated by severe PH, despite inferior hemodynamic results.

Transesophageal echocardiography (TEE) is desirable in the setting of complex anatomy and to screen for left atrial thrombus, especially in patients at risk , such as those with atrial fibrillation, stasis of blood in the left atrium, or prior embolic events.

To detect thrombus in the left atrium or left atrial appendage, transesophageal echocardiography should be performed before performing PBMV. If thrombus is found, PBMV should be postponed and the patient should be started on warfarin with the prothrombin time–international normalized ratio (INR) controlled at a relatively higher level for 3 to 6 months, after which transesophageal echocardiography should be repeated to confirm the disappearance of the clot.

If the thrombus has disappeared, PBMV can then be safely performed, or if the thrombus remains, surgical intervention on the mitral valve along with removal of the thrombus should be recommended.

Complications of PBMV techniques include failure to relieve stenosis, creation of mitral regurgitation, perforation with hemopericardium, and systemic embolization. Immediate surgery may be required in approximately 1% of procedures for resolution of technical complications such as hemopericardium or creation of severe mitral regurgitation. When there is insufficient resolution or recurrence of stenosis, repeat balloon valvuloplasty or elective mitral valve replacement can be performed. Most patients with immediate procedural success have continued good functional results at 10 years after treatment.

Currently, there are at least 500 groups working on percutaneous approaches to mitral valve repair in China and until 2008, there are 60,000 patients received PBMV. Because it provides favorable initial results and promising late outcomes, the stepwise Inoue balloon is now considered the standard technique as the design of the balloon allows a fast, safe, and effective dilatation in China.

Percutaneous Balloon Aortic Valvuloplasty (PBAV)

Following successful percutaneous dilation of pulmonary and mitral valves, the first adult Percutaneous Balloon Aortic Valvuloplasty (PBAV) was performed by Alain Cribier in France in 1985. There are two approaches with this technique. The classic retrograde approach has been used most commonly but may present difficulty with crossing a severely stenotic valve or complications caused at the arterial entry site by insertion of large-caliber devices.

The antegrade approach is a more recent alternative, in which left atrial access is obtained via the femoral vein using standard transseptal puncture, following which a balloon flotation catheter and guidewire are advanced through the mitral valve, to the left ventricular apex, and then through the aortic valve. In China, PLA General Hospital reported the first clinical application antegrade approach treatment 20 Chinese patients, including elderly population with calcific aortic stenosis (AS) and congenital bicuspid aortic valve disease. Once a guidewire has been positioned appropriately using antegrade approach, an valvuloplasty balloon then is advanced over the wire and across the stenotic valve, and it is inflated with dilute contrast material. The mechanism of action was assumed to be fracturing of calcified nodules along the leaflets with elastic expansion of the aorta. The early experience showed that PBAV was safe, but it also showed that the technique provided a far smaller increment in aortic valve area.

Early enthusiasm for the technique stemmed from its relative ease compared with surgical valve replacement, and some proponents hoped that PBAV might supplant many elective valve replacements.

However, the technique provided a far smaller increment in aortic valve area than provided by surgical valve replacement. The overall 1-year survival was 65%, and the 1-year survival free of death, aortic valve replacement, or repeat BAV was 40%. In addition, given the selected patient population, hospital mortality may be as high as 14%, with one-third having periprocedural complications, including vascular accesssite problems, arrhythmia, heart block, and stroke.

In 2007, Wang et al. working in Zhejiang University School of Medicine, reported a total of twenty one children with AS accepted the treatment of PBAV. 13 cases had more than 50% gradient reduction (81.25%), 2 had 40% - 50% gradient reduction. The follow up period ranged from 3 months to 5 years. The gradient pressures rose to more than 50 mm Hg after follow up in 3 cases and they underwent repeat balloon valvuloplasty procedure or were operated successfully. There was no moderate to severe aortic insufficiency.

The basic technique has not changed significantly since 1990, but the procedure has been aided by advances in guidewire and balloon design, as well as newer imaging modalities such as transesophageal and intracardiac echocardiography. At the present time, in China, PBAV is indicated only in select patients with severe AS and no surgical options. BAV also used for congenital valvular aortic stenosis in children and as a bridge to AVR in hemodynamically unstable patients who are at high risk for aortic valve replacement.

Present

The potential field of application for the percutaneous valve interventions techniques is vast and concerns aortic stenosis and mitral regurgitation. However, the results of contemporary valve surgery, such as operative mortality of aortic valve replacement or mitral valve repair is low, and long-term results are excellent for up to 20 years. Thus, surgery works sets a high standard for percutaneous valve intervention. Recently, developmental efforts to achieve percutaneous catheterbased therapies for cardiac valve repair and replacement have advanced rapidly. Percutaneous valvular intervention has drastically improved with the proven feasibility of percutaneous pulmonary, and aortic valve replacement, and repair of mitral regurgitation.

Two devices are now under clinical investigation for transcatheter aortic valve implantation (TAVI). One device is the Edwards-Sapien valve (Edwards Lifesciences Inc., CA USA), the other is the CoreValve Revalving System (CRS TM, CoreValve Inc., Irvine, CA, USA). The evidence suggests that this technique is feasible and provides haemodynamic and clinical improvement for up to 2 years in patients with severe symptomatic aortic stenosis at high risk or with contraindications for surgery. Direct mitral leaflet repair, a surgical approach pioneered by Alfieri in the early 1990s, edge-to-edge repair has been duplicated using percutaneous clip- and suture-based devices. This device approach has been successfully used in a phase I clinical trial in the United States, with good results reported recently. The edge-to-edge mitral valve repair can also be accomplished using the Mobius percutaneous suture device (Edwards Lifesciences Inc., Orange, Calif). Even more, kinds of simplified interventional approach to simulate surgical annuloplasty have been to work from within the coronary sinus to geometrically deform the anteroposterior dimension of the mitral annulus. Thus, the field of percutaneous valve replacement and repair is clearly developing rapidly. Transcatheter aortic and pulmonic valve replacement and a variety of mitral valve therapy approaches have been successfully performed in thousands of patients.

Transcatheter Aortic Valve Implantation (tAVI)

The transcatheter techniques for aortic valve replacement have developed for many years. The first successful percutaneous aortic stent valve implantation was performed on april 16, 2002 in a patient with critical aortic stenosis. Since then, the devices and operator techniques improved rapidly. Maybe, it could replace surgery for the treatment of aortic stenosis in the future.

In China, Percutaneous catheter-based heart valve replacemen for the treatment of valvular heart disease have been designed and studied in animal models for several years. In 2008, Zhou yongxin et al. working Tongji Hospital, Shanghai, began a series of animal studies in pursuit of successful percutaneous aortic valve replacement. The system was comprised of 0.6% glutaraldehyde solution treated for 36 hours, bovine pericardium that were sewn into a balloon expandable stent that was delivered percutaneously to the ascending aorta of Chinese mini swines through common iliac artery (Figure 2). Self-expandable nitinol stents were made by 0.2mmNi-Ti shape memory alloy (15~19mm in diameter). In vitro test showed that the closure of the percutaneous valved aortic stent leaflets was satisfactory, and the fluid flow was not restricted in the opposite direction. The devices could be released through the catheter, expanded completely, and be fixed rapidly in the tube. In vivo test, all devices were implanted in the desired position, with expanded completely and fixed rapidly in the ascending aorta(figure 3). The short-term study (animals were executed and dissected after 24 hours) in swines revealed that all the devices were fixed in the ascending aorta and there were no thrombus. The function of the percutaneous valved aortic stent is satisfactory. The size of compressed device is suitable for catheterization. It can be successfully implanted into the ascending aorta by using a retrograde method through common iliac artery.

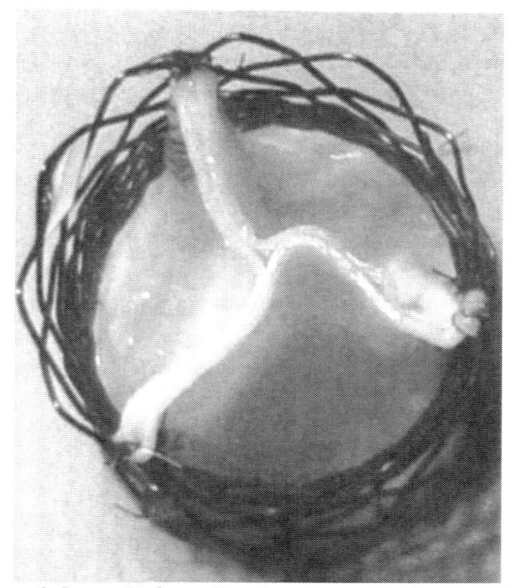

Courtesy of zhou yongxin, et al. Journal of tongji university medical science 2008;29(6):54–57.

Figure 2. Gross view of percutaneous valved stent.

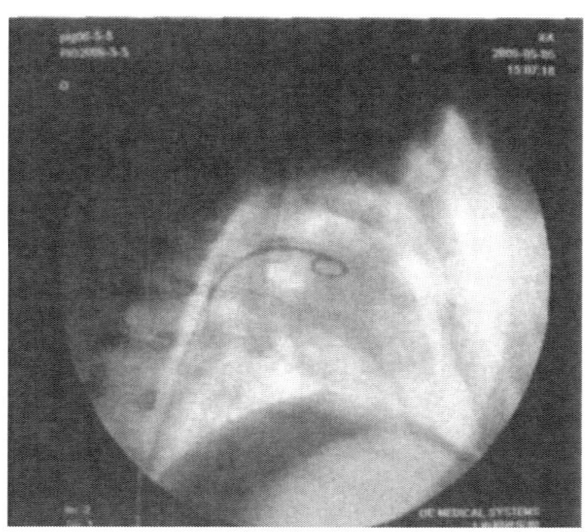

Courtesy of zhou yongxin, et al. Academic Journal of Second Military Medical University 2009;30(2):120–123.

Figure 3. X-ray of valved aortic stent placed in ascending aorta.

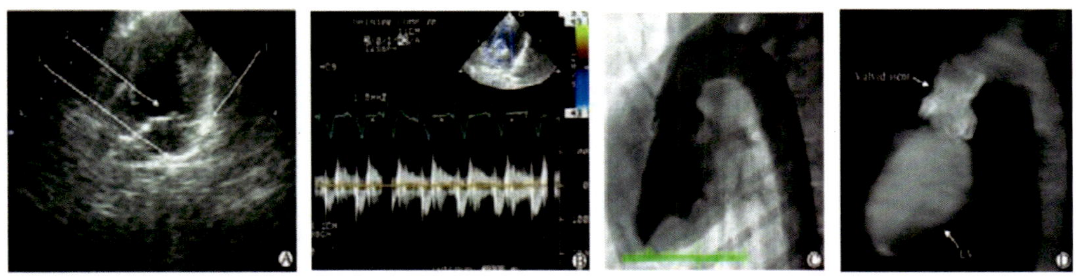

Courtesy of zhou yongxin, et al. Academic Journal of Second Military Medical University 2009;30(10):1150–53.

Figure 4. Cardiac imaging of canines implanted aortic valved stent A: Echocardiogram of aortic valved stent (1:Anterior leaflet of mitral valves; 2:Prosthetic valve; 3:Valved stent).B: Doppler echocardiogram of aortic alved stent. C: Left and right coronary angiogram in left ventriculography. D: The reconstruction image of aortic valved stent with multi-sliced CT.LV:Left ventricular.

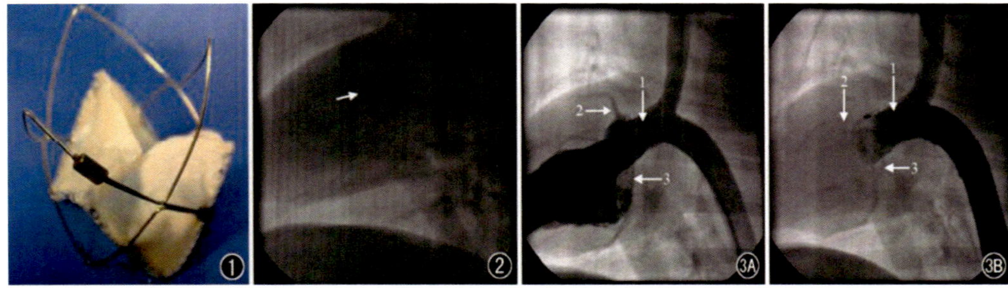

J Thorac Cardiovasc Surg. 2009 Jun;137(6):1363-9. Epub 2009 Mar 17.
Courtesy of BAI Yuan et al. Chinese Medical Journal 2009;122(6):655-658.

Figure 5-①. The W-model valved stent. ②. X-ray image of the valved stent from the left lateral projection after implantation. The image of left lateral oblique projection revealed the valved (arrow) was released in the native aorta annulus. ③. Angiography after valved stent implantation. A: Left ventriculography after device positioning showed the valved stent (arrow 1) sat in the native aortiv annulus and the orifice of coronary (arrows 2 and 3) was normal. B: The supra-aortic angiogram confirmed the stable position of the device (arrow 1) without evidence of aortic regurgitation and compromising the coronary orifice (arrows 2 and 3).

The transapical approach offers to overcome vascular access issues as well as the challenges with crossing a stenotic valve and accurate positioning. A small left anterior thoracotomy is performed, and a sheath is placed in the left ventricular apex with a purse-string suture. A guidewire is passed through the native valve under fluoroscopic guidance, and the remainder of the procedure is performed in a manner similar to the transfemoral approach. This approach was validated initially in an animal model, and has been used clinically in at least 50 patients using the Cribier-Edwards valve. While necessarily more invasive than a transfemoral approach, the shorter catheter length and antegrade approach may afford more stable control of the device for deployment.

In 2009, GU Ming-biao, et al., working in Changhai Hospital, second Military Medical University, Shanghai. used the off-pump antegrade transventricular route for aortic valved stent implantation in canines, and to observe the short-term outcomes. Fresh porcine pericardium was treated with 0.6% glutaraldehyde solution for 36 h; then it was trimmed and sutured into a valvular ring and fixed on a new self-expanding dumb-bell-shaped nickel-titanium shape-memory alloy stent. The valved stents were then implanted off-pump in 8 canines. A limited or full sternotomy approach was used to access the apex of the heart. The crimped valve was introduced through a sheath in the left ventricular apex under ultrasound guidance. The function of valved stents was evaluated with electrocardiogram, echocardiography, computed tomography and DSA angiography early and 3 months after the procedure. They successfully prepared the valved aortic stent. Five canines survived after implantation of the aortic valved stents. Angiographic and echocardiographic observation confirmed that the location and function of the stent were satisfactory, without influencing coronary blood flow and mitral valve function. CT examination showed no migration of the stent 3 months after the procedure, and there were no other prominent complications (figure 4). Their plane was supported by China National High-tech RandD Program.

There followed several reports of the efficacy of transcatheter aortic valve implantation in animal models. BAI Yuan, et al. performed successful a W-model valved stent tAVI with 14 French catheter through the right common iliac artery under guidance of fluoroscopy in six sheep. The self expanding nitinol stent with W-model contains porcine pericardium valves in its proximal part (figure 5-①). These sheep were followed up shortly after procedure with supra-aortic angiogram and left ventriculography. The procedure failed in two sheep due to coronary orifice occlusion in one case and severe aortic valve regurgitation in the other case. One sheep was killed one hour after percutaneous aortic valve replacement for anatomic evaluation. There were no signs of damage of the aortic intima, or of obstruction of the coronary orifice(figure 5-②,③). This short term in vivo study provided evidence that percutaneous aortic valve replacement with a W-model valved stent in the beating heart is possible. However, further studies are mandatory to assess safety and efficacy of this kind of valved stent in larger sample size and by longer follow-up period.

Percutaneous Pulmonary Valve Stent Implantation (PPVS)

From the earliest transcatheter valve replacement experimental study performed by Andersen and colleagues in 1992, to **Bonhoeffer and colleagues' pilot study** of percutaneous pulmonary valve replacement in a right ventricle–to–pulmonary artery prosthetic conduit with valve dysfunction in 2000, pulmonary valve replacement technology has steadily advanced. Clinically, this technique appears to offer significant benefits over standard surgical procedures for patients with congenital heart diseases requiring additional surgical intervention. Not only is the process efficacious and less traumatic, but the duration of hospital stay is shortened.

In 2008, Gang-Jun Zong, et al., Working in Changhai Hospital, piloted study of percutaneous pulmonary valve replacement in China. They performed transcatheter pulmonary valve replacement in sheep using a novel pulmonary valve stent. Fresh porcine pericardium cross-linked with 0.6% glutaraldehyde was treated with L-glutamine to eliminate glutaraldehyde toxicity and sutured onto a valve ring before mounting on a nitinol stent to construct the pulmonary valve stent. Pulmonary valve stents were implanted successfully in 8/10 (80%) sheep. Shortly after surgery, all artificial valve stents exhibited normal open and close functionality and no stenosis or insufficiency (figure 6.). Six-month follow-up revealed no evidence of valve stent dislocation and normal valvular and cardiac functionality. There was no evidence of stent fracture. Repeated valve stent implantation was well tolerated as indicated by good valvular functionality 2 months post delivery. In this study, they first introduced the delivery sheath into the pulmonary artery and then pushed the device through the sheath and into the pulmonary artery in China. However, this study had several limitations. First, the valve stent could not be completely retrieved once released. Thus, further modifications to the delivery system are needed to provide flexibility in cases of suboptimal placement and/or stent size incompatibility. Such modifications will increase the safety and reliability of this procedure. Second, the animal cohort size was small and the follow-up time was short. Last, the use of a single sheep for histologic evaluation and the lack of quantitative assessment of calcification are also limitations.

Subsequent to the report of Gang-Jun Zong, et al, Bai Y, et al in Changhai Hospital introduced the replacement of degenerated bioprosthetic valves with transcatheter reimplantation of stent-mounted pulmonary valves. The procedure was successful in 6 sheep with a homemade valved stent. Two months after the initial procedure, the 6 sheep previously implanted with a valved stent underwent the same implantation procedure of a pulmonary valved stent. All 6 sheep had successful transcatheter stent-mounted pulmonary valve replacement in the first experiment. After 2 months, reimplantation was successful in 5 sheep but failed in 1 sheep because the first valved stent was pushed to the bifurcation of the pulmonary artery by the delivery sheath. Echocardiography confirmed the stents were in the desired position during the follow-up. The remaining 5 sheep with normal valvular and cardiac functionality survived for 3 months after implantation.

In 2009, the same group reported one study describing the first successful percutaneous tricuspid valve replacements in sheep, in which 10 healthy sheep received a double-edge nitinol stent to construct the tricuspid valved stent. These sheep were follow up at 1 month and at 6 months post-implantation. Percutaneous valve implantation was successful in eight of 10 sheep. The remaining six sheep with normal valvular and cardiac functionality survived for 6 months after implantation. This study confirmed that the tricuspid stent with a valvular ring and pericardial valve can be implanted in tricuspid annulus percutaneous and the double-edge stent could substitute the native tricuspid valve chronically.

As describing in the beginning, there are two kinds of devices in transcatheter aortic valve implantation clinical investigation. One device is the Edwards-Sapien valve (Edwards Lifesciences Inc., CA USA), the other is the CoreValve Revalving System (CRS TM, CoreValve Inc., Irvine, CA, USA). The Medtronic CoreValve® System, received CE Mark in March 2007, has now been implanted in more than 1,000 patients worldwide in 32 countries outside the United States. Over two years, cardiac survival was 74 percent and no valve migrations or valve deterioration occurred. Nevertheless, until now it is not yet available in the United States for clinical trial or commercial sale or use. The Edwards Lifesciences Company received conditional Investigational Device Exemption (IDE) approval from the Food and Drug Administration (FDA) in March 2007 to initiate its PARTNER trial, a pivotal clinical trial of the Company's Edwards-Sapien valve technology. The PARTNER trial, which has two study arms, will be finished in mid-2011. In Europe, the Company has completed first-in-man procedures and initiated a small clinical feasibility study recently. In April 2010, the Company expanded the study into a CE Mark trial and expects to complete enrollment in TRITON by the end of 2010.

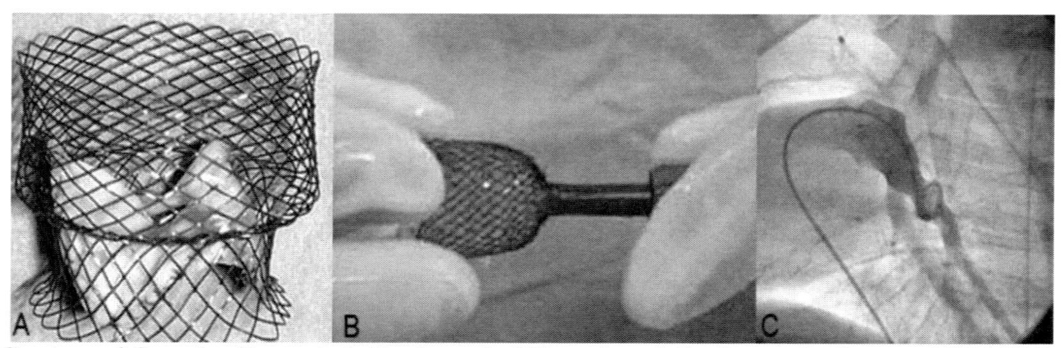

Courtesy of Gang-Jun Zong, et al. The Journal of Thoracic and Cardiovascular Surgery 2009;122(6): 655-658.

Figure 6. A. Pulmonary valve conduit-shaped stent B. Placement of valved stent into sheath. C. Image of the artificial pulmonary valve revealing good placement and no regurgitation.

In Asia, the Edwards Lifesciences Corporation completed its first compassionate use cases with the SAPIEN valve using transapical delivery systems in October 2009 only in Japan. The Company began enrolling patients in a clinical trial with its SAPIEN valve during the second quarter of 2010. The Japan clinical trial will evaluate the transfemoral and transapical delivery systems. Successful trial completion could result in an approval as early as 2013.

Until June 2010, neither the Medtronic Inc nor the Edwards Lifesciences Corporation has submitted to the State Food and Drug Administration, P.R. China (SFDA) for approval to proceed to clinical testing of transcatheter heart valve in the Chinese clinical trial sites. According a risk-based paradigm for classification of devices, percutaneous heart valve prostheses are placed in class 3, the highest risk class for devices exhibiting the most serious consequences to patients in the event of device failure. So the SFDA must assure that devices in the class perform with reasonable assurance of safety and effectiveness. Safety is preeminent in examination and is clearly defined in relation to the intended function and indication for use.

If the transcatheter heart valve is been introduced in China, the SFDA is required to evaluate the risk versus the benefit of new devices when making decisions on approvability. Obviously, a well-designed and well-carried out trial must be submitted to the SFDA for consideration. There are several ways to ensure the smoothest regulatory process. First and foremost is early collaboration with FDA to address and resolve issues regarding important aspects of the approval process. Finally, the science of clinical trial design requires innovative approaches for these innovation devices; working collaboratively with the Agency will speed the entire process.

As a cardiovascular surgeon, the authors believe that transcatheter heart valve is an effective long-term treatment alternative for many patients with severe aortic stenosis who are considered at high surgical risk or inoperable and look forward to bringing this therapy to many more patients in China.

Future

Valvular heart disease is an important cause of morbidity and mortality. Aortic stenosis and mitral regurgitation account for the majority of patients with native valve disease. Although surgical treatment provides satisfactory outcome, a large proportion of patients do not undergo a surgical intervention, because of the high estimated operative risk and multiple comorbidities. In the future, treatment options for patients with cardiovascular disease will include open surgical procedures, minimally invasive surgical intervention, and percutaneous approaches.

The field of percutaneous valve replacement and repair is clearly developing rapidly. Transcatheter aortic and pulmonic valve replacement and a variety of mitral valve therapy approaches have been successfully performed in thousands of patients. A variety of operator technique and device-related problems have been encountered and solved. Significant challenges in patient selection and clinical trial design have yet to be resolved. The patient populations may ultimately benefit most from treatment using these new technologies. Since the first-in-man TAVI by Alain Cribier in 2002, well over 1000 high risk patients with severe symptomatic AS have been treated using TAVI. The extraordinary advancements in the era of interventional cardiology have given clinicians the chance to pursue treatment options for certain diseases that previously had only surgical solutions.

Nevertheless, there are many obstacles still exist in the nonsurgical approach. Reports originate from a limited number of centers worldwide. The patients treated were mostly more than 80 years old, at high risk (e.g. Logistic EuroScore>20% and >10% with STS score in most cases) or with contraindications for surgery. Mortality at 30 days range from 5 to 18%. Acute myocardial infarction occurs in 2-11%. Coronary obstruction is less than 1%. But mild-to-moderate aortic regurgitation, mostly paravalvular is observed in ~50% of cases. This is why TAVI should be performed only in severe AS. Vascular complications, with an incidence ranging from 10 to 15%, remain a significant cause of mortality and morbidity. Stroke ranges from 3 to 9%. Finally, artrioventricular block occurs in 4-8%, necessitating pacemaker implantation in up to 24% with self-expandable devices. Long-term results up to 2 years show a survival rate of 70~80% with a significant improvement in clinical condition in most cases.

On the other hand, surgical AVR has had an illustrious history for 40 years, with low mortality, continued improvement in operative and perioperative patient management techniques, and increased valve durability. Cardiovascular surgeons can state unequivocally that surgical AVR in symptomatic patients with severe aortic stenosis both relieves symptoms and prolongs life. So it is premature to consider using it in patients who are good surgical candidates.

Accordingly, the currently available results obtained with TAVI suggest that these techniques are targeted at high-risk patients and there must be a long way to extend to the lower risk group in the future. The clinical trial landscape is also still under active discussion; if these percutaneous techniques are to be seen as an alternative to traditional surgical methodologies in low-risk to medium-risk patients, new techniques will need to demonstrate similar hemodynamic effects, safety, and durability to the current highly refined surgical techniques.

In China, we will also need to solve training issues and evaluate our outcomes, with additional assessments of cost effectiveness and quality of life. Although there remains much to do, these early results suggest that the future of percutaneous valve replacement holds great promise and benefit for our patients with valve disease. Today, these techniques are targeted at high-risk patients but they may be extended to the lower risk patients in the future. The procedure also requires the close cooperation of a team of speacialists in valve disease, including clinical cardiologists, echocardiographists, interventional cardiologists, cardiac surgeons, and anaesthesiologists. In the future, these creative new percutaneous approaches may change the face of Chinese patients' valve therapy.

References

Actis-Dato, GM, Caimmi P, Di-Rosa, E, et al. Correlation between malfunction of a bioprosthesis and deformation of a valve stent. Comparison of three different valve models. *Minerva Cardioangiol*. 1998; 46(4):97-101.

Alain Cribier, Helene Eltchaninoff, Assaf Bash, et al. Percutaneous Transcatheter Implantation of an Aortic Valve Prosthesis for Calcific Aortic Stenosis-First Human Case DescriptionCirculation. 2002;106:3006-3008.

Alan Zajarias, Alain G. Cribier, St. Louis, Rouen. Outcomes and Safety of Percutaneous Aortic Valve Replacement. *J. Am. Coll. Cardiol*. 2009;53:1829–36.

Al-Attar N, Himbert D, Descoutures F, et al. Transcatheter aortic valve_*Ann. Thorac. Surg*. 2009;87(6):1757-62.

Alec Vahanian, Christophe Acar. Percutaneous valve procedures: what is the future? *Curr. Opin. Cardiol*. 2005, 20:100-106.

Alec Vahanian, Pierrelouis Michel, Bertrand Cormier. Results of percutaneous mitral commisurotomy in 200 patients. *Am. J. Cariol*. 1989;63:847.

Andersen, HR, Knudsen, LL, Hasenkam, JM. Transluminal implantation of artificial heart valves. Description of a new expandable aortic valve and initial results with implantation by catheter technique in closed chest pigs. *Euripean Heart Journal*. 1992; 13(5):704-708.

Bai Y, Zong GJ, Jiang HB, et al. Percutaneous reimplantation of a pulmonary valved stent in sheep: a potential treatment for bioprosthetic valve degeneration. *J. Thorac. Cardiovasc. Surg*. 2009 ;138(3):733-7.

Bai Y, Zong GJ, Wang HR, et al. An integrated pericardial valved stent special for percutaneous tricuspid implantation: an animal feasibility study. *J. Surg. Res.* 2010; 160(2):215-21.

Bonoeffer P, Boudjemline Y, Saliba Z, et al. transcatheter of bovine Valve in pulmonary position: a lamb study. *Circulation*. 2000;102:813-816.

Chen CR, Cheng TO, Chen JY, Zhou YL, Mei J, Ma TZ. Percutaneous balloon mitral valvuloplasty for mitral stenosis with and without associated aortic regurgitation. *Am. Heart J*. 1993;125(1):128-37.

Chen CR, Cheng TO. Percutaneous balloon mitral valvuloplasty by the Inoue technique: a multicenter study of 4832 patients in China. *Am. Heart J*. 1995;129(6): 1197-203.

Chen CR, Lo ZX, Huang ZD, et al. Percutaneous transseptal balloon mitral valvuloplasty the Chinese experience in 30 patients. *Am. Heat J*. 1988;115-937.

Chen CR, Lo ZX, Huang ZD, Inoue KJ, Cheng TO. Percutaneous transseptal balloon mitral valvuloplasty: the Chinese experience in 30 patients. *Am. Heart J.* 1988;115(5): 937-47.

Ciechi Na, Less WM, Thompson R. Functional anatomy of normal mitral valve. *J. Thor. Surg.* 1956; 32:378-398.

Cribier A, Eltchaninoff H, Tron C, et al. Early experience with percutaneous transcatheter implantation of heart valve prosthesis for the treatment of end-stage inoperable patients with calcific aortic stenosis. *J. Am. Coll. Cardiol.* 2004;43:678-703.

Cribier A, Eltchaninoff H, Tron C, et al. Early experience with percutaneous transcatheter implantation of heart valve prosthesis for the treatment of end-stage inoperable patients with calcific aortic stenosis. *J. Am. Coll. Cardiol.* 2004;43(4):698-703.

Cribier A, Litzler PY, Eltchaninoff H, et al. Technique of transcatheter_*Herz*. 2009;34(5):347-56.

Dai R, Jiang S, Huang L, et al. Percutaneous transseptal balloon valvuloplasty for dilating mitral valve stenosis (report of 200 cases). *Chin. Med. Sci. J.* 1993;8(4):191-6.

Ferrari M, Figulla HR, Schlosser M, et al. Transarterial aortic valve replacement with a self expanding stent in pigs. *Heart*. 2004;90(11):1326-31.

Gang-Jun Zong, Yuan Bai, Hai-Bin Jiang, et al. Use of a novel valve stent for transcatheter pulmonary valve replacement: An animal study. *J. Thorac. Cardiovasc. Surg.* 2009;122(6):655-658.

Georg Lutter, Reza Ardehali, Jochen Cremer, and Philipp Bonhoeffer. Percutaneous Valve Replacement: Current State and Future Prospects. *Ann. Thorac. Surg.* 2004;78: 2199-2206.

GU Ming-biao, CHEN Xiang, BAI Yuan, et al. Transapical aortic valve implantation with a new self-expanding valved stent in canines:an observation of short-term outcomes. *Acad. J. Sec. Mil. Med. Univ*,2009,30(10):1150-1153

He Qiang, Yang jian, Yi dinghua. Percutaneous transcatheter aortic valve implantation transapical approach. *Chin. J. Thorac. Cardiovasc. Surg*, 2009;25(1):4-5.

Hung JS, Chern MS, Wu JJ, et al. Short- and long-term results of catheter balloon percutaneous transvenous mitral commissurotomy. *Am. J. Cardiol.* 1991;67(9):854-62.

Inoue K et al. Non operative mitral commissurotomy by a new balloon catheter. *Jpn. Cir. J.* 1982; 46: 87.

Inoue K, Owaki T, Nakamura T, et al. Clinical application of transvenous mitral commissuratomy by a new balloon catheter. *J. Thorac. Cardiovasc. Surg.* 1984; 87: 394-398.

James J. Glazier and Zoltan G. Turi. Percutaneous Balloon Mitral Valvuloplasty. *Progress in Cardiovascular Diseases*. 1997;40(1): 5-26.

Kempfert J, Lehmann S, Linke A, et al. Latest advances in transcatheter_*Surg. Technol. Int.* 2010;19:147-54.

Kuehne, Titus, Saeed, Maythem DVM, et al. Sequential Magnetic Resonance Monitoring of Pulmonary Flow With Endovascular Stents Placed Across the Pulmonary Valve in Growing Swine. *Circulation*. 2001;104(19):2363-2368.

Lawrence H. Cohn. Cardiac Surgery In The Adult. Third Edition. the United States of America: The McGraw-Hill Companies; 2008:963-968.

Li Huatai. Clinical application of transvenous mitral commissuratomy by balloon catheter. *Chinese Medical journal*. 1988; 27:460.

Lichtenstein SV, Cheung A, Ye J, et al. Transapical transcatheter aortic valve implantation in humans: initial clinical experience. *Circulation*. 2006;114(6):591-6.

Liu F, Wu L, Huang GY, et al. Percutaneous balloon valvuloplasty for severe and critical pulmonary valve stenosis in infants under six months. Zhonghua Yi Xue Za Zhi. 2009;89(46):3253-6.

Ma C, Liu X, Hu D, Yang X, et al. Transseptal methods for percutaneous balloon valvoplasty simultaneously with radiofrequency catheter ablation. *Chin. Med. J.* (Engl). 1995;108(12):883-6.

Masakiyo Nobuyoshi, Takeshi Arita, Shin-ichi Shirai, et al. Percutaneous Balloon Mitral Valvuloplasty A Review. *Circulation*. 2009;119:e211-e219.

Michael J. Davidson, Jennifer K. White, Donald S. Baim. Percutaneous therapies for valvular heart disease. *Cardiovascular Pathology*. 2006;123– 129.

Michael Mack. Fool me once, shame on you; fool me twice, shame on me! A perspective on the emerging world of percutaneous heart valve therapy. *J. Thorac. Cardiovasc. Surg.* 2008;136:816-9.

Ofenloch JC, Chen C, Hughes JD, et al. Endoscopic venous valve transplantation with a valve-stent device. *Ann. Vasc. Surg*. 1997; 11(1):62-7.

Paul T.L. Chiam, Carlos E. Ruiz. Percutaneous transcatheter aortic valve implantation: Evolution of the technology. *Am. Heart J.* 2009;157:229-42.

Pavenik D, Wright KC, Wallace S. Development and initial experimental evaluation of a prosthetic aortic valve for transcatheter placement. *Radiology*, 1992, 183:151-154.

Pepine CJ, Gessner JH, Teldman RL. Percutaneous ballon Valvuloplasty for treating congenital plumonic valve stenosis in the adult. *Am. J. Cardiol.* 1988; 50:1442

Philipp Lurz, Louise Coats, Sachin Khambadkone, et al. Percutaneous Pulmonary Valve Implantation Impact of Evolving Technology and Learning Curve on Clinical Outcome. *Circulation*. 2008;117:1964-1972.

Rodés-Cabau J, Webb JG, Cheung A, et al. Transcatheter aortic valve *J. Am. Coll. Cardiol.* 2010;55(11):1080-90.

Shu Maoqin, He Guoxiang, Song Zhiyuan, et al. The clinical and hemodynamic results of mitral balloon valvuloplasty for patients with mitral stenosis complicated by severe pulmonary hypertension. *European Journal of Internal Medicine*. 2005;16:413-418.

Sochman J, Peregrin JH, Pavcnik D, et al. Percutaneous transcatheter aortic disc valve prosthesis implantation: a feasibility study. *Cardiovasc. Intervent. Radiol.* 2000;23(5): 384-8.

Walther T, Falk V, Borger MA, et al. Minimally invasive transapical beating heart aortic valve implantation--proof of concept. *Eur. J. Cardiothorac. Surg*. 2007;31(1):9-15.

Walther T, Simon P, Dewey T, et al. Transapical minimally invasive aortic valve implantation: multicenter experience. *Circulation*. 2007;11:116.

Wan, WK; Campbell, G, Zhang, ZF, et al. Optimizing the tensile properties of polyvinyl alcohol hydrogel for the construction of a bioprosthetic heart valve stent. *Journal of Biomedical Materials Research*. 2002;63(6): 854-861.

Wang G, Chen Lian, Liu Guoshu, et al. Percutaneous metals dilator valvuloplasty for treating mitral valve stenosis. *Chinese Medical journal* 2000;113(Suppl):256.

Wang Guangyi, Liu Hongbin, Chen Lian, et al. Mitral stenosis treated with PBMV. *Chinese Medical Journal* 2000; 113(Suppl):234

Wang W, Xie CH, Xia CS, Zhou YB, Gong FQ. Percutaneous balloon aortic valvuloplasty for congenital valvular aortic stenosis in children. Zhonghua Xin Xue Guan Bing Za Zhi. 2007;35(3):224-6.

Webb JG, Chandavimol M, Thompson CR, et al. Percutaneous aortic valve implantation retrograde from the femoral artery. *Circulation*. 2006;113(6):842-50.

Webb, JG, Munt B, Makkar RR, Naqvi, TZ, et al. Percutaneous stent-mounted valve for treatment of aortic or pulmonary valve disease. *Catheterization and Cardiovascular Interventions*. 2004;63(1):89-93.

Ye J, Cheung A, Lichtenstein SV, Nietlispach F, et al. Transapical transcatheter aortic valve implantation: follow-up to 3 years. *J. Thorac. Cardiovasc. Surg*. 2010;139(5): 1107-13.

Yip AS, Chow WH, Fu KH, Cheung KL, Li JP, Lee JS. Effect of percutaneous balloon mitral valvuloplasty on serum creatinine phosphokinase MB-isoenzyme levels. *Cathet. Cardiovasc. Diagn*. 1993;29(3):179-82.

Yu ZX, Ma YT, Yang YN, et al. Outcome of percutaneous balloon pulmonary valvuloplasty for patients with pulmonary valve stenosis. Zhonghua Xin Xue Guan Bing Za Zhi. 2009;37(11):1006-9.

Zhang L. Long-term outcome of repeat percutaneous balloon mitral valvuloplasty in patients with mitral restenosis. Zhonghua Xin Xue Guan Bing Za Zhi. 2009;37(1):49-52.

ZHOU Yong-xin, SHAO Jie, SUN Lin, LI Gang, MEI Yun-qing, WANG Yong-wu. Preparation of valved aortic stent and trans-catheter implantation to ascending aortain vivo. *Acad. J. Sec. Mil. Med. Univ*, 2009, 30(2):120-123.

Zhou yongxin, Shao jie, Sun Lin, Li Gang, Mei Yunqing, Wang Yongwu. Preparement of percuta neous valved stent in vivo. *Journal of tongji university medical science* 2008;29(6):54–57.

Zong GJ, Bai Y, Jiang HB, et al. Use of a novel valve stent for transcatheter pulmonary valve replacement: an animal study. *J. Thorac. Cardiovasc. Surg*. 2009;137(6):1363-9.

In: Percutaneous Valve Technology: Present and Future
Editors: Jose Luis Navia and Sharif Al-Ruzzeh
ISBN: 978-1-61942-577-4

Chapter XXIII

Percutaneous Mitral Valve Repair – The Role of Coronary Sinus Approach

Saif Anwaruddin and Stephen G. Ellis

Introduction

To appreciate the complexity of the mitral valve is to understand its intricate anatomical and physiologic properties. Disease of the mitral valve can be primarily valvular (rheumatic, degenerative) or secondary to other processes, particularly those affecting the myocardium. For several years now, standard of care for treatment of mitral valve disease, particularly severe mitral regurgitation, has been surgical. Surgical repair of the mitral valve has come to be regarded as a durable alternative to surgical replacement for degenerative disease [1, 2]. Evidence in favor of surgical repair has suggested improved operative mortality, long term survival and ejection fraction as compared to replacement [3]. Treatment of functional mitral regurgitaiton, however, remains a challenge. Surgical repair of functional mitral regurgitation at the time of coronary artery bypass grafting (CABG) does not appear to provide long-term improvement in symptoms or survival [4].

Several percutaneous approaches to treating mitral regurgitation have emerged as possible alternatives to surgical treatment. It remains a challenge for percutaneous therapies to match the success reported with surgical repair of degenerative valve disease. However, treatment of patients with functional mitral regurgitation remains a problem without a well-defined solution. Theoretical advantages of percutaneous methods in treating functional mitral regurgitation include obviating the need for cardiopulmonary byapass and thoracotomy in patients who may be otherwise high risk for such open surgical procedures. The disadvantages include the inability to directly visualize the valve, relying instead on angiography and echocardiography.

Table 1. Percutaneous Mitral Valve Repair Technology

Coronary Sinus Annuloplasty	
	Viacor PTMA
	Edwards MONARC
	Cardiac Dimensions CARILLON
	Cerclage annuloplasty system
Direct Valve Repair	
	Abbott eValve
	Edwards Mobius
Septal to Lateral Cinching (SLAC)	
	Ample Med, PS3
	Myocor iCoapsys
	St Jude
Direct Annuloplasty	
	Mitralign Direct Annuloplasty System
	Guided Delivery Systems AccucCnch
	QuantumCor RF ablation
	MiCardia Dynaplasty

Many percutaneous methods have been developed (Table 1) based on previous surgical techniques that have demonstrated proven benefit. Percutaneous techniques attempt to correct mitral regurgitation by directly or indirectly dealing with the valve. The MitraClip System (Abbott, Inc) is an example of a device that corrects regurgitation by an edge-to-edge percutaneous clip, analogous to the operation described by Dr. Alfieri [5]. Several methods take advantage of the anatomical relationship between the coronary sinus (CS) and the mitral valve annulus for percutaneous annuloplasty, while still others have described septal-lateral annular cinching techniques to deal with functional mitral regurgitation. Unlike surgical repair, often employing corrective procedures for both the valve and the annulus, at this time, percutaneous strategies are singular in their approach.

For purposes of this chapter, we will delve into a discussion of the current state of the art with regards to percutaneous mitral valve repair with a focus on those techniques that utilize the CS. An appreciation of the advantages and disadvantages of such techniques will require an understanding of the anatomy of the mitral valve structure itself and we will begin by reviewing anatomical relationships and how they impact the use of the device.

Anatomical Considerations and Imaging Techniques

The mitral valve consists of several components, each vital in maintaining proper function. The valve itself is a bi-leaflet structure – a posterior leaflet with three distinct scallops and a corresponding anterior leaflet. The leaflets attach to the posteromedial and anterolateral papillary muscles by way of chordae tendinae. With systole, the contraction of the ventricle results in traction of the papillary muscles leading to valve closure by transmission of that force through the chordae.

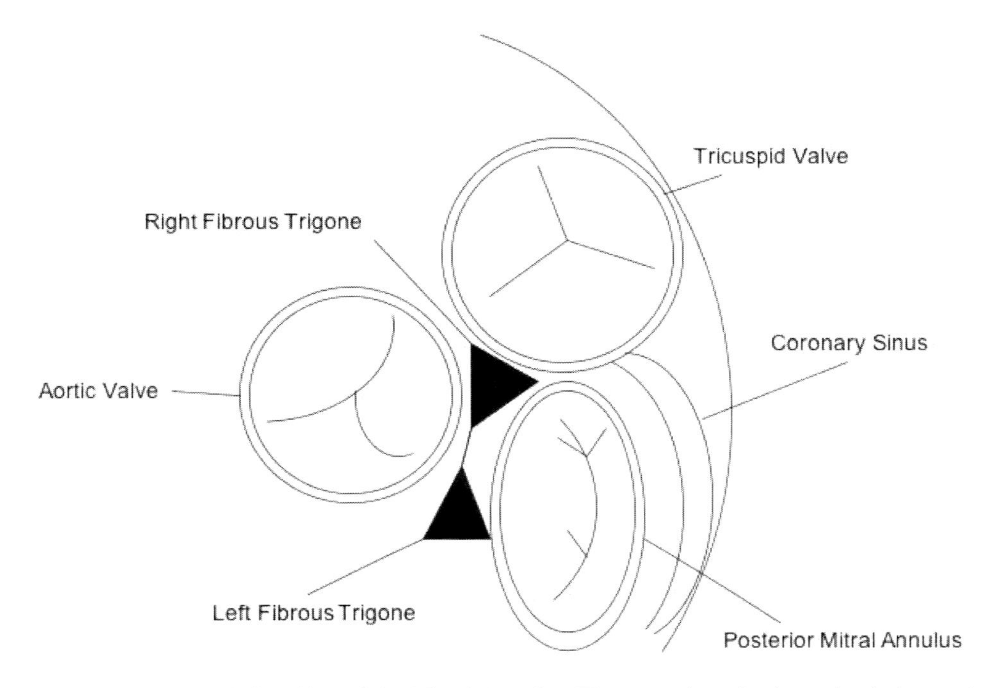

Figure 1a. Anatomical Relationships of the Mitral Annulus. The posterior mitral annulus is in proximity to the coronary sinus.

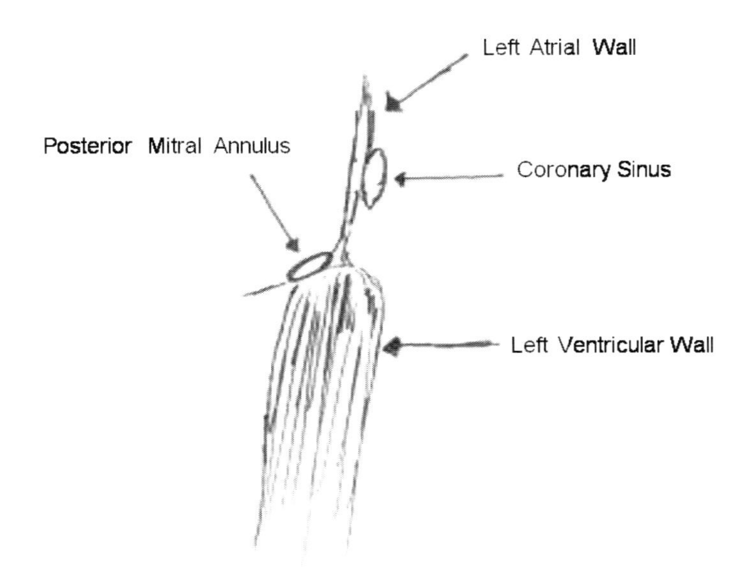

Figure 1b. The Posterior Mitral Annulus in relation to the Coronary Sinus. As can be seen from this illustration, the coronary sinus runs along the posterior left atrial wall and any coronary sinus based device will affect the posterior mitral annulus through indirect forces applied to the left atrial wall.

The leaflets attach to the base of the left atrium to a thin ovoid shaped membrane referred to as the annulus. The mitral valve annulus is a nonplanar structure [6] resembling a riding saddle, a feature conserved among several species [7]. Inability to maintain this structure may influence valve competency [8]. Surrounding the anterior portion of the annulus are two fibrous trigones (left and right).

A fibrous region between the two trigones is referred to the intertrigonal region. The anterior portion of the annulus and the aortic valve annulus are in close proximity and this region is referred to as the intervalvular fibrosa. The posterior mitral annulus is not surrounded by any fibrous tissue, however, serves to separate the ventricular from the atrial tissue (Figure 1a).

The CS runs in close proximity to the posterior mitral valve annulus and it is this anatomical relationship that allows use of the CS for percutaneous annuloplasty techniques. While echocardiography remains the standard for the diagnosis and assessment of mitral regurgitation, other imaging modalities such as cardiac computed tomography (CT) and cardiac magnetic resonance imaging (CMR) are germane to this discussion for their role in guiding intervention.

Visualization of the location of the coronary sinus and its relationship to surrounding structures, namely the posterior annulus and the left circumflex artery (LCx), is critical to planning percutaneous repair of the mitral annulus.

The spatial relationship between the coronary sinus and the mitral annulus has been studied in 61 human cadavers revealing a maximal distance between the mitral annulus and the CS to be 19 mm with a mean distance of 9.7 $\pm$ 3.2 mm [9]. Use of cardiac CT has revealed significant variability in the distance between the mitral annulus and the CS [10]. Furthermore, this analysis has also revealed, *in vivo*, that the relationship between the annulus and the CS varies in different planes with left atrial enlargement in patients with MR.

In a separate study of 105 patients, using 64-slice multi-slice CT, investigators were able to confirm the variability in the distance between the mitral annulus and the CS but were able to demonstrate that the relationship was influenced by the degree of mitral regurgitaiton [11]. This variability will likely influence the effectiveness of percutaneous annuloplasty devices that make use of the CS.

Both post mortem studies and *in vivo* imaging have confirmed that the CS does not in fact run behind the mitral annulus, but rather runs behind the left atrial wall [9, 11] (Figure 1b). The variability in the CS and mitral annulus described previously may be influenced by this relationship as left atrial enlargement and remodeling, as is often seen with chronic mitral regurgitation, can directly affect the distance between the two structures.

Use of cardiac imaging has also been important in delineating the relationship between the LCx and the CS. The use of annuloplasty devices have the potential to impinge upon the LCx [12] and careful planning must precede any device implant. Cardiac CT has again revealed that the LCx crosses between the mitral annulus and the CS in 80% of patients examined with significant variability in the location of crossover [10].

Using CT to identify the area of crossover will be important in deciding upon patient candidacy for use of a percutaneous mitral annuloplasty device.

Coronary Sinus Based Mitral Annulplasty and Percutaneous Devices

Given relative close proximity between the CS and the posterior portion of the mitral valve annulus, it is believed that percutaneous mitral annuloplasty devices placed within the coronary sinus can reduce the diameter of the mitral annulus [13]. Given the anatomical relationships discussed in the previous section, the effectivness of device reduction of annular size may be the result of indirect forces that are transmitted via the left atrial wall [9]. It remains to be seen, however, whether this will impact the long-term effectiveness of the device itself (Table 2). The efficacy of the coronary sinus based percutaneous mitral annuloplasty devices has been demonstrated in animal models of ischemic mitral regurgitation with reductions in annular diameter and degree of mitral regurgitation [14] However, these animal models are often limited in their ability to truly replicate the disease state and other associated complicating factors.

Percutaneous Transvenous Coronary Mitral Annuloplasty - Viacor PTMA

The Viacor PTMA (Viacor, Inc, Wilmington, MA) device is an annuloplasty device with two major components – a multi-lumen delivery catheter and a set of nitinol PTMA rods (Figure 2). The multi-lumen delivery catheter is used for passage of the nitinol PTMA rods, of varying stiffness, with the goal of affecting the remodeling of the coronary sinus and the posterior mitral annulus. Preclinical studies with the Viacor PTMA device have demonstrated its ability to reduce mitral regurgitation [15, 16]

Table 2. Clinical Trials of Indirect Coronary Sinus Annuloplasty Devices

Title	Device	# of patients	Comments
Dubreuil et al [17]	Viacor	4	Device temporarily placed in 3 of 4 patients with reduction in mitral regurgitation noted
Sack et al [18]	Viacor	27	Device placed successfully in 13 of 19 patients, reduction in mitral regurgitation noted, stable reduction in septal lateral annular diameter at 3 mos
Webb et al [19]	MONARC	5	Device implanted in 4 patients, reduction in mitral regurgitation noted, however follow up echo demonstrated separation of device bridge in 3 of 4 implants
Evolution I [29]	MONARC	72	Device implanted in 59 pts (82%), 64% event free survival at 3 yrs, reduction in mitral regurgitaiton and NYHA class noted
Duffy et al [21]	CARILLON	5	Device implanted in 4 pts, reduction in mitral annular dimension and mitral regurgitaiton noted, 2 devices had slippage of distal anchor
AMADEUS [22]	CARILLON	48	Device implanted in 30 pts, mitral annular to CS distance does not appear to influence effectiveness of device [23].

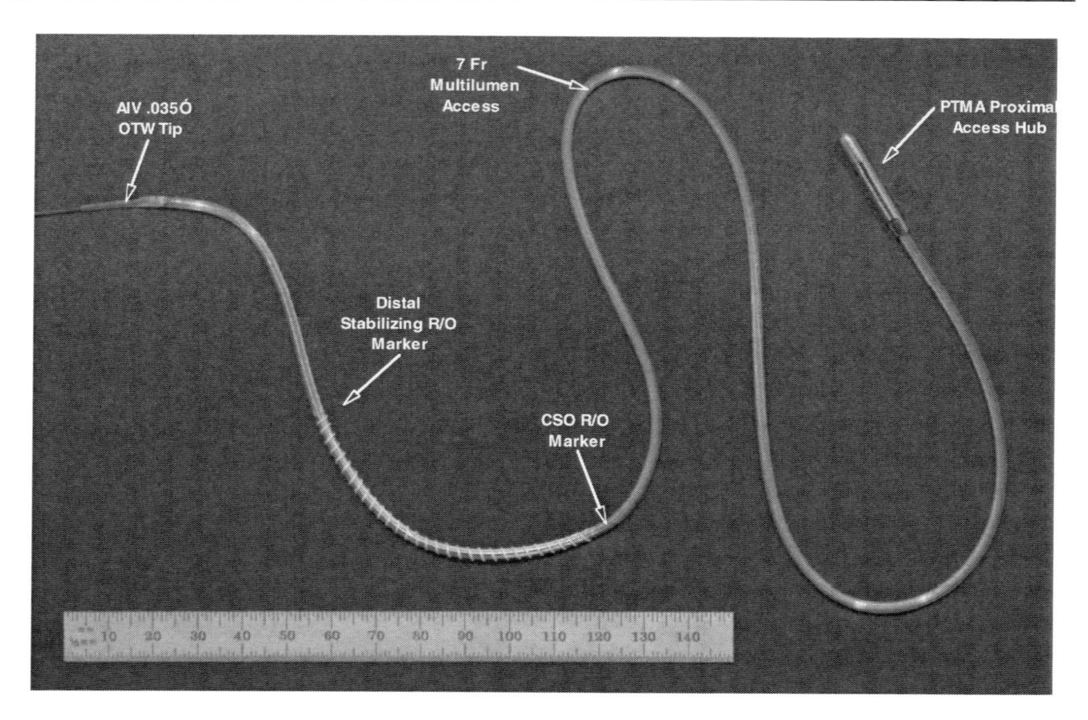

Figure 2. Viacor PTMA Device.

After venous access is obtained from either the right or left subclavian vein, an 8F coronary sinus sheath is used to engage the CS. Diagnostic venography is then performed to delineate the coronary venous anatomy. A guide wire is then used to wire the anterior interventricular vein. After the guide wire is in place, the Viacor 7F diagnostic multi-lumen sheath is then advanced over the wire into the anterior interventricular vein using fluorosocopic guidance. At this point, the nitinol PTMA rods (up to 3 at a time) are inserted through the multi-lumen sheath and simultaneous transesophageal echo (TEE) or transthoracic echo (TTE) is used to assess the impact upon mitral regurgitation. Coronary angiography is also performed to ensure no effects upon the coronary circulation. The appropriate combination of rod stiffness is used to obtain a subsequent decrease in annular diameter and mitral regurgitaiton, If there is benefit noted and there are no untoward effects (ie impingement on the coronary circulation), then the diagnostic catheter is exchanged for an implant PTMA catheter and rods of the same stiffness. At this point, the device is closed at the level of the subclavian vein and the skin is sutured over it. If needed, the device can be re-accessed to adjust rod stiffness.

The first in-man study was performed in four patients with symptomatic ischemic mitral regurgitation of at least grade 2+ [17]. The device was placed in all but 1 patient due to unfavorable CS anatomy. In the three in whom the device was placed had a reduction in MR, a mean reduction in anterior-posterior diameter of 5.1 ± 3.6 mm, and a reduction in the effective regurgitant orifice (ERO) from 0.25 ± 0.06 to 0.07 ± 0.03 cm^2. In the fourth patient, it was noted that the diagnostic device was not stable and, hence, a permanent device could not be used.

In a larger safety and feasibility study of the Viacor device (PTOLEMY-1), 27 patients with New York Heart Association (NYHA) class 2 or 3 symptoms, at least 2+ mitral regurgitation and a left ventricular fraction between 20-50% were included [18]. Of these 27, 19 patients successfully underwent the PTMA diagnostic procedure. The diagnostic procedure was deemed to be effective in 13 of the 19 and implants were subsequently placed. Device migration and lack of efficacy was cited as the reason for which 3 patients had to have implants removed. In these cases all equipment was removed percutaneously. Complications included pericardial effusion (n=1), PTMA implant fracture/removal (n=1), and LCx stent implantation (n=1). Acute TEE evaluation of post implant mitral regurgitaiton revealed a reduction from 3.2 ± 0.6 to 2.0 ± 1.0. Of note, investigators noted that echocardiography at 3 months post implant demonstrates stable and sustained reduction in septal-lateral dimensions of the mitral annulus, although not to the degree one would see with successful surgical repair. From the PTOLEMY-1 study it was clear that the use of cardiac CT guided planning was essential as part of the procedural process and ensuring secure placement of the device tip in the anterior interventricular vein was important for device stability.

There are many questions that remain with regards to this device. While this study demonstrates safety and feasibility, other issues need to be addressed, including device stability post implantation. The device is advantageous with regards to the ability to adjust device stiffness based on degree of mitral regurgitaiton and to determine safety and utility using a diagnostic device. It remains to be seen how well this device is able to reduce MR in the future. Also, with any coronary sinus based annuloplasty device, the question remains as to what effect it will have, if any, upon the remodeling. The PTOLEMY-2 trial, which is currently enrolling and will likely shed more light on the efficacy of this device (Figure 3).

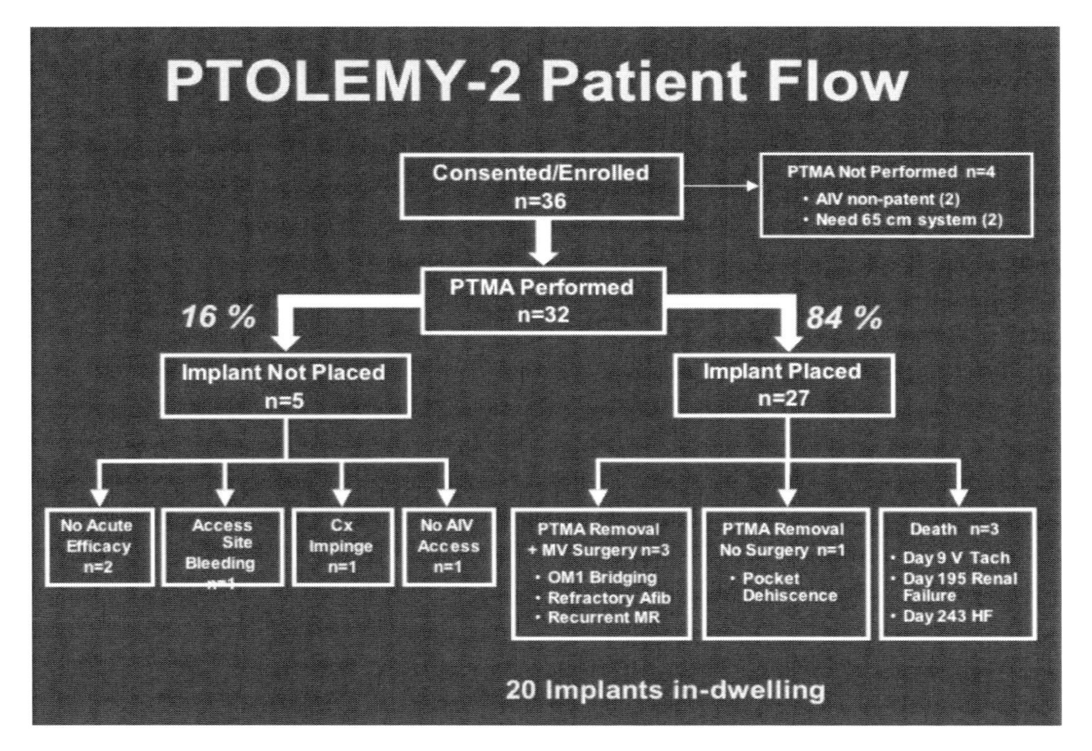

Figure 3. PTOLEMY-2 Study. Safety and Efficacy Study of the Viacor PTMA device in Europe and Canada.

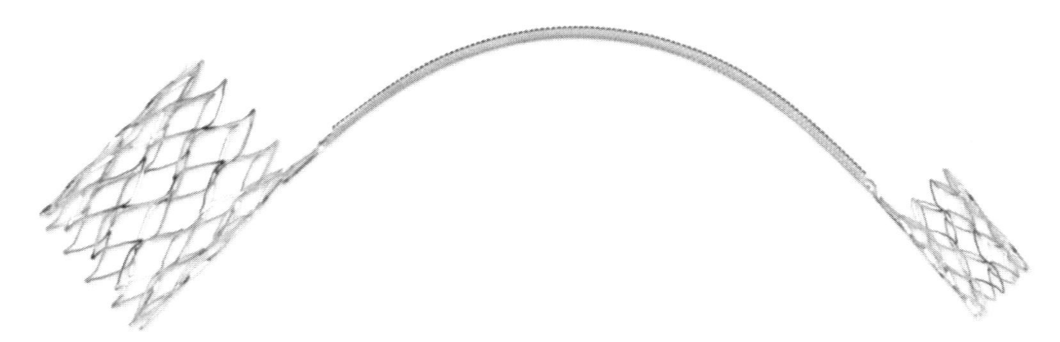

Permission for use of this image by Edwards Lifesciences, Irvine, CA.

Figure 4. MONARC PTMA System.

MONARC Percutaneous Transvenous Mitral Annuloplasty Device

The MONARC PTMA System (Edwards Lifesciences, Irvine, CA) is a nitinol-based device with two self-expanding stent-like anchors (Figure 4). The distal anchor is deployed in the distal great cardiac vein and is connected to the proximal anchor by a bridge-like segment. Within this connecting segment, there are biodegradable spacers that dissolve over time. With the device anchored in both the proximal and distal segments, over time the spacers dissolve in the connecting segment resulting in contraction of the bridge since it is a nitinol based system. Contraction should lead to shortening of the coronary sinus as well.

Access is obtained through the internal jugular vein and a sheath is placed. The coronary sinus is cannulated and wired. A measuring catheter is then used to decide upon the proper sized device. The measurement catheter is then exchanged for a 12 F delivery sheath over the wire. Left coronary angiography is also performed to assess the position of the coronary arteries relative to the great vein. The device is then delivered by first positioning and then deploying the distal anchor in the distal great cardiac vein, again, taking into account the anatomical relationship with the coronary arterial supply. Once the distal anchor is deployed, the proximal anchor is next deployed after all tension is removed from the bridge. Once both anchors are in place the device is deployed and cannot be retrieved.

An initial attempt with this PTMA system was performed using an earlier device in five patients with chronic ischemic mitral regurgitation [19]. Implantation was successful in 4 patients and mitral regurgitation was reduced in the group from grade 3.0 ± 0.7 to 1.6 ± 1.1. In the one patient in whom delivery was not successful, the procedure resulted in pericardial effusion. At follow up, it was noted that between 28-81 days, 3 of the 4 implanted devices were noted to have separation of the bridge between the two anchors. A re-iteration of this device has been made to reflect the changes described above with the biodegradable spacers.

The newer generation device, described above, is currently being trialed in the EVOLUTION I study. This trial is a multi-center, prospective, feasibility study with the primary outcome of evaluating the safety of the device in patients with functional mitral regurgitaiton of grade at least 2+ and dilated or ischemic cardiomyopathy. Patients were excluded if they were noted to have either organic mitral regurgitation, an ejection fraction < 25%, ischemia requiring revascularization, CS pacing/ICD leads, or moderate to severe mitral annular calcificaiton. The 3-year interim results of the largest study to date with a CS annuloplasty device have been presented and demonstrated a 64% event free survival in 59 of 72 patients (82%) in whom this device placed successfully placed [20]. At 3 years, the mean NYHA class decreased from 2.7 to 2.0 with a corresponding improvement in mitral regurgitation noted. The larger EVOLUTION II trial will prospectively examine the clinical safety and efficacy of the MONARC system in patients with grade 3 or higher mitral regurgitaiton.

CARILLON Miral Contour System

The third major CS annuloplasty device that is currently under investigation is the CARILLON Mitral Contour System (Cardiac Dimensions, Kirkland, WA). The CARILLON system shares some similarity with the MONARC device in that it consists of two anchors joined by a connector or ribbon.. After the device is positioned, tension can be applied to the connecting segment with the effect of shortening the CS and reducing mitral regurgitation.

Access is obtained in the catheterization laboratory via the internal jugular vein and a 9 F catheter is used to cannulate the great cardiac vein. TEE is used to assess mitral regurgitation during the implantation procedure. Coronary angiography is performed to assess for coronary atherosclerosis and to determine the relationship of the coronaries to other structures. Venography is also performed to size the vein and to ensure proper positioning in relation to the mitral valve annulus. Once sizing is confirmed, the device is deployed by retraction of the delivery catheter to allow the distal end of the nitinol device to open to its natural shape. Anchor stability is maintained by oversizing the anchors in relation to the CS. Once the distal anchor is deployed, traction is placed on the delivery sheath, which creates tension on the device, which is used to allow for tissue plication. TEE can be used to assess the effect of varying degrees of tension upon mitral regurgitation. The location of the proximal anchor is determined using a combination of TEE and fluoroscopy. Coronary angiography, again, is used to ensure that the coronary arteries are not affected. Once all conditions are satisfied, then the proximal anchor can be deployed in a fashion similar to which the distal anchor was released.

The first in human study was conducted on five patients with a dilated cardiomyopathy (EF of 30-45%), NYHA Class II or III heart failure and least 2+ mitral regurgitation [21]. With a mean age of 52.2$\pm$8.8 years, four of the five patients had successful temporary device placement. In one patient, size of the CS precluded placement. As a result of temporary deployment, the septal-lateral mitral annular dimensions decreased from 35.5$\pm$4.7 to 32.2$\pm$4.6 mm (p=0.02). A corresponding reduction in mitral regurgitation color Doppler area was noted as well (98.3$\pm$43.6 to 83.3$\pm$35.1 mm^{2}', p=0.09). In two patients, the distal anchor was noted to have slipped secondary to undersizing. All deployed devices were successfully recovered and no complications were reported. Mitral annular reduction in this study was 9%, as reported by the authors, is well below the 20-30% needed to achieve substantial improvement in mitral regurgitation.

The CARILLON Mitral Annuloplasty Device European Union Study (AMADEUS) was a prospective safety and feasibility intention-to-treat study of the CARILLON device in patients with dilated (ischemic or nonischemic) cardiomyopathy with moderate to severe mitral regurgitation, NYHA class II to IV heart failure symptoms, LV ejection fraction <40%, LV end diastolic diameter > 55mm and a 6 minute walk distance between 150-450 m [22]. 48

patients were enrolled, but only 30 patients received the implanted device. Eighteen patients did not secondary to issues relating to access, coronary artery location and insufficient mitral regurgitation. Of the 30 patients who received the device, there was noted to be a significant reduction in a variety of measures of mitral regurgitation severity at 6 months ($P<0.001$). Functional improvement was also noted with a reduction in NYHA classification from 2.9 to 1.8 at 6 months ($P<0.001$). 6-minute walk test improved from a baseline of 307 ± 87 to 403 ± 137 meters ($P<0.001$). At 30 days, the major adverse event rate was 13% with one death occurring due to complications arising from contrast-induced nephropathy.

A separate analysis from the same study reported an acute reduction in mitral regurgitation from the CARILLON device in 30 patients from grade 3.0 ± 0.6 to 2.0 ± 0.8 ($p < 0.0001$) [23]. Using multisclice CT scans from the 30 patients, there was, interestingly, no difference in the distance between the CS and the mitral annulus in the 22 patients who received a permanent implant with reduction in mitral regurgitation versus the 8 who had the device removed after there was no improvement in mitral regurgitation. This suggests that the CS/mitral annulus relationship may not be as important of a factor in determining utility of this device, although larger patients will be needed to confirm this finding.

Septal-to-Lateral Annular Cinching – Percutaneous Septal Shortening System

An increase in the septal to lateral mitral annular distance has been observed in animal models of cardiomyopathy. This has led to the development of septal-to-lateral cinching (SLAC) procedures whereby a chord is placed across the annulus and/or ventricle with the goal of shortening the annular diameter through remodeling. There are devices, which place the chord across the ventricle (iCoapsys, Myocor, Maple Grove, MN) and across the atrium (Percutaneous Septal Shortening System, PS^3, Ample Medical, Inc, Foster City, CA). The PS^3 is of interest since it utilizes the coronary sinus to anchor one end of the chord in place.

For device placement, access is via the internal jugular vein with a 12F sheath. Coronary sinus is then accessed, wired and then a great cardiac vein Magnecath is placed into the CS. Separate access is obtained via the femoral vein and a standard transseptal puncture is performed. Once the interatrial septum is crossed, a left atrial Magnecath is positioned in the left atrium until it magnetizes with the great cardiac vein Magnecath. A loop wire is then used to wire and connect the CS catheter with the left atrial catheter, and then the catheters are removed leaving the glide wire connecting the coronary sinus to the left atrium. Using the glide wire, an attachment suture is deployed and from the coronary sinus and externalized in the femoral vein. Then an Amplatzer PFO occluder is placed over the suture and deployed across the septum. Once deployed, it is used as an anchor. The tension on the suture can be adjusted for the desired amount to septal-to-lateral shortening.

Preclinical investigation demonstrated efficacy of this device in animal models of tachycardia induced cardiomyopathy [24.] The first in human study examined the safety and feasibility in two patients prior to cardiac surgery [25]. Both devices were placed successfully. In the first patient there was a 29% reduction in mean septal-to-lateral distance of 29% and a concomitant reduction in mitral regurgitation from 2+ to 1+. In the second patient a 31% reduction was noted with a decreased in mitral regurgitation from 3+ to 1+. All devices were safely removed at the time of surgery. Studies examining larger cohorts of patients will be required to make any definitive conclusions. Furthermore, it remains to be seen whether short or long term anticoagulation would be required for device in the left atrium.

The SLAC procedure is a novel method for shortening mitral annular diameter. As previously mentioned, there are several devices, which use slightly modified techniques (transventricular vs transatrial approach) to achieve the desired effect, usually involving ventricular remodeling. The long term effects of SLAC on ventricular remodeling, however, are unknown, although extreme SLAC could adversely effect left ventricular strain patterns leading to negative remodeling [26].

Discussion

The task of trying to correct functional mitral regurgitation remains a challenging one at best. The first and most fundamental question is whether or not a reduction in mitral regurgitation matters in functional mitral regurgitation. As previously mentioned, data from the surgical literature demonstrates no benefit – either symptomatic or survival [4]. Preoperative echo has demonstrated that higher mitral annular diameter and higher severity of mitral regurgitation, among others, were independent predictors of failure of surgical repair of functional mitral regurgitation [27], begging the question as to whether severity of disease and timing of repair also influences outcome. While the advent of novel percutaneous technologies has taken hold and is rapidly changing the way we consider addressing the issue, one must first ask if we are treating a symptom of a larger problem and secondly, how to go about selecting patients that will truly benefit from this procedure.

There are many obstacles that need to be overcome before these devices become a viable therapeutic option. First is to try and understand what the long-term effects of these devices will be on the natural history of the disease. Functional mitral regurgitation occurs as a result of another problem, dilated cardiomyopathy (ischemic or non ischemic). Although reducing the degree of mitral regurgitation may result in symptomatic improvement, it is unclear as to what effect it may have on the natural course of the primary disorder. Therefore, more information needs to be gathered regarding the ventricular remodeling process with these devices so as to better understand the effects upon the primary disorder. Furthermore, it remains to be seen how the anatomical relationships between the CS, the left atrial wall and the mitral annulus will influence long term efficacy and durability of these indirect annuloplasty devices.

There are many other issues to be resolved with regards to the CS mitral annuloplasty devices regarding the need for anticoagulation. In many patients with dilated cardiomyopathy and CHF, the presence of CS pacing leads may preclude placement of a device, as well (although the Viacor PTMA system has successfully been placed in patient with biventricular pacemaker). Also, these devices, unlike surgical corrective methods, are limited in that they are intended to address only one aspect of mitral regurgitation. In the future, further improvements may be obtained through the combination of both annulplasty and direct mitral valve repair techniques. Further investigation will be needed to support this hypothesis.

In the interim, many novel devices will be introduced into the mix that will likely add to or modify concepts already described. The recently published preclinical data regarding the

MRI guided "cerclage annuloplasty" is one just one example of emerging technology [28]. In closing, novel percutaneous devices hold promise in helping address the issue of functional mitral regurgitation. Larger clinical trials are underway and will likely help to clarify safety and efficacy of these devices for percutaneous mitral valve repair.

References

[1] Gillinov AM, Cosgrove DM, Blackstone EH, Diaz R, Arnold JH, Lytle BW, Smedira NG, Sabik JF, McCarthy PM, Loop FD. Durability of mitral valve repair for degenerative disease. *J. Thorac. Cardiovasc. Surg.* 1998;116:734-743.

[2] Johnston DR, Gillinov AM, Blackstone EH, Griffin B, Stewart W, Sabik JF, 3rd, Mihaljevic T, Svensson LG, Houghtaling PL, Lytle BW. Surgical repair of posterior mitral valve prolapse: implications for guidelines and percutaneous repair. *Ann. Thorac. Surg*;89:1385-1394.

[3] Enriquez-Sarano M, Schaff HV, Orszulak TA, Tajik AJ, Bailey KR, Frye RL. Valve repair improves the outcome of surgery for mitral regurgitation. A multivariate analysis. *Circulation.* 1995;91:1022-1028.

[4] Mihaljevic T, Lam BK, Rajeswaran J, Takagaki M, Lauer MS, Gillinov AM, Blackstone EH, Lytle BW. Impact of mitral valve annuloplasty combined with revascularization in patients with functional ischemic mitral regurgitation. *J. Am. Coll. Cardiol.* 2007;49:2191-2201.

[5] Maisano F, Torracca L, Oppizzi M, Stefano PL, D'Addario G, La Canna G, Zogno M, Alfieri O. The edge-to-edge technique: a simplified method to correct mitral insufficiency. *Eur. J. Cardiothorac. Surg.* 1998;13:240-245; discussion 245-246.

[6] Levine RA, Handschumacher MD, Sanfilippo AJ, Hagege AA, Harrigan P, Marshall JE, Weyman AE. Three-dimensional echocardiographic reconstruction of the mitral valve, with implications for the diagnosis of mitral valve prolapse. *Circulation.* 1989;80:589-598.

[7] Salgo IS, Gorman JH, 3rd, Gorman RC, Jackson BM, Bowen FW, Plappert T, St John Sutton MG, Edmunds LH, Jr. Effect of annular shape on leaflet curvature in reducing mitral leaflet stress. *Circulation.* 2002;106:711-717.

[8] Gorman JH, 3rd, Jackson BM, Enomoto Y, Gorman RC. The effect of regional ischemia on mitral valve annular saddle shape. *Ann. Thorac. Surg.* 2004;77:544-548.

[9] Maselli D, Guarracino F, Chiaramonti F, Mangia F, Borelli G, Minzioni G. Percutaneous mitral annuloplasty: an anatomic study of human coronary sinus and its relation with mitral valve annulus and coronary arteries. *Circulation.* 2006;114:377-380.

[10] Choure AJ, Garcia MJ, Hesse B, Sevensma M, Maly G, Greenberg NL, Borzi L, Ellis S, Tuzcu EM, Kapadia SR. In vivo analysis of the anatomical relationship of coronary sinus to mitral annulus and left circumflex coronary artery using cardiac multidetector computed tomography: implications for percutaneous coronary sinus mitral annuloplasty. *J. Am. Coll. Cardiol.* 2006;48:1938-1945.

[11] Tops LF, Van de Veire NR, Schuijf JD, de Roos A, van der Wall EE, Schalij MJ, Bax JJ. Noninvasive evaluation of coronary sinus anatomy and its relation to the mitral

valve annulus: implications for percutaneous mitral annuloplasty. *Circulation.* 2007;115:1426-1432.

[12] Maniu CV, Patel JB, Reuter DG, Meyer DM, Edwards WD, Rihal CS, Redfield MM. Acute and chronic reduction of functional mitral regurgitation in experimental heart failure by percutaneous mitral annuloplasty. *J. Am. Coll. Cardiol.* 2004;44: 1652-1661.

[13] Masson JB, Webb JG. Percutaneous mitral annuloplasty. *Coron Artery Dis.* 2009; 20:183-188.

[14] Liddicoat JR, Mac Neill BD, Gillinov AM, Cohn WE, Chin CH, Prado AD, Pandian NG, Oesterle SN. Percutaneous mitral valve repair: a feasibility study in an ovine model of acute ischemic mitral regurgitation. *Catheter Cardiovasc. Interv.* 2003;60:410-416.

[15] Daimon M, Gillinov AM, Liddicoat JR, Saracino G, Fukuda S, Koyama Y, Hayase M, Cohn WE, Ellis SG, Thomas JD, Shiota T. Dynamic change in mitral annular area and motion during percutaneous mitral annuloplasty for ischemic mitral regurgitation: preliminary animal study with real-time 3-dimensional echocardiography. *J. Am. Soc. Echocardiogr.* 2007;20:381-388.

[16] Daimon M, Shiota T, Gillinov AM, Hayase M, Ruel M, Cohn WE, Blacker SJ, Liddicoat JR. Percutaneous mitral valve repair for chronic ischemic mitral regurgitation: a real-time three-dimensional echocardiographic study in an ovine model. *Circulation.* 2005;111:2183-2189.

[17] Dubreuil O, Basmadjian A, Ducharme A, Thibault B, Crepeau J, Lam JY, Bilodeau L. Percutaneous mitral valve annuloplasty for ischemic mitral regurgitation: first in man experience with a temporary implant. *Catheter Cardiovasc Interv.* 2007;69: 1053-1061.

[18] Sack S, Kahlert P, Bilodeau L, Pierard LA, Lancellotti P, Legrand V, Bartunek J, Vanderheyden M, Hoffmann R, Schauerte P, Shiota T, Marks DS, Erbel R, Ellis SG. Percutaneous transvenous mitral annuloplasty: initial human experience with a novel coronary sinus implant device. *Circ. Cardiovasc. Interv.* 2009;2:277-284.

[19] Webb JG, Harnek J, Munt BI, Kimblad PO, Chandavimol M, Thompson CR, Mayo JR, Solem JO. Percutaneous transvenous mitral annuloplasty: initial human experience with device implantation in the coronary sinus. *Circulation.* 2006; 113:851-855.

[20] http://www.pcronline.com/Lectures/2010/Percutaneous-treatment-of-functional-mitral-repair-3-year-results-from-the-Evolution-I-study

[21] Duffy SJ, Federman J, Farrington C, Reuter DG, Richardson M, Kaye DM. Feasibility and short-term efficacy of percutaneous mitral annular reduction for the therapy of functional mitral regurgitation in patients with heart failure. *Catheter Cardiovasc. Interv.* 2006;68:205-210.

[22] Schofer J, Siminiak T, Haude M, Herrman JP, Vainer J, Wu JC, Levy WC, Mauri L, Feldman T, Kwong RY, Kaye DM, Duffy SJ, Tubler T, Degen H, Brandt MC, Van Bibber R, Goldberg S, Reuter DG, Hoppe UC. Percutaneous mitral annuloplasty for functional mitral regurgitation: results of the CARILLON Mitral Annuloplasty Device European Union Study. *Circulation.* 2009;120:326-333.

[23] Siminiak T, Hoppe UC, Schofer J, Haude M, Herrman JP, Vainer J, Firek L, Reuter DG, Goldberg SL, Van Bibber R. Effectiveness and safety of percutaneous coronary sinus-based mitral valve repair in patients with dilated cardiomyopathy (from the AMADEUS trial). *Am. J. Cardiol.* 2009;104:565-570.

[24] Rogers JH, Macoviak JA, Rahdert DA, Takeda PA, Palacios IF, Low RI. Percutaneous septal sinus shortening: a novel procedure for the treatment of functional mitral regurgitation. *Circulation.* 2006;113:2329-2334.

[25] Palacios IF, Condado JA, Brandi S, Rodriguez V, Bosch F, Silva G, Low RI, Rogers JH. Safety and feasibility of acute percutaneous septal sinus shortening: first-in-human experience. *Catheter Cardiovasc. Interv.* 2007;69:513-518.

[26] Nguyen TC, Cheng A, Tibayan FA, Liang D, Daughters GT, Ingels NB, Jr., Miller DC. Septal-lateral annnular cinching perturbs basal left ventricular transmural strains. *Eur. J. Cardiothorac. Surg.* 2007;31:423-429.

[27] Kongsaerepong V, Shiota M, Gillinov AM, Song JM, Fukuda S, McCarthy PM, Williams T, Savage R, Daimon M, Thomas JD, Shiota T. Echocardiographic predictors of successful versus unsuccessful mitral valve repair in ischemic mitral regurgitation. *Am. J. Cardiol.* 2006;98:504-508.

[28] Kim JH, Kocaturk O, Ozturk C, Faranesh AZ, Sonmez M, Sampath S, Saikus CE, Kim AH, Raman VK, Derbyshire JA, Schenke WH, Wright VJ, Berry C, McVeigh ER, Lederman RJ. Mitral cerclage annuloplasty, a novel transcatheter treatment for secondary mitral valve regurgitation: initial results in swine. *J. Am. Coll. Cardiol.* 2009;54:638-651.

[29] http://www.pcronline.com/Lectures/2010/Percutaneous-treatment-of-functional-mitral-repair-3-year-results-from-the-Evolution-I-study.

In: Percutaneous Valve Technology: Present and Future
Editors: Jose Luis Navia and Sharif Al-Ruzzeh
ISBN: 978-1-61942-577-4

Chapter XXIV

Rheumatic Mitral Valve Disease: Percutaneous Balloon Mitral Valvuloplasty, Present and Future Perspectives

Bernard Iung and Alec Vahanian

Abstract

Since it description in 1984, percutaneous mitral commissurotomy (PMC) has been widely used and its indications have been progressively widened. The Inoue technique is now the most widely used, in particular because of its ease of use and its safety, as attested by the low rates of mortality and complications seen in series from experienced centers. The most frequent complication is severe traumatic mitral regurgitation. Immediately after PMC, there is a mean doubling of mitral valve area. Good late functional results are observed in 33 to 72% of patients at 10-12 years, the wide range of rates depending on differences in patient characteristics between series. The most frequent cause of late deterioration is mitral restenosis. Analyses performed in large series have shown that the prediction of immediate and late results of PMC is multifactorial. Besides the severity of the impairment of valve anatomy, age, symptoms, atrial fibrillation and prior commissurotomy have a strong impact on patient outcome.

According to guidelines, percutaneous mitral commissurotomy is now the reference treatment for mitral stenosis with pliable valves in young patients and its efficacy has been validated in randomised trials versus surgery. Mitral stenosis in older patients with more severe impairment of valve anatomy is the most frequent presentation of mitral stenosis in industrialized countries. In this heterogeneous group, PMC should be considered in patients who have otherwise favourable characteristics. PMC can also be considered in selected asymptomatic patients, in particular in order to reduce the thromboembolic risk.

After more than 20 years, PMC is now a mature technique and has virtually replaced surgical commissurotomy in industrialised countries. PMC and valve replacement should be considered as complementary techniques applicable in the different stages and presentations of mitral stenosis.

1. Introduction

In 1984, percutaneous balloon mitral valvuloplasty, or percutaneous mitral commissurotomy (PMC) was the first percutaneous technique described as an alternative to surgery to treat valvular heart disease.[1] At the same time, important changes have occurred in the epidemiology of rheumatic heart disease, which remains the most frequent etiology of mitral stenosis. Although rheumatic heart disease is still prevalent in developing countries, a dramatic decrease in the incidence of acute rheumatic fever has led to a decrease in the prevalence of mitral stenosis in industrialised countries.[2-3] Epidemiologic changes in rheumatic heart disease have also had an impact on patient characteristics in industrialised countries, patients are now older and present with more severe valve deformity.[4]

More than 20 years of experience in a wide range of patient subsets now enables the results of PMC to be assessed accurately and predictive factors of immediate and late results to be identified with an adequate statistical power. Growing experience and improved knowledge of determinants of the results of PMC have led to progressive widening of indications and a better definition of candidates for the technique.

2. Technique

2.1. Principle

The technique of percutaneous balloon mitral commissurotomy is directly derived from surgical closed-heart commissurotomy which was proposed as early as in the 1920's by Cutler and Souttar,[5-6] but became the routine treatment only after 1950.[7] Basically, balloon commissurotomy and surgical commissurotomy act in the same way through commissural opening. Thus, experience acquired with surgical commissurotomy was helpful in defining indications for and assessing the results of PMC.

2.2. Approaches

The transvenous antegrade approach is the most widely used. After transvenous femoral puncture, transseptal catheterisation is the first and critical step in the procedure and should be performed by experienced operators since it carries a risk of cardiac perforation leading to tamponade. Transseptal catheterisation should be performed under fluoroscopy guidance using several views and under continuous pressure monitoring. In difficult cases, in particular in case of severe thoracic deformity, transesophageal echocardiographic guidance can be performed for guiding the site of the puncture in the interatrial septum.[8-9] However, intra-procedural transesophageal echocardiography requires general anesthesia. More recently, intra-cardiac echocardiography has been proposed to guide transseptal puncture.[10] Its main advantage is the absence of general anesthesia but its use is limited due to the high cost of the non-reusable probe.

The transarterial retrograde approach has also been proposed.[11] It initially comprised a transseptal catheterisation to position a guide wire to lead the retrograde progression of the balloon across the mitral valve. A pure retrograde technique without transseptal catheterisation has since been described but its use remains limited.[12]

2.3. Devices

2.3.1. Double-Balloon Technique

After the use of a singe-balloon in a few initial cases, the double-balloon technique became the first widely used technique of PMC.[13] It requires the positioning of guide wires in the apex of the ventricle, which are then used to position the balloon across the mitral valve. The most widely used combination is a cylindric and a bifoil balloon (Figure 1). The use of the double-balloon technique requires the dilatation of the interatrial septum using a peripheral angioplasty balloon.

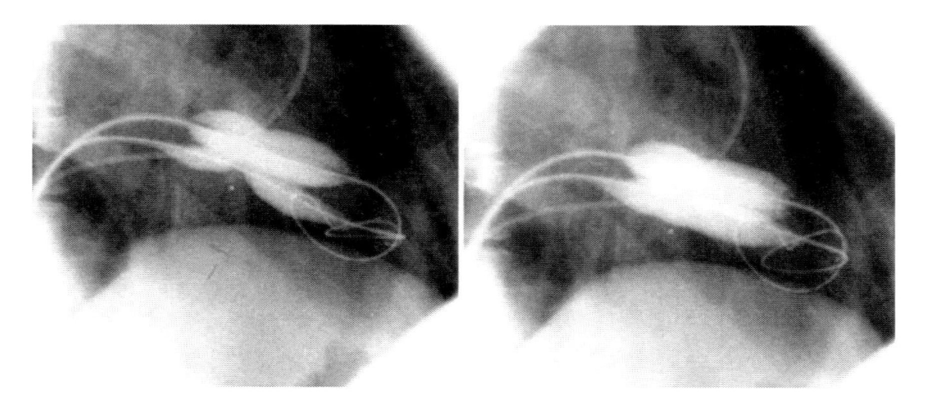

Figure 1. Fluoroscopic images recorded during a percutaneous mitral commissurotomy using the double-balloon technique.

The Multi-Track system also uses two balloons to dilate the mitral valve but requires the positioning of only one guide wire.[14].

2.3.2. Inoue Balloon

Although being the first technique of PMC to be described, the Inoue balloon became commercially available only at the beginning of the 1990's. The Inoue balloon is a single low-profile balloon which comprises three pressure-dependent parts with a specific elasticity.[1, 15] Thus, inflation begins with the distal part of the balloon, thereby allowing self positioning across the mitral valve without the need for a guide wire in the left ventricle. Sequential inflation then enables the balloon to be pulled back and stabilized in the mitral valve, and, finally, valvular dilatation to be performed (Figure 2). The initial size of the balloon, between 24 and 30 mm, is chosen according to patient height. The first inflation is performed 4 mm below the maximal balloon size and the balloon is then deflated and withdrawn into the left atrium after each inflation. The balloon size can then be increased by steps of 1 to 2 mm according to the results of the previous inflation concerning valve opening and the quantification of mitral regurgitation using intra-procedural transthoracic echocardiographic monitoring.

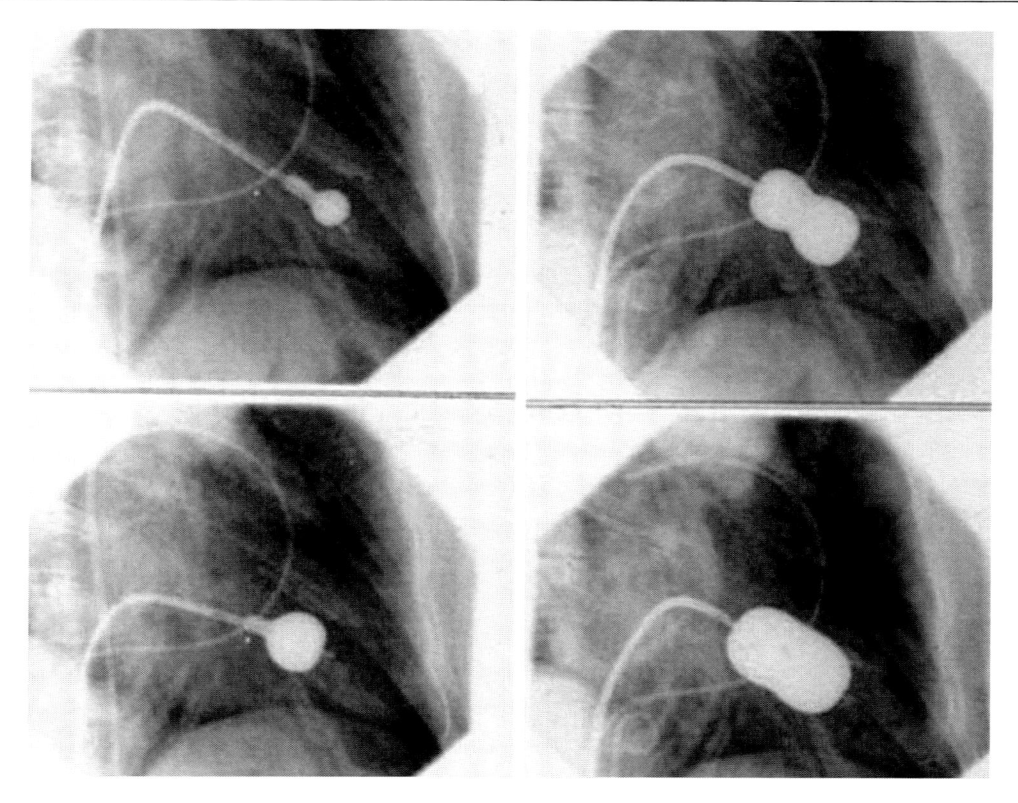

Figure 2. Fluoroscopic images recorded during a percutaneous balloon commissurotomy using an Inoue balloon. In the left panel, the distal balloon has been inflated to secure the position at the valvular level. In the middle panel, the proximal segment also has been inflated, and in the right panel, the dilating segment is briefly inflated.

The Inoue technique is now by far the most used worldwide because of its ease of use. Comparative studies suggest that the risk of complication is lower with the Inoue balloon as compared to the double-balloon technique but the immediate results do not differ significantly.[16-17] The main drawback of the Inoue balloon is its cost.

2.3.3. Metallic Commissurotome

The metallic commissurotome was developed by Dr Cribier and achieves commissural opening through the opening of two blades in a similar way to the device used for closed-heart commissurotomy.[18] The main advantage of the metallic commissurotome is that it can be sterilized and re-used. Although published experience is limited, immediate results are close to those obtained after balloon commissurotomy. The procedure is more complex than balloon commissurotomy and seems to be associated with a higher risk of tamponade.

2.4. Monitoring of the Procedure

The ability to evaluate the results of PMC in real-time is of particular importance when using the Inoue balloon, given the possibility to perform stepwise inflations. Hemodynamic evaluation of mitral valve area is not advised since it has been shown to lack accuracy in this context, in particular because of acute changes in atrio-ventricular compliance and the presence of interatrial shunt.[19-20] In addition, this requires right-heart catheterisation, which tends now to be avoided to simplify the procedure. Hemodynamic measurements of left atrial pressure and mitral valve gradient are easier to perform but their interpretation is confounded by acute changes in heart rate and cardiac output during the procedure.

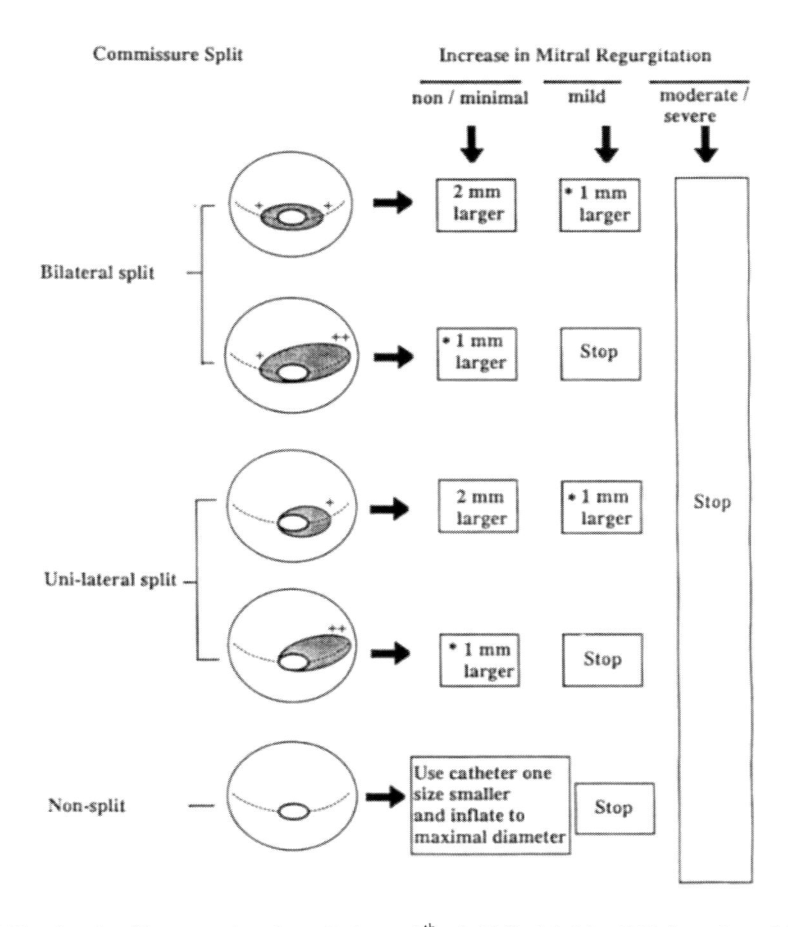

From Topol E. Textbook of interventional cardiology, 5th ed. Philadelphia, WB Saunders, 2008.

Figure 3. Decision-making during the stepwise dilation technique using the Inoue balloon, according to echocardiographic findings after each balloon inflation. +: incomplete split, ++: complete split, *: stop in cases of severely diseased valve or age > 65 years.

Thus, intra-procedural monitoring using transthoracic echocardiography is more appropriate. Half-time pressure should not be used to estimate mitral valve area since it lacks accuracy immediately after PMC for the same reasons that impair hemodynamic measurements.[21] Planimetry of the mitral orifice is reliable during the procedure and the parasternal short-axis view also enables commissural opening to be assessed, even more accurately if using a real-time three-dimensional echocardiography. Changes in the degree of mitral regurgitation can also be assessed reliably using color Doppler echocardiography. Intra-procedural echocardiography may also be helpful to promptly diagnose pericardial effusion, which is a rare but severe complication of transseptal catheterisation.

Transesophageal echocardiography is generally not considered for intra-procedural assessment of mitral valve function. The stepwise procedure is stopped when an adequate valve opening and/or complete opening of at least one commissure is obtained, without more than moderate regurgitation (Figure 3). Criteria for continuing inflations or stopping the procedure should be adapted to each individual case. Although it requires the presence of an experienced echocardiographer during the procedure, transthoracic echocardiography is the most appropriate method for intra-procedural monitoring of PMC. It also has the advantage of simplifying the invasive procedure by avoiding hemodynamic measurements.

3. Safety

A number of large single- or multi-center series enables the safety of PMC to be assessed (Table 1).[12, 22-31] As in any interventional technique, the safety of the procedure is highly dependent on the experience of the team.[22, 32] The low rate of complications in high-volume centers is obviously related to the experience of interventional cardiologists, but also to the expertise in the whole selection process. Current evidence shows that PMC is a low-risk procedure when performed on an elective basis in experienced centers.

3.1. Failure

The most frequent causes of failure of the procedure are the failure of transseptal catheterization and the inability to position or stabilize the balloon across the mitral valve. Patient-related conditions that increase the risk of failure are severe thoracic deformity, ectasy of left atrium, and severe stenosis at the level of subvalvular apparatus. Failure rate varies from 1% to 17% and is highly dependent on the experience of the interventionist. It is below 1% in experienced centers.[12, 22-24, 29-30]

3.2. Tamponade

Hemopericardium may be the consequence of atrial perforation complicating transseptal catheterisation or ventricular perforation, in particular when the technique requires the presence of guide wires in the left ventricle, as is the case with the double-balloon technique or the metallic commissurotome. Prompt echocardiographic diagnosis and management are mandatory, consisting in pericardiocentesis or surgical drainage according to the severity of the effusion and its clinical tolerance.

Table 1. Severe complications of percutaneous mitral commissurotomy

	n=	Age (years)	In-hospital death (%)	Tamponade (%)	Embolic events (%)	Severe mitral regurgitation (%)
NHLBI Registry*[22] (1987-1989)	738	54				
n < 25			2	6	4	4
25 ≤ n < 100			1	4	2	3
n ≥ 100			0.3	2	1	3
Chen et al.* [23] (1985-1994)	4832	37	0.1	0.8	0.5	1.4
Meneveau et al. [24] (1986-1996)	532	54	0.2	1.1	-	3.9
Stefanadis et al.* [12] (1988-1996)	441	44	0.2	0	0	3.4
Hernandez et al. [25] (1989-1995)	620	53	0.5	0.6	-	4.0
Ben Farhat et al. [26] (1987-1998)	654	33	0.5	0.6	1.5	4.6
Arora et al. [28] (1987-2000)	4850	27	0.2	0.2	0.1	1.4
Neumayer et al. [27] (1989-2000)	1123	57	0.4	0.9	0.9	6.0
Iung et al. [29] (1986-2001)	2773	47	0.4	0.2	0.4	4.1
Fawzy et al. [30] (1989-2004)	551	31	0	0.7	0.5	1.6
Jneid et al. [31] (1986-2000)	876	55	0.6	0.8	1.7	9.1

*: multi-center series.

3.3. Systemic Embolism

Gas embolism may occur immediately after balloon rupture and is frequently transient. The risk of fibrinocruoric embolism is decreased, but not abolished, by the systematic performance of transesophageal echocardiography before the procedure to search for the left atrial thrombus. In case of cerebral embolism, early management by a stroke center, including cerebral reperfusion is indicated to reduce the severity of sequelae.

3.4. Severe Mitral Regurgitation

Severe mitral regurgitation remains the most frequent complication of PMC. Severe regurgitation is most often the consequence of non-commissural leaflet tear, which is frequently associated with an absence of commissural opening.[33-38]

Chordal rupture may be associated or, less frequently, partial or complete papillary muscle rupture. When regurgitation is severe, functional tolerance is generally poor, as in any acute regurgitation. Severe and poorly tolerated mitral regurgitation requires early surgery. Prosthetic valve replacement is often performed, but complex valve repair may be feasible, in particular in young patients when the underlying valve deformity is not too severe.[38]

Although severe mitral regurgitation occurs more frequently in patients with unfavorable valve anatomy, it remains unpredictable in any given patient, which justifies systematic prior information regarding this risk.

Besides the severity of mitral regurgitation, accurate echocardiographic assessment of the underlying mechanism is important for patient management. Echocardiographic diagnosis of leaflet tear is an incentive for early surgery even in patients with moderate-to-severe mitral regurgitation.

Of the other hand, watchful waiting can be considered in patients with mitral regurgitation of borderline severity, which is related to excessive commissural splitting without traumatic lesion.

3.5 Atrial Septal Defect

Atrial septal defect is a consequence of transseptal catheterisation and its frequency varies widely between 10 and 90% depending on the technique used for its detection, being highest when using transesophageal echocardiography.[39] Most atrial shunts are well tolerated and do not require correction.

3.6 Vascular Complications

Transfemoral venous access is seldom the cause of vascular complications, which is an incentive for the use of pure venous access in experienced centers.[40].

3.7. Heart Block

Transient heart block occurs in 1 to 2% of the cases. Persistent conduction abnormalities requiring implantation of a permanent pacemaker are exceptional.

3.8. Emergency Surgery

Surgical intervention within the 24 hours following PMC is needed in less than 1% of cases. It is mainly the consequence of severe and poorly tolerated mitral regurgitation or, less frequently, cardiac tamponade.

3.9. Peri-procedural Death

The incidence of peri-procedural death varies from 0 to 2% (Table 1). It can be the consequence of procedural complications, in particular cardiac tamponade. Death rate is higher in patients who undergo PMC as a salvage procedure in very poor hemodynamic condition.

4. Immediate Results

4.1. Improvement of Valve Function

The effect of PMC on valve function is an increase of approximately 100% in valve area (Table 2).[12, 14, 17, 23-31] The immediate efficacy is generally assessed using a composite endpoint combining a final valve area > 1.5 cm² without severe mitral regurgitation, *i.e.* > grade 2/4, and it is observed in more than 80% of the patients in most series.

Parasternal short-axis view also enables the degree of commissural opening to be assessed, which is related to mitral valve function after PMC (Figures 4 and 5) [41].

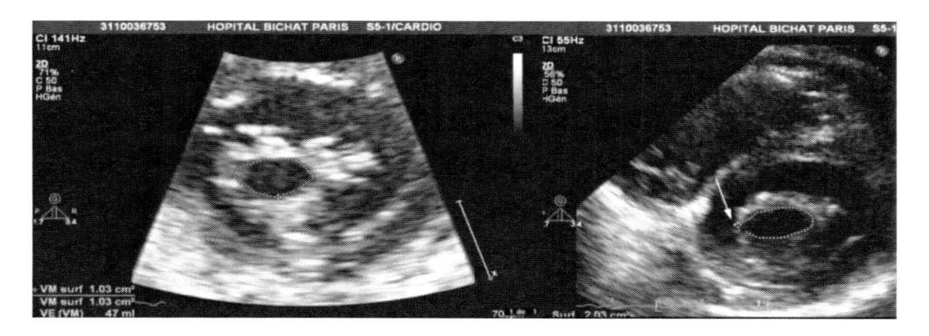

Figure 4. Unicommissural opening after percutaneous mitral commissurotomy (PMC). Parasternal short-axis view. Left panel: before PMC. Mid panel: after PMC, 2D echo. Right panel: after PMC, 3D echo. The arrow on the mid and right panel shows opening of the internal commissure. See corresponding Video 1.

Table 2. Immediate results of percutaneous mitral commissurotomy (PMC): increase in mitral valve area

	n=	Age (years)	Mitral valve area (cm^2)		Technique
			Before PMC	After PMC	
Chen et al. [23]	4832	37	1.1	2.1	Inoue balloon
Meneveau et al. [24]	532	54	1.0	1.7	Double- or Inoue balloon
Stefanadis et al. [12]	441	44	1.0	2.1	Modified single-, double-, or Inoue balloon (retrograde)
Bonhoeffer et al. [14]	100	31	0.8	2.0	Multi-track balloon
Hernandez et al. [25]	561	53	1.0	1.8	Inoue balloon
Kang et al. [17]	152	42	0.9	1.8	Inoue balloon
(randomized comparison)	150	40	0.9	1.9	Double-balloon
Ben Farhat et al. [26]	654	33	1.0	2.1	Inoue or double-balloon
Arora et al. [28]	4850	27	0.7	1.9	Inoue or double-balloon or metallic commissurotome
Neumayer et al. [27]	1123	57	1.1	1.8	Inoue balloon
Iung et al. [29]	2773	47	1.0	1.9	Inoue, single-, or double-balloon
Fawzy et al. [30]	520	31	0.9	2.0	Inoue balloon
Jneid et al. [31]	876	55	0.9	1.9	Inoue or double-balloon

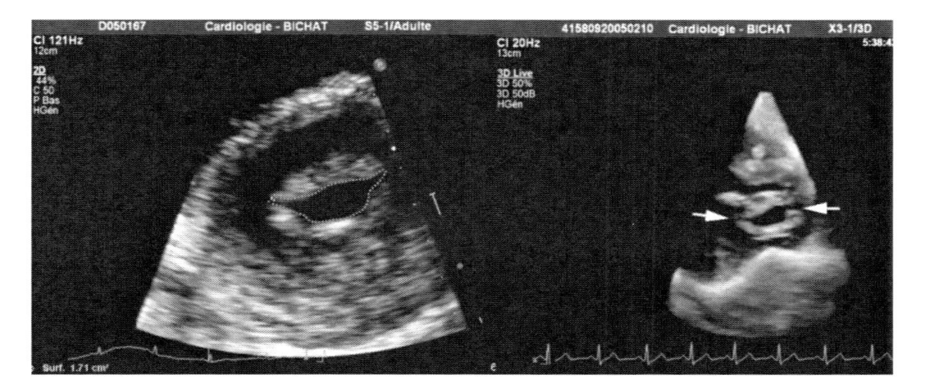

Figure 5. Bicommissural opening after percutaneous mitral commissurotomy (PMC). Parasternal short-axis view. Left panel: after PMC, 2D echo. Right panel: after PMC, 3D echo. The arrows show opening of both commissures.

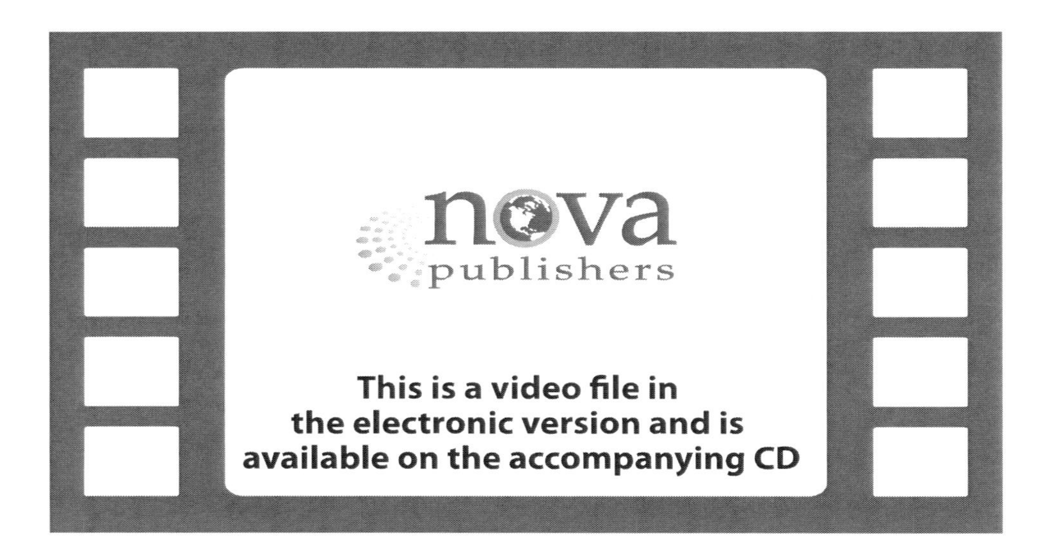

Video 1. Unicommissural opening after percutaneous mitral commissurotomy (PMC). Real time 3D transthoracic echocardiogarphy. Parasternal short-axis view.Consequences of the improvement in valve function are a decrease in left atrial and pulmonary artery pressures and a moderate increase in cardiac index. In patients with severe pulmonary hypertension and increased pulmonary vascular resistance before the procedure, the decrease in pulmonary pressure and pulmonary vascular resistance is progressive over time and may continue for several months [42].

Consequences of the improvement in valve function are a decrease in left atrial and pulmonary artery pressures and a moderate increase in cardiac index. In patients with severe pulmonary hypertension and increased pulmonary vascular resistance before the procedure, the decrease in pulmonary pressure and pulmonary vascular resistance is progressive over time and may continue for several months.[42]

Improvement in valve function and hemodynamics translate into an early improvement of exercise capacity.[43].

4.2. Predictive Factors of Immediate Results

At the beginning of the experience of PMC, it was presumed that a detailed echocardiographic analysis of mitral valve anatomy would be a reliable approach to predict the results of the procedure. However, experience from different series consistently showed that the prediction of immediate results is multifactorial. Besides valve anatomy, as assessed by the different scoring systems, other baseline patient characteristics have a strong and independent contribution to the prediction of immediate results: age, previous commissurotomy, symptoms as assessed by the NYHA functional class, presence of atrial fibrillation, valve area, associated mitral regurgitation, pulmonary hypertension, and tricuspid regurgitation.[33, 44-48] The technique used may have an impact on immediate results, but to a lesser extent than patient characteristics.[17, 24, 33] The evaluation of the predictive ability of multivariate models showed that they had a good sensitivity but a low specificity. The practical consequences of this are that models combining patient characteristics could not be used to reliably predict poor immediate results.[33, 47] The possibility of good immediate results in patients presenting with a relatively low probability of good immediate results is consistent with experimental findings and clinical experience (Figure 6).[49].

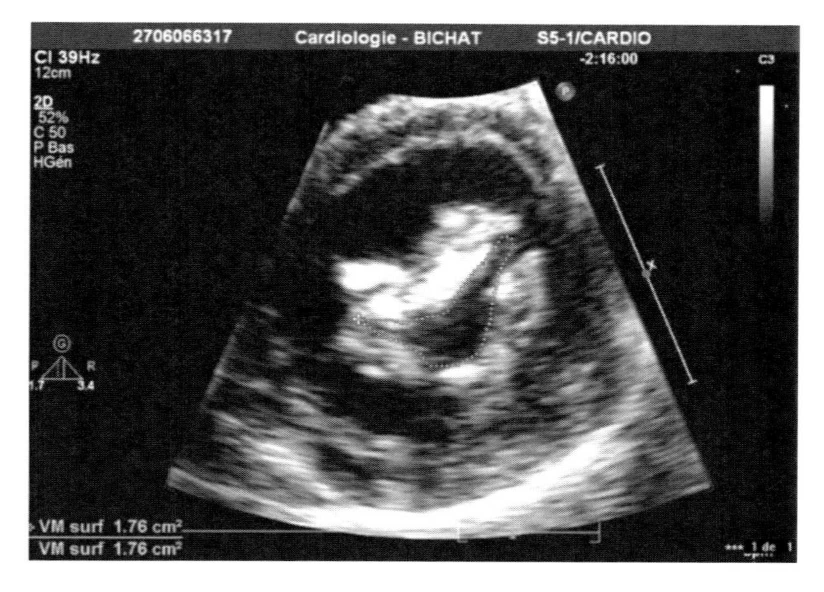

Figure 6. Complete opening of external commissure and partial opening of internal commissure after percutaneous mitral commissurotomy of a calcified valve. Parasternal short-axis view.

5. Long-Term Results

5.1. Clinical Outcome

Late results of PMC are summarized in Table 3.[12, 24-26, 30, 48, 50-54] Long-term results are available, although a few series report more than 15-year follow-up. Discrepancies between event rates are related to differences in patient characteristics. Event-free survival rates are higher in series from developing countries, where patients are younger and present with less severe valve deformity than in industrialised countries.

Table 3. Late results after balloon mitral commissurotomy

	n=	Age (years)	Maximum follow-up (years)	Event-free survival (%)
Cohen et al. [50]	146	59	5	51*
Dean et al. (NHLBI registry) [51]	736	54	4	60*
Orrange et al. [52]	132	44	7	65*
Meneveau et al. [24]	532	54	7.5	52**
Stefanadis et al. [12]	441	44	9	75**
Hernandez et al. [25]	561	53	7	69**
Iung et al. [53]	1024	49	10	56**
Ben Farhat et al. [26]	654	34	10	72**
Palacios et al. [48]	879	55	12	33**
Fawzy et al. [30]***	520	31	17	31**
Song et al. [54]	402	44	9	90*

*: survival without intervention
**: survival without intervention and in New York Heart Association class I or II
***: patients with good immediate results

Survival rates are high. However, natural history of mitral stenosis is characterized by a relatively low mortality, apart from patients in NYHA class IV.[55-58] Thus, late results of PMC are generally assessed by composite endpoints combining survival, absence of valvular reintervention, and, in certain series, functional status. Event-free survival rates range between 35 and 70% after 10 to 15 years.

5.2. Causes of Late Deterioration

The reasons for clinical deterioration should be analysed according to the quality of immediate results of PMC. After poor immediate results, the absence of significant improvement in valve function or the occurrence of severe mitral regurgitation require early mitral surgery in most cases (Figure 7).

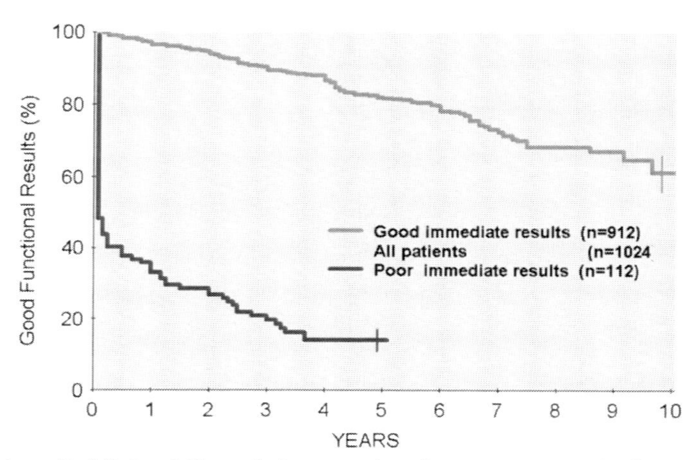

From Iung B, Garbarz E, Michaud P, et al. Late results of percutaneous mitral commissurotomy in a series of 1024 patients. Analysis of late clinical deterioration: frequency, anatomical findings, and predictive factors. Circulation 1999;99:3272-3278 [53].

Figure 7. Good functional results (survival considering cardiovascular-related deaths with no need for mitral surgery or repeat dilatation and in NYHA functional class I or II) after balloon mitral commissurotomy in 1024 patients.

On the other hand, after an initially successful PMC, progressive mitral restenosis is the most frequent cause of late functional deterioration (Figure 8).[25, 54, 59-60] Restenosis rates are more difficult to assess than clinical outcome since they require standardized echocardiographic follow-up, which is difficult to organize, particularly in large series with a long follow-up. Another limitation in the assessment of restenosis rates is the lack of a uniform definition of restenosis. Finally, as for clinical endpoints, restenosis rates are dependent on patient characteristics. After an initially successful PMC, late worsening of mitral regurgitation is rare and often combined with restenosis, so that mitral regurgitation is only rarely the main reason for re-intervention.[53]

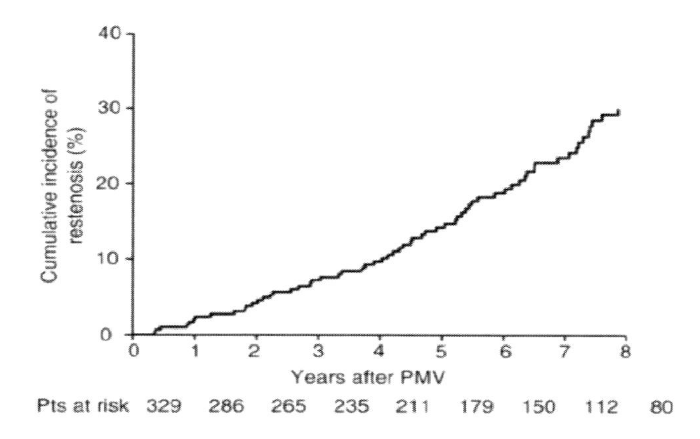

From Song JK, Song JM, Kang DH, et al. Restenosis and adverse clinical events after successful percutaneous mitral valvuloplasty: immediate post-procedural mitral valve area as an important prognosticator. Eur Heart J 2009;30:1254-1262 [54].

Figure 8. Cumulative incidence of restenosis after successful percutaneous mitral valvuloplasty.

Repeat valvular intervention may also be needed because of the progression of rheumatic heart disease on the aortic valve, either isolated or associated with mitral restenosis.

5.3. Predictive Factors of Long-Term Results

The identification of predictive factors of long-term results in patients who had good immediate results from PMC has the advantage of analysing a homogeneous mechanism of late deterioration, *i.e.* restenosis. As for immediate results, the prediction of late results of PMC is multifactorial. Besides the impairment of valve anatomy, other baseline patient characteristics are associated with late deterioration in multivariate analyses; the most consistently identified being older age, severe symptoms, and atrial fibrillation (Figure 9).[24, 26, 48, 53, 61-62] Certain series also identified male gender, previous commissurotomy, or pulmonary hypertension as predictors of poor late results. The technique used does not seem to have a significant influence on long-term results [17, 53].

The quality of immediate results of PMC also has a strong impact on late outcome.[24-26, 48, 52-54] Not surprisingly, clinical deterioration occurs more rapidly in patients who had a smaller post-procedural mitral valve area. Besides valve area, a high post-procedural mitral gradient is also an independent predictive factor of poor late functional results. The presence of moderate mitral regurgitation after PMC is a significant but weak predictive factor of poor late functional results.

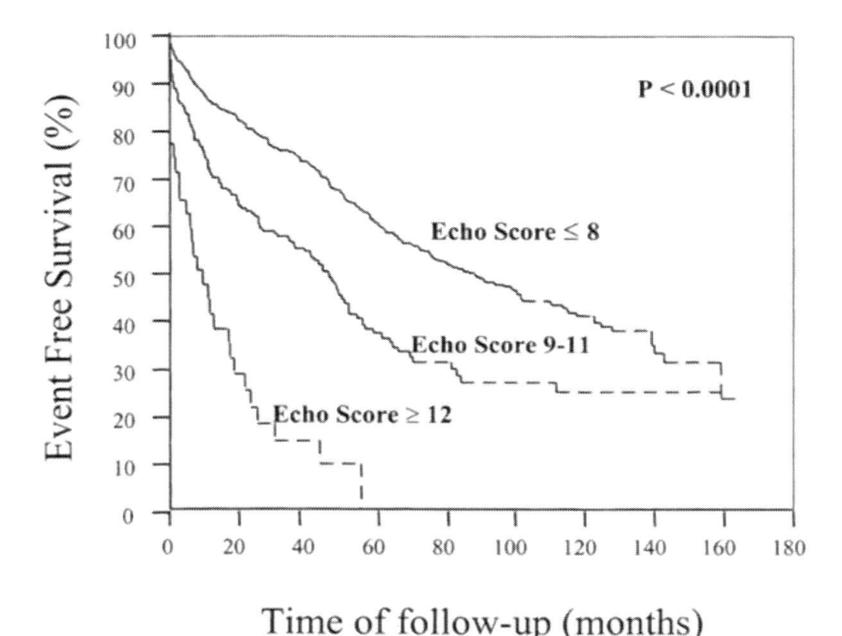

From Palacios IF, Sanchez PL, Harrell LC, et al. Which patients benefit from percutaneous mitral balloon valvuloplasty ? Prevalvuloplasty and postvalvuloplasty variables that predict long-term outcome. Circulation 2002;105:1465-1471 [48].

Figure 9. Event-free survival (alive and free of mitral valve replacement or redo balloon mitral commissurotomy) after balloon mitral commissurotomy according to echo score.

5.4. Comparison with Surgical Commissurotomy

The comparison of observational series may be biased by the confounding impact of differences in patient characteristics.

Randomized series analysing mid-term results (3 to 7 years) following percutaneous or surgical commissurotomy consistently showed that PMC achieved results at least as good as surgical commissurotomy.[63-65] In a series comparing the three techniques, the echocardiographic results of PMC were better than those of closed-heart commissurotomy and comparable to those of open-heart commissurotomy after a 7-year follow-up.[65] However, randomized series included a majority of young patients with favorable mitral valve anatomy and their conclusions cannot be extended beyond this population. There are no randomized comparisons for older patients with more severe valve deformities, who represent the most frequent presentation of mitral stenosis in industrialized countries. A recent non-randomized comparison suggested that open-heart commissurotomy may provide better long-term functional results than PMC in patients with severe valve deformity, but the multiplicity of confounding factors limit the relevance of this finding.[66].

6. Patient Selection

6.1. Patient Evaluation

Besides diagnosis, clinical assessment of a patient with mitral stenosis aims in particular to analyse the consequences of mitral stenosis, *i.e.* symptom severity, a history of embolism, and cardiac rhythm.[67]

Transthoracic echocardiography is the most important investigation for the choice of treatment strategy. The assessment of the severity of mitral stenosis is based on planimetry using the parasternal short-axis view, which is the reference measurement but requires expertise and may be difficult in patients with poor acoustic window or severe valve deformity.[68-69] Real-time three-dimensional echocardiography is helpful for improving the accuracy of planimetry, in particular for less experienced echocardiographers.[70-72] Doppler pressure half-time is less reliable because it also depends on confounding factors, in particular chamber compliance and associated aortic regurgitation. Discrepancies with planimetry are more marked in patients aged over 60, in those in atrial fibrillation, and immediately after PMC [21, 73-74] Mitral gradient is easy to measure by Doppler but is also highly dependent on hemodynamic conditions, in particular cardiac output (Figure 10). In most cases, the conjunction of planimetry, pressure half-time and mean gradient enables the severity of mitral stenosis to be defined (Figure 11).[69] In the rare cases where these measurements cannot be conclusive, mitral valve area can be assessed using continuity equation or flow convergence.[75-76] Systolic pulmonary artery pressure is more a marker of the consequences of mitral stenosis than of its severity.

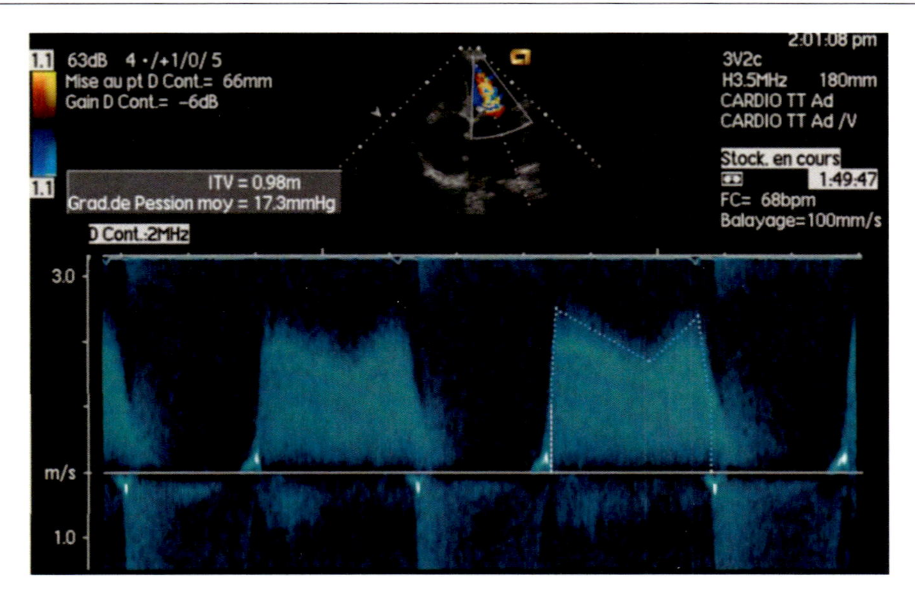

Figure 10. Mean gradient as assessed by continuous-wave Doppler. Mean gradient is 17 mmHg (same patient as in Figure 9).

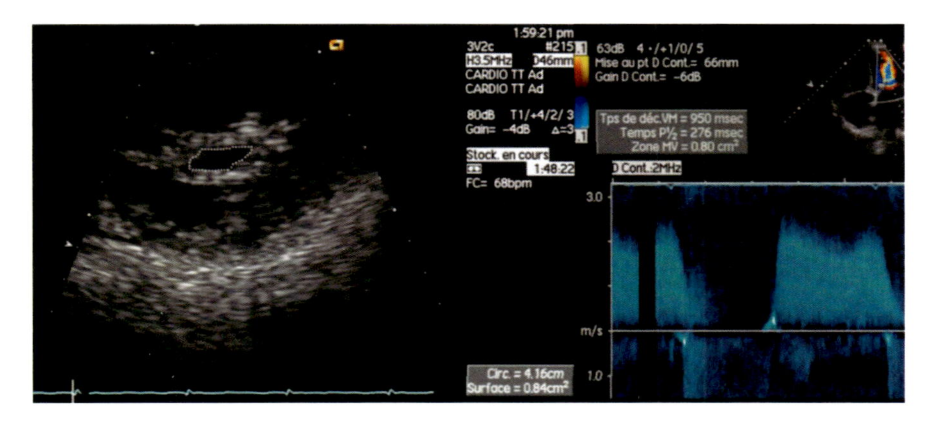

Figure 11. Consistency between the two most widely used methods to assess the severity of mitral stenosis. Valve area is estimated 0.84 cm² using 2D planimetry (left panel) and 0.80 cm² using Doppler pressure half-time (right panel).

The other main application of echocardiography is the evaluation of valve anatomy. The suitability for PMC depends on different anatomic features of the mitral valve apparatus: leaflet thickening, leaflet pliability (Figure 12), degree of involvement of the subvalvular apparatus (chordal thickening and all shortening) (Figure 13), and presence of calcification. These features are usually combined in a scoring system. The most widely used is the Wilkins score, which ranks each component between 1 and 4 and adds them together to obtain a score between 4 and 16 (Table 4).[77] **Another approach is Cormier's score which consists in an** overall approach to the mitral apparatus defining three classes (Table 5).[78] The three classes of Cormier's score correspond to the most appropriate surgical alternative: class 1 corresponds to indications for closed-heart commissurotomy, class 2 to open-heart commissurotomy, class 3 to prosthetic valve replacement. More detailed scores have been described in order to refine the prediction of immediate results of PMC.[79-82] Some of them include a detailed assessment of the impairment of commissural areas, which is likely to influence the results of PMC.[80, 83-84] However, these scoring systems have been tested only in small populations and no large series have demonstrated a better ability to predict the results of PMC. In addition, the complexity of more detailed scores raises concerns regarding their current use and their reproducibility.

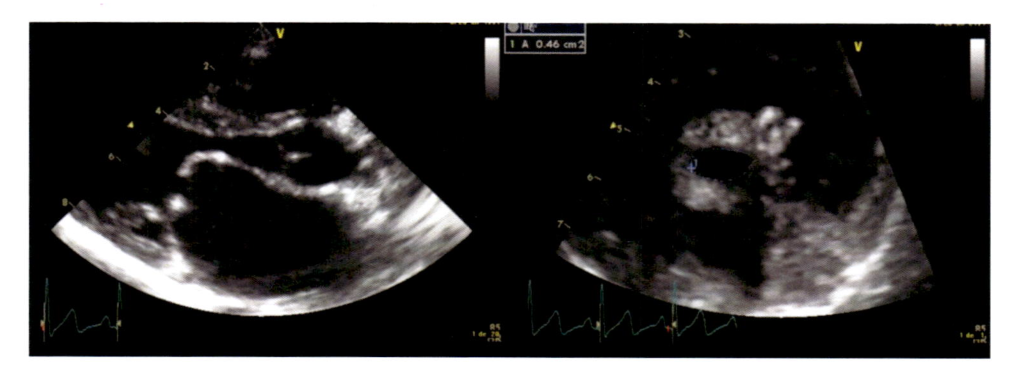

Figure 12. Echocardiographic assessment of severe mitral stenosis (valve area 0.5 cm²). Transthoracic echocardiography, parasternal long-axis (left panel) and short-axis (right panel) views. Leaflets are thickened on long- and short axis views. Anterior leaflet is pliable on the long-axis view. Both commissures are fused. See corresponding Videos 2 and 3.

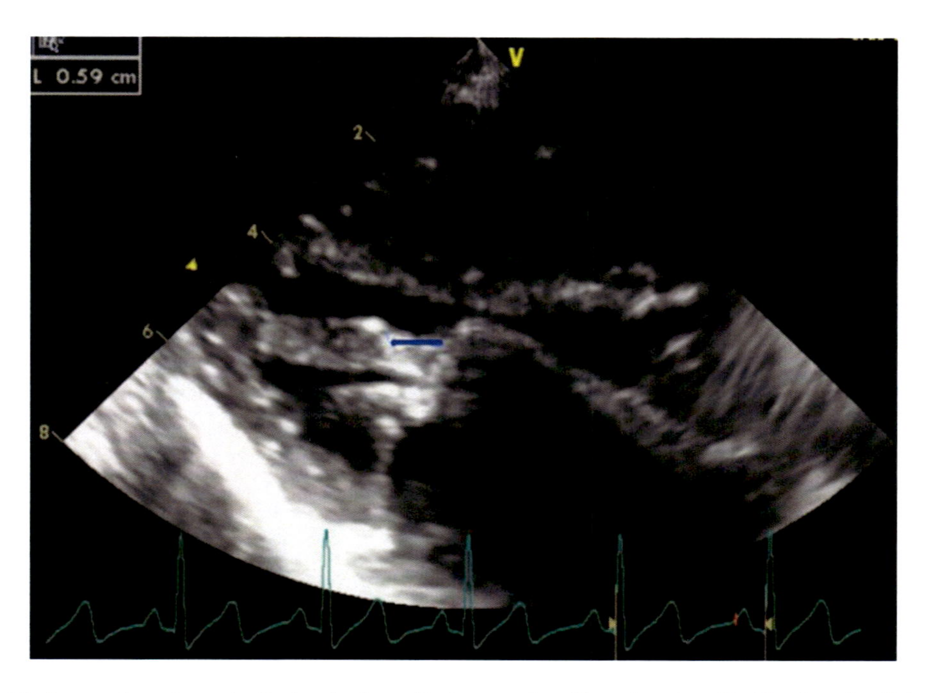

Figure 13. Severe impairment of subvalvular mitral apparatus (Cormier class 2). The length of chordae is 6 mm as assessed from the parasternal long-axis view in transthoracic echocardiography.

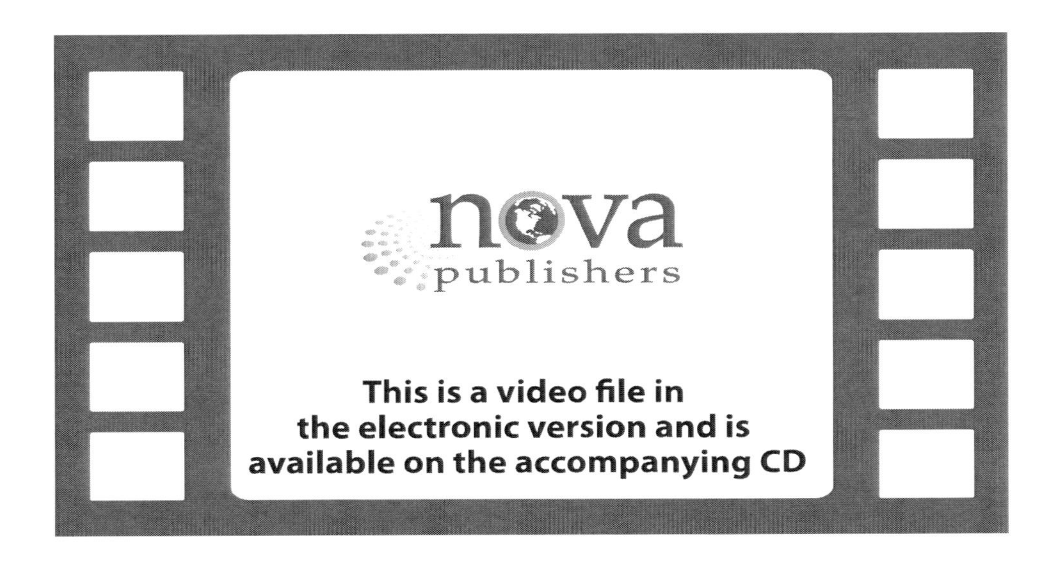

Video 2. Echocardiographic assessment of severe mitral stenosis. Transthoracic echocardiography, parasternal long-axis view.

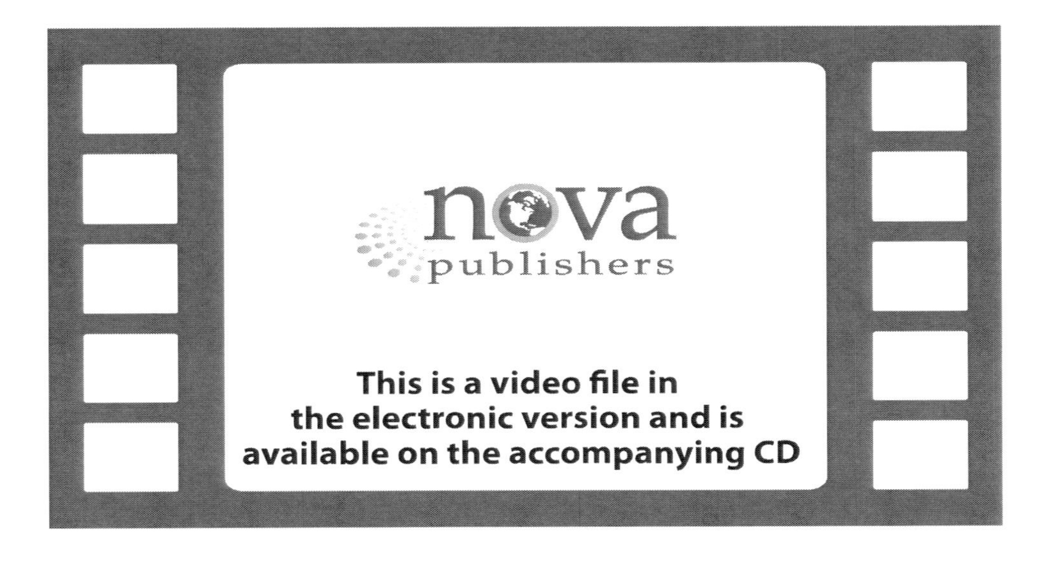

Video 3. Echocardiographic assessment of severe mitral stenosis. Transthoracic echocardiography, parasternal long-axis short-axis view.

Table 4. Assessment of mitral valve anatomy according to the Wilkins score [77]

Grade	*Mobility*	Thickening	Calcification	Subvalvular Thickening
1	Highly mobile valve with only leaflet tips restricted	Leaflets near normal in thickness (4-5 mm)	A single area of increased echo brightness	Minimal thickening just below the mitral leaflets
2	Leaflet mid and base portions have normal mobility	Midleaflets normal, considerable thickening of margins (5-8 mm)	Scattered areas of brightness confined to leaflet margins	Thickening of chordal structures extending to one of the chordal length
3	Valve continues to move forward in diastole, mainly from the base	Thickening extending through the entire leaflet (5-8 mm)	Brightness extending into the mid portions of the leaflets	Thickening extended to distal third of the chords
4	No or minimal forward movement of the leaflets in diastole	Considerable thickening of all leaflet tissue (> 8-10 mm)	Extensive brightness throughout much of the leaflet tissue	Extensive thickening and shortening of all chordal structures extending down to the papillary muscles

The total score is the sum of the four items and ranges between 4 and 16.

Table 5. Assessment of mitral valve anatomy according to the Cormier score [33, 78]

Echocardiographic group	Mitral valve anatomy
Group 1	Pliable noncalcified anterior mitral leaflet and mild subvalvular disease (i.e., thin chordae $\geq$ 10 mm long)
Group 2	Pliable noncalcified anterior mitral leaflet and severe subvalvular disease (i.e., thickened chordae $<$ 10 mm long)
Group 3	Calcification of mitral valve of any extent, as assessed by fluoroscopy, whatever the state of subvalvular apparatus

Echocardiography is also useful for assessing combined aortic or tricuspid valve disease and to quantitate left atrial enlargement. Left ventricular function is generally preserved but may be altered in rare cases.

Transesophageal echocardiography is not a routine examination although it may be used to assess valve anatomy in patients with poor acoustic window. Its main indication is to rule out the presence of left atrial thrombosis before performing PMC (Figure 14). The assessment of left atrial spontaneous contrast contributes to risk-stratification for thromboembolism [85].

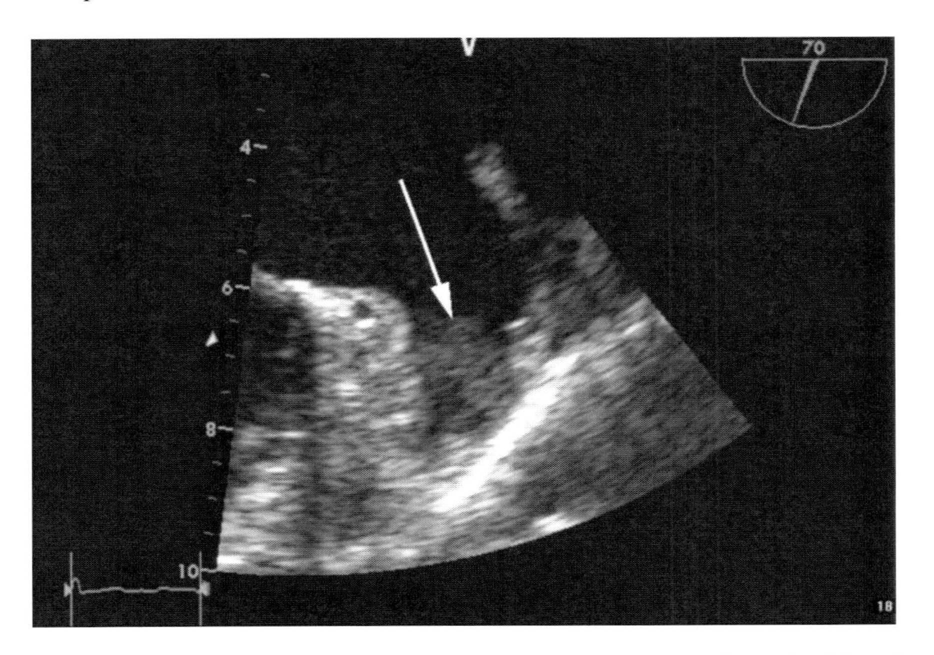

Figure 14. Left atrial appendage thrombus (arrow). Transesophageal echocardiography. Thrombus is located in the left appendage.

Exercise echocardiography is mainly considered in asymptomatic patients [86].

The other imaging techniques, such as computed tomography or magnetic resonance imaging may be used to measure mitral valve area.[87-88] They are not used routinely but may be helpful in the rare cases when echocardiographic examination is not conclusive.

Cardiac catheterization is no longer considered as the reference method for assessing the severity of mitral stenosis.[89-90] Right-heart catheterization remains useful in patient with severe pulmonary hypertension, in particular to assess pulmonary vascular resistance.

6.2. Elements of Decision-Making for Intervention

6.2.1. Severity of Mitral Stenosis

PMC is only considered in patients with severe mitral stenosis. The progression from moderate to severe mitral stenosis is slow and highly variable from one patient to another.[91-93] Therefore, the risk of an interventional procedure, even if low, is not justified at this stage to prevent the evolution toward severe stenosis. In practice, intervention is only considered in patients with a mitral valve area <1.5 cm^2, this threshold being interpreted according to patient body size, mitral gradient, and clinical tolerance.[89-90].

6.2.2. Symptoms and Risk Factors for Complications

In patients with severe mitral stenosis, the presence of symptoms is an indication for intervention. The choice between PMC and surgery depends on the suitability for PMC and contra-indications or risks inherent to PMC or surgery.

On the other hand, in asymptomatic patients with severe mitral stenosis, intervention is seldom indicated. The absence of systematic indication for intervention is justified by the low progression rate toward symptoms in studies on natural history. However, certain patients may be candidates to a low-risk intervention if they have an increased risk of thromboembolic or hemodynamic complications. The indication for PMC in patients at increased thromboembolic risk is supported by the effect of PMC on markers of the thromboemebolic risk, such as indices of left atrial function, left atrial spontaneous contrast, left atrial appendage velocities, and markers of activated coagulation.[94-97]. PMC may also limit the risk of atrial fibrillation [98]. A prospective but non randomized study showed that the performance of PMC was associated with a significant decrease of late thromboembolic risk.[99].

6.2.3. Contra-indications for Percutaneous Mitral Commissurotomy or Surgery

Left atrial thrombus is usually a contraindication for PMC,[89-90] although some small series have suggested that it could be attempted under transesophageal echocardiographic guidance when the thrombus is located in the left atrial appendage.[100-101] Our opinion, however, is that there is not enough evidence for the safety of this approach. Left atrial thrombus is not a definite contraindication since it can disappear after optimisation of anticoagulant therapy. Thus, PMC can be reconsidered after 2 to 6 months if a new transesophageal echocardiography shows the disappearance of the thrombus.[102] This strategy is particularly indicated if the patient is clinically stable, if valve anatomy is suitable for PMC, and if prior anticoagulant therapy was suboptimal.

More than mild mitral regurgitation generally contraindicates PMC. It can be nevertheless considered in patients with moderate mitral regurgitation, provided valve anatomy is favorable. Severe regurgitation is of course a definite contraindication.

Massive or bicommissural mitral valve calcification is a contraindication for PMC. In patients who have previously undergone balloon or surgical commissurotomy, the persistence of complete opening of one or both commissures indicates that restenosis is due to valve rigidity and is an indication for mitral valve replacement (Figure 15).

Other severe valvular disease or coronary heart disease requiring surgery contraindicate PMC and should lead to the consideration of combined surgical treatment. The only exception is severe tricuspid regurgitation which does not contra-indicate PMC, provided it is of functional origin and not associated with a severe enlargement of right heart cavities. On the other hand, the combination of severe mitral stenosis with other moderate valvular disease favors the use of PMC in order to postpone multiple valve surgery.

Definite contraindications for surgery are rare. The assessment of operative risk using validated scores is of importance since PMC may be favoured over surgery in patients with high expected operative risk, even in the presence of unfavorable characteristics.

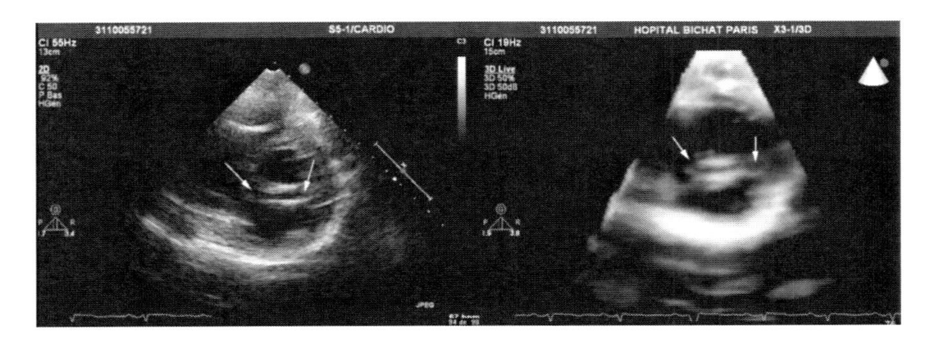

Figure 15. Mitral restenosis with persistent opening of both commissures. Parasternal short-axis view. Left panel: 2D echo. Right panel: 3D echo. The arrows show opening of both commissures. See corresponding Video 4.

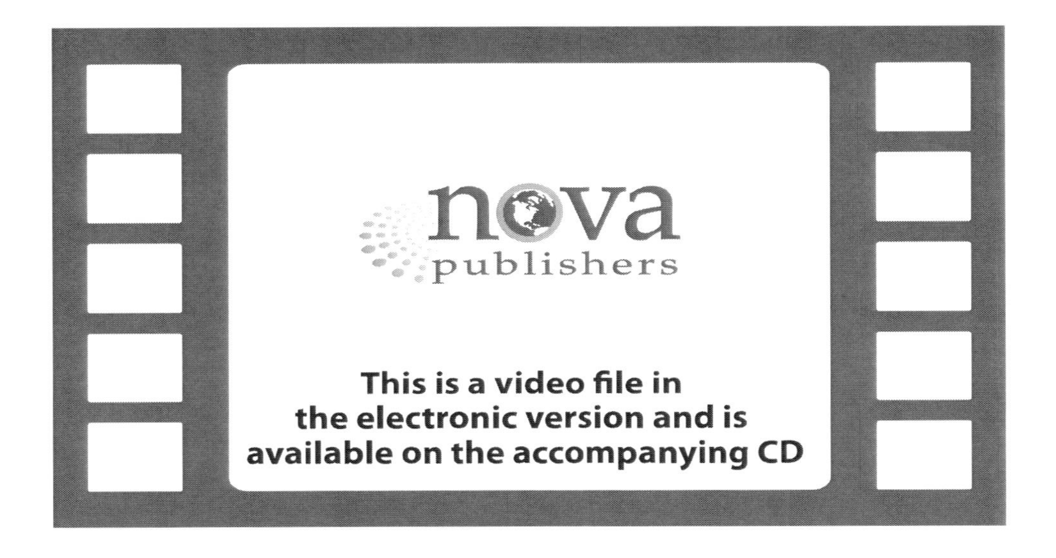

Video 4. Mitral restenosis with persistent opening of both commissures. Parasternal short-axis view.

6.3. Guidelines

Current guidelines propose treatment strategies to integrate the different patient characteristics and select the most appropriate intervention on mitral stenosis.[89-90].

6.3.1. Symptomatic Patients

Severe, symptomatic, mitral stenosis, is a class I indication for intervention according to guidelines (Figures 16 and 17) [89-90]. In these patients, the problem is the choice of the most appropriate technique. Favorable patient characteristics for PMC have been defined according to the identification of predictive factors of good immediate and late results.

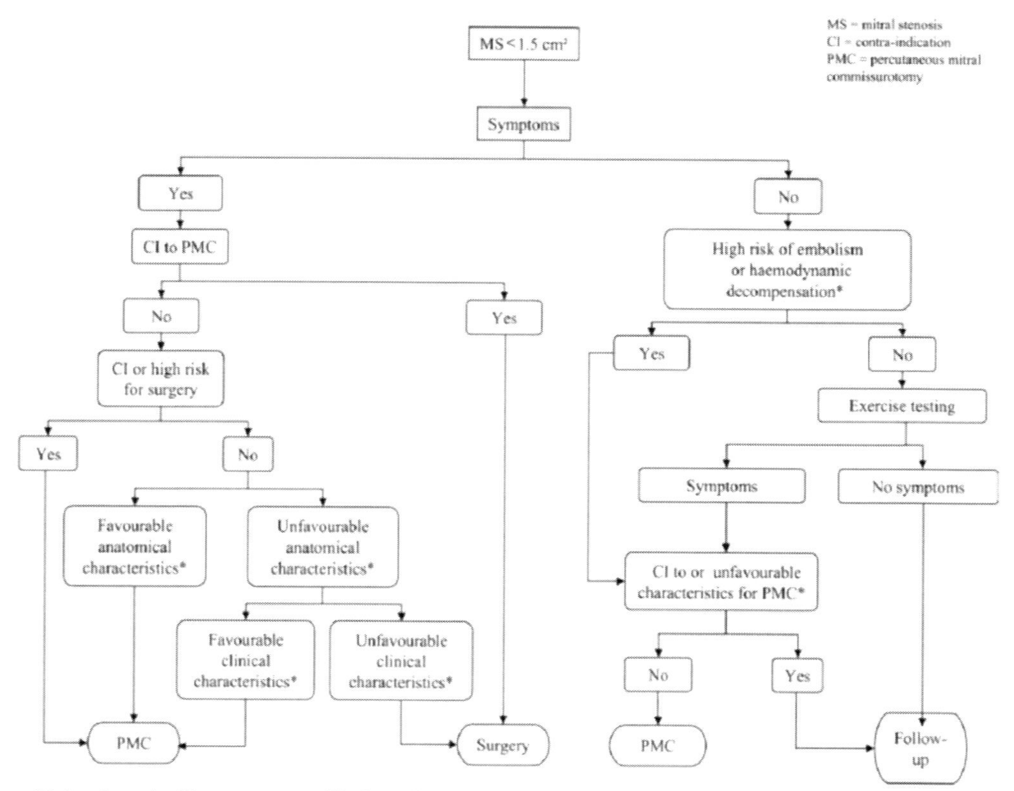

From Vahanian A, Baumgartner H, Bax J, et al. Guidelines on the management of valvular heart disease. Eur Heart J 2007;28:230-268 [89].

Figure 16. Indications for balloon mitral commissurotomy in patients with mitral stenosis. ESC guidelines (*: see Table 6 for definitions).

Echocardiographic assessment of valve anatomy is an important factor. Given the evidence from observational and randomised series, PMC is definitely the preferred treatment in patients with favorable valve anatomy, i.e. with a Wilkins Score ≤ 8 or a Cormier class 1.

In patients with less favorable valve anatomy (Wilkins Score >8 or Cormier class 2 or 3), who represent the majority of patient with mitral stenosis in industrialized countries, PMC should be widely considered in patients whose clinical characteristics are favorable.

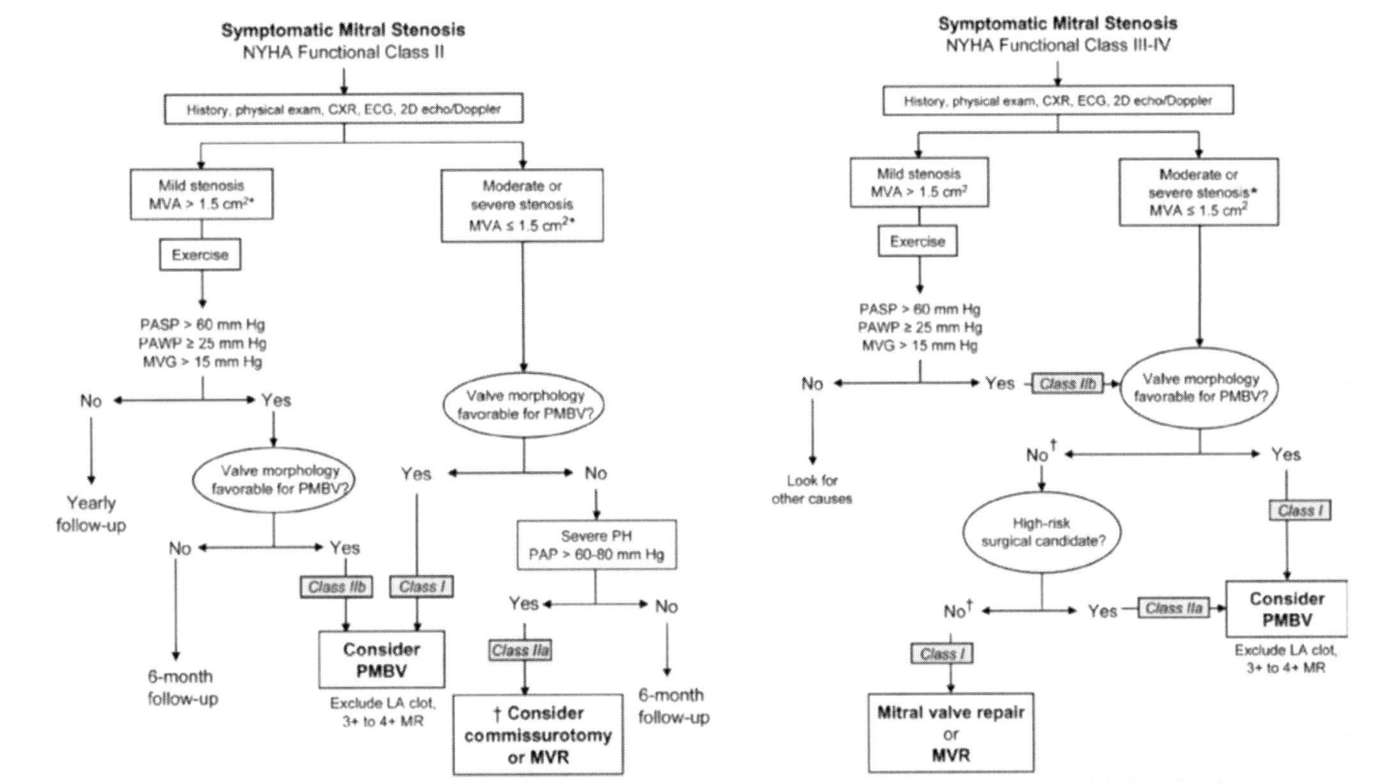

From Bonow RO, Carabello BA, Chatterjee K, et al. 2008 Focused update incorporated into the ACC/AHA 2006 guidelines for the management of patients with valvular heart disease. Circulation 2008;118:e523-661 [90].

Figure 17. Indications for balloon mitral commissurotomy in symptomatic patients with mitral stenosis. ACC/AHA Guidelines.

Table 6. Indications for percutaneous mitral commissurotomy in mitral stenosis with valve area ≤ 1.5 cm^2, according to the Guidelines of the European Society of Cardiology [89]

	Class
Symptomatic patients with favorable characteristics* for percutaneous mitral commissurotomy	IB
Symptomatic patients with contra-indication or high risk for surgery	IC
As initial treatment in symptomatic patients with unfavorable anatomy but otherwise favorable clinical characteristics*	IIaC
Asymptomatic patients with favorable characteristics* and high thromboembolic risk or high risk of haemodynamic decompensation:	
- previous history of embolism	IIaC
- dense spontaneous contrast in the left atrium	IIaC
- recent or paroxysmal atrial fibrillation	IIaC
- systolic pulmonary pressure > 50 mmHg at rest	IIaC
- need for major non-cardiac surgery,	IIaC
- desire of pregnancy	IIaC

*: Favorable characteristics for percutaneous mitral commissurotomy can be defined by the absence of several of the following unfavorable characteristics:
- Clinical characteristics: old age, history of commissurotomy, NYHA class IV, atrial fibrillation, severe pulmonary hypertension,
- Anatomic characteristics: echo score >8, Cormier score 3 (Calcification of mitral valve of any extent, as assessed by fluoroscopy), very small mitral valve area, severe tricuspid regurgitation.

The final decision should be individualised and take into account the risk of surgery and the long-term drawbacks of mitral prostheses, since most patients with unfavorable valve anatomy undergo valve replacement.[103-105] Among patients with unfavorable anatomical conditions, PMC is particularly attractive in young patients in sinus rhythm since good late results can be expected and the possibility of postponing valve replacement is particularly relevant. On the other hand, in the elderly with advanced heart disease, straightforward surgery can be considered if its risk is not expected to be prohibitive. The experience of the team should also be taken into account and this concerns local resources in interventional cardiology as well as valvular surgery.

6.3.2. Asymptomatic Patients

Indications for PMC in asymptomatic patients with severe mitral stenosis should be discussed on an individual basis (Table 6). Guidelines recommend considering PMC in patients who have an increased risk of thromboembolic events or of haemodynamic decompensation (Figures 16 and 18).

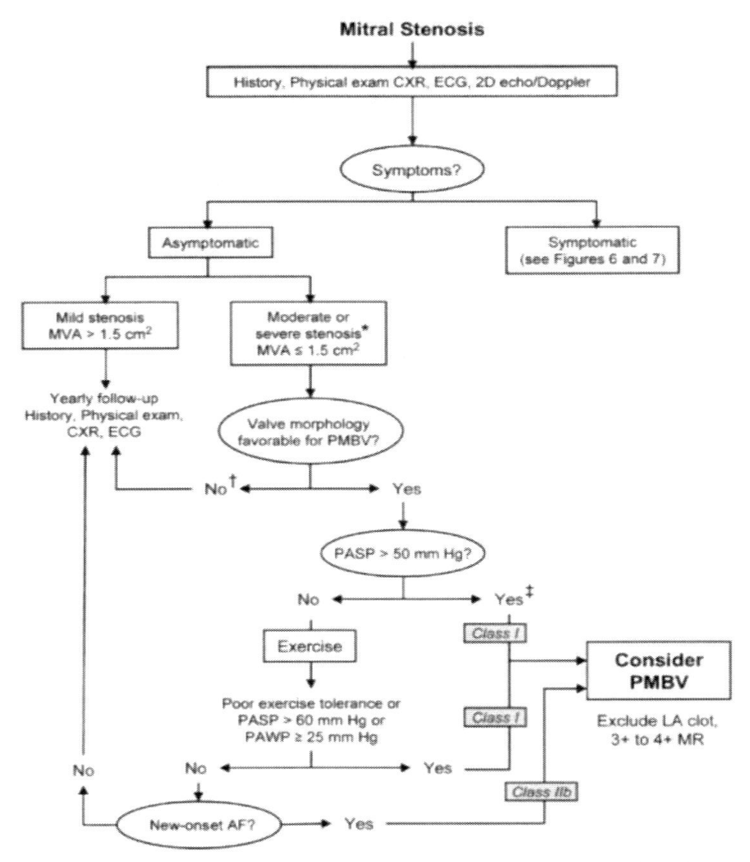

From Bonow RO, Carabello BA, Chatterjee K, et al. 2008 Focused update incorporated into the ACC/AHA 2006 guidelines for the management of patients with valvular heart disease. Circulation 2008;118:e523-661 [90].

Figure 18. Indications for balloon mitral commissurotomy in asymptomatic patients with mitral stenosis. ACC/AHA guidelines.

Risk factors for thromboembolism are previous thromboembolism, atrial fibrillation, left atrial dense spontaneous echo contrast, and left atrial enlargement. These factors are indications for anticoagulant therapy. They may also lead to the consideration of PMC to further decrease the thromboemblic risk. Among asymptomatic patients at increased risk of hemodynamic decompensation, particular attention should be given to young women who wish to be pregnant.[89-90].

6.4. Particular Situations

6.4.1. Pregnancy

Pregnancy carries a high risk of decompensation of severe mitral stenosis, even if well tolerated before pregnancy.[106] The risk of cardiac complication is further increased during delivery, so that intervention may be necessary during pregnancy. Surgery under cardiopulmonary bypass is associated with high fetal mortality (20-30%).[107] Thus, PMC is of particular interest when an intervention is required on mitral stenosis during pregnancy. Anatomical conditions are often favorable in young women. There is now evidence that PMC can be performed safely during pregnancy, in particular with a good fetal tolerance and no detectable harmful effects of radiation, provided specific precautions are taken.[108-109] The procedure should be kept as short as possible and the Inoue balloon is useful in this setting. Echocardiographic monitoring enables cardiac catheterisation and ventricular angiography to be avoided. The abdomen of the mother should be wrapped by a lead apron to reduce fetal exposure to radiation. Since transesophageal echocardiography may be poorly tolerated in pregnant women, it can be performed immediately before PMC under general anesthesia.

Given the ever present risk of complications with an interventional procedure, PMC should not be considered systematically in pregnant women with mitral stenosis, but only in those who remain symptomatic or have pulmonary hypertension despite optimal therapy, relying mainly on beta-blockers.[89, 110].

6.4.2. Elderly

Unlike other valvular diseases, mitral stenosis is seldom encountered in the elderly. In the Euro Heart Survey, only 18% of patients with mitral stenosis were older than 70 and 1.5% older than 80.[111] Mitral stenosis in the elderly may be of rheumatic origin but is characterised by an increasing frequency of degenerative aetiologies.[89] The management of mitral stenosis in the elderly should therefore pay a particular attention to the analysis of its mechanism and aetiology. Degenerative mitral stenosis is due to valvular rigidity and/or calcification without commissural fusion. These patients are clearly not candidates for PMC, even if surgery is at high-risk due to patient age and technical difficulties when there is extensive annular calcification.

Valve calcification is also frequent in rheumatic mitral stenosis in the elderly, but is generally associated with commissural fusion. PMC may thus be considered, either as a curative treatment in patients without extensive calcification, or even as a palliative treatment in patients with severe calcification but in whom surgery carries a prohibitive risk.[89-90]

Despite unfavorable anatomic conditions, PMC gives good immediate results in approximately 3 out of 4 elderly patients. However, secondary deterioration occurs more frequently than in younger patients.[112-115].

6.4.3. Patients with Previous Mitral Commissurotomy

Patients with prior surgical or percutaneous commissurotomy accounted for 31% of all patients with mitral stenosis in the Euro Heart Survey.[111] Patient selection should take into account the mechanism of valve restenosis. PMC cannot be considered when restenosis is due to valvular rigidity with persistent commissural opening. Real-time three-dimensional echocardiography is helpful to assess the degree of commissural fusion.[72] When restenosis is due to refusion of both commissures, PMC can be considered according to the same selection process as in other patients (Figure 19). [116] Immediate and late results of PMC for mitral restenosis are satisfying [116-119]. In our experience, they enable mitral surgery to be postponed of at least 8 years in half of the patients after surgical commissurotomy [116].

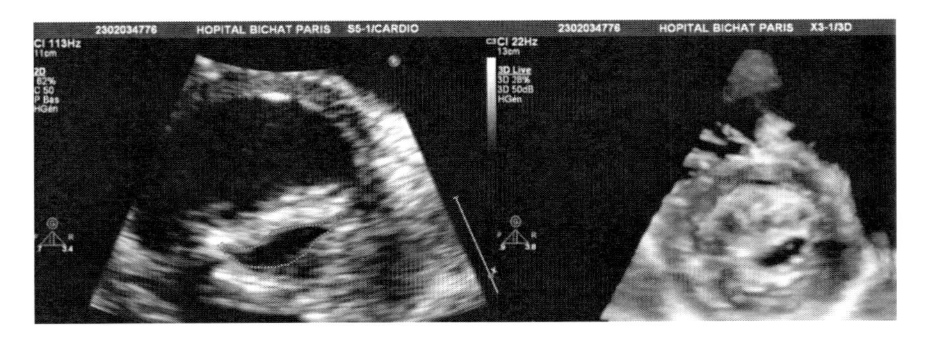

Figure 19. Mitral restenosis with refusion of both commissures. Parasternal short-axis view. Left panel: 2D echo. Right panel: 3D echo. See corresponding Video 5.

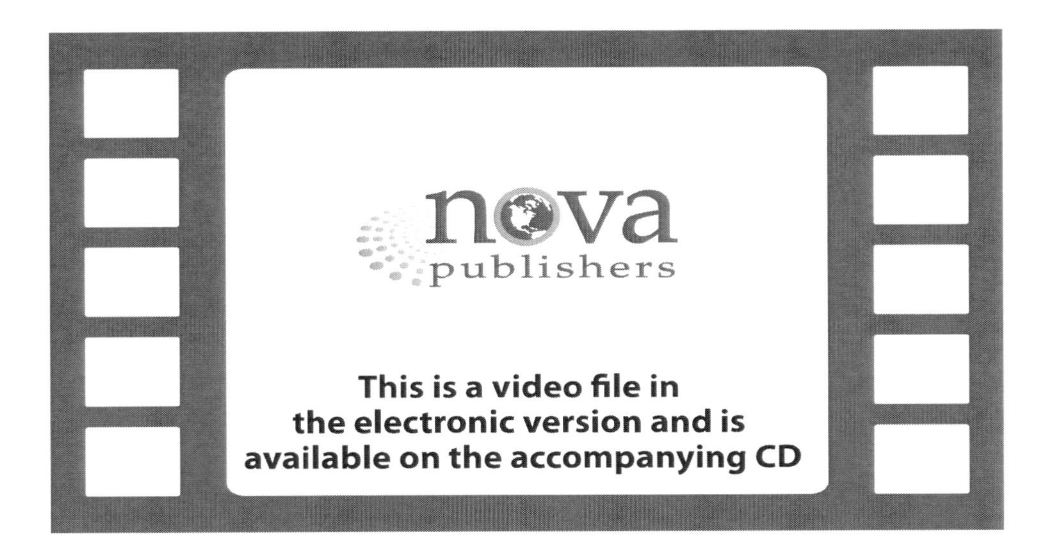

Video 5. Mitral restenosis with refusion of both commissures. Parasternal short-axis view.

Decision-making is the same in patients presenting with restenosis after previous PMC. The possibility to repeat PMC is particularly attractive in young patients to avoid the need for iterative thoracotomy.[120-121].

7. Current Use of PMC and Future Perspectives

7.1. Developing Countries

The most important field of application of PMC should be developing countries, where the prevalence of rheumatic heart disease remains high, in particular in young patients. The prevalence of rheumatic heart disease in school-age children is estimated between 1 and 6 per 1000 in Asia and between 3 and 14% in Africa.[122-123] Recent data based on systematic echocardiographic examination show that the true prevalence is approximately tenfold higher.[124] Although prevention strategies exist for rheumatic heart disease, it is likely that its prevalence will remain high, at least at mid-term, since the implementation of prevention is hampered by socio-economic conditions.[125]

The use of PMC is particularly attractive in young patients, in whom it gives good results and can be repeated in case of mitral restenosis, thereby enabling valve replacement to be postponed for several decades and avoiding multiple redo surgical interventions.[126-127] The current use of PMC in developing countries is, however, restricted because of economical constraints related to the cost of the devices. This explains why closed-heart commissurotomy remains widely used in certain developing countries.[128] Therefore, the future development of PMC in developing countries depends mainly on the possibility to afford the cost of the device rather than on technical improvements.

7.2. Industrialised Countries

The experience acquired with large series and the identification of predictive factors of immediate and late results have led to a progressive widening of indications of PMC from young patients with favorable valve anatomy to older patients with more severe valve deformities. In the experience of our team over a 15-year period between 1986 and 2001, there was a progressive increase in mean age from 43 to 51 years and an increase in the percentage of patients with unfavorable valve anatomy.[29] The procedure was also performed at an earlier stage, as attested by the increase in the percentage of patients in NYHA class I or II from 17 to 43%. Despite changing patterns, the percentages of good immediate results remained stable over time.

In the Euro Heart Survey, PMC accounted for 34% of all interventional procedures performed to treat mitral stenosis, while surgical commissurotomy represented only 4%.[3, 111] Practically, the choice is now PMC or prosthetic valve replacement in most patients with mitral stenosis.

Despite marked differences in patient characteristics, PMC is an effective treatment in the different presentations of mitral stenosis encountered worldwide.[129]

In industrialised countries, continuing evaluation of the results of PMC is necessary to refine its indications in a heterogeneous population of patients with mitral stenosis and non-optimal valve anatomy. More detailed analysis of valve deformity using echocardiography or alternative imaging techniques may contribute to improving the prediction of immediate and late results. However, attempts to refine echocardiographic scores have shown the limitations of an approach based on the assessment of valvular anatomy alone. Widely applicable and highly reproducible scoring systems should be integrated with other patient characteristics, which have been shown to be strong determinants of immediate and late outcome, in particular in patients with non favorable valve anatomy (Figure 20).[130] Testing the predictive ability of models with different patient characteristics, including valve anatomy, may contribute to improved patient selection for PMC.

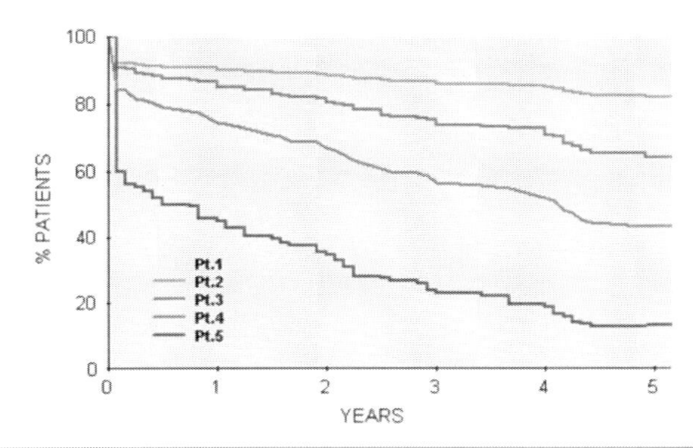

Patient	Age (yrs)	NYHA class	Rhythm	Calcification	Valve Area (cm^2)
1	< 50	II	sinus	1	1.25 - 1.5
2	< 50	II	sinus	2	1 - 1.25
3	50 - 70	III	sinus	2	1.25 - 1.5
4	50 - 70	III	A. fib	2	1.25 - 1.5
5	≥ 70	III	A. fib	3	0.75 - 1

From Iung B, Garbarz E, Doutrelant L, et al. Late results of percutaneous mitral commissurotomy for calcific mitral stenosis. the advantage of an individual assessment for patient selection. Am J Cardiol 2000;85:1308-1314 [130].

Figure 20. Predicted probability of good immediate results (valve area ≥ 1.5 cm² without regurgitation > grade 2/4) and good late functional results (survival with no intervention and in NYHA functional class I or II) after balloon mitral commissurotomy in calcified mitral stenosis, according to patient characteristics. The extent of calcification is graded from 1 (small nodule) to 4 (extensive calcification).

Conclusion

After more than 20 years, PMC is now a mature technique as attested by the number of series evaluating long-term results in a variety of patient subsets, its role in the treatment of mitral stenosis in contemporary guidelines, and its wide use worldwide. PMC has virtually replaced surgical commissurotomy in industrialised countries and its respective indications with surgery are now more clearly defined in non-optimal candidates to the technique. PMC and surgery now appear as complementary techniques, which should be used appropriately in the different stages and presentations of mitral stenosis.

The recent interest in new percutaneous techniques in the treatment of valvular disease highlights the need for continuing evaluation of new techniques to improve the selection process of patients towards surgery or less invasive techniques.

References

[1] Inoue, K; Owaki, T; Nakamura, T; Kitamura, F, Miyamoto, N. Clinical application of transvenous mitral commissurotomy by a new balloon catheter. *J Thorac Cardiovasc Surg*. 1984 Mar;87:394-402.

[2] Nkomo, VT; Gardin, JM; Skelton, TN; Gottdiener, JS; Scott, CG, Enriquez-Sarano, M. Burden of valvular heart diseases: a population-based study. *Lancet*. 2006 Sep 16;368:1005-1011.

[3] Iung, B; Baron, G; Butchart, EG; Delahaye, F; Gohlke-Barwolf, C; Levang, OW, et al. A prospective survey of patients with valvular heart disease in Europe: The Euro Heart Survey on Valvular Heart Disease. *Eur Heart J*. 2003 Jul;24:1231-1243.

[4] Carroll, JD, Feldman, T. Percutaneous mitral balloon valvotomy and the new demographics of mitral stenosis. *JAMA*. 1993 Oct 13;270:1731-1736.

[5] Cutler, EC, Levine, SA. Cardiotomy and valvulotomy for mitral stenosis: experimental observations and clinical notes concerning an operated case with recovery. *Boston Medical and Surgical Journal*. 1923;188:1023.

[6] Souttar, S. The surgical treatment of mitral stenosis. *Br Med J*. 1925603.

[7] Bailey, CP. The surgical treatment of mitral stenosis (mitral commissurotomy). *Dis Chest*. 1949 Apr;15:377-397.

[8] Park, SH; Kim, MA, Hyon, MS. The advantages of On-line transesophageal echocardiography guide during percutaneous balloon mitral valvuloplasty. *J Am Soc Echocardiogr*. 2000 Jan;13:26-34.

[9] Perk, G; Lang, RM; Garcia-Fernandez, MA; Lodato, J; Sugeng, L; Lopez, J, et al. Use of real time three-dimensional transesophageal echocardiography in intracardiac catheter based interventions. *J Am Soc Echocardiogr*. 2009 Aug;22:865-882.

[10] Liang, KW; Fu, YC; Lee, WL; Liu, TJ; Wang, KY; Hsueh, CW, et al. Intra-cardiac echocardiography guided trans-septal puncture in patients with dilated left atrium undergoing percutaneous transvenous mitral commissurotomy. *Int J Cardiol*. 2007 May 2;117:418-421.

[11] Stefanadis, C; Stratos, C; Pitsavos, C; Kallikazaros, I; Triposkiadis, F; Trikas, A, et al. Retrograde nontransseptal balloon mitral valvuloplasty. Immediate results and long-term follow-up. *Circulation*. 1992 May;85:1760-1767.

[12] Stefanadis, CI; Stratos, CG; Lambrou, SG; Bahl, VK; Cokkinos, DV; Voudris, VA, et al. Retrograde nontransseptal balloon mitral valvuloplasty: immediate results and intermediate long-term outcome in 441 cases--a multicenter experience. *J Am Coll Cardiol*. 1998 Oct;32:1009-1016.

[13] Al Zaibag, M; Ribeiro, PA; Al Kasab, S, Al Fagih, MR. Percutaneous double-balloon mitral valvotomy for rheumatic mitral-valve stenosis. *Lancet*. 1986 Apr 5;1:757-761.

[14] Bonhoeffer, P; Esteves, C; Casal, U; Tortoledo, F; Yonga, G; Patel, T, et al. Percutaneous mitral valve dilatation with the Multi-Track System. *Catheter Cardiovasc Interv*. 1999 Oct;48:178-183.

[15] Vahanian, A; Cormier, B, Iung, B. Percutaneous transvenous mitral commissurotomy using the Inoue balloon: international experience. *Cathet Cardiovasc Diagn*. 1994;Suppl 2:8-15.

[16] Bassand, JP; Schiele, F; Bernard, Y; Anguenot, T; Payet, M; Ba, SA, et al. The double-balloon and Inoue techniques in percutaneous mitral valvuloplasty: comparative results in a series of 232 cases. *J Am Coll Cardiol*. 1991 Oct;18:982-989.

[17] Kang, DH; Park, SW; Song, JK; Kim, HS; Hong, MK; Kim, JJ, et al. Long-term clinical and echocardiographic outcome of percutaneous mitral valvuloplasty: randomized comparison of Inoue and double-balloon techniques. *J Am Coll Cardiol*. 2000 Jan;35:169-175.

[18] Cribier, A; Rath, PC, Letac, B. Percutaneous mitral valvotomy with a metal dilatator. *Lancet*. 1997 Jun 7;349:1667.

[19] Segal, J; Lerner, DJ; Miller, DC; Mitchell, RS; Alderman, EA, Popp, RL. When should Doppler-determined valve area be better than the Gorlin formula?: Variation in hydraulic constants in low flow states. *J Am Coll Cardiol*. 1987 Jun;9:1294-1305.

[20] Petrossian, GA; Tuzcu, EM; Ziskind, AA; Block, PC, Palacios, I. Atrial septal occlusion improves the accuracy of mitral valve area determination following percutaneous mitral balloon valvotomy. *Cathet Cardiovasc Diagn*. 1991 Jan;22:21-24.

[21] Thomas, JD; Wilkins, GT; Choong, CY; Abascal, VM; Palacios, IF; Block, PC, et al. Inaccuracy of mitral pressure half-time immediately after percutaneous mitral valvotomy. Dependence on transmitral gradient and left atrial and ventricular compliance. *Circulation*. 1988 Oct;78:980-993.

[22] Complications and mortality of percutaneous balloon mitral commissurotomy. A report from the National Heart, Lung, and Blood Institute Balloon Valvuloplasty Registry. *Circulation*. 1992 Jun;85:2014-2024.

[23] Chen, CR, Cheng, TO. Percutaneous balloon mitral valvuloplasty by the Inoue technique: a multicenter study of 4832 patients in China. *Am Heart J*. 1995 Jun;129:1197-1203.

[24] Meneveau, N; Schiele, F; Seronde, MF; Breton, V; Gupta, S; Bernard, Y, et al. Predictors of event-free survival after percutaneous mitral commissurotomy. *Heart*. 1998 Oct;80:359-364.

[25] Hernandez, R; Banuelos, C; Alfonso, F; Goicolea, J; Fernandez-Ortiz, A; Escaned, J, et al. Long-term clinical and echocardiographic follow-up after percutaneous mitral valvuloplasty with the Inoue balloon. *Circulation*. 1999 Mar 30;99:1580-1586.

[26] Ben-Farhat, M; Betbout, F; Gamra, H; Maatouk, F; Ben-Hamda, K; Abdellaoui, M, et al. Predictors of long-term event-free survival and of freedom from restenosis after percutaneous balloon mitral commissurotomy. *Am Heart J*. 2001 Dec;142:1072-1079.

[27] Neumayer, U; Schmidt, HK; Fassbender, D; Mannebach, H; Bogunovic, N, Horstkotte, D. Early (three-month) results of percutaneous mitral valvotomy with the Inoue balloon in 1,123 consecutive patients comparing various age groups. *Am J Cardiol*. 2002 Jul 15;90:190-193.

[28] Arora, R; Kalra, GS; Singh, S; Mukhopadhyay, S; Kumar, A; Mohan, JC, et al. Percutaneous transvenous mitral commissurotomy: immediate and long-term follow-up results. *Catheter Cardiovasc Interv*. 2002 Apr;55:450-456.
[29] Iung, B; Nicoud-Houel, A; Fondard, O; Hafid, A; Haghighat, T; Brochet, E, et al. Temporal trends in percutaneous mitral commissurotomy over a 15-year period. *Eur Heart J*. 2004 Apr;25:701-707.
[30] Fawzy, ME; Shoukri, M; Al Buraiki, J; Hassan, W; El Widaal, H; Kharabsheh, S, et al. Seventeen years' clinical and echocardiographic follow up of mitral balloon valvuloplasty in 520 patients, and predictors of long-term outcome. *J Heart Valve Dis*. 2007 Sep;16:454-460.
[31] Jneid, H; Cruz-Gonzalez, I; Sanchez-Ledesma, M; Maree, AO; Cubeddu, RJ; Leon, ML, et al. Impact of pre- and postprocedural mitral regurgitation on outcomes after percutaneous mitral valvuloplasty for mitral stenosis. *Am J Cardiol*. 2009 Oct 15;104:1122-1127.
[32] Tuzcu, EM; Block, PC, Palacios, IF. Comparison of early versus late experience with percutaneous mitral balloon valvuloplasty. *J Am Coll Cardiol*. 1991 Apr;17:1121-1124.
[33] Iung, B; Cormier, B; Ducimetiere, P; Porte, JM; Nallet, O; Michel, PL, et al. Immediate results of percutaneous mitral commissurotomy. A predictive model on a series of 1514 patients. *Circulation*. 1996 Nov 1;94:2124-2130.
[34] Varma, PK; Theodore, S; Neema, PK; Ramachandran, P; Sivadasanpillai, H; Nair, KK, et al. Emergency surgery after percutaneous transmitral commissurotomy: operative versus echocardiographic findings, mechanisms of complications, and outcomes. *J Thorac Cardiovasc Surg*. 2005 Sep;130:772-776.
[35] Zimmet, AD; Almeida, AA; Harper, RW; Smolich, JJ; Goldstein, J; Shardey, GC, et al. Predictors of surgery after percutaneous mitral valvuloplasty. *Ann Thorac Surg*. 2006 Sep;82:828-833.
[36] Choudhary, SK; Talwar, S, Venugopal, P. Severe mitral regurgitation after percutaneous transmitral commissurotomy: underestimated subvalvular disease. *J Thorac Cardiovasc Surg*. 2006 Apr;131:927; author reply 927-928.
[37] Hernandez, R; Macaya, C; Banuelos, C; Alfonso, F; Goicolea, J; Iniguez, A, et al. Predictors, mechanisms and outcome of severe mitral regurgitation complicating percutaneous mitral valvotomy with the Inoue balloon. *Am J Cardiol*. 1992 Nov 1;70:1169-1174.
[38] Acar, C; Jebara, VA; Grare, P; Chachques, JC; Dervanian, P; Vahanian, A, et al. Traumatic mitral insufficiency following percutaneous mitral dilation: anatomic lesions and surgical implications. *Eur J Cardiothorac Surg*. 1992;6:660-663; discussion 663-664.
[39] Cequier, A; Bonan, R; Serra, A; Dyrda, I; Crepeau, J; Dethy, M, et al. Left-to-right atrial shunting after percutaneous mitral valvuloplasty. Incidence and long-term hemodynamic follow-up. *Circulation*. 1990 Apr;81:1190-1197.
[40] Gupta, S; Schiele, F; Xu, C; Meneveau, N; Seronde, MF; Breton, V, et al. Simplified percutaneous mitral valvuloplasty with the Inoue balloon. *Eur Heart J*. 1998 Apr;19:610-616.
[41] Messika-Zeitoun, D; Blanc, J; Iung, B; Brochet, E; Cormier, B; Himbert, D, et al. Impact of degree of commissural opening after percutaneous mitral commissurotomy on long-term outcome. *JACC Cardiovasc Imaging*. 2009 Jan;2:1-7.

[42] Krishnamoorthy, KM; Dash, PK; Radhakrishnan, S, Shrivastava, S. Response of different grades of pulmonary artery hypertension to balloon mitral valvuloplasty. *Am J Cardiol*. 2002 Nov 15;90:1170-1173.

[43] Tanabe, Y; Oshima, M; Suzuki, M, Takahashi, M. Determinants of delayed improvement in exercise capacity after percutaneous transvenous mitral commissurotomy. *Am Heart J*. 2000 May;139:889-894.

[44] Abascal, VM; Wilkins, GT; O'Shea, JP; Choong, CY; Palacios, IF; Thomas, JD, et al. Prediction of successful outcome in 130 patients undergoing percutaneous balloon mitral valvotomy. *Circulation*. 1990 Aug;82:448-456.

[45] Herrmann, HC; Ramaswamy, K; Isner, JM; Feldman, TE; Carroll, JD; Pichard, AD, et al. Factors influencing immediate results, complications, and short-term follow-up status after Inoue balloon mitral valvotomy: a North American multicenter study. *Am Heart J*. 1992 Jul;124:160-166.

[46] Feldman, T; Carroll, JD; Isner, JM; Chisholm, RJ; Holmes, DR; Massumi, A, et al. Effect of valve deformity on results and mitral regurgitation after Inoue balloon commissurotomy. *Circulation*. 1992 Jan;85:180-187.

[47] Cruz-Gonzalez, I; Sanchez-Ledesma, M; Sanchez, PL; Martin-Moreiras, J; Jneid, H; Rengifo-Moreno, P, et al. Predicting success and long-term outcomes of percutaneous mitral valvuloplasty: a multifactorial score. *Am J Med*. 2009 Jun;122:581 e511-589.

[48] Palacios, IF; Sanchez, PL; Harrell, LC; Weyman, AE, Block, PC. Which patients benefit from percutaneous mitral balloon valvuloplasty? Prevalvuloplasty and postvalvuloplasty variables that predict long-term outcome. *Circulation*. 2002 Mar 26;105:1465-1471.

[49] Reifart, N; Nowak, B; Baykut, D; Satter, P; Bussmann, WD, Kaltenbach, M. Experimental balloon valvuloplasty of fibrotic and calcific mitral valves. *Circulation*. 1990 Mar;81:1005-1011.

[50] Cohen, DJ; Kuntz, RE; Gordon, SP; Piana, RN; Safian, RD; McKay, RG, et al. Predictors of long-term outcome after percutaneous balloon mitral valvuloplasty. *N Engl J Med*. 1992 Nov 5;327:1329-1335.

[51] Dean, LS; Mickel, M; Bonan, R; Holmes, DR, Jr.; O'Neill, WW; Palacios, IF, et al. Four-year follow-up of patients undergoing percutaneous balloon mitral commissurotomy. A report from the National Heart, Lung, and Blood Institute Balloon Valvuloplasty Registry. *J Am Coll Cardiol*. 1996 Nov 15;28:1452-1457.

[52] Orrange, SE; Kawanishi, DT; Lopez, BM; Curry, SM, Rahimtoola, SH. Actuarial outcome after catheter balloon commissurotomy in patients with mitral stenosis. *Circulation*. 1997 Jan 21;95:382-389.

[53] Iung, B; Garbarz, E; Michaud, P; Helou, S; Farah, B; Berdah, P, et al. Late results of percutaneous mitral commissurotomy in a series of 1024 patients. Analysis of late clinical deterioration: frequency, anatomic findings, and predictive factors. *Circulation*. 1999 Jun 29;99:3272-3278.

[54] Song, JK; Song, JM; Kang, DH; Yun, SC; Park, DW; Lee, SW, et al. Restenosis and adverse clinical events after successful percutaneous mitral valvuloplasty: immediate post-procedural mitral valve area as an important prognosticator. *Eur Heart J*. 2009 May;30:1254-1262.

[55] Rowe, JC; Bland, EF; Sprague, HB, White, PD. The course of mitral stenosis without surgery: ten- and twenty-year perspectives. *Ann Intern Med*. 1960 Apr;52:741-749.

[56] Olesen, KH. The natural history of 271 patients with mitral stenosis under medical treatment. *Br Heart J.* 1962 May;24:349-357.

[57] Horstkotte, D; Niehues, R, Strauer, BE. Pathomorphological aspects, aetiology and natural history of acquired mitral valve stenosis. *Eur Heart J.* 1991 Jul;12 Suppl B:55-60.

[58] Chandrashekhar, Y; Westaby, S, Narula, J. Mitral stenosis. *Lancet.* 2009 Oct 10;374:1271-1283.

[59] Wang, A; Krasuski, RA; Warner, JJ; Pieper, K; Kisslo, KB; Bashore, TM, et al. Serial echocardiographic evaluation of restenosis after successful percutaneous mitral commissurotomy. *J Am Coll Cardiol.* 2002 Jan 16;39:328-334.

[60] Langerveld, J; Thijs Plokker, HW; Ernst, SM; Kelder, JC, Jaarsma, W. Predictors of clinical events or restenosis during follow-up after percutaneous mitral balloon valvotomy. *Eur Heart J.* 1999 Apr;20:519-526.

[61] Shaw, TR; Sutaria, N, Prendergast, B. Clinical and haemodynamic profiles of young, middle aged, and elderly patients with mitral stenosis undergoing mitral balloon valvotomy. *Heart.* 2003 Dec;89:1430-1436.

[62] Leon, MN; Harrell, LC; Simosa, HF; Mahdi, NA; Pathan, A; Lopez-Cuellar, J, et al. Mitral balloon valvotomy for patients with mitral stenosis in atrial fibrillation: immediate and long-term results. *J Am Coll Cardiol.* 1999 Oct;34:1145-1152.

[63] Turi, ZG; Reyes, VP; Raju, BS; Raju, AR; Kumar, DN; Rajagopal, P, et al. Percutaneous balloon versus surgical closed commissurotomy for mitral stenosis. A prospective, randomized trial. *Circulation.* 1991 Apr;83:1179-1185.

[64] Reyes, VP; Raju, BS; Wynne, J; Stephenson, LW; Raju, R; Fromm, BS, et al. Percutaneous balloon valvuloplasty compared with open surgical commissurotomy for mitral stenosis. *N Engl J Med.* 1994 Oct 13;331:961-967.

[65] Ben Farhat, M; Ayari, M; Maatouk, F; Betbout, F; Gamra, H; Jarra, M, et al. Percutaneous balloon versus surgical closed and open mitral commissurotomy: seven-year follow-up results of a randomized trial. *Circulation.* 1998 Jan 27;97:245-250.

[66] Song, JK; Kim, MJ; Yun, SC; Choo, SJ; Song, JM; Song, H, et al. Long-term outcomes of percutaneous mitral balloon valvuloplasty versus open cardiac surgery. *J Thorac Cardiovasc Surg.* 2010 Jan;139:103-110.

[67] Rahimtoola, SH; Durairaj, A; Mehra, A, Nuno, I. Current evaluation and management of patients with mitral stenosis. *Circulation.* 2002 Sep 3;106:1183-1188.

[68] Faletra, F; Pezzano, A, Jr.; Fusco, R; Mantero, A; Corno, R; Crivellaro, W, et al. Measurement of mitral valve area in mitral stenosis: four echocardiographic methods compared with direct measurement of anatomic orifices. *J Am Coll Cardiol.* 1996 Nov 1;28:1190-1197.

[69] Baumgartner, H; Hung, J; Bermejo, J; Chambers, JB; Evangelista, A; Griffin, BP, et al. Echocardiographic assessment of valve stenosis: EAE/ASE recommendations for clinical practice. *Eur J Echocardiogr.* 2009 Jan;10:1-25.

[70] Zamorano, J; Cordeiro, P; Sugeng, L; Perez de Isla, L; Weinert, L; Macaya, C, et al. Real-time three-dimensional echocardiography for rheumatic mitral valve stenosis evaluation: an accurate and novel approach. *J Am Coll Cardiol.* 2004 Jun 2;43:2091-2096.

[71] Sebag, IA; Morgan, JG; Handschumacher, MD; Marshall, JE; Nesta, F; Hung, J, et al. Usefulness of three-dimensionally guided assessment of mitral stenosis using matrix-array ultrasound. *Am J Cardiol*. 2005 Oct 15;96:1151-1156.

[72] Messika-Zeitoun, D; Brochet, E; Holmin, C; Rosenbaum, D; Cormier, B; Serfaty, JM, et al. Three-dimensional evaluation of the mitral valve area and commissural opening before and after percutaneous mitral commissurotomy in patients with mitral stenosis. *Eur Heart J*. 2007 Jan;28:72-79.

[73] Karp, K; Teien, D; Bjerle, P, Eriksson, P. Reassessment of valve area determinations in mitral stenosis by the pressure half-time method: impact of left ventricular stiffness and peak diastolic pressure difference. *J Am Coll Cardiol*. 1989 Mar 1;13:594-599.

[74] Messika-Zeitoun, D; Meizels, A; Cachier, A; Scheuble, A; Fondard, O; Brochet, E, et al. Echocardiographic evaluation of the mitral valve area before and after percutaneous mitral commissurotomy: the pressure half-time method revisited. *J Am Soc Echocardiogr*. 2005 Dec;18:1409-1414.

[75] Nakatani, S; Masuyama, T; Kodama, K; Kitabatake, A; Fujii, K, Kamada, T. Value and limitations of Doppler echocardiography in the quantification of stenotic mitral valve area: comparison of the pressure half-time and the continuity equation methods. *Circulation*. 1988 Jan;77:78-85.

[76] Messika-Zeitoun, D; Fung Yiu, S; Cormier, B; Iung, B; Scott, C; Vahanian, A, et al. Sequential assessment of mitral valve area during diastole using colour M-mode flow convergence analysis: new insights into mitral stenosis physiology. *Eur Heart J*. 2003 Jul;24:1244-1253.

[77] Wilkins, GT; Weyman, AE; Abascal, VM; Block, PC, Palacios, IF. Percutaneous balloon dilatation of the mitral valve: an analysis of echocardiographic variables related to outcome and the mechanism of dilatation. *Br Heart J*. 1988 Oct;60:299-308.

[78] Vahanian, A; Michel, PL; Cormier, B; Vitoux, B; Michel, X; Slama, M, et al. Results of percutaneous mitral commissurotomy in 200 patients. *Am J Cardiol*. 1989 Apr 1;63:847-852.

[79] Miche, E; Bogunovic, N; Fassbender, D; Baller, D; Gleichmann, U; Mannebach, H, et al. Predictors of unsuccessful outcome after percutaneous mitral valvulotomy including a new echocardiographic scoring system. *J Heart Valve Dis*. 1996 Jul;5:430-435.

[80] Fatkin, D; Roy, P; Morgan, JJ, Feneley, MP. Percutaneous balloon mitral valvotomy with the Inoue single-balloon catheter: commissural morphology as a determinant of outcome. *J Am Coll Cardiol*. 1993 Feb;21:390-397.

[81] Padial, LR; Freitas, N; Sagie, A; Newell, JB; Weyman, AE; Levine, RA, et al. Echocardiography can predict which patients will develop severe mitral regurgitation after percutaneous mitral valvulotomy. *J Am Coll Cardiol*. 1996 Apr;27:1225-1231.

[82] Nobuyoshi, M; Hamasaki, N; Kimura, T; Nosaka, H; Yokoi, H; Yasumoto, H, et al. Indications, complications, and short-term clinical outcome of percutaneous transvenous mitral commissurotomy. *Circulation*. 1989 Oct;80:782-792.

[83] Cannan, CR; Nishimura, RA; Reeder, GS; Ilstrup, DR; Larson, DR; Holmes, DR, et al. Echocardiographic assessment of commissural calcium: a simple predictor of outcome after percutaneous mitral balloon valvotomy. *J Am Coll Cardiol*. 1997 Jan;29:175-180.

[84] Sutaria, N; Shaw, TR; Prendergast, B, Northridge, D. Transoesophageal echocardiographic assessment of mitral valve commissural morphology predicts outcome after balloon mitral valvotomy. *Heart*. 2006 Jan;92:52-57]

[85] Black, IW; Hopkins, AP; Lee, LC, Walsh, WF. Left atrial spontaneous echo contrast: a clinical and echocardiographic analysis. *J Am Coll Cardiol*. 1991 Aug;18:398-404.

[86] Picano, E; Pibarot, P; Lancellotti, P; Monin, JL, Bonow, RO. The emerging role of exercise testing and stress echocardiography in valvular heart disease. *J Am Coll Cardiol*. 2009 Dec 8;54:2251-2260.

[87] Lin, SJ; Brown, PA; Watkins, MP; Williams, TA; Lehr, KA; Liu, W, et al. Quantification of stenotic mitral valve area with magnetic resonance imaging and comparison with Doppler ultrasound. *J Am Coll Cardiol*. 2004 Jul 7;44:133-137.

[88] Messika-Zeitoun, D; Serfaty, JM; Laissy, JP; Berhili, M; Brochet, E; Iung, B, et al. Assessment of the mitral valve area in patients with mitral stenosis by multislice computed tomography. *J Am Coll Cardiol*. 2006 Jul 18;48:411-413.

[89] Vahanian, A; Baumgartner, H; Bax, J; Butchart, E; Dion, R; Filippatos, G, et al. Guidelines on the management of valvular heart disease: The Task Force on the Management of Valvular Heart Disease of the European Society of Cardiology. *Eur Heart J*. 2007 Jan;28:230-268.

[90] Bonow, RO; Carabello, BA; Chatterjee, K; de Leon, AC, Jr.; Faxon, DP; Freed, MD, et al. 2008 Focused update incorporated into the ACC/AHA 2006 guidelines for the management of patients with valvular heart disease: a report of the American College of Cardiology/American Heart Association Task Force on Practice Guidelines (Writing Committee to Revise the 1998 Guidelines for the Management of Patients With Valvular Heart Disease): endorsed by the Society of Cardiovascular Anesthesiologists, Society for Cardiovascular Angiography and Interventions, and Society of Thoracic Surgeons. *Circulation*. 2008 Oct 7;118:e523-661.

[91] Dubin, AA; March, HW; Cohn, K, Selzer, A. Longitudinal hemodynamic and clinical study of mitral stenosis. *Circulation*. 1971 Sep;44:381-389.

[92] Gordon, SP; Douglas, PS; Come, PC, Manning, WJ. Two-dimensional and Doppler echocardiographic determinants of the natural history of mitral valve narrowing in patients with rheumatic mitral stenosis: implications for follow-up. *J Am Coll Cardiol*. 1992 Apr;19:968-973.

[93] Sagie, A; Freitas, N; Padial, LR; Leavitt, M; Morris, E; Weyman, AE, et al. Doppler echocardiographic assessment of long-term progression of mitral stenosis in 103 patients: valve area and right heart disease. *J Am Coll Cardiol*. 1996 Aug;28:472-479.

[94] Stefanadis, C; Dernellis, J; Stratos, C; Tsiamis, E; Vlachopoulos, C; Toutouzas, K, et al. Effects of balloon mitral valvuloplasty on left atrial function in mitral stenosis as assessed by pressure-area relation. *J Am Coll Cardiol*. 1998 Jul;32:159-168.

[95] Cormier, B; Vahanian, A; Iung, B; Porte, JM; Dadez, E; Lazarus, A, et al. Influence of percutaneous mitral commissurotomy on left atrial spontaneous contrast of mitral stenosis. *Am J Cardiol*. 1993 Apr 1;71:842-847.

[96] Porte, JM; Cormier, B; Iung, B; Dadez, E; Starkman, C; Nallet, O, et al. Early assessment by transesophageal echocardiography of left atrial appendage function after percutaneous mitral commissurotomy. *Am J Cardiol*. 1996 Jan 1;77:72-76.

[97] Zaki, A; Salama, M; El Masry, M; Abou-Freikha, M; Abou-Ammo, D; Sweelum, M, et al. Immediate effect of balloon valvuloplasty on hemostatic changes in mitral stenosis. *Am J Cardiol*. 2000 Feb 1;85:370-375.

[98] Krasuski, RA; Assar, MD; Wang, A; Kisslo, KB; Pierce, C; Harrison, JK, et al. Usefulness of percutaneous balloon mitral commissurotomy in preventing the

development of atrial fibrillation in patients with mitral stenosis. *Am J Cardiol.* 2004 Apr 1;93:936-939.

[99] Chiang, CW; Lo, SK; Ko, YS; Cheng, NJ; Lin, PJ, Chang, CH. Predictors of systemic embolism in patients with mitral stenosis. A prospective study. *Ann Intern Med.* 1998 Jun 1;128:885-889.

[100] Chen, WJ; Chen, MF; Liau, CS; Wu, CC, Lee, YT. Safety of percutaneous transvenous balloon mitral commissurotomy in patients with mitral stenosis and thrombus in the left atrial appendage. *Am J Cardiol.* 1992 Jul 1;70:117-119.

[101] Shaw, TR; Northridge, DB, Sutaria, N. Mitral balloon valvotomy and left atrial thrombus. *Heart.* 2005 Aug;91:1088-1089.

[102] Silaruks, S; Thinkhamrop, B; Kiatchoosakun, S; Wongvipaporn, C, Tatsanavivat, P. Resolution of left atrial thrombus after 6 months of anticoagulation in candidates for percutaneous transvenous mitral commissurotomy. *Ann Intern Med.* 2004 Jan 20;140:101-105.

[103] Hammermeister, K; Sethi, GK; Henderson, WG; Grover, FL; Oprian, C, Rahimtoola, SH. Outcomes 15 years after valve replacement with a mechanical versus a bioprosthetic valve: final report of the Veterans Affairs randomized trial. *J Am Coll Cardiol.* 2000 Oct;36:1152-1158.

[104] Oxenham, H; Bloomfield, P; Wheatley, DJ; Lee, RJ; Cunningham, J; Prescott, RJ, et al. Twenty year comparison of a Bjork-Shiley mechanical heart valve with porcine bioprostheses. *Heart.* 2003 Jul;89:715-721.

[105] Vahanian, A, Palacios, IF. Percutaneous approaches to valvular disease. *Circulation.* 2004 Apr 6;109:1572-1579.

[106] Hameed, A; Karaalp, IS; Tummala, PP; Wani, OR; Canetti, M; Akhter, MW, et al. The effect of valvular heart disease on maternal and fetal outcome of pregnancy. *J Am Coll Cardiol.* 2001 Mar 1;37:893-899.

[107] Arnoni, RT; Arnoni, AS; Bonini, RC; de Almeida, AF; Neto, CA; Dinkhuysen, JJ, et al. Risk factors associated with cardiac surgery during pregnancy. *Ann Thorac Surg.* 2003 Nov;76:1605-1608.

[108] Iung, B; Cormier, B; Elias, J; Michel, PL; Nallet, O; Porte, JM, et al. Usefulness of percutaneous balloon commissurotomy for mitral stenosis during pregnancy. *Am J Cardiol.* 1994 Feb 15;73:398-400.

[109] de Souza, JA; Martinez, EE, Jr.; Ambrose, JA; Alves, CM; Born, D; Buffolo, E, et al. Percutaneous balloon mitral valvuloplasty in comparison with open mitral valve commissurotomy for mitral stenosis during pregnancy. *J Am Coll Cardiol.* 2001 Mar 1;37:900-903.

[110] Oakley, C; Child, A; Iung, B; Presbitero, P, Tornos, P. Expert consensus document on management of cardiovascular diseases during pregnancy. *Eur Heart J.* 2003 April;24:761-781.

[111] Iung, B; Baron, G; Tornos, P; Gohlke-Barwolf, C; Butchart, EG, Vahanian, A. Valvular heart disease in the community: a European experience. *Curr Probl Cardiol.* 2007 Nov;32:609-661.

[112] Tuzcu, EM; Block, PC; Griffin, BP; Newell, JB, Palacios, IF. Immediate and long-term outcome of percutaneous mitral valvotomy in patients 65 years and older. *Circulation.* 1992 Mar;85:963-971.

[113] Iung, B; Cormier, B; Farah, B; Nallet, O; Porte, JM; Michel, PL, et al. Percutaneous mitral commissurotomy in the elderly. *Eur Heart J.* 1995 Aug;16:1092-1099.
[114] Sutaria, N; Elder, AT, Shaw, TR. Long term outcome of percutaneous mitral balloon valvotomy in patients aged 70 and over. *Heart.* 2000 Apr;83:433-438.
[115] Hildick-Smith, DJ; Taylor, GJ, Shapiro, LM. Inoue balloon mitral valvuloplasty: long-term clinical and echocardiographic follow-up of a predominantly unfavourable population. *Eur Heart J.* 2000 Oct;21:1690-1697.
[116] Iung, B; Garbarz, E; Michaud, P; Mahdhaoui, A; Helou, S; Farah, B, et al. Percutaneous mitral commissurotomy for restenosis after surgical commissurotomy: late efficacy and implications for patient selection. *J Am Coll Cardiol.* 2000 Apr;35:1295-1302.
[117] Kim, JB; Ha, JW; Kim, JS; Shim, WH; Kang, SM; Ko, YG, et al. Comparison of long-term outcome after mitral valve replacement or repeated balloon mitral valvotomy in patients with restenosis after previous balloon valvotomy. *Am J Cardiol.* 2007 Jun 1;99:1571-1574.
[118] Davidson, CJ; Bashore, TM; Mickel, M, Davis, K. Balloon mitral commissurotomy after previous surgical commissurotomy. The National Heart, Lung, and Blood Institute Balloon Valvuloplasty Registry participants. *Circulation.* 1992 Jul;86:91-99.
[119] Fawzy, ME; Hassan, W; Shoukri, M; Al Sanei, A; Hamadanchi, A; El Dali, A, et al. Immediate and long-term results of mitral balloon valvotomy for restenosis following previous surgical or balloon mitral commissurotomy. *Am J Cardiol.* 2005 Oct 1;96:971-975.
[120] Iung, B; Garbarz, E; Michaud, P; Fondard, O; Helou, S; Kamblock, J, et al. Immediate and mid-term results of repeat percutaneous mitral commissurotomy for restenosis following earlier percutaneous mitral commissurotomy. *Eur Heart J.* 2000 Oct;21:1683-1689.
[121] Pathan, AZ; Mahdi, NA; Leon, MN; Lopez-Cuellar, J; Simosa, H; Block, PC, et al. Is redo percutaneous mitral balloon valvuloplasty (PMV) indicated in patients with post-PMV mitral restenosis? *J Am Coll Cardiol.* 1999 Jul;34:49-54.
[122] Carapetis, JR. Rheumatic heart disease in Asia. *Circulation.* 2008 Dec 16;118:2748-2753.
[123] Essop, MR, Nkomo, VT. Rheumatic and nonrheumatic valvular heart disease: epidemiology, management, and prevention in Africa. *Circulation.* 2005 Dec 6;112:3584-3591.
[124] Marijon, E; Ou, P; Celermajer, DS; Ferreira, B; Mocumbi, AO; Jani, D, et al. Prevalence of rheumatic heart disease detected by echocardiographic screening. *N Engl J Med.* 2007 Aug 2;357:470-476.
[125] Soler-Soler, J, Galve, E. Worldwide perspective of valve disease. *Heart.* 2000 Jun;83:721-725.
[126] Gamra, H; Betbout, F; Ben Hamda, K; Addad, F; Maatouk, F; Dridi, Z, et al. Balloon mitral commissurotomy in juvenile rheumatic mitral stenosis: a ten-year clinical and echocardiographic actuarial results. *Eur Heart J.* 2003 Jul;24:1349-1356.
[127] Fawzy, ME; Stefadouros, MA; Hegazy, H; Shaer, FE; Chaudhary, MA, Fadley, FA. Long term clinical and echocardiographic results of mitral balloon valvotomy in children and adolescents. *Heart.* 2005 Jun;91:743-748.

[128] Aggarwal, N; Suri, V; Goyal, A; Malhotra, S; Manoj, R, Dhaliwal, RS. Closed mitral valvotomy in pregnancy and labor. *Int J Gynaecol Obstet*. 2005 Feb;88:118-121.

[129] Marijon, E; Iung, B; Mocumbi, AO; Kamblock, J; Thanh, CV; Gamra, H, et al. What are the differences in presentation of candidates for percutaneous mitral commissurotomy across the world and do they influence the results of the procedure? *Arch Cardiovasc Dis*. 2008 Oct;101:611-617.

[130] Iung, B; Garbarz, E; Doutrelant, L; Berdah, P; Michaud, P; Farah, B, et al. Late results of percutaneous mitral commissurotomy for calcific mitral stenosis. *Am J Cardiol*. 2000 Jun 1;85:1308-1314.

Endovascular Stents

In: Percutaneous Valve Technology: Present and Future
ISBN: 978-1-61942-577-4
Editors: Jose Luis Navia and Sharif Al-Ruzzeh

Chapter XXV

Aortic Stent Grafts

Turki B. Albacker and Eric E. Roselli

Introduction

The development of minimally invasive endovascular technology has initiated a paradigm shift in the treatment of thoracic aortic disease. A fundamental understanding of the science and engineering of endovascular stent grafts is key to their appropriate implementation in practice. Furthermore, the rapid influx of new devices requires practitioners to make their decisions based on the relative strengths and weaknesses of the various products. Shape, wire thickness, coating, graft material selection, and imaging are just a few of the factors to consider in stent graft design. The ideal stent graft and delivery system would include the following characteristics: easy pushability, trackability, a high expansion ratio, low profile, and the ability to negotiate tight lesions and a tortuous course. The material needs to be biocompatible and resistant to thrombosis, stenosis, migration, and external compression. Although current designs continue to show significant advancements, there are clearly no ideal stent grafts. Each device has merits and drawbacks that need to be tailored to a specific clinical application.

History

Dotter developed the first arterial stent in 1969, and his technique was directed at the treatment of arterial occlusive disease. In 1976, Parodi began development of a device for endovascular treatment of abdominal aortic aneurysms [1]. Two initial prototypes were hindered by a high failure rate. Simultaneously, other researchers were attempting endovascular aneurysm repair in animal renal artery and aortic models. Palmaz then made a significant breakthrough with his balloon expandable stent [2]. With this technology, Parodi was able to renew his endovascular project in 1988. The balloon expandable stent of Palmaz was attached to knitted Dacron grafts, which Parodi used in his report of the first series of successful endovascular aneurysm repairs in humans [3]. Other surgeons were working on aortic stent-grafts at the same time [4]. However, the first stent grafts were awkward and difficult to use [5].

Evolution of Aortic Stent Grafts

The first experiences with endovascular aortic stent-grafts in the early 1990s were associated with significant complications including inability to deploy the stent-graft, conversion to open surgery, and aneurysm rupture. By the mid-1990s, improved homemade and commercially available stent-grafts started to appear. These devices could achieve aneurysm exclusion with low morbidity and mortality. Devices, procedural techniques, and patient selection have evolved substantially since the initial endovascular procedure described by Parodi et al in 1991 [3]. In 2004 and 2005, the results of a randomized trial comparing endovascular aneurysm repair with open surgery for infra-renal aneurysms concluded that endovascular aneurysm repair was superior to open surgical repair in fit patients with respect to aneurysm-related death at 30 days and persisted through 4 years of follow-up [6-8]. Longer follow-up results, however, raised concerns about durability due to late stent fractures, migration, and aneurysm ruptures. In the large EUROSTAR registry of stent-grafts for abdominal aneurysms the secondary intervention rate reached almost 40 percent at 4 years, but these results were achieved with earlier generation devices [9]. Gradually, these problems have been addressed, and in the recent UK multi-centre randomized controlled trial of endovascular versus open aneurysm repair, the secondary intervention rate was reduced to 20 per cent in the endovascular group 4 years following surgery [8].

Thoracic Endovascular Stent-Grafts

Similar technologies to those used for abdominal aneurysms have been adapted to treat thoracic aortic pathology. Similar yet less convincing evidence with lower risks of morbidity and comparable mortality as compared to open repair through 1 year of follow-up supports their use [10].

The Gore TAG Thoracic Endograft

The Gore TAG thoracic endograft (Figure 1) received Food and Drug Administration (FDA) approval in March 2005, making it the first commercially available thoracic endograft in the United States. A unique feature of the Gore stent-graft system is that it is self-contained on the deliver system with the graft axially compressed onto the end of the delivery catheter and constrained by a PTFE corset laced with PTFE suture. The suture runs the length of the catheter and is attached to a deployment knob [11]. When the constraining suture is released the device opens from the center first then out to both ends simultaneously. This mechanism of expansion reduces the windsock effect and helps to improve the accuracy of delivery. Furthermore, deployment does not require delivery of the sheath above the diaphragm. The initial version of this device was porous and associated with type IV endoleaks pressurizing the aneurysm sac from flow across the graft material membrane. The current PTFE graft has a 30-micron inter-nodal distance similar to the pore size of conventional PTFE grafts used for peripheral vascular reconstructions, which has limited the issue of excessive porosity. The ends of the device have a scalloped contour to enhance graft contact with the aortic wall over a wide range of aortic tortuousities and angulations. The scalloped projections are covered with PTFE, and their length is directly proportional to the diameter of the graft. The device is very flexible radially and longitudinally.

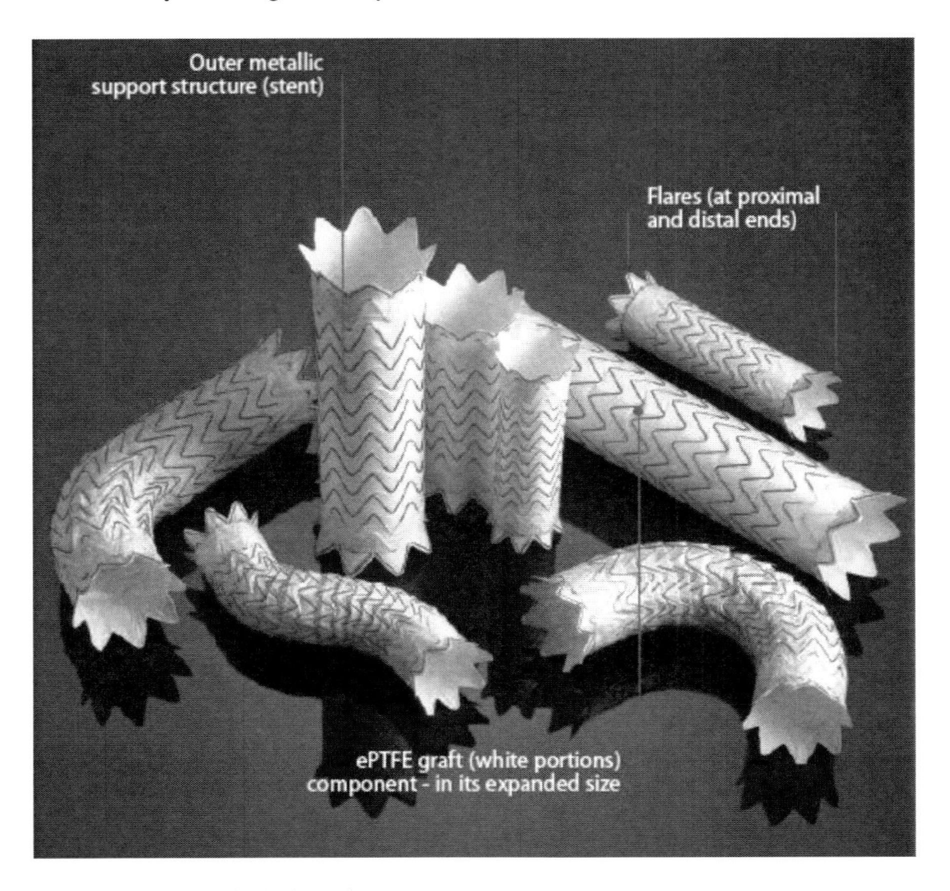

Figure 1. GOR TAG Thoracic Endograft.

Available devices range in diameter from 26 to 45 mm in increments of 2-3 mm, and in length from 10 to 20 cm. Depending on the diameter of the device they require a delivery sheath ranging in diameter from 20-24 Fr. The devices maybe be used in a modular fashion telescoping one within the next in either a proximal first or distal first manner. When placing a larger device within a smaller one, they must be within two sizes of each other (e.g. a 37 mm device may be placed within a 31 mm or 34 mm device but not into a 28 mm device). This flexibility allows for creating a tapered repair with differing diameters at proximal and distal ends, which may be tapered, or reverse tapered. The stability of the devices requires an overlap of at least 3 cm when placing a larger device within a smaller one and 5cm when placing same size grafts within each other.

The next generation system, the C-TAG is designed to be more conformable to the aortic arch where many patients require proximal landing zone stability. Furthermore, the nitinol frame has been enhanced to increase radial force at the ends to address the issue of the rare but devastating complication of device collapse that has been reported to occur in patients where the device is oversized for the intended vessel diameter.

Also, the proximal flared components extend a shorter distance from the area of circumferential fabric coverage. Other iterations of this system, which are under investigation, include a device with a branch for the left subclavian artery.

Medtronic Endografts

Since the first implant in Australia in 1996, Medtronic Vascular (Santa Rosa, California) has been the market leader in sales of thoracic endografts worldwide. The Talent device was approved for commercial use in the United States in 2008. The third generation Valiant device was first introduced in Europe in 2005, and represents an improved version of the Talent device.

The TALENT Device

The Talent device is a preloaded stent graft incorporated into its own delivery system (CoilTrac). It is composed of a polyester graft (Dacron; C.R. Bard, Haverhill, Pennsylvania) sewn to a self-expanding nitinol wire frame skeleton. Radiopaque "figure-of-8" markers are sewn to the graft material to aid in visualization during fluoroscopy.

The CoilTrac delivery system is push rod based. Preloaded onto an inner catheter, the Talent device is deployed by pulling back an outer catheter, allowing the device to self-expand and contour to the aorta. A balloon may be used to ensure proper apposition of the graft to the aneurysmal aorta after deployment.

The Talent device is a modular system; ranging in diameter from 22 to 46 mm but the lengths of the devices are fixed around 11 cm ranging from 112 to 116 mm. To accommodate the size differences often found between the proximal and distal portions of the aorta, tapered grafts are available with a four-millimeter difference in diameter between proximal and distal ends.

All of the tapered devices are larger on the proximal end than the distal end. Four configuration categories are available: proximal main, proximal extension, distal main, and distal extension.

The extension pieces are shorter at around 5.5 cm. The distal configurations are offered with or without a bare-spring design (FreeFlo), which allows placement of the device across the origins of the celiac artery distally for infra-celiac fixation [11]. All of the proximal main pieces have a bare stent, which allows for supra-subclavian extension into the arch. The proximal bare stent on the Talent device has five peaks with a significant amount of radial force (Figure 2).

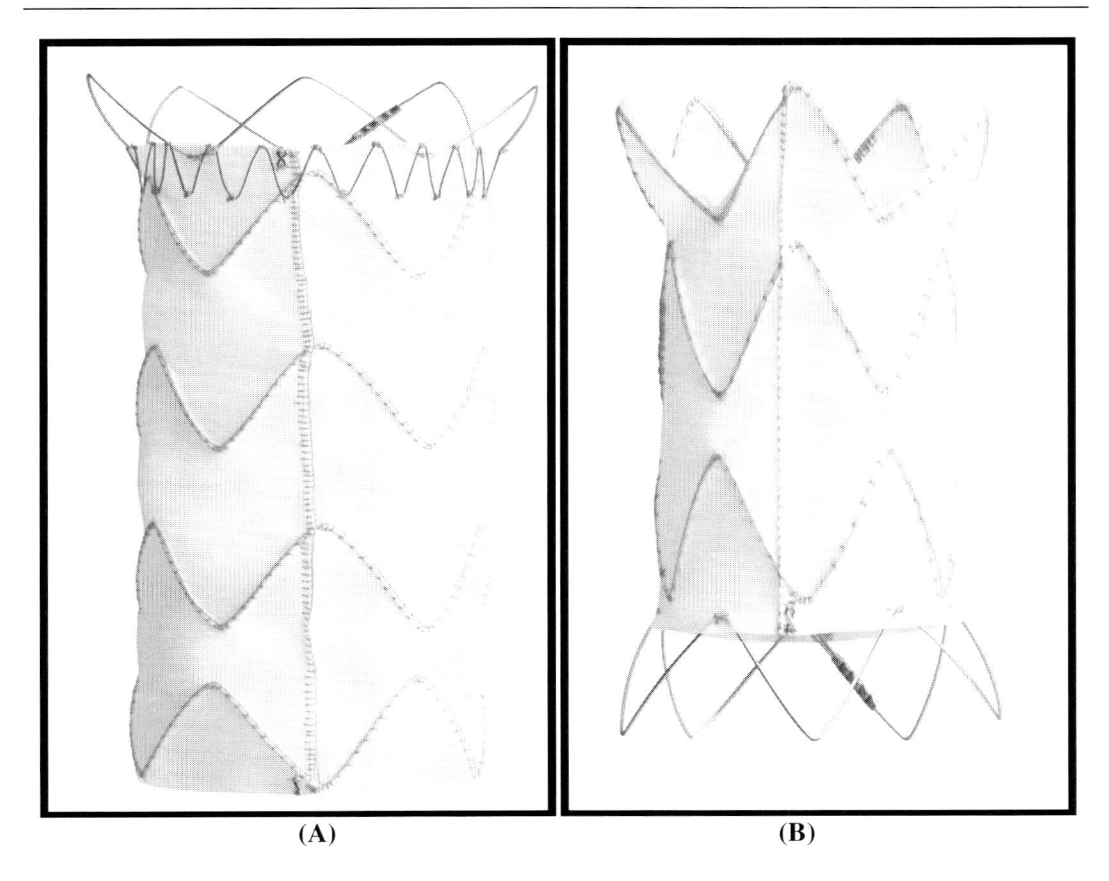

Figure 2. Medtronic Talent Thoracic Endograft. A) Proximal component, B) Distal component.

The VALIANT Device

The Valiant device is a modified design based on the experience with the Talent device. Like its predecessor, the Valiant device is also a preloaded stent-graft made of the same polyester graft built onto a self-expanding nitinol skeleton. Modifications have been made to improve trackability, conformability, and deployment. First, device lengths have been increased to a maximum of 230 mm. Because the device is a self-contained system, each piece requires individual deployment through the access vessel, resulting in repeated catheter exchanges in the artery.

Longer lengths minimize device exchanges needed during deployment when treating an extended length of thoracic aorta. Second, the connecting bar has been removed in the Valiant device for improved conformability, especially in the arch. Third, the number of bare springs at the proximal and distal ends of the device has been increased from 5 to 8 to improve circumferential force distribution and fixation along the aortic wall. Critics of the 5-spoked design cite cases where proximal dissection has occurred due to focal trauma from the bare stents.

Finally, the delivery system has been modified. to provide a more comfortable deployment mechanism.

As opposed to a simple pullback unsheathing mechanism, deployment of the new delivery system (Xcelerant) includes a gearing, ratchet-like mechanism in the handle to allow easy deployment. The amount of force required to deploy the device is reduced significantly without compromising the precision of the deployment. Like the Talent device, the Valiant device is a modular design.

Eighty-eight different configurations are available, ranging in diameter from 24 to 46 mm and covering lengths from 100 mm to 230 mm. The delivery systems ranges in diameter from 20-25 Fr. Four configuration categories are available: proximal FreeFlo straight component, proximal closed-web straight component, proximal closed-web tapered component, and distal bare-spring straight component [11].

Cook Zenith Endografts

The Cook Zenith TX1 and TX2 thoracic endovascular grafts (Cook Inc, Bloomington, Indiana) were developed in the context of a worldwide collaborative effort based on open and endovascular experience.

The devices, commercially available in Australia since 2001 and in Europe and Canada since 2004, are founded on the platform of the Zenith abdominal aortic aneurysm graft. The design consists of self-expanding stainless steel Z-stents and full thickness polyester fabric (Figure 3). The Zenith endograft is introduced through a preloaded catheter with trigger wires for graduated deployment.

The proximal and distal ends of the stent-grafts have terminal barbs to provide a mode of active fixation in addition to the radial force of the stents. The Z-stents on either end of the devices are internal to optimize sealing of the cloth to the aorta and adjacent devices. The remaining stents are external. The graft material is flush with the edge of the stents on both ends of the proximal components. The distal components have a bare uncovered stent to allow extended fixation across the celiac artery. The stents are attached to the fabric with large gaps (6 mm, 8 mm, or 10 mm, depending on device diameter) to provide flexibility of the device.

The diameter ranges from 22 to 42 mm and the lengths range from 127 mm to 216 mm. Unique to the Zenith system is the staged delivery. After introducing and releasing the proximal component out of the delivery catheter the proximal most stent is not fully expanded until the trigger wire is released. This allows for fine adjustments in the positioning before the bare metal barbs are released. The devices are used in a modular fashion and also come in a tapered configuration with a 4mm reduction in diameter from proximal to distal. . Extension cuffs are also available in shorter lengths (77 to 80 mm), with or without barbs. The sheath has a hydrophilic coating and is braided and exceptionally flexible and kink-resistant. Sheath size is from 20 F to 24 F, depending on the maximal stent diameter. The latest delivery mechanism has been modified to release the most proximal stent in such a way as to conform more closely to the curve of the distal aortic arch.

Next generation Zenith LP devices are currently under investigation and are significantly reduced in diameter (LP=low profile) with delivery systems ranging in size from 16-18 Fr. To allow for this change, the new stent graft has nitinol stents instead of stainless steel and slightly thinner graft material. Because of the elastic properties of the nitinol, this device will have a proximal uncovered stent. Diameter and length measurements are unchanged.

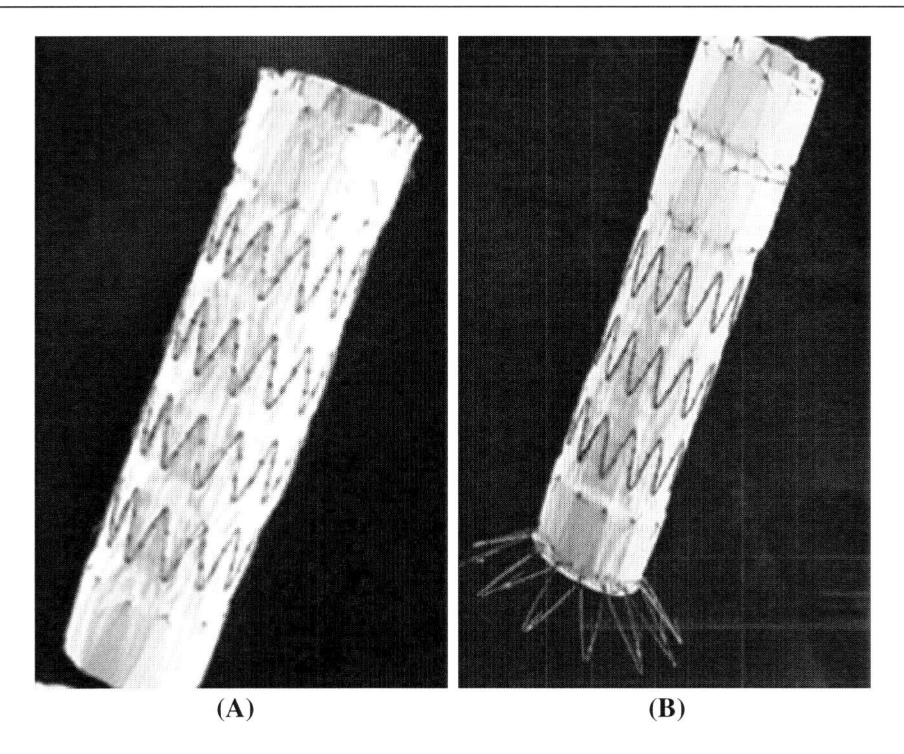

Figure 3. COOK ZENITH Thoracic Endograft. A) Proximal componenet, B) Distal component.

Bolton Relay Stent Graft

The latest player in the thoracic stent graft field is the Bolton Relay stent graft. This device is currently available under CE mark and has recently completed patient enrollment in the United States pivotal trial. It is a modular system comprised of self-expanding nitinol stents attached to woven Dacron.

The delivery system is unique in that it is made up of an inner fabric sheath surrounding the device contained within a more conventional sheath. The device has a ratcheted multi-step method of deployment such that the main sheath outermost sheath is first delivered into the distal thoracic aorta. The inner and more flexible fabric sheathed portion surrounding the device itself are then advanced more proximally into the area of interest and released separately.

A final top cap mechanism allows for final release of the proximal barest metal stent (Figure 4). The devices are available in a range of diameters between 22 and 46 mm and lengths up to 200 mm. The portfolio includes a tapered configuration and the delivery sheaths range in diameter from 20-25 Fr.

Next generation systems include a more low profile delivery sheath and investigational devices include branched graft systems and modified systems targeting the more proximal aortic arch and ascending aorta.

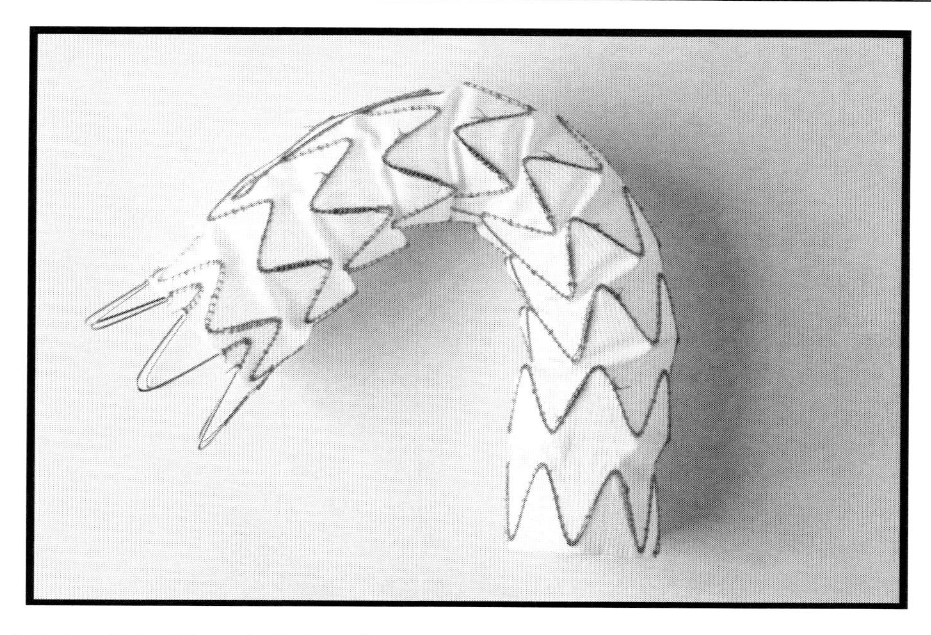

Figure 4. Bolton Relay Thoracic Endograft.

Graft Choice

All of the commercially available thoracic stent grafts are designed to treat focal aneurysms of the descending aorta with at least 2 cm of normal caliber and parallel contoured vessel landing zones at either end to allow for adequate fixation and sealing. Choice of devices is mostly user specific and related to experience but unique aspects of each device may drive the choice of one over the others. The proximal bare metal stent of the Talent device allows for extended coverage across the origin of the left subclavian or even left common carotid artery in cases where there is a short proximal neck. On the other hand, some have argued that the placement of bare metal stents in fragile proximal aorta may lead to retrograde aortic dissection. When placing a stent graft into the aortic arch with a very short landing zone it may be important to have the flush edge of fabric of the Zenith device to land at the intended site whereas the covered flares of the TAG device may compromise target vessel flow if they partially cover the origin. All of the devices are flexible enough to handle most tortuous segments of the aorta. The TAG device offers the additional advantage of being delivered sheathless to accommodate marginal caliber, calcified or tortuous access vessels. The variable graft lengths of the TAG and Zenith devices make it more efficient to treat patients with long aneurysms. In certain applications, such as aortic dissection, the relative radial force exerted by the prosthesis may be an important consideration. The radial strength of the TAG device is the lowest, the Talent is the highest, and the Zenith is intermediate. In the setting of aortic dissection, the lower hoop strength of the TAG may allow adequate coverage of the entry site without causing an iatrogenic secondary tear in the thin fragile dissection flap. On the other hand, the greater radial force of the Talent may be beneficial in cases of chronic dissection to optimize expansion of the true lumen diameter but the use of these devices in the setting of chronic aortic dissection with aneurysm is controversial [12].

Finally, diameter limitations are important. If the landing zone is 40-42 mm then only the largest Talent or Relay devices are indicated for adequate seal. The TAG is now also available in a 45 mm version. In the setting of traumatic transection the aortic diameter is often small and so the smallest TAG (26 mm) or Zenith (28 mm) devices may be excessively oversized whereas the Talent and Relay devices are available in smaller diameters.

Applications

It is clear that the ideal endovascular prosthesis is not yet available and it is unreasonable to expect that one device will be capable of optimally addressing all combinations of aortic pathologies, etiologies, morphologies, and vascular anatomy. The individual aspects of each case may dictate selection of the best-suited prosthesis from a medley of devices, and new iterations of available devices indicated for particular indications are currently undergoing investigation. In the following section a discussion of the various applications will be addressed from the simplest to the more controversial and investigational. Innovations in surgical approach and device design will be examined throughout.

Aneurysms of the Descending Thoracic Aorta

The indication for stent-grafting of a descending thoracic aortic aneurysm at the present time should be based on a predicted operative risk that is clearly lower than the risk of either conventional open repair or optimal medical management. It is well documented that isolated open replacement of the supra-diaphragmatic descending aorta can be safely accomplished in experienced centers, with mortality below 4% and prevalence of paraplegia of 2% to 4% across a wide range of patient ages. However, the morbidity of such a large operation may be prohibitive in high-risk patients. It is reasonable to conclude that for patients older than age 75 and patients with severe COPD; stent-grafting is the treatment of choice. Aneurysm morphology is also an important factor to consider when deciding for endovascular stenting. The short-term results of stent-grafting of saccular aneurysms are encouraging in several small series [13-17], and it may be ideally suited for these localized aneurysms because the aorta above and below the aneurysm is often relatively normal and a good landing zone for the stent-graft. The same is true for fusiform aneurysm involving the mid-descending thoracic aneurysm and those where there is a relatively long segment of healthy aorta on either side of the aneurysm.

Controversy exists as to when the limits of fixation should be breached. Although it is reasonable to cover the left subclavian artery in emergency or urgent indications with only slightly elevated risk, it is recommended to revascularize the left subclavian in situations of elective planned coverage. It is especially important for patients with patent internal mammary to coronary bypass grafts, or a dominant left vertebral artery. Furthermore, in patients with extensive aneurysmal disease who may have had previous aortic replacement or anticipated need for extensive aortic repair the risk of spinal cord injury may be elevated if the left subclavian collaterals are compromised. When extensive aortic replacement is expected, these patients should also undergo subclavian artery revascularization with left carotid to subclavian bypass, or arterial transposition reconstruction.

Similarly, largely anecdotal evidence has suggested that the celiac artery may be covered if necessary but the risk of visceral ischemia is more than negligible. In such situations consideration should be given to open repair, hybrid repair, or transfer of care to a center with access to branched graft technology (see below). If endovascular repair with celiac artery coverage is required in an emergency, thorough assessment of the superior mesenteric artery system and gastro-duodenal collaterals should be undertaken to more accurately assess the risk of celiac sacrifice. Rescue plans for open celiac revascularization should also be considered and these potential complications should be discussed with the patient and their family preoperatively.

Penetrating Aortic Ulcers

Early and midterm results of stent-grafting for penetrating ulcers are encouraging [18-23] primarily because they represent localized aortic pathology. When penetrating aortic ulceration is associated with intramural hematoma it should be treated as an acute aortic dissection. When it involves the proximal aorta, open aortic repair is recommended and when it involves the distal aorta it should be treated with best medical therapy when uncomplicated and endovascular stent grafting when associated with complications. Close follow-up with imaging is necessary in these patients as they are prone to develop saccular aneurysms.

Acute Traumatic Aortic Transections

In most trauma centers endovascular techniques have supplanted the open repair techniques to treat this life-threatening injury. Although it is estimated that most traumatic aortic transections die in the field due to exsanguination, those who survive the transport and resuscitation often have multiple injuries, which may be compounded by the increased morbidity of an open repair. Several series have been published documenting the safety and feasibility of the endovascular approach. In one multicenter study, 30 patients with chest trauma and multiple injuries (mean severity score = 62) underwent endovascular stent-grafting, with 100% successful implantation [24]. Two patients (6.7%) later died, 1 patient suffered a stroke (3.3%), and 1 (3.3%) had partial stent collapse. During a follow-up mean of 11.6 months, no endoleaks, migrations, or late pseudoaneurysms were observed. It is important to note that it is frequently necessary to cover the left subclavian artery to achieve an adequate proximal seal. In addition, device over sizing by more than 20% is contraindicated because the stent-graft may fold on itself and obstruct the aorta. Because many of these patients are young, the aorta is relatively small in diameter. This complication was more prevalent with the earlier experience when the TAG device was the only one commercially available and implanters were forced to place excessively oversized devices. With the availability of additional devices in smaller diameters and an increased awareness this complication has hopefully been eliminated.

It is also important to remember that the long-term durability of current stent graft technology is unknown, particularly in younger patients, especially one who has not yet reached full maturity. Further investigations are required to address these issues, but in the emergency setting of acute traumatic transection associated with multi-organ injury, endovascular repair is the first line treatment [25]. In the event that a survivor develops late complications associated with the stent graft they may undergo elective open reconstruction at a later date when it can be done more safely.

Acute Distal Aortic Dissections

Although none of the commercially available devices in the U.S. are indicated for use in dissections, there is growing worldwide experience with the procedure in this setting [26-30]. Patients presenting with acute type B dissection complicated by rupture or malperfusion are especially good candidates for TEVAR [31-32]. The goal of therapy in these patients is to improve distal perfusion and end-organ compromise. Successful management is predicated on obliteration of false lumen flow by placement of the prosthesis within the true lumen and complete fabric coverage across the primary entry tear of the intima. Stent-graft coverage closes proximal communication to the false lumen, and its flow is markedly reduced or eliminated. Additionally, radial force holding the true lumen open optimizes true lumen flow downstream. This treatment corrects any dynamic branch vessel obstruction within seconds after stent-graft placement. Stagnant blood in the thoracic aortic false lumen clots, and in the majority of patients, progressive thrombosis of the false lumen proceeds distally at least within the treated segment. In the event that there is static obstruction from false lumen thrombus formation near the origin of a branch vessel, additional stenting of the target vessels may be indicated. Over a period of weeks to months, the affected aorta will remodel and heal usually within the treated segment and sometimes beyond. The extent of this healing process is variable and based on the size of the aorta, branch vessel distribution off the aortic lumens, and the amount of residual retrograde perfusion. Depending on how much of this secondary goal of aortic remodeling is achieved, the late sequelae of aortic dissection may be reduced.

Initial results from the INSTEAD randomized trial [33] directed at the treatment of *un*complicated acute aortic dissection, the risks of the procedure are such that there was only benefit in a select group of patients. Although there was no significant difference between those randomized to stent grafts versus those getting best medical therapy, the patients who crossed-over from best medical therapy to receive the device faired well. Current recommendations are to limit the use of stent grafts in the setting of acute distal aortic dissection to patients who are complicated by malperfusion or otherwise demonstrate characteristics suggestive of late complications. The ADSORB trial is currently ongoing in Europe to readdress this question with a modification in device design [34].

Technically it is important to plan these procedures carefully because of the proximity of the primary entry tear to the aortic arch vessels and the fragility of the aorta in the acute setting. Retrograde dissection to the ascending aorta has been reported in as many as 3% of patients treated with TEVAR for acute dissection. Adequate sizing with a feasible landing zone is important and balloon dilatation should be avoided. Device selection may be based on more than one measurement, but the most important is the diameter of the non-dissected aorta immediately proximal to the entry tear. This is a good estimate of the original size of the proximal involved segment prior to the dissection. This measurement, plus an oversize factor of 10-20% to ensure secure anchoring and a tight circumferential seal, is the approximation most frequently used. It is important to implant a device that is long enough to cover the entry tear and extend around the curvature of the aortic isthmus. Typically this requires the use of a device at least 15 cm long. Others have argued that the repair should extend to the level of the celiac artery to promote remodeling of the aorta. Longer extension of the aortic repair into the distal one-third of the descending thoracic aorta, however, may increase the risk of spinal cord ischemia [28].

An investigational device based on the Zenith system is currently being evaluated to address some of these concerns. The Zenith dissection device has a proximal component very much like the existing system to cover the proximal entry tear. Beyond this, a flexible bare metal frame component without fabric is delivered into the more distally dissected aorta to provide expansile force upon the true lumen and promote healing of the downstream false lumen. These bare metal segments can be extended across the visceral branch vessels into the abdominal aorta if needed.

Subacute and Chronic Dissections

In chronic dissection, the most common late complication is false lumen aneurysmal enlargement. In survivors of the acute phase, there are usually many fenestrations between the true and the false channel, which allow the false lumen to remain pressurized. Even if a large primary or secondary intimal tear is successfully covered with a stent-graft and most of the false lumen clots there is usually a persistent dissection in the abdominal portion of the aorta. Furthermore, the small compressed true lumen and chronically scarred, thick, and less mobile dissection flap are less amenable to remodeling back into their pre-dissection state after stent grafting. Unless all of the false lumen heals, it is unlikely that stent-grafting can reliably prevent aortic rupture in cases of chronic aortic dissection over a time span extending beyond ten years. However, recent report of patients undergoing distal open aortic repair for chronic dissection also demonstrates less than desirable late outcomes with a freedom of death or reoperation of only around 50% [35]. Therefore, although the endovascular treatment of patients with chronic aortic dissection is controversial, it may be a reasonable option in patients at high risk for open surgery especially those with poor respiratory function or chronic renal dysfunction.

A meta-analysis performed by Eggebrecht and colleagues summarized the results of 39 published studies of endovascular stent-grafting in 609 patients with aortic dissection [36]. Of these, more than 42% had a subacute or chronic dissection, but the actual fraction of patients with acute (<14 days) dissections could not be determined accurately because of ambiguity in terminology used by various authors. Procedural success was achieved in 96%, with only 2.3% of patients requiring in-hospital surgical conversion. Overall, complications occurred less frequently in patients with chronic dissections than in those undergoing stent-graft placement for acute dissection (9% versus 22%, $p = 0.005$). Prevalence of neurologic complications was remarkably low: stroke, 1.2% and paraplegia, 0.5%. Operative mortality was significantly lower for those with chronic versus acute dissection (3% versus 10%, $p = 0.015$), with a trend toward better 1-year survival (93% versus 87%, $p = 0.088$). The long-term outcomes provided by future randomized studies will be of interest regarding the role of stent-grafting in these patients.

Treatment of Thoracoabdominal Aortic Aneurysms with Fenestrated and Branch Devices

Durable endovascular repair of the descending thoracic aorta requires fixation and seal in a parallel walled and normal segment of aorta. In some patients, achieving this goal requires extending aortic coverage into the aortic arch or visceral segment using custom-designed fenestrated or branched devices. Fenestrated stent-graft devices are currently approved for treatment of juxta-renal aneurysms in Europe and are currently available as part of an investigational study in the US (Figure 5). This technology has been expanded to devices used to treat thoracic aneurysms requiring fixation within the aortic arch or visceral segment of the aorta. Additionally, several case reports of homemade devices similar in design concept have been published.

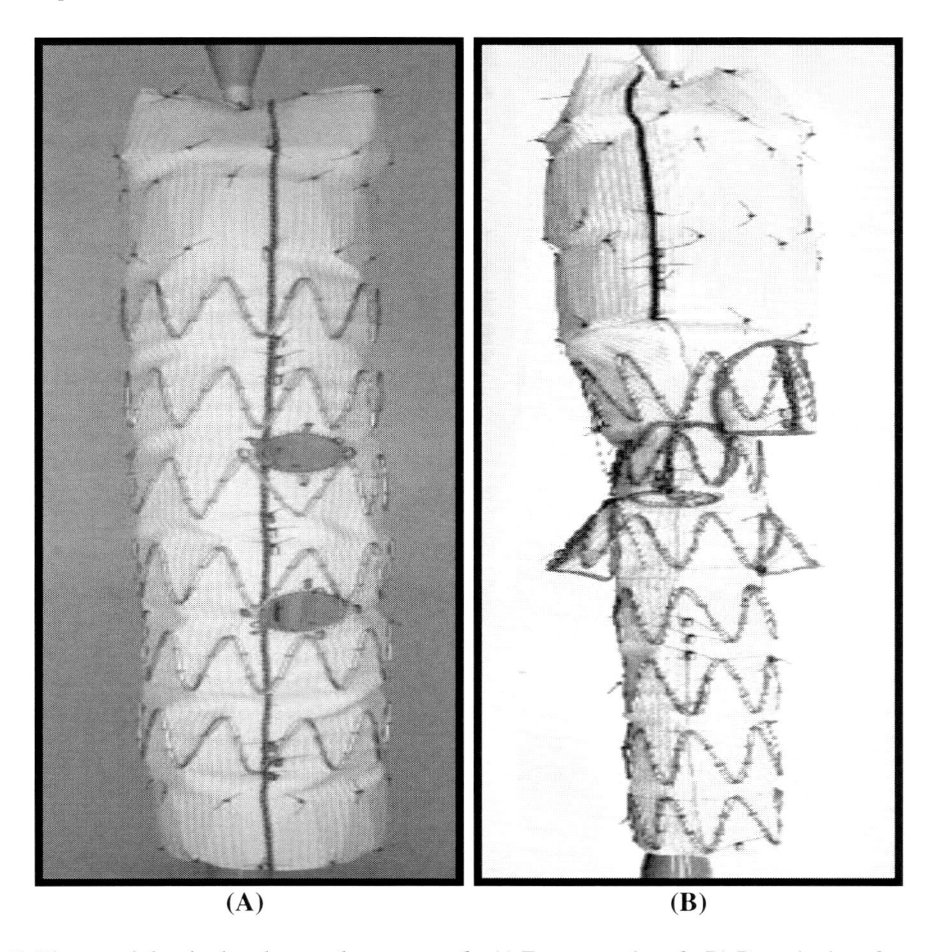

Figure 5. Thoracoabdominal endovascular stent graft. A) Fenestrated graft, B) Branched graft.

Current indications for use are for those patients with thoracic aneurysmal disease who would be at high risk for open surgical repair (usually owing to comorbid conditions) and whose anatomy is unsuitable for currently available commercial devices [37]. The proximal and distal extent of aneurysmal disease, fixation and sealing zones, luminal diameters, and precise relationships between the arch or visceral vessels are determined using three dimensional CT imaging techniques to plan the device design. Devices are modular in design, and the Zenith endograft system currently forms the basis of these devices. The main body of the device is first delivered into position in the aorta and the fenestrations or branches aligned with the target vessels. This main body component is then partially deployed without being completely released and access is obtained from the contralateral femoral artery into the branch vessels through the main device. The main body is then completely deployed and mated with a balloon expandable stent (fenestrated), balloon expandable stent-graft (reinforced fenestrated branch), or a self-expanding stent-graft (directional helical branch) for each of the target vessels. A given device may incorporate a combination of types of fenestrations and branches based on patient anatomy.

The advantages of branches over reinforced fenestrations include improved mating stent graft joint integrity and the potential to minimize the angle between the aorta and target vessel. However, a number of distinct disadvantages of this approach exist. The first relates to the need to achieve an aortic seal well above the branch origin.

This means that the amount of covered aorta, particularly in the setting of a type IV thoracoabdominal aneurysm, may exceed the amount of diseased aorta. This may result in a higher risk of paraplegia [38]. The second disadvantage relates to the need for space within the aneurysmal sac to accommodate all of the branches. If an aneurysm is not filled with thrombus, adequate room is generally available to deploy the device, cannulate the target arteries, and place mating stent grafts. However, in the setting of a small lumen (< 34 mm), the aorta can easily become overcrowded.

It has been suggested that the aortic component may be tapered through the visceral segment to create additional space and then reexpanded distal to the visceral segment. This especially becomes an issue when trying to use these devices in patients with chronic dissections where the true lumen may be too small in diameter to accommodate the precise placement of the custom made device.

In a recently reported series of 119 patients receiving fenestrated devices to treat juxtarenal aneurysms successful deployment was achieved in all, with no acute vessel loss. There was 1 death within 30 days, and actuarial survival was 92%, 83%, and 79% at 12, 24, and 36 months, respectively.

There were no ruptures or conversions, and a single aneurysm growth secondary to a type II endoleak was later successfully treated. At 24 months, aneurysm size had decreased by more than 5 mm in 77% of patients [39]. Outcomes for the investigational branched devices used to treat high-risk, thoracoabdominal aortic aneurysm at the Cleveland Clinic has also been reported in the first 73 patients [37]. Clear benefits of this approach included limited pulmonary complications, less pain, decreased transfusion requirements, shorter lengths of stay, and more rapid recoveries.

Only 2 of 73 patients developed paraplegia, both of which ultimately required tracheostomies, after endovascular repair. Given a preoperative need for supplemental home oxygen in 20% of the patients and the fact that nearly half of all patients had been diagnosed with severe chronic obstructive pulmonary disease, the lack of major pulmonary issues is impressive. The overall mean length of stay was 9 days, and only 5 days for the more than half of patients who did not suffer any complications.

Mycotic Aneurysms

Stent grafts have been used to manage patients with mycotic aneurysms as evidenced by many reports describing successful short-term results in very small numbers of patients. However, the concept of leaving a foreign body in an infected artery violates the surgical principles of treating infection. Nonetheless, many of these patients are too sick to undergo the extensive open surgical repair and so endovascular therapies have been utilized with limited success. Mostly stent grafts have been used in patients with infections as a temporary measure in patients with life threatening complications from the infection such as rupture and associated sepsis. Patients who have had a reasonable outcome have been those with aorto-pulmonary fistulas due to communication with the lung parenchyma. Patients with aorto-esophageal or central airway communication fair poorly with endovascular treatment because of the severity of their illness. Once they are stabilized they may then be candidates for definitive open repair.

Aneurysms Involving the Aortic Arch

The most important concern when treating disease involving the aortic arch is protecting the brain from malperfusion and embolization. Arch aneurysms pose several issues for endovascular treatment in addition to the presence of supra-aortic branch vessels. The ascending aorta is often dilated limiting its use as a proximal landing zone. The device needs to be deliverable through multiple segments of tortousity and into the hemodynamically stressed environment of the proximal aorta with precise accuracy. Finally the device needs to tolerate the stresses imposed upon it while it resides within the 270 degrees of curvature of the aorta.

Hybrid Stent-Grafting

Hybrid procedures refer to those which utilized both open and endovascular surgical techniques. For patients with disease involving both the aortic arch and descending thoracic aorta, a two staged technique including first stage elephant trunk procedure; followed by endovascular completion helps to minimize the trauma of two open operations (Figure 6). During insertion of the elephant trunk graft as the first procedure, cardiac pathology, such as coronary artery or valvular disease, as well as aneurysmal disease of the ascending aorta and aortic arch, can be concomitantly treated. Patients who would otherwise be poor risks for an open second-stage procedure because of comorbid disease, lung pathology, or adhesions can undergo a safer repair. Second-stage procedures using a thoracic endograft can be done earlier after the first stage than open operation because of lower morbidity. Key points during the initial repair are that the elephant trunk graft should be no longer than 15 cm, and the end of the graft is marked with metal clips to permit easy identification [40]. The size of the elephant trunk should be as large as possible to permit sealing of a stent graft matched to the later distal landing zone. In the recently presented series comparing open to endovascular elephant trunk completion at the Cleveland Clinic, we demonstrated no significant difference in survival or major complications despite the endovascular group being older and more symptomatic. The endovascular patients tended to have less severe sequelae of their perioperative complications but the survival was excellent in both groups in intermediate term follow-up [41].

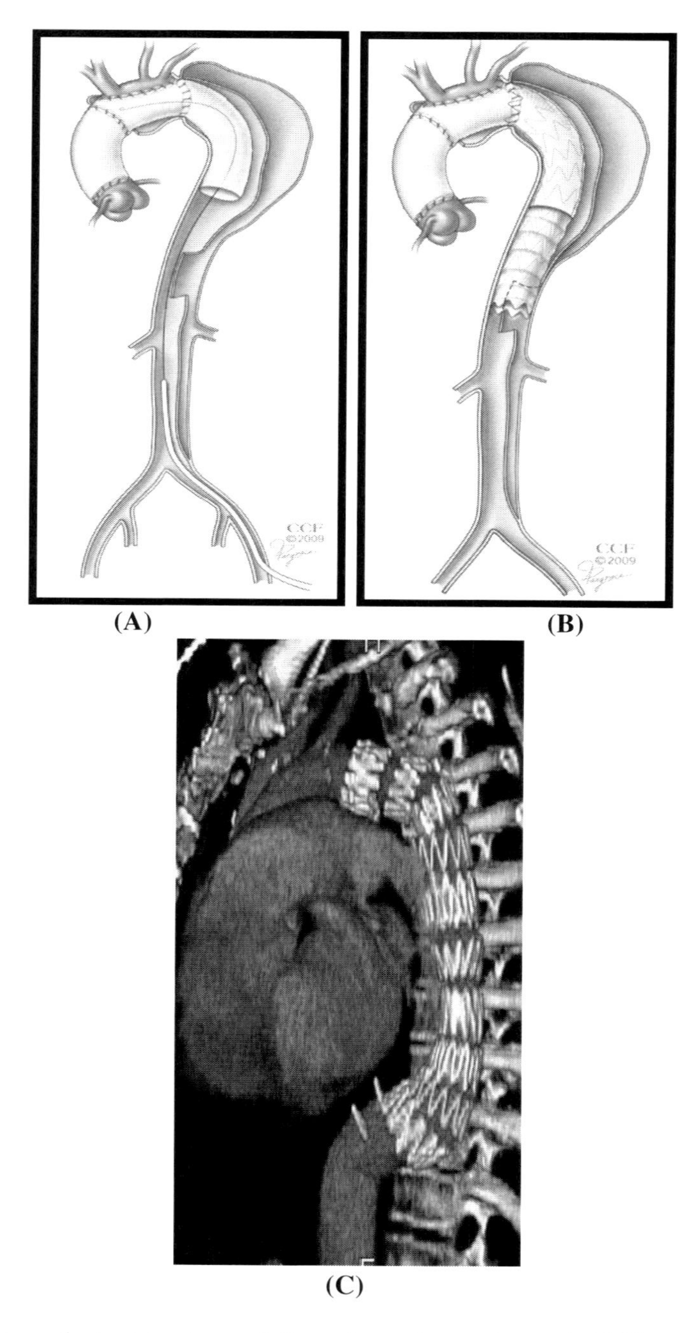

Figure 6. Second stage elephant trunk completion using endovascular graft. A) Diagramatic representation of 1st stage elephant trunk, including distal descending aortic fenestration B) Diagramatic representation of endovascular 2nd stage elephant trunk completion. C) 3D reconstructed CT scan of the chest showing the end results of endovascular 2nd stage elephant trunk completion.

Hybrid repairs can also be done by first creating an extra-anatomic bypass from the ascending aorta to the brachiocephalic vessels followed by endovascular coverage extending proximally in to the arch (Figure 7).

The endovascular portion of the repair can be done at the same time as the bypass or in a staged manner, and the device can be delivered in the usual retrograde fashion or antegrade [42].

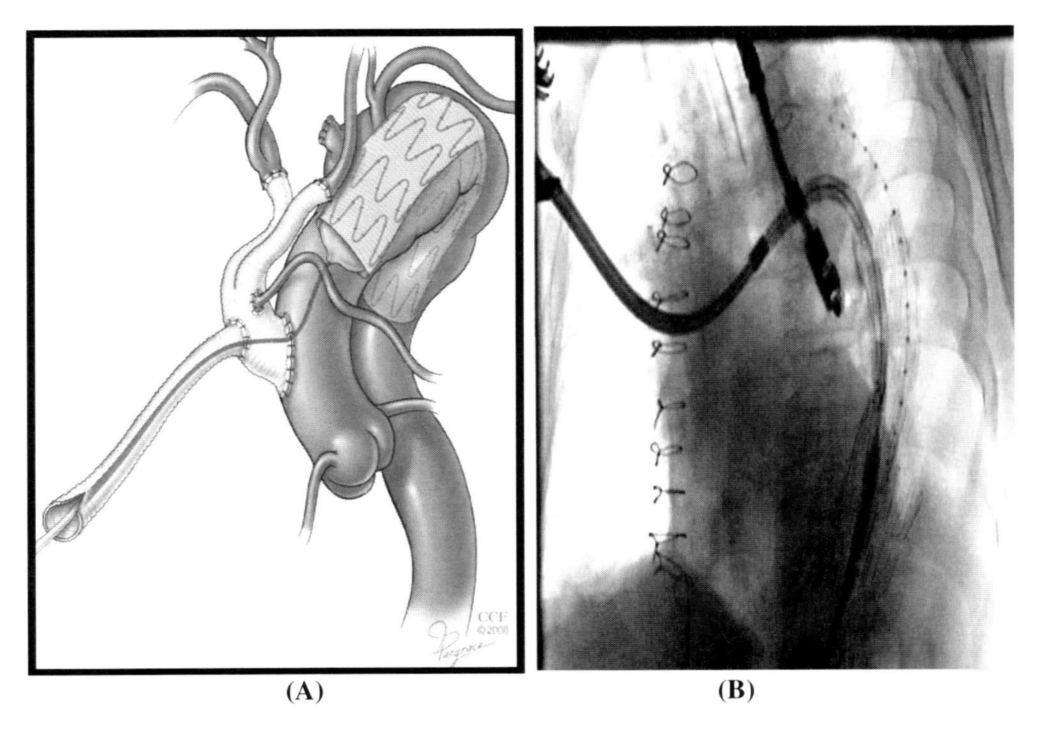

Figure 7. Hybrid Repair of aortic arch and descending aortic aneurysm with debranching of the aortic arch branches from the ascending aorta. A) Diagramatic representation of the Hybrid repair. B) Flouroscopic image of the endovascular graft insertion through the ascending aorta to axillary conduit.

Use of the so-called frozen elephant truck is another hybrid approach to complex multi-segment thoracic aortic disease in which the stent graft device is placed directly in the descending aorta under hypothermic circulatory arrest and sutured to the aorta proximally (Figure 8). This technique has proven to be especially interesting for the one-stage extended aortic repair of patients with acute type A dissection.

This technique permits the removal of the primary entry tear in the ascending aorta or the aortic arch, and the restoration of flow to the true lumen throughout the arch and upper descending aorta. Consequently, such a repair will avoid long-term distal complications of aortic dissection [43].

These procedures still pose a significant risk to patients due to their complexity and the comorbid conditions of the patients but they have been invaluable for use in patients who otherwise would not be reasonable candidates for conventional repair.

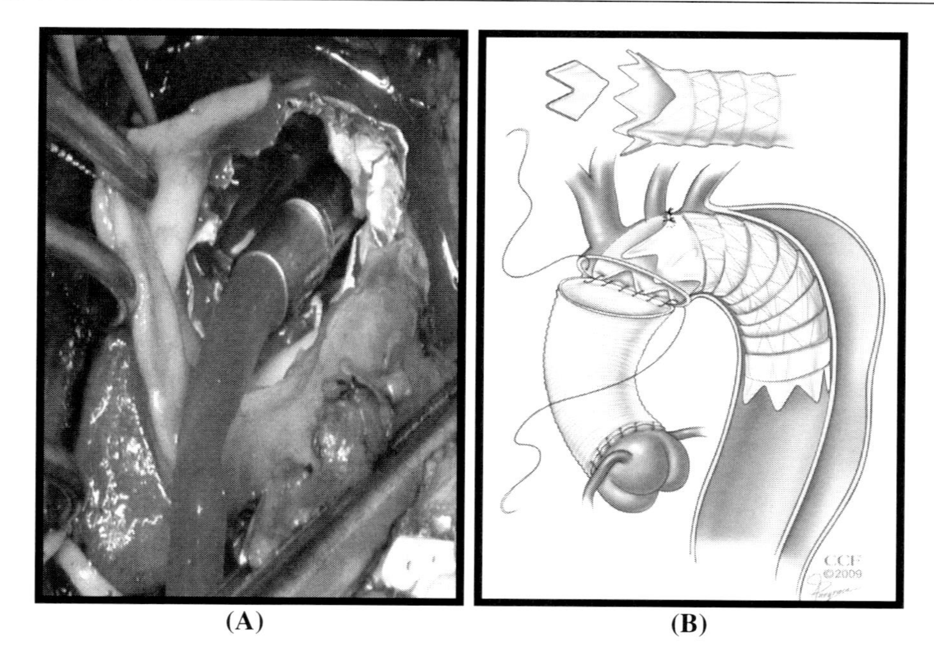

Figure 8. Frozen Elephant Trunk. A) Intraoperative picture of the endovascular stent inserted antegradely in the descending thoracic aorta. B) Diagramatic representation of the Frozen Elephant Trunk Technique.

Branched Grafts for the Arch

Currently much research is being directed at developing branched graft devices for the aortic arch much as has been done for the thoracoabdominal aorta. Patients are actively being enrolled for investigational use of one such device at a handful of sites internationally and in the United States as part of an investigator sponsored device exemption trial.

Ascending Aortic Disease

Stent grafts have been used with limited success in high-risk patients with ascending aortic disease such as focal pseudoaneurysms and chronic dissection. Other approaches have included the placement of septal defect closure devices across the intimal defect of such processes. Investigational delivery systems are directed at providing a more accurate deployment of devices in these harsh hemodynamic environments. Trans-apical delivery approaches have been performed to make the aorta more accessible. Future plans include the marriage of stent grafts to trans-catheter aortic valve devices. The majority of patients with ascending disease, however, have a fusiform pattern to their disease and so with the current designs the landing zones are severely limited.

Endovascular Stenting for Patients with Connective Tissue Disease

Patients with Marfan syndrome or other connective tissue disorders deserve special consideration. There are a few reports of short-term success after endovascular stent-grafting of the descending thoracic aorta in patients with Marfan syndrome [44-45]; however, there is limited information regarding the impact of persistent radial forces of a stent-graft in the abnormal and weak aorta of patients with these conditions. Furthermore, these patients are usually young, and because the current long-term durability of available stent-grafts is unknown. Consequently, stent-grafting in patients with Marfan syndrome or other known connective tissue disorders is generally not recommended unless operative intervention is clearly indicated and the risk of conventional open surgical repair is deemed exceptionally high risk. On the other hand, many of these patients are prone to develop aneurysmal degeneration of their entire aorta. Due to the association of spinal cord injury to extent of repair, patients are best treated by limiting repair to the at risk segments [46]. As such, many patients with Marfan and other connective tissue disorders will require multiple operations over a lifetime. The endovascular techniques do serve an important role in these patients by combining the minimally invasive stent graft repair with open repairs by landing the device into the graft material which is not at the same risk as the patient's native vulnerable aorta.

Device Related Complications

Endoleaks

Endoleaks occur less frequently after thoracic aortic repair than abdominal repairs. Important endoleaks occur more commonly at proximal or distal attachment sites (type 1 endoleak), where there is an incomplete seal between the graft and the proximal or distal aneurysm neck. These require immediate attention as they may be life-threatening [47]. Endoleaks from retrograde aortic branch vessel flow into the aneurysm from collateral channels (type 2 endoleak), on the other hand are rarely troublesome. Oversizing of the stent-graft is an important consideration. It has been found that oversizing up to 20 per cent greater than the outside diameter of the native vessel is beneficial in reducing the rate of endoleaks [48]. It is also important for the device to have a parallel lie within the aorta and the newer version of thoracic stent grafts are being developed to be more conformable to the curve of the aorta at the level of the isthmus.

Migration

Migration of aortic stent-grafts is usually detected after the first two years due to a number of forces at play [49]. It may either be a function of the device itself or the ongoing disease process at work in the patient's aorta. Migration is a risk factor for subsequent aneurysm rupture. Three factors affecting the deployed stent-graft are the internal diameter of the vessel, the starting position of the graft and the diameter of curvature of the aortic arch. The drag force on a stent-graft will depend critically on the internal diameter and the starting position of stent-graft deployment. Larger internal diameter leads to larger drag force and the stent-graft deployed at the more distal position may be associated with diminished drag force [50]. One method of resisting migration incorporates a series of hooks or barbs in order to engage the aortic wall.

Stent Occlusion

The tortuous nature of the aorta and iliac arteries may result in stent-graft kinking and occlusion. Many first-generation stent-grafts were unsupported throughout their length (e.g. the Chuter and Ancure stent-grafts). Fully supported stent-grafts were introduced to prevent this problem and have significantly reduced the incidence of iliac limb occlusion.

Conclusion

New iterations of stent graft devices and delivery systems are continuously being developed to improve upon the existing systems with regard to safety, simplification of the technical aspects of the procedures and providing durable repairs. Computerized sizing algorithms have been developed that require minimal physician interaction to generate accurate device designs. Imaging protocols for planning and follow-up are directed at reducing the harmful effects of radiation exposure. Continued innovations will lead to disease specific devices and make the entire aorta and its varied disease processes amenable to endovascular therapy. Endovascular techniques of repair in the thoracic aorta still carry the potential for devastating complications such as paraplegia and ultimately the hope is for a better biologic understanding of these diseases, which may direct therapy to be more prophylactic than is currently practiced.

References

[1] Parodi, J. C. Endovascular repair of abdominal aortic aneurysms. *Adv. Vascular Surg.*, 1993, 1, 85–106.

[2] Palmaz, J. C. Balloon-expandable intravascular stent. *Am. J. Roentgenology*, 1988, 150, 1263–1269.

[3] Parodi, J. C., Palmaz, J. C., and Barone, H. D. Transfemoral intraluminal graft implantation for abdominal aortic aneurysms. *Ann. Vascular Surg.*, 1991, 5, 491–499.

[4] Volodos, N. L., Karpovich, I. P., Troyan, V. I., Kalashnikova, Yu. V., Shekhanin, V. E., Ternyuk, N. E., Neoneta, A. S., Ustinov, N. I., and Yakovenko, L. F. Clinical experience of the use of self-fixing synthetic prostheses for remote endoprosthetics of the thoracic and the abdominal aorta and iliac arteries through the femoral artery and as intra-operative endoprosthesis for aorta reconstruction. *Vasa Suppl.*, 1991, 33, 93–95.

[5] Sidawy A, Sumpio B, Depalma R: In: The Basic Science of Vascular Diseases. New Haven: Futura Publishing Company, 1997, p 576.

[6] Greenhalgh RM, Brown LC, Kwong GP, Powell JT, Thompson SG. Comparison of endovascular aneurysm repair with open repair in patients with abdominal aortic aneurysm (EVAR trial 1), 30-day operative mortality results: randomized controlled trial. *Lancet*. 2004;364:843– 848.

[7] Prinssen M, Verhoeven EL, Buth J, Cuypers PW, van Sambeek MR, Balm R, Buskens E, Grobbee DE, Blankensteijn JD; Dutch Randomized Endovascular Aneurysm Management Team (DREAM) Trial Group. A randomized trial comparing conventional and endovascular repair of abdominal aortic aneurysms. *N Engl J Med*. 2004;351:1607–1618.

[8] EVAR Trial Participants. Endovascular aneurysm repair versus open repair in patients with abdominal aortic aneurysm (EVAR trial 1): randomized controlled trial. *Lancet*. 2005;365:2179 –2186.

[9] Laheij, R. J., Buth, J., Harris, P. L., Moll, F. L., Stelter, W. J., and Verhoeven, E. L. Need for secondary interventions after endovascular repair of abdominal aortic aneurysms. Intermediate-term follow-up results of a European collaborative registry (EUROSTAR). *Br.J.Surg*., 2000, 87, 1666–1673.

[10] Makaroun MS, Dillavou ED, Kee ST, Sicard G, Chaikof E, Bavaria J, Williams D, Cambria RP, Mitchell RS. Endovascular treatment of thoracic aortic aneurysms: results of the phase II multicenter trial of the GORE TAG thoracic endoprosthesis. *J Vasc Surg*. 2005;41:1–9.

[11] Svensson LG, Kouchoukos NT, Miller DC, Section Authors: Bavaria JE, Coselli JS, Curi MA, Eggebrecht H, Elefteriades JA, Erbel R, Gleason TG, Lytle BW, Mitchell RS, Nienaber CA, Roselli EE, Safi HJ, Shemin RJ, Sicard GA, Sundt III TM, Szeto WY, Wheatley III G. Expert Consensus Document on the Treatment of Descending Thoracic Aortic Disease Using Endovascular Stent-Grafts. Ann Thorac Surg 2008;85:S1– 41

[12] Dake, Michael D. Endovascular stent-grafts for thoracic aqneurysms and dissections. *Advanced therapy in cardiac surgery*. Chapter 39.

[13] Riesenman PJ, Farber MA, Mendes RR, et al. Endovascular repair of lesions involving the descending thoracic aorta. *J Vasc Surg* 2005;42:1063–74.

[14] Lamme B, de Jonge IC, Reekers JA, de Mol BA, Balm R.Endovascular treatment of thoracic aortic pathology: feasibility and mid-term results. *Eur J Vasc Endovasc Surg* 2003;25:532–9.

[15] Semba CP, Sakai T, Slonim SM, et al. Mycotic aneurysms of the thoracic aorta: repair with use of endovascular stentgrafts. *J Vasc Interv Radiol* 1998;9:33– 40.

[16] Lepore V, Lonn L, Delle M, et al. Endograft therapy for diseases of the descending thoracic aorta: results in 43 high-risk patients. *J Endovasc Ther* 2002;9:829 –37.

[17] Krohg-Sorensen K, Hafsahl G, Fosse E, Geiran OR. Acceptable short-term results after endovascular repair of diseases of the thoracic aorta in high risk patients. *Eur J Cardiothorac Surg* 2003;24:379–87.

[18] Demers P, Miller DC, Mitchell RS, Kee ST, Chagonjian L, Dake MD. Stent-graft repair of penetrating atherosclerotic ulcers in the descending thoracic aorta: mid-term results. *Ann Thorac Surg* 2004;77:81– 6.

[19] Czerny M, Cejna M, Hutschala D, et al. Stent-graft placement in atherosclerotic descending thoracic aortic aneurysms: midterm results. *J Endovasc Ther* 2004;11:26 – 32.

[20] Brandt M, Hussel K, Walluscheck KP, et al. Stent-graft repair versus open surgery for the descending aorta: a case-control study. *J Endovasc Ther* 2004;11:535– 8.

[21] Schoder M, Cartes-Zumelzu F, Grabenwoger M, et al. Elective endovascular stent-graft repair of atherosclerotic thoracic aortic aneurysms: clinical results and midterm follow-up. *AJR Am J Roentgenol* 2003;180:709 –15.

[22] Eggebrecht H, Baumgart D, Schmermund A, et al. Penetrating atherosclerotic ulcer of the aorta: treatment by endovascular stent-graft placement. *Curr Opin Cardiol* 2003;18:431–5.

[23] Brittenden J, McBride K, McInnes G, Gillespie IN, Bradbury AW. The use of endovascular stents in the treatment of penetrating ulcers of the thoracic aorta. *J Vasc Surg* 1999; 30:946 –9.

[24] Tehrani HY, Peterson BG, Katariya K, et al. Endovascular repair of thoracic aortic tears. *Ann Thorac Surg* 2006;82:873–78.

[25] Estrera AL, Gochnour DC, Azizzadeh A, et al. Progress in the treatment of blunt thoracic aortic injury: 12-year single-institution experience. *Ann Thorac Surg*. 2010;90:64-71.

[26] Uchida N, Ishihara H, Shibamura H, et al: Midterm results of extensive primary repair of the thoracic aorta by means of total arch replacement with open stent graft placement for an acute type A aortic dissection. *J Thorac Cardiovasc Surg* 131:862-867, 2006.

[27] Jakob H, Tsagakis K, Tossios P, et al: Combining classic surgery with descending stent grafting for acute DeBakey Type I dissection. *Ann Thorac Surg* 86:95-102, 2008.

[28] 28. Dobrilovic N, Elefteriades JA: Stenting the descending aorta during repair of type A dissection: technology looking for an application? *J Thorac Cardiovasc Surg* 131:777-778, 2006.

[29] Tsai TT, Fattori R, Trimarchi S, et al: Long-term survival in patients presenting with type B acute aortic dissection. Insights from the International Registry of Acute Aortic Dissection. *Circulation* 114:2226-2231, 2006

[30] Tsai TT, Trimarchi S, Nienaber CA: Acute aortic dissection: perspectives from the International Registry of Acute Aortic Dissection. *Eur J Vasc Endovasc Surg* 37:149-159, 2009

[31] Szeto WY, McGarvey M, Pochettino A, Moser GW, Hoboken A, Cornelius K, Woo EY, Carpenter JP, Fairman RM, Bavaria JE. Results of a new surgical paradigm: Endovascular repair for acute complicated type B aortic dissection. *Annals of Thoracic Surgery* 86(1):87-94, July 2008.

[32] Subramanian S, Roselli EE. Thoracic aortic dissection: long-term results of endovascular and open repair. *Semin Vasc Surg*. 2009 Jun;22(2):61-8.

[33] Nienaber CA, Rousseau H, Eggebrecht H, et al. Randomized comparison of strategies for type B aortic dissection: the INvestigation of STEnt grafts in Aortic Dissection (INSTEAD) trial. *Circulation* 2009;120:2519 –28.

[34] Tang DG, Dake MD: TEVAR for acute uncomplicated aortic dissection: Immediate repair versus medical therapy. *Semin Vasc Surg* 22:145-151, 2009.

[35] Roselli EE, Pujara AC, Vargas Abello LM, Burke JM, Hernandez AV, Greenberg RK, Nowicki ER, Blackstone EH, Svensson LG, Lytle BW. Open Repair of Chronic Distal Aortic Dissection: Contemporary Analysis of Outcomes and Implications for Disease Management. Personal communication - submitted for peer review.

[36] Eggebrecht H, Nienaber CA, Neuhauser M, et al. Endovascular stent-graft placement in aortic dissection: a metaanalysis. *Eur Heart J* 2006;27:489 –98.

[37] Roselli EE, Greenberg RK, Pfaff K, Francis C, Svensson LG, Lytle BW. Endovascular treatment of Thoracoabdominal aortic aneurysm. *J Thorac Cardiovasc Surg* 2007;133:1474– 82.

[38] Greenberg RK, Resch T, Nyman U, Lindh M, Brunkwall J, Brunkwall P, Malina M, Koul B, Lindblad B, Ivancev K. Endovascular repair of descending thoracic aortic aneurysms: an early experience with intermediate-term follow-up. *J Vasc Surg*. 2000;31:147–156.

[39] O'Neill S, Greenberg RK, Haddad F, Resch T, Sereika J, Katz E. A prospective analysis of fenestrated endovascular grafting: intermediate-term outcomes. *Eur J Vasc Endovasc Surg*. 2006; 32: 115–123

[40] Svensson LG, Kim KH, Blackstone EH, et al. Elephant trunk procedure: newer indications and uses. *Ann Thorac Surg* 2004;78:109 –16.

[41] Roselli EE, Subramanian S, Anderson J, et al. Endovascular Versus Open Elephant Trunk Completion for Extensive Aortic Disease. Presented at the 36th Annual Meeting of the Western Thoracic Surgical Association; June, 2010; Ojai, CA, USA.

[42] Roselli EE, Soltesz EG, Mastracci T, et al. Antegrade Delivery of Stent Grafts to Treat Complex Thoracic Aortic Disease. *Ann Thorac Surg* 2010 Aug;90(2):539-46.

[43] Lima B, Roselli E, Pujara A, et al. Single-Stage and "Reverse" Frozen Elephant Trunk Repairs for Extensive Thoracic Aortic Disease and complications after previous stentgrafting. Presented at the 57th Annual Meeting of the Southern Thoracic Surgical Association; November, 2010; Orlando, FL, USA.

[44] Fleck TM, Hutschala D, Tschernich H, et al. Stent graft placement of the thoracoabdominal aorta in a patient with Marfan syndrome. *J Thorac Cardiovasc Surg* 2003;125: 1541–3.

[45] Rocchi G, Lofiego C, Biagini E, et al. Transesophageal echocardiography-guided algorithm for stent-graft implantation in aortic dissection. *J Vasc Surg* 2004;40:880 –5.

[46] Greenberg RK, Lu Q, Roselli EE, et al. Contemporary analysis of descending thoracic and thoracoabdominal aneurysm repair: a comparison of endovascular and open techniques. *Circulation*. 2008 Aug 19;118(8):808-17.

[47] Michael D. Dake. Endovascular stent-grafts for thoracic aqneurysms and dissections. *Advanced therapy in cardiac surgery*. Chapter 39

[48] Mohan, I. V., Laheij, R. J., and Harris, P. L. and EUROSTAR Collaborators. Risk factors for endoleak and the evidence for stent-graft oversizing in patients undergoing endovascular aneurysm repair. *Eur. J. Vascular Endovascular Surg.*, 2001, 21, 344–349.

[49] Greenberg RK, et al. Beyond the aortic bifurcation: branchedendovascular grafts for thoracoabdominal and aortoiliac aneurysms. *J Vasc Surg* 2006;43: 879–86.

[50] Lam SK, Fung GSK, Cheng SWK, Chow KW. A computational study of the biomechanical factors related to stent-graft models in the thoracic aorta. *Med Biol Eng Comput* (2008) 46:1129-1138.

Tricuspid Valve

In: Percutaneous Valve Technology: Present and Future ISBN: 978-1-61942-577-4
Editors: Jose Luis Navia and Sharif Al-Ruzzeh

Chapter XXVI

Cardiology Perspective of Tricuspid Valve Disease – The Potential Role of Percutaneous Valve Technology

Deborah H. Kwon and Allan L. Klein

Abstract

Percutaneous valve techniques have been emerging of the past several years, including percutaneous replacement of aortic and pulmonic valves as well as multiple techniques regarding repairing the mitral valve for functional or degenerative mitral regurgitation. Patients are rarely referred for surgical correction of isolated tricuspid valve disease, and surgical correction of the tricuspid regurgitation often takes place only when patients are undergoing other planned open heart procedures. Therefore, patients usually do not undergo tricuspid valve operations until they have advanced to symptomatic right heart failure. The evolution of percutaneous tricuspid valve techniques which mimic those which have been developed for the mitral valve may play an important role in the management of patients with tricuspid valve disease.

Normal Tricuspid Valve Anatomy and Physiology

The tricuspid valve separates the right atrium from the right ventricle and typically is comprised of three leaflets, anterior, septal and posterior leaflets as well as two papillary muscles and their associated chordae tendinae. (Figure 1). In comparison to the mitral valve annulus, the tricuspid valve annulus is slightly apically displaced. This anatomical finding can help distinguish the tricuspid valve from the mitral valve in many complex congenital diseases where situs is uncertain. The apical displacement of the tricuspid valve creates a small area in which the left ventricle is separated from the right atrium by the membranous septum. Disruption of this space can result in a left ventricular to right atrial shunt (Gerbode defect).

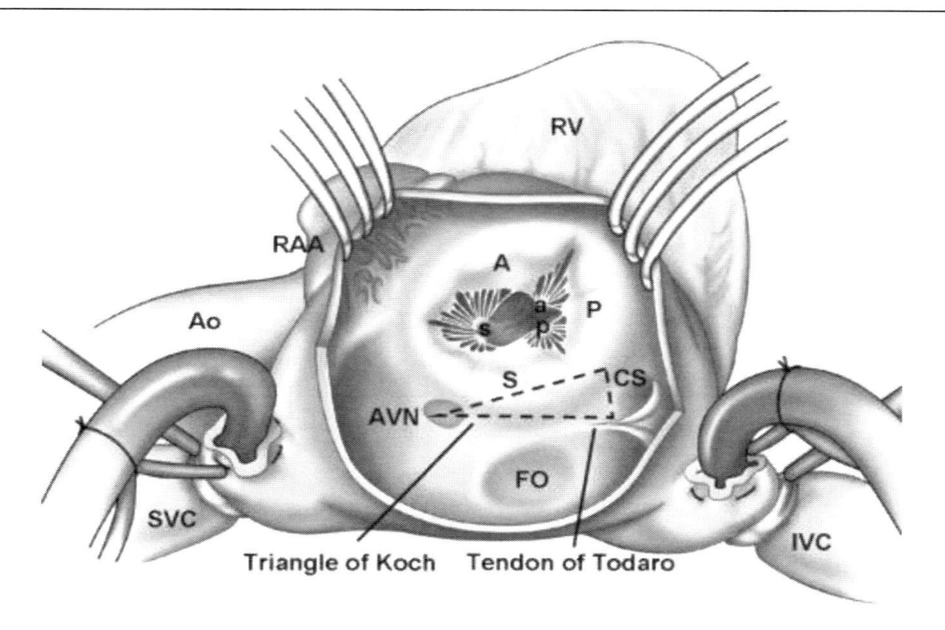

Figure 1. Surgical perspective of the tricuspid valve complex. The tricuspid valve consists of three leaflets: anterior (A), posterior (P), and septal (S). There are 2 main papillary muscles, anterior (a) and posterior (p). The septal papillary muscle (s) is rudimentary, and chordae tendinae arise directly from the ventricular septum. Relevant adjacent structures include the atrioventricular node (AVN), coronary sinus ostium (CS), and the tendon of Todaro, which form the triangle of Koch. Ao indicates aorta; FO, foramen ovale; IVC, inferior vena cava; SVC, superior vena cava; RAA, right atrial appendage; and RV, right ventricle [1].

The tricuspid valve leaflets are not symmetric, and the anterior leaflet is the largest of the leaflets, and the septal leaflet is the smallest leaflet. The posterior leaflet has multiple scallops. The anterior papillary muscle typically supplies chordae to the anterior and posterior leaflets. The medial papillary muscle typically supplies chordae to the posterior and septal leaflets. Although there is no septal papillary muscle, the septal wall provides chordae to the anterior and septal leaflets. Accessory chordae may be present which can arise from the right ventricular free wall and moderator band. When the right ventricle dilates or becomes dysfunctional, these accessory chordae can impair proper leaflet coaptation, resulting in significant tricuspid regurgitation [1, 2].

Imaging

Tricuspid Valve

Transthoracic Echocardiography

The tricuspid valve is best visualized from the long and short axis parasternal, apical four chamber, and subcostal views. The tricuspid valve leaflet anatomy can be quite variable, but the anterior leaflet is typically the most anatomically constant echocardiographic feature.

The septal and anterior leaflets typically are best seen in the parasternal long axis (right ventricular inflow) view. See Figure 2,3. The posterior leaflet is best seen in the parasternal short axis view at the level of the aortic valve, and is the leaflet adjacent to the RV free wall.

The leaflet imaged adjacent to the aortic root can be either the septal or anterior leaflet. The anterior and septal leaflets are also seen in the apical four chamber view, with the anterior leaflet adjacent to the RV free wall and the septal leaflet adjacent to the interventricular septum. Doppler echocardiography can be used to determine the presence of regurgitation or stenosis.

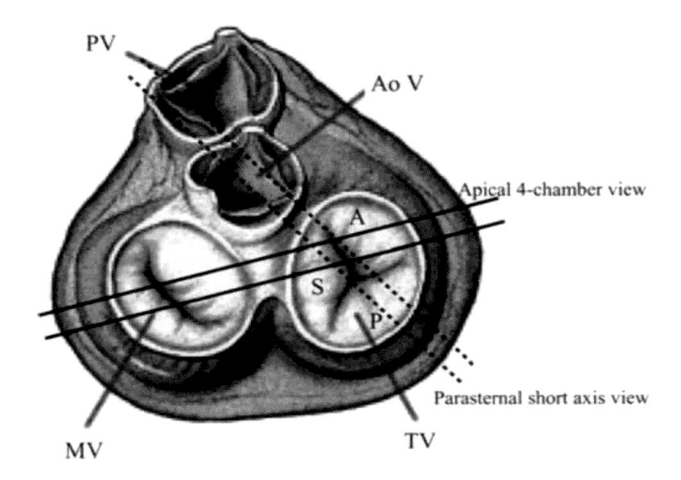

Figure 2. Surgical view of the heart valves demonstrating the range of the two-dimensional echocardiographic 4-chamber and short-axis planes [3].

Two dimensional (2-D) transthoracic echocardiography (TTE) is usually the best modality to visualize the tricuspid valve. The tricuspid valve is routinely evaluated using the long and short axis parasternal, apical four chamber, and subcostal views. The normal tricuspid valve thickness is less than or equal to 3 mm. In the 2-D parasternal long axis view, the septal and anterior leaflets are generally visualized. In the parasternal short axis view at the level of the aortic valve, the posterior leaflet is imaged along the right ventricular free wall and either the septal or anterior leaflet is imaged adjacent to the aortic root. In the apical four chamber view, the anterior and septal leaflets are visualized [3-7].

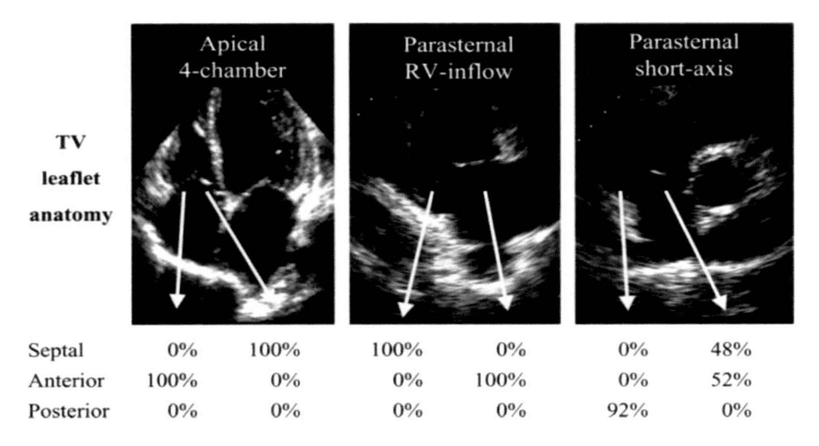

	Apical 4-chamber		Parasternal RV-inflow		Parasternal short-axis	
Septal	0%	100%	100%	0%	0%	48%
Anterior	100%	0%	0%	100%	0%	52%
Posterior	0%	0%	0%	0%	92%	0%

Figure 3. Identification of the tricuspid valve leaflets seen on two-dimensional imaging. Below the 2D images, percentage of leaflet identification in each standard view depending the RT3DE images [3].

Careful examination of the tricuspid valve annulus and leaflets may identify if the etiology of TR is from primary structural abnormalities of the leaflets and chordae or from secondary myocardial dysfunction and dilatation. Dilation of the tricuspid annulus occurs in the anterior/posterior aspect and often results in leaflet mal-coaptation. TTE may reveal prolapse of the tricuspid valve, endocarditis, rheumatic heart disease, or Ebstein's anomaly. The tricuspid valve annulus is slightly apically displaced when compared to the mitral valve annulus. This feature is useful in identifying the tricuspid valve in many congenital conditions (such as Ebstein's anomaly). See Figure 4.

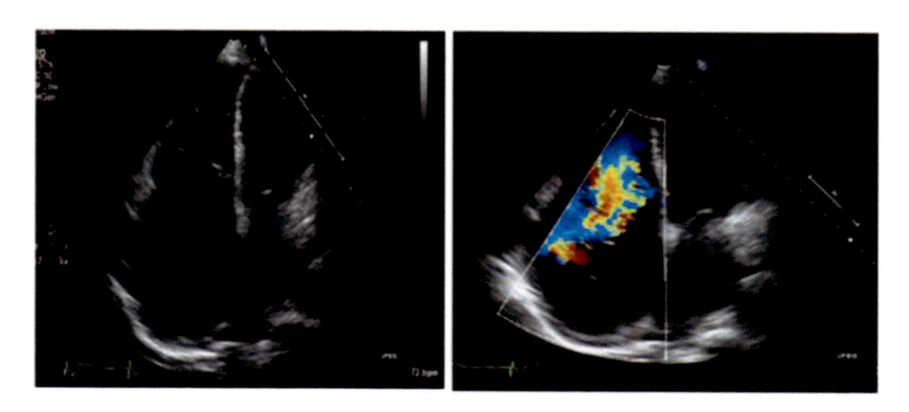

Figure 4. Ebstein's anomaly.

Transesophageal Echocardiography

The tricuspid valve is usually more difficult to visualize with transesophageal echocardiography (TEE) than with TTE since it is a thinner structure that is farther from the TEE transducer than the TTE probe. In addition, aortic or mitral valve prostheses or calcium can result in shadowing artifacts, further obscuring optimal visualization of the tricuspid valve by TEE.

The best imaging planes to visualize the tricuspid valve are: the mid-esophageal view at 0°, 30°, 60°, and transgastric views. Similar to the apical 4 chamber view with TTE, the septal and anterior leaflets are usually seen at the mid-esophageal view at 0°. Retroflexion of the probe can bring the posterior leaflet into view. The tricuspid valve also be seen in the transgastric view by turning the probe clockwise from the mitral valve short axis view (0°) or from the left ventricular long axis view (90°).

Tricuspid regurgitation jet velocity is best measured in a view in which the ultrasound beam and the regurgitant jet are most parallel, often between 30° and 60° in the mid-esophageal view. In the transgastric position, the tricuspid valve is brought into view by turning the probe clockwise from the mitral valve short axis view (0°) or left ventricular long axis view (90°).

On the 2-D echocardiogram (using TTE or TEE), the presence and degree of TR can be evaluated by inspection of RV size and function, right atrial size and function, the tricuspid valve, and the inferior vena cava.

Two-dimensional echocardiography using TTE or TEE enables identification of the specific features of tricuspid stenosis. Doming of the tricuspid valve is pathognomonic for tricuspid stenosis and is seen in the parasternal long-axis view or in the apical four-chamber view. Other 2-D echocardiographic features of tricuspid stenosis include restricted mobility of the leaflets, reduced separation of the leaflet tips, reduction in the diameter of the tricuspid annulus, thickening and calcification of the leaflets. Although leaflet thickening is seen, the degree of thickening and calcification is generally less pronounced than in rheumatic mitral stenosis.

3 Dimensional Echocardiography

3-dimensional echocardiography (3DE) can be used to provide more comprehensive assessment of the complex geometry of the tricuspid valve annulus, commissures, and leaflet anatomy. (Figure 5, 6). A recent study demonstrated the non-planar, elliptical shape of the tricuspid annulus [8]. (See Figure 7). Patients with significant functional tricuspid valve regurgitation were found to have a more planar annulus, rather than the more elliptical shape seen in normal patients.

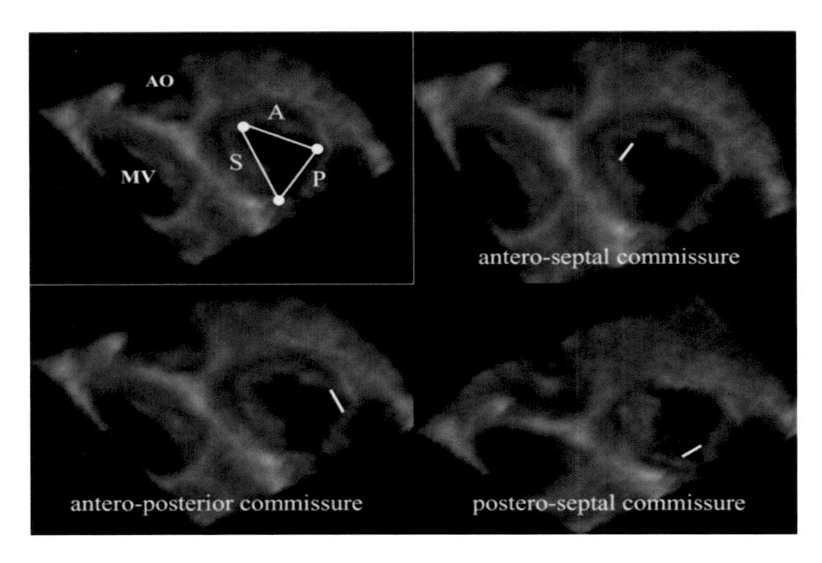

Figure 5. Triangular shape TV area and commissural views [3].

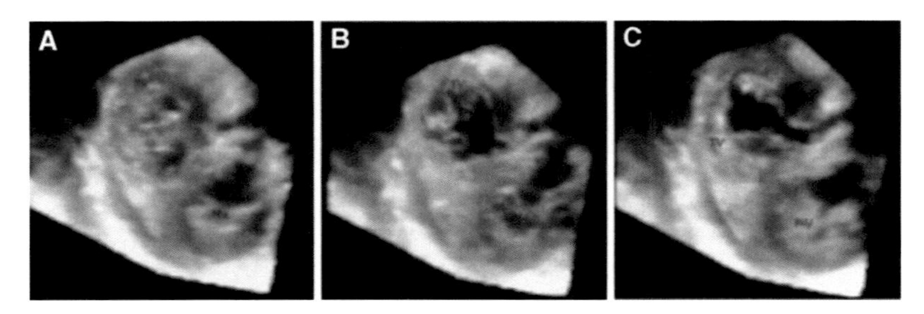

Figure 6. Visualization of the 3 TV leaflets during valve closure (A), at early diastole (B), and at late diastole (C) [3].

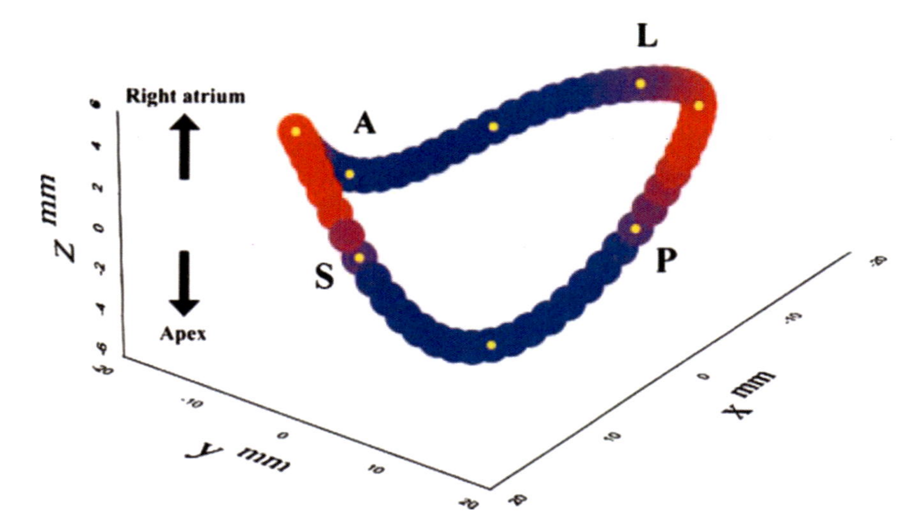

Figure 7. The reconstructed ring shape for tricuspid annuloplasty, based on the average results obtained in healthy subjects at the time of minimum TA area. The positive *x-y-z* axis indicates the respective directions toward the septum, the posterior wall, and the right atrium. At the yellow dot, the average of each of the manually selected TA locations is shown. The reconstructed TA locations were color coded by assigning shades of red to points located above the best-fit plane toward the atrium and shades of blue to points located below the best-fit plane toward the apex. A indicates anterior; L, lateral; P, posterior; and S, septum [8].

Furthermore, just as 3DE has been shown to be useful in patients with mitral valve disease, 3DE can also help to assess and evaluate other mechanisms of tricuspid disease, such as prolapse, perforation, and endocarditis. Additional studies have demonstrated the utility of real-time three-dimensional echocardiography for more complete and accurate assessment of the tricuspid valve annulus and leaflet morphology. Real time 3D echo overcomes the inability to correctly identify the three tricuspid leaflets by traditional 2D echocardiography. Three-dimensional echo may also prove to be useful in planning surgical tricuspid valve interventions. It has been shown to be highly reproducible, providing real time anatomical and functional measurements [3, 9, 10].

Evaluation of Stenosis Severity

Although two-dimensional echocardiography using TTE or TEE enables the identification and characterization of tricuspid stenosis (TS), planimetry of the tricuspid valve area usually cannot be obtained [11]. Therefore, Doppler echocardiography is essential for quantifying the degree of tricuspid stenosis [9]. TS is present when there is diastolic flow acceleration on the atrial side of the valve and an increased pressure half-time. The mean tricuspid diastolic gradient can be estimated from the tricuspid inflow time velocity integral by applying the modified Bernoulli equation. Though estimating tricuspid valve area using echocardiography is not as well-established as estimating mitral valve area, the same methods for calculating mitral valve area, such as pressure half-time, the continuity equation, and proximal isovelocity surface area, can be applied to the tricuspid valve [10]. The severity of TS can also be determined by the mean and end-diastolic gradients. Significant TS results in a mean gradient of 3-5mmHg and an end-diastolic gradient of 1-3mmHg [11]. Tricuspid valve area in cm^2 can be calculated by the following equation: 190/pressure half-time [12]. A tricuspid valve with valve area less than 1 cm, with elevated mean and end-diastolic gradients, is considered severely stenotic and may need surgical intervention.

Evaluation of Regurgitant Severity

The severity of TR is determined using a semi-quantitative approach. Jet area, proximal flow acceleration, and the width of the vena contracta are used to quantify the severity of TR. If the TR jet is central, the Nyquist limit should be set at 50 - 60 cm/sec. A jet area of <5 cm2 suggests mild TR, 5 to 10 cm2 suggests moderate TR, and >10 cm2 suggests severe TR.

Proximal flow acceleration refers to the effect of increasing blood velocity as regurgitant blood approaches the regurgitant orifice from the ventricular side of the valve. This phenomenon is seen as a series of concentric roughly hemispheric isovelocity shells of decreasing surface area and increasing surface velocity using color Doppler. The peak measurable blood velocity is limited by the relatively low sampling rate of color Doppler. When flow velocity exceeds the aliasing velocity (Va) (Nyquist limit), color reversal occurs. This convergence signal is referred to as the proximal isovelocity surface area (PISA) [13]. At a given aliasing velocity, the radius (r) of PISA increases with increasing regurgitant volume. The effective regurgitant orifice area (EROA) can be calculated by dividing the flow rate through the regurgitant orifice (which is estimated as the product of the surface area of the hemisphere (2πr2) and Va) by the peak velocity of the regurgitant jet (PkVreg):

EROA = (2πr2 * Va)/PkVreg

An EROA of ≥40 mm2 is a criterion of severe regurgitation in both TR and MR [1, 19].

The PISA method is not as accurate in quantifing eccentric jets as compared to central jets. Although PISA is widely used to quantify the severity of MR, it has limitations in its applicability to the assessment of TR due to the greater difficulty in visualizing a measurable contour of flow convergence [13]. The 2003 ASE guideline recommendations include PISA radius as a parameter for grading TR severity, although the guidelines note that such quantification is rarely needed clinically given the availability of other methods, such as the width of the vena contracta [13]. At a Nyquist limit of 28 cm/sec, a TR PISA radius of ≤0.5 cm is categorized as mild, a radius of 0.6 to 0.9 cm is moderate, and a radius of >0.9 cm is severe.

The vena contracta is the narrowest width of the color flow regurgitant jet as it flows downstream from the valve orifice. The vena contracta width correlates with other echocardiographic measures of TR severity and with clinical evidence of TR [13-15]. TR is severe if the vena contracta width is >0.7 cm at a Nyquist limit of 50 to 60 cm/sec [13].

Early diastolic peak velocity (peak E) and velocity time integral of right ventricular inflow is increased in proportion to TR severity. A tricuspid peak E of ≥ 0.65 m/sec is consistent with the presence of severe TR [16, 23]. The presence of an A-wave dominant tricuspid inflow pattern virtually excludes the likelihood that the TR is severe.

TR jet contour is also used to grade TR. The continuous Doppler flow pattern of the TR jet is usually a symmetric, reflecting the relative equality of rates of flow acceleration and deceleration. However, severe TR, the large regurgitant volume flows into the right atrium during systole and overwhelms the ability of atrial capacitance or compliance to maintain low pressure. Therefore, a rapid rise in atrial late systolic pressure occurs. This rise or V-wave results in early equilibration of right atrial and right ventricular pressures. This is illustrated by an asymmetric early peaking triangular regurgitant wave form. Therefore, mild TR is associated with a parabolic shape, moderate TR is associated with a variable contour, and severe TR is associated with a triangular early peaking jet [13, 16].

Furthermore, the strength of the Doppler signal is proportional to the number of red blood cells regurgitating into the right atrium. Therefore, the relative density of the regurgitant signal reflects the magnitude of the regurgitant fraction. As a result, sparse TR jets usually indicate mild TR and dense TR jets indicate moderate or severe TR [13].

Hepatic vein systolic flow reversal is an important criterion for severe TR. However, systolic flow reversal may not be accurate when atrial fibrillation is present. If severe TR is suspected, but the echocardiographic findings are not consistent with this suspicion, agitated saline or other ultrasound contrast agents can be used to enhance the tricuspid regurgitation jet signal and visualization of hepatic vein flow reversal [9]. Other findings which aid in the confirmation of the presence of severe TR include: RV and RA enlargement, dilated tricuspid annulus, paradoxical interventricular septal movement, reflecting the increased volume within the right ventricle (diastolic overload), and a dilated IVC with systolic flow reversal.

Assessment of the Inferior Vena Cava Size

The inferior vena cava (IVC) and hepatic veins can be best imaged in the subcostal view. The inferior vena cava size and respiratory variation is used to estimate right atrial pressure. The IVC diameter should be measured at end-expiration and just proximal to the junction of the hepatic veins that lie approximately 0.5 to 3.0 cm proximal to the ostium of the right atrium. The American Society of Echocardiography recently released revised 2009 guidelines in the assessment of right atrial pressures [17]. An IVC diameter of < 2.1 cm that collapses >50% with a sniff suggests a normal RA pressure of 3 mm Hg (range, 0-5 mm Hg), whereas an IVC diameter > 2.1 cm that does not collapses <50% with a sniff suggests a high RA pressure of 15 mm Hg (range, 10-20 mm Hg). In indeterminate cases in which the IVC diameter and collapse do not fit this paradigm, an intermediate value of 8 mm Hg (range, 5-10 mm Hg) may be used, or, preferably, secondary indices of elevated RA pressure should be integrated. In severe TR, the vena cava expands in systole and retrograde V waves are often present. Pulsed wave and color Doppler imaging of the IVC can also demonstrate alterations in IVC and hepatic vein flow due to severe TR. Generally, blood flow toward the heart during both phases of the cardiac cycle in these vessels. During inspiration, the normally dominant systolic inflow signal is exaggerated. Retrograde IVC flow occurs only briefly after atrial contraction under normal conditions. However, systolic reversal in these vessels indicates severe TR The normally dominant systolic component of flow may be blunted or reversed and, this abnormality is accentuated during inspiration [18, 19].

Pathophysiology

Tricuspid Regurgitation

Tricuspid regurgitation (TR) gives rise to a flow of blood back into the right atrium during systole. As the right atrium is usually compliant, there are no significant hemodynamic consequences with mild or moderately severe TR. However, if TR is severe, the right atrial and venous pressure rises and can result in the signs and symptoms of right sided heart failure such as edema and hepatic congestion. Furthermore, reduced forward flow can lead to impaired perfusion of the kidneys and other vital organs.

Tricuspid regurgitation (TR) can be classified as (a) primary/ intrinsic valve pathology or (b) secondary or functional [20, 21]. See Table 1. Secondary TR is due to right ventricular hypertension, dilatation, and dysfunction. Although the tricuspid leaflets are typically normal in patients with functional TR, incomplete leaflet closure is often due geometric alteration of the tricuspid annulus. Such geometric alteration is not completely understood, but altered tricuspid annulus size and shape, right ventricular remodelling, and displacement of papillary muscles which lead to leaflet tethering all contribute to the distortion of the tricuspid valve apparatus.[22] TR is usually secondary to conditions affecting the left heart and which results in annular dilatation and leaflet tethering.

Table 1. Etiologogy of Tricuspid Regrugitation

Functional/secondary causes of TR	**Primary Causes of TR**
Left sided heart failure * Coronary artery disease * Mitral stenosis or regurgitation * Aortic stenosis or regurgitation	Congenital causes of TR — Cleft valve generally in association with atrioventricular canal defect — Ebstein's anomaly (See Figure 4)
Primary pulmonary disease cor pulmonale, pulmonary embolism, pulmonary hypertension of any cause	Rheumatic
Left to right shunt atrial septal defect, ventricular septal defect, anomalous pulmonary venous return	Myxomatous
Eisenmenger syndrome	Endomyocardial Fibrosis
Stenosis of the pulmonic valve or pulmonary artery	Endocarditis
Right ventricular dilatation	Carcinoid disease (See Figure 9)
Right ventricular dysfunction Cardiomyopathy, myocarditis, RV ischemia, endomyocardial fibrosis, arrhythmogenic right ventricular dysplasia Hyperthyroidism	Trauma/ Pacemaker or ICD leads resulting in perforation or leaflet restriction (See Figure 8)
	Other: Connective Tissue Disorders Autoimmune Disease Medications

Primary tricuspid valve pathology leading to significant TR is much less common. Various congenital anomalies and acquired diseases can alter the tricuspid valve morphology leading to valve incompetence. Causes of primary TR are listed in Table 1.

Ebstein Anomaly

The anatomy of the tricuspid valve in Ebstein's anomaly is highly variable. The tricuspid valve leaflets are malformed and partly attached to the fibrous tricuspid valve annulus and the right ventricular endocardium. The anterior leaflet is the largest leaflet and is usually attached to the tricuspid valve annulus. The posterior and septal leaflets are usually vestigial or absent. If these leaflets are present, the free edges are usually displaced into the body of the right ventricle or the apex, leading to "atrialization" of the right ventricle. The tricuspid valve is often referred to as "sail-like" or funnel-shaped and is almost always incompetent, and sometimes stenotic [33].

Ebstein's anomaly is confirmed by the presence of apical displacement of the septal tricuspid valve leaflet (by $\geq$ 8 mm/m^2 body surface area compared to the position of the mitral valve) demonstrated in the apical four chamber view. A dilated right ventricle with an atrialized portion of the ventricle should be identified based upon the position of the tricuspid annulus. Paradoxical septal motion is typically present due to right ventricular volume overload induced by tricuspid regurgitation [23, 24].

Ebstein's anomaly is classified as mild, moderate, or severe depending on the extent of apical displacement of the valve leaflets, degree of tricuspid regurgitation, and degree of right-sided cardiac chamber dilation and dysfunction [25]. Such classification helps to risk-stratify patients with Ebstein's anomaly as prognosis has been shown to be dependent upon the degree of apical displacement of the tricuspid annulus and the severity of the regurgitation [26].

Rheumatic Heart Disease

TR due to rheumatic involvement is usually associated with mitral and aortic valve pathology.[27] Diffuse fibrous thickening, commisural fusion, fused chordae, or calcific deposits develop. The subvalvular apparatus may occasionally be mildly thickened by fibrous tissue. Rheumatic involvement of the tricuspid valve usually results in a combination of TR and TS. Rheumatic disease is the most common cause of pure tricuspid regurgitation due to deformation of the leaflets.

Endocarditis

Endocarditis of the tricuspid valve can lead to significant tricuspid regurgitation. Precipitating factors that contribute to infection of the valve include alcoholism, intravenous drug use, neoplasms, infected indwelling catheters, extensive burns, and immune deficiency disease. Patients with tricuspid valve endocarditis usually present with pneumonia from septic pulmonary emboli rather than with symptoms of right heart failure.

Prolapse (Floppy, Redundant)

The incidence of floppy tricuspid valve varies from 0.3-3.2%. Tricuspid valve prolapse is associated with mitral valve prolapse and rarely is isolated to the tricuspid valve [11, 27]. Tricuspid valve prolapse may lead to significant tricuspid regurgitation and even to a flail valve leaflet. See Figure 8.

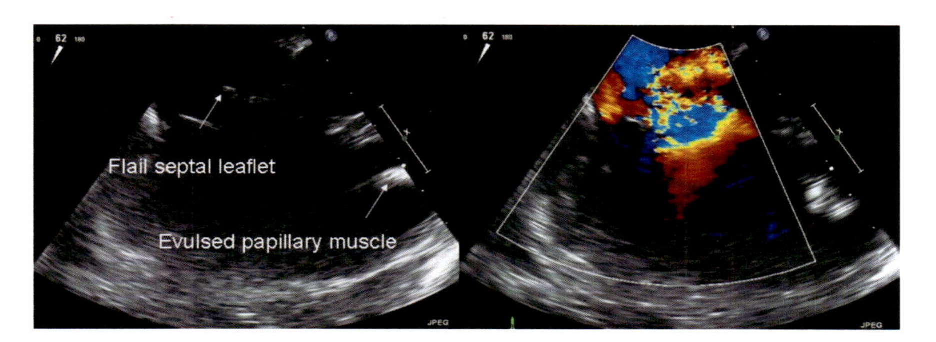

Figure 8. Severe tricuspid regurgitation due to a flail septal leaflet due to an evulsed RV papillary muscle caused by ICD lead implantation.

Carcinoid

Pure TR can occur as part of the carcinoid heart syndrome. Carcinoid heart disease is characterized by plaque-like deposits of fibrous tissue. The valves and endocardium of the right side of the heart are most often affected [28, 29], because inactivation of humoral substances by the lung protect the left heart. Fibrous white plaques form on the ventricular aspect of the tricuspid valve and endocardium, and cause the valve to adhere to the RV wall. The leaflets become restricted, preventing proper coaptation of the leaflets does during systole, and resulting in tricuspid regurgitation [30]. See Figure 9.

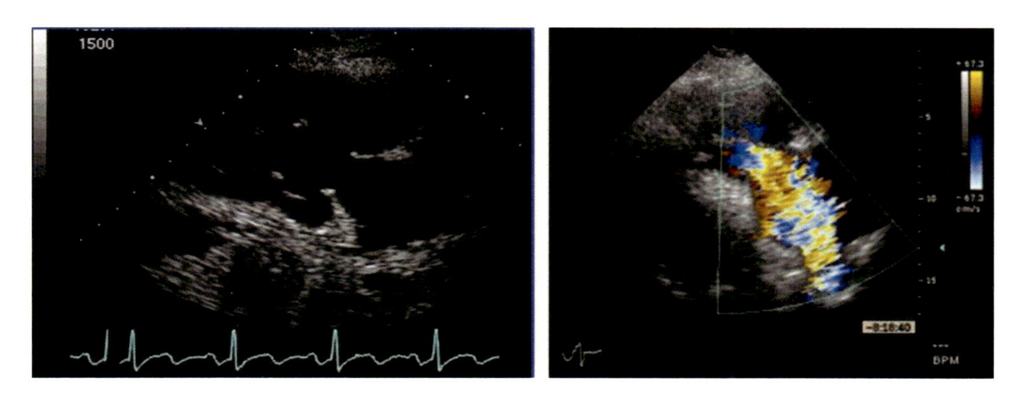

Figure 9. Severe tricuspid regurgitation due to carcinoid, resulting in fixed, thickened, tethered, and dysfunctional valve leaflets.

Papillary Muscle Dysfunction

Papillary muscle dysfunction may result from RV ischemia or infarction, fibrosis, or infiltrative processes.

Trauma

Trauma to the right ventricle may damage the structures of the tricuspid valve, resulting in insufficiency of the structure [31]. Trauma can be associated with stab wounds or projectile destruction of the valve. However, trauma may be external such as blunt chest wall injury with disruption of chordal structures. Iatrogenic trauma can result from damage with a pacemaker lead, a stiff guide wire, or radiofrequency ablation for treatment of arrhythmias or due to inadvertent damage to the tricuspid apparatus at the time of endomyocardial biopsy. Iatrogenic causes of TR are often unrecognized as the functional consequences are slow to develop and the regurgitation is often progressive.

Connective-Tissue Diseases

Patients with Marfan syndrome or other connective-tissue diseases (eg, osteogenesis imperfecta, Ehlers-Danlos syndrome) may have tricuspid regurgitation. Typically, dysfunction of other valves is also observed in the same patient. The etiology of the regurgitation can be attributed to a floppy tricuspid valve and a mildly dilated tricuspid valve annulus.

Autoimmune Diseases

Endocarditis in systemic lupus erythematosus or rheumatoid arthritis can also result in TR.

Medications

Medications that activate serotoninergic pathways may cause valvular lesions similar to those observed with carcinoid. Other medications such as methysergide, pergolide, and fenfluramine have also been associated with tricuspid regurgitation [32, 33].

Tricuspid Stenosis

Tricuspid stenosis(TS) results from inadequate excursion of the valve leaflets due to alterations in the structure of the tricuspid valve. Tricuspid stenosis leads to a persistent diastolic pressure gradient between the right atrium and right ventricle. This gradient increases when blood flow across the tricuspid valve increase (inspiration and exercise) and decreases when blood flow decreases (expiration). A mean pressure gradient of 2 mmHg establishes the diagnosis of TS. A gradient as low as 5 mmHg usually leads to an elevated mean right atrial pressure. As a result, most patients with significant TS have jugular venous distension, ascites, and peripheral edema.

There are four main causes of TS: rheumatic heart disease, carcinoid heart disease, congenital TS or tricuspid atresia, and endocarditis. The most common etiology is rheumatic fever, and tricuspid valve involvement occurs universally with mitral and aortic valve involvement [34-37]. Other rare causes are listed in the table below.

Rheumatic tricuspid stenosis results from diffuse thickening of the leaflets and occurs, with or without fusion of the commissures. The chordae tendineae may be thickened and shortened; however, calcification of the valve rarely occurs. The leaflet tissue is composed of dense collagen and elastic fibers and leads to significant distortion of the normal leaflet layers [34, 35, 38].

Carcinoid heart disease can occasionally result in TS. The carcinoid fibrous white plaques located on the valvular and mural endocardium lead to thickened, rigid leaflets which are restricted in mobility. This usually results in significant tricuspid regurgitation. Fibrous tissue proliferation on the atrial and ventricular surfaces of the valve structure can lead to a reduced valve orifice area [28, 29].

Congenital tricuspid stenosis or tricuspid atresia can manifest as incompletely developed leaflets, shortened or malformed chordae, small annuli, abnormal size and number of the papillary muscles, or any combination of these defects [39, 40]. Other cardiac anomalies are usually present [41].

Bacterial endocarditis of the tricuspid valve usually results in significant regurgitation. However, significant TS occasionally results when large vegetations obstruct the orifice usually in the setting of an infected permanent pacemaker lead or a prosthetic valve.

Unusual causes [36, 37, 42] of stenosis include: Fabry disease, giant blood cysts, right atrial or metastatic tumor, endomyocardial fibrosis, or systemic lupus erythematosus.

Diagnostic Evaluation

Evaluation of Right Ventricular Function

Careful evaluation of the right ventricle is necessary in determining the chronicity and severity of the right sided valvular lesions. This involves evaluation of wall thickness, shape, ventricular cavity size and content, as well as regional and global contractile function. The right ventricle presents challenges to imaging with echocardiography due to its anterior position and complex shape.

The right ventricle plays an important role in the morbidity and mortality of patients presenting with signs and symptoms of cardiopulmonary disease. However, the systematic assessment of right heart function is not uniformly carried out. Because most of the attention has been given to the evaluation of the left heart, there is a paucity of ultrasound studies providing normal reference values of right heart size and function. Recently, the American Society of Echocardiography (ASE) published guidelines regarding the assessment of the right heart. They recommend routine assessment of right ventricular (RV) size, right atrial (RA) size, RV systolic function (fractional area change, Tissue/pulsed Doppler, and tricuspid annular plane systolic excursion), and systolic pulmonary artery (PA) pressure (SPAP) as well as an estimate of RA pressure on the basis of inferior vena cava (IVC) size and collapse [17]. Normalized values are listed in Table 1.

The RV size is best estimated at end-diastole from an apical 4-chamber view, with an view demonstrating the maximum diameter of the right ventricle without foreshortening. RV Diameter > 42 mm at the base and > 35 mm at the mid level, and a longitudinal dimension > 86 mm indicates RV dilation.

The apical 4-chamber view also allows assessment of the RA dimensions (Figure 3). RA area > 18 cm2, RA length > 53 mm, and RA diameter > 44mm indicate at end-diastole RA enlargement.

Cardiac MRI can also provide precise assessment of the right ventricle, allowing for volumetric analysis and assessment of the chamber size and ejection fraction [17].

Table 2. [17]

Variable	Abnormal
Chamber Dimensions	
RV basal diameter	>4.2cm
RV subcostal wall thickness	>0.5cm
RVOT PSAX distal diameter	>2.7cm
RVOT PLAX proximal diameter	>3.3cm
RA major dimension	>5.3cm
RA minor dimension	>4.4cm
RA end-systolic area	>18cm^2
Systolic Function	
TAPSE	<1.6cm
Pulsed Doppler peak velocity at the annulus	<10cm/s
Pulsed Doppler MPI	>0.40
Tissue Doppler MPI	>0.55
FAC %	<35%
Diastolic function	
E/A ratio	<0.8 or >2.1
E/E' ratio	> 6
Deceleration time	<120 ms

FAC – Fraction area change; MPI, myocardial performance index; PLAX, parasternal long-asix; PSAX, parasternal short-asxi, RA, right atrium; RV, right ventricle; RVD, right ventricular diameter, RVOT, right ventricular outflow tract; TAPSE, tricuspid annular plane systolic excursion.

Determining Optimal Time of Intervention

Significant TR can progress over time and lead to symptoms of right heart failure, biventricular failure, and death [43]. A large retrospective study of 5223 patients demonstrated that patients with moderate and severe TR had worse survival than for those with no TR, independent of echo-derived pulmonary artery systolic pressure, left ventricular ejection fraction, inferior vena cava size, and right ventricular size and function [44].

It is unclear whether surgical correction of TR in patients with elevated PASP is indicated. Due to the lack of clear evidence, the guidelines offer only Class III recommendations for asymptomatic patients with PASP < 60mmHg (with level of evidence C) (Table 4) [45]. Although theoretically, the correction of TR could alleviate unfavorable volume overload of the right ventricle, there is no clear evidence that correcting TR in the setting of pulmonary hypertension prevents right ventricular dilation and development of right heart failure.

Although pulmonary artery hypertension from any cause can lead to the development of secondary tricuspid regurgitation, not all patients with pulmonary hypertension develop significant tricuspid regurgitation. Mutlak et al, studied 2139 subjects with either mild, moderate, or severe pulmonary hypertension and found that although , increasing PASP was independently associated with greater degrees of TR (odds ratio, 2.26 per 10 mm Hg increase), many patients with high PASP had only mild TR (65.4% of patients with PASP 50 to 69 mm Hg and 45.6% of patients with PASP >70 mm Hg had only mild TR) [60]. In this study, atrial fibrillation, pacemaker leads, and right heart enlargement, were also significantly associated with TR severity. The authors concluded that the cause of TR in patients with pulmonary hypertension is only partially related to an increase in trans-tricuspid pressure gradient, with remodeling of the right heart in response to elevated PASP as the major mechanism responsible for TR in these patients.

Although there are relatively few existing studies, there is evidence of strong impact of TR on clinical outcome. Patients with moderate and severe TR have been shown to have worse survival, independent of left ventricular ejection fraction or pulmonary artery pressure [44]. In addition, significant TR has been shown to be associated with poor prognosis in patients with mitral stenosis after percutaneous balloon valvuloplasty [46] and with a reduction in exercise capacity after mitral valve surgery [47]. Furthermore, in 60 patients with flail tricuspid leaflet due to trauma, significant increases in atrial fibrillation, heart failure, and death were observed [48]. TR has also been shown to be an independent predictor of increased mortality in 1400 patients with left ventricular systolic dysfunction [49].

However, the impact of surgical correction of tricuspid regurgitation on long-term outcomes is still unknown. Recently, a study of >2000 patients demonstrated that 34% of patients had moderate or severe TR at 3 months post surgery, which increased to 45% of patients at 5 years, irrespective of the mode of repair [50]. Risk factors of recurrent TR include higher grade of pre-operative TR, female gender, mitral valve replacement, and left ventricular dysfunction. One study of 39 patients demonstrated the importance of both right and left ventricular function in addition to tricuspid valve tethering, in predicting the durability of tricuspid repair [51].

Although these prior studies have not include comprehensive evaluation of RV function before and after tricuspid valve repair, a recent study prospectively enrolled patients with isolated severe TR to identify preoperative predictors of clinical outcomes after surgery. Kim, et al demonstrated that RV end systolic area was a reliable indicator of good postoperative outcome on multivariable analysis. In this study, there was a relatively high operative mortality of 9.8% and a poor event-free survival rate of 75% during a median follow-up period of 32 months. These results are disappointing because left-sided valve surgeries have shown operative mortality rates as low as 1% to 2% in many cardiac centers [52]. However, operative mortality and event-free survival were much improved in patients with preserved RV systolic function in this study. In patients with preoperative RV ESA< 20 cm^2, operative mortality and 2-year event-free survival rate were 0% and 91%, respectively. These findings imply that RV function strongly impacts outcomes in patients with severe tricuspid regurgitation [53]. Three-dimensional echocardiography and cardiac magnetic resonance imaging may offer a better assessment of RV volume and systolic function, and further studies with these new imaging modalities should be conducted.

Over time, severe tricuspid regurgitation can lead to congestive hepatopathy, resulting in hepatocyte dysfunction, atrophy, and eventually cardiac cirrhosis (fibrosis) due to elevated pressures and volume overload transmitted from the right heart to the liver. Liver dysfunction can also occur due to ischemic hepatopathy secondary to decreased cardiac output [54]. In general, most patients with cardiac cirrhosis present late in the disease state, at which time they may be too high risk for surgical intervention, given their coagulopathic state and low likelihood of improvement of right ventricular function. Therefore, it is essential to identify these patients before they progress to end-stage right heart failure.

Symptomatic Severe TR

In patients with severe TR and symptoms of right heart failure, the underlying cause for the TR should be ascertained and optimally treated. If the TR continues to be severe, or the patient is undergoing mitral valve repair/replacement, patients can undergo tricuspid annuloplasty. Patients with intrinsic tricuspid valve pathology may require tricuspid valve replacement if the valve is not amenable to repair. Because of the increased incidence of mechanical prosthetic valve thrombosis in this low-flow position, a bioprosthetic valve is preferable.

Asymptomatic Severe TR

Patients with severe TR and no symptoms or echocardiographic signs of right heart failure can be treated medically. The underlying cause for the TR again should be determined and optimally treated. If the patient is undergoing mitral valve repair/replacement, it is reasonable to also repair the tricuspid valve at that time. However, if TR is the sole valvular lesion, the patient can be treated medically with diuretics as needed, but will need to be followed closely with to look for signs of RV dilation or failure. Once this occurs, the patient may benefit from tricuspid annuloplasty or replacement as patients with severe TR and signs of RV failure have worse outcomes [46].

Symptomatic Moderate TR

Patients with moderate TR and symptoms of right heart failure should be optimally medically treated. Thorough investigations for other causes of RV failure should be conducted and addressed. There are no current guidelines for surgical intervention in patients with moderate TR regardless of symptoms. Therefore, tricuspid annuloplasty or replacement should only be considered if the patient is undergoing open heart surgery for other reasons, or has severe, refractory symptoms despite optimal medical therapy.

Symptomatic Severe TS

Patients with signs and symptoms of systemic venous hypertension and congestion should be considered for balloon valvotomy. Patients with symptoms and transvalvular pressure gradients of $\geq$ 3 mmHg and valve areas < 1.5 cm2 can be referred for this intervention. Valvotomy is contraindicated in patients with moderate or severe TR. Valve area usually increases from < 1.0 cm2 to almost 2.0 cm2. Residual TS usually still persists, however, the increase in valve area is usually sufficient to produce a significant reduction in the transvalvular pressure gradient and right atrial pressure as well as symptoms [5, 56]. Tumor masses, vegetations, and thrombi are also contraindications to valvotomy. Patients with the previously stated conditions or with intrinsic valve disease with severely altered tricuspid valve morphology should undergo a tricuspid replacement with a bioprosthetic valve.

Asymptomatic Severe TS

In the treatment of tricuspid stenosis, the underlying cause of the valvular pathology should be assessed and treated appropriately. Treat bacterial endocarditis with the appropriate antibiotics as determined by the sensitivity of the organisms cultured. Restore sinus rhythm if any cardiac arrhythmias are present. Decrease right atrial volume overload with diuresis and salt restriction. If TS remains severe and the patient exhibits echocardiographic signs of right heart failure valvotomy or tricuspid replacement may be reasonable.

Symptomatic Moderate TS

As stated above, the underlying cause of the valvular pathology should be assessed and treated appropriately. Endocarditis and cardiac arrhythmias should be treated appropriately. If the patient's symptoms persist and/or the patient exhibits echocardiographic signs of right heart failure valvotomy may be reasonable.

Selecting and Guiding Therapy

Medical Therapy

Mild TR do not warrant medical therapy as these findings are physiologic. More significant tricuspid regurgitation is most often secondary to left sided heart disease or pulmonary hypertension. Therefore, the mainstay of medical therapy is to treat the underlying cause to prevent progression to right ventricular failure. When right heart failure is present, diuretics and restoration of sinus rhythm are the focus of medical therapy.

Surgical Valve Repair/Replacement

Surgical valve repair is always preferred given the low-flow state of the right side of the heart and the theoretic risk of thrombosis of prosthetic valves. Because the septal wall leaflet is relatively small and fixed, it usually is spared when the tricuspid annulus dilates. Therefore, the septal annulus is typically used for tricuspid annular sizing algorithms [57, 58]. With functional TR, the main surgical strategies are to insert annular bands (rigid or flexible), which reduce the annular size with the aim of improving leaflet coaptation. Other forms of tricuspid repair include: Alfieri-type repairs [58, 59]; partial purse-string suture techniques to reduce the anterior posterior portions of the annulus (DeVega-style technique) [60]; and posterior annular bicuspidalization (placing a pledget-supported mattress suture from the anteroposterior commissure to the posteroseptal commissure along the posterior annulus) [64, 61].

Surgical valve replacement should only be performed when the valve cannot be repaired. Patients with severely altered tricuspid valve morphology should undergo a valve replacement. Historically, bioprosthetic valves are the valves of choice given theoretic high likelihood of thrombosis of mechanical valves, given the relatively low-flow state of the right heart. However, a recent meta-analysis has demonstrated that the thrombosis rate of mechanical tricuspid valves is extremely low (<1% per year). Furthermore, there was no significant difference in overall survival in patient with bioprosthetic tricuspid valves vs. mechanical valves [62].

Percutaneous Approaches to the Tricuspid Valve

Although tricuspid valve repair/replacement should be performed surgically in the setting of concomitant left sided valvular disease or significant coronary artery disease, percutaneous approaches may be attractive alternative options for patients with isolated tricuspid disease. As correction of isolated tricuspid regurgitation has been shown to result in improved RV function [63], percutaneous approaches to the tricuspid valve may offer an alternative strategy to those who are too high risk for surgical repair/replacement.

There have been recent advancements in the realm of percutaneous strategies for addressing tricuspid valve disease. Although annular dilatation, is the most common scenario leading to significant tricuspid regurgitation, exacerbation of right heart failure, right atrial dilatation and arrhythmia, no percutaneous tricuspid annuloplasty techniques have been developed. Because of the complex morphology of the tricuspid valve, a transcatheter approach to repair of this valve using an annuloplasty ring has not been attempted. This is likely due to the complex geometry of the tricuspid annulus and the lack of a suitable approach and anatomical anchor for a percutaneous annuloplasty ring.

Placement of a surgical Alfieri stitch has been reported for treatment of tricuspid regurgitation [58, 59]. Therefore, just as an percutaneous approach to the mitral valve using an E-clip has been developed, this percutaneous technique could potentially be translated to the tricuspid valve. However, because of the complex tri-leaflet morphology of the tricuspid valve, this technique would be much more technically challenging.

However, percutaneous valve replacement has been performed in animals. There have been a few case reports of percutaneous tricuspid valve procedures in humans. Roberts, et al. [64] describe implantation of a percutaneous transjugular TVR with a 22-mm percutaneous Medtronic Melody pulmonary valve in a 28-year-old woman with a history of bioprosthetic tricuspid valve replacement (27-mm Medtronic Mosaic valve, Minneapolis, Minn) for tricuspid endocarditis, who presented 9 years later with progressive New York Heart Association Class III right-sided heart failure caused by severe tricuspid valve stenosis, mean tricuspid transvalvular gradient of 16 mm Hg, with mild tricuspid regurgitation. Internal valve diameter was estimated at 21 mm, using 3D transesophageal echo images.

The procedure was performed in the cardiac catheterization laboratory under general anesthesia through the right jugular approach. A percutaneous balloon tricuspid valvuloplasty was performed to confirm device sizing, The inflation of the 20-mm balloon resulted in only transient amelioration of the pressure gradient across the valve. The percutaneous Medtronic Melody pulmonary valve was deployed using a 22-mm Ensemble delivery system. Figure 9 The transvalvular mean gradient decreased acutely from 13 mm Hg to 3.6 mm Hg. Mild tricuspid regurgitation was observed and was unchanged from before the procedure. The procedure was complicated by a minor neck hematoma, but was otherwise uncomplicated. Her symptoms improved and her functional class decreased from NYHA Class III to I.

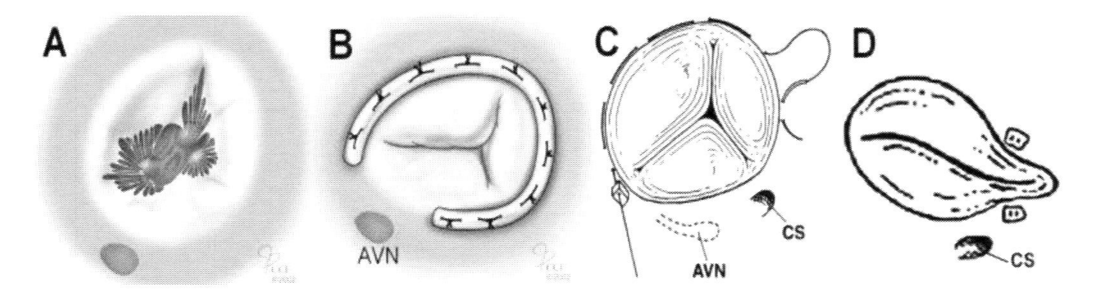

Figure 10. Predominant surgical repair techniques for functional tricuspid regurgitation (TR). The main surgical approaches for correcting functional TR in the presence of a dilated annulus are shown. (A) Dilated tricuspid annulus with abnormal circular shape, failure of leaflet coaptation, and resultant TR. Note that in functional TR, dilation occurs primarily along the mural portion of the tricuspid annulus, above the right ventricular free wall. (B) Rigid or flexible annular bands are used to restore a more normal annular size and shape (ovoid), thereby reducing or eliminating TR. The open ring shown spares the atrioventricular node (AVN), thus reducing the incidence of heart block. (C) DeVega–style suture annuloplasty in which a purse-string suture technique is used to partially plicate the annulus and reduce annular circumference and diameter. (D) Suture bicuspidalization is performed by placement of a mattress suture from the anteroposterior to the posteroseptal commissures along the posterior annulus. CS indicates coronary sinus [1].

On the other hand, Boccuzzi, et al report successful percutaneous balloon valvuloplasty in a 26-year-old woman with severe tricuspid stenosis and Ebstein's anomaly [65]. The patient had a mean diastolic gradient across her tricuspid valve was 13mmHg, with a peak gradient of 19mmHg and moderate tricuspid regurgitation. Percutaneous transcatheter balloon valvuloplasty elected to reduce the gradient across the tricuspid valve despite the moderate valvular regurgitation. Balloon valvuloplasty was performed with a 20x45mm crystal balloon inflated at nominal pressure. Two inflations were performed. After the balloon valvuloplasty (Figure 10,11), the mean diastolic gradient across the tricuspid valve decreased from 9mm to 4mmHg. The right ventriculogram done after the procedure showed a mild worsening of the tricuspid. However, the patient's symptoms improved immediately, and the leg edema disappeared in a few days. Predischarge transthoracic echocardiography demonstrated a persistent reduction in mean diastolic gradient across the tricuspid valve to 4 mmHg, which was also confirmed at 1-month follow-up.

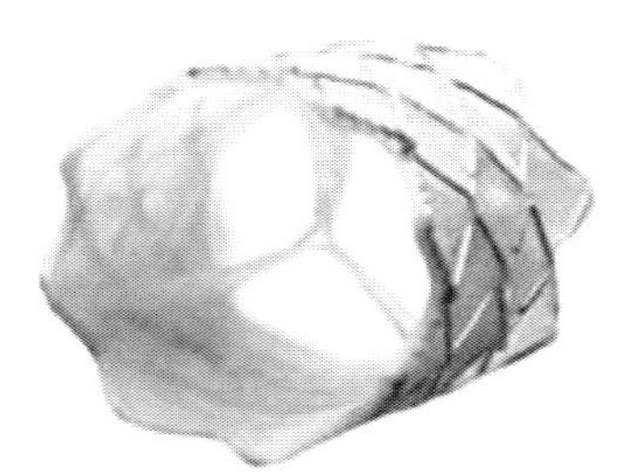

Figure 11. Medtronic Melody pulmonary valve.

Boudjemline, et al have reported successful insertion of a novel percutaneous tricuspid valve [66]. This valve was comprised of a bovine jugular venous valve mounted to two self-expanding nitinol disks. Figure 12 and 13. The device was delivered via an 18F sheath in the right internal jugular vein in normal sheep. Complications that were reported in this study include entrapment of the device in tricuspid cordae, leading to its incomplete valve opening, and a significant paravalvular leak in a separate animal. This device has not yet advanced to human studies.

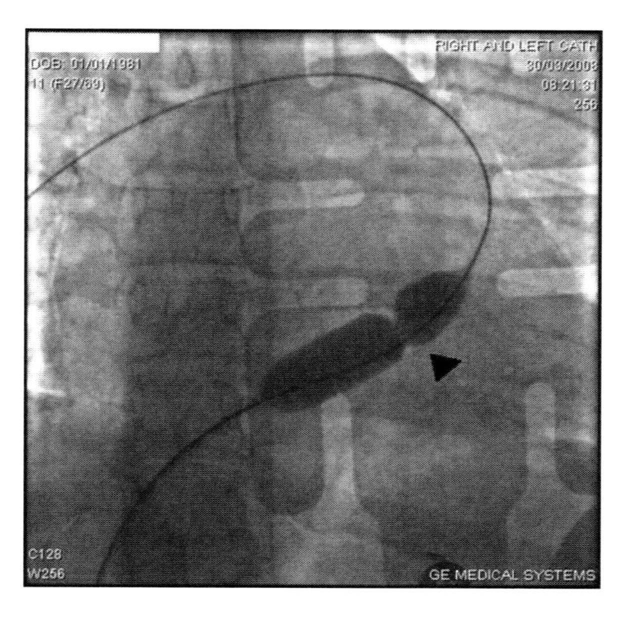

Figure 12. Fluoroscopic image in the anterior posterior view demonstrates the balloon's waist (black arrow) during the inflation in the stenotic valve [65].

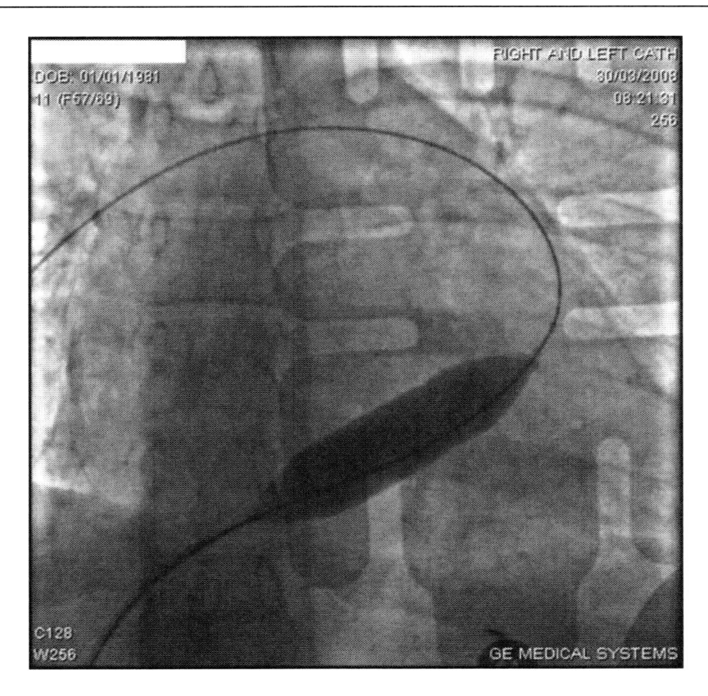

Figure 13. Balloon valvuloplasty was performed with a 20_45mm crystal balloon inflated at nominal pressure[65].

In addition, Lauten, et al performed percutaneous implantation of valved stents in the inferior vena cava (IVC) and superior vena cava (SVC) in sheep with severe tricuspid regurgitation due to papillary muscle and chrodae avulsion [67]. Two self-expanding nitinol stents containing a porcine pulmonary valve were then percutanesously implanted in the IVC and SVC. Figure 14 and 15 Implantation was performed through the right jugular vein via a 21 F catheter under fluoroscopic guidance. After deployment of the IVC and the SVC valve, there was a significant improvement in cardiac output and venous regurgitation. The authors concluded that the implantation of one or two valves in central venous position is technically feasible and functional replacement of the insufficient tricuspid valve leads to an increase in CO [67].

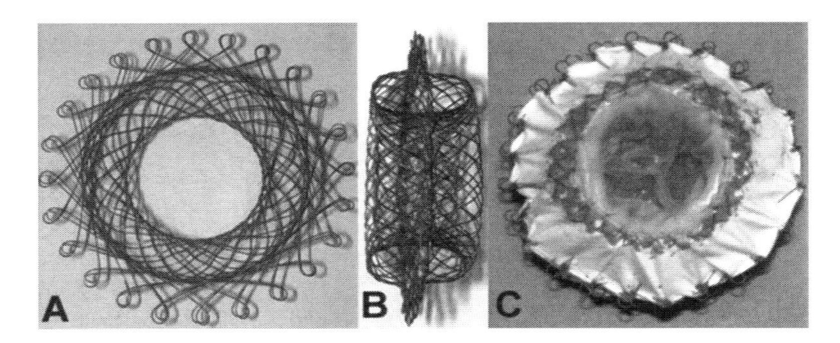

Figure 14. (A, B, C) En face and lateral views of the newly designed stent before its covering **(A and B)**, after its covering by a polytetrafluoroethylene membrane and the suture of the valve in the central tubular part **(C)**. The stent is shown from the ventricular side with a valve in closed position [66].

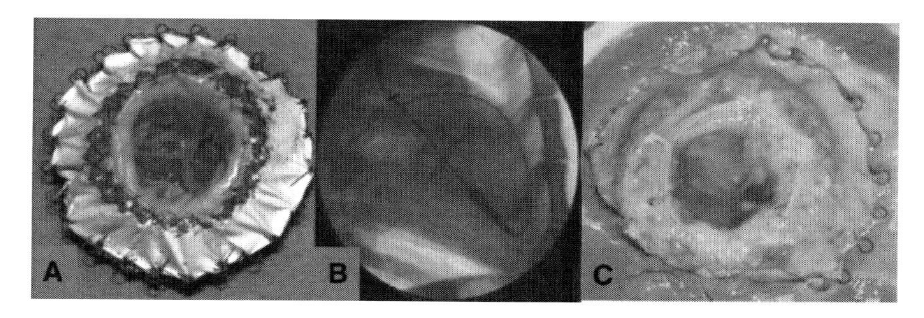

Figure 15. Percutaneous tricuspid valve replacement. (A) Novel nitinol stent-based percutaneous tricuspid valve. An 18-mm bovine jugular venous valve is mounted in the central part of the stent, with a polytetrafluoroethylene membrane sutured to the ventricular disk to assist in sealing. B, Percutaneous tricuspid valve delivered in an ovine model via an 18F sheath in the internal jugular vein under fluoroscopic and echocardiographic guidance. C, Gross appearance of valve explanted at 1 month after implantation showing neoendocardial coverage of the stent (atrial view) [66].

Obstacles for percutaneous approaches to the tricuspid valve include the lack of stable adjacent structures for device placement (i.e coronary sinus and its relationship to the mitral valve). Furthermore, the relatively low-flow state in the right heart may promote thrombus formation, and may require anti-platelet/anticoagulant therapy. The close proximity of the coronary sinus ostium, atrioventricular node, and inferior vena cava to the tricuspid valve result in much more technical difficulties in successfully deploying percutaneous devices. However, as technology continues to advance, solutions for these obstacles may arise and make percutaneous devices more feasible in the future.

Conclusion

Because reoperation for recurrent TR carry high mortality rates, and recurrence of tricuspid regurgitation after surgical repair is common, few patients are offered reoperation. Percutaneous approaches to tricuspid valve disease could attractive alternative solution. In addition, the less invasive strategies may allow earlier mechanical treatment of TR than is currently practiced. There are many challenges and obstacles to emerging percutaneous approaches, however with the advancement of cardiac imaging and percutaneous devices, advancement in this area is likely to continue.

References

[1] Rogers JH, Bolling SF. The tricuspid valve: current perspective and evolving management of tricuspid regurgitation. *Circulation* 2009;119(20):2718-25.

[2] Silver MD, Lam JH, Ranganathan N, Wigle ED. Morphology of the human tricuspid valve. *Circulation* 1971;43(3):333-48.

[3] Anwar AM, Geleijnse ML, Soliman OI, McGhie JS, Frowijn R, Nemes A, et al. Assessment of normal tricuspid valve anatomy in adults by real-time three-dimensional echocardiography. *Int J Cardiovasc Imaging* 2007;23(6):717-24.

[4] Brown AK, Anderson V. Two dimensional echocardiography and the tricuspid valve. Leaflet definition and prolapse. *Br Heart J* 1983;49(5):495-500.
[5] Tei C, Shah PM, Cherian G, Trim PA, Wong M, Ormiston JA. Echocardiographic evaluation of normal and prolapsed tricuspid valve leaflets. *Am J Cardiol* 1983;52(7):796-800.
[6] Otto CM. Textbook of clinical echocardiography, 3rd Edition. 2004.
[7] Tajik AJ, Seward JB, Hagler DJ, Mair DD, Lie JT. Two-dimensional real-time ultrasonic imaging of the heart and great vessels. Technique, image orientation, structure identification, and validation. *Mayo Clin Proc* 1978;53(5):271-303.
[8] Fukuda S, Saracino G, Matsumura Y, Daimon M, Tran H, Greenberg NL, et al. Three-dimensional geometry of the tricuspid annulus in healthy subjects and in patients with functional tricuspid regurgitation: a real-time, 3-dimensional echocardiographic study. *Circulation* 2006;114(1 Suppl):I492-8.
[9] Cheitlin MD, Armstrong WF, Aurigemma GP, Beller GA, Bierman FZ, Davis JL, et al. ACC/AHA/ASE 2003 guideline update for the clinical application of echocardiography--summary article: a report of the American College of Cardiology/American Heart Association Task Force on Practice Guidelines (ACC/AHA/ASE Committee to Update the 1997 Guidelines for the Clinical Application of Echocardiography). *J Am Coll Cardiol* 2003;42(5):954-70.
[10] Fawzy ME, Mercer EN, Dunn B, al-Amri M, Andaya W. Doppler echocardiography in the evaluation of tricuspid stenosis. *Eur Heart J* 1989;10(11):985-90.
[11] Shah PM, Raney AA. Tricuspid valve disease. *Curr Probl Cardiol* 2008;33(2):47-84.
[12] Perez JE, Ludbrook PA, Ahumada GG. Usefulness of Doppler echocardiography in detecting tricuspid valve stenosis. *Am J Cardiol* 1985;55(5):601-3.
[13] Zoghbi WA, Enriquez-Sarano M, Foster E, Grayburn PA, Kraft CD, Levine RA, et al. Recommendations for evaluation of the severity of native valvular regurgitation with two-dimensional and Doppler echocardiography. *J Am Soc Echocardiogr* 2003;16(7):777-802.
[14] Shapira Y, Porter A, Wurzel M, Vaturi M, Sagie A. Evaluation of tricuspid regurgitation severity: echocardiographic and clinical correlation. *J Am Soc Echocardiogr* 1998;11(6):652-9.
[15] Simpson IA, Shiota T, Gharib M, Sahn DJ. Current status of flow convergence for clinical applications: is it a leaning tower of "PISA"? *J Am Coll Cardiol* 1996;27(2):504-9.
[16] Imanishi T, Nakatani S, Yamada S, Nakanishi N, Beppu S, Nagata S, et al. Validation of continuous wave Doppler-determined right ventricular peak positive and negative dP/dt: effect of right atrial pressure on measurement. *J Am Coll Cardiol* 1994;23(7):1638-43.
[17] Rudski LG, Lai WW, Afilalo J, Hua L, Handschumacher MD, Chandrasekaran K, et al. Guidelines for the echocardiographic assessment of the right heart in adults: a report from the American Society of Echocardiography endorsed by the European Association of Echocardiography, a registered branch of the European Society of Cardiology, and the Canadian Society of Echocardiography. *J Am Soc Echocardiogr*;23(7):685-713; quiz 786-8.

[18] Danicek V, Sagie A, Vaturi M, Weisenberg DE, Rot G, Shapira Y. Relation of tricuspid inflow E-wave peak velocity to severity of tricuspid regurgitation. *Am J Cardiol* 2006;98(3):399-401.

[19] Skjaerpe T, Hatle L. Diagnosis of tricuspid regurgitation. Sensitivity of Doppler ultrasound compared with contrast echocardiography. *Eur Heart J* 1985;6(5):429-36.

[20] Waller BF, Howard J, Fess S. Pathology of tricuspid valve stenosis and pure tricuspid regurgitation--Part III. *Clin Cardiol* 1995;18(4):225-30.

[21] Waller BF, Moriarty AT, Eble JN, Davey DM, Hawley DA, Pless JE. Etiology of pure tricuspid regurgitation based on anular circumference and leaflet area: analysis of 45 necropsy patients with clinical and morphologic evidence of pure tricuspid regurgitation. *J Am Coll Cardiol* 1986;7(5):1063-74.

[22] Fukuda S, Song JM, Gillinov AM, McCarthy PM, Daimon M, Kongsaerepong V, et al. Tricuspid valve tethering predicts residual tricuspid regurgitation after tricuspid annuloplasty. *Circulation* 2005;111(8):975-9.

[23] Gussenhoven EJ, Stewart PA, Becker AE, Essed CE, Ligtvoet KM, De Villeneuve VH. "Offsetting" of the septal tricuspid leaflet in normal hearts and in hearts with Ebstein's anomaly. Anatomic and echographic correlation. *Am J Cardiol* 1984;54(1):172-6.

[24] Shiina A, Seward JB, Edwards WD, Hagler DJ, Tajik AJ. Two-dimensional echocardiographic spectrum of Ebstein's anomaly: detailed anatomic assessment. *J Am Coll Cardiol* 1984;3(2 Pt 1):356-70.

[25] Attenhofer Jost CH, Connolly HM, Dearani JA, Edwards WD, Danielson GK. Ebstein's anomaly. *Circulation* 2007;115(2):277-85.

[26] Khan IA. Ebstein's anomaly of the tricuspid valve with associated mitral valve prolapse. *Tex Heart Inst J* 2001;28(1):72.

[27] Frater R. Tricuspid insufficiency. *J Thorac Cardiovasc Surg* 2001;122(3):427-9.

[28] Lundin L, Norheim I, Landelius J, Oberg K, Theodorsson-Norheim E. Carcinoid heart disease: relationship of circulating vasoactive substances to ultrasound-detectable cardiac abnormalities. *Circulation* 1988;77(2):264-9.

[29] Pellikka PA, Tajik AJ, Khandheria BK, Seward JB, Callahan JA, Pitot HC, et al. Carcinoid heart disease. Clinical and echocardiographic spectrum in 74 patients. *Circulation* 1993;87(4):1188-96.

[30] Simula DV, Edwards WD, Tazelaar HD, Connolly HM, Schaff HV. Surgical pathology of carcinoid heart disease: a study of 139 valves from 75 patients spanning 20 years. *Mayo Clin Proc* 2002;77(2):139-47.

[31] Luo GH, Ma WG, Sun HS, Xu JP, Sun LZ, Hu SS. Correction of traumatic tricuspid insufficiency using the double orifice technique. *Asian Cardiovasc Thorac Ann* 2005;13(3):238-40.

[32] Pritchett AM, Morrison JF, Edwards WD, Schaff HV, Connolly HM, Espinosa RE. Valvular heart disease in patients taking pergolide. *Mayo Clin Proc* 2002;77(12):1280-6.

[33] Connolly HM, Crary JL, McGoon MD, Hensrud DD, Edwards BS, Edwards WD, et al. Valvular heart disease associated with fenfluramine-phentermine. *N Engl J Med* 1997;337(9):581-8.

[34] Daniels SJ, Mintz GS, Kotler MN. Rheumatic tricuspid valve disease: two-dimensional echocardiographic, hemodynamic, and angiographic correlations. *Am J Cardiol* 1983;51(3):492-6.

[35] Hauck AJ, Freeman DP, Ackermann DM, Danielson GK, Edwards WD. Surgical pathology of the tricuspid valve: a study of 363 cases spanning 25 years. *Mayo Clin Proc* 1988;63(9):851-63.

[36] Waller BF. Morphological aspects of valvular heart disease: *Part II. Curr Probl Cardiol* 1984;9(8):1-74.

[37] Waller BF. Morphological aspects of valvular heart disease: *Part I. Curr Probl Cardiol* 1984;9(7):1-66.

[38] Roguin A, Rinkevich D, Milo S, Markiewicz W, Reisner SA. Long-term follow-up of patients with severe rheumatic tricuspid stenosis. *Am Heart J* 1998;136(1):103-8.

[39] Cohen ML, Spray T, Gutierrez F, Barzilai B, Bauwens D. Congenital tricuspid valve stenosis with atrial septal defect and left anterior fascicular block. *Clin Cardiol* 1990;13(7):497-9.

[40] Tennstedt C, Chaoui R, Korner H, Dietel M. Spectrum of congenital heart defects and extracardiac malformations associated with chromosomal abnormalities: results of a seven year necropsy study. *Heart* 1999;82(1):34-9.

[41] Lev M, Liberthson RR, Joseph RH, Seten CE, Eckner FA, Kunske RD, et al. The pathologic anatomy of Ebstein's disease. *Arch Pathol* 1970;90(4):334-43.

[42] Acikel M, Erol MK, Yekeler I, Ozyazicioglu A. A case of free-floating ball thrombus in right atrium with tricuspid stenosis. *Int J Cardiol* 2004;94(2-3):329-30.

[43] McCarthy PM, Bhudia SK, Rajeswaran J, Hoercher KJ, Lytle BW, Cosgrove DM, et al. Tricuspid valve repair: durability and risk factors for failure. *J Thorac Cardiovasc Surg* 2004;127(3):674-85.

[44] Nath J, Foster E, Heidenreich PA. Impact of tricuspid regurgitation on long-term survival. *J Am Coll Cardiol* 2004;43(3):405-9.

[45] Bonow RO, Carabello BA, Kanu C, de Leon AC, Jr., Faxon DP, Freed MD, et al. ACC/AHA 2006 guidelines for the management of patients with valvular heart disease: a report of the American College of Cardiology/American Heart Association Task Force on Practice Guidelines (writing committee to revise the 1998 Guidelines for the Management of Patients With Valvular Heart Disease): developed in collaboration with the Society of Cardiovascular Anesthesiologists: endorsed by the Society for Cardiovascular Angiography and Interventions and the Society of Thoracic Surgeons. *Circulation* 2006;114(5):e84-231.

[46] Sagie A, Schwammenthal E, Newell JB, Harrell L, Joziatis TB, Weyman AE, et al. Significant tricuspid regurgitation is a marker for adverse outcome in patients undergoing percutaneous balloon mitral valvuloplasty. *J Am Coll Cardiol* 1994;24(3):696-702.

[47] Groves PH, Lewis NP, Ikram S, Maire R, Hall RJ. Reduced exercise capacity in patients with tricuspid regurgitation after successful mitral valve replacement for rheumatic mitral valve disease. *Br Heart J* 1991;66(4):295-301.

[48] Messika-Zeitoun D, Thomson H, Bellamy M, Scott C, Tribouilloy C, Dearani J, et al. Medical and surgical outcome of tricuspid regurgitation caused by flail leaflets. *J Thorac Cardiovasc Surg* 2004;128(2):296-302.

[49] Koelling TM, Aaronson KD, Cody RJ, Bach DS, Armstrong WF. Prognostic significance of mitral regurgitation and tricuspid regurgitation in patients with left ventricular systolic dysfunction. *Am Heart J* 2002;144(3):524-9.

[50] Navia JL, Nowicki ER, Blackstone EH, Brozzi NA, Nento DE, Atik FA, et al. Surgical management of secondary tricuspid valve regurgitation: annulus, commissure, or leaflet procedure? *J Thorac Cardiovasc Surg*;139(6):1473-1482 e5.

[51] Fukuda S, Gillinov AM, McCarthy PM, Stewart WJ, Song JM, Kihara T, et al. Determinants of recurrent or residual functional tricuspid regurgitation after tricuspid annuloplasty. *Circulation* 2006;114(1 Suppl):I582-7.

[52] Gammie JS, O'Brien SM, Griffith BP, Ferguson TB, Peterson ED. Influence of hospital procedural volume on care process and mortality for patients undergoing elective surgery for mitral regurgitation. *Circulation* 2007;115(7):881-7.

[53] Kim YJ, Kwon DA, Kim HK, Park JS, Hahn S, Kim KH, et al. Determinants of surgical outcome in patients with isolated tricuspid regurgitation. *Circulation* 2009;120(17):1672-8.

[54] Deloche A, Guerinon J, Fabiani JN, Morillo F, Caramanian M, Carpentier A, et al. [Anatomical study of rheumatic tricuspid valve diseases: Application to the study of various valvuloplasties]. *Ann Chir Thorac Cardiovasc* 1973;12(4):343-9.

[55] Orbe LC, Sobrino N, Arcas R, Peinado R, Frutos A, Blazquez JR, et al. Initial outcome of percutaneous balloon valvuloplasty in rheumatic tricuspid valve stenosis. *Am J Cardiol* 1993;71(4):353-4.

[56] Ribeiro PA, Al Zaibag M, Al Kasab S, Idris M, Halim M, Abdullah M, et al. Percutaneous double balloon valvotomy for rheumatic tricuspid stenosis. *Am J Cardiol* 1988;61(8):660-2.

[57] Yiwu L, Yingchun C, Jianqun Z, Bin Y, Ping B. Exact quantitative selective annuloplasty of the tricuspid valve. *J Thorac Cardiovasc Surg* 2001;122(3):611-4.

[58] Castedo E, Canas A, Cabo RA, Burgos R, Ugarte J. Edge-to-Edge tricuspid repair for redeveloped valve incompetence after DeVega's annuloplasty. *Ann Thorac Surg* 2003;75(2):605-6.

[59] Castedo E, Monguio E, Cabo RA, Ugarte J. Edge-to-edge technique for correction of tricuspid valve regurgitation due to complex lesions. *Eur J Cardiothorac Surg* 2005;27(5):933-4; author reply 934-5.

[60] Devega N. La anulopastia selective, reguable y permanente. *Revista Espanola de Cardiologia* 1972;25:6-9.

[61] Ghanta RK, Chen R, Narayanasamy N, McGurk S, Lipsitz S, Chen FY, et al. Suture bicuspidization of the tricuspid valve versus ring annuloplasty for repair of functional tricuspid regurgitation: midterm results of 237 consecutive patients. *J Thorac Cardiovasc Surg* 2007;133(1):117-26.

[62] Kunadian B, Vijayalakshmi K, Balasubramanian S, Dunning J. Should the tricuspid valve be replaced with a mechanical or biological valve? *Interact Cardiovasc Thorac Surg* 2007;6(4):551-7.

[63] Mukherjee D, Nader S, Olano A, Garcia MJ, Griffin BP. Improvement in right ventricular systolic function after surgical correction of isolated tricuspid regurgitation. *J Am Soc Echocardiogr* 2000;13(7):650-4.

[64] Roberts P, Spina R, Vallely M, Wilson M, Bailey B, Celermajer DS. Percutaneous tricuspid valve replacement for a stenosed bioprosthesis. *Circ Cardiovasc Interv*;3(4):e14-5.

[65] Boccuzzi G, Gigli N, Cian D, Vullo C, Bonomini L, Ribichini F, et al. Percutaneous transcatheter balloon valvuloplasty for severe tricuspid valve stenosis in Ebstein's anomaly. *J Cardiovasc Med* (Hagerstown) 2009;10(6):510-5.
[66] Boudjemline Y, Agnoletti G, Bonnet D, Behr L, Borenstein N, Sidi D, et al. Steps toward the percutaneous replacement of atrioventricular valves an experimental study. *J Am Coll Cardiol* 2005;46(2):360-5.
[67] Lauten A, Figulla HR, Willich C, Laube A, Rademacher W, Schubert H, et al. Percutaneous caval stent valve implantation: investigation of an interventional approach for treatment of tricuspid regurgitation. *Eur Heart J*;31(10):1274-81.
[68] Bonow RO, Carabello BA, Chatterjee K, de Leon AC, Jr., Faxon DP, Freed MD, et al. 2008 focused update incorporated into the ACC/AHA 2006 guidelines for the management of patients with valvular heart disease: a report of the American College of Cardiology/American Heart Association Task Force on Practice Guidelines (Writing Committee to revise the 1998 guidelines for the management of patients with valvular heart disease). Endorsed by the Society of Cardiovascular Anesthesiologists, Society for Cardiovascular Angiography and Interventions, and Society of Thoracic Surgeons. *J Am Coll Cardiol* 2008;52(13):e1-142.

Appendix

Table 1. PISA method for quantifying TR

1. Area of hemispheric PISA = $2\Pi r^2$ (r = radius of the hemisphere)
2. Flow through PISA = Area · Velocity or $2\Pi r^2 \cdot V_A$ (V_A = aliasing velocity based on the color Doppler scale)
3. Flow through PISA = Flow through regurgitation orifice, based on Continuity Principle
4. Flow through Regurgitation Orifice = ROA · V_R (ROA = Regurgitation Orifice Area; V_R = Regurgitation Velocity)
5. Thus, as per step 3: $2\Pi r^2 \cdot V_A$ = ROA · V_R or ROA = $2\Pi r^2 \cdot V_A/V_R$

Table 2. Simplified method of quantifying regurgitant orifice area (ROA)

1. ROA = $2\Pi r^2 \cdot V_A/V_R$ or $6.28r^2 \cdot V_A/V_R$
2. Measure tricuspid regurgitation velocity, which in absence of pulmonary (or right ventricular) hypertension, would be between 2.0 and 3.0 m/s
3. Adjust V_A to be approximately 1/12th of V_R Thus, if, for example, TR velocity = 3.0 m/s, select V_A at approximately 25 to 30 cm/s
4. ROA = $6.28r^2 \cdot 1/12 = 0.5r^2$
5. Measure PISA radius and estimate ROA

Table 3. Echo Doppler Quantification of TR

PISA radius method with adjusted aliasing scale	Severity of tricuspid regurgitation
PISA radius	
=1-4 mm	Mild
=5-8 mm	Moderate
= >9 mm	Severe

Color flow jet in RA	IVC flow profile	Severity of regurgitation
<2 cm	Normal	Mild
2-4 cm	Normal	Moderate
>4 cm	Systolicreversal	Severe

** Shah PM, Raney AA.Tricuspid valve disease.
Curr Probl Cardiol. 2008 Feb;33(2):47-84.

Table 4. Indications for Surgical intervention for TR in adults [68]

CLASS I

1. Tricuspid valve repair is beneficial for severe TR in patients with MV disease requiring MV surgery. *(Level of Evidence: B)*

CLASS IIa

1. Tricuspid valve replacement or annuloplasty is reasonable for severe primary TR when symptomatic. *(Level of Evidence: C)*
2. Tricuspid valve replacement is reasonable for severe TR secondary to diseased/abnormal tricuspid valve leaflets not amenable to annuloplasty or repair. *(Level of Evidence: C)*

CLASS IIb

Tricuspid annuloplasty may be considered for less than severe TR in patients undergoing MV surgery when there is pulmonary hypertension or tricuspid annular dilatation. *(Level of Evidence: C)*

CLASS III

1. Tricuspid valve replacement or annuloplasty is not indicated in asymptomatic patients with TR whose pulmonary artery systolic pressure is less than 60 mm Hg in the presence of a normal MV. *(Level of Evidence: C)*
2. Tricuspid valve replacement or annuloplasty is not indicated in patients with mild primary TR. *(Level of Evidence: C)*

In: Percutaneous Valve Technology: Present and Future ISBN: 978-1-61942-577-4
Editors: Jose Luis Navia and Sharif Al-Ruzzeh

Chapter XXVII

Transcatheter Tricuspid Valve Technology

Nicolas A. Brozzi, Eric E. Roselli, Sharif Al-Ruzzeh and Jose L. Navia

Introduction

Tricuspid valve pathology has a prevalence of 0.8% in the United States of America, significantly less than mitral valve pathology that may be present in up to 2,4% of patients [1]. Most patients with tricuspid valve disease are asymptomatic and receive medical treatment upon development of symptoms, Only 8000 patients receive surgical treatment of the tricuspid valve every year [2].

Tricuspid valve anatomy and function are most frequently affected by pathologic processes that involve other structures of the heart. Historically, most tricuspid valve pathology in adult patients was considered secondary to left heart valve disease leading to changes in right ventricular dimensions and function. It was assumed that tricuspid valve function would improve after treatment of the original left-sided pathology [3]. This concept has been modified after recent studies reported that tricuspid valve pathology persists, and in many cases progresses even after adequate treatment of left heart valve pathology [4, 5]. Treatment of tricuspid valve disease concomitant with left side heart valve disease can improve functional results and long term survival of these patients.

Independent of the etiology of tricuspid valve disease, the indication for surgical treatment is based on the degree of hemodynamic compromise generated by valvular dysfunction. Surgical treatment of tricuspid valve disease has been shown to be associated with increased mortality, but it is most frequently performed simultaneously to the surgical treatment of left side valvular disease, and as such may be a marker for more advanced bi-ventricular dysfunction [6, 7]. However, the surgical correction of tricuspid valve disease has also been shown to improve postoperative recovery and offers clinical and survival benefits to patients with multiple valve disease.

Persistence of tricuspid valve pathology with progressive dysfunction of the right ventricle represents a negative prognostic factor that affects the quality of life and survival of patients. Those patients that require cardiac reoperations for progression of tricuspid valve pathology generally present late in the course of disease after years of medical treatment and are at high risk for surgical mortality [8].

Patients with severe right ventricular dysfunction are especially vulnerable to the fluid shifts and other hydrodynamic sequelae of open heart surgery. This is particularly true for patients requiring reoperations with the potential for associated bleeding and transfusions. These patients are expected to reap the most benefit from a less invasive approach.

Transcatheter valve intervention is a less invasive approach to treating valvular heart diseases. Transcatheter replacement of both the pulmonary and aortic valves have been shown to be safe, and many devices have been implanted in the last decade [9, 10].

A decade has passed since the initial reports of transcatheter valve implants for aortic valve stenosis. Early clinical trials have shown good results in high-risk patients and it's approval for commercial use in the U.S. is expected to result in a 5 fold increase of their application over the following 3-5 years. Recently, the attention has focused on the development of transcatheter techniques for atrioventricular valves [11, 12].

Several transcatheter approaches have been employed to repair the mitral valve in humans as well, including a clip that can bring the free edge of the leaflets together to increase leaflet coaptation, and a band that can be implanted inside the coronary sinus to correct the dilatation of the mitral valve annulus [13, 14]. Several groups have made significant progress toward the development of valves that can be implanted percutaneously in the mitral position, but the experience is limited to feasibility animal studies.

In contrast to the increased attention paid to the other valves, reported experience for the treatment of tricuspid valve insufficiency to date has been limited mostly to animal models with percutaneous implant of stented valves [15]. The initial experiences look promising, but several challenges will need to be resolved before the transcatheter approach becomes an available option for clinical practice.

This chapter will review the anatomic characteristics and functional dynamics of the tricuspid valve, the current therapeutic options, the pioneering experiences with transcatheter valve implantation, and the potential and limitations for development of catheter-based therapies in the future.

Functional Anatomy of the Tricuspid Valve:

The tricuspid valve constitutes the atrio-ventricular valve of the right heart, located between the right atrium and right ventricle. Its three leaflets are designated as anterior, posterior and septal leaflets, that are in continuity by their base with the right atrio-ventricular groove and attached to chordae tendinae by their ventricular surface that precludes their systolic protrusion into the right atrium. The tricuspid valve is not limited by a true fibrous annulus but the base of the tricuspid leaflets are in continuity with the right atrial and ventricular myocardium. Only the medial aspect of the annulus related to the base of the septal leaflet is a component of the fibrous skeleton of the heart. This anatomic characteristic explains the dependence of tricuspid valve function on the hydrodynamic state of the right ventricle and the tendency for early dilatation and insufficiency in patients with increasing pulmonary pressures and right ventricular dysfunction. Papillary muscles vary in number and shape, but most often a prominent anterior papillary muscle is recognized along with varying number of smaller additional papillary muscles arising from the septo-marginalis trabeculae. The chordae tendinae of the tricuspid leaflets are divided into primary and secondary order chordae that generally attach to the head of the papillary muscles and the ventricular surface of the anterior and posterior leaflets. Additionally, third order chordae may be found going from the interventricular septum toward the septal leaflet. (Figure 1).

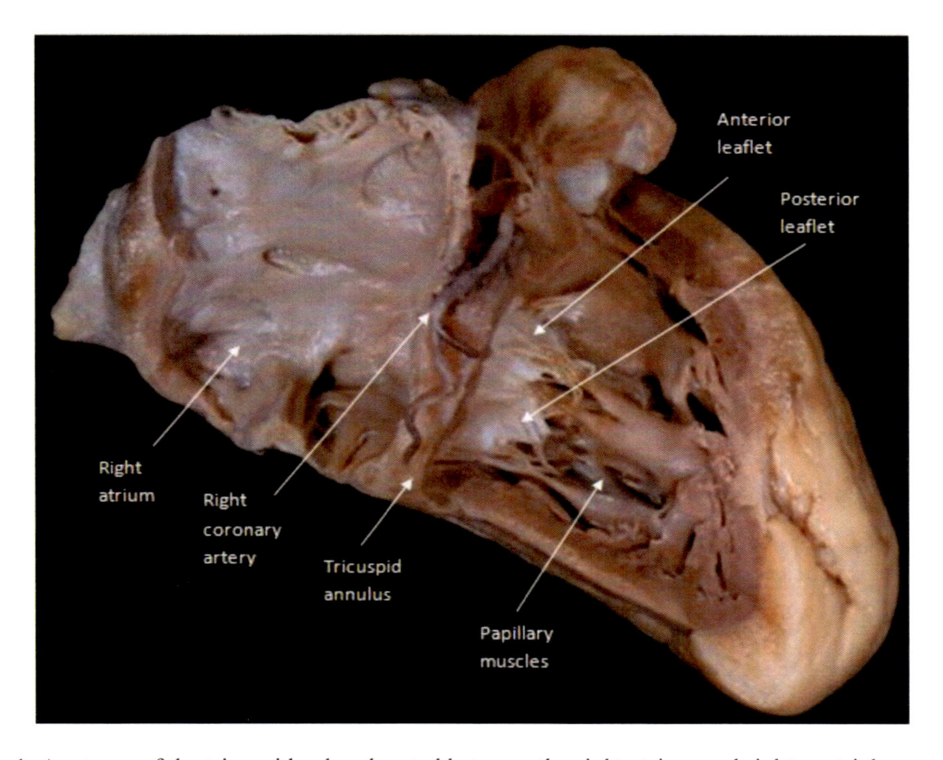

Figure 1. Anatomy of the tricuspid valve, located between the right atrium and right ventricle.

The annular orifice area of the normal tricuspid valve is about 20% larger that the mitral annulus, and the average diameter measured by two-dimensional echocardiography is 3.0 to 3.5 cm in the adult. The annulus expands in diastole providing for the inflow to occur at a lower velocity and lower pressure drop and constricts during midsystole in order to increase leaflet coaptation and tricuspid valve competence [16].

Secondary Tricuspid Regurgitation

Secondary tricuspid valve regurgitation is frequent in patients with long standing left sided-valve disease, particularly in the setting of severe pulmonary hypertension and atrial fibrillation [17]. Uncorrected, moderate, or severe tricuspid regurgitation is associated with progressive heart failure and premature death [18]. Even if corrected, recurrence or progression of tricuspid regurgitation is related to lower long-term survival.

Multiple mechanisms have been implicated in the generation of tricuspid regurgitation in patients with right ventricular dilatation and/or dysfunction secondary to pulmonary hypertension or left side heart disease. As the right ventricle dilates the annulus enlarges considerably even in the absence of substantial tricuspid regurgitation [19]. Recent 3-D echocardiographic studies suggest that as the tricuspid annulus dilates, it looses convexity and flattens potentially altering the normal papillary muscle to leaflet and annulus relationship and resulting in functional regurgitation [20]. Dilatation of the right ventricle also pulls the papillary muscles and the chordae tendinae back and away tethering the leaflets. This mechanism compromises coaptation and has been implicated as a major role in the generation of tricuspid regurgitation [21]. Paradoxical movement of the interventricular septum can also affect the septal leaflet and contribute to tricuspid insufficiency. Most current surgical procedures for correction of tricuspid valve insufficiency address one or two anatomic levels, and this may be one of the reasons for a suboptimal long-term result with high recurrence of regurgitation.

The optimal surgical technique to eliminate tricuspid regurgitation remains challenging [22]. Techniques employed *today* concomitantly with left-sided heart valve surgery address tricuspid regurgitation at 3 anatomic levels—annulus, commissure, and leaflet. The degree to which these alone or in combination are successful in sustained elimination of tricuspid regurgitation is suboptimal, with over 12% of recurrence of TR during long term follow up even with the best techniques. (Figure 2).

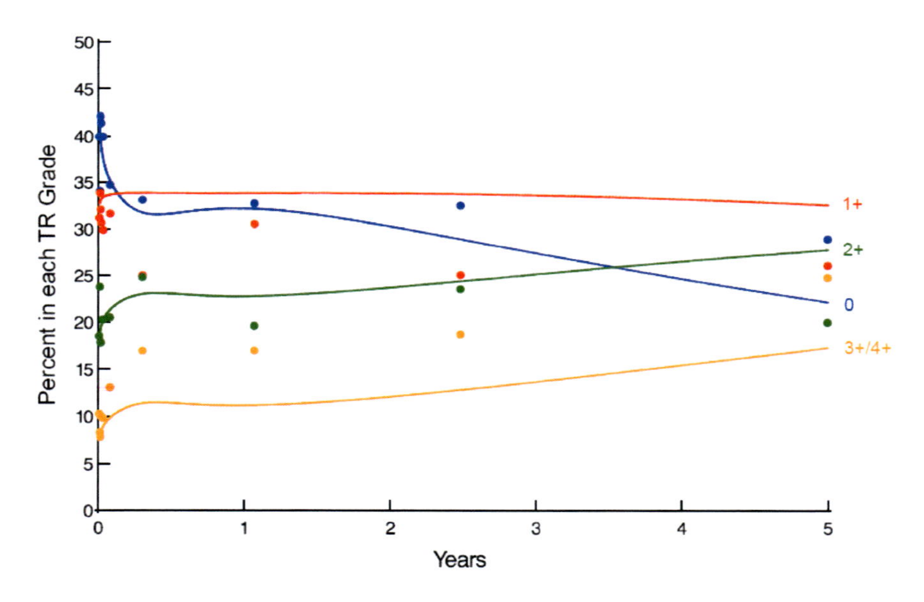

Figure 2. Tricuspid valve insufficiency recurrence after surgical repair [23].

In the largest series reporting long-term follow up comparing different techniques for repair of secondary tricuspid regurgitation, Navia et al concluded that there is not a definitive surgical solution for tricuspid insufficiency and proposed that this might be related to the fact that changes in the anatomy of the tricuspid valve are related to the anatomical changes of the right ventricle and atrium. As the right heart chambers dilate, the tricuspid annulus also dilates decreasing leaflet coaptation. Most current surgical techniques employ annuloplasty rings alone or associated with additional techniques of leaflet plication in order to improve valve competence. The authors proposed more attention be directed at additional anatomic levels such as the papillary muscles or the right ventricular wall itself in order to correct additional mechanisms of tricuspid insufficiency such as leaflet tethering, and to optimize long-term surgical results.

The long-term survival after tricuspid valve repair is reduced independent of the surgical technique employed with an average survival of 60% at 5 years. (Figure 3).

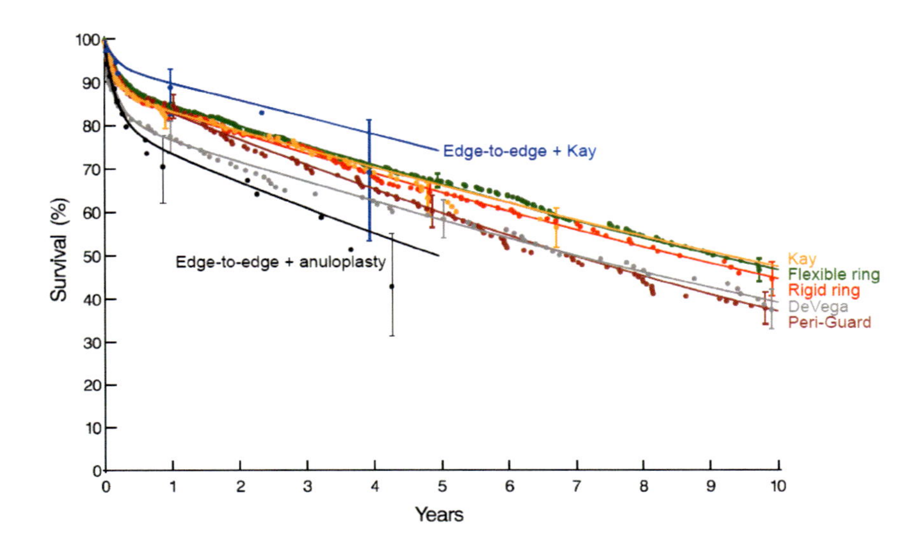

Figure 3. Long-term survival after tricuspid valve repair with different surgical techniques [24].

The recurrence of tricuspid valve insufficiency is usually related to progression of right heart failure and congestion, and is associated with decreased quality of life and compromised long-term survival. The progressive deterioration of right ventricular function in this subgroup of patients is reflected by the high risk for mortality when they undergo cardiac reoperations, and it is estimated that only 2% of patients undergo additional surgery for correction of tricuspid insufficiency. These patients could obtain significant benefit from the development of new technologies for percutaneous treatment of tricuspid insufficiency.

Diagnostic Studies of Tricuspid Valve

Evaluation of right ventricular function and shape is an important clinical marker in several cardiac disorders, that is, congestive heart failure, congenital heart disease, pulmonary hypertension, and overall right chamber volume and/or pressure overload.

Two dimensional echocardiography provides important information regarding ventricular function, dimensions and valvular function, but the images that can be obtained on the right ventricle and tricuspid valve are usually limited due to the proximity of these structures to the chest wall (TTE) and the distance from the esophagus (TEE) [25].

With the development of real time three dimensional echocardiography it is now possible to examine the atrioventricular valves by the transthoracic approach in views from the ventricles or the atria within a short period of time [26]. Real time three dimensional echocardiography allows volume quantification without any geometric assumption and has been validated in comparison with different other techniques, including cardiac magnetic resonance imaging [27]. It also provides images of the three leaflets of the tricuspid valve allowing for a more precise assessment of the valvular function. (Figure 4).

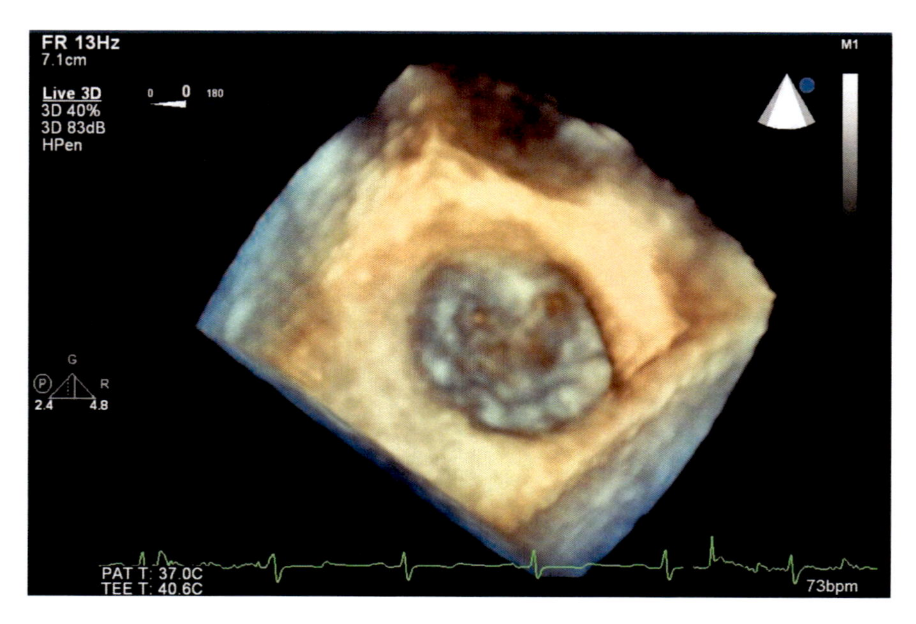

Figure 4. Real time three dimensional echocardiography allows for a more complete evaluation of right ventricle and tricuspid valve.

Recently, magnetic resonance imaging has been showed to provide precise images of the heart and cardiac structures, allowing for a dynamic evaluation of the heart, but even magnetic resonance imaging has limitations caused by rapidly moving structures, such as valve leaflets, and by implant artifacts.

Current Percutaneous Approaches for Tricuspid Valve Insufficiency

Several approaches have been described to treat tricuspid valve insufficiency in animal models by implanting tissue valves anchored to the tricuspid valve annulus or at the level of the superior and inferior vena cavae. Limited experience in humans has been reported in the literature.

Bai et al. [28] described the implantation of a porcine pericardial trileaflet semilunar valve mounted on a nitinol ring and assembled in a double-edge stent constructed from nitinol wire. The double edge stents were constructed with a waist diameter of 22 and 26 mm, in continuity with the ventricular and atrial disks 6 mm larger than the waist that provide for a secure anchor of the stent to the tricuspid annulus after deployment while avoiding compression of the atrio-ventricular node or the conduction bundle to prevent potential blockade of the conduction system. (Figure 5) The valvular ring with pericardial valve is integrated to the stent that was implanted in 10 healthy sheep under fluoroscopic guidance. (Figure 6) These sheep were periodically evaluated by 64-slice CT imaging and echocardiographic examination for a period of up to 6 months validating the feasibility of percutaneous implantation of the valved stent in tricuspid position.

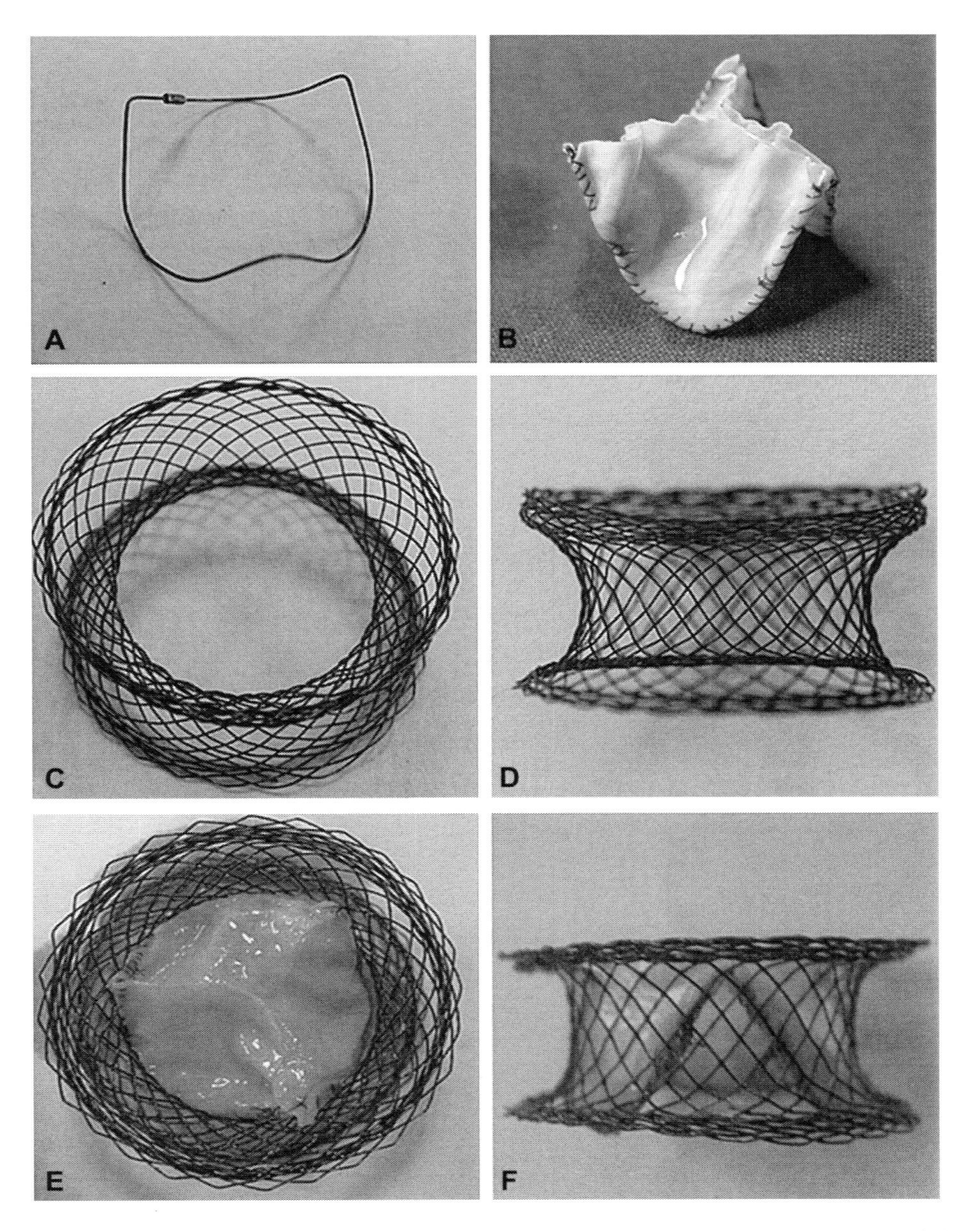

Figure 5. Assembly of the valved stent. The nitinol valvular ring (A) was sutured with pericardial valve to form unidirectional trileaflet valve(B).The double-edge stent constructed from nitinol wire (C) en face view; (D) the lateral view. The valvular ring with pericardial valve was integrated to the stent (E: the ventricular side-view of tricuspid stent; (F) the lateral view).

Under general anesthesia, the authors first performed right atrial-graphy via the femoral vein to identify the position and diameter of native tricuspid valve. Then a super-stiff guidewire and multipurpose catheter were advanced into the pulmonary artery through the right external jugular vein, and exchanged for a 16F delivery system. The tricuspid stented valve was inserted into the delivery system and advanced to the desired position under fluoroscopic guidance to be deployed by pulling back the external sheath. (Figure 6) As the sheath was retrieved the ventricular disk opened and the delivery system was pulled back to position the disk on the ventricular side of the tricuspid annulus. Further retrieval of the sheath released the waist and the atrial disk that ultimately anchored the stented valve in position by sandwiching the tricuspid annulus between both disks.

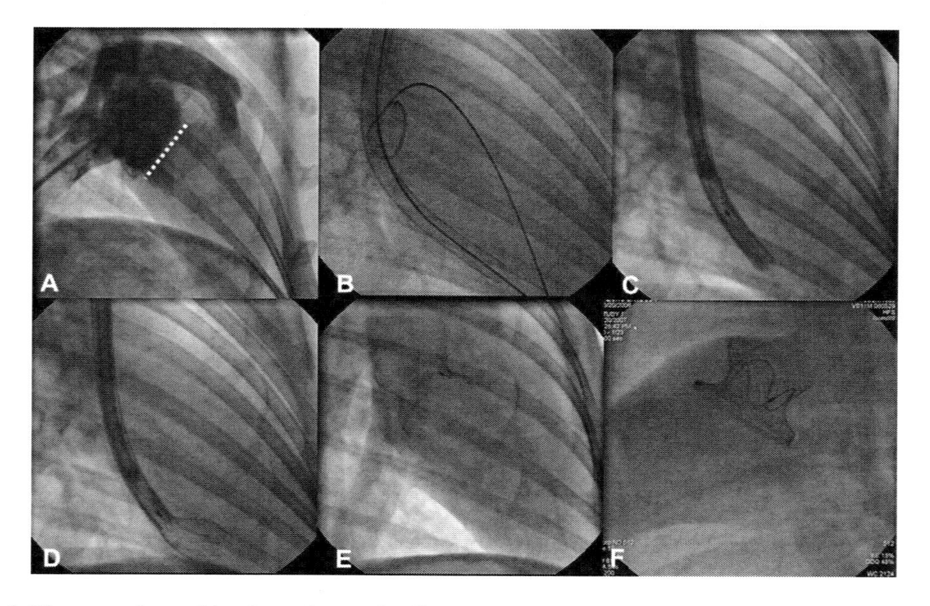

Figure 6. The procedure of implantation under fluoroscopic Guidance. (A) The angiogram of right atrium at the right anterior oblique 27° and cranial 4° plane, the native tricuspid annulus became a line when the contrast eject to right ventricle from right atrium in right ventricular early-diastolic period. (The white dashed line designates the native tricuspid annulus). (B) The delivery system was advanced over a wire placed in the pulmonary artery. (C) The stent was pushed forward toward to the tricuspid annulus. (D) The stent's distal edge was first deployed gradually in the right ventricle. (E) The stent was completely deployed and anchored the tricuspid annulus. (F) View of the device from the left lateral projection after implantation.

Two deaths occurred periprocedurally related to cardiac arrhythmias, two animals were sacrificed during the first postoperative month and 6 were followed up for 6 months. No significant persistent atrio-ventricular block or ventricular arrhythmias were observed, no significant change was observed between pre and postoperative right heart pressures, and no moderate or significant tricuspid regurgitation developed in any of the animals. Only one of them presented a paravalvular leakage at one month evaluation. The autopsy studies showed that the native tricuspid valves were stuck between the annulus and stent and the tricuspid stent was anchored to the tricuspid annulus, with the atrial edge of the stent remaining far away from the coronary sinus. In contrast to the pioneering report by Boudjemline et al. [29] of a tricuspid valved stent covered by politetrafluoroethilene (PTFE) membrane on the ventricular side, Bai et al relied on implanting a larger size valved stent and observed paravalvular leak in only one case. Furthermore, by avoiding the use of PTFE membrane, the delivery system could be reduced to a 14F catheter.

An alternative approach was described by Lauten et al. [30] who implanted two separate valves in each of the superior and inferior vena cava to block the distal transmission of right ventricular pressures to the body. (Figure 7)

The authors performed experimental procedures in 13 sheep creating acute grade III-IV tricuspid regurgitation by percutaneous avulsion of the papillary muscles and chordae tendinae with a wire blade. Using a 21 F right jugular vein introducer, under fluoroscopic guidance, two self-expanding nitinol stents containing a porcine pulmonary valve were then implanted in the inferior and superior vena cava, each at 2 cm from the corresponding vein orifice in the right atrium. (Figure 8).

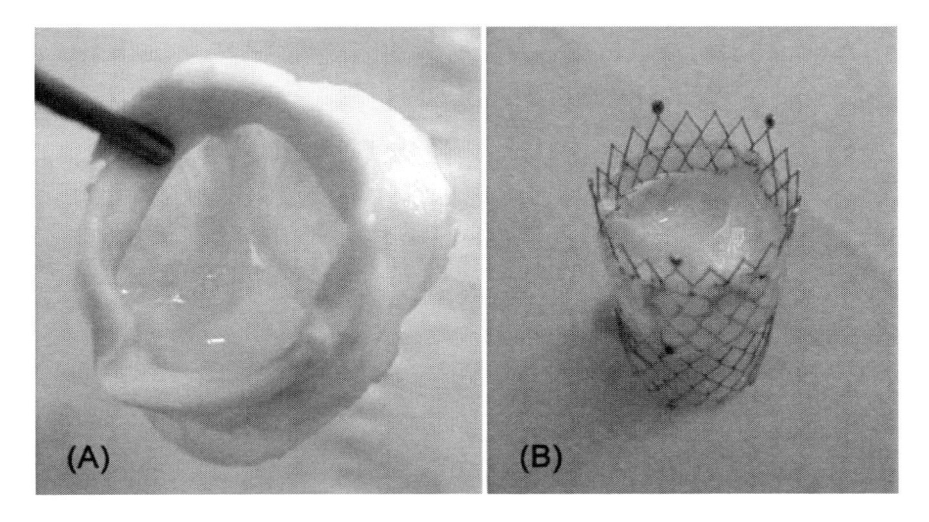

Figure 7. Self-expanding prosthetic valve. (A) Porcine pulmonary valve after pressure fixation in formalin and glutaraldehyde. Valves were carefully trimmed to remove excessive tissue and facilitate crimping into the delivery catheter. (B) Valves were then mounted to self-expanding nitinol stents of 28 or 26 mm in diameter. A pericardial sleeve was sutured around the outer surface of the stent to facilitate perivalvular sealing.

The authors reported significant hemodynamic changes after generating the acute tricuspid insufficiency, with prominent ventricular wave in the right atrium and inferior vena cava with increase in pressure from 10.1±3.14 and 9.6±3.47 mmHg to 16.2±2.33 and 16.2±2.82 mmHg, respectively.

Cardiac output significantly decreased from 5.15±1.69 to 2.9±1.16 L/min. After implantation of both valves, a significant reduction of the v-wave in the inferior vena cava was observed, whereas no major changes of right atrial and ventricular pressure were recorded, and cardiac output increased to 4.2±0.84 L/min during the 1 hour observational period.

A further increase in the cardiac output to 7.9±1.3 L/min was recorded during pharmacological stress testing by epinephrine injection. (Figure 9).

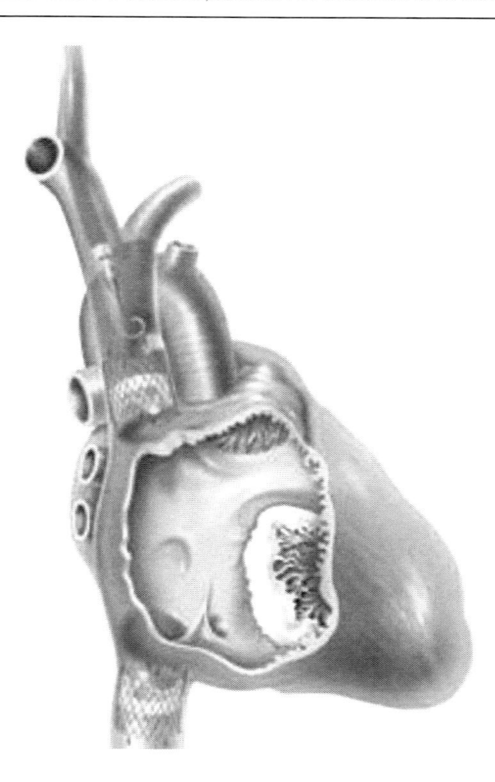

Figure 8. Position of both full expanded valves after release in the superior and inferior vena cava. Note that the right atrium continues to receive the volume overload generated by tricuspid regurgitation.

This study documented the hemodynamic changes generated by acute tricuspid insufficiency and showed the feasibility to partially reverse these changes, specifically improving cardiac output, by heterotopic tricuspid valve replacement via implantation of self-expanding stented valves into the inferior and superior vena cava. While this approach may prevent distal organs congestion and blunt fluid overload, the effects of persistent high right atrial pressures resulting from the tricuspid regurgitation are not resolved and may lead to the development of arrhythmias.

Current commercially available percutaneous devices are constructed for transcatheter aortic valve implantation in calcified aortic stenosis, relying on fixation in a rigid aortic annulus. The high venous wall elasticity and low pressure gradients prevailing in the venous system requires a specific stent design to ensure fixation as well as the use of tissue valves with optimal hemodynamic characteristics for application in the venous circulation. This characteristic of the vena cavae is particularly important in the chronically diseased state where the vessels may be dilated to nearly 4 cm in diameter. This poses serious challenges to the creation of stents because axial force is inversely proportional to diameter. Understanding the shortcomings of the heterotopic approach, a novel device utilizing commercially available materials was constructed at Cleveland Clinic by Greenberg et al. who deployed it in the inferior vena cava for compassionate use in a patient with severe biventricular dysfunction, previous heart surgery and hostile mediastinum secondary to radiation heart disease. This constitutes the only human transcatheter valve implantation in man for tricuspid valve disease. The device is unique in its design in that the stents used for fixation of the entire construct are separated from the site of valve fixation by mounting a commercially available stentless aortic valve onto a Dacron "neo-annulus". The bulk of the device required a large bore (30 F) sheath but it was successfully deployed into the inferior vena cava and the patient experienced symptomatic improvement [31]. Further work with next generation versions of these heterotopic approaches continues.

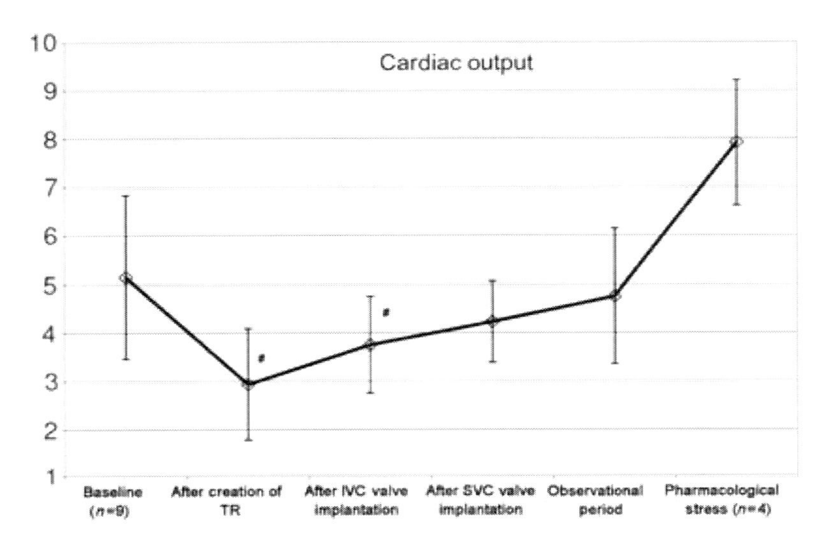

Figure 9. Cardiac output values during the creation of acute tricuspid insufficiency and later implantation of percutaneous valves in both vena cava.

Conclusion

Tricuspid valve disease continues to present a challenging problem to cardiovascular specialists particularly in patients who develop tricuspid insufficiency associated with left heart valve disease or severe right ventricular dysfunction. When reoperation for tricuspid insufficiency recurrence or progression is necessary, patients are at especially elevated surgical risk which may preclude them from receiving open surgery. These factors have led researchers to explore alternative transcatheter approaches for patients with severe tricuspid insufficiency and congestive heart failure, including percutaneous implantation of a stented valve both in the orthotopic tricuspid position or the heterotopic approach with devices in or near both vena cavae. To date pioneering animal experiences and a single first-in-man experience have demonstrated the feasibility of the concept but further progress and investigation is needed to better understand the disease process and the device-patient interface.

References

[1] Singh JP, Vans JC, Levy D. Prevalence and clinical determinants of mitral, tricuspid and aortic regurgitation (the Framingham Study). *Am J Cardiol* 1999;83:897-902.

[2] Stuge O, Liddicoat J. Emerging opportutunities for cardiac surgeons within structutural heart disease. *J Thorac Cardiovasc Surg* 2006;132:1258-61.

[3] Branwald NS, Ross J, Morrow AG. Conservative management of tricuspid regurgitation in patients undergoing mitral valve replacement. *Circulation* 1967;35:I6-9.

[4] Porter A, Shapira Y, Wurzel M, et al. Tricuspid regurgitation late after mitral valve replacement: clinical and echocardiographic evaluation. *J Heart valve Dis* 1999;8:57-62.

[5] King RM, Shaff HV, Danielson GK, et al. Surgery for tricuspid regurgitation late after mitral valve replacement: National Cardiac surgery Database. Ann Thorac Surg. 1999,67:943-51.

[6] Frater R. Tricuspid insufficiency. *J Thorac CArdiovasc Surg* 2003;125(3):S9-11.

[7] Jamieson WR, Edwards FH, Shwartz M, et al. Risk stratification for cardiac valve replacement: National Cardiac Surgery Database. *Ann Thorac Surg* 1999;67:943-51.

[8] Groves PH, Ellis FH. Late tricuspid regurgitation following mitral valve surgery. *J Heart valve Dis* 1992;1:80-6.

[9] Bonhoeffer P, Boudjemline , Saliba Z, et al. Percutaneous replacement of pulmonary valve in a right ventricle to pulmonary artery prosthetic conduit with valve dysfunction. *Lancet* 2000;356:1403.

[10] Cribier A, Eltchaninoff H, Bash A, et al. Percutaneous transcatheter implantation of an aortic valve prosthesis for calccific aortic stenosis: First human case description. *Circulation* 2002;106:3006.

[11] Boudjemline Y, Agnoletti G, Bonnet D, et al. Steps toward the percutaneous replacement of atrioventricular valves. An experimental study. *J Am Coll Cardiol* 2005;46:360.

[12] Zegdi R, Khabbaz Z, Borenstein N, et al. A repositionable valved stent for endovascular treatment of deteriorated bioprostheses. *J Am Coll Cardiol* 2006;48:1365.

[13] Feldman T, Kar S, Rinalde M, et al. Percutaneous mitral repair with the MitraClip System. Safety and Midterm Durability in the Initial EVEREST cohort. *J Am Coll CArdiol* 2009;54:686-94.

[14] Byrne MJ, Kaye DM, Mathiis M, et al. Percutaneous mitral annular reduction provides continued benefit in an ovine model of dilated cardiomyopathy. *Circulation* 2004;110:3088-92.

[15] Rogers JH, Bolling SF. The tricuspid valve: Current perspective and evolving management of tricuspid regurgitation. *Circulation* 2009;119:2718-25.

[16] Tei C, Pilgrim JP, Shah PM, et al. The tricuspid valve annulus: study of size and motion in normal subjects and in patients with tricuspid regurgitation. *Circulation* 1982;66(3):665-71.

[17] Sagie A, Freitas N, Chen MH, et al. Echocardiographic assessment of mitral stenosis and its associated valvular lesions in 205 patients and lack of association with mitral valve prolapse. J Am Soc Echocardiogr 1997;10:141-8.

[18] Matsuyama K, Matsumoto M, Sugita T, et al. Predictors of residual tricuspid regurgitation after mitral valve surgery. *Ann Thorac Surg* 2003;75:1826-8.

[19] Dreyfus GD, Corbi PJ, Chan KMJ, et al. Secondary tricuspid regurgitation or dilatation: which should be the criteria for surgical repair? *Ann Thorac Surg* 2005;79:127-32.

[20] Ton-Nu TT, Levine RA, Handschumacher MD, et al. Geometric determinants of functional tricuspid regurgitation: insights from 3-dimensional echocardiography. *Circulation* 2006;114: 143-9.

[21] Fukuda S, Song JM, Gillinov AM, et al. Tricuspid valve tethering predicts tricuspid regurgitation after tricuspid annuloplasty. *Circulation* 2005;111:975-9.

[22] McCarthy PM, Bhudia SK, Rajeswaran J, et al. Tricuspid valve repair: durability and risk factors for failure. *J Thorac Cardiovasc Surg* 2004;127:674-85.

[23] Navia JL, Nowicki ER, Blackstone EH, Brozzi NA, et al. Surgical management of secondary tricuspid valve regurgitation: Annulus, commissure, or leaflet procedure? *J Thorac Cardiovasc Surg* 2010;139:1473-82

[24] Navia JL, Nowicki ER, Blackstone EH, Brozzi NA, et al. Surgical management of secondary tricuspid valve regurgitation: Annulus, commissure, or leaflet procedure? *J Thorac Cardiovasc Surg* 2010;139:1473-82

[25] Meluzin J, Spinarov´a L, Hude P, et al: Prognostic importance of various echocardiographic right ventricular functional parameters in patients with symptomatic heart failure. *J Am Soc Echocardiogr* 2005;18:435–444.

[26] Schnabel R, Khaw A, von Bardeleben RS, et al. Assessment of the tricuspid valve morphology by transthoracic real-time-3-D-echochardiography. *Echocardiography* 2005;22(1):15-23.

[27] De Castro S, Cavarretta E, Milan A, et al. Usefulness of tricuspid annular velocity in identifying global RV dysfunction in patients with primary pulmonary hypertension: A Comparison with 3D Echo-derived right ventricular ejection fraction. *Echocardiography* 2008;25(3):289-93.

[28] Bay Y, Zong GJ, Wang HR, et al. An integrated pericardial valved stent special for percutaneous tricuspid implantation: An animal feasibility study. *Journal of Surgical Research* 2010;160:215-21.

[29] Boudjemline Y, Agnoletti G, Bonnet D, et al. Steps toward the percutaneous replacement of atrioventricular valves. *J Am Coll Cardiol* 2005;46:360-5.

[30] Lauten A, Figulla HR, Willich C, et al. Percutaneous caval stent valve implantation: investigation of an interventional approach for treatment of tricuspid regurgitation. *European Heart Journal* 2010;31:1274-81.

[31] Roselli EE, Greenberg RK, Lytle BW. Endovascular tricuspid valve replacement for high risk patients. Presented at 4th Annual At the Heart of Evolution Meeting. Marseille, France, November 11th 2006.

Pulmonary Valve

In: Percutaneous Valve Technology: Present and Future ISBN: 978-1-61942-577-4
Editors: Jose Luis Navia and Sharif Al-Ruzzeh

Chapter XXVIII

Percutaneous Pulmonary Valve Technology

Stephen A. Hart and Richard A. Krasuski

Abstract

Pulmonic valve disease is ubiquitous across age, gender and ethnicity. The pulmonary valve is unique in that the incidence of congenital cases far outnumbers the incidence of acquired cases.

The most prevalent pulmonary valve disease is pulmonary stenosis (PS), either isolated or in concert with other congenital heart disease. The treatment for PS has a storied history dating back to 1913 with the first ever intracardiac surgery. Over the past century interventions on the pulmonary valve have undergone a remarkable evolution progressing from closed, "blind" surgical valvotomy to open surgical valvotomy and finally percutaneous balloon valvuloplasty, all with excellent procedural and long term outcomes.

A frequent consequence of pulmonary valve intervention is pulmonary valve regurgitation. Although once thought to be a benign entity, pulmonary insufficiency and chronic ventricular volume overload will cause the right ventricle to fail given enough time. A burgeoning population of patients who underwent surgical repair of congenital heart disease now require additional interventions as adults, primarily on their right ventricular outflow tract.

Percutaneous bioprosthetic pulmonary valves offer a new minimally invasive strategy of managing this complex patient population. This chapter will review the history of pulmonic valve interventions and discuss current technology in percutaneous pulmonary valve treatments.

Introduction

The pulmonic valve is unique among its counterparts in that congenital lesions, although rare, far outnumber valve pathology secondary to acquired conditions such as endocarditis, carcinoid heart disease and pulmonary hypertension. Congenital diseases of the pulmonary valve may be broadly categorized as stenotic, insufficient or a combination of the two.

Pulmonary Stenosis

Congenital pulmonic stenosis (PS) may occur at, above or below the pulmonary valve, with majority of the cases occurring at the level of the valve. Valvular PS constitutes approximately 8% of all congenital heart disease [1]. Pulmonary stenosis typically occurs as an isolated lesion, though it can coexist with other congenital heart defects such as double outlet right ventricle, single ventricle and d- or l-transposition of the great arteries. Genetic contributions to PS are highly likely as familial disease is frequent [2, 3]. It is also part of a variety of syndromes that can affect the embryological development of the pulmonic valve, such as Noonan syndrome, neurofibromatosis, Williams syndrome, 22q11 deletion syndromes (such as DiGeorge syndrome) and Alagille syndrome [4-8].

Patients with mild PS are asymptomatic and survive well into adulthood [9]. Right ventricular hypertrophy results from more than mild stenosis and becomes quite evident with severe stenosis. Severe stenosis also promotes the development of ischemic fibrosis related to poor coronary perfusion of the thickened muscle [10]. Symptoms, including fatigue and dyspnea, tend to develop late; and congestive heart failure typically occurs around the fourth decade if left untreated, but may occur much earlier for very severe PS [11]. Exercise tolerance is depressed in patients with PS, due in part to the inability to significantly increase cardiac output [12].

Valvular PS accounts for 80 to 90% of all lesions causing right ventricular outflow tract (RVOT) obstruction and its inheritance rate is estimated between 1.7% and 3.6% [13, 14]. There are 3 clinically significant morphologies for valvular PS:

1) Dome shaped: This abnormality is characterized by bowing of the valve toward the pulmonary trunk. Vestigial valve leaflets are fused along their commissures and there is a central opening. When there is no central opening, the patient is said to have pulmonary atresia. Although the valve leaflets are fused, they retain normal mobility. Post-stenoic dilation of the pulmonary trunk is also present due to turbulent flow distal to the valve and intrinsic arterial wall abnormalities. Blood flow through the valve tends to favor the left pulmonary artery because of its less acute takeoff from the pulmonary trunk compared with the right pulmonary artery. Significant calcification of this type of PS may be seen in adult patients.
2) Dysplastic: This abnormality is characterized by a poorly mobile valve with marked myxomatous thickening. Typically seen in Noonan syndrome, this subtype accounts for about 20% of valvular PS. Other segments along the RVOT may also be narrowed when the pulmonic valve is dysplastic.
3) Unicuspid/bicuspid: The unicuspid or bicuspid pulmonary valve is generally associated with tetralogy of Fallot. It is also present less frequently in isolation.

Isolated subvalvular or infundibular PS is an uncommon cardiac abnormality. It accounts for 0.4% of patients with congenital heart disease, and is responsible for less than 10% of all

RVOT obstruction [15]. It is more likely to be associated with tetralogy of Fallot or double-chambered right ventricle [16, 17]. Other causes of subvalvular PS include infundibular hypertrophy, protrusion of right sinus of Valsalva into the RVOT, aneurysm of the membranous ventricular septum into the RVOT or intra- and extra- cardiac mass lesions in the RVOT such as sarcoma [18].

Supravalvular PS or pulmonary arterial stenosis is caused by narrowing of any portion of the pulmonary arteries including the pulmonary trunk, the pulmonary arterial bifurcation or the pulmonary branches. The so called "hourglass pattern" of narrowing is due to stenosis at the commissural ridge of the valve and is actually a form of valvular PS. Other pulmonary supravalvular lesions may range from single focal lesions to diffuse hypoplasia. Supravalvular PS is associated with Alagille and Keutel syndromes and pulmonary artery stenosis is seen with congenital rubella and Williams syndrome [4, 5, 19, 20].

Recurrent pulmonary stenosis is not infrequent following surgical intervention on the RVOT. Bioprosthetic valved conduits placed between the right ventricle and pulmonary artery often require reintervention for stenosis or insufficiency later in life [21]. Stenosis of conduits placed for surgical correction of tetralogy of Fallot is also common and homograft stenosis following the Ross procedure may occur in up to 20% of treated patients [22, 23].

In patients with significant PS, the right ventricular pressure reaches its maximum as pulmonary artery pressure is still rising to its maximum. That is to say, peak RV pressure occurs *before* peak PA pressure. This can have significant implications on the method used to assess PS severity. The two most utilized methods for assessing PS severity are echocardiography and heart catheterization (Figure 1), both of which have limitations. Echocardiography has the advantage of being noninvasive, though its utility is adversely impacted by imaging limitations such as obesity, lung disease and an inability to properly position the patient. Additionally Doppler measurements of outflow velocity can be inaccurate, as the complexity of RVOT anatomy invalidates the assumptions of the simplified Bernoulli equation. When imaging is adequate, however, echo can be most helpful in assessing the morphology of the valve and clarifying the location of the stenosis. Quantification of stenosis is performed using continuous wave Doppler. The gradient is measured through the systolic ejection period, and the peak and mean pressures are typically reported.

Catheterization can also assess the severity of PS. It. is most accurately performed by inserting 2 venous catheters and measuring the right ventricular and pulmonary artery pressures simultaneously using 2 pressure transducers. Traditionally the "peak to peak" pressure is reported. This is calculated by measuring the difference between the peak right ventricular systolic and the peak pulmonary artery systolic pressure. A recent study demonstrated that the catheterization derived peak-to-peak pressure best correlates with the *mean* pressure measured using echo in the outpatient setting. The peak velocity by echo would have overestimated the cath peak-to-peak measurement in this study by almost 20mmHg. It remains controversial if simultaneously measured echo and cath gradients would have the same characteristics [24, 25].

One must exercise extreme caution when evaluating the impact of "peak gradients" that are recorded in the literature, because either method (catheterization or echocardiography) may be implied. By convention valvular PS is considered "mild" when the peak gradient across the valve by echo is <30mmHg, moderate when the gradient is 30-50mmHg and severe when the gradient is >50mmHg [26].

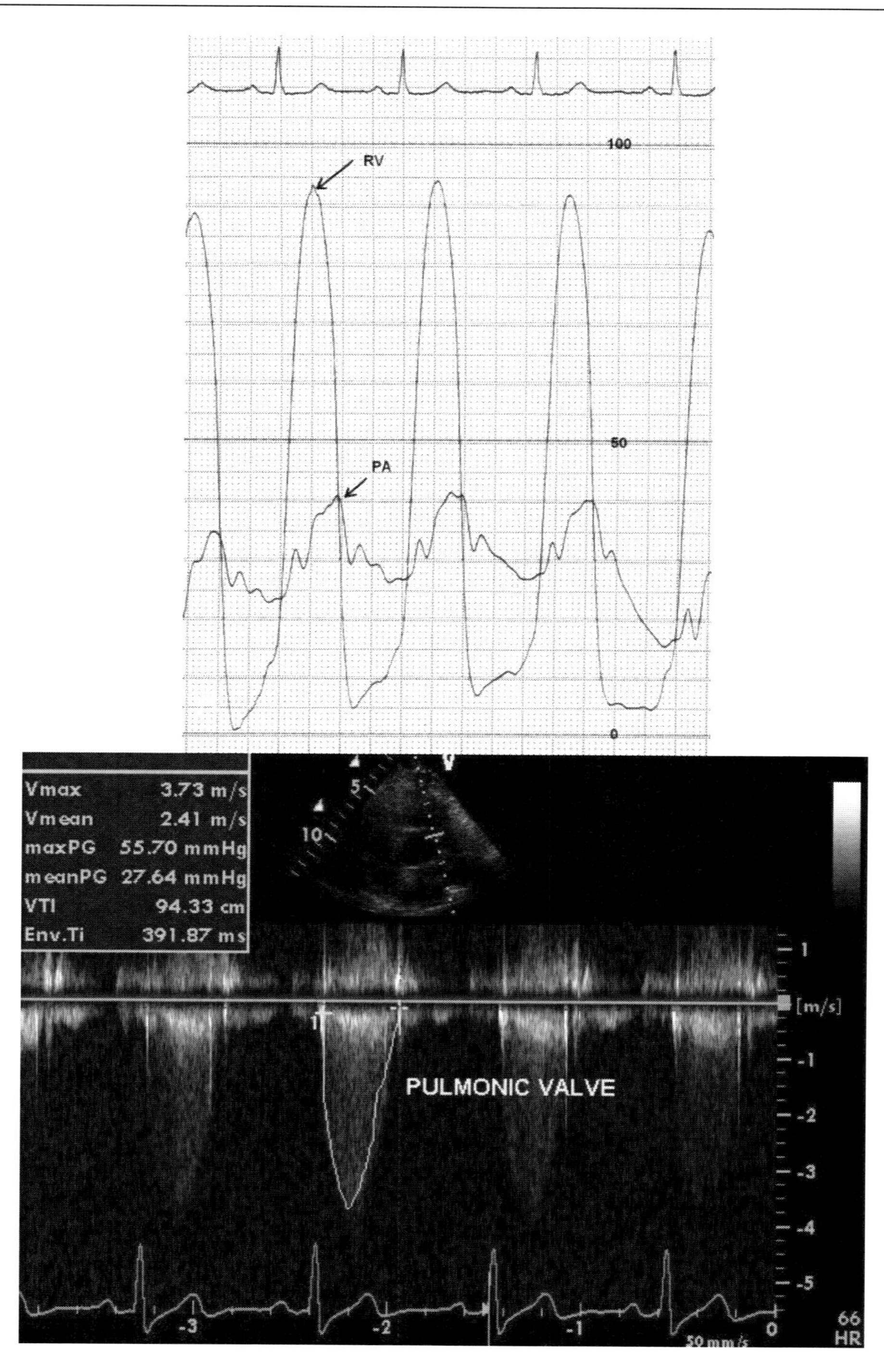

Figure 1. Methods of measuring the pulmonic valve gradient. Above is a simultaneous recording of the right ventricular and pulmonary artery systolic pressure in the catheterization laboratory. The peak-to-peak gradient in this case measures 53 mm Hg. Below the continuous Doppler signal is assessed in the parasternal short axis view on echocardiography. The peak gradient is measured at 56 mm Hg with a mean of 28 mm Hg. PA = pulmonary arterial pressure tracing; RV = right ventricular pressure tracing.

Pulmonary Insufficiency

Many individuals exhibit trivial to mild pulmonary insufficiency (PI), which is considered to be normal. Insufficiency may be present concomitantly with PS, but rarely does it become severe in this setting. Though it is far more likely for PI to occur as a consequence after PS intervention, it does occur as a native congenital lesion. Congenital PI is usually accompanied by additional lesions such as a form of tetralogy of Fallot with absent valve leaflets. Idiopathic PI is strongly associated with pulmonary artery dilation, which may be severe; the pathophysiology of this relationship is poorly understood.

The consequence of long standing PI has been well documented. Chronic volume and/or pressure overload on the right ventricle initiates a cascade leading toward heart failure including ventricular dilation, hypertrophy, ischemia and fibrosis [27]. Exercise intolerance, arrhythmia generation and sudden cardiac death are also attendant risks in this setting [28-32]. Epidemiological studies have demonstrated that right heart failure is an inevitable consequence of PI and typically occurs after 4 decades [33].

Pulmonary Valve Interventions – A Historical Perspective

The treatment for pulmonary stenosis is straightforward – relief of obstruction. This simple concept has undergone a remarkable evolution in technique from the first 'blind' procedure in 1913 to the transcatheter delivery of bioprosthetic valves today.

The first recorded attempt at relief of PS came from Paris in 1913 by Doyen. He attempted to excise the stenotic pulmonic valve of a cyanotic adolescent using a tenatome introduced through the right ventricle [34]. In doing so, he performed the first intracardiac surgery for an intrinsic cardiac defect. Although the patient survived the immediate post-operative period, they expired the day following surgery. Autopsy demonstrated that the patient did have PS, but unfortunately not in the location that was originally believed. The ensuing years saw improved diagnostic techniques for PS, but the next step forward in treatment did not occur for another 3 decades.

In 1944, Blalock performed the first so-called Blalock-Taussig shunt for tetralogy of Fallot which was largely developed by Helen Taussig and Vivian Thomas [35]. The procedure involves anastamosis of the right subclavian artery to the right pulmonary artery, resulting in augmented pulmonary blood flow. This procedure bypassed the stenotic pulmonary valve all-together and avoided the complications inherent to ventriculotomy. Treatment of PS and tetralogy of Fallot was revolutionized, and a once fatal diagnosis now had a legitimate treatment. Other shunt procedures developed by Potts, Waterston, Cooley and Davidson were also developed to bypass stenotic pulmonary valves and improve pulmonary blood flow, but these procedures were not widely adopted due to the technical challenge of balancing pulmonary and systemic blood flows through the shunt [36-39].

In the late 1940's Brock and Sellors independently developed successful methods to divide stenotic pulmonary valves using the transventricular approach first attempted by Doyen [40, 41]. They incised the valve with specially designed cutting tools introduced through a small right ventriculotomy and then mechanically expanded the stenotic valve. The technical success of this procedure was improved with the use of a rubber sleeve sutured directly to the pulmonary artery which allowed the passage of a finger into the vessel without interruption of blood flow [42]. This made digital assessment and guidance of valvotomy possible. Temporary venous occlusion enabled brief visual inspection of the valve and swift open valvotomy. This was refined with the advent of deep hypothermia, which gave the surgeon more time to complete the procedure [43-45]. Often, no thought was given to pulmonary incompetence, which was believed to be "inconsequential" at the time [46]. Improvements in extracorporeal oxygenation and cardiopulmonary bypass techniques that were first developed in the mid 1950's ushered in a new era of cardiothoracic surgery, and open valvuloplasty became firmly established as the treatment of choice for PS.

The next advance in PS treatment didn't occur until 1979 when Semb performed pulmonary valvuloplasty via cardiac catheterization [47]. The late 1960's and early 70's saw the development and refinement of cardiac catheterization and balloon angioplasty. Angioplasty proliferated and began replacing surgical treatments for a variety of vascular lesions. Rashkind took the techniques of angioplasty one step further and developed the so-called Rashkind procedure for the early palliation of d-transposition of the great arteries [48]. After advancing a balloon across the foramen ovale into the left ventricle, a balloon was inflated and forcibly withdrawn across the atrial septum tearing that structure. This same technique inspired Semb in 1979. He dilated a balloon distal to a stenotic pulmonary valve and withdrew it across the valve relieving the stenosis. A more controlled "static" form of balloon valvulopasty was developed by Kan and White in 1982 [49]. Their system utilized a fluid filled balloon that was positioned across the valve and gave the operator control over the extent of the valvuloplasty. Percutaneous valvuloplasty soon became the treatment of choice for valvular PS and remains an important treatment modality for valvular heart disease.

Surgical Valvotomy

A half century of surgical experience has led to excellent procedural and long term outcomes following surgically repaired PS. The First and Second Joint Study on the Natural History of Congenital Heart Disease (NHS-1 and NHS-2) provided long term outcomes data on valvular PS [9, 50, 51]. On enrollment to NHS-1, patients were categorized based on peak to peak gradients (<25mmHg, trivial; 25 to 49 mmHg, mild; 50 to 79mmHg, moderate; ≥80mmHg, severe). Approximately half of the cohort was managed medically and the other half surgically. At the conclusion of NHS-2, the 25-year survival was estimated at 95.7±0.9% regardless of PS severity or treatment modality compared with 96.6% for an age and sex matched, healthy control population. Most patients who were diagnosed as having mild stenosis or worse eventually needed pulmonary valve intervention. During the NHS-2 follow-up period the average maximum gradient across the pulmonary valve was 17.1mmHg in the medically managed group and only 9.6mmHg in the surgical group, but the improved gradient appeared to have come at the expense of increased pulmonic insufficiency. PI occurred in 56% of surgically managed patients compared to 11% of medically managed patients. Of those with PI though, only 14% were considered to have "severe" regurgitation and only 5% required repeat surgery.

NHS-2 showed that PS is a very well tolerated lesion and patients with a mild gradient on presentation or a mild gradient after valvotomy have an excellent prognosis. However, the effects of mild PS or chronic PI on the right heart might not have become apparent after only 25 years of follow-up. Earing and colleagues expanded on NHS-2 with a longer study following patients over a median of 34 years following surgical treatment of isolated pulmonary valve stenosis [52]. They found similar procedural success as NHS-1, but the extra decade of follow-up in this study elucidated a growing problem. Fifty three percent of the cohort underwent eventual reoperation, the majority of which were for pulmonary valve insufficiency. Furthermore they found a positive correlation between the incidence of reintervention and time from initial surgery, highlighting the consequence of long standing PI.

Balloon Valvuloplasty

Percutaneous balloon valvuloplasty (PBV) has been available for only half as long as surgical valvotomy, but has produced similarly impressive results, and is now the treatment of choice for patients with domed valvular PS. Indications for PBV are mixed. The original indications for PBV were similar to those used for surgical valvotomy, with a peak-to-peak gradient of 50mmHg used as the cut-off for intervention. Recently published guidelines use much lower gradients, as low as 30mmHg peak-to-peak in symptomatic patients for class I indications. The rationale for using lower gradients is that natural history studies following PBV show that many patients in the mild-moderate category will eventually need pulmonary valve intervention, and earlier valvuloplasty has demonstrated better results [26, 53]. Debate over the appropriate cut-off still exists and some advocate using a peak-to-peak pulmonary gradient of 50mmHg as a cut-off regardless of symptoms [54].

With decades of experience at hand, successful balloon dilation now occurs in over 90% of patients undergoing the procedure [55, 56]. Procedural deaths occur in far less than 1% of patients [57]. BPV has a number of immediate effects on hemodynamics and valve function. The peak-to-peak gradient and right ventricular systolic pressure drop with minimal, if any, increase in peak pulmonary artery pressure. The valve becomes more mobile and less doming occurs. Although there is minimal change in cardiac output, the right ventricular function may improve, accompanied by reduction in tricuspid valve regurgitation over time [58-60]. An important acute complication with BPV (or surgical valvotomy) is the so-called “suicide right ventricle,” which may be seen immediately following the procedure [61]. If infundibular hypertrophy or stenosis is present prior to valvuloplasty, a dramatic reduction in end systolic pressure can result in acutely worsened right ventricular outflow obstruction. This physiology is similar to what is seen in the left ventricular in patients with hypertrophic obstructive cardiomyopathy. Intravascular volume expansion and beta-blockade are useful treatments in this scenario, with eventual resolution of this problem as the infundibular stenosis regresses during follow-up [55, 62].

Outcomes following PBV have been uniformly excellent. One of the first long-term studies by McCrindle and Khan followed 46 patients for a mean of 4.6 years following PBV. The pulmonary gradient dropped from 70mmHg at baseline to 23 mmHg immediately following the procedure and 20mmHg at the end of the follow-up period [60]. Another early study followed 20 patients for a mean of 5.3 years and found the long-term residual gradient to be 24mmHg with no evidence of restenosis [63]. The largest study published on the topic comes from the Valvuloplasty and Angioplasty of Congenital Anomalies (VACA) registry [59]. This cohort of 533 patients was followed for a median of 8.7 years. Twenty three percent had evidence of restenosis (>35mmHg) and 16.8% eventually required reintervention. This study defined risk factors for restenosis which include a small pulmonary annulus diameter, high residual gradient immediately following PBV, small balloon diameter to annulus ratio and young age at intervention.

The next important study focused on adults and adolescents instead of a primarily pediatric population like its predecessors. The cohort studied by Chen and colleagues showed a decrease in pulmonary gradient from 107mmHg at baseline to 50mmHg immediately following valvuloplasty, and this dropped further to 30mmHg at a mean of 6.9 years after the procedure [64]. The late improvement seen was likely the result of regression of infundibular stenosis. Rao and colleagues published a study following 85 patients for an average of 7 years, the longest to date [65]. Of the 82 patients followed at the 2 year interval, 9 (11%) had restenosis (defined as a gradient >50mmHg). No additional restenosis was seen in the 80 patients followed for greater than 2 years. They reported survival free from reintervention as 94%, 89%, 88% and 84% at 1, 2, 5 and 10 years, respectively. They also cautioned that the majority of patients had evidence of pulmonary insufficiency, which has been described by most other groups as well.

Many of these retrospective studies began collecting data in the early 1980's, just when pulmonary valvuloplasty became widely available. Since that time there has been a shift in technique from using balloons sized to the pulmonary valve annulus to using oversized balloons. It should be expected, therefore, that the procedural results and long-term restenosis rates should be even better today than these studies have shown. The most recently published long-term study following PBV determined the restenosis rate to be just 4.8% after a mean of 6.4 years [55].

Balloon valvuloplasty does not produce the same dramatic reductions in pulmonary gradients seen in patients undergoing surgical valvotomy. In a recent study, patients udergoing PBV had a reduction from 66 to 22 mmHg at 5.4 years following the procedure, while patients undergoing surgery had a redution from 65 to 13mmHg at 9.8 years [66]. Moderate PI occurred in 44% of the surgical cohort but only 11% of the PBV cohort. The restenosis rate for the surgical cohort was 6% while the restenosis rate in the PBV cohort was 14%. Despite the better gradient and lower incidence of reintervention, the authors conclude that PBV is still preferred because it is less invasive, less expensive and requires a shorter hospital stay.

Despite favorable outcomes with balloon interventions, there are circumstances in which surgical intervention is required. Surgical therapy is recommended for patients with severe PS and with a hypoplastic pulmonary annulus, severe pulmonary regurgitation, subvalvular PS and supravalvular PS. Surgery is also preferred for most dysplastic pulmonary valves, when there are other congenital or valvular lesions or when a surgical Maze procedure is also required [26].

Balloon Valvuloplasty Technique

Balloon Valvuloplasty relieves pulmonic gradients by splitting the commissures of the fused leaflets and rarely by leaflet tearing or avulsion of the valve cusps. Without the need for a trans-septal left heart catheterization and lack of encroachment on the systemic arterial bed, pulmonary balloon valvuloplasty (PBV) is significantly less technically challenging than balloon mitral or aortic valvuloplasty procedures. More expanded procedural details for percutaneous balloon valvuloplasty are available elsewhere [54, 67]. An overview of valvuloplasty techniques will be discussed below highlighting technological advancements.

Femoral venous access is obtained for right heart catheterization and a femoral arterial line is placed for continuous hemodynamic monitoring. Right ventricular outflow anatomy, stenosis severity and valve annulus diameter are determined with a right ventricular cineangiogram (Figure 2). Typically lateral and anteroposterior projections are used to obtain an image of the outflow tract with the pulmonary valve in cross section (on edge). The valve is measured at the "hinge point" located at the base of the valve sinus at end systole. This dimension is critical for balloon sizing.

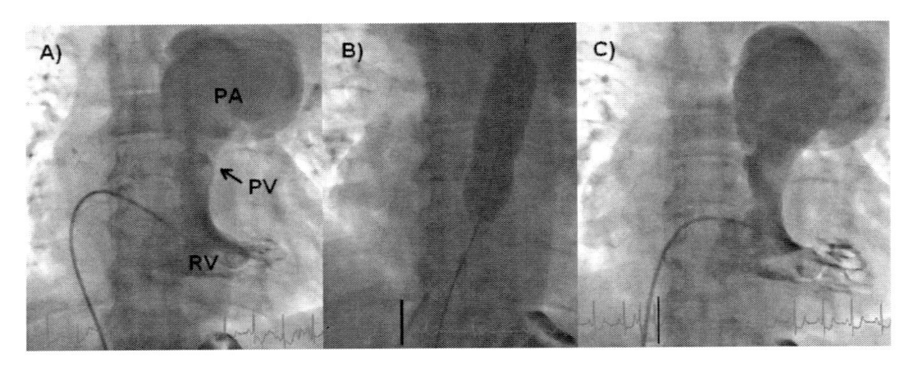

Figure 2. Percutaneous balloon valvuloplasty in a patient with severe pulmonic stenosis and a grossly dilated main pulmonary artery. A) Right ventriculogram during systole demonstrating a domed pulmonic valve with severely narrowed outflow into a very dilated main pulmonary artery. B) Balloon dilatation of the pulmonic valve using a Z-Med II® balloon (NuMED Inc; Hopkinton, NY). C) Repeat right ventriculogram after balloon dilatation demonstrating better leaflet excursion with improved outflow into the pulmonary artery. PA = pulmonary artery; PV = pulmonic valve; RV = right ventricle.

Single Balloon Technique

A very floppy tipped wire is used to cross the pulmonary valve after which an end-hole catheter is advanced into the distal left (preferred) or right pulmonary artery. A stiff guide wire with a floppy tip is then exchanged in preparation for the balloon catheter. The balloon size should yield a balloon to annulus ratio of 1.2-1.4:1. Using a ratio greater than 1.5:1 has not been proven superior to 1.2-1.4:1 and may predispose to rupture of the RVOT [67, 68]. Similarly, a ratio <1.2:1 is a risk factor for recurrent stenosis. Of note some authors have suggested 1.2 or 1.25:1 to be the "ideal" ratio to balance the risk of restenosis with the risk of valve insufficiency, [54, 69, 70] but we have not found this to be the case. In very tight PS or in neonates, sequential dilation starting with a smaller balloon may be used to prevent occlusion of blood flow across the pulmonary valve with the deflated balloon [71, 72]. The length of the balloon is chosen so as not interfere with distal or proximal structures, but ensure uniform inflation across the valve annulus. The balloon catheter is then carefully advanced across the exchange wire.

Once fluoroscopy markers on the balloon are lined up with the valve, the balloon is inflated. When the "waist" of the balloon appears around the valve, proper balloon placement should be confirmed. Inflation continues until the waist disappears or the maximum recommended balloon inflation pressure is reached, whichever comes first. Total inflation time should not exceed 10 seconds. The process may be repeated as necessary to achieve successful dilation. The right ventricular pressure should be dramatically reduced and the residual gradient across the valve should be minimal. If a gradient persists, it is likely that the infundibulum is creating a dynamic obstruction, as discussed above ("the suicide right ventricle"). Alternatively the valve might be dysplastic. Dysplastic valves tend to be elastic and simply "spring" back to their native shape when the balloon is deflated. This valve subtype generally necessitates a surgical intervention to truly abolish the stenosis, although successful balloon valvuloplasty of dysplastic valves using a balloon to annulus ratio of 1.4-1.5:1 has been reported [25, 68]. Current teaching, however, defines a dysplastic valve as a valve which does not dilate appropriately with the properly performed balloon valvuloplasty.

The Inoue balloon developed for percutaneous mitral dilatation in rheumatic patients has also been used for pulmonary valvuloplasty by some (Figure 3), but has never been widely adopted. The advantage of this balloon is its hourglass shape, which aids in proper placement and stability during balloon inflation [64, 73]. The disadvantage is that it is difficult to maneuver into the outflow tract as the exchange wire is not designed for use within the pulmonic anatomy.

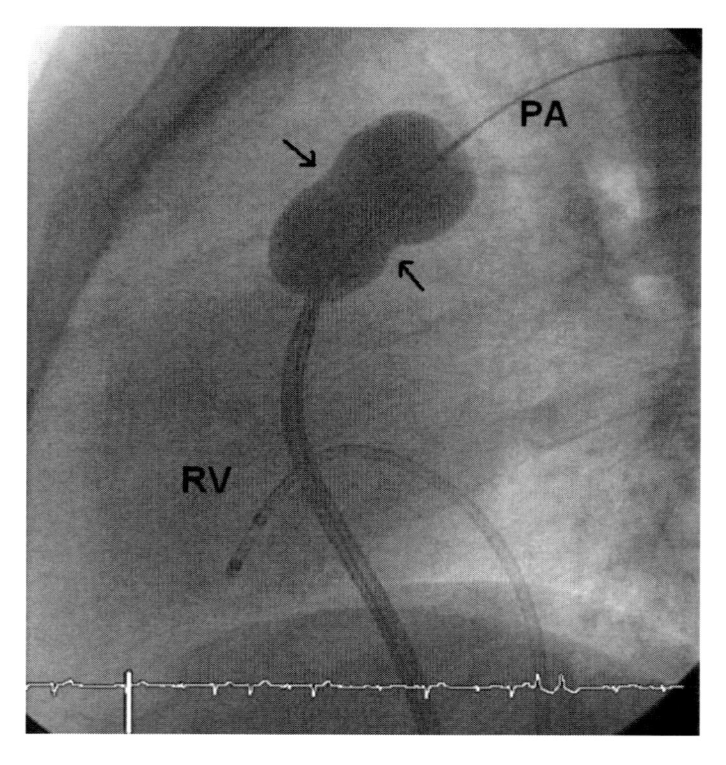

Figure 3. Lateral projection of a percutaneous balloon valvuloplasty performed using an Inoue balloon (Toray International America Inc.; Houston, TX). A catheter is positioned in the right ventricle to continuously measure the right ventricular pressure and assess the valve gradient between inflations. The Inoue balloon has a unique hourglass design and inflates distally first, proximally second and lastly at the waist (designated by the arrows) which allows for more stable positioning. PA = pulmonary artery; RV = right ventricle.

Double Balloon Technique

While the single balloon technique is straightforward, there are inherent limitations. The pulmonary valve annulus is typically large compared to body size and is more compliant than other valves. This requires a large balloon for adequate dilation (up to 1.4:1 compared with 1.0:1 for aortic valvuloplasty). Larger balloons require larger catheters which traumatize peripheral access sites. Balloon inflation also completely occludes the RVOT, which can cause hemodynamic instability and a significant vagal response. The double balloon technique ameliorates some of these hazards. Smaller balloons are more easily advanced into position and only partially occlude the RVOT when inflated, but require additional skill (and hands) to maneuver. The techniques for double balloon valvuloplasty are similar to those discussed for the single balloon technique, except in duplicate and with an additional venous access. Ideally the balloons are rotated within the valve annulus by 90° during sequential inflation-deflation dilation attempts to dilate all aspects of the valve annulus.

Balloon sizing for double balloon valvuloplasty is less straightforward than for single balloon technique. Rao and colleagues proposed the following equation to account for the ellipse formed by two adjacent circles, where D1 and D2 are the diameters of the respective balloons:

$$Effective\ Diameter = \frac{D_1 + D_2 + \frac{\pi(D_1 + D_2)}{2}}{\pi} \quad [74]$$

This equation simplifies to: $Effective\ Diameter = 0.82(D_1 + D_2)$ [75]. Others have suggested circumference as a better means of estimating the dilating effect with multiple balloons [76]. Experience has shown that simply using a combined diameter to annulus ratio of 1.4-1.6:1 is practical and produces results at least as good as single balloon technique [68, 77, 78].

Triple Balloon Technique

The advantages of double balloon valvuloplasty can be further extended to triple balloon valvuloplasty for patients with a very large pulmonary valve annulus. Even though this technique requires yet another venous access, the sheaths are all relatively small, which induces less trauma to the venous system. In the first report of triple balloon technique, effective balloon diameters to annulus diameters were chosen to be 1.2-1.3:1 [79]. In this series the mean pulmonary gradient was reduced from 44 to 12mmHg without procedural complications. The use of bifoil and trefoil balloons has also been reported for pulmonary valvuloplasty [80]. The advantage of using this technique is that only a single balloon guide wire is used (instead of two or three), but having all the balloons mounted together requires a large introduction sheath and limits its use. This design has not gained popularity over standard multi-balloon pulmonary valvuloplasty.

Pulmonary Valve Stenting

Pulmonary valve stent placement is generally reserved for stenotic right ventricular to pulmonary artery (RV-PA) conduits. A completely new RVOT is required for a variety of congenital lesions including pulmonary atresia with intact ventricular septum, transposition complexes and truncus arteriosus. A replacement RVOT may also be necessary when coronary anatomy prevents RVOT surgery, as part of a Rastelli procedure or as a treatment for post-surgical PI. A RV-PA conduit may palliate these lesions with acceptable results. The original conduits were made of Dacron, which was later replaced with PTFE to prevent early calcification. Conduits may also include prosthetic valves such as homografts (allographic human aortic or pulmonary valves) or heterographs (xenographic bovine jugular vein valves). The major drawback to bioprosthetic valved conduits is their short life-span after implantation (approximately 10 years) [23, 81-83]. Biological material is subject to immunological reactions that cause degradation and calcification [84, 85]. Conduits become stenotic and/or regurgitant as a consequence of inevitable structural breakdown. In addition, young patients may outgrow their conduit and require repeat surgery.

Conduit stenosis was initially treated with balloon angioplasty following the success of PBV for valvular PS. This technique had far less impressive results than PBV and balloon rupture and fragmentation were common [21, 86, 87]. The next logical step was the use of balloon expandable stents, which have been shown to prolong the time to surgical reintervention [23, 88-92]. In a study of 242 patients, the gradient across the RV-PA conduit was reduced from 59 to 27mmHg after stent placement [93]. This cohort was followed for an average of 4 years and median freedom from conduit surgery was 2.7 years (3.9 years for those greater than 5 years old). One hundred twenty six patients underwent repeat catheterizations, many of whom had stent redilation (66%) or placement of additional stents (33%). Another study has shown freedom from surgical reintervention of more than 4 years, but this cohort had less severe disease at baseline [94].

Stent fractures have been reported to occur in up to 40% of cases [93]. The relatively elastic RVOT and cyclic stress caused by compression between the beating heart and the sternum likely cause fatigue fractures. Even though some stent fragments may embolize to the distal pulmonary arterial bed, they typically do not cause hemodynamic compromise or other adverse events.

Another drawback of stenting stenosed conduits is that the patient is left with wide open PI. The attendant risks of right ventricular volume overload have generally not been seen in these patients. This is probably because most, if not all, undergo surgical valve replacement within a few years of the procedure, well before signs of volume overload may become apparent.

Percutaneous Pulmonary Valves

The next major advance in treating pulmonary valve disease has been the development of percutaneous pulmonary valves (PPV). Treatment for PS, be it surgical or percutaneous, often trades a pressure overloaded ventricle for a volume overloaded ventricle as a result of procedural related PI. Percutaneous pulmonary valves offer a novel solution to this problem by relieving the obstruction without resultant PI. To date, two types of percutaneous valves have been successfully implanted in the pulmonary position: the Melody valve and the Sapian valve.

The first PPV was the Melody valve implanted in 2000 by Bonhoeffer and colleagues [95]. The Melody valve consists of a valved bovine jugular vein stitched to a platinum-iridium balloon expandable stent (Figure 4). The delivery system accepts a crimped Melody valve under a protective sheath and is inflated using a balloon-in-balloon system. Two design modifications have been added for the current generation Melody valves. Gold has been added to the weld points to prevent stent fractures and the bovine jugular vein is now sutured to the stent along its entire length to prevent the so called "hammock effect," where blood is trapped between the stent and the vein graft [96, 97]. The implantation site of the Melody, however, must be between 14 and 22mm in dilated diameter, precluding its use in dilated RVOTs.

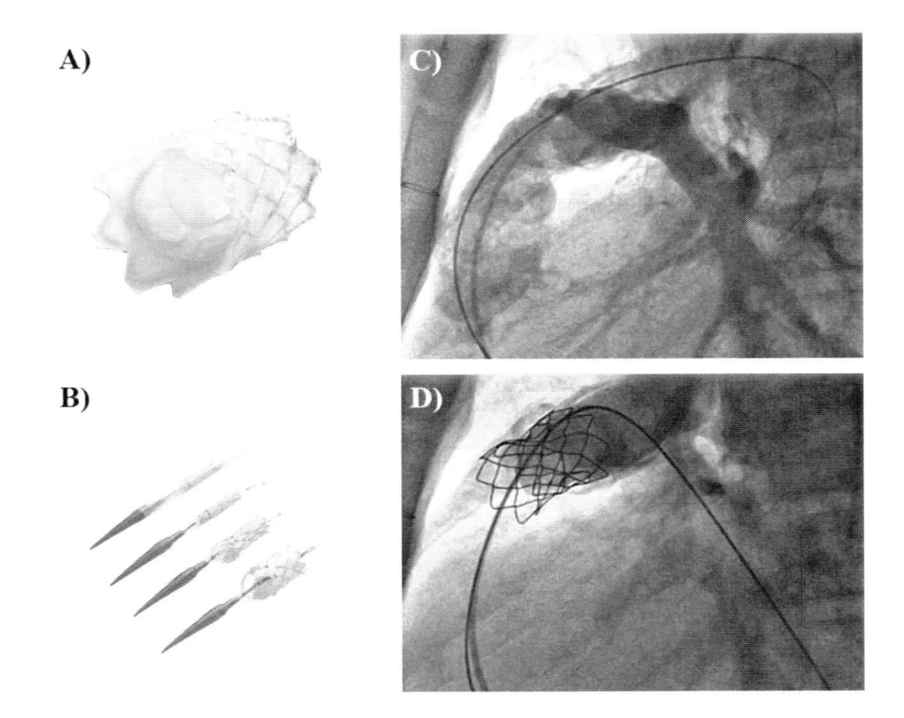

Figure 4. A) The Melody® transcatheter pulmonary valve (Medtronic; Minneapolis, MN.) shown in expanded form and B) in various steps of expansion through balloon inflation. C) Pulmonary angiography to help guide catheter delivery of the valve into the right ventricular outflow tract (angiogram also demonstrates severe pulmonic valve insufficiency) and D) a fully expanded valve with angiography demonstrating near complete resolution of pulmonic valve insufficiency.

The Sapian valve, originally developed for use in the aortic position, was successfully implanted in the pulmonary position in 2006 [98]. This valve is a tri-leaflet valve made from bovine pericardium. Although this valve has been implanted in well over 1500 patients in the aortic position, its use in the pulmonary position has been limited and feasibility trials are currently enrolling [99].

Melody Delivery Technique

Percutaneous pulmonary valves are delivered under general anesthesia. Arterial and venous access are obtained in the usual fashion. Femoral access is preferred to accept the required 22-French dilator, but jugular access is also acceptable. Right heart catheterization is performed to obtain pressure measurements and to delineate the RVOT and pulmonary arterial anatomy. The exact RVOT diameter can be measured with a sizing balloon at this stage if there is any question of a borderline large conduit. Coronary angiography is performed to ensure that the coronary anatomy will not be adversely impacted by the stent. Predilitation of severely stenosed conduits may also be performed at this stage to better accept the delivery catheter. Similar to PBV, a floppy tipped wire is used to cross the RV-PA conduit after which an end-hole catheter is advanced into a distal pulmonary artery. A stiff guide wire with a floppy tip is then exchanged in preparation for the Melody Ensemble. The valved stent is crimped down over a double balloon (balloon-in-balloon) catheter ensuring proper orientation. Blue stitching on the downstream edge of the stent must line up with the blue tip of the delivery catheter. The catheter is then advanced into position with the aid of contrast injected through a side hole. The inner balloon is inflated followed by the outer balloon. Once in position, repeat hemodynamic measurements may be collected.

Melody Experience

The initial experience implanting PPVs has been promising and results of the first trial were published by Bonhoeffer and colleagues in 2005 [97]. Inclusion criteria for the study included previous RVOT reconstruction with a RV-PA conduit, RVOT dysfunction severe enough to warrant surgical intervention as evidenced by right ventricular hypertension (defined as 2/3rds systemic pressure), significant PI, right ventricular dilation or right ventricular failure. There were 59 eligible participants, 58 of whom were successfully implanted with the Melody valve. One patient's anatomy prohibited advancement of the Melody delivery catheter. Immediately following implantation, right ventricular systolic pressure fell from 64 to 50mmHg and the RVOT gradient fell from 33 to 20mmHg. The investigators reported that no patient demonstrated more than mild PI after valve implantation. Cardiac magnetic resonance imaging was performed before and after valve implantation in 28 of 58 patients (48%). The PI fraction and right ventricular end diastolic volume improved significantly, and in 13 patients PI was completely abolished. There were 3 adverse events requiring conversion to surgery and 7 minor events, all treated conservatively and with no attendant mortality. Stent dislodgment from the delivery catheter occurred in 2 patients requiring conversion to open homograft replacement and 1 patient experienced conduit dissection after predilation with PBV. Although a valve was successfully implanted, the patient required a blood transfusion and surgery for drainage of right hemothorax.

The Melody experience in the United States has paralleled the European experience [100]. In the first published series, PPV was planned in 34 patients and successfully implanted in 30. Conduit gradients were reduced from 37 to 17mmHg and no patient was left with more than mild PI. At 6 month follow-up, the gradient remained low (22mmHg by Doppler echocardiography) and PI fraction was 3%. Freedom from reintervention at 15 months was estimated to be 90%. The Toronto experience, published in 2010, has had similar results and this group reports freedom from reintervention at 91%, 80% and 80% at 1, 2 and 3 years, respectively [101, 102].

A limitation of currently published studies is the lack of consensus indications for PPVs. Surgical pulmonary valve replacement is currently one of the most debated topics in congenital heart disease, and it is expected that indications for PPV will be similarly debated for years to come.

Percutaneous pulmonary valves are subject to stent fracture, similar to that experienced with bare metal stents. In the first 123 patients undergoing PPV implantation, 26 (21.1%) experienced stent fracture [103]. In this early study freedom from stent fracture was estimated to be 85%, 75% and 69% at 1, 2 and 3 years, respectively. At initial follow-up most patients were completely asymptomatic, but 6 of 26 (23%) experienced adverse outcomes. One patient's valve dislodged and embolized to the right pulmonary artery, while the remaining 5 had loss of valve integrity necessitating reintervention. Three patients with clinically silent stent fractures subsequently lost valve integrity requiring reintervention. At the conclusion of the follow-up period, freedom from stent fracture requiring intervention was estimated to be 96%, 93% and 87% at 1, 2 and 3 years, respectively. The investigators identified risk factors for stent fracture in their cohort, which included implantation into a native RVOT, implantation into a non-calcified RVOT and presence of PPV recoil during balloon deflation.

Stent fracture is likely to be due to cyclical loading. More compliant conduits impart greater loads on the stent, which is likely why native and non-calcified conduits fair worse. Nordmeyer and collegues, however, suggest that not all PPVs undergo cyclic stress [103]. They site observations where circumferential conduit calcification appears confluent with a patient's sternum, and the position of the valve does not change during the cardiac cycle. While immobile, the valve is surely sustaining cyclic stresses imposed by the beating heart. Although these stresses may be smaller in magnitude and may be directed differently (asymmetrical, torsional, etc.) compared to a freely mobile valve, fatigue fracture likely remains a long-term risk. Pre-stenting the RVOT with a bare metal stent is an attractive method to increase the rigidity of the RVOT prior to PPV placement and prevent stent fracture [96].

A unique benefit to PPVs is that in the event of failure, another valve can be easily implanted within the first. This technique was shown to be successful in 20 patients who suffered early valve failure or residual obstruction [104]. A second PPV was implanted at a mean of 16 months following the first valve and no adverse events were recorded. It is reasonable to assume that percutaneous bioprosthetic valves will have a similar lifespan to that of currently available bioprosthetic valves implanted surgically (~10 years). Valve-in-valve techniques could prevent the need for repeat surgical procedures.

The next advance in percutaneous pulmonary valve technology will likely be the development of PPVs for use in large or dilated RVOTs. Current generation PPVs cannot be implanted in RVOTs greater than 22mm (Melody) and 26mm (Sapian), generally limiting their use to within surgically placed RV-PA conduits. Many patients undergoing RVOT dysfunction have large and dilated anatomy, and these patients must still be managed surgically when right ventricular dysfunction occurs. Development of percutaneously deployed "reducers" or "fillers" are currently underway, and will likely soon expand PPV technology to a much broader patient population [105, 107].

Conclusion

Percutaneous pulmonary valve interventions have seen a dramatic evolution over the last century, fueled by very innovative technologies. The scientific achievements made in the field have undoubtedly improved the natural history of pulmonic valve disease in the general population. Treatment for congenital heart disease continues to improve and the prevalence of late pulmonary valve dysfunction will continue to grow. As the percutaneous pulmonary valve experience matures, this technology will soon become the standard of care for many patients.

References

[1] Hoffman JI, Kaplan S. The incidence of congenital heart disease. *J Am Coll Cardiol.* 2002; 39: 1890-1900.

[2] McCarron WE, Perloff JK. Familial congenital valvular pulmonic stenosis. *Am Heart J.* 1974; 88: 357-359.

[3] Sanchez Cascos A. Genetics of pulmonic stenosis. *Acta Cardiol.* 1972; 27: 316-330.

[4] Towbin JA, Belmont J. Molecular determinants of left and right outflow tract obstruction. *Am J Med Genet.* 2000; 97: 297-303.

[5] Kumar A, Stalker HJ, Williams CA. Concurrence of supravalvular aortic stenosis and peripheral pulmonary stenosis in three generations of a family: a form of arterial dysplasia. *Am J Med Genet.* 1993; 45: 739-742.

[6] Lin AE, Basson CT, Goldmuntz E, Magoulas PL, McDermott DA, McDonald-McGinn DM, McPherson E, Morris CA, Noonan J, Nowak C, Pierpont ME, Pyeritz RE, Rope AF, Zackai E, Pober BR. Adults with genetic syndromes and cardiovascular abnormalities: clinical history and management. *Genet Med.* 2008; 10: 469-494.

[7] Shaw AC, Kalidas K, Crosby AH, Jeffery S, Patton MA. The natural history of Noonan syndrome: a long-term follow-up study. *Arch Dis Child.* 2007; 92: 128-132.

[8] Silberbach M, Lashley D, Reller MD, Kinn WF,Jr, Terry A, Sunderland CO. Arteriohepatic dysplasia and cardiovascular malformations. *Am Heart J.* 1994; 127: 695-699.

[9] Nadas AS. Report from the Joint Study on the Natural History of Congenital Heart Defects. IV. Clinical course. Introduction. *Circulation.* 1977; 56: I36-8.

[10] Hoffman JI. The natural history of congenital isolated pulmonic and aortic stenosis. *Annu Rev Med.* 1969; 20: 15-28.

[11] Greene DG, Baldwin ED. Pure congenital pulmonary stenosis and idiopathic congenital dilatation of the pulmonary artery. *Am J Med.* 1949; 6: 24-40.

[12] Jonsson B, Lee SJ. Haemodynamic effects of exercise in isolated pulmonary stenosis before and after surgery. *Br Heart J.* 1968; 30: 60-66.

[13] Driscoll DJ, Michels VV, Gersony WM, Hayes CJ, Keane JF, Kidd L, Pieroni DR, Rings LJ, Wolfe RR, Weidman WH. Occurrence risk for congenital heart defects in relatives of patients with aortic stenosis, pulmonary stenosis, or ventricular septal defect. *Circulation.* 1993; 87: I114-20.

[14] Nora JJ, Nora AH. Recurrence risks in children having one parent with a congenital heart disease. *Circulation.* 1976; 53: 701-702.

[15] Shyu KG, Tseng CD, Chiu IS, Hung CR, Chu SH, Lue HC, Tseng YZ, Lien WP. Infundibular pulmonic stenosis with intact ventricular septum: a report of 15 surgically corrected patients. *Int J Cardiol.* 1993; 41: 115-121.

[16] Fox D, Devendra GP, Hart SA, Krasuski RA. When 'blue babies' grow up: What you need to know about tetralogy of Fallot. *Cleve Clin J Med.* 2010; 77: 821-828.

[17] Cabrera A, Martinez P, Rumoroso JR, Alcibar J, Arriola J, Pastor E, Galdeano JM. Double-chambered right ventricle. *Eur Heart J.* 1995; 16: 682-686.

[18] Kurup V, Perrino A,Jr, Barash P, Hashim SW. Infundibular pulmonary stenosis. *Anesth Analg.* 2007; 104: 507-508.

[19] Cormode EJ, Dawson M, Lowry RB. Keutel syndrome: clinical report and literature review. *Am J Med Genet.* 1986; 24: 289-294.

[20] Rowe RD. Cardiovascular disease in the rubella syndrome. *Cardiovasc Clin.* 1973; 5: 61-80.

[21] Lloyd TR, Marvin WJ,Jr, Mahoney LT, Lauer RM. Balloon dilation valvuloplasty of bioprosthetic valves in extracardiac conduits. *Am Heart J.* 1987; 114: 268-274.

[22] Laforest I, Dumesnil JG, Briand M, Cartier PC, Pibarot P. Hemodynamic performance at rest and during exercise after aortic valve replacement: comparison of pulmonary autografts versus aortic homografts. *Circulation.* 2002; 106: I57-I62.

[23] Powell AJ, Lock JE, Keane JF, Perry SB. Prolongation of RV-PA conduit life span by percutaneous stent implantation. Intermediate-term results. *Circulation.* 1995; 92: 3282-3288.

[24] Silvilairat S, Cabalka AK, Cetta F, Hagler DJ, O'Leary PW. Outpatient echocardiographic assessment of complex pulmonary outflow stenosis: Doppler mean gradient is superior to the maximum instantaneous gradient. *J Am Soc Echocardiogr.* 2005; 18: 1143-1148.

[25] Mullins CE, Ludomirsky A, O'Laughlin MP, Vick GW,3rd, Murphy DJ,Jr, Huhta JC, Nihill MR. Balloon valvuloplasty for pulmonic valve stenosis--two-year follow-up: hemodynamic and Doppler evaluation. *Cathet Cardiovasc Diagn.* 1988; 14: 76-81.

[26] Warnes CA, Williams RG, Bashore TM, Child JS, Connolly HM, Dearani JA, del Nido P, Fasules JW, Graham TP,Jr, Hijazi ZM, Hunt SA, King ME, Landzberg MJ, Miner PD, Radford MJ, Walsh EP, Webb GD. ACC/AHA 2008 Guidelines for the Management of Adults with Congenital Heart Disease: a report of the American College of Cardiology/American Heart Association Task Force on Practice Guidelines (writing committee to develop guidelines on the management of adults with congenital heart disease). *Circulation.* 2008; 118: e714-833.

[27] Frigiola A, Tsang V, Nordmeyer J, Lurz P, van Doorn C, Taylor AM, Bonhoeffer P, de Leval M. Current approaches to pulmonary regurgitation. *Eur J Cardiothorac Surg.* 2008; 34: 576-80; discussion 581-2.

[28] Meadows J, Powell AJ, Geva T, Dorfman A, Gauvreau K, Rhodes J. Cardiac magnetic resonance imaging correlates of exercise capacity in patients with surgically repaired tetralogy of Fallot. *Am J Cardiol.* 2007; 100: 1446-1450.

[29] Carvalho JS, Shinebourne EA, Busst C, Rigby ML, Redington AN. Exercise capacity after complete repair of tetralogy of Fallot: deleterious effects of residual pulmonary regurgitation. *Br Heart J.* 1992; 67: 470-473.

[30] Bouzas B, Kilner PJ, Gatzoulis MA. Pulmonary regurgitation: not a benign lesion. *Eur Heart J.* 2005; 26: 433-439.

[31] Davlouros PA, Karatza AA, Gatzoulis MA, Shore DF. Timing and type of surgery for severe pulmonary regurgitation after repair of tetralogy of Fallot. *Int J Cardiol.* 2004; 97 Suppl 1: 91-101.

[32] Risk factors for arrhythmia and sudden cardiac death late after repair of tetralogy of Fallot: a multicentre study. 2000; 356: 975-981.

[33] Shimazaki Y, Blackstone EH, Kirklin JW. The natural history of isolated congenital pulmonary valve incompetence: surgical implications. *Thorac Cardiovasc Surg.* 1984; 32: 257-259.

[34] Doyen E. Chirugie des Malformation Congenitales ou acquises du coeur. *Presse Med.* 1913; 21: 860.

[35] Blalock A, Taussig H.B. The surgical treatment of malformations of the heart in which there is pulmonary stenosis or pulmnary atresia. *JAMA.* 1945; 128: 189-202.

[36] Potts WJ, Smith S, Gibson S. Anastomoses of the Aorta to a Pulmonary Artery for Certain Types of Congenital Heart Disease. *JAMA: The Journal of the American Medical Association.* 1946; 132: 627.

[37] Waterston DJ. Treatment of Fallot's tetralogy in children under 1 year of age]. *Rozhl Chir.* 1962; 41: 181-183.

[38] Hallman GL, Yashar JJ, Bloodwell RD, Cooley DA. Intrapericardial aortopulmonary anastomosis for tetralogy of Fallot. Clinical experience. *Arch Surg.* 1967; 95: 709-716.

[39] Davidson JS. Anastomosis between the ascending aorta and the main pulmonary artery in the tetralogy of Fallot. *Thorax.* 1955; 10: 348-350.

[40] Brock RC. Pulmonary valvulotomy for the relief of congenital pulmonary stenosis; report of three cases. *Br Med J.* 1948; 1: 1121-1126.

[41] Sellors TH. Surgery of pulmonary stenosis; a case in which the pulmonary valve was successfully divided. *Lancet.* 1948; 1: 988.

[42] Sondergaard T. Valvulotomy for pulmonary stenosis performed through the main stem of the pulmonary artery utilizing a special ring clamp. *Acta Chir Scand.* 1953; 104: 362-372.

[43] Varco R. Simultaneous pulmonary valvulotomy and resection for pulmonary tuberculosis. *Surgery.* 1958; 43: 391-396.

[44] Swan H, Zeavin I. Cessation of crculation in general hypothermia. III. Techniques of intracardiac surgery under direct vision. *Ann Surg.* 1954; 139: 385-396.

[45] Lam CR, Taber RE. Simplified technique for direct vision pulmonary valvotomy. *J Thorac Cardiovasc Surg.* 1959; 38: 309-318.

[46] Glenn WW. The evolution of the treatment of isolated pulmonary valve stenosis. *Yale J Biol Med.* 1987; 60: 471-482.

[47] Semb BK, Tjonneland S, Stake G, Aabyholm G. "Balloon valvulotomy" of congenital pulmonary valve stenosis with tricuspid valve insufficiency. *Cardiovasc Radiol.* 1979; 2: 239-241.

[48] Rashkind WJ, Miller WW. Creation of an atrial septal defect without thoracotomy. A palliative approach to complete transposition of the great arteries. *JAMA.* 1966; 196: 991-992.

[49] Kan JS, White RI,Jr, Mitchell SE, Gardner TJ. Percutaneous balloon valvuloplasty: a new method for treating congenital pulmonary-valve stenosis. *N Engl J Med.* 1982; 307: 540-542.

[50] Weidman WH. Report from the Joint Study on the Natural History of Congenital Heart Defects. III. Indirect assessment of severity. Introduction. *Circulation.* 1977; 56: I13-4.

[51] Hayes CJ, Gersony WM, Driscoll DJ, Keane JF, Kidd L, O'Fallon WM, Pieroni DR, Wolfe RR, Weidman WH. Second natural history study of congenital heart defects. Results of treatment of patients with pulmonary valvar stenosis. *Circulation.* 1993; 87: I28-37.

[52] Earing MG, Connolly HM, Dearani JA, Ammash NM, Grogan M, Warnes CA. Long-term follow-up of patients after surgical treatment for isolated pulmonary valve stenosis. *Mayo Clin Proc.* 2005; 80: 871-876.

[53] Bonow RO, Carabello BA, Chatterjee K, de Leon AC,Jr, Faxon DP, Freed MD, Gaasch WH, Lytle BW, Nishimura RA, O'Gara PT, O'Rourke RA, Otto CM, Shah PM, Shanewise JS, 2006 Writing Committee Members, American College of Cardiology/American Heart Association Task Force. 2008 Focused update incorporated into the ACC/AHA 2006 guidelines for the management of patients with valvular heart disease: a report of the American College of Cardiology/American Heart Association Task Force on Practice Guidelines (Writing Committee to Revise the 1998 Guidelines for the Management of Patients With Valvular Heart Disease): endorsed by the Society of Cardiovascular Anesthesiologists, Society for Cardiovascular Angiography and Interventions, and Society of Thoracic Surgeons. *Circulation.* 2008; 118: e523-661.

[54] Rao PS. Percutaneous balloon pulmonary valvuloplasty: state of the art. *Catheter Cardiovasc Interv.* 2007; 69: 747-763.

[55] Jarrar M, Betbout F, Farhat MB, Maatouk F, Gamra H, Addad F, Hammami S, Hamda KB. Long-term invasive and noninvasive results of percutaneous balloon pulmonary valvuloplasty in children, adolescents, and adults. *Am Heart J.* 1999; 138: 950-954.

[56] Hatem DM, Castro I, Haertel JC, Rossi RI, Zielinsky P, Leboute FC, Pomar N, Winckler M, Kersten RN, Cardoso CR, Gottschall CA. Short- and long- term results of percutaneous balloon valvuloplasty in pulmonary valve stenosis]. *Arq Bras Cardiol.* 2004; 82: 221-227.

[57] Stanger P, Cassidy SC, Girod DA, Kan JS, Lababidi Z, Shapiro SR. Balloon pulmonary valvuloplasty: results of the Valvuloplasty and Angioplasty of Congenital Anomalies Registry. *Am J Cardiol.* 1990; 65: 775-783.

[58] Fawzy ME, Hassan W, Fadel BM, Sergani H, El Shaer F, El Widaa H, Al Sanei A. Long-term results (up to 17 years) of pulmonary balloon valvuloplasty in adults and its effects on concomitant severe infundibular stenosis and tricuspid regurgitation. *Am Heart J.* 2007; 153: 433-438.

[59] McCrindle BW. Independent predictors of long-term results after balloon pulmonary valvuloplasty. Valvuloplasty and Angioplasty of Congenital Anomalies (VACA) Registry Investigators. *Circulation.* 1994; 89: 1751-1759.

[60] McCrindle BW, Kan JS. Long-term results after balloon pulmonary valvuloplasty. *Circulation.* 1991; 83: 1915-1922.

[61] Kirkin JW, Connolly DC, Ellis FH,Jr, Burchell HB, Edwards JE, Wood EH. Problems in the diagnosis and surgical treatment of pulmonic stenosis with intact ventricular septum. *Circulation.* 1953; 8: 849-863.

[62] Ben-Shachar G, Cohen MH, Sivakoff MC, Portman MA, Riemenschneider TA, Van Heeckeren DW. Development of infundibular obstruction after percutaneous pulmonary balloon valvuloplasty. *J Am Coll Cardiol.* 1985; 5: 754-756.

[63] O'Connor BK, Beekman RH, Lindauer A, Rocchini A. Intermediate-term outcome after pulmonary balloon valvuloplasty: comparison with a matched surgical control group. *J Am Coll Cardiol.* 1992; 20: 169-173.

[64] Chen CR, Cheng TO, Huang T, Zhou YL, Chen JY, Huang YG, Li HJ. Percutaneous balloon valvuloplasty for pulmonic stenosis in adolescents and adults. *N Engl J Med.* 1996; 335: 21-25]

[65] Rao PS, Galal O, Patnana M, Buck SH, Wilson AD. Results of three to 10 year follow up of balloon dilatation of the pulmonary valve. *Heart.* 1998; 80: 591-595.

[66] Peterson C, Schilthuis JJ, Dodge-Khatami A, Hitchcock JF, Meijboom EJ, Bennink GB. Comparative long-term results of surgery versus balloon valvuloplasty for pulmonary valve stenosis in infants and children. *Ann Thorac Surg.* 2003; 76: 1078-82; discussion 1082-3.

[67] Rao PS. Further observations on the effect of balloon size on the short term and intermediate term results of balloon dilatation of the pulmonary valve. *Br Heart J.* 1988; 60: 507-511.

[68] Rao PS. How big a balloon and how many balloons for pulmonary valvuloplasty? *Am Heart J.* 1988; 116: 577-580.

[69] Rao PS. Late pulmonary insufficiency after balloon dilatation of the pulmonary valve. *Catheter Cardiovasc Interv.* 2000; 49: 118-119.

[70] Berman W,Jr, Fripp RR, Raisher BD, Yabek SM. Significant pulmonary valve incompetence following oversize balloon pulmonary valveplasty in small infants: A long-term follow-up study. *Catheter Cardiovasc Interv.* 1999; 48: 61-5; discussion 66.

[71] Ali Khan MA, al-Yousef S, Huhta JC, Bricker JT, Mullins CE, Sawyer W. Critical pulmonary valve stenosis in patients less than 1 year of age: treatment with percutaneous gradational balloon pulmonary valvuloplasty. *Am Heart J.* 1989; 117: 1008-1014.

[72] Wang JK, Wu MH, Lee WL, Cheng CF, Lue HC. Balloon dilatation for critical pulmonary stenosis. *Int J Cardiol.* 1999; 69: 27-32.

[73] Lau KW, Hung JS, Wu JJ, Chern MS, Yeh KH, Fu M. Pulmonary valvuloplasty in adults using the Inoue balloon catheter. *Cathet Cardiovasc Diagn.* 1993; 29: 99-104.

[74] Rao PS. Influence of balloon size on short-term and long-term results of balloon pulmonary valvuloplasty. *Tex Heart Inst J.* 1987; 14: 57-61.

[75] Narang R, Das G, Dev V, Goswami K, Saxena A, Shrivastava S. Effect of the balloon-anulus ratio on the intermediate and follow-up results of pulmonary balloon valvuloplasty. *Cardiology.* 1997; 88: 271-276.

[76] Park JH, Yoon YS, Yeon KM, Han MC, Kim CW, Oh BH, Lee YW. Percutaneous pulmonary valvuloplasty with a double-balloon technique. *Radiology.* 1987; 164: 715-718.

[77] Pedra CA, Arrieta SR, Esteves CA, Braga SL, Neves J, Cassar R, Pedra SR, Santana MV, Silva MA, Sousa JE, Fontes VF. Double balloon pulmonary valvuloplasty: multi-track system versus conventional technique. *Catheter Cardiovasc Interv.* 2006; 68: 193-198.

[78] Yeager SB. Balloon selection for double balloon valvotomy. *J Am Coll Cardiol.* 1987; 9: 467-468.

[79] Escalera RB,2nd, Chase TJ, Owada CY. Triple-balloon pulmonary valvuloplasty: an advantageous technique for percutaneous repair of pulmonary valve stenosis in the large pediatric and adult patients. *Catheter Cardiovasc Interv.* 2005; 66: 446-451.

[80] Meier B, Friedli B, von Segesser L. Valvuloplasty with trefoil and bifoil balloons and the long sheath technique. *Herz.* 1988; 13: 1-13.

[81] Bull C, Macartney FJ, Horvath P, Almeida R, Merrill W, Douglas J, Taylor JF, de Leval MR, Stark J. Evaluation of long-term results of homograft and heterograft valves in extracardiac conduits. *J Thorac Cardiovasc Surg.* 1987; 94: 12-19.

[82] Tweddell JS, Pelech AN, Frommelt PC, Mussatto KA, Wyman JD, Fedderly RT, Berger S, Frommelt MA, Lewis DA, Friedberg DZ, Thomas JP,Jr, Sachdeva R, Litwin SB. Factors affecting longevity of homograft valves used in right ventricular outflow tract reconstruction for congenital heart disease. *Circulation.* 2000; 102: III130-5.

[83] Dearani JA, Danielson GK, Puga FJ, Schaff HV, Warnes CW, Driscoll DJ, Schleck CD, Ilstrup DM. Late follow-up of 1095 patients undergoing operation for complex congenital heart disease utilizing pulmonary ventricle to pulmonary artery conduits. *Ann Thorac Surg.* 2003; 75: 399-410; discussion 410-1.

[84] Smith JD, Ogino H, Hunt D, Laylor RM, Rose ML, Yacoub MH. Humoral immune response to human aortic valve homografts. *Ann Thorac Surg.* 1995; 60: S127-30.

[85] Rajani B, Mee RB, Ratliff NB. Evidence for rejection of homograft cardiac valves in infants. *J Thorac Cardiovasc Surg.* 1998; 115: 111-117.

[86] Zeevi B, Keane JF, Perry SB, Lock JE. Balloon dilation of postoperative right ventricular outflow obstructions. *J Am Coll Cardiol.* 1989; 14: 401-8; discussion 409-12.

[87] Ensing GJ, Hagler DJ, Seward JB, Julsrud PR, Mair DD. Caveats of balloon dilation of conduits and conduit valves. *J Am Coll Cardiol.* 1989; 14: 397-400.

[88] Hosking MC, Benson LN, Nakanishi T, Burrows PE, Williams WG, Freedom RM. Intravascular stent prosthesis for right ventricular outflow obstruction. *J Am Coll Cardiol.* 1992; 20: 373-380.

[89] O'Laughlin MP, Slack MC, Grifka RG, Perry SB, Lock JE, Mullins CE. Implantation and intermediate-term follow-up of stents in congenital heart disease. *Circulation.* 1993; 88: 605-614.

[90] Ovaert C, Caldarone CA, McCrindle BW, Nykanen D, Freedom RM, Coles JG, Williams WG, Benson LN. Endovascular stent implantation for the management of postoperative right ventricular outflow tract obstruction: clinical efficacy. *J Thorac Cardiovasc Surg.* 1999; 118: 886-893.

[91] Petit CJ, Gillespie MJ, Kreutzer J, Rome JJ. Endovascular stents for relief of cyanosis in single-ventricle patients with shunt or conduit-dependent pulmonary blood flow. *Catheter Cardiovasc Interv.* 2006; 68: 280-286.

[92] Desai T, Stumper O, Miller P, Dhillon R, Wright J, Barron D, Brawn W, Jones T, DeGiovanni J. Acute interventions for stenosed right ventricle-pulmonary artery conduit following the right-sided modification of Norwood-Sano procedure. *Congenit Heart Dis.* 2009; 4: 433-439.

[93] Peng LF, McElhinney DB, Nugent AW, Powell AJ, Marshall AC, Bacha EA, Lock JE. Endovascular stenting of obstructed right ventricle-to-pulmonary artery conduits: a 15-year experience. *Circulation.* 2006; 113: 2598-2605.
[94] Sugiyama H, Williams W, Benson LN. Implantation of endovascular stents for the obstructive right ventricular outflow tract. *Heart.* 2005; 91: 1058-1063.
[95] Bonhoeffer P, Boudjemline Y, Saliba Z, Merckx J, Aggoun Y, Bonnet D, Acar P, Le Bidois J, Sidi D, Kachaner J. Percutaneous replacement of pulmonary valve in a right-ventricle to pulmonary-artery prosthetic conduit with valve dysfunction. *Lancet.* 2000; 356: 1403-1405.
[96] Lurz P, Bonhoeffer P, Taylor AM. Percutaneous pulmonary valve implantation: an update. *Expert Rev Cardiovasc Ther.* 2009; 7: 823-833.
[97] Khambadkone S, Coats L, Taylor A, Boudjemline Y, Derrick G, Tsang V, Cooper J, Muthurangu V, Hegde SR, Razavi RS, Pellerin D, Deanfield J, Bonhoeffer P. Percutaneous pulmonary valve implantation in humans: results in 59 consecutive patients. *Circulation.* 2005; 112: 1189-1197.
[98] Garay F, Webb J, Hijazi ZM. Percutaneous replacement of pulmonary valve using the Edwards-Cribier percutaneous heart valve: first report in a human patient. *Catheter Cardiovasc Interv.* 2006; 67: 659-662.
[99] Cubeddu RJ, Palacios IF. Percutaneous heart valve replacement and repair: advances and future potential. *Expert Rev Cardiovasc Ther.* 2009; 7: 811-821.
[100] Zahn EM, Hellenbrand WE, Lock JE, McElhinney DB. Implantation of the melody transcatheter pulmonary valve in patients with a dysfunctional right ventricular outflow tract conduit early results from the u.s. Clinical trial. *J Am Coll Cardiol.* 2009; 54: 1722-1729.
[101] Vezmar M, Chaturvedi R, Lee KJ, Almeida C, Manlhiot C, McCrindle BW, Horlick EM, Benson LN. Percutaneous pulmonary valve implantation in the young 2-year follow-up. *JACC Cardiovasc Interv.* 2010; 3: 439-448.
[102] Asoh K, Walsh M, Hickey E, Nagiub M, Chaturvedi R, Lee KJ, Benson LN. Percutaneous pulmonary valve implantation within bioprosthetic valves. *Eur Heart J.* 2010; 31: 1404-1409.
[103] Nordmeyer J, Khambadkone S, Coats L, Schievano S, Lurz P, Parenzan G, Taylor AM, Lock JE, Bonhoeffer P. Risk stratification, systematic classification, and anticipatory management strategies for stent fracture after percutaneous pulmonary valve implantation. *Circulation.* 2007; 115: 1392-1397.
[104] Nordmeyer J, Coats L, Lurz P, Lee TY, Derrick G, Rees P, Cullen S, Taylor AM, Khambadkone S, Bonhoeffer P. Percutaneous pulmonary valve-in-valve implantation: a successful treatment concept for early device failure. *Eur Heart J.* 2008; 29: 810-815.
[105] Basquin A, Pineau E, Galmiche L, Bonnet D, Sidi D, Boudjemline Y. Transcatheter valve insertion in a model of enlarged right ventricular outflow tracts. *J Thorac Cardiovasc Surg.* 2010; 139: 198-208.
[106] Boudjemline Y, Agnoletti G, Bonnet D, Sidi D, Bonhoeffer P. Percutaneous pulmonary valve replacement in a large right ventricular outflow tract: an experimental study. *J Am Coll Cardiol.* 2004; 43: 1082-1087.
[107] Mollet A, Basquin A, Stos B, Boudjemline Y. Off-pump replacement of the pulmonary valve in large right ventricular outflow tracts: a transcatheter approach using an intravascular infundibulum reducer. *Pediatr Res.* 2007; 62: 428-433.

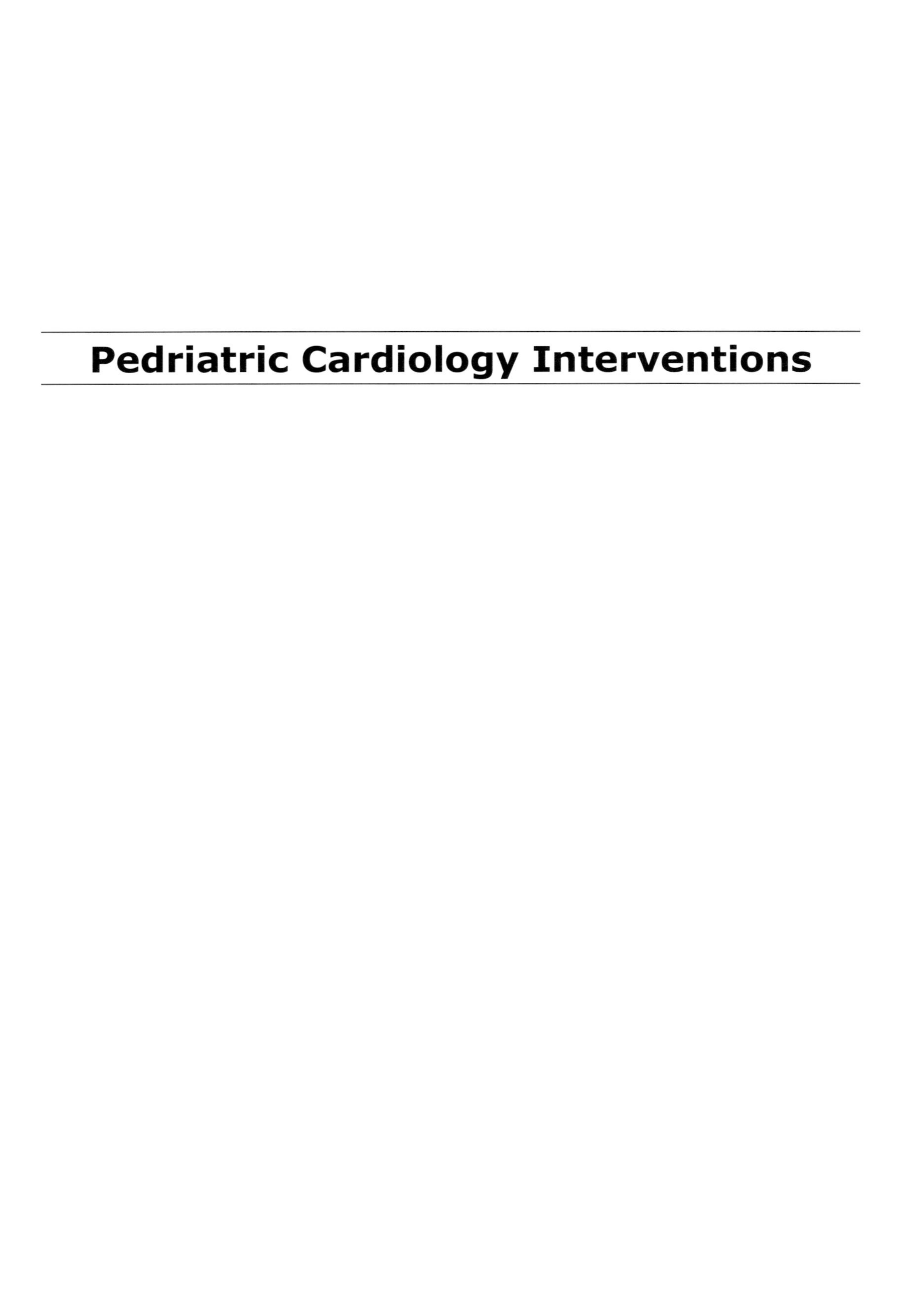

Pedriatric Cardiology Interventions

In: Percutaneous Valve Technology: Present and Future ISBN: 978-1-61942-577-4
Editors: Jose Luis Navia and Sharif Al-Ruzzeh

Chapter XXIX

Pediatric Percutaneous Interventions: Present and Future Perspectives

Lourdes R. Prieto

Abstract

The field of catheter based intervention for congenital heart lesions spans nearly half a century beginning with the Rashkind balloon atrial septostomy first performed in 1966 [1], shortly followed by the first successful percutaneous closure of the patent ductus by Porstmann in 1967 [2]. About a decade later in 1976 King and Mills reported the first transcatheter closure of an atrial septal defect in a human [3]. The widespread application of this procedure would have to wait over two decades of intense technical development. Balloon dilation of a stenotic pulmonary valve, described by Kan in 1982, was the first percutaneous intervention to gain wide acceptance as the first line of treatment for a congenital cardiac lesion [4]. From this relatively straightforward procedure to the recent development of transcatheter pulmonary valve replacement [5], this chapter will review the current state of the art and future directions of pediatric cardiac intervention.

Percutaneous Closure of the Patent Ductus Arteriosus

Following Porstmann's initial description of a "plug" to close the patent ductus arteriosus (PDA), several devices were developed including the Rashkind double-umbrella occluder, which required relatively large delivery systems and were somewhat cumbersome to implant [2,6]. The introduction of coils for PDA closure by Cambier et al in 1992 simplified the procedure and was highly successful for closing relatively small PDA's < 2.5 mm in diameter [7]. Successful closure of moderate to large PDA's up to 11 mm in diameter has been accomplished with the development of the Amplatzer Duct Occluder (ADO I), a nitinol frame device with polyester fiber packing, resulting in excellent closure rates and low incidence of complications [8] (Figures 1A-C). However, this device could not always be implanted in very small patients with large PDA's due to excessive protrusion into the aorta or the left pulmonary artery. In addition, deployment is limited to a transvenous approach, and there is not sufficient flexibility in the device configuration to allow closure of all the different morphological types of PDA [9]. The recently introduced new version of this device (ADO II), with two low profile discs connected by an articulated waist and elimination of the polyester fiber packing, has enabled closure of moderate to large PDA's in very small infants [10-13] (Figures 2A-C). The manufacturer's recommendation for minimum patient weight is 6 kg, but infants weighing as little as 3 kg have undergone PDA closure with this device [10]. The waist diameter ranges from 3 to 6 mm, allowing closure of PDA's with minimal diameters no larger than 5.5 mm. Based on Krichenko's classification of ductal anatomy only aortopulmonary window type PDA's may not be amenable to closure with this device. Very small infants with very large PDA's continue to be at risk for left pulmonary artery or aortic obstruction caused by the retention discs. Aortic and pulmonary artery angiography can be performed with the device fully deployed but not released, and the device recaptured and removed if significant obstruction is detected. A smaller device if available can be tried, but some patients, most often premature babies, still require surgical closure. The ADO II device received CE Mark approval in 2008, and at the time of this writing a clinical trial evaluating its safety and efficacy is underway in the United States. For the future, additional design changes and a greater range of available sizes may further expand the patient size and ductal morphology amenable to percutaneous closure.

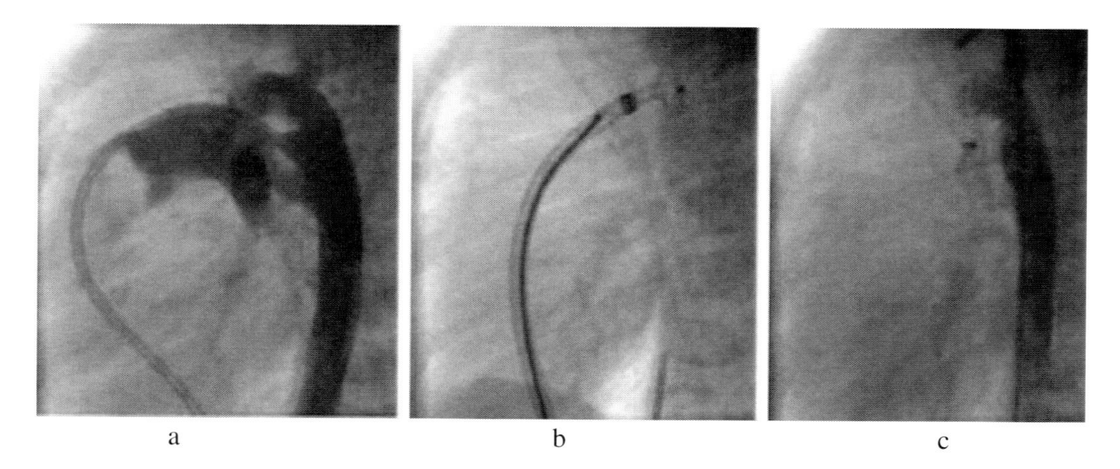

Figure 1. A. Angiography in the descending aorta in the lateral projection shows a moderate to large patent ductus with dense opacification of the main and branch pulmonary arteries. Note the venous catheter has been advanced across the PDA. B. Deployment of the retention disc (aortic end) of the ADO I device from a transvenous approach. C. Angiography in the descending aorta following ADO I deployment demonstrates complete PDA closure (ADO = Amplatzer duct occluder, PDA = patent ductus arteriosus).

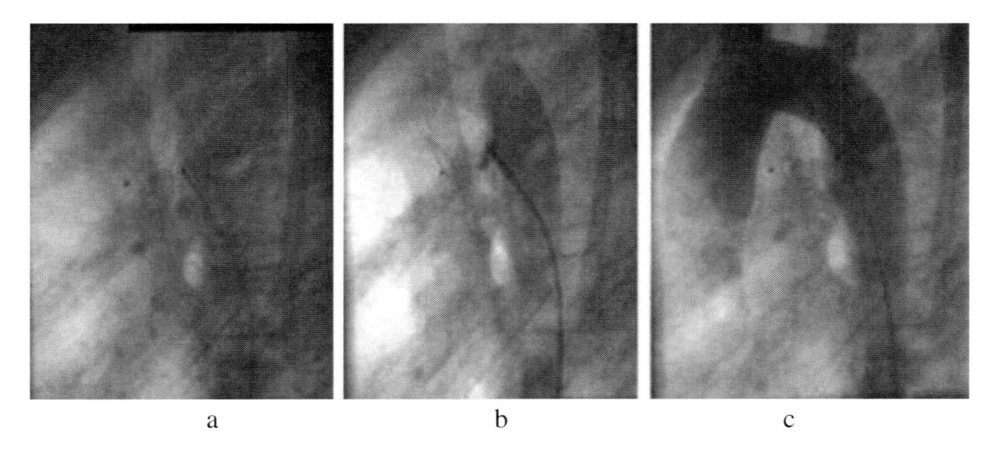

Figure 2. A. Deployment of the ADO II device from a retrograde approach as seen in the lateral projection. The pulmonary and aortic discs are both deployed and the intervening waist is across the PDA, but the device is still attached to the delivery wire. B. Angiography prior to release ensures adequate position. C. Angiography in the descending aorta following ADO II deployment demonstrates complete PDA closure (ADO = Amplatzer duct occluder, PDA = patent ductus arteriosus).

Pulmonary Valvuloplasty

Balloon dilation of the pulmonary valve, first reported in 1982, is the first line of treatment for congenital pulmonary valve stenosis [4]. Excellent immediate and long-term results have been reported in children with typical pulmonary valve stenosis with a very low incidence of reintervention, provided an adequate balloon to annulus ratio (BAR) is used [14-19]. Generally the recommended BAR is 1.2 – 1.4, with lower ratios resulting in suboptimal outcome. Patients with dysplastic pulmonary valves do not respond nearly as well and typically require a BAR closer to 1.4, with adequate relief of obstruction reported in 35% to 65% of these patients [15,17,18]. Soon after introduction of balloon pulmonary valvuloplasty in children the procedure was successfully performed in neonates with critical pulmonary valve stenosis [20] (Figures 3A-B). Since that early report, technical advances including availability of low profile balloons, preformed catheters, and high torque wires have increased the success and safety of the procedure, also considered the first line of treatment in neonates. The baby is stabilized with a prostaglandin E1 infusion to maintain the ductus open before and during the procedure. An open ductus enables the wire to be advanced across the pulmonary valve to the descending aorta for greater stability. The wire can also be externalized as a "wire rail" via the femoral artery, facilitating advancement of a balloon across the very tiny pulmonary valve orifice [21]. In contrast to older children, 25–30% of neonates have residual or recurrent obstruction requiring reintervention, most often within the first year of life [22-26]. Repeat valvuloplasty is often successful with long-term relief, but 15-20% ultimately requires surgery due to either annular hypoplasia and/or subvalvar stenosis.

Severe pulmonary regurgitation is uncommon following pulmonary valve dilation, and milder degrees are well tolerated at least in intermediate term follow-up. There is, however, increasing evidence that more than mild regurgitation may result in detrimental effects on the right ventricle and decreased exercise capacity in the longer term, even in patients with isolated congenital pulmonary valve stenosis [27]. Risk factors for moderate or severe regurgitation include younger age, smaller body surface area and larger BAR, particularly when ≥ 1.4 [17,28]. It may be prudent, particularly in neonates and in patients with typical pulmonary valve morphology, to aim for a BAR closer to 1.2 and not exceeding 1.3 [29,30]. For those few patients who may require pulmonary valve replacement late after pulmonary valvuloplasty, percutaneous pulmonary valve implantation may become a feasible alternative.

Percutaneous Pulmonary Valve Replacement

One of the most exciting developments in pediatric intervention over the past decade has been the introduction of the percutaneous pulmonary valve (PPV), first implanted in a human in 2000 [5]. A significant number of patients with congenital heart disease require surgically placed conduits from the right ventricle (RV) to the pulmonary artery (PA), often at a very early age. These conduits have a limited lifespan due to development of stenosis, regurgitation or both, with detrimental effects on the right ventricle. Over the course of a lifetime multiple operations are needed to replace dysfunctional conduits. Bare metal stenting of stenotic RV to PA conduits has been performed at the expense of creating wide open pulmonary regurgitation [31,32]. The PPV has the potential to extend the life of these conduits, and decrease the number of open heart procedures performed on these patients.

The Melody percutaneous pulmonary valve (Medtronic Inc., Minneapolis, Minnesota) consists of a bovine jugular venous valve sawn to a platinum-iridium balloon expandable stent (Figure 4, Video 1). The delivery system is 22 Fr, which is acceptable for children weighing at least 20 kg. The current device can be dilated to a diameter of 18, 20 or 22 mm. Certain anatomic features must be met by the right ventricular outflow tract (RVOT) "landing zone" to allow successful deployment and adequate valve function. The current iteration of the valve is limited primarily to patients with an RV to PA conduit ≥ 16 mm and ≤ 22 mm in diameter at the time of surgical implantation, as opposed to a native or patched RVOT (Figures 5A,B). Balloon sizing of the RVOT is performed to determine suitability, and the balloon waist must be ≥ 14 and ≤ 20 mm. At the time of this writing, over a thousand of these valves have been implanted worldwide. The valve has received CE Mark, and is approved for use in the United States under HDE guidelines. The majority of patients who have benefited from this procedure are postoperative tetralogy of Fallot patients who have undergone one or multiple surgical pulmonary valve replacement(s) with a homograft or bioprosthetic valve [33]. Other patients treated with PPV implantation include those with truncus arteriosus or aortic valve disease post Ross operation [34].

The largest series reported to date with a mean follow-up of 28.4 months documents very good valve function with 70% freedom from reoperation at 70 months [35]. This series includes the learning curve from the first 50 patients undergoing the procedure, and improvement in patient selection, implantation technique and design of the device have further improved these results. A significant reduction in the RV pressure and RVOT gradient, and relief of pulmonary regurgitation was achieved with low morbidity.

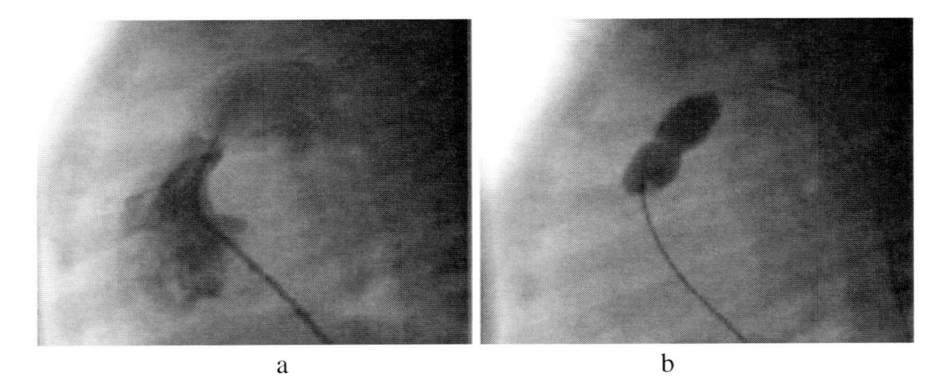

Figure 3. A. Right ventricular angiogram in the lateral projection demonstrates the stenotic pulmonary valve in a neonate with critical pulmonary valve stenosis. B. Balloon inflation across the pulmonary valve shows the typical waist in the middle of the balloon. Note the wire position across the patent ductus in the descending aorta.

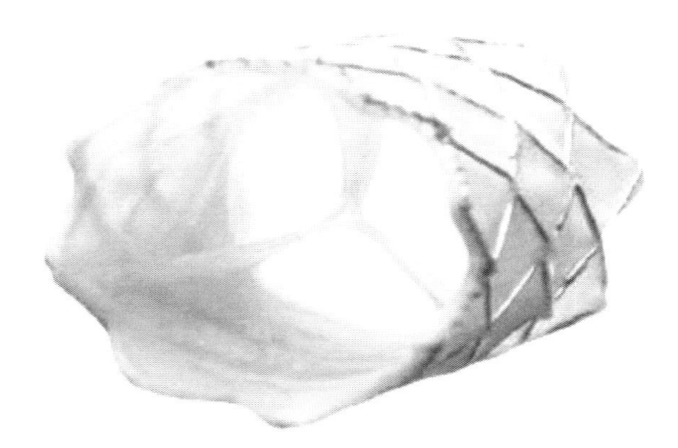

Figure 4. Melody percutaneous pulmonary valve consists of a bovine jugular venous valve sawn to a platinum-iridium balloon expandable stent.

Very few deaths have occurred directly as a result of the procedure, most importantly related to coronary artery compression. The current protocol calls for careful evaluation of the coronary arteries and their proximity to the RV to PA conduit by cardiac MRI before the procedure. In addition, aortic root angiography or selective coronary angiography is performed while maintaining a fully inflated balloon across the conduit prior to valve implantation. If coronary artery compression results the valve is not implanted. Another serious complication is conduit (usually homograft) rupture, and to date no specific risk factors for this fortunately rare complication have been found. It is recommended that the final diameter of a high pressure balloon or of the valve not exceed the original conduit diameter by more than 10%. This complication can be effectively treated in the catheterization laboratory by simultaneous pericardiocentesis and/or thoracentesis, auto/exogenous transfusion, and insertion of either a covered stent or of the PPV itself. The PPV is a covered stent by virtue of the jugular venous tube that contains the valve and is sawn to the stent. Alternatively urgent surgical intervention may be required [36].

In mid term follow-up pressure gradients have shown mild increase overtime, while the valve has remained remarkably competent even in patients followed as long as 5-10 years. A significant problem that can result in stenosis has been stent fractures, reported to occur in about 20% of cases. Risk factors for stent fractures include implantation into a native RVOT, lack of calcification of the conduit, and recoil of the PPV following balloon deflation [37,38]. In the hope of decreasing stent fractures, some operators are pre-stenting the conduits prior to valve implantation, with the thought that reinforcing the landing zone will decrease compressive stresses on the valve. Preliminary results suggest that pre-stenting does lower the risk of stent fractures [39,40]. Patients with stent fractures who develop significant obstruction requiring reintervention can undergo placement of a second PPV (37,41).

The Edwards SAPIEN transcatheter valve has also been implanted in RVOT conduits in a small number of patients at the time of this writing. The device is the same as the Cribier Edwards transcatheter aortic valve, for which there is extensive experience in high risk elderly patients with severe aortic stenosis [42]. This valve consists of three bovine pericardial leaflets sawn to a stainless steel balloon expandable stent. The delivery system (22 and 24 Fr) is a little bulkier than that of the Melody valve. The valve is available in 23 and 26 mm diameters, and 14.5 and 16 mm lengths. At a median follow-up of 10 months for 7 patients reported in 2010 the valves were functioning well and no stent fractures had been observed [43]. Conduits had to be 18 – 30 mm in size at the time of surgical implantation, and significant conduit narrowing had to be present for the valve to be implanted. Pre-stenting with a bare metal stent to a diameter 2-3 mm less than the final valve diameter was always performed given the relatively short length of this valve. This valve allows implantation in patients with larger conduits, but follow-up is more limited than for the Melody valve at this time. The valve has received CE Mark, while in the United States a feasibility trial has been completed, and further investigation is underway with the goal of receiving HDE.

At present both percutaneous pulmonary valves are suitable for delivery in surgically implanted conduits within the size constraints mentioned above, which account for only about 15% of patients with pulmonary valve dysfunction. The biggest challenge for the future is the larger group with native outflow tracts, most commonly post-operative Tetralogy of Fallot patients, whose dilated and distensible pulmonary trunks preclude safe implantation of the available devices. A great deal of work currently taking place promises new technology in valve design that will hopefully allow extension of percutaneous pulmonary valve implantation to the majority of patients in need of a functional pulmonary valve [44,45].

Aortic Valvuloplasty

Severe aortic valve stenosis is a progressive disease typically requiring repeat interventions for either recurrent stenosis or progressive aortic insufficiency following either surgical or percutaneous palliation. Balloon dilation of the aortic valve, initially reported by Lababidi et al in 1984 [46], has become the procedure of choice for initial treatment of moderate to severe congenital aortic valve stenosis in the majority of centers. It has also been shown to be effective for recurrent stenosis after either balloon dilation or surgical valvotomy, as long as there is less than moderate aortic insufficiency [47]. Balloon aortic valvuloplasty has both delayed surgical intervention [48] and reduced the number of open heart surgical procedures in this patient population.

The procedure is performed in most instances from a retrograde approach via the femoral artery. It is helpful to place a catheter in the left ventricle from a venous approach through an atrial communication or transseptal puncture for continuous monitoring of left ventricular pressure. A left ventriculogram delineates the valve anatomy and location of the stenotic orifice to guide introduction of the wire across it. An ascending aortogram should be performed to evaluate the degree of aortic insufficiency before intervention. Various catheters can be used to direct a soft wire across the aortic valve; frequently angled catheters such as coronary catheters work well. A stiffer wire is then placed across the valve for balloon dilation. In older children and adolescents simultaneous inflation of 2 balloons (double balloon technique) minimizes the size of the required arterial sheath thus decreasing vascular complications (Figure 6).

The initial balloon to annulus ratio is chosen to be 0.9 (for double balloons the effective balloon diameter is used). Generally a reduction in the gradient to about 50% of the initial gradient, or a peak to peak gradient of < 40 mmHg, is aimed for. If this is not achieved with the initial dilation an ascending aortogram is performed to evaluate the degree of aortic insufficiency, and if less than moderate a slightly larger balloon is used, not to exceed a balloon/annulus ratio of 1.0 [49]. Intracardiac echocardiography can also be used to evaluate the degree of aortic insufficiency, decreasing the number of angiograms and the radiation exposure. Some studies have shown a correlation between balloon:annulus ratio and a significant increase in aortic insufficiency, but this has not been a consistent finding [47,49,50]. In some cases exceeding the balloon:annulus ratio to slightly > 1.0 may be justified.

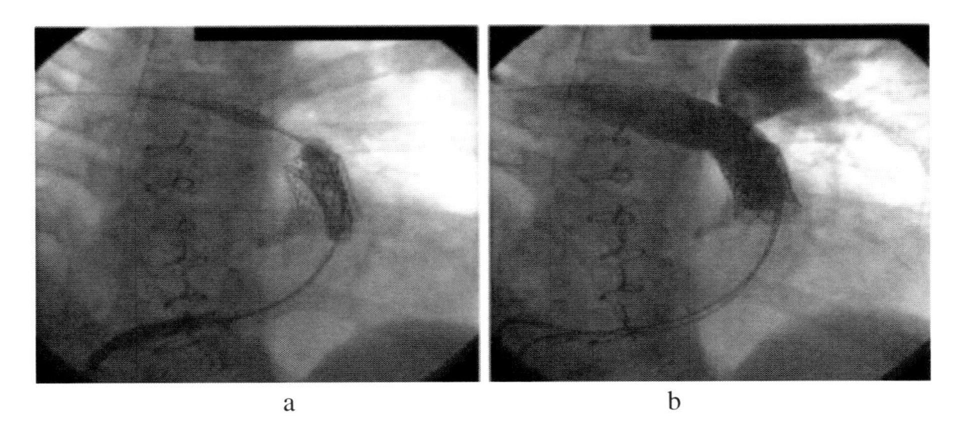

a b

Figure 5. A. Deployment of the Melody percutaneous pulmonary valve in a patient with truncus arteriosus status post prior surgical pulmonary valve replacement with a 20 mm homograft. The inner balloon is fully inflated and the outer balloon is beginning to be inflated. Two stents were placed in the homograft prior to pulmonary valve insertion to reinforce the landing zone. B. Main pulmonary artery angiogram following Melody valve implantation shows a well expanded and completely competent valve.

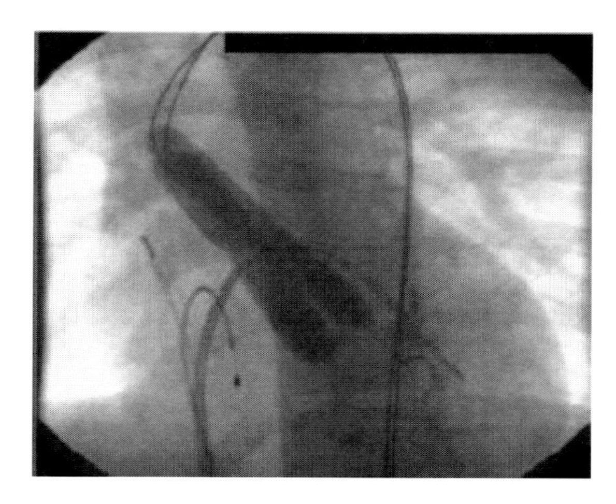

Figure 6. Aortic valvuloplasty using the double balloon technique. Note the waist in the middle of the balloons at the level of the valve annulus. Also note the ventricular pacing wire in the right ventricle for rapid ventricular pacing during balloon inflation and the intracardiac echocardiography probe in the right atrium to assess for aortic insufficiency during the procedure.

In older children and adolescents cardiac contractions during inflation can result in significant movement of the balloons across the aortic valve, making it difficult to maintain the balloon in optimal position, and potentially causing damage to the valve or myocardium. Rapid ventricular pacing during balloon inflation stabilizes balloon position by transiently decreasing cardiac output [51]. A pacing rate that decreases the blood pressure by about 50% from baseline has been found to work well [52].

Neonates with critical aortic valve stenosis are also treated with balloon dilation in most centers, and results have been shown to be comparable to surgical valvotomy [53]. The approach in the majority is also retrograde from the femoral artery, but the carotid artery and umbilical arteries have also been used. Antegrade approach via the femoral vein through an interatrial communication and across the mitral valve is another option when crossing the valve retrograde proves difficult, but care must the taken not to injure the mitral valve.

Complications are in the order of 5% outside of the neonatal period, most commonly rhythm disturbances and vascular problems at the access site. More serious complications such as leaflet evulsion or myocardial perforation can occur but are rare. Severe aortic insufficiency immediately after valvuloplasty requiring surgical intervention has been reported to occur in 0-1% of patients [47,54]. Neonates have a higher risk of complications, in the order of 10-15%. Similarly mortality is rare in older children, but about 15% in neonates within 30 days of the procedure. However a significant proportion of these infants in most studies have succumbed due to inadequate left heart structures and/or endocardial fibroelastosis [53].

Although reintervention is common, 10 year survival free from aortic valve surgery has been reported to be around 60% for patients undergoing valvuloplasty at < 1 month of age, and around 70% for older patients [48,50,55]. Freedom from either surgical or catheter reinterventions is about 50% at 10 years in children [50], and 50% at 5 years in neonates [53,56]. Transcatheter aortic valve implantation is currently being performed in adult patients with severe aortic stenosis who are high risk surgical candidates, but it is not yet feasible in the pediatric population [57].

Coarctation Angioplasty or Stenting

Despite nearly 3 decades since the first report of percutaneous balloon angioplasty of aortic coarctation in 1982 [58], the role of balloon dilation and/or stent angioplasty in the treatment of this lesion is still evolving, with many questions yet to be answered. It is widely accepted that neonates and infants with native coarctation of the aorta should undergo surgical intervention due to the very high incidence of recurrent obstruction in this age group following balloon dilation [59]. It is also widely accepted that teenagers and adults with newly diagnosed coarctation can generally undergo stenting as a first line of treatment. The approach to patients beyond infancy but who are not yet close to fully grown varies with institutional philosophy. The absence of long-term, randomized studies comparing surgery to transcatheter treatment modalities result in the lack of a standardized approach, while retrospective short and mid-term data reveals some of the pros and cons of the different available therapies.

The use of stents in small children is generally avoided due to inability to implant a stent that can be later dilated to adult size to keep up with the patient's growth. Implantation of a low-profile stent that can be accommodated by the vascular structures of a small child would result in the creation of a fixed obstruction over time as the healthy aorta grows around the stent. Elimination of this obstruction would require surgical stent removal and extensive aortic reconstruction, a situation that should certainly be avoided. Balloon angioplasty is therefore the transcatheter treatment generally considered in this group of patients.

Balloon angioplasty has been shown to achieve a similar immediate relief of obstruction in comparison to surgery, with comparable complication rates. However, recurrent stenosis is more common, hovering around 25% in contrast to 5-10% after surgery [60,61]. The reported rate of aneurysm formation varies greatly from one series to another ranging from 0-43%, owing in part to differences in the definition of an aneurysm, lack of standardized imaging protocols and variable lengths of follow-up. Some of the aneurysms became apparent as late as 6-8 years after ballooning [61,62]. Long-term follow-up studies are needed to determine the true incidence and clinical significance of aneurysms.

Technically balloon dilation of aortic coarctation is relatively straightforward. A wire is positioned in the ascending aorta from a femoral arterial approach. It is important to make accurate measurements of the aortic arch, isthmus, coarctation site and descending aorta at the level of the diaphragm. A balloon diameter is chosen equal to the size of the healthy aorta proximal to the coarctation and generally not exceeding the coarctation diameter by more than a 4:1 ratio. If a residual gradient of more than 10-20 mmHg persists a larger balloon can be used typically not exceeding the diameter of the aorta at the diaphragm.

Stent angioplasty for coarctation of the aorta was first introduced in the mid 1990s by Charles Mullins [63,64]. Several studies have documented excellent relief of the obstruction with residual gradient less than 20 mmHg or increase in the coarctation to descending aorta diameter ratio of > 0.8 in 98% of patients [65-69]. The absence of recoil allows use of a balloon that is equal to the final desired diameter and not greater, theoretically resulting in less aortic wall disruption than may be caused by balloon angioplasty. The patient should be large enough to allow placement of a stent that can be dilated to adult size either at the time of deployment or at subsequent catheterizations. There are currently 2 approved stent series that can be expanded to 26 mm, the normal mean diameter of an adult male aorta. The Johnson and Johnson (Cordis) Palmaz XL 10 series (3110, 4010, 5010) is designed to expand to a minimum of 10 mm, and can be later expanded to a maximum of 25-28 mm. There will be some shortening at these larger diameters that the operator must be aware of. The second line approved in 2002 is the EV3 IntraStent LD Max series (EV3, Bloomington, MN). It has an open cell design reducing the degree of shortening, and more rounded cell edges at the stent's ends than the Palmaz series, theoretically decreasing aortic injury as the stent expands. The stent can also be enlarged to 24-26 mm, and has slightly less radial strength than the Palmaz series. Available lengths are 16, 26 and 36 mm. In addition to these large stents the Palmaz Genesis XD series (Cordis) may be appropriate for some patients due to its greater flexibility, facilitating advancement around curves. The maximum expanded diameter of this stent is 18-20 mm, however many patients with coarctation appear to have some degree of generalized aortic hypoplasia and their aorta will not grow beyond this size. All of these stents must be manually mounted on the appropriate sized balloon in a way that minimizes the risk of slippage of the stent off the balloon. The BIB balloon (balloon in balloon, NuMED, Hopkinton, New York) is preferred by most operators as it allows gradual expansion of the stent and ability to reposition after inflating the inner balloon, followed by inflation to the intended diameter by the outer balloon (Figures 7A-C).

The balloon size is chosen to be equal to the diameter of the distal transverse arch or the descending aorta at the level of the diaphragm, whichever smaller. A stiff wire is positioned across the coarctation from a retrograde approach and a long sheath advanced proximal to the coarctation. The balloon and stent combination is advanced inside the sheath to the coarctation segment. The sheath is withdrawn and stent positioning prior to deployment is checked by injection of contrast via the sheath or via a second arterial catheter.

The overall complication rate for this procedure is in the order of 5-10%, and includes aortic wall injury including catastrophic aortic rupture, stent migration, balloon rupture, cerebrovascular accident, peripheral embolic events, and injury to the vascular access sites [66]. To minimize the risk of aortic rupture a staged approach is sometimes elected with intentional partial dilation of the stent at the initial implantation and further dilation to the final intended diameter 6-12 months later. Patients with near atresia and older patients, known to be at higher risk of aortic rupture, are suitable candidates for staged approach. Alternatively, implantation of a covered stent would significantly decrease, although not completely eliminate, the risk of rupture. Covered stents are not yet approved in the United States, but will likely receive approval in the near future upon completion of the Coarctation of the Aorta Stent Trial (COAST). Institutions currently participating in this trial have access to covered stents and can, under specific circumstances, request to use one on an emergent basis.

Intermediate term followup for stent angioplasty demonstrates a very low incidence of in-stent restenosis [70]. Reported reintervention rates as high as 40% include patients with intentional staged approach and therefore do not reflect recurrent stenosis. Late aneurysm formation has been reported in up to 6% of patients [71]. The risk of aortic wall injury on follow-up was noted to be higher when the balloon to coarctation ratio exceeded 3.5 and when pre-stenting balloon angioplasty was performed [65].

Transcatheter therapy is generally offered as the first line of treatment for recurrent coarctation (recoarctation) following surgery at any age, with the exception of patients with extended aortic arch hypoplasia. However, prospective studies comparing surgery and transcatheter therapy for recoarctation are lacking. The choice of balloon angioplasty or stent placement follows the patterns discussed above.

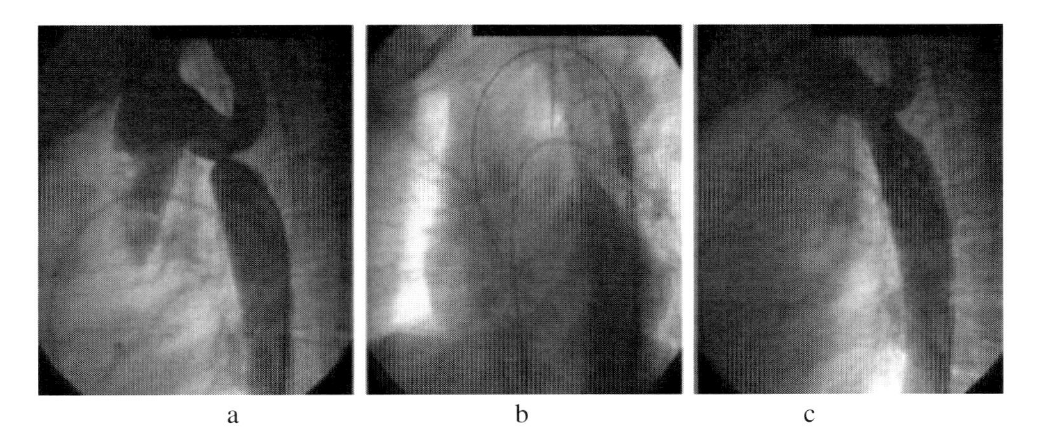

Figure 7. A. Angiography in the descending aorta in the lateral projection shows a discrete coarctation in the typical location just below the left subclavian artery. B. Inflation of the inner balloon of a BIB balloon partially deploys the stent and allows further assessment of positioning before full deployment. C. Angiography post stenting shows excellent relief of the coarctation.

A significant limitation to percutaneous treatment of coarctation is the creation of a fixed obstruction by placement of a stent in a growing patient that cannot be dilated to adult size. The concept of biodegradable stents to provide temporary scaffolding, and allow further growth of the vessel or further percutaneous intervention as the patient reaches adult size, has received considerable attention. Clinical trials with biodegradable stents from several materials including polymers and magnesium alloys in coronary or peripheral arteries have not demonstrated superiority over existing stents in those settings, where adaptation to growth is not the limiting factor [72]. However, further development of this technology may play an important role in growing infants and children. Use of a biodegradable magnesium stent to temporarily relieve a critical recoarctation in a newborn has been reported [73]. Other stent designs such as the Growth Stent [74,75], made of two separate longitudinal halves of stainless steel connected with bioabsorbable sutures, will continue to extend the interventional repertoire for percutaneous treatment of this and other lesions to younger patients.

Percutaneous Atrial Septal Defect Closure

The last decade has seen an explosion in feasibility and technical advances of percutaneous atrial septal defect closure (ASD). Percutaneous closure is now the procedure of choice over surgical closure for the majority of atrial septal defects in both children and adults, with experienced centers successfully closing over 80% of all ASD's [76]. There are currently 3 FDA approved devices in the United States for ASD closure: The Amplatzer septal occluder (ASO; AGA Medical Corp., Golden Valley, MN), the Helex septal occluder (W. L. Gore and Associates, Flagstaff, Arizona) and the Amplatzer cribriform septal occluder (ASO; AGA Medical Corp., Golden Valley, MN). Several other devices are available outside the United States, and development of new devices continues to be a very active field.

Although each device has different technical attributes in general the procedure is carried out in a similar fashion. In addition to fluoroscopy either transesophageal echocardiogram (TEE) or intracardiac echocardiography (ICE) is used to evaluate the anatomy of the ASD and to guide closure [77]. Choice of the type and size of device depends on the size and the anatomic features of the defect. In addition to the static diameter of the ASD obtained in multiple echocardiographic views the majority of operators use the "stop-flow" balloon stretched diameter to size the defect. The atrial septal defect is crossed from a femoral venous approach with an end hole catheter and the left superior pulmonary vein is accessed. A stiff wire is positioned in the vein and used to advance a balloon sizing catheter across the atrial septal defect. While interrogating the septum with color Doppler the balloon is inflated only until shunting through the defect is eliminated by disappearance of color flow [78]. The diameter of the balloon at the point of contact with the ASD rims represents the "stop-flow" stretched diameter. Typically a mild waist in the balloon will be visible by both fluoroscopy and TEE or ICE. Depending on the device a delivery sheath is advanced over the wire into the left atrium or the device and delivery sheath ensemble is advanced together across the ASD. The device is then deployed according to specific recommendations.

The first device to obtain FDA approval was the Amplatzer Septal Occluder in December 2001 [79] (Figures 8A,B). The device is made of nitinol and consists of two expandable discs with a connecting waist. The left atrial disc is slightly larger than the right atrial disc since the direction of flow through an ASD is from left to right. A polyester mesh inside the nitinol frame enhances thrombogenicity. The delivery sheath ranges from 8 to 12 French depending on the size of the device. Although the device comes with its own delivery sheath, some operators prefer to either modify the sheath or use specially shaped sheaths that allow a more parallel approach of the left atrial disc to the septum [80-82]. Closure is achieved by the central waist which self centers at the ASD and exerts a radial force against the defect rims. The left and right atrial discs flatten against the surrounding septum stabilizing the device in place. Available sizes range from 4-38 mm (central waist diameter) in the United States, and up to 40 mm in other countries.

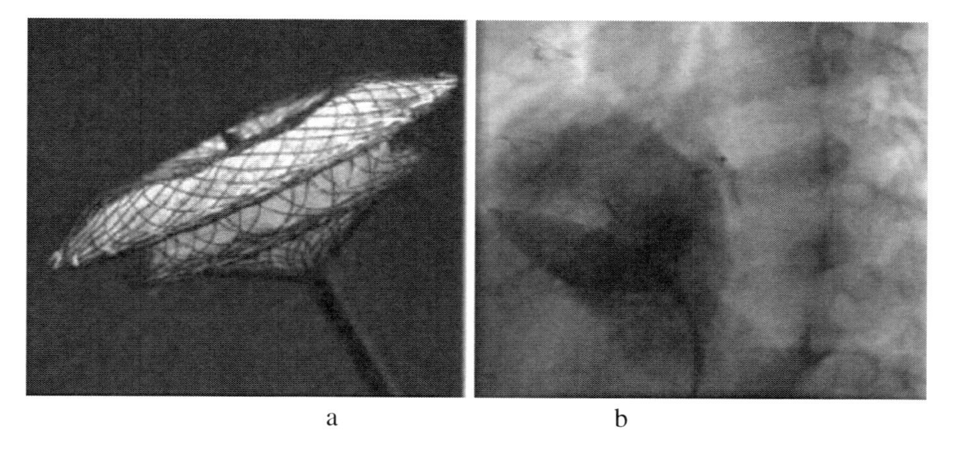

a b

Figure 8. A. Amplatzer Septal Occluder is a memory shaped nitinol device consisting of two expandable discs connected by a central waist. A polyester mesh inside the nitinol frame promotes closure. B. Right atrial angiogram shows no residual shunt across an atrial septal defect closed with an Amplatzer device. Note the ICE probe in the right atrium. (ICE = intracardiac echocardiography).

The device size is chosen to be equal to or within 1-2 mm of the "stop-flow" stretched ASD diameter, meaning that ASD's with a stretched diameter as large as 38 mm can theoretically be closed percutaneously. However, other considerations must be taken into account, including the total septal length to accommodate the device in smaller patients and the available rims around the defect. It is generally accepted that a rim is adequate if it measures more than 5 mm. Of all the available devices, the ASO is the most likely to allow closure of an ASD even when some of the rims are relatively deficient. Specifically, when the antero-superior (also known as retro-aortic) rim is deficient the device can obtain stable position by straddling the aorta. Deficiency of the postero-inferior rim is the most problematic for all devices and such ASD's typically require surgical closure [81]. Several techniques have been described to increase the success of ASD closure even in patients with very large or anatomically challenging ASD's, such as deployment of the left atrial disc within the left or right upper pulmonary vein followed by release of the waist and right atrial disc while simultaneously withdrawing the left atrial disc towards the septum [80]. Care must be taken not to injure the pulmonary vein with this maneuver. A balloon-assisted technique to support the left atrial disc of the Amplatzer device during deployment may also facilitate closure of large ASD's [83].

The Helex device, approved by the FDA in 2006, is a low profile double disc occluder made of polytetrafluoroethylene bonded to a nitinol wire frame (Figures 9A-E). It is available in 15-35 mm diameters in 5 mm increments. It is a relatively pliable, non-self centering device and can be delivered through a 9 French sheath. It has the additional safety feature of a retrieval cord that allows removal following implantation if the device does not appear to be adequately positioned or there is a significant residual shunt. The recommended device to stretched ASD diameter ratio is 2:1. This device is therefore not suitable for large ASD's with "stop-flow" diameter > about 18 mm. However, its lower profile makes it well suited for small to medium sized ASD's, particularly in young children.

The Amplatzer Multi-Fenestrated Septal Occluder ("Cribriform" Occluder) was also approved by the FDA in 2006. As its name implies, it is designed specifically for closure of multiple fenestrations in the atrial septum [84]. It is available in four sizes (18, 25, 30, and 35 mm). It is similar to the Amplatzer septal occluder described above, but the central connecting waist is narrow and the two discs are equal in size. This design allows the device to be placed through a relatively small hole while the discs cover other adjacent holes. The Helex device has also proven to be a good device for closure of fenestrated ASD's.

Multiple studies have documented excellent results for percutaneous ASD closure comparable to those of surgical closure [76,79,85-87]. Although a small amount of residual shunting can be present either through or around the device immediately after deployment the majority decrease in size or completely disappear on follow-up as endothelialization of the device occurs. Clinical success, typically defined as complete closure or small, hemodynamically insignificant residual shunts ≤ 3 mm in diameter, is achieved in about 98% of patients by 12 months of follow-up. Major complications such as device embolization, heart block, and cerebrovascular accidents are rare, occurring in less than 5% of patients in most large series.

An important, although exceedingly rare complication, is erosion of the atrial wall by the device resulting in pericardial effusion or frank tamponade. As of the time of this writing the incidence of this complication is approximately 0.1% for the Amplatzer device [88], while it has not been reported to occur with the Helex device. About 80% of these perforations occur in patients with deficient anterosuperior (aortic) rim and occur at the roof of the right or left atrium or in the atrial junction with the aorta resulting in either hemopericardium or aortic fistula. It has been speculated that oversizing the device may be causative, and the manufacturer advises against using a device that is ≥ 1.5 times the static (unstretched) diameter of the ASD. However, there is variability in the experience of the interventional community with regards to the mechanism of perforation. Some feel that undersizing the device such that it does not straddle the aorta carries a higher risk due to greater motion of the device relative to the heart and increased friction between the edge of the device and the atrial roof or aorta [89].

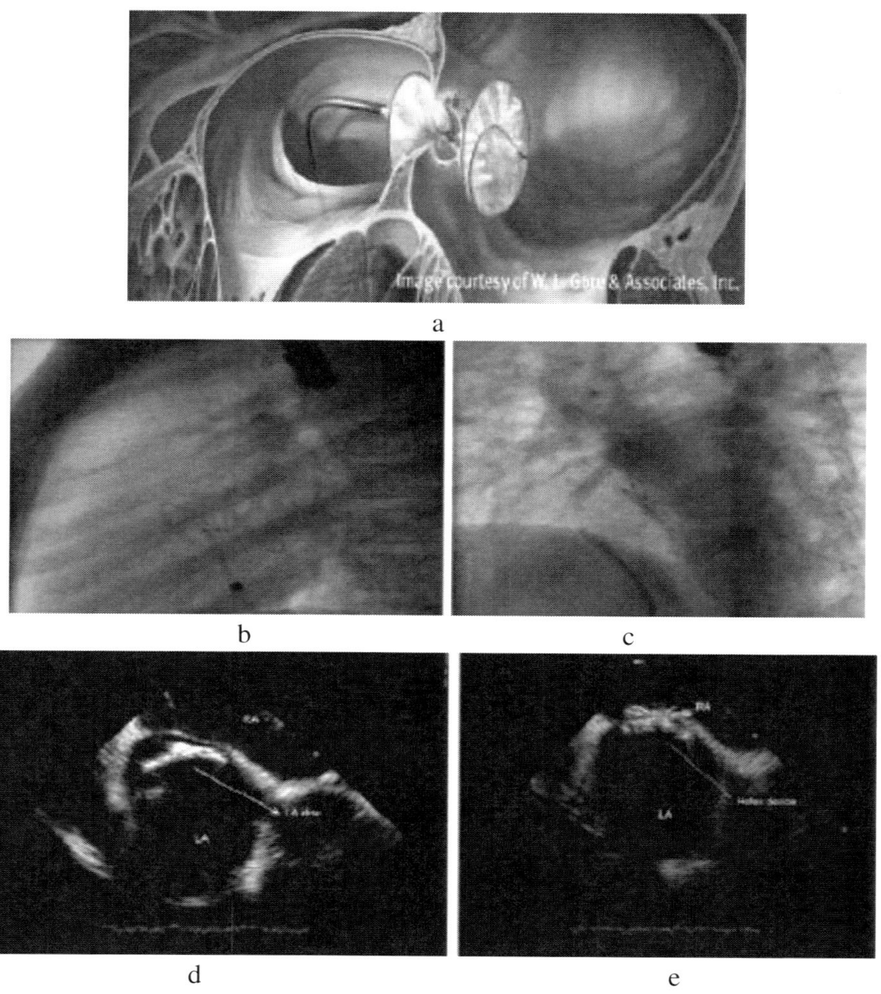

Image courtesy of W. L. Gore and Assosiates, Inc.

Figure 9. A. Helex septal occluder is a double disc occluder made of polytetrafluoroethylene bonded to a nitinol wire frame. B. Both discs of the Helex device have been formed. The device is still attached to the control catheter via a thread, allowing removal if needed because of malposition or significant residual shunting. C. Recirculation phase of a right atrial angiogram showing opacification of the left atrium and complete ASD closure with the Helex septal occluder. D. Intracardiac echocardiography guiding placement of a Helex device shows the left atrial disc approaching the septum. E. Intracardiac echocardiography shows the fully released Helex device. (LA = left atrium, RA = right atrium).

Improving the results of percutaneous ASD closure and minimizing complications continues to be an area of intense research. There is a great deal of interest in developing biodegradable devices in the hope of diminishing long-term complications and allowing future transseptal access for left heart catheterization or treatment of arrhythmias originating on the left side of the heart. A biodegradable device would decrease the risk of long-term thrombogenicity or any chronic tissue reaction to a foreign body. Most importantly, the long-term risk of erosion may be eliminated. The BioSTAR device (NMT Medical, Boston, MA) is a partially resorbable implant already in existence. It consists of a stainless steel double umbrella framework with a nitinol ring connecting the ends of the 8 arms. Two discs of acellular porcine collagen are attached to the wire frame and are completely absorbed within 6 months of implantation, leaving only the wire frame behind. A new generation of this device (BioTREK, NMT Medical) is undergoing preclinical trials at the time of this writing.

The BioSTAR device, which follows the family of clamshell-type devices (CardioSEAL, STARFlex; NMT Medical) is limited to small to medium-size ASD's and requires an adequate anterosuperior rim to avoid prolapse of the left atrial disc into the right atrium [90]. Further research should be aimed at creating more versatile biodegradable devices capable of closing larger defects.

Future advances in echocardiographic imaging of the atrial septum in the form of three-dimensional reconstruction would enhance the interventionalist's ability to deal with complex anatomy, such as multiple defects. It would also improve our understanding of the relationship between the device and adjacent cardiac structures. This technology has now been coupled with a transesophageal probe that allows on line display of the three-dimensional septal anatomy. Progress is still needed in improving temporal resolution. Improved training of echocardiographers in this area should allow more widespread clinical use of this valuable technology [91].

Percutaneous Ventricular Septal Defect Closure

Percutaneous closure of ventricular septal defects was first attempted in 1988 with the same class of clamshell-type devices originally intended for closure of atrial septal defects [92]. More recently Amplatzer devices specifically designed for VSD closure have become available. Despite this, a relatively small minority of ventricular septal defects are closed percutaneously at this time. The anatomy of the ventricular septum presents a greater challenge both in obtaining adequate positioning across the VSD for device delivery and in avoiding impingement of important structures such as the conduction system or the intracardiac valves. Unlike ASD's, large VSD's resulting in congestive heart failure and pulmonary hypertension require closure in infancy, therefore patient size is an important limiting factor to percutaneous VSD closure. Even in larger patients the procedure requires a high level of technical expertise and should only be performed in specialized centers with high volume and pediatric cardiothoracic surgical backup.

In a discussion of percutaneous VSD closure it should be emphasized that the natural history of ventricular septal defects needs to be well understood for adequate selection of patients [93]. Asymptomatic patients with moderate to large, but pressure restrictive VSD's can be observed even in the presence of significant left ventricular dilation early in life. The vast majority of these patients will experience spontaneous progressive decrease in left ventricular dimensions during childhood. There is no recommendation at this time to close ventricular septal defects only to decrease the small risk of bacterial endocarditis in the absence of sufficient evidence demonstrating that the risk of closure, whether surgical or transcatheter, is smaller than the risk of endocarditis [94].

One of the most important roles of transcatheter VSD devices is in closure of hemodynamically significant muscular ventricular septal defects, which are sometimes difficult for the surgeon to visualize or which may require ventriculotomy for the surgical approach (95). A small percentage of these patients have multiple muscular ventricle septal defects, or what is referred to as Swiss cheese septum. These patients can be extremely challenging for the surgeon, and although also extremely challenging for the interventional cardiologist, percutaneous closure of at least the most significant VSD's can sometimes be the best approach.

Although data remains relatively limited percutaneous closure of post-operative residual ventricular septal defects is a valuable option in sometimes very ill or complex patients (Figures 10A-D). These defects are often in areas difficult to reach by the surgeon, and require a second open heart procedure to close surgically at a time when myocardial function may be compromised by persistence of a hemodynamic burden following cardiopulmonary bypass [95,96].

In most circumstances deployment of a VSD device is best accomplished by creation of an arteriovenous wire loop. The VSD is crossed from the left ventricle with the aid of an angled catheter. An exchange length guidewire is advanced across the VSD into the right ventricle and into a branch pulmonary artery. The wire is snared in the pulmonary artery and exteriorized via either the right internal jugular or the femoral vein. If the VSD is located in the mid, posterior or apical septum the right internal jugular vein is chosen and for anterior muscular or perimembranous VSD's the femoral vein provides a better course. The delivery sheath is then advanced from the vein over the wire across the VSD and positioned in the left ventricle. The device is then deployed according to protocol for the specific device. Retrograde delivery can also be performed depending on the anatomy if the patient size allows placement of the required sheath in the artery. Delivery of the device should be guided by both fluoroscopy and transesophageal echocardiography.

Two devices are currently approved by the FDA for closure of muscular ventricular septal defects. The CardioSEAL device, from the family of clamshell-type devices, is a self expandable device with a double umbrella design. Each umbrella has four metal arms joined in the center and covered with a woven Dacron fabric. Knauth et al reported the largest series to date of VSD closure with this device [95]. More than 90% of the patients had either complete closure or significant decrease in the VSD size. Device arm fractures were observed in about 15% of devices, with a higher frequency in the larger devices, but were not associated with clinical problems. The complication rate was not insignificant, with approximately half the patients having a moderately serious or serious event. However, many of these included transient hemodynamic instability during these complex procedures with no permanent sequelae. Explantation of the device was necessary in 8% of the patients due to malposition, embolization or a significant residual shunt. There was one death directly related to device closure.

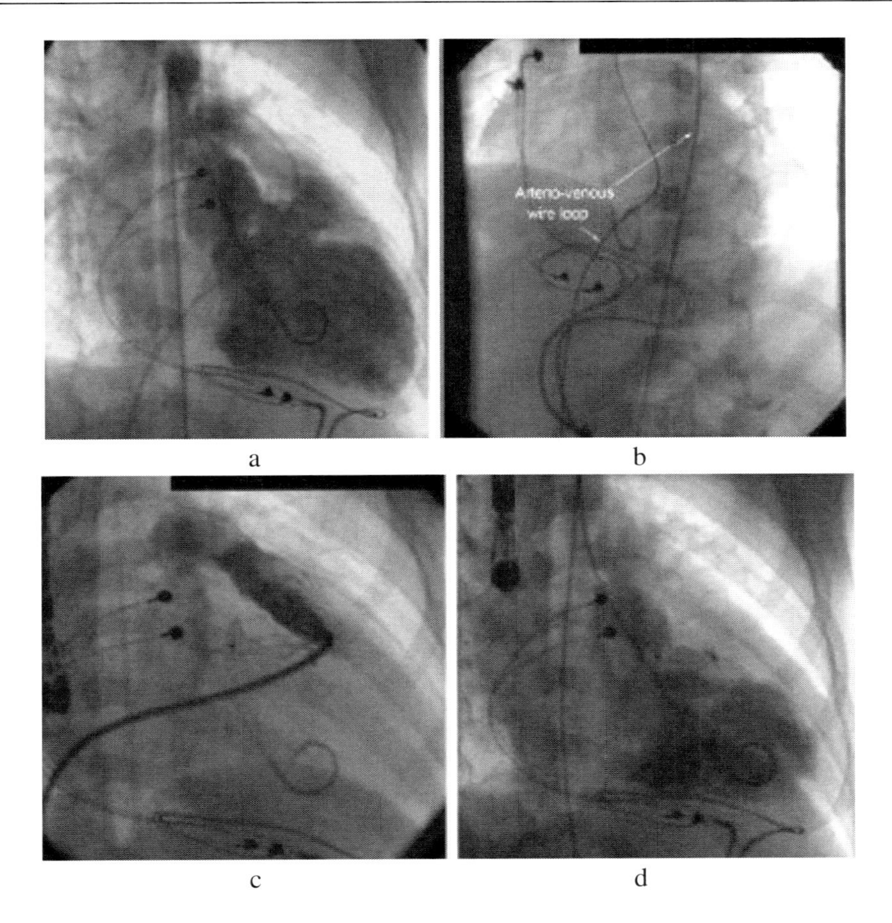

Figure 10. A. Left ventricular angiogram in a patient with congenitally corrected transposition status post double switch procedure shows a significant residual ventricular septal defect with opacification of the main and branch pulmonary arteries. B. Arteriovenous wire loop to allow insertion of the delivery sheath from the venous side across the VSD. The VSD was crossed retrograde from the left ventricle, the wire was snared in the main pulmonary artery and brought down to the IVC. C. Injection of contrast via the delivery sheath to check device position after deployment of the left ventricular disc while forming the right ventricular disc. D. Left ventricular angiogram after release of the VSD device shows no significant residual shunting. (IVC = inferior vena cava, VSD = ventricular septal defect).

The second approved device is the Amplatzer muscular VSD occluder. Similar to the Amplatzer ASD device, it is made of nitinol wire with a polyester mesh inside. The waist is 7 mm long to accommodate the ventricular musculature, and the left and right ventricular discs are 8 mm larger than the connecting waist. It is available in 4-16 mm diameter (which refers to the waist) and requires a 6-9 French sheath for delivery. The device is chosen to be 1-2 mm larger than the VSD diameter as measured by TEE at end diastole.

Excellent results have been reported by large centers with successful deployment in 85-95% of patients and closure rates of 90-95% [97,98]. Severe complications do occur in 7-10% of patients including device embolization, valve regurgitation, arrhythmias, perforation, hemolysis and complete heart block. Complications are associated with younger age and lower weight of the patient at the time of the procedure.

The Amplatzer perimembranous VSD device was developed more recently and has undergone initial clinical trials, but has not received FDA approval [99]. It is also made of nitinol wire with a polyester mesh inside to promote thrombosis. The device is asymmetric with the aortic end of the left ventricular disc only 0.5 mm larger than the waist in order to avoid impingement on the aortic valve, and the other end 5.5 mm larger than the waist. The right ventricular disc is 2 mm larger on either side. A 2 mm rim of tissue below the aortic valve is required to be able to implant this device. In the initial trials patients had to weigh at least 8 kg in order to be included. Although good closure rates have been reported by large centers [100] complete heart block occurs in about 5-6 % of patients in most series and is associated with younger age [99,100]. It can occur during or early after the procedure, but can also be a late event as long as 20 months post device deployment. Rare reports of late sudden death may be related to late onset of complete heart block. In some patients new aortic insufficiency has been observed after deployment of this device. Given these potential complications, particularly in younger patients, surgical closure of perimembranous VSD's remains the procedure of choice in the majority of patients at the time of this writing.

Outside the United States Nit-Occlud coils (pfm medical, Cologne, Germany), originally designed for closure of PDA's [101], have been used to close small to moderate muscular and perimembranous VSD's with good results [102]. The device is made of nitinol coils in a cone-in-cone configuration. A new, stiffer version of the device with the addition of polyester fibers covering its distal end is currently being evaluated in clinical trials for closure of muscular and perimembranous VSD's ≤ 7 mm in diameter. Patients must be older than 24 months for inclusion, and the rim of the VSD must be at least 3 mm from the aortic annulus. The deployment technique is as described above with formation of an arteriovenous loop and advancement of the delivery sheath from the venous side. The presence of some aneurysmal tissue at the VSD is advantageous for anchoring this device. Complete heart block associated with this device has not been described, but clinical experience is relatively limited.

Future advances in VSD closure techniques should focus on development of devices with less potential for impingement on intracardiac valves or on the conduction system. Improved visualization of the complex 3-dimensional anatomy of the ventricular septum and surrounding structures with such modalities as 3-dimensional TEE or MRI to guide the procedure would be a great advantage [103,104]. The development of MRI compatible catheters, wires and other interventional equipment is currently an area of ongoing research [105].

Pulmonary Artery Stenosis

Interventional work on the branch pulmonary arteries runs across the gamut of congenital cardiac lesions including tetralogy of Fallot, single ventricle, and syndromes associated with pulmonary artery stenosis such as William's syndrome (Figures 11 A, B). The ability of the interventional cardiologist to reach peripheral pulmonary arteries not accessible to the surgeon plays an important role in improving the outcome of either definitive treatment or palliation of multiple congenital cardiac lesions.

Balloon angioplasty is the transcatheter procedure of choice in small peripheral pulmonary arteries, or when patient size precludes stent implantation due to inability to expand a small stent to adult size. Exact definition of the anatomy by selective angiography in the stenotic branch is imperative. Access to a stenotic pulmonary artery branch can sometimes be challenging, particularly in patients with complex congenital heart disease and prior surgery involving the right ventricular outflow tract, systemic to pulmonary artery shunts, or surgically reconstructed pulmonary arteries. Angled catheters and high torque wires can be very useful. When dilation of multiple peripheral stenoses is to be performed, it is helpful to maintain a long sheath in the proximal pulmonary artery for post dilation angiography, and to ease multiple exchanges of wires and catheters.

The availability of high pressure balloons that can reach as high as 20-25 atmospheres, and more recently cutting balloons [106] has improved the results of pulmonary artery balloon angioplasty over the past decade, but a restenosis rate of about 30% is still observed [107,108]. For conventional (as opposed to "cutting") balloon angioplasty, generally a balloon is chosen that is 3 – 4 times the diameter of the stenotic segment and no more than 1.5 times the diameter of the distal vessel. A successful dilation has been arbitrarily defined as an increase of 50% or more in vessel diameter, or a decrease of more than 20% in systolic right ventricular to aortic pressure ratio [109]. Acute success with currently available balloons is around 70-80% [108]. Vessels resistant to high pressure balloon angioplasty may respond to either cutting balloon angioplasty alone, or cutting balloon angioplasty followed by high pressure ballooning. Cutting balloons, available in diameters from 4 to 8 mm, have three or four microsurgical blades with a cutting depth of 0.15 mm mounted longitudinally at 90 degree angles to the balloon. The cuts made by the blades create sites for the tear to enlarge when further dilated with a high pressure balloon. Success rates as high as 90% have been reported for resistant vessels treated with cutting balloons [110]. Repeat dilation for recurrent stenosis can be performed, and it is often possible to use larger balloons if there has been interim growth of the distal vessel. Although repeat procedures for peripheral pulmonary artery stenosis are not infrequent, ultimately significant gains in vessel diameter can be achieved.

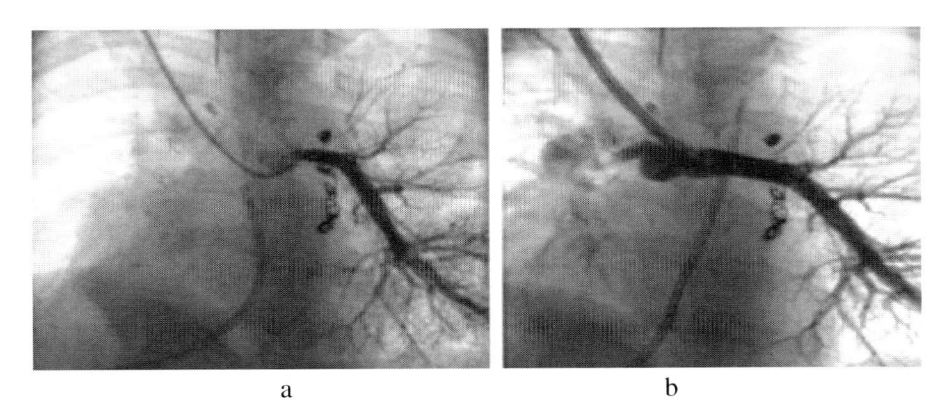

Figure 11. A. Left pulmonary angiogram in a patient with single ventricle status post cavopulmonary anastamosis shows significant proximal left pulmonary artery stenosis. Note the hemiazygous vein, which was decompressing the cavopulmonary anastamosis and causing increased cyanosis, was closed with coils. B. After stent placement in the left pulmonary artery there is marked improvement with no residual stenosis.

Excellent results have been reported for pulmonary artery stenting in larger patients [111,112]. The Palmaz Genesis series of unmounted balloon expandable stents have excellent radial strength and are typically flexible enough to maneuver the curves associated with delivery to a stenotic pulmonary artery branch. Another important feature of these stents is that they can be redilated to larger diameters (as large as18 mm) at subsequent procedures to accommodate for somatic growth. A long sheath must first be placed past the stenotic segment, and after manually mounting the stent on the balloon the balloon-stent assembly is advanced to the stenosis. The balloon diameter is chosen to match the distal vessel. Acute success is almost always achieved with stent implantation, with increases of more than 100% in stenosis diameter and greater than 75% reduction in pressure gradient [113-115]. In mid to long-term follow-up a small amount of neo-intimal proliferation about 1 mm in diameter is observed within the stent, but the incidence of significant restenosis has been found to be only 2 - 4% [112,115]. Stent redilation, most often performed to enlarge the stent to accommodate for somatic growth, has been shown to be effective [116].

Premounted stents can be delivered directly over a wire without placement of a long sheath across the stenosis, and require smaller sheaths than manually mounted stents. They would be a better option in smaller children, in whom placement of a large, long sheath in a pulmonary artery can be associated with hemodynamic instability, or may be prohibitive due to the required sheath size. However, these stents are limited in the final diameter that can be achieved at subsequent dilations, and therefore can result in a fixed stenosis with somatic growth. A new premounted stent, the Valeo Biliary Lifestent (Edward Lifesciences, Irvine, CA), may allow dilation to adult size pulmonary arteries, although dilation to such diameters (18-20 mm) has only been tested outside the body [117]. It has less radial strength than the Palmaz series, and an open cell design that may be subject to more intimal proliferation. Clinical experience with this stent is very limited at this time.

Significant complications of percutaneous treatment of pulmonary artery stenosis, reported to occur in 5-15% of patients in various series, include exanguination from vessel rupture, pulmonary hemorrhage, pulmonary edema from acute increase in perfusion, and pulmonary artery aneurysm. Limited follow-up on these aneurysms suggests that they tend to remain the same or decrease in size over time, and not cause significant clinical sequelae [109]. Of note, patients with isolated congenital pulmonary artery stenosis, such as seen in William's syndrome, are at higher risk of complications and derive less benefit both acutely and long-term from pulmonary artery intervention [115,118].

Improving balloon and stent technology, such as drug eluting balloons and stents, and importantly absorbable stents, may further improve the results of pulmonary artery interventions, particularly in smaller patients.

Pulmonary Vein Stenosis

Congenital pulmonary vein stenosis remains one of the most difficult problems faced by pediatric cardiologists, and mortality remains high regardless of treatment modality [119]. Although immediate improvement can be seen with balloon angioplasty, recurrent stenosis occurs in the vast majority of patients. Restenosis following stent implantation is nearly universal. Repeated interventions with increasingly larger balloons, or repeated dilation of stents to relatively large diameters may achieve reasonable mid-term results in some patients [120], but no series has reported acceptable long-term results. Maximizing the stent size has been associated with good outcomes in acquired post-ablation pulmonary vein stenosis [121], but the pathology underlying congenital pulmonary vein stenosis is different and the response is likely to be less favorable. Cutting balloon angioplasty has also been disappointing [122]. Drug eluting balloons or larger drug eluting stents may be beneficial, but are untested beyond very short follow-up [123,124].

Miscellaneous Procedures

Several other percutaneous pediatric interventions are commonly performed, sometimes adapting the same devices described above to other applications. Closure of abnormal vascular connections (aorto-pulmonary collaterals, veno-venous collaterals, coronary artery fistulae) can be accomplished with coils, PDA occluders, or vascular plugs also of the Amplatzer family (Figures 12 A,B). ASD devices are routinely used to close Fontan fenestrations. Perforation of the pulmonary valve plate in neonates with pulmonary atresia/intact ventricular septum and a tripartite right ventricle is currently achieved with radiofrequency energy (Figures 13A-C). New technologies on the horizon, such as ultrasound energy for tissue erosion [125,126] may increase the safety of the procedure. Such technology may also be applied to creation of a Fontan fenestration, or creation of an atrial communication in patients with left heart obstruction.

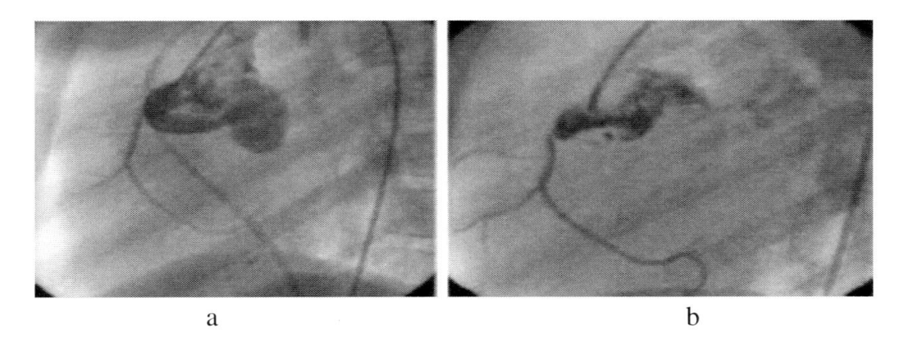

Figure 12. A. Selective angiogram in the right coronary artery shows a large proximal RCA fistula draining into the right atrium. Note the normal caliber RCA distal to the fistula. B. An ADO I has been used to close the fistula. (ADO = Amplatzer duct occluder, RCA = right coronary artery).

Fetal Interventions

Alteration in flow dynamics caused by anatomic obstruction during fetal cardiac development can lead to cardiac chamber hypoplasia, resulting in univentricular circulation. The concept of relieving such obstruction in fetal life emerged as an attempt to restore flow and theoretically allow continued growth of the cardiac structures in the hope of achieving a 2 ventricle heart. In a subset of fetuses with severe aortic stenosis detected in mid gestation, the left ventricular size is normal or enlarged, but progression to hypoplastic left heart syndrome (HLHS) has been documented. Percutaneous ultrasound guided dilation of the aortic valve in the fetus, first reported in 1991 [127], has met with mixed results. The largest series to date reported on 70 fetuses with critical aortic stenosis and evolving HLHS who underwent aortic valvuloplasty at a median gestational age of 23 weeks with 74% technical success [128]. Ultrasound guided percutaneous access to the fetal left ventricle was successful in ¾ of the patients, while a limited laparatomy was necessary in the rest. Although prenatal growth of the aortic and mitral valves was improved in comparison to a similar group of untreated fetuses, growth of the left ventricle was not improved. A biventricular outcome was ultimately achieved in 20 of the 70 patients. Complications, including fetal hemodynamic compromise and/or hemopericardium, occurred in 40% of the fetuses, and 13% did not reach viable term or preterm birth. Maternal complications were not described in this series, but appeared to be relatively minor in a prior report from the same center [129].

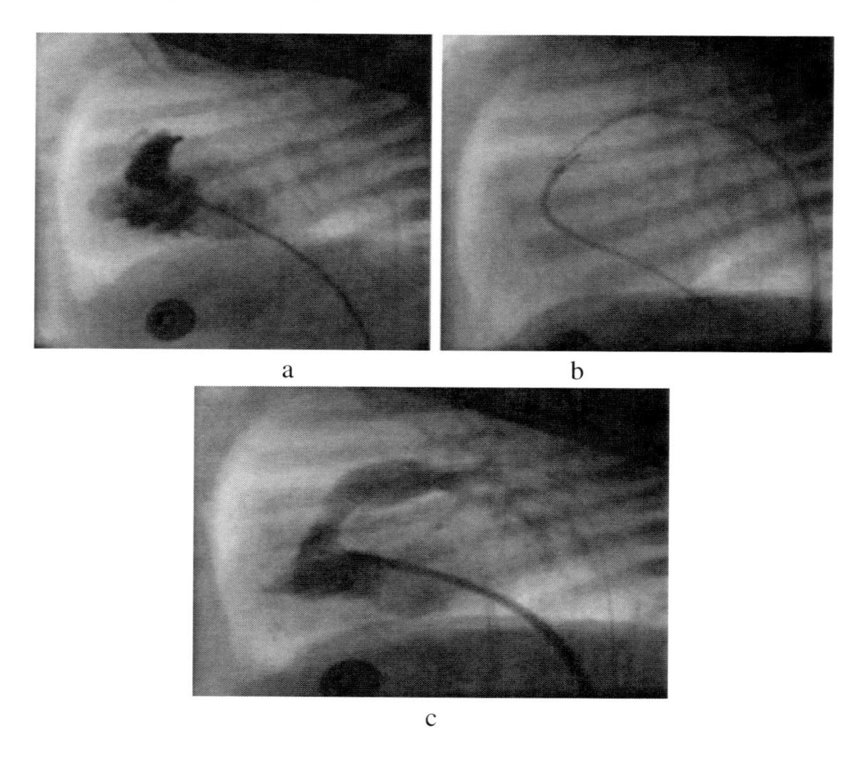

Figure 13. A. Right ventricular angiogram in a neonate with pulmonary atresia/intact ventricular septum shows the atretic pulmonary valve plate. B. A snare has been advanced retrograde from the aorta across the patent ductus and is positioned immediately above the pulmonary valve plate to guide perforation. The radiofrequency wire has crossed the atretic valve and is seen in the middle of the snare. C. Right ventricular angiogram after pulmonary valve perforation shows excellent flow into the main and branch pulmonary arteries.

Along similar lines fetal pulmonary valvuloplasty for critical pulmonary stenosis or atresia and intact ventricular septum, is aimed at improving growth of the right heart during gestation and increasing the likelihood of a biventricular outcome. First reported in 2002 in 2 fetuses with imminent hydrops [130], it has been performed in only a handful of patients to date. In a series of 10 fetuses with pulmonary atresia reported in 2009 [131], an important learning curve was demonstrated with technical failure in the first 4 attempts. In the 6 fetuses who underwent successful pulmonary valve perforation Z scores for the pulmonary valve (PV), tricuspid valve (TV) and RV increased following intervention, and 5 of the 6 have achieved (n = 4) or are on route to a biventricular circulation postnatally. Comparison with an untreated control group of fetuses with similar mid gestational Z scores for the right heart and univentricular outcome showed improved growth and higher late gestation Z scores for the PV, TV and RV in the treated group.

Fetal intervention has also been performed in fetuses with HLHS and highly restrictive or intact atrial septum, a condition requiring immediate transcatheter intervention shortly after birth and associated with a 50% mortality following the Norwood stage I operation even after successful opening of the atrial septum preoperatively. In the largest series to date, in utero atrial septoplasty was successfully performed in 19 of 21 fetuses, while 2 died within 24 hours of the procedure [132]. Of the 19 surviving fetuses 12 still required urgent left atrial decompression at birth, while 7 were stable with adequate oxygen saturations, and proceeded to stage I surgical palliation with no intervening procedure. Although survival remained poor at 42% in those requiring left atrial decompression at birth, it was significantly improved at 86% for the 7 patients who proceeded directly to a Norwood stage I procedure.

As can be gleamed from the above studies reporting data from essentially a single highly specialized center, results of fetal intervention have been mixed, and these procedures remain controversial [133]. The potential benefit of prenatal intervention must be weighed against current outcomes for surgical or hybrid procedures for the same lesions. For the future, technical advances in imaging and further miniaturization of the equipment could increase the success and safety of fetal intervention, or perhaps allow these procedures to be performed earlier in gestation when the likelihood of altering the natural history of these cardiac abnormalities may be greater. Less invasive techniques, such as controlled ultrasound tissue erosion, could decrease the morbidity of these procedures, but are experimental at this time [125,126,134]. For the moment, further advances in this field will hinge on improved selection criteria in order to optimize the risk/benefit ratio of these intrinsically high risk interventions.

Hybrid Procedures

Over the past decade intraprocedural collaboration between the interventional pediatric cardiologist and pediatric cardiac surgeon has made it possible to treat certain lesions when neither surgery nor catheter intervention alone can achieve the desired result. In some cases this collaboration has enabled less invasive treatment, or has decreased the number of procedures the patient is exposed to. Some congenital heart centers have a dedicated hybrid suite with all the equipment typically present in both a catheterization laboratory and an operating room, while in others portable equipment is brought into either the catheterization laboratory or the surgical suite depending on the procedure. Extensive use of imaging, including transesophageal echocardiography, fluoroscopy and angiography is often required.

One of the first applications of this technique was in patients with muscular VSD's, where surgical visualization in the arrested heart is sometimes difficult. Closure of muscular VSD's in small patients, or those with vascular access problems due to previous catheterizations, has been successfully performed via a perventricular approach on the beating heart [135-137]. Closing the VSD in this manner in patients with associated lesions requiring surgical intervention decreases time on cardiopulmonary bypass. Transesophageal echocardiography is used to guide the procedure. A subxiphoid minimally invasive incision is sufficient unless other lesions need to be treated surgically. A purse-string suture is placed by the surgeon and the right ventricle is punctured with a small needle, choosing the puncture site to give the most direct route to the VSD. A guidewire is then passed via the needle across the VSD, and a short sheath introduced into the LV cavity over the wire. Delivery of the device is then performed in the same manner as described in the previous section on percutaneous VSD closure. Similarly, peratrial closure of ASD's can be accomplished in infants with large, hemodynamically significant ASD's and significant lung disease rendering them poor surgical candidates, such as premature babies with bronchopulmonary dysplasia [138]. Another application of hybrid techniques, described as far back as 1993, includes intraoperative pulmonary artery stenting in patients with limited vascular access, or when the anatomy of the pulmonary vasculature precludes percutaneous access to the stenotic branch [139,140].

The most commonly performed hybrid procedure at this time is stenting of the patent ductus concomitant with pulmonary artery banding for neonates with hypoplastic left heart syndrome [140-143] (Figures 14A,B). Performed at a limited number of centers, the procedure is usually reserved for babies who are especially high risk for the Norwood stage I operation. These risks include prematurity, very low birth weight, shock on presentation, intracranial hemorrhage, or co-existing significant non-cardiac anomalies. The procedure is performed via a median sternotomy. Pulmonary artery bands are first applied by the surgeon, followed by stenting of the PDA by the cardiologist. Stenting is accomplished via a short sheath placed in the main pulmonary artery by the surgeon. A self-expanding, 8 mm diameter x 20 mm long stent is most often used. Stent placement is guided by hand injection angiograms through the sheath, which also allows visualization of the pulmonary artery bands.

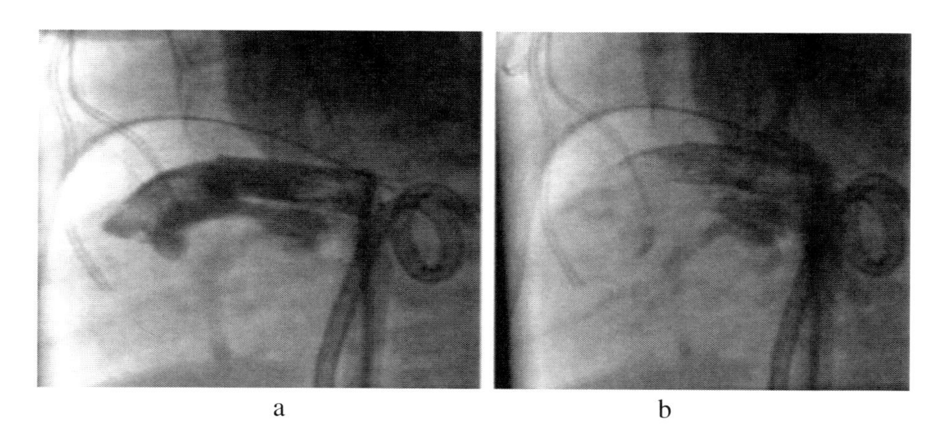

Figure 14. A. Angiogram in the descending aorta in the lateral projection in an infant with hypoplastic left heart syndrome status post hybrid procedure shows a stent maintaining the ductus arteriosus widely patent. Below the stent the banded branch pulmonary arteries are opacified. B. Same angiogram shows unobstructed retrograde flow across the stent into the native aortic arch. A pigtail catheter is draining a left pleural effusion.

A steep learning curve characterizes not just the technical aspects of the initial procedure, but also the meticulous care of these patients post procedure until they reach the next stage of their palliation [143]. The second stage consists of a complex surgical procedure including extensive aortic arch reconstruction, removal of the PDA stent and pulmonary artery bands, atrial septectomy and creation of a bidirectional cavopulmonary anastamosis. Data on mid to long-term outcome is still being gathered, but survival beyond stage 2 has been reported to be in the range of 70-80% in experienced centers, and appears comparable to the classic Norwood pathway in those series when similar patient groups are compared [144-146]. Percutaneous completion of the Fontan procedure has been performed in some of these patients by anastomosing the right pulmonary artery to the SVC and then excluding it by placing a pericardial patch within the right atrium at the time of the second stage operation. The patch can then be perforated at a later time and a covered stent deployed to direct flow from the IVC to the pulmonary arteries [147]. Other groups have also reported percutaneous Fontan completion, but the techniques are still being perfected [148,149].

Lastly, percutaneous valve implantation may be limited by the size of the required sheath, or by inability of these relatively stiff devices to negotiate the convoluted course from the access site to the outflow tract. Direct access to the heart provided by the surgeon is sometimes the best alternative [150]. In the future, development of robotic or thoracoscopic techniques may facilitate these and other intracardiac procedures. Ongoing collaboration to bring together the expertise of multiple specialists, and changes in training philosophy to provide the necessary exposure across the disciplines, will take pediatric intervention to a new level for the benefit of our patients.

References

[1] Rashkind, W. J., Miller, W. W. Creation of an atrial septal defect without thoracotomy. A palliative approach to complete transposition of the great arteries. *JAMA* 1966 Jun. 13;196(11):991-992.

[2] Porstmann, W., Wierny, L., Warnke, H. The closure of the patent ductus arteriosus without thoractomy. (preliminary report)]. *Thoraxchir. Vask. Chir.* 1967 Apr.;15 (2):199-203.

[3] King, T. D., Thompson, S. L., Steiner, C., Mills, N. L. Secundum atrial septal defect. Nonoperative closure during cardiac catheterization. *JAMA* 1976 Jun. 7;235(23):2506-2509.

[4] Kan, J. S., White, R. I.,Jr, Mitchell, S. E., Gardner, T. J. Percutaneous balloon valvuloplasty: a new method for treating congenital pulmonary valve stenosis. *N Engl. J. Med.* 1982 Aug. 26;307(9):540-542.

[5] Bonhoeffer, P., Boudjemline, Y., Saliba, Z., Merckx, J., Aggoun, Y., Bonnet, D. et al. Percutaneous replacement of pulmonary valve in a right-ventricle to pulmonary-artery prosthetic conduit with valve dysfunction. *Lancet* 2000 Oct. 21;356(9239):1403-1405.

[6] Rashkind, W. J., Mullins, C. E., Hellenbrand, W. E., Tait, M. A. Nonsurgical closure of patent ductus arteriosus: clinical application of the Rashkind PDA Occluder System. *Circulation* 1987 Mar.;75(3):583-592.

[7] Cambier, P. A., Kirby, W. C., Wortham, D. C., Moore, J. W. Percutaneous closure of the small (less than 2.5 mm) patent ductus arteriosus using coil embolization. *Am. J. Cardiol.* 1992 Mar. 15;69(8):815-816.

[8] Pass, R. H., Hijazi, Z., Hsu, D. T., Lewis, V., Hellenbrand, W. E. Multicenter USA Amplatzer patent ductus arteriosus occlusion device trial: initial and one-year results. *J. Am. Coll. Cardiol.* 2004 Aug. 4;44(3):513-519.

[9] Krichenko, A., Benson, L. N., Burrows, P., Moes, C. A., McLaughlin, P., Freedom, R. M. Angiographic classification of the isolated, persistently patent ductus arteriosus and implications for percutaneous catheter occlusion. *Am. J. Cardiol.* 1989 Apr. 1;63(12):877-880.

[10] Thanopoulos, B., Eleftherakis, N., Tzannos, K., Stefanadis, C. Transcatheter closure of the patent ductus arteriosus using the new Amplatzer duct occluder: initial clinical applications in children. *Am. Heart J.* 2008 Nov.;156(5):917.e1-917.e6.

[11] Bhole, V., Miller, P., Mehta, C., Stumper, O., Reinhardt, Z., De Giovanni, J. V. Clinical evaluation of the new Amplatzer duct occluder II for patent arterial duct occlusion. *Catheter Cardiovasc. Interv.* 2009 Nov. 1;74(5):762-769.

[12] Forsey, J., Kenny, D., Morgan, G., Hayes, A., Turner, M., Tometzki, A. et al. Early clinical experience with the new Amplatzer Ductal Occluder II for closure of the persistent arterial duct. *Catheter Cardiovasc. Interv.* 2009 Oct. 1;74(4):615-623.

[13] Thanopoulos, B. V., Eleftherakis, N., Tzannos, K., Stefanadis, C., Giannopoulos, A. Further experience with catheter closure of patent ductus arteriosus using the new Amplatzer duct occluder in children. *Am. J. Cardiol.* 2010 Apr. 1;105(7):1005-1009.

[14] Stanger, P., Cassidy, S. C., Girod, D. A., Kan, J. S., Lababidi, Z., Shapiro, S. R. Balloon pulmonary valvuloplasty: results of the Valvuloplasty and Angioplasty of Congenital Anomalies Registry. *Am. J. Cardiol.* 1990 Mar. 15;65(11):775-783.

[15] McCrindle, B. W., Kan, J. S. Long-term results after balloon pulmonary valvuloplasty. *Circulation* 1991 Jun.;83(6):1915-1922.

[16] O'Connor, B. K., Beekman, R. H., Lindauer, A., Rocchini, A. Intermediate-term outcome after pulmonary balloon valvuloplasty: comparison with a matched surgical control group. *J. Am. Coll. Cardiol.* 1992 Jul.;20(1):169-173.

[17] Masura, J., Burch, M., Deanfield, J. E., Sullivan, I. D. Five-year follow-up after balloon pulmonary valvuloplasty. *J. Am. Coll. Cardiol.* 1993 Jan.;21(1):132-136.

[18] McCrindle, B. W. Independent predictors of long-term results after balloon pulmonary valvuloplasty. Valvuloplasty and Angioplasty of Congenital Anomalies (VACA) Registry Investigators. *Circulation* 1994 Apr.;89(4):1751-1759.

[19] Garty, Y., Veldtman, G., Lee, K., Benson, L. Late outcomes after pulmonary valve balloon dilatation in neonates, infants and children. *J. Invasive Cardiol.* 2005 Jun.;17(6):318-322.

[20] Tynan, M., Jones, O., Joseph, M. C., Deverall, P. B., Yates, A. K. Relief of pulmonary valve stenosis in first week of life by percutaneous balloon valvuloplasty. *Lancet* 1984 Feb. 4;1(8371):273.

[21] Latson, L., Cheatham, J., Froemming, S., Kugler, J. Transductal guidewire "rail" for balloon valvuloplasty in neonates with isolated critical pulmonary valve stenosis or atresia. *Am. J. Cardiol.* 1994 Apr. 1;73(9):713-714.

[22] Colli, A. M., Perry, S. B., Lock, J. E., Keane, J. F. Balloon dilation of critical valvar pulmonary stenosis in the first month of life. *Cathet. Cardiovasc. Diagn.* 1995 Jan.;34(1):23-28.

[23] Gournay, V., Piechaud, J. F., Delogu, A., Sidi, D., Kachaner, J. Balloon valvotomy for critical stenosis or atresia of pulmonary valve in newborns. *J. Am. Coll. Cardiol.* 1995 Dec.;26(7):1725-1731.

[24] Tabatabaei, H., Boutin, C., Nykanen, D. G., Freedom, R. M., Benson, L. N. Morphologic and hemodynamic consequences after percutaneous balloon valvotomy for neonatal pulmonary stenosis: medium-term follow-up. *J. Am. Coll. Cardiol.* 1996 Feb.;27(2):473-478.

[25] Weber, H. S. Initial and late results after catheter intervention for neonatal critical pulmonary valve stenosis and atresia with intact ventricular septum: a technique in continual evolution. *Catheter Cardiovasc. Interv.* 2002 Jul.;56(3):394-399.

[26] Karagoz, T., Asoh, K., Hickey, E., Chaturvedi, R., Lee, K. J., Nykanen, D. et al. Balloon dilation of pulmonary valve stenosis in infants less than 3 kg: a 20-year experience. *Catheter Cardiovasc. Interv.* 2009 Nov. 1;74(5):753-761.

[27] Harrild, D. M., Powell, A. J., Tran, T. X., Geva, T., Lock, J. E., Rhodes, J. et al. Long-term pulmonary regurgitation following balloon valvuloplasty for pulmonary stenosis risk factors and relationship to exercise capacity and ventricular volume and function. *J. Am. Coll. Cardiol.* 2010 Mar. 9;55(10):1041-1047.

[28] Fedderly, R. T., Lloyd, T. R., Mendelsohn, A. M., Beekman, R. H. Determinants of successful balloon valvotomy in infants with critical pulmonary stenosis or membranous pulmonary atresia with intact ventricular septum. *J. Am. Coll. Cardiol.* 1995 Feb.;25(2):460-465.

[29] Latson, L. A. Critical pulmonary stenosis. *J. Interv. Cardiol.* 2001 Jun.;14(3):345-350.

[30] Rao, P. S. Percutaneous balloon pulmonary valvuloplasty: state of the art. *Catheter Cardiovasc. Interv.* 2007 Apr. 1;69(5):747-763.

[31] Peng, L. F., McElhinney, D. B., Nugent, A. W., Powell, A. J., Marshall, A. C., Bacha, E. A., et al. Endovascular stenting of obstructed right ventricle-to-pulmonary artery conduits: a 15-year experience. *Circulation* 2006 Jun. 6;113(22):2598-2605.

[32] Lurz, P., Nordmeyer, J., Muthurangu, V., Khambadkone, S., Derrick, G., Yates, R. et al. Comparison of bare metal stenting and percutaneous pulmonary valve implantation for treatment of right ventricular outflow tract obstruction: use of an x-ray/magnetic resonance hybrid laboratory for acute physiological assessment. *Circulation* 2009 Jun. 16;119(23):2995-3001.

[33] Asoh, K., Walsh, M., Hickey, E., Nagiub, M., Chaturvedi, R., Lee, K. J. et al. Percutaneous pulmonary valve implantation within bioprosthetic valves. *Eur. Heart. J.* 2010 Jun.;31(11):1404-1409.

[34] Nordmeyer, J., Lurz, P., Tsang, V. T., Coats, L., Walker, F., Taylor, A. M. et al. Effective transcatheter valve implantation after pulmonary homograft failure: a new perspective on the Ross operation. *J. Thorac. Cardiovasc. Surg.* 2009 Jul.;138(1):84-88.

[35] Lurz, P., Coats, L., Khambadkone, S., Nordmeyer, J., Boudjemline, Y., Schievano, S. et al. Percutaneous pulmonary valve implantation: impact of evolving technology and learning curve on clinical outcome. *Circulation* 2008 Apr. 15;117(15):1964-1972.

[36] Kostolny, M., Tsang, V., Nordmeyer, J., Van Doorn, C., Frigiola, A., Khambadkone, S. et al. Rescue surgery following percutaneous pulmonary valve implantation. *Eur. J. Cardiothorac. Surg.* 2008 Apr.;33(4):607-612.

[37] Nordmeyer, J., Khambadkone, S., Coats, L., Schievano, S., Lurz, P., Parenzan, G., et al. Risk stratification, systematic classification, and anticipatory management strategies for

stent fracture after percutaneous pulmonary valve implantation. *Circulation* 2007 Mar. 20;115(11):1392-1397.

[38] Schievano, S., Taylor, A. M., Capelli, C., Lurz, P., Nordmeyer, J., Migliavacca, F. et al. Patient specific finite element analysis results in more accurate prediction of stent fractures: application to percutaneous pulmonary valve implantation. *J. Biomech.* 2010 Mar. 3;43(4):687-693.

[39] Lurz, P., Gaudin, R., Taylor, A. M., Bonhoeffer, P. Percutaneous pulmonary valve implantation. *Semin. Thorac. Cardiovasc. Surg. Pediatr. Card. Surg. Annu.* 2009:112-117.

[40] Nordmeyer, J., Lurz, P., Khambadkone, S., Schievano, S., Jones, A., McElhinney, D. B. et al. Pre-stenting with a bare metal stent before percutaneous pulmonary valve implantation: acute and 1-year outcomes. *Heart* 2011 Jan.;97(2):118-123.

[41] Nordmeyer, J., Coats, L., Lurz, P., Lee, T. Y., Derrick, G., Rees, P. et al. Percutaneous pulmonary valve-in-valve implantation: a successful treatment concept for early device failure. *Eur. Heart J.* 2008 Mar.;29(6):810-815.

[42] Webb, J. G., Pasupati, S., Humphries, K., Thompson, C., Altwegg, L., Moss, R. et al. Percutaneous transarterial aortic valve replacement in selected high-risk patients with aortic stenosis. *Circulation* 2007 Aug. 14;116(7):755-763.

[43] Boone, R. H., Webb, J. G., Horlick, E., Benson, L., Cao, Q. L., Nadeem, N. et al. Transcatheter pulmonary valve implantation using the Edwards SAPIEN transcatheter heart valve. *Catheter Cardiovasc. Interv.* 2010 Feb. 1;75(2):286-294.

[44] Mollet, A., Basquin, A., Stos, B., Boudjemline, Y. Off-pump replacement of the pulmonary valve in large right ventricular outflow tracts: a transcatheter approach using an intravascular infundibulum reducer. *Pediatr. Res.* 2007 Oct.;62(4):428-433.

[45] Capelli, C., Taylor, A. M., Migliavacca, F., Bonhoeffer, P., Schievano, S. Patient-specific reconstructed anatomies and computer simulations are fundamental for selecting medical device treatment: application to a new percutaneous pulmonary valve. Philos. Transact. *A Math. Phys. Eng. Sci.* 2010 Jun. 28;368(1921):3027-3038.

[46] Lababidi, Z., Wu, J. R., Walls, J. T. Percutaneous balloon aortic valvuloplasty: results in 23 patients. *Am. J. Cardiol.* 1984 Jan. 1;53(1):194-197.

[47] Ewert, P., Bertram, H., Breuer, J., Dahnert, I., Dittrich, S., Eicken, A. et al. Balloon valvuloplasty in the treatment of congenital aortic valve stenosis - A retrospective multicenter survey of more than 1000 patients. *Int. J. Cardiol.* 2010 Feb. 10.

[48] Fratz, S., Gildein, H. P., Balling, G., Sebening, W., Genz, T., Eicken, A. et al. Aortic valvuloplasty in pediatric patients substantially postpones the need for aortic valve surgery: a single-center experience of 188 patients after up to 17.5 years of follow-up. *Circulation* 2008 Mar. 4;117(9):1201-1206.

[49] McCrindle, B. W. Independent predictors of immediate results of percutaneous balloon aortic valvotomy in children. Valvuloplasty and Angioplasty of Congenital Anomalies (VACA) Registry Investigators. *Am. J. Cardiol.* 1996 Feb. 1;77(4):286-293.

[50] Moore, P., Egito, E., Mowrey, H., Perry, S. B., Lock, J. E., Keane, J. F. Midterm results of balloon dilation of congenital aortic stenosis: predictors of success. *J. Am. Coll. Cardiol.* 1996 Apr.;27(5):1257-1263.

[51] Daehnert, I., Rotzsch, C., Wiener, M., Schneider, P. Rapid right ventricular pacing is an alternative to adenosine in catheter interventional procedures for congenital heart disease. *Heart* 2004 Sep.;90(9):1047-1050.

[52] Mehta, C., Desai, T., Shebani, S., Stickley, J., De Giovanni, J. Rapid ventricular pacing for catheter interventions in congenital aortic stenosis and coarctation: effectiveness, safety, and rate titration for optimal results. *J. Interv. Cardiol.* 2010 Feb.;23(1):7-13.

[53] McCrindle, B. W., Blackstone, E. H., Williams, W. G., Sittiwangkul, R., Spray, T. L., Azakie, A. et al. Are outcomes of surgical versus transcatheter balloon valvotomy equivalent in neonatal critical aortic stenosis? *Circulation* 2001 Sep. 18;104(12 Suppl. 1):I152-8.

[54] Justo, R. N., McCrindle, B. W., Benson, L. N., Williams, W. G., Freedom, R. M., Smallhorn, J. F. Aortic valve regurgitation after surgical versus percutaneous balloon valvotomy for congenital aortic valve stenosis. *Am. J. Cardiol.* 1996 Jun. 15;77(15):1332-1338.

[55] Kuhn, M. A., Latson, L. A., Cheatham, J. P., Fletcher, S. E., Foreman, C. Management of pediatric patients with isolated valvar aortic stenosis by balloon aortic valvuloplasty. *Cathet. Cardiovasc. Diagn.* 1996 Sep.;39(1):55-61.

[56] McElhinney, D. B., Lock, J. E., Keane, J. F., Moran, A. M., Colan, S. D. Left heart growth, function, and reintervention after balloon aortic valvuloplasty for neonatal aortic stenosis. *Circulation* 2005 Feb. 1;111(4):451-458.

[57] Leon, M. B., Smith, C. R., Mack, M., Miller, D. C., Moses, J. W., Svensson, L. G. et al. Transcatheter aortic-valve implantation for aortic stenosis in patients who cannot undergo surgery. *N Engl. J. Med.* 2010 Oct. 21;363(17):1597-1607.

[58] Singer, M. I., Rowen, M., Dorsey, T. J. Transluminal aortic balloon angioplasty for coarctation of the aorta in the newborn. *Am. Heart J.* 1982 Jan.;103(1):131-132.

[59] Galal, M. O., Schmaltz, A. A., Joufan, M., Benson, L., Samatou, L., Halees, Z. Balloon dilation of native aortic coarctation in infancy. *Z Kardiol.* 2003 Sep.;92(9):735-741.

[60] Fletcher, S. E., Nihill, M. R., Grifka, R. G., O'Laughlin, M. P., Mullins, C. E. Balloon angioplasty of native coarctation of the aorta: midterm follow-up and prognostic factors. *J. Am. Coll. Cardiol.* 1995 Mar. 1;25(3):730-734.

[61] Rodes-Cabau, J., Miro, J., Dancea, A., Ibrahim, R., Piette, E., Lapierre, C. et al. Comparison of surgical and transcatheter treatment for native coarctation of the aorta in patients > or = 1 year old. The Quebec Native Coarctation of the Aorta study. *Am. Heart J.* 2007 Jul.;154(1):186-192.

[62] Cowley, C. G., Orsmond, G. S., Feola, P., McQuillan, L., Shaddy, R. E. Long-term, randomized comparison of balloon angioplasty and surgery for native coarctation of the aorta in childhood. *Circulation* 2005 Jun. 28;111(25):3453-3456.

[63] Morrow, W. R., Smith, V. C., Ehler, W. J., VanDellen, A. F., Mullins, C. E. Balloon angioplasty with stent implantation in experimental coarctation of the aorta. *Circulation* 1994 Jun.;89(6):2677-2683.

[64] Pedulla, D. M., Grifka, R. G., Mullins, C. E., Allen, D. Endovascular stent implantation for severe recoarctation of the aorta: case report with angiographic and 18-month clinical follow-up. *Cathet. Cardiovasc. Diagn.* 1997 Mar.;40(3):311-314.

[65] Forbes, T. J., Moore, P., Pedra, C. A., Zahn, E. M., Nykanen, D., Amin, Z. et al. Intermediate follow-up following intravascular stenting for treatment of coarctation of the aorta. *Catheter Cardiovasc. Interv.* 2007 Oct. 1;70(4):569-577.

[66] Forbes, T. J., Garekar, S., Amin, Z., Zahn, E. M., Nykanen, D., Moore, P. et al. Procedural results and acute complications in stenting native and recurrent coarctation

of the aorta in patients over 4 years of age: a multi-institutional study. *Catheter Cardiovasc. Interv.* 2007 Aug. 1;70(2):276-285.

[67] Hamdan, M. A., Maheshwari, S., Fahey, J. T., Hellenbrand, W. E. Endovascular stents for coarctation of the aorta: initial results and intermediate-term follow-up. *J. Am. Coll. Cardiol.* 2001 Nov. 1;38(5):1518-1523.

[68] Harrison, D. A., McLaughlin, P. R., Lazzam, C., Connelly, M., Benson, L. N. Endovascular stents in the management of coarctation of the aorta in the adolescent and adult: one year follow up. *Heart* 2001 May;85(5):561-566.

[69] Rosenthal, E., Qureshi, S. A., Tynan, M. Stent implantation for aortic recoarctation. *Am. Heart J.* 1995 Jun.;129(6):1220-1221.

[70] Suarez de Lezo, J., Pan, M., Romero, M., Segura, J., Pavlovic, D., Ojeda, S. et al. Percutaneous interventions on severe coarctation of the aorta: a 21-year experience. *Pediatr. Cardiol.* 2005 Mar.-Apr.;26(2):176-189.

[71] Qureshi, A. M., McElhinney, D. B., Lock, J. E., Landzberg, M. J., Lang, P., Marshall, A. C. Acute and intermediate outcomes, and evaluation of injury to the aortic wall, as based on 15 years experience of implanting stents to treat aortic coarctation. *Cardiol. Young* 2007 Jun.;17(3):307-318.

[72] Peters, B., Ewert, P., Berger, F. The role of stents in the treatment of congenital heart disease: Current status and future perspectives. *Ann. Pediatr. Cardiol.* 2009 Jan.;2(1):3-23.

[73] Schranz, D., Zartner, P., Michel-Behnke, I., Akinturk, H. Bioabsorbable metal stents for percutaneous treatment of critical recoarctation of the aorta in a newborn. *Catheter Cardiovasc. Interv.* 2006 May;67(5):671-673.

[74] Ewert, P., Riesenkampff, E., Neuss, M., Kretschmar, O., Nagdyman, N., Lange, P. E. Novel growth stent for the permanent treatment of vessel stenosis in growing children: an experimental study. *Catheter Cardiovasc. Interv.* 2004 Aug.;62(4):506-510.

[75] Ewert, P., Peters, B., Nagdyman, N., Miera, O., Kuhne, T., Berger, F. Early and mid-term results with the Growth Stent--a possible concept for transcatheter treatment of aortic coarctation from infancy to adulthood by stent implantation? *Catheter Cardiovasc. Interv.* 2008 Jan. 1;71(1):120-126.

[76] Butera, G., Romagnoli, E., Carminati, M., Chessa, M., Piazza, L., Negura, D. et al. Treatment of isolated secundum atrial septal defects: impact of age and defect morphology in 1,013 consecutive patients. *Am. Heart J.* 2008 Oct.;156(4):706-712.

[77] Hijazi, Z., Wang, Z., Cao, Q., Koenig, P., Waight, D., Lang, R. Transcatheter closure of atrial septal defects and patent foramen ovale under intracardiac echocardiographic guidance: feasibility and comparison with transesophageal echocardiography. *Catheter Cardiovasc. Interv.* 2001 Feb.;52(2):194-199.

[78] Carlson, K. M., Justino, H., O'Brien, R. E., Dimas, V. V., Leonard, G. T.,Jr, Pignatelli, R. H. et al. Transcatheter atrial septal defect closure: modified balloon sizing technique to avoid overstretching the defect and oversizing the Amplatzer septal occluder. *Catheter Cardiovasc. Interv.* 2005 Nov.;66(3):390-396.

[79] Du, Z. D., Hijazi, Z. M., Kleinman, C. S., Silverman, N. H., Larntz, K., Amplatzer Investigators. Comparison between transcatheter and surgical closure of secundum atrial septal defect in children and adults: results of a multicenter nonrandomized trial. *J. Am. Coll. Cardiol.* 2002 Jun. 5;39(11):1836-1844.

[80] Knirsch, W., Dodge-Khatami, A., Valsangiacomo-Buechel, E., Weiss, M., Berger, F. Challenges encountered during closure of atrial septal defects. *Pediatr. Cardiol.* 2005 Mar.-Apr.;26(2):147-153.

[81] Mathewson, J. W., Bichell, D., Rothman, A., Ing, F. F. Absent posteroinferior and anterosuperior atrial septal defect rims: Factors affecting nonsurgical closure of large secundum defects using the Amplatzer occluder. *J. Am. Soc. Echocardiogr.* 2004 Jan.;17(1):62-69.

[82] Kutty, S., Asnes, J. D., Srinath, G., Preminger, T. J., Prieto, L. R., Latson, L. A. Use of a straight, side-hole delivery sheath for improved delivery of Amplatzer ASD occluder. *Catheter Cardiovasc. Interv.* 2007 Jan.;69(1):15-20.

[83] Dalvi, B. V., Pinto, R. J., Gupta, A. New technique for device closure of large atrial septal defects. *Catheter Cardiovasc. Interv.* 2005 Jan.;64(1):102-107.

[84] Numan, M., El Sisi, A., Tofeig, M., Gendi, S., Tohami, T., El-Said, H. G. Cribriform amplatzer device closure of fenestrated atrial septal defects: feasibility and technical aspects. *Pediatr. Cardiol.* 2008 May.;29(3):530-535.

[85] Jones, T. K., Latson, L. A., Zahn, E., Fleishman, C. E., Jacobson, J., Vincent, R. et al. Results of the U.S. multicenter pivotal study of the HELEX septal occluder for percutaneous closure of secundum atrial septal defects. *J. Am. Coll. Cardiol.* 2007 Jun. 5;49(22):2215-2221.

[86] Wilson, N. J., Smith, J., Prommete, B., O'Donnell, C., Gentles, T. L., Ruygrok, P. N. Transcatheter closure of secundum atrial septal defects with the Amplatzer septal occluder in adults and children-follow-up closure rates, degree of mitral regurgitation and evolution of arrhythmias. *Heart Lung Circ.* 2008 Aug.;17(4):318-324.

[87] Knepp, M. D., Rocchini, A. P., Lloyd, T. R., Aiyagari, R. M. Long-term follow up of secundum atrial septal defect closure with the Amplatzer septal occluder. *Congenit. Heart Dis.* 2010 Jan;5(1):32-37.

[88] Amin, Z., Hijazi, Z. M., Bass, J. L., Cheatham, J. P., Hellenbrand, W. E., Kleinman, C. S. Erosion of Amplatzer septal occluder device after closure of secundum atrial septal defects: review of registry of complications and recommendations to minimize future risk. *Catheter Cardiovasc. Interv.* 2004 Dec.;63(4):496-502.

[89] El-Said, H. G., Moore, J. W. Erosion by the Amplatzer septal occluder: experienced operator opinions at odds with manufacturer recommendations? *Catheter Cardiovasc. Interv.* 2009 Jun. 1;73(7):925-930.

[90] Morgan, G., Lee, K. J., Chaturvedi, R., Benson, L. A biodegradable device (BioSTAR) for atrial septal defect closure in children. *Catheter Cardiovasc. Interv.* 2010 Aug. 1;76(2):241-245.

[91] Perk, G., Lang, R. M., Garcia-Fernandez, M. A., Lodato, J., Sugeng, L., Lopez, J. et al. Use of real time three-dimensional transesophageal echocardiography in intracardiac catheter based interventions. *J. Am. Soc. Echocardiogr.* 2009 Aug.;22(8):865-882.

[92] Lock, J. E., Block, P. C., McKay, R. G., Baim, D. S., Keane, J. F. Transcatheter closure of ventricular septal defects. *Circulation* 1988 Aug.;78(2):361-368.

[93] Kleinman, C. S., Tabibian, M., Starc, T. J., Hsu, D. T., Gersony, W. M. Spontaneous regression of left ventricular dilation in children with restrictive ventricular septal defects. *J. Pediatr.* 2007 Jun.;150(6):583-586.

[94] Gersony, W. M., Hayes, C. J., Driscoll, D. J., Keane, J. F., Kidd, L., O'Fallon, W. M. et al. Bacterial endocarditis in patients with aortic stenosis, pulmonary stenosis, or ventricular septal defect. *Circulation* 1993 Feb.;87(2 Suppl.):I121-6.

[95] Knauth, A. L., Lock, J. E., Perry, S. B., McElhinney, D. B., Gauvreau, K., Landzberg, M. J. et al. Transcatheter device closure of congenital and postoperative residual ventricular septal defects. *Circulation* 2004 Aug. 3;110(5):501-507.

[96] Dua, J. S., Carminati, M., Lucente, M., Piazza, L., Chessa, M., Negura, D. et al. Transcatheter closure of postsurgical residual ventricular septal defects: early and mid-term results. *Catheter Cardiovasc. Interv.* 2010 Feb. 1;75(2):246-255.

[97] Carminati, M., Butera, G., Chessa, M., De Giovanni, J., Fisher, G., Gewillig, M. et al. Transcatheter closure of congenital ventricular septal defects: results of the European Registry. *Eur. Heart J.* 2007 Oct.;28(19):2361-2368.

[98] Holzer, R., Balzer, D., Cao, Q. L., Lock, K., Hijazi, Z. M., Amplatzer, Muscular Ventricular Septal Defect Investigators. Device closure of muscular ventricular septal defects using the Amplatzer muscular ventricular septal defect occluder: immediate and mid-term results of a U.S. registry. *J. Am. Coll. Cardiol.* 2004 Apr. 7;43(7):1257-1263.

[99] Fu, Y. C., Bass, J., Amin, Z., Radtke, W., Cheatham, J. P., Hellenbrand, W. E. et al. Transcatheter closure of perimembranous ventricular septal defects using the new Amplatzer membranous VSD occluder: results of the U.S. phase I trial. *J. Am. Coll. Cardiol.* 2006 Jan. 17;47(2):319-325.

[100] Butera, G., Carminati, M., Chessa, M., Piazza, L., Micheletti, A., Negura, D. G. et al. Transcatheter closure of perimembranous ventricular septal defects: early and long-term results. *J. Am. Coll. Cardiol.* 2007 Sep. 18;50(12):1189-1195.

[101] Tometzki, A., Chan, K., De Giovanni, J., Houston, A., Martin, R., Redel, D. et al. Total UK multi-centre experience with a novel arterial occlusion device (Duct Occlud pfm). *Heart* 1996 Dec.;76(6):520-524.

[102] Sievert, H., Qureshi, S. A., Wilson, N., Hijazi, Z. editors. Percutaneous Interventions for Congenital Heart Disease. London, England: *Informa Healthcare*; 2007.

[103] Rickers, C., Seethamraju, R. T., Jerosch-Herold, M., Wilke, N. M. Magnetic resonance imaging guided cardiovascular interventions in congenital heart diseases. *J. Interv. Cardiol.* 2003 Apr.;16(2):143-147.

[104] Moore, P. MRI-guided congenital cardiac catheterization and intervention: the future? *Catheter Cardiovasc. Interv.* 2005 Sep.;66(1):1-8.

[105] Qiu, B., Gao, F., Karmarkar, P., Atalar, E., Yang, X. Intracoronary MR imaging using a 0.014-inch MR imaging-guidewire: toward MRI-guided coronary interventions. *J. Magn. Reson. Imaging* 2008 Aug.;28(2):515-518.

[106] Bergersen, L. J., Perry, S. B., Lock, J. E. Effect of cutting balloon angioplasty on resistant pulmonary artery stenosis. *Am. J. Cardiol.* 2003 Jan. 15;91(2):185-189.

[107] Rosario, J., Eiriksson, H., Rome, J. J. Frequency of restenosis after balloon pulmonary arterioplasty and its causes. *Am. J. Cardiol.* 2000 Dec. 1;86(11):1205-1209.

[108] Baerlocher, L., Kretschmar, O., Harpes, P., Arbenz, U., Berger, F., Knirsch, W. Stent implantation and balloon angioplasty for treatment of branch pulmonary artery stenosis in children. *Clin. Res. Cardiol.* 2008 May;97(5):310-317.

[109] Rothman, A., Perry, S. B., Keane, J. F., Lock, J. E. Early results and follow-up of balloon angioplasty for branch pulmonary artery stenoses. *J. Am. Coll. Cardiol.* 1990 Apr.;15(5):1109-1117.

[110] Bergersen, L. J., Perry, S. B., Lock, J. E. Effect of cutting balloon angioplasty on resistant pulmonary artery stenosis. *Am. J. Cardiol.* 2003 Jan. 15;91(2):185-189.

[111] McMahon, C. J., El Said, H. G., Vincent, J. A., Grifka, R. G., Nihill, M. R., Ing, F. F. et al. Refinements in the implantation of pulmonary arterial stents: impact on morbidity and mortality of the procedure over the last two decades. *Cardiol. Young* 2002 Oct.;12(5):445-452.

[112] Law, M. A., Shamszad, P., Nugent, A. W., Justino, H., Breinholt, J. P., Mullins, C. E. et al. Pulmonary artery stents: long-term follow-up. *Catheter Cardiovasc. Interv.* 2010 Apr. 1;75(5):757-764.

[113] Fogelman, R., Nykanen, D., Smallhorn, J. F., McCrindle, B. W., Freedom, R. M., Benson, L. N. Endovascular stents in the pulmonary circulation. Clinical impact on management and medium-term follow-up. *Circulation* 1995 Aug. 15;92(4):881-885.

[114] Shaffer, K. M., Mullins, C. E., Grifka, R. G., O'Laughlin, M. P., McMahon, W., Ing, F. F. et al. Intravascular stents in congenital heart disease: short- and long-term results from a large single-center experience. *J. Am. Coll. Cardiol.* 1998 Mar. 1;31(3):661-667.

[115] McMahon, C. J., El Said, H. G., Vincent, J. A., Grifka, R. G., Nihill, M. R., Ing, F. F. et al. Refinements in the implantation of pulmonary arterial stents: impact on morbidity and mortality of the procedure over the last two decades. *Cardiol. Young* 2002 Oct.;12(5):445-452.

[116] Ing, F. F., Grifka, R. G., Nihill, M. R., Mullins, C. E. Repeat dilation of intravascular stents in congenital heart defects. *Circulation* 1995 Aug. 15;92(4):893-897.

[117] Stern, H. J., Baird, C. W. A premounted stent that can be implanted in infants and re-dilated to 20 mm: introducing the Edwards Valeo Lifestent. *Catheter Cardiovasc. Interv.* 2009 Nov. 15;74(6):905-912.

[118] Geggel, R. L., Gauvreau, K., Lock, J. E. Balloon dilation angioplasty of peripheral pulmonary stenosis associated with Williams syndrome. *Circulation* 2001 May 1;103(17):2165-2170.

[119] Latson, L. A., Prieto, L. R. Congenital and acquired pulmonary vein stenosis. *Circulation* 2007 Jan. 2;115(1):103-108.

[120] Tomita, H., Watanabe, K., Yazaki, S., Kimura, K., Ono, Y., Yagihara, T. et al. Stent implantation and subsequent dilatation for pulmonary vein stenosis in pediatric patients: maximizing effectiveness. *Circ. J.* 2003 Mar.;67(3):187-190.

[121] Prieto, L. R., Schoenhagen, P., Arruda, M. J., Natale, A., Worley, S. E. Comparison of stent versus balloon angioplasty for pulmonary vein stenosis complicating pulmonary vein isolation. *J. Cardiovasc. Electrophysiol.* 2008 Jul.;19(7):673-678.

[122] Peng, L. F., Lock, J. E., Nugent, A. W., Jenkins, K. J., McElhinney, D. B. Comparison of conventional and cutting balloon angioplasty for congenital and postoperative pulmonary vein stenosis in infants and young children. *Catheter Cardiovasc. Interv.* 2010 Jun. 1;75(7):1084-1090.

[123] Mueller, G. C., Dodge-Khatami, A., Weil, J. First experience with a new drug-eluting balloon for the treatment of congenital pulmonary vein stenosis in a neonate. *Cardiol. Young* 2010 Aug.;20(4):455-458.

[124] Dragulescu, A., Ghez, O., Quilici, J., Fraisse, A. Paclitaxel drug-eluting stent placement for pulmonary vein stenosis as a bridge to heart-lung transplantation. *Pediatr. Cardiol.* 2009 Nov.;30(8):1169-1171.

[125] Xu, Z., Ludomirsky, A., Eun, L. Y., Hall, T. L., Tran, B. C., Fowlkes, J. B. et al. Controlled ultrasound tissue erosion. IEEE Trans Ultrason. *Ferroelectr. Freq. Control.* 2004 Jun.;51(6):726-736.

[126] Fujisaki, M., Chiba, T., Enosawa, S., Dohi, T., Takamoto, S. Cardiac intervention using high-intensity focused ultrasound: creation of interatrial communication in beating heart of an anesthetized rabbit. *Ultrasound Obstet. Gynecol.* 2010 Nov.;36(5):607-612.

[127] Maxwell, D., Allan, L., Tynan, M. J. Balloon dilatation of the aortic valve in the fetus: a report of two cases. *Br. Heart J.* 1991 May;65(5):256-258.

[128] McElhinney, D. B., Marshall, A. C., Wilkins-Haug, L. E., Brown, D. W., Benson, C. B., Silva, V. et al. Predictors of technical success and postnatal biventricular outcome after in utero aortic valvuloplasty for aortic stenosis with evolving hypoplastic left heart syndrome. *Circulation* 2009 Oct. 13;120(15):1482-1490.

[129] Tworetzky, W., Wilkins-Haug, L., Jennings, R. W., Van der Velde, M. E., Marshall, A. C., Marx, G. R. et al. Balloon dilation of severe aortic stenosis in the fetus: potential for prevention of hypoplastic left heart syndrome: candidate selection, technique, and results of successful intervention. *Circulation* 2004 Oct. 12;110(15):2125-2131.

[130] Tulzer, G., Arzt, W., Franklin, R. C., Loughna, P. V., Mair, R., Gardiner, H. M. Fetal pulmonary valvuloplasty for critical pulmonary stenosis or atresia with intact septum. *Lancet* 2002 Nov. 16;360(9345):1567-1568.

[131] Tworetzky, W., McElhinney, D. B., Marx, G. R., Benson, C. B., Brusseau, R., Morash, D. et al. In utero valvuloplasty for pulmonary atresia with hypoplastic right ventricle: techniques and outcomes. *Pediatrics* 2009 Sep.;124(3):e510-8.

[132] Marshall, A. C., Levine, J., Morash, D., Silva, V., Lock, J. E., Benson, C. B. et al. Results of in utero atrial septoplasty in fetuses with hypoplastic left heart syndrome. *Prenat. Diagn.* 2008 Nov.;28(11):1023-1028.

[133] Pavlovic, M., Acharya, G., Huhta, J. C. Controversies of fetal cardiac intervention. *Early Hum. Dev.* 2008 Mar.;84(3):149-153.

[134] Lee, L. A., Simon, C., Bove, E. L., Mosca, R. S., Ebbini, E. S., Abrams, G. D. et al. High intensity focused ultrasound effect on cardiac tissues: potential for clinical application. *Echocardiography* 2000 Aug.;17(6 Pt 1):563-566.

[135] Amin, Z., Berry, J. M., Foker, J. E., Rocchini, A. P., Bass, J. L. Intraoperative closure of muscular ventricular septal defect in a canine model and application of the technique in a baby. *J. Thorac. Cardiovasc. Surg.* 1998 Jun.;115(6):1374-1376.

[136] Bacha, E. A., Cao, Q. L., Starr, J. P., Waight, D., Ebeid. M. R., Hijazi, Z. M. Perventricular device closure of muscular ventricular septal defects on the beating heart: technique and results. *J. Thorac. Cardiovasc. Surg.* 2003 Dec.;126(6):1718-1723.

[137] Bacha, E. A., Cao, Q. L., Galantowicz, M. E., Cheatham, J. P., Fleishman, C. E., Weinstein, S. W. et al. Multicenter experience with perventricular device closure of muscular ventricular septal defects. *Pediatr. Cardiol.* 2005 Mar.-Apr.;26(2):169-175.

[138] Diab, K. A., Cao, Q. L., Bacha, E. A., Hijazi, Z. M. Device closure of atrial septal defects with the Amplatzer septal occluder: safety and outcome in infants. *J. Thorac. Cardiovasc. Surg.* 2007 Oct.;134(4):960-966.

[139] Mendelsohn, A. M., Bove, E. L., Lupinetti, F. M., Crowley, D. C., Lloyd, T. R., Fedderly, R. T. et al. Intraoperative and percutaneous stenting of congenital pulmonary artery and vein stenosis. *Circulation* 1993 Nov.;88(5 Pt 2):II210-7.

[140] Holzer, R., Marshall, A., Kreutzer, J., Hirsch, R., Chisolm, J., Hill, S. et al. Hybrid procedures: adverse events and procedural characteristics--results of a multi-institutional registry. *Congenit. Heart Dis.* 2010 May-Jun.;5(3):233-242.
[141] Gibbs, J. L., Wren, C., Watterson, K. G., Hunter, S., Hamilton, J. R. Stenting of the arterial duct combined with banding of the pulmonary arteries and atrial septectomy or septostomy: a new approach to palliation for the hypoplastic left heart syndrome. *Br. Heart J.* 1993 Jun.;69(6):551-555.
[142] Akintuerk, H., Michel-Behnke, I., Valeske, K., Mueller, M., Thul, J., Bauer, J. et al. Stenting of the arterial duct and banding of the pulmonary arteries: basis for combined Norwood stage I and II repair in hypoplastic left heart. *Circulation* 2002 Mar. 5;105(9):1099-1103.
[143] Galantowicz, M., Cheatham, J. P. Lessons learned from the development of a new hybrid strategy for the management of hypoplastic left heart syndrome. *Pediatr. Cardiol.* 2005 Mar.-Apr.;26(2):190-199.
[144] Caldarone, C. A., Benson, L., Holtby, H., Li, J., Redington, A. .N, Van Arsdell, G. S. Initial experience with hybrid palliation for neonates with single-ventricle physiology. *Ann. Thorac. Surg.* 2007 Oct.;84(4):1294-1300.
[145] Pizarro, C., Derby, C. D., Baffa, J. .M., Murdison, K. A., Radtke, W. A. Improving the outcome of high-risk neonates with hypoplastic left heart syndrome: hybrid procedure or conventional surgical palliation? *Eur. J. Cardiothorac. Surg.* 2008 Apr.;33(4):613-618.
[146] Galantowicz, M., Cheatham, J. P., Phillips, A., Cua, C. L., Hoffman, T. M., Hill, S. L. et al. Hybrid approach for hypoplastic left heart syndrome: intermediate results after the learning curve. *Ann. Thorac. Surg.* 2008 Jun.;85(6):2063-70; *discussion* 2070-1.
[147] Galantowicz, M., Cheatham, J. P. Fontan completion without surgery. Semin. Thorac. Cardiovasc. *Surg. Pediatr. Card. Surg. Annu.* 2004;7:48-55.
[148] Hausdorf, G., Schneider, M., Konertz, W. Surgical preconditioning and completion of total cavopulmonary connection by interventional cardiac catheterisation: a new concept. *Heart* 1996 Apr.;75(4):403-409.
[149] Konstantinov, I. E., Benson, L. N., Caldarone, C. A., Li, J., Shimizu, M., Coles, J. G. et al. A simple surgical technique for interventional transcatheter completion of the total cavopulmonary connection. *J. Thorac. Cardiovasc. Surg.* 2005 Jan.;129(1):210-212.
[150] Simpson, K. E., Huddleston, C. B., Foerster, S., Nicholas, R., Balzer, D. Successful subxyphoid hybrid approach for placement of a melody percutaneous pulmonary valve. *Catheter Cardiovasc. Interv.* 2011 Jan. 13.

Economy and Marketing

In: Percutaneous Valve Technology: Present and Future ISBN: 978-1-61942-577-4
Editors: Jose Luis Navia and Sharif Al-Ruzzeh

Chapter XXX

Transcatheter Aortic Valve Implantation (TAVI): Bringing a Medical Device to Market

Thomas A. Vassiliades, Jr., John Liddicoat and Martin T. Rothman

Introduction

Valve repair/replacement and coronary artery bypass grafting are the most common cardiac surgical procedures performed today. Historically, aortic valve replacement has required open heart surgery, disqualifying many patients for whom the risks of such surgery are too great. Partly for this reason, the surgical heart valve market is in decline as more patients requiring valve replacement fall into a high-risk category.

Recent advances in transcatheter aortic valve implantation (TAVI), however, have brought the benefits of aortic valve replacement to those higher risk patients. The TAVI procedure is performed with fluoroscopic and echocardiographic guidance by an interdisciplinary team that includes cardiac surgeons, cardiologists, and anesthesiologists. Typically, it is performed in a setting where both catheter-based and surgical facilities can be immediately accessed.

How does a device such as TAVI make its way from "promising idea" into the surgical repertoire? This chapter provides an overview of the risks, challenges, and opportunities inherent in bringing a device to market together with a perspective on the subject from Medtronic, a leader in the field of structural heart disease.

Make or Buy?

In the beginning, there is an idea. It is an idea for an innovative therapy that could help improve the health of millions around the world. Device manufacturers large and small investigate it and ask: Is it feasible? How much will it cost to develop? Does the market potential justify the investment? Some will decide to pursue the idea; others will give it a pass. As the idea gains traction over time, manufacturers may reconsider their earlier decisions. Not wanting to cede a promising new market to competitors, they continue their questioning: Is it economically and technically feasible to develop this technology internally? Does it make more sense to recruit personnel with the knowledge to further the technology? Should we outright acquire a smaller company that leads in the technology's development?

What is the best solution? Make it or buy it?

Do Your Homework

Every medical device company has in place a due diligence process to help in deciding whether to acquire new technology or invest in its internal development. Experts from the relevant business areas analyze the potential investment from their unique perspectives to ensure that it is a good fit. For example, the intellectual properties (IP) attorney may find that the intellectual property is not valid or cannot be enforced, so the investment is not made. Research and development (R&D) may determine that the device can be built but marketing finds that the market is not large enough to justify the investment.

Medtronic's due diligence process on the transcatheter valve market began years ago, when the earliest technology was developed. The company made quarterly assessments to determine if in-house development should continue or if outside technology should be acquired to speed the process. All along, Medtronic invested its own resources for internal development but ultimately determined that it was economically more prudent to acquire CoreValve than continue in-house development.

Medtronic's Structural Heart Division's goal is to develop internally about 70% of its product innovation. Outside parties assist with development of the remaining 30%. This model is consistent with those of other world-class companies such as Merck, Johnson and Johnson, and Abbott.

Many factors influence a company's decision to develop a technology internally or acquire it externally. The primary factor is a company's core competencies and whether there is a strategic interest in a technology that lies outside these competencies. Acquiring another company to create a foundational competence is one method that Medtronic and other companies use to supplement internal innovation.

Another factor that some companies assess is the cultural fit of the acquisition within the acquiring company. For example, Medtronic is a mission driven corporation that scrutinizes this aspect of an acquisition to ensure its fit within Medtronic. If it is not deemed a good fit, it will likely pass on the acquisition, even though the company is a good opportunity in every other aspect.The competitive landscape also influences the decision. Market assessment may indicate that a company with the core competence to develop an important new technology does not have the ability to respond quickly enough to the rapidly growing market for that technology. TAVI is a good example of this as the market developed much faster than many manufacturers anticipated. In the early stages, none of the major valve companies invested heavily in internal development programs since TAVI was perceived as a disruptive technology.

Disruptive technologies are those that differ radically from the current standard of practice. Coronary stents in the mid 1990s, for example, were disruptive since they replaced open-heart bypass grafts. Laparoscopic surgery is another example. When the technique appeared in the late 1980s, surgeons were faced with repairing gall bladders laparoscopically rather than with familiar open surgery.Disruptive technologies often are developed within a start-up company. Among the reasons for this are the risk profiles associated with many innovative technologies:

1. Early clinical results may not be entirely positive.
2. First generation devices may be too experimental.

Larger companies tend to be more conservative, particularly from the standpoint of product exposure. If a larger company introduces an innovation that proves disappointing, the company's reputation and credibility suffer. Moreover, the quality systems larger companies have in place typically do not allow experimental procedures to be performed. Because of their relatively low industry profile, incubator companies such as Percutaneous Valve Therapies (PVT) or CoreValve, Inc. are better suited to advance disruptive technologies.

Why Acquire?

As smaller companies advance novel technology, larger companies may decide to acquire them because they can more innovatively work through final design challenges that new technology often presents. Larger companies generally have the funding and infrastructure needed for the required preclinical and clinical testing, as well as the resources to market the product and train clinicians in its use.

In the 1990s, Medtronic investigated the possibility of delivering a heart valve through a catheter and concluded that, although it might have value, no engineering time could be devoted to the concept. At this stage in the technology's development, many clinicians were skeptical about its practicality and efficacy. Since several start-up companies were already working on developing the technology, PVT being one of them, Medtronic decided to invest $5 million in PVT to help advance the technology. In 2005, Edwards Lifesciences made a $150 million offer to buy PVT. Medtronic, believing PVT to be a high-risk venture, declined to join the bidding. Since acquiring PVT, we believe Edwards has spent an estimated $450 million to bring the PVT valve to its current state.

In time, the market for TAVI technology accelerated and Medtronic initiated a transcatheter aortic valve program of its own. Despite significant strides in its internal development program, Medtronic made the decision to acquire CoreValve to accelerate its entry into the market.

At the time of Medtronic's CoreValve acquisition, Edwards' product development was five years further along than Medtronic's internal efforts. It was strategically important for Medtronic to get into the market as quickly as possible, and the CoreValve acquisition provided the necessary boost. Today, Medtronic and Edwards share the transcatheter market outside of the United States.

Today, many companies are entering the TAVI marketplace. St. Jude Medical has an internal program. In addition, there are more than 10 start-up companies developing the technology, hoping to be acquired by one of the major medical companies wishing to accelerate its time to market.

Make Versus Buy: Pros and Cons

When considering an acquisition, a company must carefully analyze the strategic and economic implications. The economic analysis weighs the value of the project if carried out internally as opposed to the value if done via acquisition. The company looks at whether it has access to the required intellectual property and, if not, how much it would cost to develop alternate intellectual property. It assesses how long it will take to bring the product to market, and how much it will cost to develop the technology's knowledge base compared to hiring people who possess the knowledge base needed to carry the project forward.

Once calculated, these costs are compared to the estimated price for buying the technology outright, and time-to-market is assessed relative to the technology's price premium. All other things being equal, the final decision often hinges on the timing of access to market.

During this assessment process, a company must answer some difficult questions before a final decision can be made:

1. If we make the product, will we be able to get to market in time?
2. Can we design and manufacture the optimal product versus buying something that requires further development and refinement?
3. Can in-house strengths, such as knowledge of the FDA regulatory process and other development issues, be leveraged to the ultimate benefit of the patient?
4. Can we make a product as good as a product we could buy?
5. Do we have the time or internal R&D funds to conduct a new program without impinging on existing project requirements?

In developing novel technologies, smaller companies or start-ups typically have less oversight and fewer controls in place, so they are able to take more risks than larger companies. Larger companies are more risk averse because they may have a slate of legacy products to protect. They have a lot more to lose if they fail.

Another important factor that larger companies must consider is how new technology will affect, possibly even cannibalize, existing business. The patient population for TAVI was ineligible for open-heart surgery and their life expectancy was less than 2 years. TAVI technology, therefore, would not affect existing business. However, once TAVI's efficacy is proven in a younger or healthier patient population, existing business could be vulnerable. It is essential that a company consider both the short-term and long-term implications of new technologies on existing product lines. Medtronic, for example, maintains an internal development program for all its heart valve devices. The goal is to maintain competitive advantage in each patient population market without having one device impinge on the market of another.

But first, a company must establish a presence in a market. The CoreValve acquisition enabled Medtronic to progress faster, enhancing its time to market. By combining CoreValve's technology with its own, Medtronic was able to improve the standard of care much more quickly than would have been possible without the acquisition. Without the CoreValve acquisition, Medtronic would have been third or fourth to market. The gap would have been difficult to close without a product clearly superior to competitive devices.

The "make it versus buy it" analysis in this situation indicated that Medtronic needed to continue its own development, joining **that effort with CoreValve's capabilities**. In turn, Medtronic's ability to leverage the TAVI product would have been almost impossible for CoreValve to do on its own given the financial issues affecting the market in 2008 and 2009.

Product Development

Most of the time and expense involved in device development is spent before the product undergoes clinical investigation and regulatory review. Table 1 shows the time to market for identical products in the U.S. and Europe.

The development process is categorized into phases, starting with Phase 0 and moving thorough Phase 3.

European Union (EU) Pivotal Study

Once the device design has been stabilized and the therapy protocol is understood, the EU pivotal study is initiated. An EU pivotal study evaluates the safety of a given device and typically takes approximately two years. After the agency reviews the data and receives satisfactory answers to any questions occasioned by the data, CE Mark approval is extended to the device. An FDA pivotal study can be run concurrently or it can be initiated after the EU study has begun. Manufacturers are usually able to start marketing their device in Europe with less supporting data than is required in the U.S. Often, results from the European clinical experience can be used in the first phase of the FDA study.

U.S. Pivotal Study

Running concurrently with or subsequent to the EU pivotal study, the U.S. pivotal study takes from three to five years to complete. For a device such as transcatheter valves, where clinical interest is high and a substantial unserved market exists, study enrollment will be rapid, resulting in a study time closer to three years.

Premarket Approval (PMA)

For a Class III device associated with a high level of risk, such as the transcatheter valve, premarket approval must be granted before it is released for clinical use. A PMA review requires submission of clinical data to establish safety and efficacy of the device, and support the claims made by the manufacturer for the device. The review panel consists of professionals thoroughly familiar with the clinical applications for which the device is intended. In order to gather the relevant clinical data, an Investigational Device Exemption (IDE) must be obtained so that clinical studies may be conducted. See the Regulatory Process section for details.

From start to finish, bringing a novel Class III device to market can take up to 13 years and cost from several million dollars to close to one billion dollars.

Table 1. Development timeline for a novel product, from concept through commercialization. Red arrows show best case, blue arrows show worst case. Stars represent product development milestones

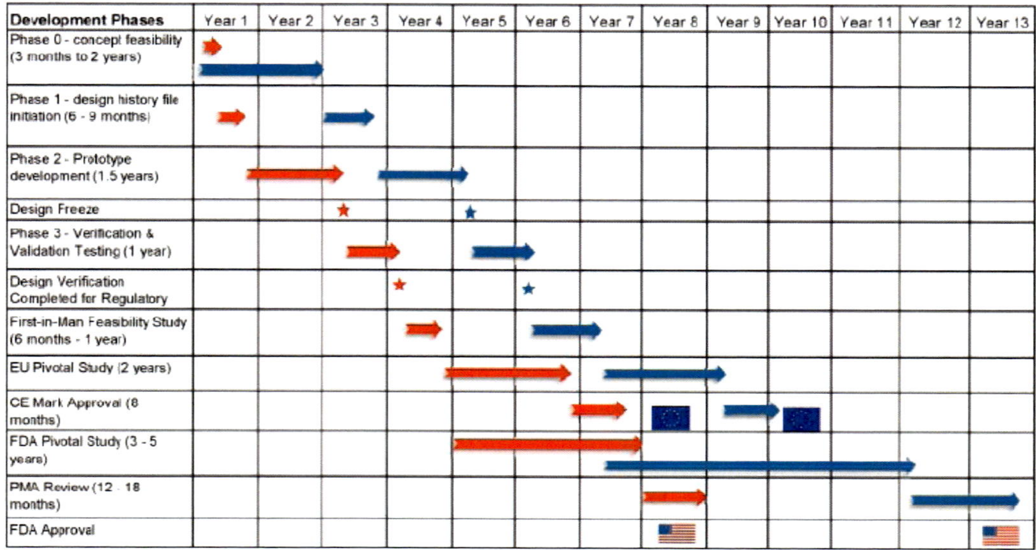

Phase 0: The process begins with investigation into the feasibility of a given concept. When it is determined that a product can, indeed, be made (a transcatheter valve, for example), discussions are held with potential customers to better understand their needs. This phase can take as little as three months or as long as several years, depending on the device's complexity.

Phase 1: The design history is initiated during this phase. Design histories, required by the regulatory body that will approve the device, document the manufacturer's quality and manufacturing processes. During this phase, audits are routinely conducted to verify that each segment of the process is followed and documented. Customer inputs captured during Phase 0 are ranked to create a Customer Requirements document, the principal deliverable for this phase.

Phase 2: Prototypes are built during Phase 2. The goal is to capture 100% of customer requirements, though the percentage typically achieved is closer to 80-85%. After the design has met the highest percentage of customer requirements, has sufficient structural integrity, and has met internal development standards, a design freeze is implemented, which indicates that the manufacturer is confident the device meets essential customer requirements and can be reliably built and reproduced.

Phase 3: The device is tested and built in a controlled environment during this phase, which includes a design verification build. Device sampling, varying in size from 10 to 60, is tested according to prospectively identified criteria. If the device passes the verification build, clinical builds are started. If it fails, design modifications are made and the verification build begins again. Devices produced during the clinical build are used in the first clinical implants. During the first-in-man feasibility portion of this stage, manufacturers learn as much as possible about the device's short-term safety performance. This information dictates if further design modifications must be made before a broader patient population is exposed to the product. First-in-man feasibility is generally completed in six to 12 months.

The Tortoise or the Hare?

Bringing a device such as TAVI from Phase 0 through FDA approval can take up to ten years and cost millions of dollars. Do smaller companies have an advantage? Smaller companies usually focus on driving a single product through the process and thus are able to devote virtually all of their resources to that end. One might conclude that this makes them more nimble, better able to react to challenges and quicker to overcome obstacles. Larger corporations, on the other hand, often have several projects in different phases of development. They must share available capital, technical, and intellectual resources among these programs, thus slowing the pace at which progress can be made.

This scenario may hold true through Phase 0 and Phase 1, when smaller companies focus all their resources on innovation and information gathering. But at Phase 2, the process begins to even out. A novel therapy like TAVI is complicated, and the many interactions it will have in clinical application must be evaluated. A larger company with a history of developing Class III devices will know where the weak links and pitfalls are. Experience, in this case, helps the larger company perform the steps leading to design freeze more efficiently and faster.

Yet, in the end, it seems that smaller companies commercialize their devices faster than larger companies. This is partially true. Regulatory requirements in the U.S. can add years to the process of bringing a device to market. For this reason, it is estimated that 75% of first clinical use testing of cardiovascular devices is done outside the U.S., reducing the time to product launch by six to twelve months. Consequently, smaller firm concentrates on the European Union (EU) market, going quickly from feasibility to first-in-man study to CE Mark, so that revenue can begin to flow and the company's financial viability is not threatened. At this point, the smaller company will often look for an exit, which usually involves selling the technology (or the company itself) to a larger company. The larger company then assumes the task of moving the product through the FDA process, leveraging its larger test capabilities and its experience in regulatory process and execution.

Appearance Versus Reality

The clinical world may perceive that innovation in device development springs almost exclusively from smaller companies. This perception derives from a strategy startups and small companies use to attract venture capital investment. Often startup companies will show their latest developments to clinicians, knowing that venture capitalists look to these industry opinion leaders to assess whether a new technology is viable.

It is true that small companies do a greater share of the feasibility work in the industry. According to the Dartmouth Device and Drug Development Symposium held in October 2003, "… most new device categories are typically developed by venture-backed start-up companies ... [The] preclinical stage … may consume $10 to $20 million before the device is ready for clinical testing. These capital requirements exceed the means of most angel syndicates and are typically obtained from venture capital firms in the form of equity financing."[1]

Larger companies are more deliberate in obtaining clinical input on therapy concepts. They are interested in protecting their intellectual property and therefore do not showcase a technology too early in the process. For large companies, obtaining outside funding is not as critical as ensuring that the investment they are making is properly targeted.

Once a device is approved for clinical use, larger companies are better equipped to put thousands of units into the distribution chain, whereas smaller companies may struggle to produce 100. With TAVI, for example, Medtronic can produce 10,000 devices, sell them, and thereby help treat 10,000 patients with no other therapy alternative.

New technologies like TAVI generate a lot of excitement and anticipation. But the road to market is long. Only two transcatheter devices have been commercialized, neither of them in the U.S. In the aortic device market, 12 to 15 active programs are moving toward the commercialization stage. In the transcatheter mitral market, much larger and more difficult than the aortic market, no devices have been commercialized for replacement and only one product has been commercialized for repair. Twenty to 25 companies are actively pursuing the transcatheter mitral replacement market.

The Regulatory Process

In contrast to bringing a pharmaceutical to market in the United States, introducing a medical device is somewhat clearer. The U.S. Food and Drug Administration (FDA) has three classifications for medical devices based on the degree of risk a device presents to a patient. Class I presents the least amount of risk; Class III presents the greatest amount of risk. TAVI falls into Class III.

The FDA has set seven regulatory requirements for manufacturers of devices destined for distribution in the U.S.

1. Establishment Registration: Owners or operators of places of business (called establishments) that are involved in the production and distribution of medical devices intended for use in the United States are required to register annually with the FDA.
2. Medical Device Listing: After registering the establishment, the company must create listings for devices produced or processed at this facility.
3. Premarket Notification 510(k), Unless Exempt, or Premarket Approval (PMA): Class III devices such as TAVI require PMAs. They are high-risk devices that pose a significant risk of illness or injury to the patient population.
4. Investigational Device Exemption (IDE) for Clinical Studies: An investigational device exemption (IDE) allows the device to be used in a clinical study in order to collect safety and effectiveness data required to support a Premarket Approval (PMA) application. Clinical studies with devices of significant risk must be approved by FDA and by an Institutional Review Board (IRB) before the study can begin.
5. Quality System (QS) Regulation: The quality system regulation includes requirements related to the methods used in and the facilities and controls used for: designing, purchasing, manufacturing, packaging, labeling, storing, installing and servicing of medical devices.

6. Labeling: Labeling includes labels on the device as well as descriptive and informational literature that accompanies the device.
7. Medical Device Reporting (MDR): Incidents in which a device may have caused or contributed to a death or serious injury must to be reported to FDA under the Medical Device Reporting program. The goal of this regulation is to detect and correct problems in a timely manner.

In addition to the above requirements, TAVI, considered a novel Class III device, must be reviewed by a scientific panel before it receives FDA approval. Bringing a novel device such as TAVI through the development and approval processes typically costs hundreds of millions of dollars.

Many attempts have been made to create a global regulatory process for medical device approval. Despite these efforts, three distinct regulatory models exist:

1. United States (FDA approval)
2. European Union (CE mark)
3. Japan

Other medical device regulations exist (e.g., India, Korea, China, Taiwan, Singapore, Brazil) but the three models listed above are well established and represent a large portion of the device market.

In the United States, The Center for Devices and Radiological Health (CDRH) of the FDA regulates medical devices. This organization's mandate is to promote and protect public health by ensuring that safe and effective medical devices become available in a timely manner. Devices are classified in a three-tiered system according to perceived risk. This classification system defines CDRH's standards for demonstrating a devices safety and effectiveness:[1]

1. Class I (lowest risk) – subject to general controls such as published standards for labeling, manufacturing, post-market studies, and reporting.
2. Class II (higher risk) – general controls are insufficient for reasonable assurance of safety and effectiveness; however, sufficient information is available to establish special controls. Special controls may include performance standards, design controls, and post-market studies. Most Class II devices require FDA clearance of a premarket notification application (PMA) or 510(k) prior to product marketing.
3. Class III (highest potential risk) – these devices are either life sustaining or supporting, are important for preventing impairment of human health, or present a high risk of illness or injury. Class III devices usually require Premarket Approval, which generally requires clinical data demonstrating reasonable assurance of device safety and effectiveness in the target population, before they can be marketed.

The FDA Approval Process

TAVI is a Class III device and is therefore subject to the most stringent FDA scrutiny. All devices in this class must obtain Premarket Approval (PMA), the FDA process of scientific and regulatory review that evaluates a device's safety and effectiveness.

PMA applications must show, through documentation and in-depth analysis of clinical and non-clinical studies, that the benefits a device provides outweigh its risks. The data to substantiate claims made for a device are gathered through non-clinical and clinical studies.

Non-clinical studies typically include information on microbiology, toxicology, immunology, biocompatibility, the results of animal tests, and other applicable laboratory procedures. These tests must themselves be run according to the FDA's Good Laboratory Practice for Nonclinical Laboratory Studies guidelines.

Clinical studies demonstrate the device's safety and efficacy through clinical application. Gathering data for this portion of the PMA application takes a significant length of time. The submission must include:

1. Study protocols.
2. Safety and effectiveness data.
3. Data detailing adverse reactions/complications.
4. Information on device failures and replacements.
5. Patient information.
6. Documentation of patient complaints.
7. Data tabulations from all cohort subjects.
8. Statistical analysis results.

The clinical study, when well-designed and executed, actually meets several objectives. First, it satisfies the major portion of the FDA's PMA application requirements. Second, through publication in a citable, peer-reviewed journal, it provides physicians with information about safety, effectiveness, and patient indications. To achieve these objectives, a study must:

1. Clearly define the patient population for the device.
2. Define the control group.
3. Have an adequate sample size.
4. Define relevant primary and secondary endpoints.
5. Define inclusion/exclusion criteria.

The pilot phase of a clinical study, generally limited to fewer than 100 patients treated in two to three centers, is designed to evaluate a device's safety and help define the pivotal trial.

The pivotal trial itself is designed to define the patient populations for which the device is safe and effective. Novel device studies may require a patient cohort of 1,000 or more from 30 to 50 clinical sites and the trial may last one to two years. Appropriate follow-up frequency typically extends for an additional year after treatment.

For novel devices such as TAVI, with limited short-term data and virtually no long-term data, results of prospective randomized controlled studies are required for PMA application.

The FDA approval process begins with a panel track PMA review, during which a panel of 13 experts provides device feedback and make an approval recommendation to the FDA. The panel may also recommend restricted indications for use. While the FDA is not required to accept the panel's recommendation, it typically does.

Accurate device labeling is another important FDA requirement. The manufacturer must provide descriptive labels on the product itself, or on its packaging. Labeling may include instructions for use, service instructions, warnings and cautions against uses that may be dangerous to health, and include information that may be necessary for the protection of others. The labeling requirement also stipulates that descriptive and informational literature accompany the device to the end user.

Once FDA approval has been granted, the FDA and the manufacturer will design a post-market study to evaluate end-points and determine the length of follow-up duration since long-term results are of particular interest to the FDA.

European Union (EU) CE Mark Approval Process

While some process similarities exist, there are significant differences between the EU and U.S. regulatory processes that affect the time and cost of launching novel medical device technology. The EU approval pathway is often faster thanks to set guidelines for how specific types of products such as stents or heart valves are to be tested.

The EU process incorporates vertical and horizontal standards. Vertical standards are specific to a device type. Horizontal standards apply to all devices. Novel devices, such as CoreValve, however, do not fit comfortably into any of the known testing categories. Consequently the manufacturer must show that bench testing was rigorous enough to demonstrate a level of safety that warrants its implantation in humans.

The approval criteria for Class III devices are another major difference between the EU and FDA regulatory processes. The FDA requires manufacturers to demonstrate safety and effectiveness, which typically requires a prospective, randomized controlled clinical trial. For the EU process, the manufacturer need only demonstrate safety and that the device performance is consistent with its stated intended use.[1] This difference greatly impacts the size and scope of the required clinical studies.

Notified bodies (NBs) are independent commercial organizations that implement regulatory control over medical devices. They are central to the EU system and are authorized to issue the CE Mark. Authorities within each EU member state designate, monitor and audit the NBs, and a manufacturer may choose any of the more than 50 NBs to evaluate the device for which approval is sought, the only stipulation being that the NB chosen is approved to evaluate the device class under review.

After reviewing the U.S. and EU regulatory approval processes, the Dartmouth Device and Drug Development Symposium concluded that "... the demonstration of safety and efficacy for a new medical device is a long, arduous, and expensive developmental path from early concept to introduction into clinical practice ... understanding [the differences between the U.S. and European regulatory environments] helps explain why much early device testing takes place outside the U.S., and why the introduction of new devices into clinical practice is usually significantly delayed in the U.S. when compared with Europe." The authors observed that "... these factors account for the 1- to 3-year delays in the introduction of new device technologies into general clinical practice in the U.S. as compared with Europe."[1]

Japan's Approval Process

Device approval in Japan is governed by the Pharmaceuticals and Medical Devices Agency (PMDA). Like its European and U.S. counterparts, the PMDA is responsible for reviewing the efficacy, safety, and quality of medical devices. All applications for medical device marketing approval must be submitted in Japanese. The language barrier, combined with a complex registration process, makes Japan one of the most time-consuming and expensive markets in which to gain medical device approval.

Clinical data to support an approval application in Japan must be developed from Japanese people. The PMDA does not accept clinical study data from outside Japan, adding significant time, expense, and difficulty to the approval process.

For foreign manufacturers, complying with Japan's Pharmaceutical Affairs Law (PAL) of 2005 can be challenging. Few English language documents have been issued by the Ministry of Health, Labor and Welfare (MHLW) and its division, the Pharmaceutical and Medical Devices Agency (PMDA). A foreign manufacturer first must go through the process of becoming a Marketing Authorization Holder (MAH). Manufacturing facilities outside of Japan are required to obtain Foreign Manufacturer Accreditation rather than a Manufacturer License.

Japan's device classification system has four rather than three classes of devices, and determining a device's classification is another complex process. To obtain market approval for a medical device, the MAH must register the device using these guidelines:

1. Pre-market submission (Todokede) – Class I or general medical devices – no assessment by the PMDA is required.
2. Pre-market certification (Ninsho) – Class II or specified controlled medical devices – a pre-Market Approval application with a Registered Certification Body (RCB) must be filed to obtain certification. This process is similar to using a Notified Body in Europe.
3. Pre-market Approval (Shonin) – Class II III and IV or highly controlled medical devices – a Pre-market Approval Application must be filed with the PMDA to obtain their approval. Class II devices that are not Specified Controlled Devices are also subject to Pre-market Approval.

TAVI Approval Process

Both the FDA and the EU required a controlled trial for CoreValve's TAVI technology since it was a novel device.

In the EU, a controlled trial to establish safety and performance is not always required. But with novel technologies like TAVI, manufacturers do not always know at the outset what the regulatory requirements will be. In the case of the CoreValve ® product, the manufacturer and the regulatory authorities worked together to determine what information was required to demonstrate safety and performance before commencing the clinical trial.

Business Model Development

A well-constructed business model is essential to maximizing the potential of a new technology. Whether the technology is novel, as with TAVI, or mature, clinicians often tend to under- appreciate a manufacturer's resource constraints and its need to prioritize investment spending in order to maximize efficiency.

An effective business model must address several key questions:

1. How will the new technology be acquired and developed?
2. How will internal resources be applied to developing the new technology?
3. How will the new technology affect existing product lines?
4. Will the return on the new technology justify the expense of developing it?
5. What level of clinician training will be required to successfully implement the new technology?
6. What are the reimbursement possibilities for the new technology?

Medtronic has products ranging from $10 catheters to $30,000 transcatheter heart valves. It is important to decide budget allocation over all these products in order to maintain a competitive edge in all market categories. For many products, funds have to be invested in next-generation product development. Typically, next-generation ideas outstrip the available budget, so judicious trade-offs must be made. Wall Street has an expectation that companies such as Medtronic will grow at a certain rate, and this too must be taken into account. The company must be managed so that it is deemed a worthy stock investment. For that to happen, a balance must be struck between developing technology internally and acquiring it from outside. Large companies such as Medtronic grow through investing in technology with significant potential. This is not possible in every business segment. Consequently, large companies seek growth opportunities substantial enough to average out across their entire business range.

Sources of Ideas

Many of the best ideas come from customers. Medtronic maintains close contact with its customer base through regular meetings where market, product trends and potential are discussed and pertinent questions posed:

1. What will the next "best technology" be?
2. Will physicians adopt new technology?
3. What is an acceptable level of new device learning versus maintaining current product usage?
4. What new therapies are needed to supplement existing options?

Ideas from physicians and others are funneled to the appropriate company division (R&D, sales, marketing) for further consideration. Each division assesses ideas differently. R&D, for example, may examine iterations that could be made to an existing product while evaluating intellectual properties being developed in the field. Marketing may examine market movement, procedural numbers, which patient demographic is receiving treatment, which patient demographic needs treatment not yet available. Analysis of unmet needs is a vital part of any business process development.

Getting Ahead in the World

Acquisition does not always halt internal development. The acquisition of CoreValve gave Medtronic a well-developed technology platform supported by solid clinical data, enabling the company to move further along their internal development pathway.

While both the Medtronic and Edwards TAVI devices were released almost simultaneously in Europe, it appears that Edwards will receive FDA approval first. There are advantages and disadvantages to being second in market. The obvious disadvantage is that if the first-to-market device is well-accepted, convincing clinicians to switch product preference may be difficult. But, the second-to-market company can observe the first company's progress, learn from any problems, and make appropriate product adjustments. Also, a significant investment is required to educate the market about a novel therapy, and second-to-market companies benefit from the first company's pioneering educational efforts.

Importance of Physician Education

Assessing market needs often goes beyond product development. A novel device involves much more than simply making it clinically available. Transcatheter valves are a complex, intricate product with their use indicated for a specific patient population. Clinicians need to be educated on identifying which patients will benefit most from the product, how the product is most effectively administered, and the unique changes the implanted product may engender in patients. Education and training are key components in marketing new therapies, particularly when the therapy can impact a patient's life as significantly as TAVI. Historically, manufacturers voluntarily provide a level of clinician training rather than a regulatory body mandating it. For the CoreValve product, education extends to requiring proctors be present in the initial cases. CoreValve training and education programs in Europe are very well defined. After a site has been selected to use the CoreValve product, Medtronic conducts didactic and simulated hands-on training at its European training facility. Following this training, clinicians perform a prescribed number of cases at their home facilities with proctor involvement. Medtronic provides proctoring for as long as a clinician wants it, often for more than 10 cases. After clinicians have have successfully completed their proctored cases, they are certified to perform TAVI implantation on their own. Medtronic's clinical specialists, however, attend each procedure until the clinician is deemed ready to "solo." This long and intense course of training and proctoring allows a high quality of the therapy to be provided.

Clinical Evidence and Post-Marketing Studies

Even after a novel device has been through pilot studies, pivotal studies, received CE and FDA approval, the data collection process does not stop. In fact, it picks up speed. If the device is successful, more and more patients will receive the therapy, and more and more safety and performance data will be available. Post-marketing studies are essential to helping a company ensure clinical acceptance of its device and to foster the market's growth. Continued clinical evidence documents a product's performance in the targeted patient population and can be used to define expanded indications for FDA submission. Today, the CoreValve ® product is indicated for patients unable to undergo surgical valve replacement or for patients at high risk if they undergo surgery. A post-market study may reveal that patients at moderate risk may also benefit from the therapy. On-going clinical studies can also be used to evaluate whether surgeons are optimizing the device implant technique. Information from these studies may help to define best practices in relation to procedures and patient management.

Reimbursement

In any business model for medical devices, reimbursement is a critical factor. Companies must assess whether their clinical studies will generate sufficient evidence to prove performance superior to currently accepted therapies. Among the factors that must be considered:

1. Will the new technology add ancillary costs or eliminate existing ancillary costs?
2. What are the anticipated cost offsets of the new technology compared to the standard of care?
3. Is Medicare's current DRG assignment and payment adequate for this technology?
4. Will new codes need to be established for this therapy?

Without properly considering reimbursement implications from every angle, a novel device therapy could very well face a bleak future in the marketplace. And with the time, money, and energy expended in its development that is the least desirable outcome.

Wall Street's Perspective

Investors in smaller, privately held firms closely monitor every step of the development process. They have a very direct interest in the company's success. Setbacks and delays can seriously diminish a technology's eventual return on investment.

A larger, publicly held corporation, such as Medtronic, is subject to broader scrutiny from internal management, its board of directors, and Wall Street.

Wall Street brokers look closely at the development process of a publicly-held company's new technology. They examine the myriad business decisions that were made along the way, analyze the business model and assess the market potential of the new product. They ask whether all of these factors together enhance the company's standing in the marketplace and add to its bottom line. A favorable Wall Street rating can help a large company maintain its ability to develop and refine its products, thereby securing its competitive posture.

In the case of TAVI, Wall Street agreed that acquisition of CoreValve, Inc. was a sound business decision, giving Medtronic a crucial edge in claiming a portion of an expanding market.

Conclusion

As we have shown, developing a disruptive technology, such as TAVI, from idea to clinical procedure is a long and expensive process. For this device's target patient population, it is quite literally a matter of life and death. No step in the development process can be trivialized, and best practices must be followed every step of the way. From feasibility testing, through engineering and regulatory approval, to marketing and clinician training, the best interests of the end users—the patients—must be foremost in everyone's mind.

Because this process is so lengthy and costly, it requires the resources of a large, experienced company to see it through—a company with the resources to conduct clinical trials and with the experience to accurately fulfill regulatory requirements. Also integral to the success of such a device is the innovation that smaller companies and start-ups can inject into the equation—the ability to take risks, the freedom to invent and experiment with new, untested technology. It is a somewhat symbiotic process: resources and experience coupled with creativity and innovation.

In the end, bringing medical devices to market is a business. It is an industry devoted to helping people live longer, healthier lives. To continue that pursuit, device manufacturers must stay in business so that they can continually refine their existing products and assist in developing new therapies. To do that, they must carefully monitor and allocate their resources to maximize their profits. The medical device industry is an intricate interplay of engineering, marketing, medicine, and accounting. It may be unseemly to mention devotion to patient health and maximized profits in the same paragraph, but it is the profits that keep the innovation coming and make possible the devotion to patient care.

Reference

[1] Kaplan, A. V., Baim, D. S., Smith, J. J. et al. Medical Device Development: From Prototype to Regulatory Approval, *Circulation.* 2004:109:3068-3072. CoreValve is a registered trademark of Medtronic, Inc.

In: Percutaneous Valve Technology: Present and Future ISBN: 978-1-61942-577-4
Editors: Jose Luis Navia and Sharif Al-Ruzzeh

Chapter XXXI

From Starr-Edwards to SAPIEN™: The History of Transcatheter Aortic Valve Replacement

Francis G. Duhay and Sarah Huoh

Introduction

To understand the history of transcatheter valve technology, it is important first to gain a perspective of the advancements in surgery and interventional cardiology that provided its foundation – valves, stents and balloons. Much as today's portable computing technologies trace their lineage to the supercomputers of the 1960s that once occupied entire rooms, transcatheter heart valves arose from purposeful, incremental innovation. In this context, the clinical reality of transcatheter aortic valve replacement (TAVR) could only have been achieved "by standing on the shoulders of giants."

This chapter will review the evolution of the Edwards SAPIEN™ THV (Transcatheter Heart Valve) by first exploring the history of surgical heart valve prostheses, which still remain the standard of care for the treatment of many valvular heart conditions. The history of percutaneous diagnostic and therapeutic cardiovascular catheterization then will be summarized, culminating in the rebirth of a procedure long abandoned – balloon aortic valvuloplasty – so that the foundations of transcatheter aortic valve replacement can be best understood. Transcatheter aortic valve replacement will then be reviewed, from concept and experimentation, to the historic undertaking of the first-in-man procedure in 2002. Finally, in these challenging times of growing regulatory and third-party payer scrutiny over medical devices, it is mandatory to make the case for clinical value. To this end, the final section will summarize the two pivotal clinical trials (PARTNER Cohorts A and B) from the standpoint of safety, efficacy, quality of life and health economics.

1. Epidemiology, Natural History and Undertreatment of Aortic Stenosis

Degenerative valvular heart diseases are common in industrial countries and increase with age. In population-based epidemiologic studies, the prevalence of aortic stenosis in individuals over 75 years of age is 2.8%, and is second only to mitral regurgitation in frequency (Nkomo VT, Gardin JM, TN Skelton). In the U.S., the estimated incidence of symptomatic severe aortic stenosis is 97,000 cases per year. The accepted gold standard for the treatment of aortic stenosis is surgical valve replacement, which is associated with excellent clinical outcomes in selected patients. The number of aortic valve replacements performed in the U.S. is approximately 68,000 operations per year (Healthcare Cost and Utilization Project (HCUP) 2008). However, for multiple reasons, many patients are not referred to cardiac surgeons for consideration for valve replacement or, if referred, choose not to undergo the procedure.

The natural history of degenerative calcific aortic stenosis is associated with a long latent period during which worsening mechanical obstruction and consequent pressure overload of the left ventricle progresses while the patient remains essentially asymptomatic. The primary symptoms of aortic stenosis, which ensue most commonly in the seventh and eighth decades of life, are angina pectoris, syncope and heart failure. In those patients in whom the aortic stenosis remains untreated, the prognosis generally is poor once these symptoms are manifested. Indeed, survival curves demonstrate that the interval between the onset of symptoms and death is approximately five years for angina, three years for syncope and two years for heart failure (Figure 1).

Several studies have tried to address the potential size of the untreated population with aortic stenosis. The Euro Heart Survey included 216 patients aged >75 years with symptomatic aortic stenosis (aortic valve area (AVA) ≤ 0.6 cm^2/m^2 or mean aortic valve gradient (AVG) ≥ 50 mm Hg) (Iung B, Cachier A, Baron G). Of these patients, 33 percent (72 or 216) did not undergo surgical valve replacement. The main reasons given were advanced age (≥ 80 years) and poor left ventricular function. Three often cited studies by Pellika *et al.* (Pellika PA, Serrano ME, Nishimura RA), Charlson *et al.* (Charlson E, Legedza ATR, Hamel MB), and Bouma *et al.* (Bouma BJ, van den Brink RB, van der Meulen JHP) were based on retrospective review of echocardiographic databases.

Although each study defined severe aortic stenosis differently (Pellika, aortic jet velocity ≥ 4.0 m-sec^{-1}; Charlson, AVA < 0.8 cm^2 or mean AVG ≥ 50 mm Hg; Bouma, AVA ≤ 1.0 cm^2 or peak AVG ≥ 50 mm Hg), the frequency of untreated aortic stenosis reported was remarkably consistent –30 percent (90 of 297), 35 percent (43 of 124), and 40 percent (56 of 140), respectively.

Further, in addition to advanced age and poor left ventricular function, a third important factor predictive of non-operative management was the presence of severe comorbid conditions. As the coexistence of these clinical features can contribute to significantly higher rates of mortality and complications after surgical valve replacement, many investigators began to explore the possibility of a less intrusive approach to achieve anatomic relief of aortic stenosis. Moreover, if the true rate of untreated aortic stenosis in the U.S. population is between 30 percent and 40 percent, then the number of potential candidates benefiting from this procedure could be approximately 40,000 patients per year.

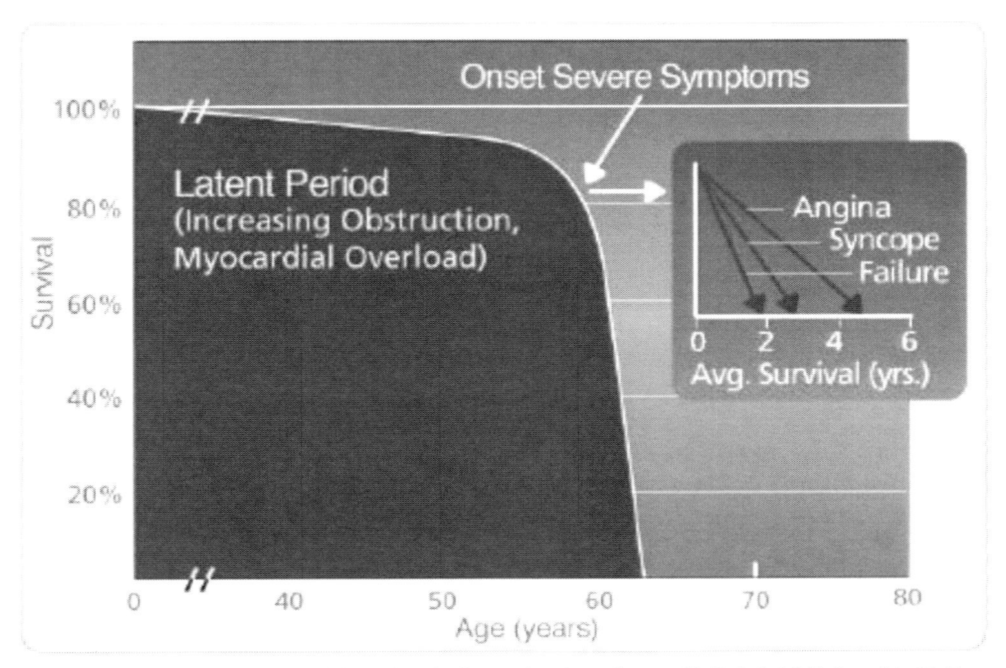

Adopted from Ross, J. Jr, Braunwald, E. Aortic Stenosis. *Circulation* 1968 Jul.;38(1 Suppl.):61-7.

Figure 1. Natural history of severe aortic stenosis after symptom onset.

2. The Rise of Prosthetic Heart Valves

Before the advent of open heart surgery, early attempts to address valvular diseases involved extracardiac approaches. In the late 1940s, Dr. Charles Hufnagel, Professor of Experimental Surgery at Georgetown Medical Center, developed an artificial heart valve to address aortic regurgitation. Using a methyl methacrylate (Plexiglas) tube, a substance known to resist blood coagulation, he experimented with a simple caged ball design (Figure 2).

To preserve blood flow to the head, neck and upper extremities during the requisite period of aortic clamping, Dr. Hufnagel chose to implant the valve in the descending aorta just beyond the origin of the left subclavian artery (Hufnagel CA, Harvey WP, Rabil PJ).

In this location, he calculated that 75 percent of the total regurgitant flow could be prevented. Because of the risk of pressure necrosis to the aortic wall caused by rigid circumferential sutures, the methacrylate tube was secured at each aortic end by means of a "multiple-point" fixation ring (Hufnagel CA, Harvey WP, Rabil PJ). These distributed the pressure at discrete intervals along the entire circumference of the aorta, rather than continuously.

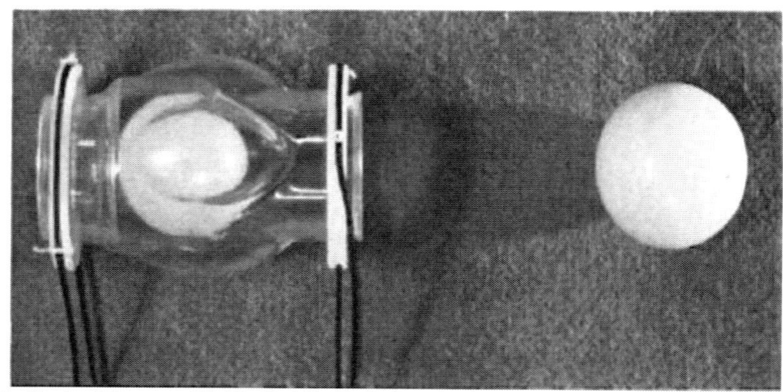

Ref.: Hufnagel, C. A., Harvey, W. P., Rabil, P. J. Surgical correction of aortic insufficiency. *Surgery*, 1954;35:673-683.

Figure 2. The Hufnagel valve was a simple caged ball valve design composed of a polyethylene ball and a methyl methacrylate (Plexiglas) tube, secured at each end by a "multiple point" fixation ring.

In September 1952, Dr. Hufnagel began his first clinical series of 23 patients with aortic regurgitation (Hufnagel CA, Harvey WP, Rabil PJ). The operative mortality rate in the first 10 cases was 40 percent, but decreased to 15 percent over the next 13 cases. Of significance, there was no ECG evidence of myocardial ischemia during or after operation. This approach allowed rapid and sutureless implantation of a valve without the need for cardiopulmonary bypass. Subsequently, more than 200 Hufnagel valves were implanted in patients with aortic insufficiency (Gott VL, Alejo DE, Cameron DE). Some valves have functioned up to 30 years without evidence of structural deterioration (Gott VL, Alejo DE, Cameron DE). Although the long-term outcomes were excellent, with the development of cardiopulmonary bypass the reality of orthotopic (subcoronary) aortic valve replacement was within reach.

The key to unlocking the door on the field of valve replacement surgery was the development and widespread clinical use of the heart-lung machine, which enabled open-heart operations. One year after Dr. Hufnagel's landmark report, Dr. John Gibbon, Jr., Professor of Surgery at Jefferson Medical College, performed the first successful open-heart operation using a heart-lung machine (Gibbon JH Jr.). Cardiopulmonary bypass was used for a total 26 minutes in the case of a teenage girl in need of closure of a large secundum atrial septal defect (Gibbon JH Jr.). This operation represented the culmination of more than 20 years of intensive research investigation. Since then, "generations of cardiac surgeons have been able to operate on millions of human hearts with alacrity, efficiency, and consistency to correct … cardiac valve disorders in the young and old" (Cohn LH).

In March 1960, Dr. Dwight Harken, at the Peter Bent Brigham Hospital, performed the first aortic valve replacement using a caged ball prosthetic valve (Harken-Soroff) in a patient with severe aortic stenosis (Harken DE, Soroff HS, Taylor WJ). There were only two survivors among the first seven patients, and both eventually required valve reoperations, one at three years for a paravalvular leak, and the other at 22 years for infectious endocarditis. Of note, several years later, during testimony to Congress on the safety of medical devices, Dr. Harken famously responded, "A device is safe when it is safer than the condition it corrects and is the best available." (Harken DE)

In 1958, Miles Lowell Edwards, a retired 60-year-old electrical engineer – who held a patent for a centrifugal fuel-booster pump for rapidly climbing aircraft during World War II

(Starr A 2007) – approached Dr. Albert Starr, a young heart surgeon at the University of Oregon, with an ambitious plan to build an artificial heart. Dr. Starr persuaded the determined Edwards to start with the mitral valve. (Matthew AM)

Based loosely on the Hufnagel design, the Starr-Edwards caged ball valve was composed of four thick, methyl methacrylate (Lucite) struts, later changed to Stellite-21 (a mixture of cobalt, chromium, molybdenum, and nickel) in 1961, surrounding a silicone elastomer ball (Figure 3). After extensive experimentation in dogs, Dr. Starr and Edwards progressed to humans using, as Dr. Starr recounts, "an interdisciplinary team to select patients for operation and to provide continuous care postoperatively. The team included cardiologists, anesthesiologists, nephrologists, hematologists, neurologists, and even a psychiatrist" (Starr A 2010) – a precursor to the multidisciplinary heart team of today.

On September 21, 1960, Dr. Starr performed the first successful mitral valve replacement using a caged ball prosthetic valve (Starr-Edwards, Edwards Lifesciences, Irvine, CA) in a 52-year-old truck dispatcher with severe calcific mitral stenosis, the result of childhood rheumatic fever (Starr A 2007) (Figure 4). This patient recovered completely and newspapers nationwide hailed it as the "Miracle Heart Surgery Success."(Matthews AM).

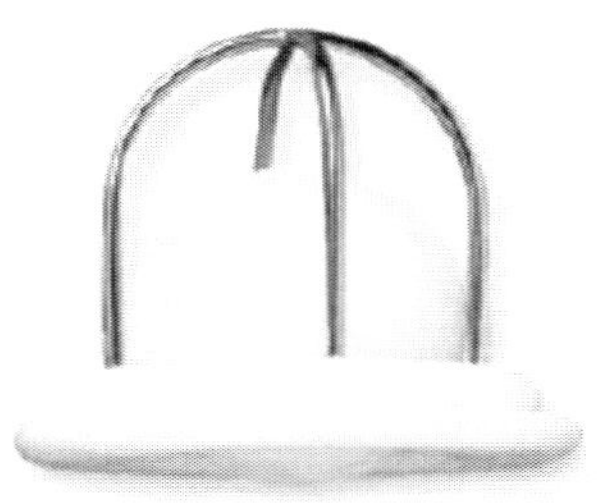

Ref.: Courtesy of Edwards Lifesciences archive (Edwards Lifesciences, Irvine, C. A).

Figure 3. Starr-Edwards caged ball valve. Over 250,000 valves implanted in patients worldwide.

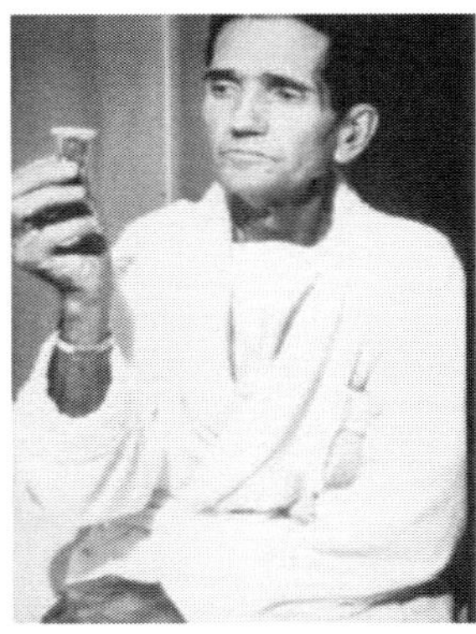

Ref.: Courtesy of Edwards Lifesciences archive (Edwards Lifesciences, Irvine, C. A).

Figure 4. After losing his first patient to massive air embolism, Dr. Albert Starr performed the first successful mitral valve replacement in the world on Philip Admunson, a 52-year-old man with severe calcific mitral stenosis, using the Starr-Edwards caged ball prosthesis.

The patient remained in good health for 15 years when he died, not from his heart condition but from injuries suffered after falling from a ladder (Kouchoukos NT). After a visit to Dr. Harken in Boston, where Dr. Starr observed an aortic valve replacement, he and Edwards modified the mitral design to accommodate the aortic valve.

Forty years after the Starr-Edwards valve was introduced, more than 250,000 patients have received the valve worldwide, with remarkable durability extending beyond 30 years. Indeed, Gödje and colleagues, reporting on 415 patients operated on using the Starr-Edwards prostheses between 1963 and 1977, demonstrated no echocardiographic abnormalities in 52 percent of aortic valves and 68 percent of mitral valves, after follow-up of 4,254 patient-years (Gödje OL, Fischlein T, Adelhard K).

The team of Dr. George Magovern, Professor of Surgery at the University of Pittsburgh, and Harry Cromie, an engineer, were perhaps decades ahead of their time as they set out to develop a prosthetic valve that would enable surgeons to perform a more rapid valve replacement (Magovern GJ, Kent EM, and Cromie HW). The Magovern-Cromie caged ball valve featured a double-barbed anchoring ring with a snap-on mechanism that sandwiched the native annulus to facilitate sutureless valve anchoring (Figure 5).

According to Dr. Magovern, his motivation was to "simplify the method of fixation, lessen [cardiopulmonary] bypass time and reduce thrombus formation." The first implants occurred in 1962 and, subsequently, 728 patients were treated over the next 26 years (Gott VL, AlejoDE, Cameron DE). In general, the disadvantages of the caged ball prostheses included low-grade hemolysis from the repetitive impact of the ball on the cage, and less than optimal valve hemodynamics if the height of the cage was either too tall or too short. These provided the impetus for the development of disk prostheses.

As recalled by Dr. Viking Björk, Professor and Chairman of Surgery at the Karolinska Institute, Stockholm, Sweden, the development of the tilting disk valve was inspired by the need to address the gaps in valve technologies of the 1960s. Where one valve design would advance the field by addressing vulnerabilities exposed by another – such as the Starr-Edwards caged ball prosthesis solving the problem of ruptured plastic valve cusps – it invariably came with a price, such as higher valve gradients.

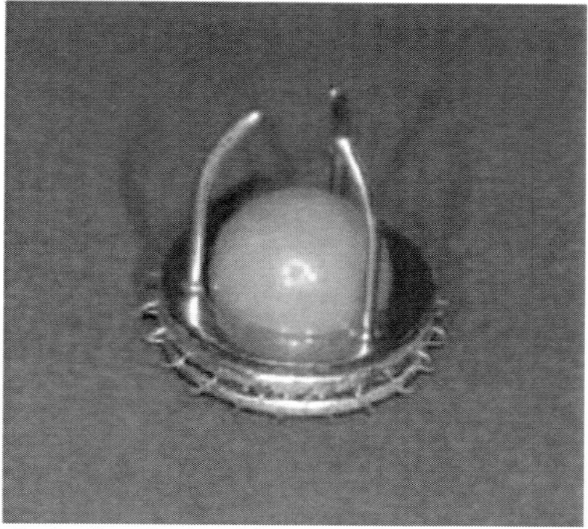

Ref.: Zlotnick, A. Y. A perfectly functioning Magovern-Cromie sutureless prosthetic aortic valve 42 years after implantation. *Circulation*, 2008;117:e1-e2.

Figure 5. The sutureless Magovern-Cromie caged ball valve.

In a 1984 report, Dr. Björk reflected: "In 1968, together with an American engineer, Donald P. Shiley, a free-floating disc valve was developed that opened in the aortic position to 60-degrees. The disc was composed of Delrin™ (Dupont, Inc.) polyacetal plastic. On 16 January 1969, I implanted this valve in a patient for the first time. Many patients are still in good health at present after more than 14 years with these valves." (Gott VL, Alejo DE, Cameron DE)

The original Björk-Shiley tilting disc valve prosthesis was modified in 1971 by an iteration in which the original disc material was changed from Delrin™ to an extremely durable carbon material (pyrolytic carbon), because of the propensity of the former to absorb water, which alters the disc shape (Gott VL, Alejo DE, Cameron DE). This flat, circular design achieved tremendous worldwide success, with nearly 300,000 aortic and mitral Björk-Shiley valve prostheses implanted between 1969 and 1986 (Gott VL, AlejoDE, Cameron DE).

In 1977, Dr. Karl Victor Hall, Professor and Chairman of Surgery at the Rikshospitalet, Oslo, Norway, and Robert Kaster, an electrical engineer, jointly developed the Hall-Kaster tilting disc valve prosthesis. The circular disc occluder, composed of pyrolytic carbon, had a central hole through which a thin metal strut guided its opening and closing (Gott VL, Alejo DE, Cameron DE). The two struts were attached to the circular metal ring, which was covered by a sewing cuff made of expanded PTFE. In 1987, medical device manufacturer Medtronic Inc. (Minneapolis, MN) acquired the Hall-Kaster valve prosthesis, and marketed a slightly modified version as the Medtronic-Hall tilting disc valve prosthesis. The Medtronic-Hall model is the most commonly used tilting-disc valve in the US.

A true collaborative effort, the bileaflet valve prosthesis by St. Jude Medical, Inc. (St. Paul, MN) was the product of engineers Xinon (Chris) Posis and Donald Hanson, Dr. Demetre Nicolof, a cardiovascular surgeon at the University of Minnesota, Jack Bokros, the discoverer pyrolytic carbon in 1963, and Manny Villafana, businessman and medical device veteran (Gott VL, Alejo DE, Cameron DE). In an effort to achieve a lower profile than the bulky caged ball designs, the St. Jude valve prosthesis was conceived as a low-profile and lightweight device made entirely of pyrolytic carbon. Its unique leaflet pivot mechanism was comprised of the leaflet-tabs rotating in a "butterfly recess" in the inner wall of the valve housing (Emery RW, Mettler E, Nicoloff DM) (Figure 6).

In October 1997, Dr. Nicolof implanted the first St. Jude bileaflet valve prosthesis. By far the most popular mechanical valve prosthesis, the St. Jude valve has been implanted in over one million patients worldwide (Gott VL, Alejo DE, Cameron DE).

In parallel to the evolution of modern mechanical valve prostheses, was an effort to develop valves composed primarily of biologic tissue. The major drivers in this field were the availability of cadaveric tissue and cost, as mechanical valves were not yet being manufactured on a large scale. In 1956, Dr. Gordon Murray was the first to implant valved aortic homografts in the descending aorta, akin to a biologic Hufnagel valve, to treat severe aortic insufficiency (Ross DN 1962).

Although the Starr-Edwards caged ball valve prosthesis had been reported in 1960, it was not yet available in the United Kingdom, where many patients with valvular heart disease were left untreated. Consequently, in 1962, Mr. Donald Ross, at Guy's Hospital, London, UK, performed the first orthotopic aortic valve replacement using a freeze-dried homograft in a patient with severe aortic stenosis (Ross DN 1962).

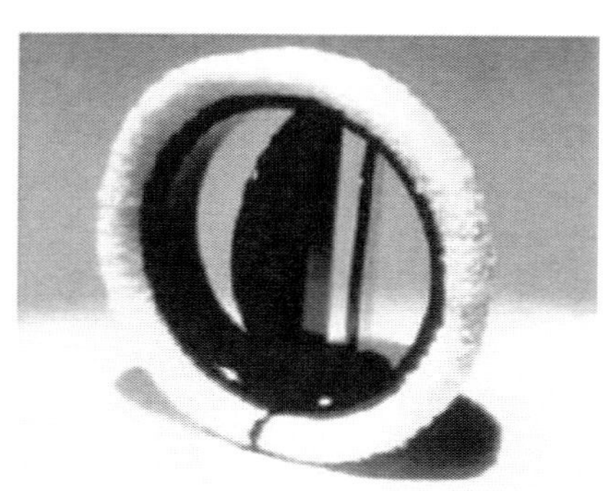

Ref.: Gott, V. L., Alejo, D. E., Cameron, D. E. Mechanical heart valves: 50 years of evolution. *Ann. Thorac. Surg. 2003*;76:S2230-2239.

Figure 6. The St. Jude Medical bileaflet valve prosthesis.

This successful operation was followed one week later by Sir Brian Barratt-Boyes, at Green Lane Hospital, Auckland, New Zealand, who reported his series of homograft valve replacement in 44 patients with aortic valvular insufficiency and stenosis (Barratt-Boyes BG). The putative advantages of homografts included superior hemodynamic function, extremely low rates of thromboembolism and hemolysis, and relative immunity to leaflet calcification and prosthetic valve endocarditis. On the other hand, the disadvantages included the relative lack of availability of cadaveric hearts, operative technical complexity, potential transmission of disease, and the absence of robust durability data.

In response to a devastating stroke that afflicted one of his patients, an artist, three months after mechanical valve replacement, Dr. Alain Carpentier, Professor of Surgery at the l'Hôpital Broussais, Paris, France, set forth to develop a xenograft valve prosthesis. "A clot had formed at the site of the valve and migrated to the brain, causing serious damage. The same valve that saved the patient had now affected the quality of his life to a point in which he could not paint anymore. At that very moment, I decided to devote my research to the challenge of valve thrombogenicity," Dr. Carpentier wrote (Carpentier A 2007).

Based on his experience with homograft valves during his residency, Dr. Carpentier knew of their potential benefits to patients, but a change in French law prevented the harvest of cadaveric valves within a reasonable time frame. Consequently, he turned to pigs. At first, he tried mercury-based solutions to ameliorate the immune reaction observed during valve implantation. However, the mercury-treated porcine leaflets still incited marked inflammation and collagen denaturation in some patients. This impelled Dr. Carpentier to return to the lab bench to better understand the fundamental mechanisms at play.

By 1968, Dr. Carpentier felt he had found a solution. By preserving porcine tissue with glutaraldehyde, instead of mercury, he could block collagen denaturation and the immune-mediated inflammatory response by lessening tissue antigenicity. He mounted the glutaraldehyde-preserved valves onto a stainless steel frame to facilitate implantation in his first series of patients (Carpentier A, Deloche A, Relland J) (Figure 7). Building on this success, Dr. Carpentier later developed an anti-calcification treatment process to extend tissue valve durability. His next major contribution was achieved in the 1980s, when Dr. Carpentier introduced bovine pericardium to construct a bioprosthetic valve with better hemodynamic performance than even a porcine valve crafted by nature. Many years of diligent research investigation culminated in the Carpentier-Edwards PERIMOUNT valve in 1991 (Frater, RWM) (Figure 8).

3. Balloon Aortic Valvuloplasty Redux

While developments in surgical aortic valve replacement enabled surgeons to resolve the debilitating symptoms of valve disease, there were still many patients who were not suitable candidates for operation. The first proposed therapeutic alternative that emerged for the treatment of aortic valve stenosis was balloon aortic valvuloplasty (BAV) in the 1980s.

Experimentation with catheter-based techniques for accessing the heart traces back to the 1920s, when surgical resident Dr. Werner Forssmann, from Eberswald, Germany, inserted a catheter into his own antecubital vein and advanced it 65 cm into his right atrium, documenting its final resting position on x-ray. At the time, manipulation of the human heart was fraught with risk and often ended in patient death; Dr. Forssmann proved that the heart could be accessed safely – although he was summarily dismissed for his actions and never returned to cardiology.

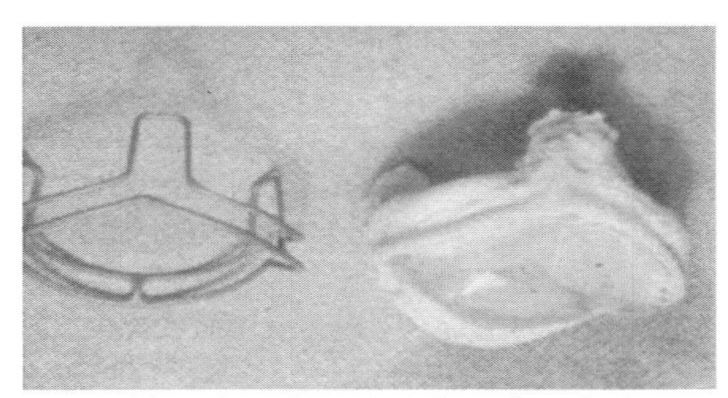

Ref.: Carpentier, A. The surprising rise of nonthrombogenic valvular surgery. *Nature Medicine*, 2007;13: xvii-xx.

Figure 7. Dr. Alain Carpentier's first (homemade) glutaraldehyde-treated porcine valve implanted in a human. Left, Teflon-covered stainless steel frame was used to support the valve. Right, frame covered with Dacron fabric to facilitate fixation and tissue in-growth. The porcine valve was sewn to the frame, which preserved full motion of the leaflets.

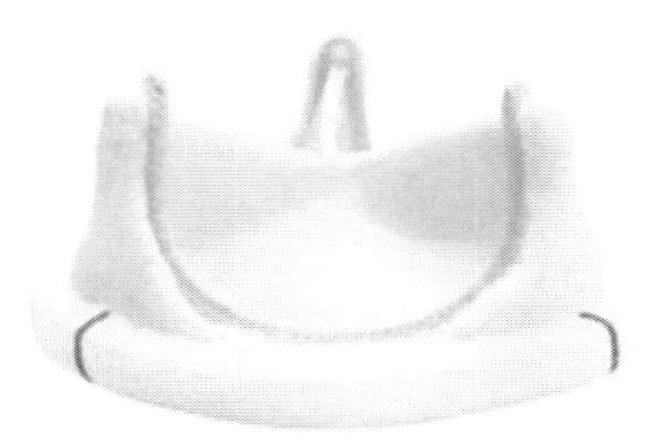

Ref.: Courtesy of Edwards Lifesciences, Irvine, C. A.

Figure 8. Modern Carpentier-Edwards PERIMOUNT valve (model 6900).

From this early effort, Dr. André Frédéric Cournand and Dr. Dickinson W. Richards, at Bellevue Hospital, New York, in 1941 refined the technique of cardiac catheterization and introduced it into the clinical realm. The three shared the Nobel Prize in Medicine in 1956, "for their discoveries concerning heart catheterization and pathological changes in the circulatory system".

In the early years the applications of cardiac catheterization were for purely *diagnostic* rather than *therapeutic* purposes. The 1950s and early 1960s witnessed new applications of diagnostic catheterization, with Dr. Henry A. Zimmerman developing left heart catheterization in 1950, Dr. Ivar Seldinger introducing the catheter-over-a-needle technique in 1953, and Dr. Mason Sones, a pediatric cardiologist, developing selective coronary angiography in 1958 by accidentally injecting contrast into the right coronary artery. In 1964, Dr. Charles Dotter and Dr. Melvin Judkins, at the University of Oregon, introduced the technique of transluminal angioplasty in their report of 11 cases of atherosclerotic obstruction of the superficial femoral or popliteal arteries (Dotter CT and Judkins MP). This was achieved by inserting a guidewire across the stenotic lesion and dilating it using a series of tapered, radiopaque Teflon catheters.

The transition of cardiac catheters from purely diagnostic to therapeutic applications occurred in 1966. Dr. William Rashkind, from Children's Hospital of Philadelphia, is considered the first to perform therapeutic balloon dilatation (Rashkind WJ and Miller WW). His efforts were focused on alleviating hypoxemia by creating an atrial septal defect in infants with transposition of the great vessels. Later, in 1969, Dr. Dotter conducted studies in dogs using percutaneous intravascular scaffolding devices, or stents, made from stainless steel coil springs, to provide structural support of the femoral or popliteal arteries (Dotter CT).

Dr. Dotter's technique of transluminal angioplasty inspired Dr. Andreas Grüntzig, from the University Hospital in Zurich, Switzerland, to develop a double-lumen dilatation catheter with a nonelastic balloon to facilitate the angioplasty procedure. In May of 1977, Dr. Grüntzig performed the first coronary angioplasty in three patients undergoing coronary artery bypass surgery at St. Mary's Hospital in San Francisco (Gruntzig AR, Myler RK, Hanna ES), and in 1979, he reported his landmark series of percutaneous transluminal coronary angioplasty in 50 patients (Gruntzig AR, Senning A, Siegenthaler WE). It was Dr. Grüntzig's introduction of the flexible balloon catheter combined with the historical success of surgical mechanical dilation of stenotic heart valves that enabled therapeutic balloon valvuloplasty.

Dr. Jean Kan, of Johns Hopkins University, applied balloon dilatation to treat diseased pulmonary valves. In treating an eight-year-old child with congenital pulmonic stenosis, Dr. Kan conducted the first successful percutaneous balloon pulmonic valvuloplasty via the right femoral vein using a 9 Fr introducer sheath (Kan JS, White RI, Mitchell SE). The polyethylene balloon was 14 mm by 40 mm, inflated to 45 psi, with an inflation-deflation cycle lasting 20-30 seconds, and required less than 10 seconds of complete occlusion. Dr. Kan's success with the pulmonic valve created possibilities to treat other valves of the heart. Indeed, within two years of Dr. Kan's publication, Dr. Kanji Inoue, from Kochi Municipal Hospital, Kochi, Japan, reported his experience with percutaneous transseptal balloon mitral valvuloplasty in six patients with mitral stenosis (Inoue K, Owaki T, Nakamura T). The balloon was composed of double layers of rubber tubing, between which nylon mesh was inserted as reinforcement (Figure 9).

The modern era of balloon aortic valvuloplasty began in 1985 with the work of Dr. Alain Cribier, from Hôpital Charles Nicolle, Rouen, France. Dr. Cribier performed the first adult percutaneous balloon aortic valvuloplasty in three elderly patients with severe aortic stenosis (Cribier A, Eltchaninoff H, Tron C). The balloons were 40 mm long, and the injection of 10 mL of saline achieved pressures of up to 6-8 atm (Cribier A, Saoudi N, Berland J) (Figure 10). Three serial inflations, each lasting 20-60 seconds, were performed with maximum diameters of eight, 10, and 12 mm, respectively. This led to an immediate reduction in the peak systolic aortic pressure gradient from 75 to 33 mm Hg, and an increase in valve area from 0.5 to 0.8 cm^2 (Cribier A, Eltchaninoff H, Tron C). This technique was rapidly adopted and saw explosive growth in the two years after Dr. Cribier's first case report. However, despite immediate relief of symptoms, the combination of early restenosis in the majority of patients and the lack of long-term survival benefit led to a rapid decline in the use of BAV (NHLBI Balloon Valvuloplasty Registry Participants; Lieberman EB, Bashore TM, Hermiller JB; Otto CM, Mickel MC, Kennedy JW). Accordingly, balloon aortic valvuloplasty became a palliative procedure limited to patients who were poor candidates for surgical valve replacement, or as a bridge to surgery. Until the introduction of transcatheter aortic valve replacement, BAV was the only percutaneous treatment option available for prohibitive or high risk patients with symptomatic severe aortic stenosis.

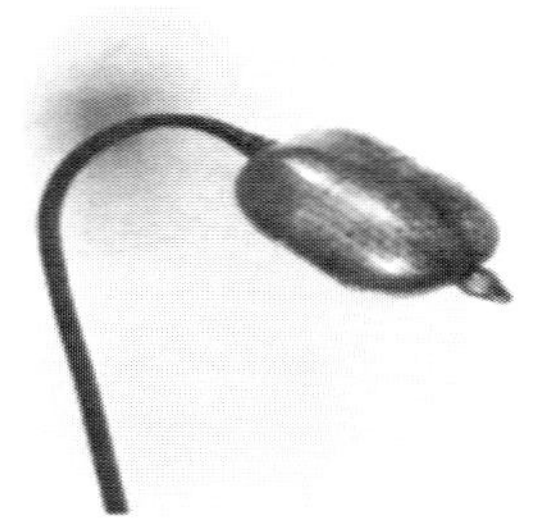

Ref.: Inoue, K., Owaki, T., Nakamura, T. Clinical application of transvenous mitral commissurotomy by a new balloon catheter. *J. Thorac. Cardiovasc. Surg.* 1984;87:394-402.

Figure 9. Inoue percutaneous transseptal balloon mitral valvuloplasty catheter.

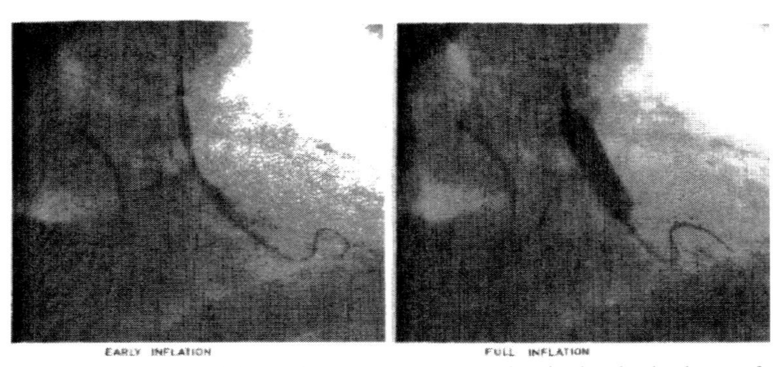

Ref.: Cribier, A., Saoudi N, Berland J, *et al* Percutaneous transluminal valvuloplasty of acquired aortic stenosis in elderly patients: An alternative to valve replacement? *Lancet* 1986;1(8472):63-67.

Figure 10. Correct position of the valvuloplasty balloon centered across the stenotic aortic valve during early and full inflation. Indentation, or "dog-bone", of the balloon is seen during early inflation and disappears at full inflation.

4. The Transcatheter Heart Valve: An "Overnight Success" Decades in the Making

To many it may come as a surprise that a temporary transcatheter heart valve was first developed shortly after Dr. Harken's first successful aortic valve replacement in 1960. Bearing similarities to Dr. Hufnagel's caged ball valve from the 1950s, which was implanted in the descending thoracic aorta, Dr. Hywel Davies, from Guy's Hospital, London, United Kingdom, delivered a catheter-mounted cone-shaped "parachute" valve into the descending aorta (Davies H). Introduced through the femoral artery, the "parachute" valve was designed to provide temporary support in patients with decompensated heart failure due to aortic insufficiency. This was followed by Dr. S.D. Moulopoulos, from Athens University, Athens, Greece, and Dr. S.J. Phillips, from Sinai Hospital, Detroit, Michigan, who each reported successful animal studies using a series of catheter-mounted aortic valves during the 1970s (Moulopoulos SD, Anthopoulos L, Stametelopoulos; Phillips SJ, Ciborski M, Freed PS). These temporary valves were positioned in the ascending aorta and came in a variety of designs, including a wind sock, umbrella, and a "balloon-on-a-stick."

The first two operated passively, opening and closing in synchrony with each heart beat, while the latter was electronically actuated much like an intraaortic balloon pump. Importantly, neither Dr. Moulopoulos nor Dr. Phillips incorporated any anchoring elements into their valves, which limited these devices to only short-term use because of they were mounted on the end of a catheter that extended outside the body.

The introduction of a percutaneous heart valve that could be implanted permanently awaited the development of devices to treat vascular restenosis after angioplasty. In 1989, several years after Dr. Ulrich Sigwart's landmark report in 1986 of the first intracoronary stent (Sigwart U, Puel J, Mirkovitch V), the concept of suspending a valve within a scaffold was born. Dr. Henning-Rud Andersen and his colleagues, from Skejby University Hospital, Aarhus, Denmark, inspired by the advances in transluminal balloon-expandable vascular stents, were the first to attach a xenograft aortic valve onto a stainless steel stent (Andersen HR, Knudsen LL, Hasenkam JM 1990). Harvesting the aortic valve from freshly slaughtered pigs, he sutured the valve to a metallic frame using 45 to 50 interrupted fine sutures (Andersen HR, Knudsen LL, Hasenkam JM 1992). The carrier balloon was a standard 12 Fr three-foiled BAV catheter (o.d. 31 mm).

In one embodiment, the fully collapsed external diameter of the frame was 12 mm and, when fully expanded, 32 mm. Once the valved frame was manually compressed on the balloon catheter, it was introduced into the abdominal aorta of pigs through a 41 Fr introducer sheath. Advanced by catheter into the ascending aorta, it was positioned at the level of the native aortic valve annulus and deployed by balloon expansion (Figure 11; Andersen HR, Knudsen LL, Hasenkam JM 1992). The valved frame was intentionally hyper-expanded to ensure secure anchoring. Many years later, valve oversizing would also become appreciated as an important technique to reduce paravalvular leakage in the clinical setting.

From prototypes built on the bench, the next major step in the evolution of transcatheter heart valves was to demonstrate proof-of-concept and feasibility in a large series of animals.

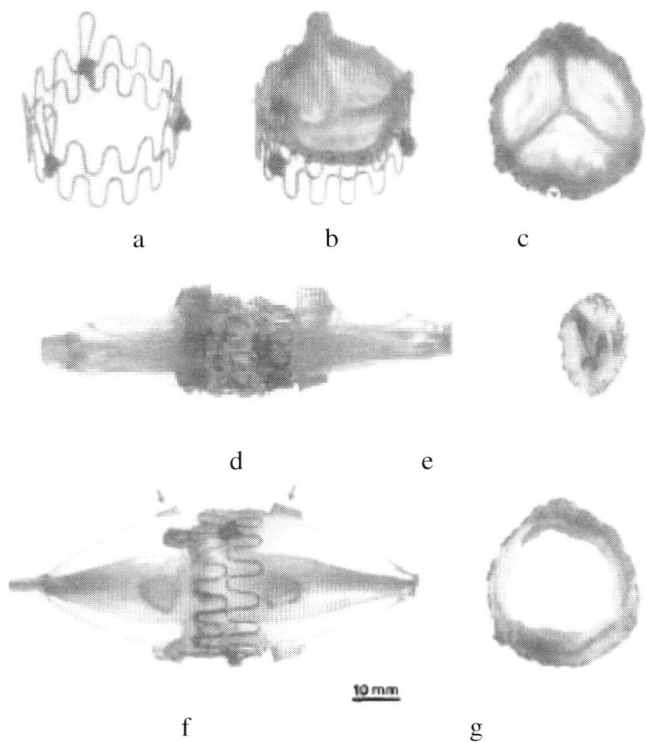

Ref.: Andersen, H. R., Knudsen, L. L., Hasenkam, J. M. Transluminal implantation of artificial heart valves. *Eur. Heart J.* 1992;13:704-708.

Figure 11. The world's first transcatheter valve designed by Dr. Henning-Rud Andersen and his colleagues. (a) A three-leaflet porcine aortic valve was mounted inside the frame and attached to the frame by sutures (b) and (c). Before implantation the valved stent was collapsed onto a deflated balloon dilatation catheter (d) and (e). The valved stent was subsequently expanded by balloon inflation (f) and (g).

Consequently, Dr. Andersen in 1990 reported his first series in abstract form, which described successful valve implantation in 10 anesthetized pigs – five in the descending aorta, two in the ascending aorta, and three in the subcoronary aortic root (Andersen HR, Knudsen LL, Hasenkam JM 1990). Of significance, this was achieved without thoracotomy or cardiopulmonary bypass. His first paper was published in 1992, which detailed his experience in seven additional pigs (Andersen HR, Knudsen LL, Hasenkam JM 1992). This report was noteworthy as it was also the first to warn of potential hazards associated with aortic transcatheter valve implantation, including coronary artery obstruction, observed in two of four pigs, and paravalvular regurgitation, documented in two of seven. Moreover, Dr. Andersen expressed concern about the risk of vascular injury due to the large caliber of the access sheath (41 Fr), as well as the durability of the compressed porcine valve. Clearly, 20 years later, these cautionary statements have not lost their relevance, but standard commercial development has since, and continues to, optimize the device components.

Within a few years of Dr. Andersen's successful valve implants in animals, early attempts also were made to develop a percutaneous mechanical valve. In 1992, Dr. Dusan Pavcnik, from the University of Texas M.D. Anderson Cancer Center, Houston, Texas, demonstrated in 12 dogs the feasibility of transcatheter implantation of a self-expanding caged ball valve in the subcoronary aortic position (Pavcnik D, Wright KC, Wallace S). The prosthesis was comprised of three parts – a cage, ring and ball. The cage was essentially a modified Gianturco self-expanding stainless steel Z-stent, which was closed at the outflow end by several lengths of wire, giving a total height of 2.2 cm. The ring was made of stainless steel wire coiled in a spring-like configuration and covered with expandable nylon mesh; it was attached to the cage by means of stainless steel tubing. The ball was a detachable latex balloon filled with radiopaque silicone connected to a 60-cm long 5 Fr catheter. Successful subcoronary implantation was accomplished through the right common carotid artery using an 11 Fr or 12 Fr introducer sheath, and he observed excellent immediate valve function. Working in collaboration with Dr. Pavcnik, Dr. Jan Šochman, from Prague, Czech Republic, reported the successful implantation of a percutaneous tilting disc valve in six pigs with acute aortic insufficiency (Šochman J, Peregrin JH, Roček M). The frame was comprised of a flexible circular disc of silicone elastomer attached to a nitinol stent by a crossbar tie. It was introduced through the right common carotid artery using a 12 Fr sheath, and deployed in the supracoronary ascending aorta. Unlike Dr. Pavcnik's caged ball design, however, this device was intended as short-term support in patients with decompensated aortic insufficiency while awaiting conventional surgical valve replacement.

While most investigators were focused on aortic insufficiency, a few directed their attention to other valve-related conditions such as the problem of failed right ventricular (RV) to pulmonary artery (PA) conduits in children after congenital surgical repair. Dr. Phillip Bonhoeffer and Dr. Younes Boudjemline, from Hôpital Necker Enfants Malades, Paris, France, began their research efforts by successfully implanting a valve in the pulmonic valve position through the internal jugular vein in seven sheep (Bonhoeffer P, Boudjemline Y, Saliba Z. Circulation 2000). This balloon-expandable valve was constructed from fresh bovine jugular vein, which contained a functional valve, sutured to a platinum-iridium frame (Figure 12, Bonhoeffer P, Boudjemline Y, Saliba Z. Circulation 2000). Autopsy findings confirmed that the ends of the valve frame were embedded into the pulmonary arterial wall and the right ventricular outflow tract. Based on these compelling results, Dr. Bonhoeffer performed the first successful percutaneous valve implantation in a human in September 2000 (Bonhoeffer P, Boudjemline Y, Saliba Z. Lancet 2000). His patient, a 12-year-old boy suffering from a failed RV to PA valved conduit secondary to progressive fibrocalcific obstruction, was treated using an 18-mm bovine jugular vein valve delivered over an 18-mm balloon catheter through the right femoral vein using an 18 Fr sheath. Under fluoroscopy, the frame was deployed by balloon inflation at the site of conduit obstruction. No complications were observed, and good valve function was documented by echocardiography. After one month of follow-up, the child was in New York Heart Association class I. In 2002, Dr. Bonhoeffer extended his experience to seven children and one adult with failed RV to PA valved conduits (Bonhoeffer P, Boudjemline Y, Qureshi SA). Under general anesthesia, the percutaneous balloon-expandable valve was introduced through the right femoral vein using an 18 Fr or 20 Fr sheath. All patients were successfully treated without any complications. With Dr. Bonhoeffer's initial clinical success, a new therapeutic option to treat these challenging patients was born.

Nitinol, an alloy with temperature-sensitive shape memory properties, was commonly used in peripheral vascular stents during the 1990s.I Its application in transcatheter valves was demonstrated by Dr. Šochman's transcatheter mechanical valve reported in 2000.

Its first appearance as the main component of a tissue valve can be attributed to Dr. Georg Lutter, from the University of Kiel, Kiel, Germany, in 2002 (Lutter G, Kuklinski D, Berg G). In his original study, a porcine aortic valve was mounted to a self-expanding nitinol frame; the outer diameter of which ranged from 15 to 23 mm, and the length ranged from 21 to 28 mm (Lutter G, Kuklinski D, Berg G). Inserted into 14 pigs through a 22 Fr sheath using the left iliac artery or infrarenal aorta, six valves were implanted in the descending aorta and eight in the ascending aorta. Other investigators published their experiences with nitinol-based frames, including Dr. Christoph Huber, from the Centre Hospitalier Universitaire Vaudois CHUV, Lausanne, Switzerland, and Dr. Markus Ferrari, from Friedrich-Schiller University, Erlanger, Germany (Huber CH, Nasratulla M, Augstburger M; Ferrari M, Figulla HR, Schlosser M). Incidentally, in his 2004 paper, Dr. Huber gave the first description of an animal study for the transapical approach to the aortic valve in a series of five pigs using an equine pericardial valve sutured onto a self-expanding nitinol frame (Huber CH, Tozzi P, Corno AF).

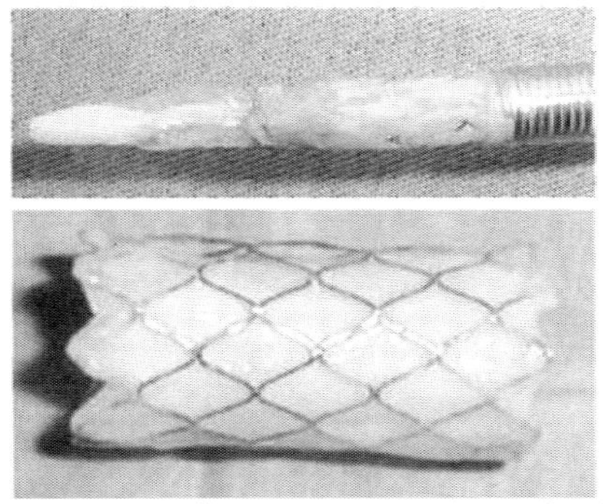

Ref.: Bonhoeffer, P., Boudjemline, Y., Saliba, Z. Transcatheter implantation of a bovine valve in pulmonary position. *Circulation* 2000;102:813-816.

Figure 12. Dr. Bonhoeffer's bovine jugular vein valve. Top, valved stent collapsed and front-loaded onto a 16 Fr Mullins sheath.

Later that same year, Dr. Ferrari reported successful nitinol valve implantation in the subcoronary aortic position in six pigs (Ferrari M, Figulla HR, Schlosser M).

Mirroring the fruitful collaborative efforts that produced the Starr-Edwards mechanical and Carpentier-Edwards bioprosthetic valves, the achievement of the first clinically successful percutaneous aortic heart valve replacement involved several individuals. Dr. Alain Cribier first recognized the need for a percutaneous solution to severe aortic stenosis after his pioneering efforts in developing balloon aortic valvuloplasty were met with mid-term outcomes that were less than satisfactory. After searching across the medical device industry for a suitable corporate partner – and confronting waves of skepticism – a business venture was founded in 1999 linking engineering and business skill with Dr. Cribier's formidable clinical experience. The founding of Percutaneous Valve Technologies was among the first commercial efforts focused on developing a transcatheter heart valve, and was a partnership of Dr. Cribier, Dr. Martin Leon, Stan Rabinovich, and Stanton Rowe, the first two being interventional cardiologists and the latter two seasoned businessmen and early-stage medical device veterans. The team successfully optimized many valve design features: radial strength requirements, the attachment mechanism of the valve, and valve materials, just to name a few. Remarkably, in less than 2½ years, this team effort resulted in the first human implant.

Many reasons were given to argue why transcatheter heart valve implantation for severe aortic stenosis should not be attempted. These included bulky leaflet calcification predisposing to coronary artery obstruction or liberating a lethal dose of embolic debris; noncompliant leaflets and annulus promoting irregular valve expansion with poor leaflet coaptation; and, asymmetric calcium deposits exacerbating paravalvular leakage. Hence, the cardiology and cardiac surgery community took a keen interest when Dr. Alain Cribier, Rouen, France, performed the first successful aortic transcatheter valve implantation on April 16, 2002, in a 57-year-old man with severe calcific aortic stenosis (0.6 cm^2)(Cribier A, Eltchaninoff H, Bash A). The presence of cardiogenic shock (systolic blood pressure 80 mm Hg and ejection fraction 14%) and subacute leg ischemia (status post aorto-bifemoral bypass) excluded the patient from conventional valve replacement. The valved stent was a tri-leaflet bovine pericardial valve mounted on a balloon-expandable stainless steel frame (length 14 mm, o.d. 21-23 mm) (Figure 13), and was the archetype of the Edwards SAPIEN™ THV. A percutaneous, antegrade transseptal approach was employed through the right femoral vein using a 24 Fr sheath. Dr. Cribier used BAV as an integral step in the TAVR procedure to achieve pre-dilation of the stenotic aortic valve and facilitate accurate transcatheter valve position. Immediate valve assessment demonstrated a mean gradient of 9 mm hg, and a valve area of 1.6 cm^2. Two years later, Dr. Cribier published a series of six patients with severe aortic stenosis treated between April 2002 and August 2003 (Figure 14, Cribier A, Eltchaninoff H, Tron C). The bovine pericardial valve was successfully implanted in five of six patients, with no residual gradient, a mean valve area of 1.7 cm^2, and no cases of coronary artery obstruction. With Dr. Cribier's successful clinical series, a new era of transcatheter aortic valve replacement was born.

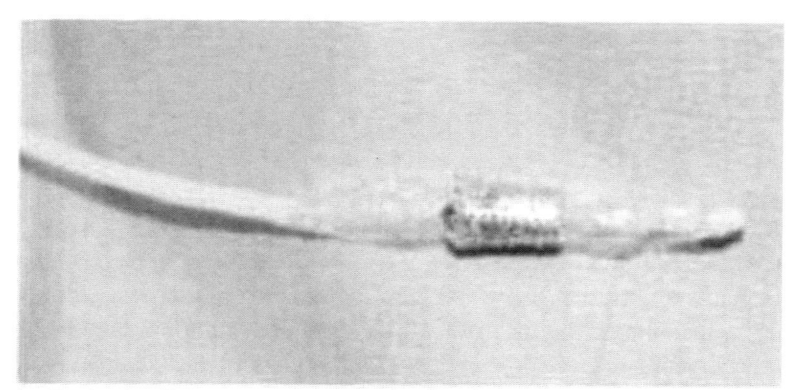

Ref.: Cribier, A., Eltchaninoff, H., Bash, A. Percutaneous transcatheter implantation of an aortic valve prosthesis for calcific aortic stenosis: First human case. *Circulation* 2002;106:3006-3008.

Figure 13. Dr. Cribier's tri-leaflet bovine pericardial valved stent mounted on a collapsed 30-mm balloon.

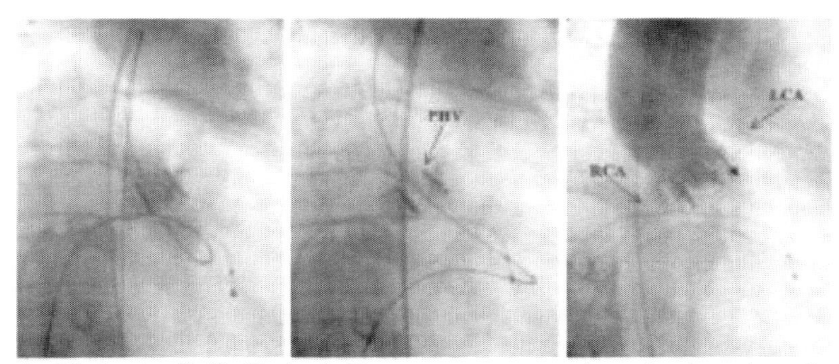

Ref.: Cribier, A., Eltchaninoff, H., Bash, A. Percutaneous transcatheter implantation of an aortic valve prosthesis for calcific aortic stenosis: First human case. *Circulation* 2002;106:3006-3008.

Figure 14. Positioning and deployment of the balloon-expandable transcatheter valve. Left, after the crimped valve on balloon is centered within the stenotic aortic valve annulus, the valve is balloon-expanded. Middle, it is perfectly positioned 50:50 within the native aortic annulus, pushing aside the calcific leaflets. Right, aortography demonstrates no transvalvular regurgitation and mild paravalvular regurgitation (arrow). Both coronary ostia are patent. LCA, left coronary artery; RCA, right coronary artery.

5. Proving Clinical Value

Today, the ever rising share of GDP devoted to health care expenditures have forced governmental regulatory agencies and third-party payers to critically examine the value they are receiving for their health care dollar. Accordingly, it is imperative that transcatheter aortic valve replacement establish evidence of value, whether through improvements in clinical efficacy and safety, quality of life, or cost savings to the health care system.

Evidence of value can be derived from carefully designed clinical studies to determine feasibility, safety and effectiveness. The world's first transcatheter aortic valve implanted into a human by Dr. Cribier was manufactured by a small, privately held medical technology company called Percutaneous Valve Technologies (PVT)(Cribier A, Eltchaninoff H, Bash A). In January 2004, PVT was acquired by global heart valve manufacturer Edwards Lifesciences (Irvine, CA) and the valve was renamed the Cribier-Edwards Aortic Bioprosthesis, then later the Edwards SAPIEN™ Transcatheter Heart Valve (THV) (Figure 15).

During the evolution of the Edwards SAPIEN™ valve, Edwards invested in no fewer than nine clinical trials and registries, entitled (1) Registry of Endovascular Critical Aortic Stenosis Treatment (RECAST); (2) Initial Registry of Endovascular Implantation of Valves in Europe (iREVIVE); (3) REVIVE II; (4) Transapical Surgical Delivery of the Cribier-Edwards Aortic Bioprosthesis Clinical Feasibility (TRAVERCE); (5) Registry of Endovascular Implantation of Valves II (REVIVAL II); (6) Placement of Aortic Transcatheter Valves in Europe (PARTNER EU); (7) SAPIEN™ Aortic Bioprosthesis European Outcome Registry (SOURCE); (8) PARTNER IDE; and, (9) Placement of Aortic Balloon Expandable Transcatheter Valves Trial in Europe (PREVAIL EU). All studies were prospective, in multiple centers, and the clinical outcomes were independently adjudicated. The first six listed studies were designed to assess feasibility. European CE Mark was conferred in August and December 2007 for the transfemoral (TF) and transapical (TA) delivery systems, respectively, and, starting in November 2007, 32 centers began enrolling patients into the SOURCE commercial registry.

The first valve implant in the U.S. occurred in the REVIVAL I study on March 10, 2005 by Dr. William O'Neill. REVIVAL I compared the Edwards SAPIEN™ THV to balloon aortic valvuloplasty (BAV) alone, and included both retrograde (via the femoral artery) and antegrade (via the femoral vein) approaches using a 23 mm valve (Kodali SK, O'Neill WW, Moses JW). After the first seven implants, the study was halted to implement design modifications and to institute a comprehensive training program. These modifications included the addition of a 26 mm valve size, a new retrograde delivery catheter, replacement of equine pericardial tissue with bovine pericardium, and treatment of valve leaflets with a proprietary anti-calcification regimen (ThermaFix™, Edwards Lifesciences, Irvine, CA). The protocol was redrafted as the REVIVAL II study, a non-randomized study involving only the retrograde TF approach in 55 patients. The first REVIVAL II subject was enrolled on December 15, 2005.

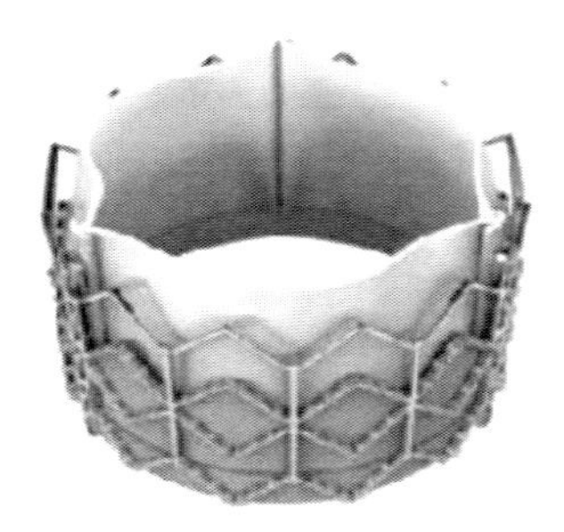

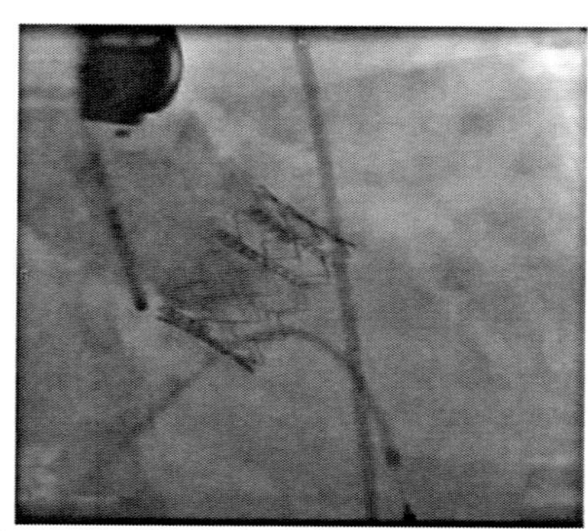

Ref.: Left, courtesy of Edwards Lifesciences, Irvine, C. A. Right, Leon, M. B., Smith, C. R., Mack, M. J. Transcatheter aortic-valve implantation for aortic stenosis in patients who cannot undergo surgery. *N Engl J. Med.*, 2010, 363, 1397-1607.

Figure 15. Edwards SAPIEN™ THV (Transcatheter Heart Valve).

After TF enrollment was completed, the TA approach was proposed for individuals with inadequate vessel size or significant tortuosity or occlusive disease, which precluded the transfemoral approach. As the TA arm of REVIVAL II was nearing completion, the U.S. Food and Drug Administration (FDA) allowed Edwards to start the pivotal PARTNER IDE Trial. The Placement of Aortic Transcatheter Valves (PARTNER) IDE Trial was a prospective, multicenter, randomized, active-treatment controlled clinical trial comparing transcatheter aortic valve replacement with standard therapy in high-risk patients with aortic stenosis (Leon MB, Smith CR, Mack MJ; Smith CR, Leon MB, Mack MJ).

The PARTNER Trial -- Cohort B

The purpose of Cohort B of The PARTNER Trial was to determine whether transfemoral TAVR was safer and more effective than standard medical therapy in patients with symptomatic, severe aortic stenosis who could not undergo surgery (Leon MB, Smith CR,

Mack MJ). Inoperability was determined by at least two surgeons, and defined as a predicted risk of death or serious irreversible morbidity at 30 days of 50% or more. Subjects were excluded for bicuspid or noncalcified aortic valves, acute myocardial infarction within one month of treatment, coronary disease needing revascularization, ejection fraction < 20%, severe mitral regurgitation, severe renal insufficiency and stroke or transient ischemic attack (TIA) within six months of treatment. The primary endpoint was the rate of death from any cause.

Quality of life (QOL) was evaluated using three validated instruments: Kansas City Cardiomyopathy Questionnaire (KCCQ), a heart failure-specific QOL tool; SF-12, a general physical and mental health assessment; and, EQ-5D, a general instrument to assess utilities and quality adjusted life years. Finally, cost effectiveness was determined by calculating the cost per life-year gained based on observed survival, QOL, health care resource use and hospital billing data. Lifetime analysis was based on projections of survival, quality-adjusted survival and costs beyond 12 months.

Between May 2007 and March 2009, 358 patients were enrolled at 21 sites (18 in the US; two in Canada; and one in Germany) and randomized to transfemoral TAVR (n = 179) and standard therapy (n = 179)(Leon MB, Smith CR, Mack MJ). Standard therapy included BAV in 83.8% of patients. Patients were followed for a median of 1.6 years. Baseline characteristics in the two groups were generally well balanced (Table 1, Leon MB, Smith CR, Mack MJ). At one year, the rate of death from any cause was 30.7% for TAVR versus 50.7% for standard therapy (HR 0.55; 95% CI, 0.40 to 0.74; $P < 0.001$) (Figure 16). Beyond 30 days, the causes of death after TAVR were cardiovascular in 11.2% (mainly heart failure, sudden death and stroke), and non-cardiovascular in 14.5% (mainly infection, cancer and kidney disease). At 30 days, the rate of stroke and TIA was 6.7% for TAVR versus 1.7% for standard therapy ($P < 0.05$); and, at one year, 10.6% for TAVR versus 4.5% for standard therapy ($P < 0.05$).

At one year, 74.8% of patients receiving TAVR versus 42.0% of patients receiving standard therapy were asymptomatic or had mild symptoms (NYHA functional class I or II) ($P < 0.001$). With TAVR, the mean valve area increased from 0.6 ± 0.2 cm^2 at baseline to 1.5 ± 0.5 cm^2 at 30 days ($P < 0.001$), and the mean aortic valve gradient decreased from 44.5 ± 15.7 mm Hg to 11.1 ± 6.9 mm Hg ($P < 0.001$). These hemodynamic improvements were maintained at one year. Moderate or severe paravalvular regurgitation was present in 10.5% after TAVR at one year.

Quality of life was significantly improved after TAVR versus standard therapy: KCCQ improved by 24.5 absolute percentage points ($P < 0.001$), equivalent to an improvement in two NYHA functional classes; and, the SF-12 Physical improved by 4.7 absolute percentage points ($P < 0.01$), comparable to a 10-year reduction in effective age. TAVR was associated with index admission costs averaging $78,000 (2010 US dollars). Given an increased life expectancy of about 1.9 years compared to standard therapy, the incremental cost-effectiveness ratio was $50,200 per life-year gained – well within accepted values for commonly used cardiovascular therapies.

In conclusion, Cohort B of The PARTNER Trial demonstrated that standard therapy did not alter the dismal natural history of aortic stenosis – tragically, more than 50% of patients were dead at one year (Leon MB, Smith CR, Mack MJ). Transfemoral TAVR was superior to standard therapy in reducing death from any cause.

Table 1. Baseline Characteristics of the Patients and Echocardiographic Findings

Characteristic	TAVR[1] (N=179)	Standard Theraphy[1] (N=179	P Value
Age, yrs	83.1 ± 8.6	83.2 ± 8.3	0.95
Male sex, no. (%)	82 (45.8)	84 (46.9)	0.92
STS score[2]	11.2 ± 5.8	12.1 ± 6.1	0.14
Logistic EuroSCORE[3]	26.4 ± 17.2	30.4 ± 19.1	0.04
NYHA class, no. (%)			0.68
II	14 (7.8)	11 (6.1)	
III or IV	165 (92.2)	168 (93.9)	
Coronary artery disease, no. (%)	121(67.6)	133 (74.3)	0.20
Previous myocardial infarction, no./ total no. (%)	33/177 (18.6)	47/178 (26.4)	0.10
Previous intervention, no./ total no. (%)			
CABG	58/155 (37.4)	73/160 (45.6)	0.17
PCI	47/154 (30.5)	39/157 (24.8)	0.31
Ballon aortic valvuloplasty	25/154 (16.2)	39/160 (24.4)	0.09
Cerebrovascular disease, no./ total no. (%)	48/175 (27.4)	46/167 (27.5)	1.00
Peripheral vascular disease, no./ total no. (%)	54/178 (30.3)	45/179 (25.1)	0.29
COPD, no. (%)			
Any	74 (41.3)	94 (52.5)	0.04
Oxygen-dependent	38.(21.2)	46.(25.7)	0.38
Creatinine >2mg/dl, no./ total no. (%)	10/178 (5.6)	17/178 (9.6)	0.23
Atrial fibrillation, no./ total no. (%)	28/85 (32.9)	39/80 (48.8)	0.04
Permanent pacemaker, no./ total no. (%)	35/153 (22.9)	31/159 (19.5)	0.49
Pulmonary hypertension, no./ total no. (%)	50/118 (42.4)	53/121 (43.8)	0.90
Frailty[4], no./ total no. (%)	21/116 (18.1)	33/118 (28.0)	0.09
Extensively calcified aorta, no. (%)	34 (19.0)	20 (11.2)	0.05
Deleterious effects of chest-wall irradiation, no. (%)	16 (8.9)	15 (8.4)	1.00
Chest-wall deformity, no. (%)	15 (8.4)	9 (5.0)	0.29
Liver disease, no. (%)	6/177 (3.4)	6/178 (3.4)	1.00
Echocardiographic findings			
Aortic-valve area, cm^2	0.6 ± 0.2	0.6 ± 0.2	0.97
Mean aortic-valve gradient, mm Hg	44.5 ± 15.7	43.0 ± 15.3	0.39
Mean LVEF (%)	53.9 ± 13.1	51.1 ± 14.3	0.06
Moderate[5] or severe mitral regurgitation, no./ total no. (%)	38/171 (22.2)	38/165 (23.0)	0.90

[1] Plus-minus values are means ± SD. CABG denotes coronary artery bypass grafting, CPD chronic obstructive pulmonary disease, LVEF left ventricular ejection fraction, NYHA New York Heart Assosiation, PCI percutaneous coronary intervention, and TAVR transcatheter aortic valve replacement.

[2] The Society of Thoracic Surgeons (STS) score measures patient risk at the time of cardiovascular surgery on a scale that ranges from 0% to 100%, with higher numbers indicating greater risk. An STS score higher than 100% indicates very high surgical risk.

[3] The logistic European System for Cardiac Operative Risk Evaluation (EuroSCORE), which measures patien risk at the time of cardiovascular surgery, is calculated with the use of a logistic-regretion equation. Scores range from 0% to 100%, with higher scores indicaring greater risk. A logistic EuroSCORE higher than 20% indicates very high surgical risk.

[4] Frailty was determined by the surgeons according to prespecified criteria.

[5] Moderate or severe mitral regurgitation was defined as regurgitation of grade 3+ or higher.

Ref.: Leon, M. B., Smith, C. R., Mack, M. J. Transcatheter aortic-valve implantation for aortic stenosis in patients who cannot undergo surgery. N Engl. J. Med. 2010;363:1397-1607.

Indeed, at one year, only five patients needed to be treated with TAVR to prevent one death. TAVR led to better improvement in heart failure symptoms and better quality of life. On the other hand, there were important complications associated with TAVR, including adverse neurological events, major vascular complications and major bleeding events. Finally, TAVR frequently was associated with trace or mild paravalvular regurgitation.

The PARTNER Trial -- Cohort A

The purpose of Cohort A of The PARTNER Trial was to compare the safety and effectiveness of TAVR, with either the TF or TA approach, to surgical aortic valve replacement (AVR) in high-risk, operable patients with symptomatic, severe aortic stenosis (Smith CR, Leon MB, Mack MJ). All patients were considered eligible for conventional surgical AVR. High risk was defined as a risk of death of at least 15% at 30 days, or a Society of Thoracic Surgeons (STS) predicted risk of mortality of 10% or higher. Of note, the decision to pursue TF or TA in a given patient was based on whether the peripheral arteries could accommodate the large caliber sheaths required for the TF approach (22 Fr for the 23 mm valve and 24 Fr for the 26 mm valve). The primary endpoint was the rate of death from any cause at one year.

Between May 2007 and August 2009, 699 patients were enrolled at 25 sites (22 in the US; two in Canada; and one in Germany)(Smith CR, Leon MB, Mack MJ). Four hundred and ninety two patients were deemed suitable for TF and 207 for TA. Patients in each arm were then randomly assigned to undergo TAVR or surgical AVR. Accordingly, 244 patients were assigned to TF, 104 to TA and 351 to AVR. Median follow-up was 1.4 years. As compared to the TF arm, the TA arm had significantly more patients with prior CABG, cerebrovascular disease and peripheral vascular disease. Of note, 38 patients assigned to AVR and four patients assigned to TAVR did not receive the assigned procedure. The main reason was withdrawal from the study or a decision not to undergo surgical AVR in 28 of 38 patients. The mortality rate from any cause at 30 days was 3.3% for TAVR versus 6.2% for AVR (P = 0.13).

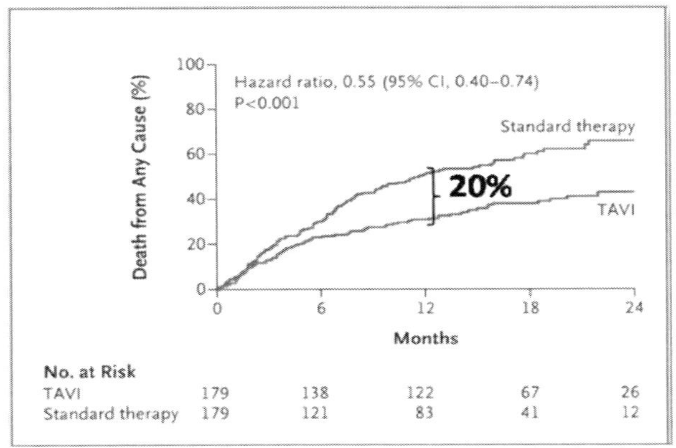

Ref.: Leon, M. B., Smith, C. R., Mack, M. J. Transcatheter aortic-valve implantation for aortic stenosis in patients who cannot undergo surgery. *N Engl. J. Med.* 2010;363:1397-1607.

Figure 16. Kaplan-Meier survival curves for all-cause mortality at one year.

At one year, the rate of death from any cause was 24.2% for TAVR versus 26.8% for AVR (P = 0.44). The difference of -2.6% absolute percentage points was within the prespecified noninferiority margins of 7.5 percentage points (P = 0.001 for noninferiority).

At 30 days, the rate of stroke and TIA was 5.5% for TAVR versus 2.4% for AVR (P < 0.05); and, at one year, 8.3% for TAVR versus 4.3% for AVR (P < 0.05). At 30 days, the rate of major vascular complications was higher for TAVR than AVR, 11.0% versus 3.2%, respectively (P < 0.001), but the rate of major bleeding events was lower, 9.3% versus 19.5%, respectively (P < 0.001).

At one year, both groups saw equivalent improvement in NYHA functional class. Patients receiving TAVR experienced a significantly shorter length of stay in the ICU, three days versus five days after AVR (P < 0.001), and a shorter index hospitalization, eight days versus 12 days after AVR (P < 0.001). Moderate or severe paravalvular regurgitation was present in 12.2% for TAVR versus 0.9% for surgical AVR at 30 days, and 6.8% versus 1.9%, respectively, at one year.

In conclusion, Cohort A of The PARTNER Trial demonstrated that among patients with severe aortic stenosis who were at high risk for surgical AVR, TAVR was equivalent to AVR with respect to death from any cause at one year (Smith CR, Leon MB, Mack MJ). Surgical AVR was associated with more frequent major bleeding events and new-onset atrial fibrillation; whereas, TAVR had more frequent adverse neurological events and major vascular complications.

6. Toward the Future

On July 20, 2011, the FDA convened a Circulatory System Devices Advisory Panel to evaluate the Premarket Approval (PMA) application for the Edwards SAPIEN™ THV in patients with symptomatic severe aortic stenosis who are deemed inoperable for surgical AVR. After a rigorous review of the findings from Cohort B of The PARTNER Trial, the Panel voted on whether the benefits outweighed the risks in the prespecified patient group. The final tally was 9 to 0 in favor, with one abstention (Dooren, JC).

The evolution of transcatheter aortic valve replacement continues today, and there is still much to be learned as clinical experience is gained throughout the world. Legitimate questions exist about appropriate patient selection and procedure management. Physicians continue to strive to reduce the rates of procedural complications – mainly stroke, vascular access issues and atrioventricular block. Uncertainty lingers about long-term valve performance and the natural history of paravalvular leak, particularly if evidence supports expanded indication into patients with longer life expectancies. Yet, the benefit-risk calculus is overwhelmingly positive. Transcatheter aortic valve replacement offers significant benefit to patients with severe aortic stenosis who, on the basis of advanced age, poor left ventricular function or severe comorbid conditions, are at prohibitive or extremely high risk for death and serious complications after surgical AVR. The history of transcatheter heart valves is studded with resolute surgeons and interventionalists, incisive engineers and courageous patients who helped advance the science of heart valves, vascular stents and balloons over the last 50 years. Many of these ideas flew in the face of fiercely entrenched surgical wisdom. For these intrepid pioneers, the words of Victor Hugo provide inspiration: "There is nothing so powerful as an idea whose time has come."

References

Andersen, H. R., Knudsen, L. L., Hasenkam, J. M. Transluminal catheter implantation of a new expandable artificial cardiac valve in the aorta [abstract #P1132]. *Eur. Heart J.* 1990;11(suppl.): 224a.

Andersen, H. R., Knudsen, L. L., Hasenkam, J. M. Transluminal implantation of artificial heart valves. *Eur. Heart J.* 1992;13:704-708.

Bach, D. S. Prevalence and characteristics of unoperated patients with severe aortic stenosis. *J. Heart Valv. Dis.* 2011;20:284-291.

Barratt-Boyes, B. G. Homograft aortic valve replacement in aortic incompetence and stenosis. *Thorax.* 1964;19:131-150.

Bavaria, J. E., Szeto, W., Roche, L. A. The impact of a transcatheter valve program: outcome of nearly 600 referrals (abstract #27). Southern Thoracic Surgical Association 57th Annual Meeting, November 5, 2010.

Ben-Dor, I., Pichard, A. D., Satler, L. F. Clinical profile, treatment assignment and clinical outcome of patients with severe aortic stenosis. *Am. J. Cardiol.* 2010;105:857-861.

Ben-Dor, I., Pichard, A. D., Satler, L. F. Complications and outcome of balloon aortic valvuloplasty in high-risk or inoperable patients. *JACC Interv.* 2010;3:1150-1156.

Bjork, V. O. A new tilting disc valve prosthesis. *Scand. J. Thorac. Cardiovasc. Surg.* 1969;3:1-10.

Bollati, M., Tizzani, E., Moretti, C. The future of new aortic valve replacement approaches. *Future Cardiol.* 2010;6:351-360.

Bonhoeffer, P., Boudjemline, Y., Qureshi, S. A. Percutaneous insertion of the pulmonary valve. *J. Am. Coll. Cardiol.* 2002;39:1664-1669.

Bonhoeffer, P., Boudjemline, Y., Saliba, Z. Transcatheter implantation of a bovine valve in pulmonary position. *Circulation* 2000;102:813-816.

Bonhoeffer, P., Boudjemline, Y., Saliba, Z. Percutaneous replacement of pulmonary valve in a right-ventricle to pulmonary-artery prosthetic conduit. *Lancet* 2000;356:1403-1405.

Boudjemline, Y., Bonhoeffer, P. Percutaneous implantation of a valve in the descending aorta in lambs. *Eur. Heart J.* 2002;23:1045-1049.

Boudjemline, Y., Bonhoeffer, P. Steps toward percutaneous aortic valve replacement. *Circulation* 2002;105:775-778.

Boudjemline, Y., Bonhoeffer, P. Percutaneous valve insertion: A new approach? *J. Thorac. Cardiovasc. Surg.* 2003;125:741-743.

Boudjemline, Y., Bonhoeffer, P. Percutaneous heart valve replacement in animals. *Circulation* 2004;109:e61.

Boudjemline, Y., Bonnet, D., Sidi, D. Percutaneous implantation of a biological valve in the aorta to treat aortic valve insufficiency. *Med. Sci. Monit.* 2002;8:BR113-116.

Bouma, B. J., Van den Brink, R. B., Van der Meulen, J. H. P. To operate or not on elderly patients with aortic stenosis: the decision and its consequences. *Heart* 1999;82:143-148.

Campbell, J. M. An artificial aortic valve. *J. Thorac. Cardiovasc. Surg.* 1958;19:312.

Carpentier, A., Deloche, A., Relland, J. Six-year follow-up of glutaraldehyde-preserved homografts. *J. Thorac. Cardiovasc. Surg.* 1974;68:771-782.

Carpentier, A. The surprising rise of nonthrombogenic valvular surgery. *Nature Medicine* 2007;13:xvii-xx.

Charlson, E., Legedza, A. T. R., Hamel, M. B. Decision making and outcomes in severe symptomatic aortic stenosis. *J. Heart Valv. Dis.* 2006;15:312-321.

Cheng, T. O. The history of balloon valvuloplasty. *J. Intervent. Cardiol.* 2000;13:365-373.

Cobanoglu, A., Grunkemeier, G. L., Aru, G. M. Mitral replacement: Clinical experience with a ball-valve prosthesis. *Ann. Surg.* 1986;202:376-383.

Cohn, L. H. Fifty years of open heart surgery. *Circulation* 2003;107:2168-2170.

Cribier, A., Eltchaninoff, H., Bash, A. Percutaneous transcatheter implantation of an aortic valve prosthesis for calcific aortic stenosis: First human case. *Circulation* 2002;106:3006-3008.

Cribier, A., Eltchaninoff, H., Tron, C. Early experience with percutaneous transcatheter implantation of heart valve prosthesis. *J. Am. Coll. Cardiol.* 2004;43:698-703.

Cribier, A., Saoudi, N., Berland, J. Percutaneous transluminal valvuloplasty of acquired aortic stenosis in elderly patients. *Lancet* 1986;1:63-67.

Davies, H. Catheter-mounted valve for temporary relief of aortic insufficiency. *Lancet* 1965;1:250.

Dewey, T. M., Brown, D. L., Das, T. S. High-risk patients referred for transcatheter aortic valve implantation: management and outcomes. *Ann. Thorac. Surg.* 2008;86:1450-1457.

Dooren, J. C. FDA Panel Backs Proposed Edwards Transcatheter Heart Valve [online]. 2011 July 20. Available from http://online.wsj.com/article/BT-CO-20110720-717666.html?KEYWORDS=edwards+lifesciences+and+fda.

Dotter, C. T. Transluminally-placed coilspring endarterial tube grafts. *Invest. Radiol.* 1969;4:329-332.

Dotter, C. T., Judkins, M. P. Transluminal treatment of arteriosclerotic obstruction: Description of a new technique. *Circulation* 1964;30:654-670.

Emery, R. W., Mettler, E., Nicoloff, D. M. A new cardiac prosthesis: The St. Jude Medical cardiac valve. *Circulation* 1979;60:I48-I54.

Ferrari, M., Figulla, H. R., Schlosser, M. Transarterial aortic valve replacement with a self expanding stent in pigs. *Heart* 2004;90:1326-1331.

Frater, R. W. M. The Carpentier-Edwards Pericardial Aortic Valve Intermediate Results UPDATE 1998. *Ann. Thorac. Surg.* 1998;66:2153–2154.

Gibbon, J. H., Jr. Application of a mechanical heart and lung apparatus to cardiac surgery. *Minn. Med.* 1954;37:171-180.

Gödje, O. L., Fischlein, T., Adelhard, K. Thirty-year results of Starr-Edwards prostheses in the aortic and mitral position. *Ann. Thorac. Surg.* 1997;63:613-619.

Gott, V. L., Alejo, D. E., Cameron, D. E. Mechanical heart valves: 50 years of evolution. *Ann. Thorac. Surg.* 2003;76:S2230-2239.

Gruntzig, A. R., Myler, R. K., Hanna, E. S. Coronary transluminal angioplasty [abstract #319]. *Circulation* 1977;84:55-56.

Gruntzig, A. R., Senning, A., Siegenthaler, W. E. Nonoperative dilatation of coronary artery stenosis: Percutaneous transluminal coronary angioplasty. *N Engl. J. Med.* 1979;301:61-68.

Harken, D. E. Heart valves. Ten commandments and still counting. *Ann. Thorac. Surg.* 1989;48: 18-19.

Harken, D. E., Soroff, H. S., Taylor, W. J. Partial and complete prostheses in aortic insufficiency. *J. Thorac. Cardiovasc. Surg.* 1960;40:744-747.

Hopkins, R. A. Ross' first homograft replacement of the aortic valve. *Ann. Thorac. Surg.* 1991;52: 1190-1193.

Huber, C. H., Nasratulla, M., Augstburger, M. Ultrasound navigation through the heart for off-pump aortic valved stent implantation. *J. Endovasc. Ther.* 2004;11:503-510.

Huber, C. H., Tozzi, P., Corno, A. F. Do valved stents compromise coronary flow? *Eur. J. Cardiothorac. Surg.* 2004;25:754-759.

Hufnagel, C. A., Harvey, W. P., Rabil, P. J. Surgical correction of aortic insufficiency. *Surgery* 1954;35:673-683.

Inoue, K., Owaki, T., Nakamura, T. Clinical application of transvenous mitral commissurotomy by a new balloon catheter. *J. Thorac. Cardiovasc. Surg.* 1984;87:394-402.

Iung, B., Cachier, A., Baron, G. Decision making in elderly patients with severe aortic stenosis: why are so many denied surgery? *Eur. Heart J.* 2005;26:2714-2720.

Kan, J. S., White, R. I., Mitchell, S. E. Percutaneous balloon valvuloplasty: a new method for treating congenital pulmonary valve stenosis. *N Engl. J. Med.* 1982;307:540-542.

Kapadia, S. R., Goel, S. S., Svensson, L. Characterization and outcome of patients with severe symptomatic aortic stenosis referred for PAVR. *J. Thorac. Cardiovasc. Surg.* 2009;137:1430-1435.

Kodali, S. K., O'Neill, W. W., Moses, J. W. Early and late (one year) outcomes following transcatheter aortic valve implantation from the US REVIVAL trial. *Am. J. Cardiol.* 2011;107:1058-1064.

Kouchoukos, N. T. Dr. Albert Starr: A Historical Commentary [online]. 2010. Available from: http://www.sts.org/news/dr-albert-starr-historical-commentary.

Lababidi, Z., Wu, J. R. Percutaneous balloon pulmonary valvuloplasty. *Am. J. Cardiol.* 1983;52:560-562.

Leon, M. B., Smith, C. R., Mack, M. J. Transcatheter aortic-valve implantation for aortic stenosis in patients who cannot undergo surgery. *N Engl. J. Med.* 2010;363:1397-1607.

Libby, P., Bonow, R., Zipes, P. *Braunwald's Heart Disease.* 8th Edition. Philadelphia, PA: Saunders El Sevier; 2008.

Lieberman, E. B., Bashore, T. M., Hermiller, J. B. Balloon aortic valvuloplasty in adults: failure of procedure to improve long-term survival. *Am. Coll. Cardiol.* 1995;26:1522-1528.

Lutter, G., Ardehali, R., Cremer, J. Percutaneous valve replacement: Current state and future prospects. *Ann. Thorac. Surg.* 2004;78:2199-2206.

Lutter, G., Kuklinski, D., Berg, G. Percuateneous aortic valve replacement: An experimental study. *J. Thorac. Cardiovasc. Surg.* 2002;123:768-776.

Maass, D., Zollikofer, C. L., Largiadèr, F. Radiological follow-up of transluminally inserted vascular endoprostheses. *Radiology* 1984;152:659-663.

Magovern, G. J., Kent, E. M. and Cromie, H. W. Sutureless artificial heart valves. *Circulation* 1963;27:2784-2788.

Matthews A. M. The Development of the Starr-Edwards Heart Valve. *Tex. Heart Inst. J.* 1998;25(4):282-93.

Moazami, N., Bessler, M., Argenziano, M. Transluminal aortic valve placement. *ASAIO J.* 1996;42:M381-M385.

Moulopoulos, S. D., Anthopoulos, L., Stametelopoulos, S. Catheter mounted aortic valves. *Ann. Thorac. Surg.* 1971;11:423-430.

NHLBI Balloon Valvuloplasty Registry Participants. Percutaneous balloon aortic valvuloplasty. *Circulation* 1991;84:2383-2397.

Nkomo, V. T., Gardin, J. M., Skelton, T. N. Burden of valvular heart disease: a population-based study. *Lancet* 2006;368:1005-1011.

Norman, A. F. The first mitral valve replacement [letter]. *Ann. Thorac. Surg.* 1991;51:525-526.

Nossaman, B. D., Scruggs, B. A., Nossaman, V. E. History of right heart catheterization : 100 years of experimentation and methodology development. *Cardiol. Rev.* 2010;18:94-101.

Otto, C. M., Mickel, M. C., Kennedy, J. W. Three-year outcome after balloon aortic valvuloplasty. Insights into prognosis of valvular aortic stenosis. *Circulation* 1994;89:642-650.

Paniagua, D., Induni, E., Ortiz, C. Percutaneous heart valve in the chronic in vitro testing model. *Circulation* 2002;106:e51-e52.

Pavcnik, D., Uchida, B., Timmermans, H. Square stent: A new self-expandable endoluminal device and its application. *Cardiovasc. Intervent. Radiol.* 2001;24:207-217.

Pavcnik, D., Wright, K. C., Wallace, S. Development and initial experimental evaluation of a prosthetic aortic valve for transcatheter placement. *Radiology* 1992;183:151-154.

Pellika, P. A. Serrano, M. E., Nishimura, R. A. Outcome of 622 adults with asymptomatic hemodynamically significant aortic stenosis. *Circulation* 2005;111:3290-3295.

Phillips, S. J., Ciborski, M., Freed, P. S. A temporary catheter-tip aortic valve. *Ann. Thorac. Surg.* 1976;21:134-137.

Rashkind, W. J., Miller, W. W. Creation of an atrial septal defect without thoracotomy. *JAMA* 1966;196:173-174.

Ross, J. Jr., Braunwald, E. Aortic stenosis. *Circulation* 1968;38 (1 Suppl.):61-67.

Ross, D. N. Homograft replacement of the aortic valve. *Lancet* 1962;2:487.

Ross, D. N. Replacement of aortic and mitral valves with a pulmonary autograft. *Lancet* 1967;2:956-958.

Sigwart, U., Puel, J., Mirkovitch, V. Intravascular stents to prevent occlusion and restenosis after transluminal angioplasty. *N Engl. J. Med.* 1987;316:701-706.

Smith, C. R., Leon, M. B., Mack, M. J. Transcatheter and surgical aortic-valve replacement in high-risk patients. *N Engl. J. Med.* 2011;364:2191-2202.

Sochman, J., Peregrin, J. H., Roček, M. Percutaneous transcatheter one-step mechanical aortic disc valve prosthesis implantation. *Cardio Vasc. Intervent. Radiol.* 2006;29:114-119.

Starr, A. Mitral replacement: Clinical experience with a ball-valve prosthesis. *Ann. Surg.* 1961;154:726-740.

Starr, A. A cherry blossom moment in the history of heart valve replacement. *J. Thorac. Cardiovasc. Surg.* 2010;140:1226-1229.

Starr, A. The artificial heart valve. *Nature Medicine* 2007;13:xii-xvi.

Varadarajan, P., Kapoor, N., Bansal, R. C. Clinical profile and natural history of 453 nonsurgically managed patients with severe AS. *Ann. Thorac. Surg.* 2006;82:2111-2115.

Zlotnick, A. Y. A perfectly functioning Magovern-Cromie sutureless prosthetic aortic valve 42 years after implantation. *Circulation* 2008:117;e1-e2.

"Any views or opinions expressed are solely those of the authors and don"t necessarily represent those of Edwards Lifesciences."

Index

#

A

B

C

D

E

F

G

H

I

N

O

P

Q

R

S

T

U

V

W

X

Y

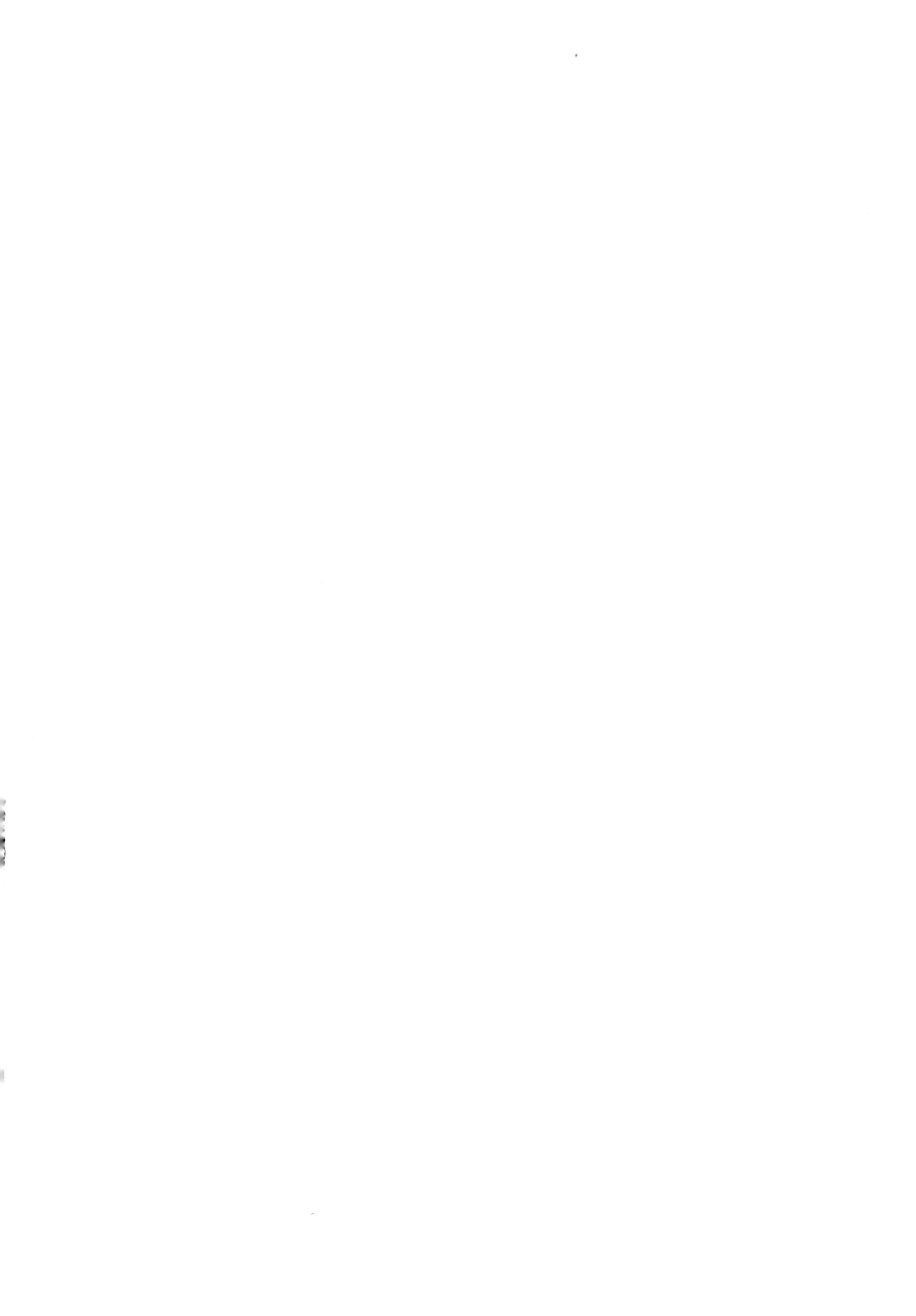

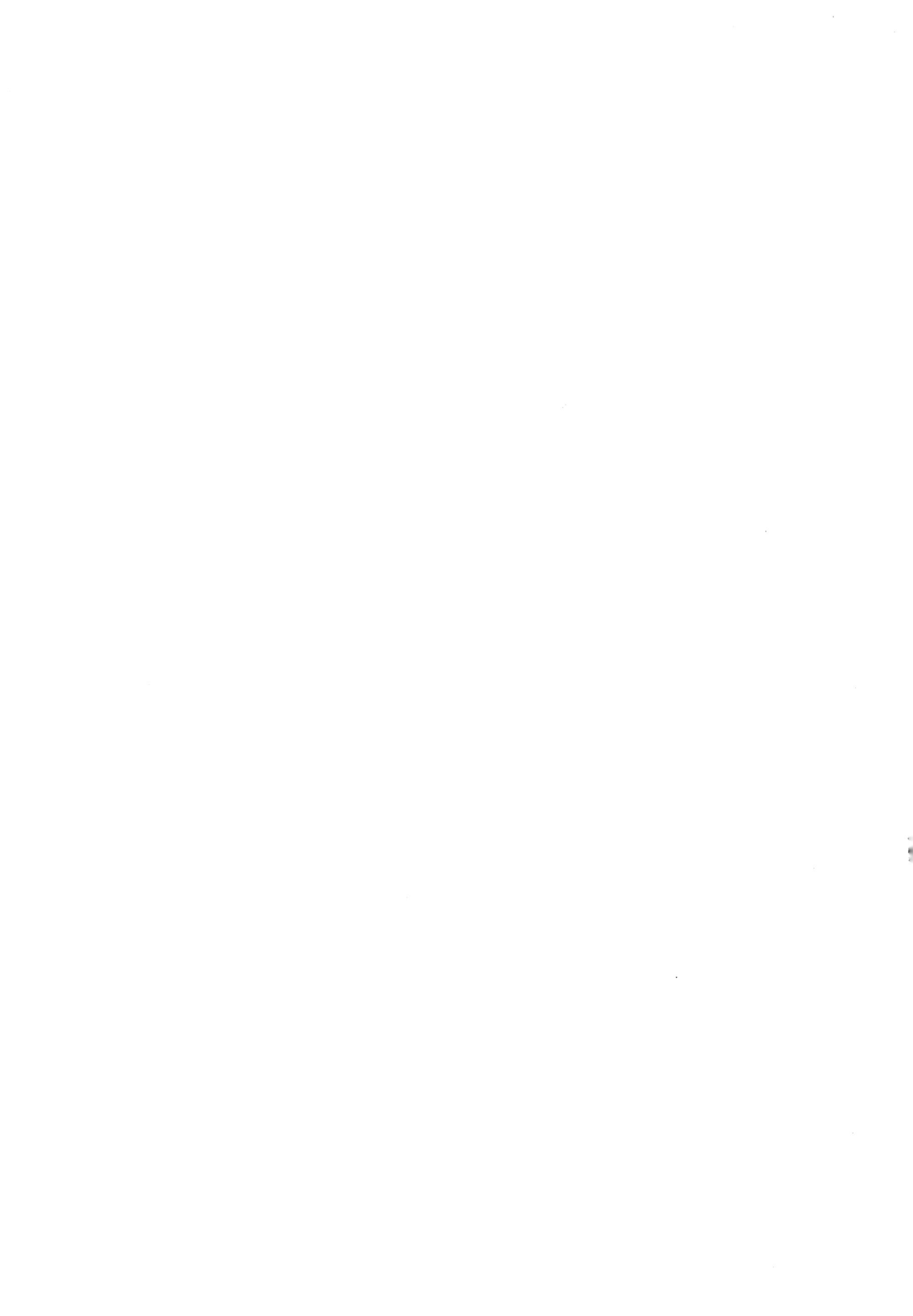